Pathophysiological Phenomena in Nursing

HUMAN RESPONSES TO ILLNESS

second edition

Pathophysiological Phenomena in Nursing

HUMAN RESPONSES TO ILLNESS

VIRGINIA CARRIERI-KOHLMAN, DNSc, RN
Professor and Coordinator
Critical Care/Trauma Program
Department of Physiological Nursing
University of California, San Francisco
San Francisco, California

ADA M. LINDSEY, PhD, RN, FAAN
Dean and Professor
School of Nursing
University of California, Los Angeles
Los Angeles, California

CLAUDIA M. WEST, MS, RN
Associate Clinical Professor
Department of Physiological Nursing
University of California, San Francisco
San Francisco, California

W.B. SAUNDERS COMPANY
A Division of Harcourt Brace & Company
Philadelphia   London   Toronto   Montreal   Sydney   Tokyo

second edition

W.B. SAUNDERS COMPANY
A Division of
Harcourt Brace & Company

The Curtis Center
Independence Square West
Philadelphia, PA 19106

Library of Congress Cataloging-in-Publication Data

Pathophysiological phenomena in nursing: human responses to
illness / [edited by] Virginia Carrieri-Kohlman, Ada M. Lindsey,
Claudia M. West.—2nd ed.

p.   cm.

ISBN: 0–7216–3494-X

1. Nursing.   2. Physiology, Pathological.   I. Carrieri-Kohlman,
Virginia.   II. West, Claudia M.
[DNLM: 1. Disease—nurses' instruction.   2. Nursing
Care.   3. Stress—nurses' instruction.   QZ 160 P297]

RT65.P27 1993
616—dc20
DNLM/DLC   92–49314

PATHOPHYSIOLOGICAL PHENOMENA IN NURSING:
HUMAN RESPONSES TO ILLNESS   ISBN 0–7216–3494–X

Last digit is the print number: 9   8   7   6   5   4   3   2

Contributors

Melissa C. Behnke, M.N., R.N.
Consultant in Oncology Nursing,
Ashland, Kentucky.
Anorexia

**Virginia Carrieri-Kohlman,
D.N.Sc., R.N.**
Professor and Coordinator, Critical
Care/Trauma Program, Department
of Physiological Nursing, University
of California, San Francisco, School
of Nursing. Clinical Associate,
University of California Medical
Center, San Francisco.
*The Conceptual Approach; Dyspnea;
Stress Response*

Janet DiJulio, M.S.N., R.N.
Nursing Manager, Petersen Cancer
Treatment Center, Stanford
University Hospital, Palo Alto,
California.
Nausea, Vomiting, and Retching

Helen L. Dulock, D.N.Sc., R.N.
Assistant Professor, Coordinator,
Perinatal-Neonatal Program, School
of Nursing, Emory University,
Atlanta, Georgia.
Apnea

Gayle Giboney Page, D.N.Sc., R.N.
Postdoctoral Research Fellow,
University of California, Los
Angeles.
Stress Response

**Marcia Grant, D.N.Sc., R.N.,
F.A.A.N.**
Assistant Director, Nursing
Research Department, City of Hope
National Medical Center, Duarte,
California.
Anorexia

Pat Halliburton, M.S., R.N.
Associate Clinical Professor,
University of California, San
Francisco, School of Nursing, San
Francisco, California.
*Nausea, Vomiting, and Retching;
Immunosuppression*

Cheryl Hubner, M.S., R.N.
Critical Care Clinical Nurse
Specialist, Intensive Care Unit,
Veterans Administration Medical
Center, San Francisco. Lecturer,
Department of Physiological
Nursing, University of California
School of Nursing, San Francisco.
Altered Clotting

**Susan Janson-Bjerklie, D.N.Sc.,
R.N., F.A.A.N.**
Professor, Department of
Physiological Nursing, and Adjunct
Professor, Department of Medicine,
University of California, San
Francisco. Clinical Associate,
University of California, San
Francisco.
Dyspnea

Christine E. Kasper, Ph.D., R.N.
Assistant Professor, School of
Nursing, University of California,
Los Angeles.
Skeletal Muscle Atrophy

Dorothy M. Lanuza, Ph.D., R.N., F.A.A.N.
Associate Professor, Department of Medical-Surgical Nursing, Niehoff School of Nursing, Loyola University. Nurse Scientist, Foster G. McGaw Hospital, Loyola University Medical Center, Chicago, Illinois.
Circadian Rhythm Disorders

Patricia Larson, D.N.Sc., R.N.
Associate Professor, Oncology Graduate Program, School of Nursing, University of California, San Francisco.
Nausea, Vomiting, and Retching

Ada M. Lindsey, Ph.D., R.N., F.A.A.N.
Dean and Professor, School of Nursing, University of California, Los Angeles.
The Conceptual Approach; Cancer Cachexia; Stress Response

Marylou Muwaswes, M.S., R.N.
Associate Clinical Professor, University of California School of Nursing, San Francisco. Clinical Nurse, University of California Hospitals, San Francisco.
Alterations in Consciousness; Edema

Mary H. Palmer, Ph.D., R.N., C., F.A.A.N.
Staff Fellow, Laboratory of Clinical Therapeutics, National Center for Nursing Research, Baltimore, Maryland.
Urinary Incontinence

Rebecca Phillips, M.S., R.N., C.C.R.N.
Clinical Nurse Specialist, Critical Care Nursing, Northridge Hospital Medical Center, Northridge, California.
Hypothermia

Barbara F. Piper, D.N.Sc., R.N., F.A.A.N., O.C.N.
Clinical Nurse, Oncology Unit, University of California, San Francisco, and Mount Zion Medical Center, San Francisco.
Fatigue

Kathleen Puntillo, D.N.Sc., R.N.
Professor of Nursing, Sonoma State University, Rohnert Park, California.
Pain

Connie R. Robinson, Ph.D., R.N.
Consultant, Neurophysiology and Sleep, Dedham, Massachusetts.
Impaired Sleep

Mary Jane Sauvé, D.N.Sc., R.N.
Assistant Research Nurse, University of California, San Francisco, School of Nursing. Principal Investigator/Project Director, Kaiser Permanente Medical Center, Santa Rosa, California.
Cardiac Dysrhythmias

Phylita Skov, R.N., M.S.
Assistant Clinical Professor, University of California, San Francisco, School of Nursing, San Francisco, California.
Edema

Nancy Stotts, Ed.D., M.N.
Associate Professor, University of California, San Francisco. Clinical Associate, University of California Hospitals, Department of Nursing, San Francisco.
Impaired Wound Healing

Mary D. Tesler, M.S., R.N.
Emeritus Professor of Clinical Nursing, University of California, School of Nursing, San Francisco.
Pain

Claudia M. West, M.S., R.N.
Associate Clinical Professor,
University of California,
Department of Physiological
Nursing, San Francisco. Clinical
Associate, University of California
Medical Center, San Francisco.
The Conceptual Approach; Ischemia

Karen R. Williams, D.N.Sc., R.N.
Associate Professor of Nursing, San
Francisco State University. Staff
Nurse, Davies Medical Center, San
Francisco.
Hunger

Preface

If nursing is truly the "diagnosis and treatment of human responses to potential or actual health problems,"* then it is important that these human responses be described, that their correlates be measured, and that therapeutic trials to modulate their effects be designed. The phenomena identified in this book are examples of human responses to health problems. Some can be considered symptoms, some processes, and some clinical problems. All are phenomena within the purview of nursing practice and nursing research. The most current knowledge about each phenomenon is presented, offering a basis for developing or examining the knowledge base of nursing practice.

Chapter Format

We attempted to make the chapter organization for each phenomenon more consistent in this edition but found that the particular needs of each topic did not allow us to achieve absolute consistency. We therefore allowed contributors to follow a more general format, with deviations as necessary to convey their topic as effectively as possible. A particularly praised feature from the previous edition, "Implications for Research," is again highlighted in this edition.

New to Second Edition

The strengths of the first edition were its inclusion of phenomena commonly encountered by nurses across settings and populations; the state-of-the-art, research-based presentations of knowledge related to these physiological mechanisms; the discussions of measurement and clinical management of these phenomena; and the extensive and timely reviews of the literature related to each phenomenon. Updating the knowledge base underlying this material was our first goal. Recent explosions of knowledge related to such topics as dyspnea, immunosuppression, fatigue, and pain have radically altered our understanding of these phenomena, and the newest literature and developments at the time of writing are reflected in the second edition.

Further, we sought to broaden the scope of the book in response to suggestions from reviewers and readers of the first edition. Additional human responses of significance to nursing included in the second edition are nausea, vomiting, and retching; hypothermia; altered circadian rhythms, skeletal muscle

---

*American Nurses' Association (1980). *Nursing: A Social Policy Statement.* (Publ. No. NP-6335M) Kansas City, MO.

ix

atrophy; urinary incontinence; and cardiac dysrhythmias. We recognize, however, the impossibility of including in one volume every important pathophysiological phenomenon of interest to nurses. We have included those that occur frequently in diverse clinical populations. Again in this edition we address the continuum of each phenomenon by a discussion of the developmental aspects in each chapter.

Relation to Theory and Research

Although development of nursing knowledge in the past has emphasized the use of grand theories, nurse researchers have shown growing support for an inductive approach to theory construction at the beginning, empirical level. Our book supports this empirical level of theory construction. It is important to recognize, however, that the underlying theoretical and empirical bases are not evenly developed for each phenomenon. For some, considerable work has accumulated over a long period; for others, much less is known. An equivalent volume of research for each phenomenon is not presented here. For some phenomena there may be little or no published nursing research, and for some others the most exemplary research may not be conducted by nurses. We have, however, incorporated the best examples of research that represent the body of knowledge available for the respective phenomena.

Audience

The content and approach of this book make it useful to nurse clinicians, advanced baccalaureate and graduate nursing students, faculty, and researchers. Nurse clinicians can use the information in this book to help identify these phenomena in clients across the age and health-illness continuums and to develop, test, and implement clinical nursing therapies to prevent or alleviate these responses. Students and faculty should find this book a thoughtful attempt to create a conceptual foundation from which to teach and learn the science of nursing. Researchers can consider these chapters a baseline of conceptual, research-based information from which to design further investigations, to ask more probing questions, and to continue much needed theory development.

Our intent in the first edition was to stimulate thinking about pathophysiological phenomena and the use of a conceptual approach to organize nursing knowledge. Our purposes now are to continue and extend the dialogue on human responses by offering more current information on a broader spectrum of topics. We hope that readers will continue to benefit from our work and suggest ways in which we can make it more useful in future editions.

Contents

1

The Conceptual Approach

Virginia Carrieri-Kohlman
Ada M. Lindsey
Claudia M. West

Nursing scholars have called for a renewed focus on the development of the substantive content (or knowledge base) for nursing.[1-4] Most agree that this content must be specialty based if it is to be used by practicing clinical nurses and must add cumulatively to a multidisciplinary body of knowledge and nursing science.[2, 5, 6] Others have emphasized the need for the study of biobehavioral phenomena and the importance of developing these constructs from a nursing perspective.[7, 8] The development of structures, typologies, and classifications for the knowledge base within the discipline is important if nursing knowledge is to be made specific and visible for individuals in nursing practice.[9] The process used throughout this book is a deliberate attempt to examine the nature and substance of nursing from a conceptual perspective. The conceptual approach we propose is an excellent method for developing substantive content in nursing. Experience in using this approach has shown us that it facilitates the development of nursing substantive content for curricula and promotes the generation of research questions relevant to specialty practice.[3, 10] The focus of this text is on the development of in-depth "substance"[1] or knowledge relevant to nursing practice. The goal is to include a number of biophysiological clinical phenomena (human responses) that are of major concern to nurses and for which nurses assume a major role in assessing, monitoring, managing, and evaluating. The selected phenomena are viewed as pathophysiological clinical patient problems. All are human responses or an outcome of human responses to illness, some are symptoms, and some are processes. The level of abstraction of the phenomena varies, which shows that biological concepts as a framework for nursing are in the early phases of development. There is a need for future work related to the categorization and leveling of pathophysiological concepts within a biological process framework.

The conceptual approach used in this text provides a way of analyzing concepts without creating a set of words that seems "foreign." The language used is commonly understood by all health care professionals and has clinical meaning to them. The authors have not created a new vocabulary but rather use generally accepted terminology. The use of a structure and vocabulary that is understood by other disciplines increases the communication and interdisciplinary dialogue in the development of content around a selected phenomenon. Research findings by nurses can be communicated effectively not only to nurses but also through publications supported and read by others from related disciplines. Adequate pursuit of knowledge about these complex phenomena necessitates multidisciplinary research teams. The conceptual approach facilitates communication among team members while adding to the body of knowledge about the phenomena for the nursing discipline and practice across other disciplines.

Using a conceptual approach to view and examine phenomena helps the nurse to focus on clinical problems encountered across disease or illness categories and across populations; to ask questions about relationships of specific events or conditions that may influence the extent, progression, or remission of the clinical problem; to become more systematic in making observations about these events or conditions; to collect information about the effectiveness of nursing actions directed at the problem; and to formalize questions that serve as the basis for studies that ultimately will provide the empirical data requisite for influencing nursing practice. The American Nurses Association Social Policy Statement[11] indicates that there are two kinds of human responses: those that are reactions of individuals and groups to actual health problems and those that are expressed as concerns of individuals and groups about potential health problems. The first group is labeled *health-restoring responses* and the second, *health-supporting responses.* We have suggested that the conceptualization of human responses needs to be expanded to include those responses that are neither restoring nor supporting. It is the authors' opinion that the phenomena discussed in the chapters in this book, such as anorexia, impaired sleep, and ischemia, are human responses.[10, 12] Other authors appear to agree with the position that physiological responses are human responses and have proposed physiological variables in their categorization of human responses.[13, 14]

The concepts included have been selected from an enormous field of possibilities and do not exist as isolated clinical problems but are interrelated. As the scientific frontier is pushed forward, the importance of a specific clinical problem or human response will change. The nature of nursing practice is always evolving. The approach used in this text is flexible and open to provide a way of examining phenomena for nursing practice, curricular planning, and research within a changing health care environment.

FRAMEWORK FOR ORGANIZING PHENOMENA

Biophysiologically based life processes serve as a guide for the development and study of concepts relevant to the discipline of nursing. Life processes are those biological and psychosocial processes that combine to make up the entire individual. They are viewed as being ever-present, ongoing processes, and together are reflected in the total functioning human. The life processes rep-

resent an initial delineation and are not mutually exclusive. Selected biological life processes are listed in Table 1–1. The life processes of regulation, sensation, protection, and motion are defined in the introductory material of Sections I, II, III, and IV.

Phenomena that may result in disruptions or alterations of the naturally occurring life processes are examined within an adaptation—developmental conceptual framework.[15] Human beings are described as biological, psychological, and sociocultural in nature, constantly interacting with their environment. Assumptions regarding this interaction are that "individuals, families, groups and populations are continuously adapting and developing; development and adaptation occur together, but one or the other may predominate at a given point in time; and systems constantly adapt with a variety of outcomes extending from survival to optimum health levels."[15] The environmental and contextual factors that humans encounter are designated as developmental and situational stressors. These stressors act as stimuli to produce changes in the client system.

Stressors are stimuli that affect life processes and alter a human's adaptation and development. Various stressors, such as developmental transitions, age-related biological changes, diseases, or environmental and physiological conditions, impinge upon and produce alterations in the life processes. These alterations may be pathological or beneficial to the client system. The resultant changes place the client system at various adaptational and developmental stages throughout the life span. The changes that take place within the individual in response to developmental and situational stressors are manifested as alterations in one or more life processes.

Developmental stressors are forces that arise predictably within the individual as that person encounters the conflicts and tasks inherent in traversing developmental phases throughout the life cycle. Situational stressors are forces that arise from the internal or

TABLE 1–1   BIOLOGICAL LIFE PROCESSES

Cognition	Sensation
Generativity	Regeneration
Motion	Regulation
Protection	Nurturance
	Perception

TABLE 1–2   EXAMPLES OF INDIVIDUAL DEVELOPMENTAL STRESSORS

Identity formation
Sex role attainment
Moral attainment
Achievement of integrity and dignity
Vocational or career decisions
Age-related biological changes
Procreation
Menopause—Midlife crisis or transition
"Empty nest" syndrome—Loss of nurturing functions
Declining of physical and sensory capacities
Impending death

From the University of California, San Francisco, School of Nursing, Conceptual Framework Committee (1980). The adaptation-developmental conceptual framework—the subject component.

external environment.[15] Examples of developmental and situational stressors are listed in Tables 1–2 and 1–3, respectively.

One goal of nursing is to promote optimum adaptation and development of the client system. This goal is achieved through direct alteration or by assisting the client and his or her support system to alter both stressors and/or the responses to stressors. Nursing involves a socially sanctioned, caring relationship with clients; a temporal continuity of concern; involvement with clients in all stages and phases of the life span and in all phases of health and illness; a holistic view of mind-body relations; relationships with clients within a transactional context involving biological, psychological, and sociocultural variables; and interaction with the client's adaptive and coping responses to stressors. The paramount importance of nursing's caring relationship with the client system dictates that professional nurses anticipate and influence evolving health needs, provide leadership in health care systems, and utilize, test, and generate a scientific knowledge base to direct practice.

IDENTIFICATION OF PHENOMENA FOR STUDY

Biophysiologically based life processes can be used to organize the substantive content relevant to nursing care of the acutely ill. The following is a description of the process by which phenomena (human responses) can be selected and used for teaching, clinical practice, or research. The life processes are used as the higher level of abstraction from which to identify phenomena. For example, sensation is a life process, whereas pain and dyspnea are examples of phenomena classified under this life process. It is apparent from the list of biological life processes in Table 1–1 that they are at different levels of abstraction, as are the human responses that are derived from them. This lack of uniformity in level of abstraction reflects the current state of the formalization of these constructs and their biological complexity. Individuals representing different clinical practice specialties can be involved in the identification of phenomena, concepts, or variables that seem relevant to each life process. This initial stage of selection is dependent on the participants' theoretical knowledge, clinical expertise, and knowledge of the literature. A typical list of words that might be generated initially under the life process of sensation is given in Table 1–4. This type of listing can be completed for each life process.

CURRICULUM PLANNING AND TEACHING

Within nursing courses emphasis is on defining physiological processes or mechanisms related to a specific phenomenon; related physiological and psychosocial phenomena; situational stressors, including medical diag-

TABLE 1–3   EXAMPLES OF SITUATIONAL STRESSORS

Stressor	Examples
Physical illness or injury	Hospitalization, threats to personal safety or health
Environmental deprivation	Sensory deprivation, institutionalization, malnutrition
Economic pressures	Inadequate finances, change in financial status
Interpersonal discordance	Problems with friends, spouse, neighbors, or co-workers
Changes in life style	Relocation, divorce, retirement, immigration
Occupational stressors	Unemployment, problems at work, school, or home
Legal pressures	Arrest, lawsuit, or incarceration

From the University of California, San Francisco, School of Nursing, Conceptual Framework Committee (1980). The adaptation-developmental conceptual framework—the subject component.

TABLE 1–4 EXAMPLES OF WORDS IDENTIFIED IN RELATION TO THE LIFE PROCESS OF SENSATION*

Pain	Stickiness
Special sense deprivation:	Itchiness
blindness, taste, deafness	Nausea
Thirst	Streakiness
Hunger	Hue
Anxiety	Saturation
Touch	Loudness
Receptors	Sweetness
Comfort	Pungency
Fatigue	Cell receptor
Distress	Dyspnea
Discrimination	Stimulus
Selectivity	Threshold
Constancy	Membrane
Potential	
Perception	
Hardness	
Glossiness	

*List generated during one faculty meeting.

noses and clinical states; indicator behaviors or manifestations of the phenomenon, including both objective and subjective signs or symptoms; and suggested relevant clinical activities.

An example of defining and making operational the phenomenon of delirium categorized under the life process of cognition, is illustrated in Table 1–5. Physiological processes related to confusion include neurotransmitter failure, metabolic dysfunction, impaired energy metabolism, and electrolyte imbalance. Related physiological and psychosocial concepts include mentation, dementia, delirium, competence, isolation, and fear. Suggested situational stressors, which could be used for further study to compare and contrast the phenomenon among clients, include states such as sleep deprivation, sundowning, drug withdrawal, or medical diagnoses, including uremia, metastatic cancer, hepatic encephalopathy, and postcardiac surgery. Manifestations might include agitation, impaired perception, or hallucinations. The suggested activities, such as developing an instrument to measure confusion or identifying safety measures for the patient, can be used further to explore the phenomenon clinically, theoretically, and empirically.

At the doctoral level, physiological processes provide a framework for the study of specific phenomena. The doctoral student interested in biological science can focus on one or several biological processes. These can be combined with psychosocial processes to provide a more holistic framework for the

study of the phenomenon. Qualitative and quantitative variables that are related to the phenomena are studied across ages, cultures, illnesses, and situational stressors. An inventory of variables that cause the concept and those factors that result from the presence of the concept facilitates the review of the literature, the development of a conceptual model, and study of the phenomenon by advanced students. Doctoral students use a variety of research methods to study phenomena for dissertation research.

Alternate Ways to Examine Phenomena

We suggest that in the development of courses and teaching of the content, phenomena may be viewed in one of two ways: (1) as alterations in one normal life process or (2) as the phenomena affect all the life processes. It is helpful to use both approaches. An example of viewing the phenomena as alterations in one life process is seen in the relationship of the life process of sensation to pain. Pain is described as an alteration in sensation. The physiology of sensation and pathophysiological changes related to pain are studied. Related physiological phenomena may include reception, threshold, and tolerance to pain; referral of pain; and transmission of impulses. With an understanding of the normal physiological processes of sensation, there is subsequent examination of related physiological and psychosocial concepts such as pleasure, comfort, analgesia, isolation, anxiety, and depression. Manifestations of pain and actions to alter the pain experience also would be studied.

An example of the alternate method of viewing the effects of the phenomena across all the life processes is the relationship of pain to the life processes, for example, the effects of pain on cognition, affiliation, motion, and sensation. The approach taken is to examine the pathophysiology or changes in the salient life processes that either are a result of or contribute to the presence of that phenomenon. Within the discussion of each life process and the changes in it due to the phenomenon, manifestations that are present as a result of a disruption in the process are examined. Another example of this method is the human response of dyspnea. The effect of dyspnea on each process would be exam-

TABLE 1–5 MODEL OF EXAMINING THE PHENOMENON OF CONFUSION

Life Process: Cognition
Key Concept: Delirium

Physiological Processes	Related Physiological Concepts	Related Psychosocial Concepts
Electrolyte imbalance	Mentation	Isolation
Neurotransmitter failure	Dementia	Fear
Metabolic dysfunction	Competence	Altered trust in relationships
Impaired energy metabolism	Encoding (memory)	
	Language acquisition	
	Consciousness	

Manifestations		Suggested Situational Stressors	
Subjective	*Objective*	*Medical Diagnosis*	*Clinical States*
Agitation	Combativeness	Stroke	Sleep deprivation
Impaired perception	Disorientation	Brain trauma	Sensory alterations
Indecisiveness	Altered intellectual functions	Metastatic	Decreased trust in
Fear	Increased or decreased	carcinoma	relationships
Anxiety	electrolytes	Hepatic	Sundowning
Restlessness	Insomnia	encephalopathy	Drug withdrawal,
Hallucination (auditory,	Tremors, seizures	Emphysema	overdose
visual, tactile)	Increased vital signs	Sepsis	Intoxication
Loss of orientation	Hypoxia	Encephalitis	Metabolic disorders
Memory loss	Increased hormonal levels	Epilepsy	Cardiac surgery
Loss of image formation	Vitamin deficiencies	Uremia	Increased intracranial
	Hyperthermia		pressure
			Radiation therapy

Suggested Activities for Practice and Research
Use or develop a tool for assessing a confused patient.
Compare and contrast confused patients with varying diagnoses.
Develop a model of practice for a confused patient.
Differentiate between signs and symptoms of patients with
    functional confusion and those with organic confusion.
Develop a check list of factors causing confusion for hospitalized patients.
Develop interventions that may contribute to the safety of a confused patient.
Identify areas of research related to confusion.
Review the literature and identify areas for further study.

ined. Changes in cognition, sensation, regulation, motion, and generativity, for example, would be described, and manifestations of these processes would be discussed. Actions to decrease the phenomenon of dyspnea would be studied.

There are advantages to using either approach. The first alternative may provide more depth of knowledge about the specific human response, while the second approach might yield more information about interactions occurring across life processes in relation to the human response. It is recommended that both approaches be used for greater comprehension of each phenomenon.

For example, one of the authors has knowledge and expertise in respiratory physiology and nursing care; she has been teaching these subjects in the graduate program. The phenomenon of dyspnea under the life process of sensation is her area of research interest.

This human response is relevant across cardiopulmonary diseases and across age groups, while at the same time it is a clinical symptom frequently encountered by the nurse. In addition, examination of the phenomenon helped her to generate research questions salient to theory development and nursing care of respiratory patients. Other phenomena chosen to be representative of the human response seen commonly in cardiopulmonary specialties include ischemia, fatigue, edema, and pain. Using life processes in either of these two ways guides the student or professional nurse in thinking conceptually about phenomena related to both health and illness states.

Selection of Phenomena

The selection of pathophysiological phenomena relevant to nursing in graduate and upper division undergraduate study, research, and advanced clinical practice promotes the teaching and development of substantive content. In addition, it helps identify nursing content that can become "core," crossing a variety of clinical specialties and age groups, from neonates to the elderly. It is also important for faculty to be teaching, practicing, and directing their research endeavors in one conceptual area. Our intent was to select those phenomena that are of interest within and across clinical specialties. Finally, in the selection process, consideration should be given to ensure the inclusion of representative phenomena of critical importance to each specialty area.

In using this approach for curriculum implementation, selected phenomena can be presented in core lectures and then discussed in specialty seminars with the students. Specialty seminars allow students to focus on the specific human response as it occurs in populations for whom they provide care. For example, the phenomenon immunosuppression can be presented in lecture followed by specialty seminars in which the nursing care related to immunosuppression in populations with the clinical states of asthma, human immunodeficiency virus (HIV) seropositivity, leukemia, and malnutrition would be discussed. These represent possible topics for nursing seminars in the specialty areas of respiratory care, oncology, and gastrointestinal surgery. We have had 9 years of experience with this conceptual approach as a framework for courses at the bachelor, master, and doctorate levels. The approach has provided nursing content for lectures and seminars. In addition, doctoral students have selected conceptual areas providing both preliminary research questions and long-term research programs that are adding to the substantive knowledge in nursing.

THEORY DEVELOPMENT

This textbook was first published during an era in which nurse scholars were debating which nursing models or theories should be used to guide the development of nursing knowledge,[16–21] nursing theories were being critiqued and compared,[22–24] and the central concepts of nursing were beginning to be reexamined.[25–27] Since the mid-1980s these discussions have shifted to issues regarding the types of scientific inquiry or methods that

should be used to study nursing phenomena;[28–31] to further delineation of the important or essential concepts within the domain of the discipline, with a focus on how nursing knowledge should be structured;[25, 26, 32–34] and to the analysis and development of concepts and instruments to measure these phenomena. There has been concurrent deliberation of various methods to analyze and teach the concepts.[10, 13, 16, 32]

Discussions in the nursing literature related to the modes of inquiry center around the use of empirical methods versus phenomenological approaches, qualitative versus quantitative methods, or the "received" and "perceived" view of scientific inquiry.[16, 29, 35–37] Currently, many nurse scientists are using more than one scientific orientation to study human responses, depending on the philosophical beliefs of the researcher, the questions posed, and type of variables.[28, 38] As suggested by others,[16, 28] we believe that multiple modes of inquiry are necessary and can be used with the conceptual approach, depending on the question and theoretical level of the concept of interest. The research studies discussed throughout this book offer excellent examples of the use of multiple scientific methods to analyze and develop concepts, propositions, and middle-range theories. Diverse research methods are necessary to begin to understand the complexities of many of these concepts.

Authors have suggested alternative ways of organizing, identifying, and labeling content for the discipline.[26, 33, 34, 39] Meleis[16] proposes that concepts central to the domain of nursing are the nursing client, transitions, interaction, nursing process, environment, nursing therapeutics, and health. However, she acknowledges that the most significant concept within the domain of nursing is the recipient of care—the nursing client. Kim[32] suggests that the client, the client-nurse, practice, and environment are four domains for structuring nursing knowledge. This theorist further identifies four classes of client phenomena: essential, developmental, problematic, and health care experiential concepts. The chapters in this book are all evidence of efforts toward developing knowledge within the client domain. As correlates or stressors that impact on a phenomenon, concepts from the client-nurse, environment, and practice are also addressed.

Roy[33] has proposed an integrated metaparadigm of nursing science in which she distinguishes the understanding of life processes as basic nursing science from clinical nursing science, that is, the diagnosis and treatment of the patterning of life processes. The basic science nursing component includes life processes similar to those presented in the framework described in this chapter. Other major categories of processes include health promotion and developmental and group processes. It is suggested that the burden of operationalizing conceptual categories within these processes rests with individual programs of research. The content of this book reflects individual attempts to operationalize these concepts.

These theorists have provided greater specificity for the generally accepted central domains for nursing, that is, person, environment, health, and nursing.[25] For instance, Kim[58] includes infection, confusion, anxiety, and stress as examples of health care experiential phenomena and the pain experience and stress as client health outcomes within the client-nurse domain. However, these frameworks are still considered to be at the level of "grand" theory or remain too abstract for some to generate realistic questions and operational propositions that facilitate the development of research questions directly related to nursing practice.[10, 40]

The Nursing Diagnosis Conference Group[41] has developed a framework that uses processes to categorize nursing diagnoses accepted by the North American Nursing Diagnosis Association (NANDA) group. This classification has not been developed with explanatory theories and remains a classification of diagnoses that are not grounded in a theoretical base that can be used to guide nursing interventions. Descriptive studies have been used to describe variables surrounding diagnoses, but at the present time this classification remains a nomenclature that is used clinically to identify problems. The classification needs research-generated theory to guide future clinical intervention.[32] Because the human responses included in this text have scientific knowledge to support their description, measurement, and related nursing therapeutics, they are viewed as being different from nursing diagnoses and may be at a different level of abstraction. For example, several nursing diagnoses could be identified that would be related to the phenomenon of pain or ischemia.

RESEARCH

It is imperative that there be an intentional process of selection of clinical problems salient to practice for research investigations and that the formulation of questions and hypotheses directing study be pertinent to the development of knowledge that can direct practice.[2] Previous experience has demonstrated the difficulty that faculty, clinicians, and students have in generating nursing research questions from a broad clinical specialty such as cardiovascular nursing. Within specialties, the focus on selected phenomena promotes cluster studies resulting in knowledge development with both theoretical and practical implications for the discipline of nursing.

In an effort to develop content that is relevant to nursing practice, in the last several years there has been an increase in the use of the conceptual approach described in this book, both in research and communication of research findings.[4, 42–52] National conferences have focused on concepts such as nutrition, rest, and mobility.[42, 53] The National Institutes of Health, National Center for Nursing Research, has chosen symptom management as a priority.[54] Many of the concepts included in this book are symptoms.

It has been suggested that middle-range theories developed within conceptual areas, which are pertinent to the explanation and prediction of phenomena, will expedite the development of nursing science.[5, 55, 56] Middle-range theories similar to those discussed throughout the chapters of this book are thought to be more directly relevant than grand theories for addressing practice concerns in a nursing specialty area. Efforts to develop middle-range theories related to one phenomenon have prompted nurse researchers to conduct descriptive and correlational studies. Some nurse investigators have focused their efforts on developing instruments to measure pathophysiological concepts in order to measure these concepts and use them as variables in scientific studies.[57] Nurse researchers have described concepts across illness groups, ages, and cultures. Relationships among the phenomena of interest and demographic, psychosocial, environmental, and biological variables have been identified in correlational studies. The levels of knowledge vary across concepts. For example, the concept of pain has been studied extensively,

TABLE 1–6   DEFINITIONS OF CATEGORIES FOR CHAPTER DIVISIONS

Definition—a clear succinct orientation to the perspective from which the phenomenon is examined.

Prevalence—(of the phenomenon) the magnitude and significance in a given population.

Situational stressors—forces extended upon the individual that arise from the external environment.

Developmental stressors—forces that arise predictably within individuals as they encounter the conflicts and tasks inherent in traversing development phases of the life cycle.

Populations at risk—individuals who because of the existence of and/or their responses to various stressors have increased predisposition to the occurrence of the phenomenon.

Mechanisms—pathophysiological processes involved in the expression of the phenomenon.

Pathological consequences—potential detrimental outcomes associated with the phenomenon.

Related pathophysiological concepts—illustrations of the differences between the phenomenon and other similar phenomena.

Related psychosocial concepts—illustrations of the sets of behaviors that may contribute to or alter the expression of the pathophysiological phenomenon.

Manifestations—the objective, observable, and measurable (direct or indirect) expressions of the phenomenon and the individual's reported subjective perception.

Surveillance—process of identification and monitoring of selected parameters over time; used to evaluate the status of the phenomenon and the individual's response.

Clinical goals and therapies—primary objectives and strategies of management.

Case studies—clinical situations in which the various dimensions of the phenomenon are explored.

Research findings—illustrative and significant studies relevant to the phenomenon and its clinical management; implications for further study.

Implications for research—areas requiring additional study and/or exemplar questions for further study.

while nurses are only beginning to describe disruptions in biological rhythms in illness. When the level of knowledge has been appropriate, alternative methods of treatment have been tested; for example, cognitive-behavioral therapies and pharmacological treatments have been tested with nausea and vomiting.[45] Meleis[16] suggests that the recent work directed toward one concept is more practice oriented and integrative and represents early attempts to develop "single-domain" theories.

ORGANIZATION AND CONTENT OF CHAPTERS

Four biological life processes form the broad organizing structure for this book: regulation, sensation, protection, and motion. The particular phenomena to be included are commonly encountered in populations with acute or long-term illnesses; often found to be alterations in function involving multiple body systems; frequently seen across the boundaries of age, disease entities, and clinical states; and ultimately categorized as those for which nurses have a major role in assessing, monitoring, managing, and evaluating.

A critical and comprehensive examination of the phenomenon of each chapter includes definition, prevalence, populations at risk, developmental dimensions, physiological mechanisms, related psychosocial concepts, manifestations, surveillance, and clinical therapies. These categories are not unlike those suggested by other authors[13, 58] and are defined in Table 1–6. Authors of each chapter vary in their use of these divisions depending on the nature of the phenomenon. Case examples are used to illustrate each human response in a given clinical situation. Research from nursing and other disciplines is included to provide the foundation for the conceptual explanation of each phenomenon and to stimulate the generation of exemplar questions for further research. Areas requiring additional study are identified. The intent is to provide an approach to study human responses and clinical pathophysiological phenomena, which are of major concern in professional nursing practice, and to generate a spirit of inquiry that is essential for the development of the knowledge base for professional practice.

REFERENCES

1. Meleis, A.I. (1987). ReVisions in knowledge development: A passion for substance. Scholar Inq Nurs Pract *1*:5–19.
2. Hinshaw, A.S. (1989). Nursing science: The challenge to develop knowledge. Nurs Sci Q *2*:162–171.
3. Carrieri, V.K. (1992). Response to physiological research in dyspnea: A paradigm shift and a meta-paradigm exemplar. Scholar Inq Nurs Pract *6*:105–109.
4. Woods, N.F. (1987). Response: Early morning musing on the passion for substance. Scholar Inq Nurs Pract *1*:25–28.

5. Walker, L. (1989). The future of theory development: Generic or specialty? Commentary and response. Nurs Sci Q 2:118–119.
6. Stevenson, J.S. (1988). Nursing knowledge development: Into era II. J Prof Nurs 4:152–162.
7. Cowan, M.J. (1991). Nurse scientists: Research using a nursing and biological science model. *Nursing Research: Global Health Perspectives. 1991 International Council of Nurse Researchers Conference* (p. A411). Kansas City, MO: American Nurses' Association.
8. Hinshaw, A.S., Sigmon, H.D., & Lindsey, A.M. (1991). Interfacing nursing and biologic science. J Prof Nurs 7:264.
9. Hinshaw, A.S. (1987). Response to "Structuring the Nursing Knowledge System: A Typology of Four Domains." Scholar Inq Nurs Pract 1:11–14.
10. Lindsey, A.M. (1990). Identification and labeling of human responses. J Prof Nurs 6:143–150.
11. American Nurses' Association (1980). *A Social Policy Statement* (Pub. No. NP-63). Kansas City, MO: American Nurses' Association.
12. Carrieri, V.K., Lindsey, A.M., & West, C.M. (1986). The Conceptual Approach. In V.K. Carrieri, A.M. Lindsey, & C.M. West (eds.), *Pathophysiological Phenomena in Nursing: Human Responses To Illness* (pp. 4–10). Philadelphia: W.B. Saunders.
13. Goosen, G.M. (1989). Concept analysis: An approach to teaching physiologic variables. J Prof Nurs 5:31–38.
14. Loomis, M.E., & Wood, D.J. (1983). Cure: The potential outcome of nursing care. Image: J Nurs Scholar 15:4–7.
15. University of California, San Francisco, School of Nursing, Conceptual Framework Committee (1980). The adaptation-developmental conceptual framework—the subject component.
16. Meleis, A.I. (1991). *Theoretical Nursing: Development and Progress* (2nd ed.). Philadelphia: J.B. Lippincott.
17. King, I.M. (1988). Concepts: Essential elements of theories. Nurs Sci Q 1:22–25.
18. Orem, D.E. (1985). *Nursing: Concepts of Practice* (3rd ed.). New York: McGraw-Hill.
19. Rogers, M.E. (1987). Roger's science of unitary human beings. In R.R. Parse (ed.), *Nursing Science: Major Paradigms, Theories, and Critiques.* Philadelphia: W.B. Saunders.
20. Roy, C.L., & Andrews, H.A. (1991). *The Roy Adaptation Model: The Definitive Statement.* East Norwalk, CT: Appleton & Lange.
21. Neuman, B. (1989). *The Neuman Systems Model* (2nd ed.). Norwalk, CT: Appleton & Lange.
22. Riehl-Sisca, J.P. (1989). *Conceptual Models for Nursing Practice* (3rd ed.). Norwalk, CT: Appleton & Lange.
23. Fawcett, J. (1989). *Analysis and Evaluation of Conceptual Models of Nursing* (2nd ed.). Philadelphia: F.A. Davis.
24. Beckstrand, J. (1980). A critique of several conceptions of practice theory in nursing. Res Nurs Health 1:175–179.
25. Fawcett, J. (1983). Hallmarks of success in nursing theory development. In W.P. Chinn (ed.), *Advances in Nursing Theory Development* (pp. 3–18). Rockville, MD: Aspen Systems.
26. Meleis, A.I. (1986). Theory development and domain concepts. In P. Moccia (ed.), *New Approaches to Theory Development.* New York: National League for Nursing.
27. Shaver, J.F. (1985). A biopsychosocial view of human health. Nurs Outlook 33:186–191.
28. Gortner, S.R., & Schultz, P.R. (1988). Approaches to nursing science methods. Image: J Nurs Scholar 20:22–24.
29. Norbeck, J.S. (1987). In defense of empiricism. Image: J Nurs Scholar 19:28–30.
30. Allen, D., Benner, P., & Diekelman, N.K. (1986). Three paradigms for nursing research: Methodological implications. In P.L. Chinn (ed.), *Nursing Research Methodology: Issues and Implementation.* Rockville, MD: Aspen Systems.
31. Stevenson, J.S., & Woods, N.F. (1986). Nursing science and contemporary science: Emerging paradigms. In *Setting the Agenda for the Year 2000: Knowledge Development in Nursing.* Kansas City, MO: American Academy of Nursing.
32. Kim, H.S. (1987). Structuring the nursing knowledge system: A typology of four domains. Scholar Inq Nurs Pract 1:99–110.
33. Roy, C.L. (1988). An explication of the philosophical assumptions of the Roy Adaptation Model of Nursing. Nurs Sci Q 1:26–34.
34. Orem, D.E. (1988). The form of nursing science. Nurs Sci Q 1:75–79.
35. Walker, L.O., & Avant, K.C. (1989). *Strategies for Theory Construction in Nursing* (2nd ed.). East Norwalk, CT: Appleton & Lange.
36. Thompson, J.L. (1985). Practical discourse in nursing: Going beyond empiricism and historicism. Adv Nurs Sci 7:27–36.
37. Silva, M.C., & Rothbart, D. (1984). An analysis of changing trends in philosophies of science on nursing theory development and testing. Adv Nurs Sci 6:1–13.
38. Duffy, M.E. (1987). Methodological triangulation: A vehicle for merging quantitative and qualitative research methods. Image: J Nurs Scholar 19:130–133.
39. Scholtfeldt, R.M. (1988). Structuring nursing knowledge: A priority for creating nursing's future. Nurs Sci Q 1:35–38.
40. Lush, M.T., Janson-Bjerklie, S., Carrieri, V.K., & Lovejoy, N. (1988). Dyspnea in the ventilator-assisted patient. Heart Lung 17:528–535.
41. Carroll-Johnson, R.M. (1989). *Classification of Nursing Diagnoses: Proceedings of the Eighth Conference of North American Nursing Diagnosis Association.* Philadelphia: J.B. Lippincott.
42. Funk, S.G., Tornquist, E.M., Champagne, M.T., Copp, L.A., & Wiese, R.A. (1990). *Key Aspects of Recovery: Improving Nutrition, Rest, and Mobility.* New York: Springer Publishing.
43. Wadle, K.R. (1990). Diarrhea. Nurs Clin North Am 25:901–908.
44. Piper B.F., Lindsey, A.M., & Dodd, M.J. (1987). Fatigue mechanisms in cancer patients: Developing nursing theory. Oncol Nurs Forum 14:17–23, 1987.
45. Rhodes, V.A. (1990). Nausea, vomiting, and retching. Nurs Clin North Am 25:885–900.
46. Holtzclaw, B.J. (1990). Shivering: A clinical nursing problem. Nurs Clin North Am 25:977–986.
47. McCormick, K.A. (1991). From clinical trial to health policy—research on urinary incontinence in the adult, Part I. J Prof Nurs 7:147.
48. Walike, B.C., Walike, J.W., Hanson, R.L., Grant, M., Kubo, W., Bergstrom, N., Wong, H.L., Padilla, G., & Williams, K. (1975). Nasogastric tube feeding: Clinical complications and current progress of research. Northwest Health Team Approach 2:33–41.
49. Breslin, E.H., Roy, C., & Robinson, C.R. (1992). Physiological nursing research in dyspnea: A para-

digm shift and a metaparadigm exemplar. Scholar Inq Nurs Pract 6:81–101.

50. Norris, C.M. (1982). *Concept Clarification in Nursing* (pp. 3–45). Rockville, MD: Aspen Systems.

51. Gift, A. (1990). Dyspnea. Nurs Clin North Am 25:955–965.

52. Hart, L.K., Freel, M.I., & Milde, F.K. (1990). Fatigue. Nurs Clin North Am 25:967–976.

53. Funk, S.G., Tornquist, E.M., Champagne, M.T., Copp, L.A., & Wiese, R.A. (1989). *Key Aspects of Comfort: Management of Pain, Fatigue, and Nausea.* New York: Springer Publishing.

54. National Institutes of Health (1989). Report of the 1989 NIH Task Force on Nursing Research (NIH Publication 89–487, p. 3) Washington, DC: National Institutes of Health.

55. McLaughlin, F.E., & Marascuilo, L.A. (1990). Nursing science: The interrelationship of nursing constructs, concepts, hypothesis formulation, and measurement. In F.E. McLaughlin & Marascuilo, L.A. (eds.), *Advanced Nursing and Health Care Research.* Philadelphia: W.B. Saunders.

56. Hoeffer, B., & Murphy, S.A. (1984). *Issues in Professional Nursing Practice: Specialization in Nursing Practice.* Kansas City, MO: American Nurses' Association.

57. Frank-Stromberg, M. (ed.) (1988). *Instruments for Clinical Nursing Research.* Norwalk, CT: Appleton & Lange.

58. Kim, M.J. (1988). Physiologic responses in health and illness: An overview. Ann Rev Nurs Res 5:79–104.

I

ALTERATIONS IN REGULATION

Physiological processes are regulated by exquisitely sensitive controlling and integrating systems; when changes occur, compensatory mechanisms serve to return the processes involved to a normal range of function. The actions of these mechanisms are regulation. When the situational or developmental stressors are sufficiently great or of such prolonged duration that the compensatory mechanisms are unable to bring the processes to a normal range of function, pathological states evolve.

There are numerous examples of this very exquisite regulation of physiological processes. Maintenance of the narrow range of serum calcium, rapid changes in cardiovascular functions when an individual rises to a standing position or exercises, maintenance of blood glucose or pH levels, body temperature, and involuntary changes in respiratory rate or food intake are examples of regulation, that is, maintenance of homeostasis. The myriad of complex actions and interactions that occur to keep the individual within a normal range of physiological functioning across systems is generally referred to as *homeostatic mechanisms.*

When the specific changes are identified and the mechanisms involved and the pathological consequences are understood, it then becomes possible to determine what actions or influences nurses may have on alleviating the stressor, preventing or mediating the effects of the consequences, and monitoring parameters indicative for the clinical outcome. This kind of nursing practice requires considerable knowledge and ability to comprehend the physiologically and pathophysiologically complex interactions that occur in health and illness.

The nine chapters included in this section present phenomena that are representative of those in which alterations in regulatory processes have occurred. These pathophysiological phenomena are ischemia, cardiac dysrhythmias, circadian rhythm disorders, anorexia, cancer cachexia, hypothermia, apnea, alterations in consciousness, and urinary incontinence. These responses are observed frequently in a variety of clinical conditions and occur in all age groups.

Ischemia can occur as a response to alterations in regulation of tissue perfusion whether from a local biochemical, an obstructive, or a nervous system event. Cardiac dysrhythmias are alterations in cardiac rhythms that can result in changes in heart rate, stroke volume, and ultimately cardiac function. Circadian rhythm disorders change the individual's ability to adapt to the external temporal environment and disturb the internal circadian regulation of physiological and metabolic events. Anorexia reflects alterations in one or more of the physiological processes involved in the regulation of food intake and ultimately in maintaining energy balance. Cachexia of malignancy results from a variety of alterations ranging from decreased intake to increased metabolic rate and energy expenditure. Hypothermia may be induced deliberately or may result from disturbances in the body's thermoregulatory mechanisms and balance. Apnea reflects alterations in a number of processes involved in establishing and controlling a normal breathing pattern. Alterations in consciousness impair an individual's ability to function; regulatory processes may be severely compromised. The kind and extent of impairment and the specific processes compromised are dependent on the causative pathological processes involved. Urinary incontinence can be caused by defects in the storage of urine, alterations in urinary elimination, or disturbances in the regulation of both storage and emptying of urine.

These particular phenomena were selected as being representative of alterations in regulation. They are seen frequently, they occur in all age groups, and they are phenomena for which nurses can have a primary role in identifying, preventing, or alleviating. Nurses also have a primary role in monitoring and documenting the clinical progress of patients experiencing such responses. These professional nursing activities can occur only when there is sufficient comprehension of the phenomenon and its attendant complexities. The following chapters provide information that serves as the basis for professional nursing practice.

2

Ischemia

Claudia M. West

The phenomenon of ischemia can be manifested in any or all tissues of the body, is caused by multiple and varied processes, occurs across all ages and races, and is seen frequently by nurses in all health care settings. Given such a broad context and a large literature base, in-depth discussion of ischemia across several organ systems is not feasible. Ischemia as a general phenomenon will provide the substance for the discussion of populations at risk and of mechanisms. Myocardial ischemia will be used as the prototype to discuss manifestations, therapies, and research.

DEFINITION

Ischemia is the reversible cellular injury that occurs when tissue demand for oxygen exceeds the supply and when toxic metabolites accumulate. The imbalance in oxygen supply and demand is produced by a reduction or cessation of blood flow that results in tissue hypoxia, decreased energy substrate, and build-up of toxic metabolic wastes.[1, 2] These events result in identifiable derangements of cellular structure and function that are manifested by subsequent alterations in tissue function. Infarction is the inevitable outcome if perfusion is not re-established in a timely fashion. Because it is probable that an area of infarction is surrounded by ischemic and viable tissue,[3, 4] infarctions of various organ systems will also be considered in this chapter.

PREVALENCE

It is difficult to estimate the prevalence of ischemia, since the phenomenon is not a medical diagnosis with data available from medical records. Ischemia also is not generally thought of as an isolated entity but rather in relation to a particular tissue or organ. The list of possible medical diagnoses and clinical states is long and diverse (Table 2–1), and the prevalence of only the most commonly encountered medical diagnoses associated with ischemia of the cardiovascular system are included.

In 1988 an estimated 68.1 million Americans had one or more forms of cardiovascular disease, including 6.1 million with coronary heart disease (CHD), 3 million with angina pectoris (AP), 1.5 million with myocardial infarction (MI), and 2.9 million with stroke. CHD is the leading cause of death in the United States, accounting for 511,050 deaths annually.[5]

Approximately 500,000 persons suffer strokes each year, and 150,000 die, making this disease the third leading cause of death behind CHD and cancer. Transient ischemic attack (TIA) is the occurrence of focal neurological deficits that completely resolve in 24 hours or less. Approximately 10 per cent of strokes are preceded by TIA, and persons who have had one or more TIAs have a 36 per cent chance of having a stroke.[5]

There has been a downward trend in the incidence of both CHD and stroke in the United States over the last 40 years,[6, 7] although the decrease is greater for stroke than for CHD. Between 1978 and 1988 deaths from CHD declined by 29.2 per cent, and those from stroke declined 33.2 per cent. This decline is evident in both sexes and all races with a greater decrease in races other than white.[7] This marked downward trend

TABLE 2–1   EXAMPLES OF CLINICAL STATES AND MEDICAL DIAGNOSES ASSOCIATED WITH ISCHEMIA

A. Decreased cardiac output
    Hypovolemia: burns, hemorrhagic shock, dehydration
    Vasodilation: gram-negative sepsis, antihypertensive drug therapy
    Reduced pumping efficiency of the heart: MI, congestive cardiomyopathy, coarctation of the aorta, supraventricular or ventricular arrhythmias
B. Increased vascular resistance
    1. Obstruction of blood vessels
        Atherosclerosis: CAD, TIA, diabetes mellitus
        Thromboembolic phenomena: DIC, sickle cell anemia, bacterial endocarditis, pregnancy-induced hypertension, polycythemia
        Vasospasm: Raynaud's disease, Prinzmetal's angina
        Mechanical compression: thoracic outlet syndrome, decubitus ulcers, subdural hematoma
        Intra-arterial catheters: blood pressure monitoring
    2. Shunting of blood flow
        Shock states
        Physiological stress: postcardiotomy, major abdominal surgery
        Increased metabolic demand: exercise
        AV anastomoses: congenital AV malformations, surgical AV shunts for hemodialysis access
    3. Injury to blood vessels
        Primary: Traumatic and surgical injury
        Secondary: Leaking aortic aneurysms, periarteritis nodosa
    4. Decreased capillary-tissue ratio
        Severe tissue edema: lymphedema
        Tissue hypertrophy: left ventricular hypertrophy as in aortic stenosis, congenital coarctation of the aorta, ventricular septal defect

AV, arteriovenous; CAD, coronary artery disease; DIC, disseminated intravascular coagulation; MI, myocardial infarction; TIA, transient ischemic attack.

reflects greater public awareness and alteration of important vascular disease risk factors.[8]

Although these figures are a cause for optimism, CHD and stroke remain leading causes of death in this country and exert tremendous impact on health and disability care costs. In fiscal year 1991 an estimated $101.3 billion was spent on heart disease. This cost includes hospitalization, physician and nursing care, medications, nursing home services, and lost productivity from disability.[5] Significantly, approximately 45 per cent of MIs occur in persons below age 65 during the peak years of their functional capabilities.[5, 9] Stroke also impairs functional capacity. Approximately 70 per cent of individuals who have had a stroke cannot work[10] or must change jobs, and about one third are completely dependent on family and health institutions for their care and support.[10]

The true prevalence of ischemia is hidden in the myriad of other diseases and conditions with which it is commonly associated. The full magnitude of its occurrence can be appreciated with consideration of the etiological factors and the populations at risk.

SITUATIONAL STRESSORS AND POPULATIONS AT RISK

The various etiologic factors proposed as the causes of ischemia are factors that arise in the environment as well as predictably within the individual, that is, as a result of situational and developmental stressors. The situational stressors that result in ischemia are those clinical states or diseases that diminish tissue perfusion by either a reduction in cardiac output (such as hemorrhage) or an increase in vascular resistance (such as atherosclerosis). Developmental stressors are those that place the individual at risk for ischemia because of either the direct effect of the age of the person or the events that are more likely to occur because of the individual's age.

Clinical States and Medical Diagnoses

A classification system that is useful in categorizing the types of decreased perfusion states usually seen with ischemia is presented in Table 2–1; commonly associated clinical states and medical diagnoses are included. The categories identified are those that result in decreased cardiac output or increased vascular resistance due to obstruction of blood vessels, shunting of blood flow, injury to blood vessels, and decreased capillary-tissue ratio. The populations at risk for ischemia in each of these categories are presented in Table 2–2. This is not a complete list, and only selected populations at risk are highlighted in the following discussion.

Decreased Cardiac Output

Clinical states that lower cardiac output or mean arterial pressure (MAP) or both are hypovolemia, massive vasodilation, and reduced pumping efficiency of the heart. These clinical states are represented, respectively, by hemorrhagic shock, gram-negative sepsis, and left ventricular failure. Persons at risk for gram-negative septicemia are those who have a primary infection with a gram-negative bacillus in the lungs, genitourinary (GU) system, biliary tree, or gastrointestinal (GI) tract or those in whom enteric bacilli enter the blood stream after instrumentation or surgery of the GU or GI tract. Elderly males, neonates, and childbearing women make up the majority of this risk group.

Reduced pumping efficiency of the heart can be due to decreased left ventricular contractility or ventricular arrhythmias. Populations at risk in this category are those with congenital or acquired valvular disorders, MI, ventricular aneurysms, cardiomyopathy, or cardiac tamponade.

Increased Vascular Resistance

Obstruction of Blood Vessels. Obstruction of blood vessels results from a variety of clinical states, such as atherosclerosis, thromboembolic phenomena, the presence of an intra-arterial catheter, vasospasm, and external compression. Examples of medical diagnoses associated with these clinical states include coronary artery disease (CAD), disseminated intravascular coagulation (DIC), Prinzmetal's angina, Raynaud's disease (and phenomenon), decubitus ulcers, and subdural hematoma.

Populations at risk for obstruction of blood vessels due to atherosclerosis are the elderly, persons with a family history of atherosclerosis, men over age 40, and those with left ventricular hypertrophy,[11] cigarette smoking,[12] hypertension,[13] elevated total cholesterol,[14] elevated low-density lipoproteins (LDL) or reduced high-density lipoproteins (HDL),[15] obesity, sedentary life style,[16] or type A behavior pattern.[17, 18] Women have a lower risk of developing CHD than men at all ages, although the difference narrows significantly after age 65.[19, 20] Risk factors that are more predictive of CHD in women than in men are hypertriglyceridemia[21] and uncontrolled diabetes mellitus.[22]

Long-term use of oral contraceptives (OCs) may increase risk of heart disease.[23, 24] Recent evidence indicates that otherwise healthy women (i.e., nonsmokers, nondiabetics, and nonhypertensives) who are taking OCs currently in use (estrogen content less than 50 µg) have no excess risk of CHD.[25]

Risk factors for Prinzmetal's angina (due to coronary vasospasm) are not completely delineated, but atherosclerotic vessels seem to be hypersensitive to vasospastic stimuli such as stress and cold environmental temperature. An increasingly recognized risk factor for myocardial ischemia and stroke is cocaine and "crack" cocaine use.[26–28] Cocaine can cause coronary vasospasm, increased platelet aggregation, and acute increases in heart rate (HR) and blood pressure (BP).[26, 27] Cocaine may also accelerate coronary atherogenesis.[27]

Mechanical compression of blood vessels can result from severe tissue edema, tumors, bedrest, constrictive devices (e.g., orthopedic casts and appliances), and entrapment (e.g., compartment syndrome). Persons at risk include, respectively, those with increased capillary permeability, hypoproteinemia, lymphedema, and solid tumors; the bedridden (especially those who are immobile and incontinent and have decreased levels of consciousness, neuromuscular disability, and poor nutrition), persons with fractured limbs, and those with soft tissue trauma to the extremities. Another significant population is those persons who undergo periods of aortic occlusion with surgical clamps during vascular bypass graft procedures. They are at high risk for ischemia of distal tissues, especially the kidneys and the spinal cord.

Shunting of Blood Flow. Shunting of blood flow from peripheral tissues may occur in response to shock, physiological stress, or exercise. Arteriovenous (AV) malformations or anastomoses may be responsible for sig-

TABLE 2–2 **POPULATIONS AT RISK FOR ISCHEMIA**

Clinical States and Diagnoses	Population–Persons Who Experience
A. Decreased cardiac output	
1. Hypovolemia	Motor vehicle or industrial accidents
	Burns
	Infants
	Elderly
2. Vasodilation	Gram-negative sepsis
	● Primary infection with a gram-negative organism
	● After instrumentation or surgery of the GU or GI tract
	Therapy with a potent vasodilator
3. Reduced pumping efficiency of the heart	Decreased left ventricular contractility
	● Congenital valve disease or valve disease acquired from rheumatic fever, papillary muscle infarction, or bacterial endocarditis
	● Myocardial infarction
	● Ventricular septal defect
	● Ventricular aneurysm
	● Intrapericardial hemorrhage and tamponade
	Supraventricular and ventricular arrhythmias
	Asystole
B. Obstruction of blood vessels	
1. Atherosclerosis	Cerebral and cardiovascular disease
	● Elderly
	● Men over 40
	● Cigarette smoking
	● Hyperlipidemia
	● Use of oral contraceptives
	● Hypertension
	● Obesity
	● Sedentary life style
	● Type A behavior pattern
2. Thromboembolism	Increased blood viscosity
	● Polycythemia
	● Leukemia
	● Severe hyperglycemia
	● Dehydration
	Hypercoagulability
	● Pregnancy
	● General anesthesia
	● Immobility
	Bacterial endocarditis
	Atrial fibrillation
	Sickle cell crisis
	DIC
	● Septicemia
	● Crush injury
	● Transfusion reaction
	● Burns
	● Amniotic fluid embolism
	● Placental abruption
	Air embolism
	● Central venous or pulmonary artery catheter
	● Mechanical ventilation with high peak airway pressure
	Fat embolism
	● Long bone fractures
	● Burns
	● Contusion
	● Childbirth
	● Pump oxygenator
3. Vasospasm	Prinzmetal's angina
	Raynaud's disease and phenomenon
	Subarachnoid hemorrhge
	Cocaine use

TABLE 2–2   POPULATIONS AT RISK FOR ISCHEMIA Continued

Clinical States and Diagnoses	Population—Persons Who Experience:

4. Mechanical compression	Severe tissue edema
	  • Hypoproteinemia
	  • Lymphedema
	  • Cerebral edema
	Solid tumors
	Bed rest
	  • Decreased level of consciousness
	  • Elderly
	  • Fatigued
	  • Neuromuscular disability
	Surgical clamps
	  • Vascular bypass surgery
	Entrapment
	  • Thoracic outlet syndrome
	  • Compartment syndrome

5. Intra-arterial catheters	Arterial pressure monitoring
C. Shunting of blood flow 1. Decreased MAP	Motor vehicle or industrial accident Large surgical blood loss Burns Septic shock Cardiogenic shock Dehydration
2. Increased metabolic demand	Vigorous aerobic exercise Mild to moderate exercise of a limb with atherosclerotic occlusive disease
3. AV anastomosis	Congenital Surgical • Hemodialysis access Traumatic injury to blood vessels
D. Injury to blood vessels	Trauma or surgery Burns Leaking aneurysms Atherosclerosis Hypertension Inflammation • Vasculitis

E. Decreased capillary-tissue ratio	Severe tissue edema
	  • Lymphedema
	  • Hypoproteinemia
	Tissue hypertrophy
	  • Left ventricular hypertrophy

nificant shunting of blood flow away from tissues. They can be congenital or surgically created for the purpose of acute or chronic hemodialysis access. Populations at risk for ischemia in this situation are those with compromised blood flow distal to the AV shunt, such as those with low MAP or diabetes—often those who are in renal failure and require these types of shunts.

Injury to Blood Vessels. Injury to blood vessels may be primary, as in crushing or stabbing injuries or surgical incisions. Secondary injuries may occur, such as with a leaking aortic aneurysm or an arterial inflammatory disease, for example, periarteritis nodosa. Acquired immunodeficiency syndrome (AIDS) has been associated with a variety of vasculopathies in children and adults resulting in hemorrhagic and nonhemorrhagic strokes.[29, 30]

Decreased Capillary-Tissue Ratio. A decreased capillary-tissue ratio occurs when severe tissue edema or hypertrophy increases the tissue mass relative to its blood supply, as in lymphedema or severe left ventricular hypertrophy.[31] Populations at risk for severe tissue edema include those with lymphatic disease (e.g., scleroderma or malignancies of the lymph tissue) or hypoproteinemia (e.g., protein-losing nephropathy). Individuals at risk for severe left ventricular hypertrophy include those with congenital or acquired valve disease, coarctation of the aorta, patent ductus arteriosus, ventricular septal defects, idiopathic hypertrophic subaortic stenosis, congestive cardiomyopathy, hypertension, and congestive heart failure.

Often a particular population manifests more than one of the clinical states or diagnoses listed in Table 2–1. In addition, the presence of reduced arterial oxygen content due to hypoxemia or anemia will significantly increase the risk of ischemia.

DEVELOPMENTAL DIMENSIONS

The developmental stage of the individual may influence the risk for developing ischemia because of either the direct effect of age on the tissue or the events that are more likely to occur because of age. The direct effect of age is seen primarily in the neonatal population (less than 10 days old). It has been shown that survival of the total animal after exsanguination is much longer in the newborn than in the adult animal (20 minutes versus 20 seconds).[32] The proposed mechanisms of this phenomenon will be discussed later.

The perinatal period is one of rapidly changing oxygenation and blood flow patterns. Either a preterm or perinatal accident can exaggerate these changes, producing hypoxia or ischemia or both. Hypercapnia may also be a feature of this disturbance if there is an alteration in respiratory gas exchange (known as asphyxia). Frequently the result is variable degrees of neurological injury known as hypoxic-ischemic encephalopathy.[33]

Infants and small children are at increased risk for dehydration and hypovolemia because of their immature fluid regulatory mechanisms.[34] The elderly also are at increased risk for dehydration due to a decreased sense of thirst that may coexist with an impaired ability to respond to thirst owing to disease or debilitation. The elderly are more likely than younger individuals to be receiving chronic diuretic therapy and to suffer significant losses of water and electrolytes. The elderly predictably encounter changes in vascular compliance and vasomotor responsiveness that do not produce clinically significant reductions in perfusion in the absence of other vascular disease, such as atherosclerosis or hypertension.[35] However, the likelihood of atherosclerosis is greater in the elderly and may be severe enough to diminish perfusion markedly at times of increased demand, such as exercise, fever, or injury, or at times of decreased mean arterial pressure. There have been a number of reports of fatal and nonfatal cerebral ischemia and stroke in elderly hypertensive individuals who experienced a rapid drop in MAP (as little as 11 per cent in some) when treated with antihypertensive drugs.[36] Presumably, this was due to diminished autoregulation of cerebral blood flow and baroreceptor responsiveness in the face of a rapid fall in MAP. Coexistent carotid artery stenosis in a few individuals contributed to the cerebral hypoperfusion.

During the late stage of pregnancy and after delivery, women have an increased risk for ischemia because of hypercoagulability of the blood, putting them at risk for thromboembolic events such as MI or stroke.[37] Also, pregnancy-induced hypertension (formerly known as eclampsia) can occur and result in vascular injury, thrombosis, and significant end-organ damage.[38]

MECHANISMS

Determinants of Blood Flow

Blood flow is directly related to driving pressure (mean arterial pressure minus central venous pressure) and inversely related to arteriolar resistance.[39] Factors influencing driving pressure include blood volume, myocardial contractility, and heart rate (which also determine cardiac output). Arteriolar resistance is dependent on the net effects of systemically circulating substances, such as catecholamines, angiotensin, and prostaglandins. Substances locally released in response to a tissue's changing oxygen and energy needs (autoregulation) include carbon dioxide, potassium, lactate, adenosine, and the recently discovered endothelium-derived relaxing and contracting factors (EDRF and EDCF).[40, 41] Factors such as temperature and intraluminal pressure also influence arteriolar resistance.[39]

Autoregulation occurs within a MAP range of 70 to 175 mm Hg for most tissues.[39] Arterial pressures above or below these limits result in passive increases or decreases in the arteriolar lumen and tissue blood flow. If MAP falls below the pressure within which an arteriole can regulate its flow, the vessel diameter becomes smaller, and blood flow decreases. When intraluminal pressure becomes less than the surrounding tissue pressure, the vessel collapses and flow ceases, even though blood pressure may be greater than zero. The intraluminal pressure at which the vessel collapses is called the critical closing pressure.[42]

Tissue perfusion depends upon a delicately regulated balance between cardiac output and vascular resistance. The situational or developmental stressors that result in ischemia are those factors that reduce cardiac output or increase vascular resistance or both. The mechanisms by which these factors decrease tissue perfusion are discussed in the following sections.

Reduction in Cardiac Output

Any disease or clinical state that reduces cardiac output below a tissue's ability to compensate will result in ischemia of that tissue. Because cardiac output is a major determinant of MAP, the MAP will also be decreased, placing all tissues at risk for ischemia. Situations that result in reduced cardiac output are ones in which there is (1) a reduction in total blood volume (hypovolemia), (2) an increase in the vascular space, or (3) a reduction in the pumping efficiency of the heart. Hemorrhage, burns, and dehydration are examples of states resulting in hypovolemia. Septic shock and generalized vasodilation from vasodilator therapy result in an increase in the size of the vascular space, creating a relative hypovolemia.

Diseases or clinical states that compromise the pumping efficiency of the heart, such as congestive heart failure or ventricular arrhythmias, threaten systemic tissue perfusion. Also, because the heart is uniquely responsible for its own perfusion, a reduction in cardiac output itself propagates a vicious circle of events that can be difficult to halt: a reduction in coronary artery perfusion resulting in myocardial ischemia, which further decreases cardiac output and systemic perfusion, which further aggravates coronary artery perfusion, and so forth.

Increased Vascular Resistance

Factors that increase systemic or tissue vascular resistance will cause a low-flow state that may result in a partial or complete cessation of blood flow to most body tissues or to a localized region. The causes of increased vascular resistance can be organized under the broad categories displayed in Table 2–1.

Obstruction of Blood Vessels. Ischemia resulting from obstruction of blood vessels occurs primarily on the arterial side of the circulation, that is, arteries, arterioles, and capillaries, which deliver oxygen and nutrients to the tissues. Obstruction of the venous side of the circulation at times can cause localized ischemia. The process takes much longer than with arterial obstruction and occurs because the subsequent increase in venous hydrostatic pressure results in increases in interstitial fluid, which interfere with diffusion of nutrients and elimination of waste products. Eventually, the arterial system upstream becomes congested and obstructed as well, severely compromising the tissue it supplies. Nevertheless, venous obstruction is a much less common and less important etiology of ischemia than arterial obstruction.

Shunting of Blood Flow. One type of shunting occurs in peripheral vascular beds, such as the renal and mesenteric circulations, in response to vasoactive substances released during states of shock or physiological stress. The targeted vascular beds constrict, reducing blood flow to their respective tissues and preferentially increasing the blood available for perfusion of more critical tissues, such as the brain. This response, however, places the targeted tissues at risk for ischemia. For example, a frequent complication of shock is renal failure secondary to ischemia of the nephron.

Shunting also is the result of congenital AV malformations or traumatically or surgically created anastomoses. In the absence of collateral flow this type of shunt can result in significant loss of nutrients and oxygen to the tissue. AV malformations or anastomoses can cause pooling of blood within themselves and become a source of emboli. The malformation can also rupture, jeopardizing distal tissues. In the brain, an AV malformation can be a space-occupying lesion or can rupture and cause significant pressure and compression of other blood vessels, further compromising flow.

Injury to Blood Vessels. Any process that interrupts the integrity of nutrient blood vessels places the distal tissues at risk for ischemia. Traumatic laceration of an artery, surgical incision, chemical or thermal injury, dissection of an aneurysm, and an inflammatory process all result in interruption of the vessel wall and in abnormal hemodynamics, which compromise distal perfusion. The blood vessels themselves also are at risk for ischemia if their own nutrient supply via the vasa vasorum is interrupted. Additionally, the vessel's inflammatory response to injury results in local edema, migration of inflammatory cells, sloughing of dead cells, vasospasm, and clot formation, further jeopardizing blood flow in that area.[40]

Decreased Capillary-Tissue Ratio. The normal number and distribution of capillaries are such that the diffusion distance for oxygen, nutrients, and waste products is optimal for the requirements of the individual tissues. For example, each of the islet cells of the pancreas is in contact with several capillaries, whereas this contact is not as great in less metabolically active tissues.[40] A reduction in capillary density can result when either the number of cells relative to the capillary supply increases or tissue edema increases the distance between capillary and cell. A common example of the first case is left ventricular hypertrophy (LVH), in which the growth of myocardium has outstripped the generation of capillaries to supply it.[43] In the second case, tissue edema may be severe enough to increase significantly the diffusion distance between capillary and cell and to cause mechanical compression of blood vessels.

Energy Metabolism

Ischemia is a result of abnormalities of cellular energy metabolism due to decreased tissue perfusion. Understanding the underlying pathophysiological mechanisms and consequences of ischemia is predicated upon a basic familiarity with the normal processes of energy production. It is beyond the scope of this chapter to review in detail the physiology of cellular energy metabolism; for an in-depth review, refer to other sources.[39, 42] Several basic concepts of normal energy metabolism are presented here to provide a framework for understanding the functional changes that occur within the cell as a result of ischemia.

Figures 2–1 and 2–2 present the major features of energy metabolism within the cell. There are three primary sets of reactions: glycolysis, the tricarboxylic acid (TCA) cycle, and oxidative phosphorylation. The series of reactions up to and including the conversion of pyruvate to lactate is glycolysis; this process occurs within the cytoplasm under either aerobic or anaerobic conditions. Under aerobic conditions more pyruvate than lactate is produced, and the reverse is true under anaerobic conditions.

Glycolysis results in the net production of 2 molecules of adenosine triphosphate (ATP) per mole of blood glucose.[42] Under aerobic conditions, the pyruvate formed via glycolysis enters the mitochondria and is converted to acetylcoenzyme A (acetyl-CoA). Acetyl-CoA enters the TCA cycle (also called the Krebs citric acid cycle), which represents the second major set of reactions. The important products of the TCA cycle are ATP, hydrogen ions, and carbon dioxide. The hydrogen ions enter the electron transport chain, where the third series of reactions, known as oxidative phosphorylation, occurs (Fig. 2–2). Various proteins act as electron (hydrogen) carriers until the electrons are accepted by oxygen, the last carrier in the series.[32] For each pair of hydrogen ions transferred from one protein to the next, 2 molecules of ATP are generated.[42] The ATP is then transported out of the mitochondria into the cytoplasm by means of a special carrier located in the membrane of the mitochondria. Once in the cytoplasm ATP becomes the most important source of high energy phosphate that is available to fuel the synthesizing and transporting functions of the cell.[32]

Cellular Events in Ischemia

When perfusion to a tissue slows or completely stops, the resultant decreased oxygen and substrate delivery cause a reduction in oxidative phosphorylation and an increase in anaerobic glycolysis. Figure 2–3 is a diagram of the resulting major cellular events that constitute the process of ischemia and occur in all cells. This complex chain of events has not been completely elucidated, since these processes interact and overlap in ways that are difficult to isolate and to sequence.[1, 2]

A drastic reduction in the amount of ATP produced and the initiation of anaerobic glycolysis are the primary initiators of a complex series of reactions that, if not checked, eventually result in irreversible injury, the so-called point of no return[1] (p. 6). Reduced ATP production results in abnormalities of ion flux into and out of the cell, particularly

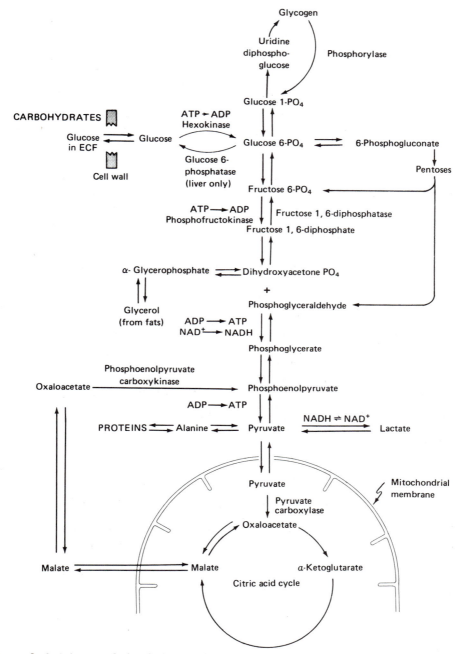

Figure 2–1. Schema of glycolysis and the tricarboxylic acid cycle. (From Ganong, W.F. [1991]. *Review of Medical Physiology* [15th ed]. San Mateo, CA: Appleton & Lange, p. 267 with permission.)

sodium (Na^+) and potassium (K^+), which normally are regulated by the Na^+-K^+ ATPase pump.[42] Calcium (Ca^{++}) and magnesium (Mg^{++}) ions are also regulated in part by similar pumps.[1] The result is increased efflux of K^+ and influx of Na^+ and possibly Ca^{++}. The transmembrane potential difference is altered, and the regulation of many cellular functions is impaired, such as nerve conduction and muscle contraction. It is likely that

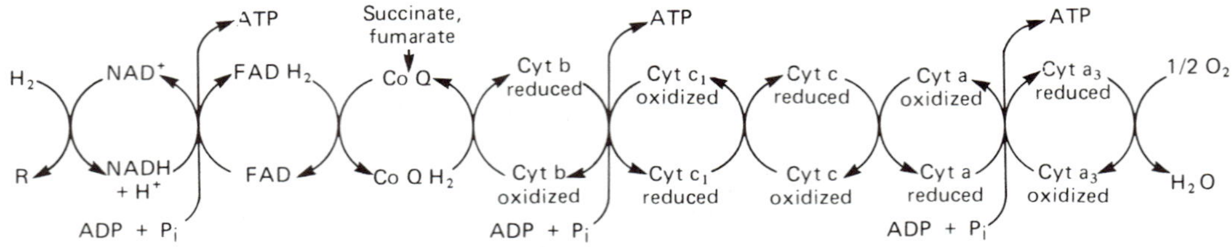

Figure 2–2. Oxidative phosphorylation via the electron transport chain. (From Ganong, W.F. [1991]. *Review of Medical Physiology* [15th ed]. San Mateo, CA: Appleton & Lange, p. 268 with permission.)

aberrations in K^+ flux are responsible in large part for the arrhythmogenesis of myocardial ischemia.[44]

With increased intracellular sodium, intracellular water increases, causing the cell and most organelles to swell. This is a very early microscopic manifestation of ischemia.[1] Accumulation of osmotically active particles such as lactate, adenosine, creatine, and inorganic phosphate contribute to excessive cellular and subcellular swelling.[45] As the swelling increases and is prolonged, organelle and cell membranes leak, causing the escape of several macromolecules[2] (e.g., lactate and adenosine) that have vasodilating properties important in increasing perfusion to the area.[40] However, as the cellular swelling progresses, compression of capillaries occurs, further compromising perfusion.[2]

Intracellular Ca^{++} increases as a result of decreased ATPase activity and opening of Ca^{++} channels in the cell membrane.[46] Larger than normal amounts of Ca^{++} within the cell cause widespread and damaging effects, either directly, by interference with the contractile proteins in the myocardium, or indirectly, by reactions influenced by the presence of increased Ca^{++}.

It is controversial whether Ca^{++} exerts its injurious effects during the period of decreased perfusion or during reperfusion.[46, 47] Differences in experimental models and measurements of intracellular Ca^{++} may account, in part, for this controversy.[48] Forman and associates[49] and Krause and associates[50] described a theoretical role for Ca^{++} injury during the period of decreased perfusion that sets up conditions for further injury with reperfusion. Intracellular calcium combines with calmodulin, a protein that is inactive until it binds with Ca^{++}. The Ca^{++}-calmodulin complex is normally responsible for many intracellular processes that are held in balance by the usually very low (about 1 μm)

and very narrow range of intracellular calcium levels.[1] During ischemia, formation of Ca^{++}-calmodulin complexes increases, and the processes they initiate are allowed to proceed without check (Fig. 2–4). Among the many destructive effects that can result are production of the oxygen free radicals, superoxide (O_2^-), hydrogen peroxide (H_2O_2), and hydroxyl radical (OH^-). These are highly reactive products of oxygen metabolism that are toxic to many biological substances. Oxygen radicals react with the protein-phospholipid structures of cellular and intracellular membranes, forming additional highly reactive free radical species that perpetuate the membrane injury.[49–51] Oxygen free radical scavengers normally produced by the cell to catabolize O_2^-, H_2O_2, and OH^- to harmless end products are rapidly depleted by the increased production of free radicals.[42, 51]

Ca^{++}-calmodulin complexes also activate phospholipases that metabolize free fatty acids in the cell membranes, particularly arachidonic acid. The products of arachidonic acid metabolism are prostaglandins, thromboxanes, and leukotrienes. These substances produce vasospasm and vasodilation in varying degrees in different vascular beds, platelet aggregation, increased neutrophil adhesion and clumping, reduced deformability of red blood cells, arteriolar and capillary endothelial leaking, and further disruption of cell membranes.[49, 50] Changes in cellular membrane structure may activate the complement system, resulting in additional neutrophil chemotaxis and adhesion. Clumping of neutrophils (leukoemboli) have been implicated in extending myocardial injury after infarction.[52]

Increased intracellular Ca^{++} also activates nucleases that damage deoxyribonucleic acid (DNA), which interferes with protein synthesis.[50] In the brain Ca^{++} stimulates the pre-

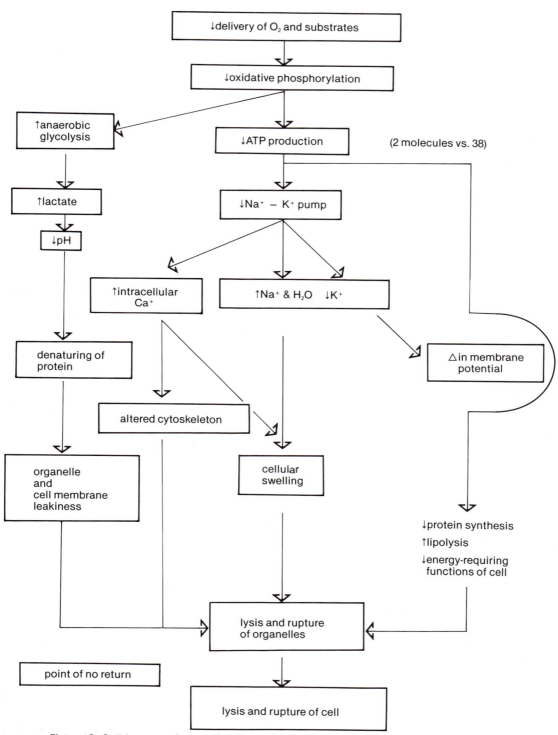

Figure 2–3. Diagram of several major cellular events that occur in ischemic injury.

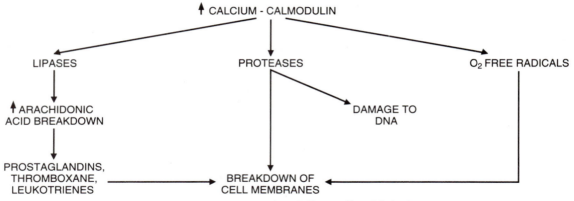

Figure 2–4. Calcium-calmodulin mediated injuries.

synaptic release of neurotransmitters that have an excitatory effect on certain postsynaptic neurons, resulting in enhanced metabolic activity and more rapid depletion of energy stores. This occurs in selectively vulnerable areas of the brain that are particularly sensitive to short periods of absent perfusion, such as different regions of the hippocampus and cerebellum.[46, 50]

As ATP stores are depleted, anaerobic glycolysis becomes the major source of energy production, while yielding increased lactate and a reduction in intracellular pH. The hydrolysis of ATP as it is metabolized for energy also contributes significantly to the hydrogen ions produced.[53] The acid pH may slow or halt glycolysis, although recent investigations using nuclear magnetic resonance (NMR) spectroscopy have found that anaerobic metabolism is limited primarily by diminishing glycogen stores.[53] The reduction in pH may have an inhibitory effect on the activities of the Ca^{++}-calmodulin complexes, at least early in ischemia[1] and thus may have a membrane-stabilizing effect by delaying some of the cellular damage.

Eventually, the low pH itself will exert damaging effects directly on the protein structures of the cell and the chromatin material within the nucleus. In the mitochondria the complex membrane system as well as the electron transport proteins are denatured. The electron transport system supplies 95 per cent of the energy required by the body under normal conditions. Therefore, significant damage to this system will result in irreversible cell damage.[1] The acid pH also inhibits the activity of many enzymes required for nearly all cellular processes.

As a result of these alterations, the entire machinery of the cell becomes depressed or nonfunctional. As the point of irreversible injury is approached within the cell, there is increasing leakiness and eventual rupture of organelles. Rupture of intracellular lysosomes in particular is thought of as the final event signaling irrevocable cell injury.[1] When the lysosomes rupture, hydrolases that digest cellular contents and surrounding tissue are released. Other intracellular enzymes are released to the surrounding tissue as well, such as aspartate aminotransferase (AST—formerly known as glutamic oxalacetic transaminase [GOT]), lactate dehydrogenase (LDH), and creatine phosphokinase (CPK), which are used as clinical indicators of infarction[54] but which may be released before infarction.[54–56]

Once the point of irreversible injury has been reached and autodigestion of the cell has begun, prostaglandins and other products of inflammation are released from the cells. Polymorphonucleocytes accumulate in the area and phagocytize the remainder of the cellular structures.[1] Over time, fibrin and collagen fibers replace the infarcted tissue, and a scar is formed. Scar tissue does not participate in the function of the organ and if large enough can seriously impair whatever normal tissue function remains. For example, the scar that forms from infarcted myocardium may expand early in the healing process and cause ventricular dilation.[57]

Perhaps the most long-standing and vital issue that remains unresolved in the study of ischemic injury is the identification of the structural, functional, and biochemical markers of irreversible injury. One way in which researchers have examined this issue has been to study the effect of a loss of perfusion on gross tissue function and key biochemical processes such as oxidative phosphorylation; the amount of time required for these functions to be lost has been approximated closely in most tissues.[58–64] Hearse[65] contends, however, that biological life of the cell (e.g., energy production) may be intact while its physiological life (e.g., ventricular contraction) is dead. Resolution of this issue will allow for monitoring the progression of ischemia and response to therapy and for deciding when therapy will have no effect.[48]

Reperfusion Injury

Reperfusion injury occurs when re-established blood flow increases delivery of oxygen, calcium, sodium, water, and leukocytes to the ischemic tissue, causing acceleration of oxygen free radical production, protease and phospholipase activation, and cell membrane damage.[48] There is explosive cellular and subcellular swelling, release of the accumulated products of anaerobic metabolism, and free radical reactions into the tissue, causing local vasodilation and hyperemia. Ischemic vascular endothelium is further injured by these substances, resulting in swelling, activation of neutrophils and platelets, vasospasm, and obstruction of capillary flow, which accounts for the nonuniform return of blood flow postreperfusion.[66] Additionally, there is washout of critical substances, such as K^+ and Mg^{++}, adenine nucleotides and phosphate, and oxygen free radical scavengers. Loss of these substances may contribute, respectively, to further alteration of nerve impulse conduction and muscle contraction, delayed restoration of ATP stores, and unchecked cellular and subcellular membrane injury.[49]

Braunwald and Kloner[67] described the concept of "stunned myocardium," which may exemplify one organ's response to reperfusion in that there is a period of hours and up to 2 weeks of myocardial depression postreperfusion. ATP levels are low, biochemical and mechanical abnormalities persist, but normal function is ultimately restored.[66, 67] Clinical evidence for stunned myocardium came as a result of the observations of subjects after a variety of revascularization procedures. For example, in the thrombolysis

trials successfully recanalized subjects gained only a modest improvement in ventricular function in the first day after thrombolysis compared with pre-thrombolysis measures. However, up to 14 to 16 days later there continued to be gradual improvement and significant recovery of ventricular function.[66] It has also been found that depressed myocardial function can be reversed by inotropic agents, indicating that the myocardium is viable and that sufficient ATP stores are present for a good contractile response.[68]

The ability to modify reperfusion injury has been demonstrated by decreased size of tissue infarction when animals are given agents before or during reperfusion that decrease O_2 radical production (e.g., allopurinol) or that decrease neutrophil activity (e.g., steroids).[49, 69] Calcium antagonists may improve recovery of myocardium when given before ischemia, although the mechanism is probably due to decreased contractility and reduction of afterload (i.e., a reduction of energy demand) rather than a decrease in Ca^{++}-mediated injuries.[70]

Several investigators currently believe that reperfusion hastens the inevitable death of already severely impaired cells,[63, 70, 71] but it is possible that reperfusion can induce irreversible injury in ischemic but viable tissue.[49, 66] The cellular mechanisms of reperfusion injury and potential therapeutic agents require continued investigation, especially in humans.

Factors Influencing Sensitivity to Ischemia

The risk and the degree of ischemia sustained by any tissue are determined by the complex interactions of time, amount of blood flow, and several factors inherent in the tissue and the organism as a whole. In general, factors that increase a tissue's sensitivity to diminished blood flow include a high metabolic rate,[1] a high dependency on aerobic energy production,[72] low or absent collateral flow,[72] and low arterial oxygen content. Tissues with low metabolic rate, good collateral flow,[72] low temperature (hypothermia),[58] or an ability to store oxygen are able to withstand relatively long periods of low or absent flow. Table 2–3 displays various tissues, factors that influence their sensitivities to ischemic injury, and the period of dimin-

TABLE 2–3 FACTORS INFLUENCING TISSUE SENSITIVITY TO ISCHEMIA AND TIME BEFORE
IRREVERSIBLE INJURY

Tissue	Influencing Factors	Irreversibility
Brain	↑ Metabolic rate • Reliance on aerobic energy production • Collateral blood flow	4 to 5 minutes[62]
Heart	↑ Metabolic rate • Reliance on aerobic energy production • ↑ O_2 extraction • ± Collateral blood flow	20 to 40 minutes[63]
Renal proximal tubule	High metabolic rate • Collateral blood flow	1 to 2 hours[1]
Liver	High metabolic rate • Collateral blood flow	65 minutes[68]
Intestinal villi	High metabolic rate • Collateral blood flow	1 hour[67]
Skeletal muscle	Large glycogen stores Collateral blood flow Can store O_2 in resting state	2 hours[64, 65]
Pulmonary alveoli	Low metabolic rate Several sources of O_2	5 hours[66]

[1]Trump et al, 1982.
[62]Modry & Chin, 1987.
[63]Haglund et al, 1987.
[64]Hasselgren, 1987.
[65]Hearse, 1984.
[66]Braunwald & Kloner, 1982.
[67]Braunwald & Kloner, 1982.
[68]Kloner et al, 1989.

ished flow before irreversible injury occurs. Additional important factors that influence sensitivity to ischemia are the age of the tissue and the blood glucose level of the organism.

Age

The influence of age on tissue sensitivity to states of inadequate perfusion is probably most evident in studies of the brains and hearts of many species of newborn animals.[32] Mechanisms proposed for the relative resistance to ischemia of newborn brains center around cerebral energy utilization. The newborn brain does not synthesize or respond to central nervous system neurotransmitters in a mature fashion, resulting in a lower cerebral metabolic rate and oxygen utilization. There is a reduced production of lactate and, therefore, less of a decrease in pH and its consequent deleterious effects.[32] Additionally, the permeability of the immature blood-brain barrier to lactate (i.e., from tissue to circulation) is six times that of the adult blood-brain barrier, thus greatly reducing the opportunity for lactate to accumulate locally in ischemic cerebral tissue.[73]

The survival of the total organism is much longer in the newborn animal than in the adult animal after an ischemic insult (20 minutes versus 20 seconds).[32] A major reason for this increased survival is that the newborn heart is also less sensitive to ischemia, and pump failure is a later occurrence than is seen in adult animals. This effect appears to be due to the presence of larger glycogen stores in newborn hearts and a concomitantly greater capacity for anaerobic glycolysis. Also, the mitochondria in newborn myocardial cells have been shown to have a greater aerobic capacity, resulting in increased electron transport.[32]

Blood Glucose

The effect of blood glucose level on the cerebral damage during global or focal reduction in blood flow is unclear.[74] The findings in animal models of ischemia and clinical studies in humans demonstrate conflicting responses to hypo- and hyperglycemia. The weight of evidence suggests that hyperglycemia in animals before or during global reductions in cerebral blood flow (e.g., cardiac arrest) increases ischemic injury and worsens neurological outcomes. Human studies of global cerebral ischemia lack sufficient data to draw any conclusions about the effect of blood glucose levels.[74]

In animal models of focal ischemia the effect of hyperglycemia differs, depending on the blood flow in and around the infarct, local metabolism, and pre-existing disease state.[74] Many studies in humans show an association between hyperglycemia and poor outcomes after stroke and head injury,[74, 75] although the study designs make it difficult to determine a cause and effect relationship.[74] The strongest association between hyperglycemia and mortality occurred with hemorrhagic stroke in a recent study of 252 patients.[76] The hypothesized mechanism for these findings is that the availability of high glucose levels allows continued anaerobic production of lactate and the subsequent acidosis-related injury. On the other hand, hypoglycemia can be just as deleterious as hyperglycemia and should be avoided.

Fasting-induced hypoglycemia in the immature animal may have a protective effect in reducing damage from a hypoxic-ischemic insult, especially if serum ketone bodies are elevated.[77] The proposed mechanisms for this observation are that the newborn brain in animals (and similarly in humans) has a decreased ability to take up and utilize glucose compared with the adult brain, thus decreasing lactate production, and that other substances can be utilized by the newborn brain to support anaerobic metabolism, such as ketone bodies, lactate, and pyruvate.[77]

PATHOLOGICAL CONSEQUENCES OF ISCHEMIA

Acute and severe ischemia will result in transient organ system failure, and, if prolonged, eventual infarction and irreversible loss of tissue function. If the area of ischemia is large or in a critical tissue, such as the bundle of His in the heart, the alteration in tissue function could cause the death of the individual.

Chronic and less severe states of ischemia will cause changes in the tissue that may be adaptive in that they allow the tissue to remain somewhat functional. Changes in the size of the affected tissue, such as hypertrophy or atrophy, are common adaptations to chronic states of absolute or relative reductions in perfusion. In tissue such as chronically ischemic myocardium there is an increase in the number of mitochondria and possibly other organelles that contributes to the increased size of individual myocytes (hypertrophy).[1] This change improves the capacity for aerobic energy production in the face of either reduced perfusion or increased oxygen demand. Some tissues respond to the same situations by reducing the size of the cells (atrophy) and, therefore, cellular energy requirements.[1] Skeletal muscle atrophy is a common manifestation of chronic arterial insufficiency in which the muscle is chronically underperfused. Resultant ischemic leg pain, weakness, and peripheral neuropathy result in relative disuse of the limb, which also contributes to muscle atrophy (see Chapter 21, Skeletal Muscle Atrophy).

Compromise of a tissue's integrity before an ischemic episode will result in less capacity of that tissue to withstand injury and possibly a more rapid onset of altered function. For example, patients with alveolar hypoventilation or overall compromise of the pulmonary circulation have a greater risk of sustaining a pulmonary infarction from an embolus than those with healthy lungs and otherwise normal pulmonary blood flow.[78]

RELATED PATHOPHYSIOLOGICAL CONCEPTS

Ischemia must be distinguished from other phenomena that closely resemble it, since decisions related to therapies and measurement of outcomes depend upon a correct initial assessment. Other related phenomena are infarction, hypoxia, and perinatal asphyxia. The major feature shared by these three phenomena with ischemia is the presence of reduced tissue oxygen. Another commonality is the similarity of the cellular injury (i.e., the reduction in energy production and the events that occur as a result).

The features that distinguish these states from ischemia are the reversibility of injury, energy substrate delivery, and washout of toxic metabolites. Infarction denotes irreversible injury and a complete absence of cellular function. If allowed to progress, ischemia, hypoxia, and asphyxia all can result in infarction. Although reversible injury and irreversible injury are clearly different, distinguishing ischemia from infarction in the clinical setting may be very difficult. Usually it is the complete reversal of the signs of abnormal organ function that are used to denote correction of ischemia before the point of infarction has been reached. However, reperfusion injury may temporarily mask the potential for returning organ function. Also, areas of infarction may have evolved during the ischemic episode that are not clinically detected. It is not uncommon for post-mortem evidence of multiple small infarcts to be apparent in nearly any organ of the body, although these infarcts were not clinically evident during life. Consequently, return of clinically normal organ function or the absence of symptoms or both are unreliable indicators that infarction has not occurred.

Hypoxia denotes a reduction in tissue oxygen, which can occur in the presence of adequate perfusion when arterial oxygen content is reduced. Energy substrate may still be delivered, and toxic metabolites may still be eliminated. As a result of lactate elimination, cellular acidosis occurs over a slower period, and glycolysis can proceed for a longer period than would be possible if perfusion were inadequate.[79] Reduced perfusion results in earlier and greater tissue injury than merely lowering the tissue oxygen tension; experiments have shown that the ischemic heart is much more susceptible to ventricular fibrillation than hearts made hypoxic but continuously perfused.[80] Additionally, the electrophysiological abnormalities occurring within the initial 20 minutes of myocardial ischemia in vivo were eradicated when this same tissue was perfused in vitro.[81] Presumably, one or more substances accumulated during the period of ischemia that caused the arrhythmia and were washed out during perfusion. Support for this conclusion is found in studies in which venous blood from ischemic myocardium produced qualitatively similar electrophysiological aberrations in isolated myocardium as those found in ischemic myocardium in vivo.[82]

Perinatal asphyxia is an impairment of gas exchange resulting in hypoxemia and hypercapnia during the perinatal period. If the hypoxemia is severe or prolonged, hypoxia will result. The hypercapnia superimposes a respiratory acidosis upon the metabolic acidosis of hypoxia, and the cellular pH becomes acidic more rapidly than with hypoxia alone; the hypoxia and acidosis can create significant neurological deficits known as hypoxic-ischemic encephalopathy.[33] In this condition energy substrate continues to be delivered for a time, allowing for some degree of aerobic and anaerobic energy production.

ASSOCIATED PSYCHOSOCIAL CONCEPTS

Coronary heart disease is a convenient model with which to illustrate some of the psychosocial concepts associated with ischemia. CHD is the result of complex physiological and psychosocial processes that act independently and in concert to produce disease. Psychosocial risk factors in the development of CHD have been identified; these include stress, job strain, anxiety, depression, type A behavior pattern (TABP), low socioeconomic status, low educational level, and lack of social support or group belonging.[17-19, 83, 84] The mechanisms underlying these last three processes are not well understood and may relate as much to availability of health care and follow-up as to physiological causes.[84]

Once a major ischemic cardiac event occurs, additional psychological and social factors influence the patient's abilities to cope with and adapt to this chronic disease. Initial anxiety followed by depression or denial is a common sequela to the acute event.[85, 86] If not resolved, depression and denial can have deleterious effects on short- and long-term outcomes, such as continued symptoms, decreased activity levels, decreased frequency of return to work, withdrawal, reinfarction, and death.[87-91] Spouses and families often have difficulty coping with and adjusting to the acute event and to recovery.[92-94] Conflicts occur between spouses and patients regarding overprotectiveness and watchfulness, adherence to treatment, activity levels, and resumption of sexual relations.[89, 95] Family support is critical to patient recovery and positive outcomes.[96]

MANIFESTATIONS AND MEASUREMENT

Ischemia of an organ system is usually accompanied by alterations in the normal functions of that organ, which may be manifested through symptoms, physical findings, and laboratory and diagnostic tests. Because the functions of the various organ systems are diverse, ischemia is manifested in varied ways.

There are a few manifestations that cross several organ systems. For example, pain is often encountered in myocardial, cerebral, pulmonary, renal, and intestinal ischemia and in ischemia of the extremities. The release of prostaglandins, lactate, and other substances is thought to be responsible for irritating peripheral fibers and transmitting pain impulses. Failure to sense pain may be due to alteration of neuronal pathways, as in diabetes mellitus or organ transplantation, differences in individuals' perceptions of pain, or lack of a sufficiently strong stimulus to reach the pain threshold.[97]

Direct observation of many ischemic tissues often reveals pallor and mottling progressing to cyanosis and ultimately a dark discoloration suggestive of necrosis. Normal color is rapidly achieved when perfusion is re-established in viable tissue.

Biochemical indicators of ischemia may be utilized. For example, lactate levels in the venous drainage of ischemic tissues exceed arterial lactate, indicating lactate production. By-products of ATP metabolism such as adenosine, inosine, and hypoxanthine are also elevated in the venous blood draining these same areas. Studies of critically ill patients have examined lactate and hypoxanthine levels and found them to be significantly elevated.[98, 99] Venous lactate had a highly significant and negative correlation with oxygen delivery and cardiac output.[98] Patients with the highest mixed venous levels of hypoxanthine had the lowest systolic blood pressure and survival.[99]

Myocardial Ischemia

The focus of this section will be a discussion of the subjective and objective manifestations of myocardial ischemia (Table 2–4).

Subjective Manifestations

Angina pectoris is the manifestation most frequently associated with myocardial ischemia. Its pathological correlate is most frequently atherosclerotic CAD, although angina may occur in the absence of significant CAD. Prinzmetal and associates[100] first proposed the association of angina with coronary artery spasm in 1959, and Maseri and coworkers[101] have since demonstrated this relationship with coronary angiography.

The association of angina with other etiologies of myocardial ischemia has also been made. Angina may be seen in children with aortic stenosis, anomalous origin of one or more coronary arteries,[102] pulmonary valvu-

TABLE 2–4 MANIFESTATIONS OF MYOCARDIAL ISCHEMIA

Subjective Manifestations
Angina with exercise, cold temperature, meals, emotional stress or at rest
Dyspnea
Nausea
Anxiety

Objective Manifestations
Physical findings
  ± Diaphoretic, cold, clammy
  ± S_3 or S_4 gallop or both
  ± Regurgitant murmurs
  ± Crackles
  ± Elevated jugular venous pressure
  ± Elevated double product
Electrocardiogram
  ST segment elevation or depression > 1 mm
  Peaked T wave or pseudonormalization of inverted T waves
  Arrhythmias
Hemodynamics
  Elevated pulmonary artery and capillary wedge pressures
  Elevated left ventricular end-diastolic pressure
  Elevated right atrial pressure
  Decreased cardiac output
  Ejection fraction < 50 per cent
Radionuclide and echocardiographic studies
  "Cold spot" on thallium-201 perfusion scan with delayed filling
  Abnormalities in wall motion on echocardiogram
Cardiac catheterization
  Confirms many of the findings listed above
  Elevated coronary sinus lactate
  Identifies significant obstructive lesions in coronary arteries and their major branches

lar stenosis, and pulmonary hypertension[103] and in adults with aortic stenosis and insufficiency,[104] hypertrophic and congestive cardiomyopathies,[43] tachyarrhythmias,[103] pulmonary hypertension,[103] and severe anemia or other impairments of oxygen carriage.[103]

The characteristic of "classic" angina due to atherosclerotic narrowing of the coronary arteries is chest pain preceded by physical or emotional stress, relieved by rest, and commonly associated with ST segment depression on the electrocardiogram (ECG).[103] The sensation is described as crushing, burning, squeezing, gripping, or pressing usually originating below the sternum and frequently radiating to the neck, jaws, or medial aspects of either or both arms. Occasionally, the pain may be felt in only one of these peripheral areas rather than substernally. The pain may be slight or severe, but it is usually moderately intense and easily tolerable and lasts for 5 to 10 minutes.[103]

"Variant" angina[100] associated with coronary artery spasm shares the same characteristics as classic angina, with the primary distinction being that variant angina usually occurs at rest and frequently during the night and early morning hours.[105] Significant overlap of rest angina and that occurring with exertion exists in the same individual.[106]

Angina does not always accompany myocardial ischemia even in the same individual,[97, 101] although angina is frequently associated with predictable levels of exercise and double product (heart rate × systolic blood pressure) within the same individual.[107] For this reason, angina is the patient's most important indicator of the safe limits of intensity and duration of exercise. Silent myocardial ischemia, in which no symptoms of ischemia are experienced, occurs in approximately 34 per cent of persons who have stable CAD.[97] In persons with unstable angina the incidence of asymptomatic ischemia (identified by ST depression on the ECG) is as high as 90 per cent, and in the post-MI population it is about 5.4 per cent with treadmill exercise.[97] When silent ischemia occurs frequently with unstable angina or after MI, the prognosis is worse.[97] Unstable angina is an increase in the frequency, intensity, and duration of angina, and its occurrence at rest when it was previously provoked by exercise is considered an ominous sign.[108]

Patients may experience a symptom profile that is atypical but characteristic of their particular ischemic episodes, such as chest pain that does not fit the usual angina picture, or, in the absence of angina, other symptoms such as dyspnea, nausea, and fatigue. These symptoms represent anginal equivalents in these patients. It is critical that the nurse help patients characterize their angina, or its equivalent, identify factors that precipitate it, and learn to distinguish it from the pain of myocardial infarction. The pain of myocardial infarction is unlike angina in that it is usually more severe, lasts for a half-hour or longer, and is not relieved by nitroglycerin.

Other subjective manifestations of ischemia that may accompany angina are dyspnea, nausea, fatigue, and anxiety.

Objective Manifestations

The most commonly used objective indicators of myocardial ischemia are ECG changes, particularly elevation or depression of the ST segment greater than 1 mm (0.1 mV) for at least three successive heart beats.[107] ST segment elevation reflects more severe, that is, transmural, ischemia[107] and is characteristic of coronary vasospasm.[109] Peaked T waves or pseudonormalization of inverted T waves may also accompany ST segment changes, although pseudonormalization of T waves alone during coronary vasospasm has been documented by angiography.[101] The changes in the ECG occur in the leads corresponding to the ischemic areas.

Diagnosis of silent ischemia is usually made by ST segment changes of at least 1 minute using two bipolar ECG leads observed during ambulatory (Holter) monitoring or at rest. Additionally, there must be a normal baseline ST, no bundle branch block, and no drugs present that alter the ST segment (such as digitalis).[97]

ST-T changes are usually absent from the resting ECG of patients with stable angina, consequently the diagnosis of ischemic heart disease is made by stressing the myocardium with dynamic exercise (e.g., a treadmill or cycle ergometer), by atrial pacing at high rates,[110] or via intravenous dipyridamole administration.[111] The stress tests are considered indicative of ischemia if angina, ST-T changes, or a significant drop in blood pressure occurs. One of the major disadvantages of treadmill testing is that the patient may become fatigued before adequate myocardial stress has been achieved, possibly yielding a false-negative test.[112] However, the absence of ST segment depression or elevation does not rule out the presence of ischemia.[112] Other ECG changes thought to increase the sensitivity of detecting ischemia include increases in R wave amplitude[113] and an increased ratio of the amount of ST depression in multiple leads to the heart rate achieved by exercise (the ST/HR slope).[114]

The exercise stress ECG is less sensitive and specific in women, resulting in large numbers of both false positives and false negatives. This may be due to differences (either greater or lesser) in coronary sensitivity to catecholamines released during exercise in women or to differences in fluid and electrolyte metabolism. Additionally, estrogen's chemical structure is similar to digitalis and possibly causes similar effects on the ECG, such as ST segment depression.[115]

Ischemia of the cardiac conduction system

causes alterations in both electrical impulse formation and conduction. The presence of several types of arrhythmias is often evident on the ECG. Ischemia increases excitability and reduces the threshold for fibrillation. It also sets up conditions for generating re-entrant arrhythmias, including supraventricular tachycardia, ventricular tachycardia, and ventricular fibrillation.[44] Ischemia of nodal or bundle of His tissue may produce conduction delays and blocks. Arrhythmias occur more frequently in patients with ST elevation than with ST depression.[116]

Certain physical findings may be apparent during the period of ischemia. The patient may appear anxious or fearful and, because of sympathetic nervous system stimulation, cold and clammy. If ventricular function is significantly compromised, there may be transient jugular venous distention, pulmonary crackles, and an S_3 or S_4 gallop rhythm, all of which denote failure of the left ventricle. Ischemia of a papillary muscle, often of the mitral valve, may result in the transient appearance of a systolic ejection murmur.[103] If the patient is undergoing hemodynamic monitoring, these physical findings may be reflected in increased pulmonary capillary wedge, pulmonary artery, and/or right atrial and jugular venous pressures,[117] depending on whether the right ventricle is involved.[118] The severity of wedge pressure elevations have been shown to correlate with the degree of ST elevations in patients with transmural ischemia.[113]

The appearance of all of these changes in heart function may be preceded by an increase, a decrease, or no change in arterial pressure and heart rate. An increase in arterial pressure or heart rate or both may precede the above signs if the ischemia is a result of a primary increase in myocardial oxygen consumption (MVO_2), such as occurs with anxiety, exercise, or digestion of a large meal.[116] If the ischemia is due to a primary reduction in coronary blood flow, such as coronary vasospasm or platelet aggregation, there will be no signs of increased oxygen demand, but there may be a resultant global ventricular dysfunction that may be reflected first in decreased arterial pressure.[101, 116]

A variety of diagnostic tests are utilized to identify areas of decreased myocardial perfusion and the associated functional effects. These include thallium-201 scans at rest or with exercise,[119] echocardiography,[120] and single-photon emission computerized tomography (SPECT).[121]

New imaging techniques are being studied that will have significant potential for differentiating ischemic from irreversibly injured myocardium. These include nuclear magnetic resonance imaging,[122, 123] positron emission tomography,[124] and nuclear magnetic resonance spectroscopy.[53] The latter two techniques have the ability to study tissue metabolism during normal and ischemic states and will contribute greatly to elucidating these complex processes.

Cardiac catheterization is used to diagnose the pathophysiological process responsible for myocardial ischemia and at the same time evaluate myocardial function and metabolism. Coronary arteriography allows visualization of the degree and extent of atherosclerotic narrowing and vasospasm.

Increased coronary sinus levels of purines, such as adenosine and hypoxanthine, have been found in a variety of populations during periods of ischemia, such as angina, stress testing, and angioplasty.[125] These markers have been identified in arterial blood also, but to a less significant level and less consistently than in coronary sinus blood.[125]

SURVEILLANCE

The occurrence of angina and its pattern, duration, and intensity; ST-T wave changes; and arrhythmias are monitored in every patient admitted to the hospital for evaluation or treatment of myocardial ischemia. The characteristics of angina and the ECG findings dictate the frequency and the time of day or night these manifestations are assessed. The cardiac monitor should be evaluated for the presence and frequency of asymptomatic ECG changes. If ECG changes are present, the nurse should note associated factors in the patient or the environment that may establish a pattern of silent ischemia in that person; that is, the relationship of ECG changes to activities, rest, visitors, anxiety, and other factors.

Deciding which leads to monitor is critical for accurate identification of ECG changes. An admission 12-lead ECG can be used to identify the leads manifesting the ischemic changes and the best leads for continuous monitoring.[126] A full 12-lead ECG should be obtained with each episode of ST segment shift noted on the visual monitor[126] or with angina.[127] This is important in accurately locating the ischemia and when trying to document the possibility of coronary vasospasm, which has a variable presentation even in the same patient.[127] A complete discussion of appropriate lead placement to capture important ECG changes during ischemia and other circumstances can be found elsewhere.[126]

A parameter that correlates with MVO_2 in patients with exertional angina is the rate-pressure product or double product: the product of the heart rate (HR) and systolic blood pressure (SBP). HR and SBP are major determinants of MVO_2 and provide an indirect index of myocardial oxygen need. Angina occurs with a predictable double product in many patients with stable angina, and the beneficial effects of therapy are evidenced by the occurrence of angina at a higher double product than that measured before therapy was initiated. Thus, monitoring this parameter will provide an objective indicator of response to exercise and therapy.

Physical findings are invaluable in establishing the presence of ischemia and its response to therapy. Increased jugular venous pressure (JVP), S_3 or S_4 gallop rhythm, a loud pulmonic sound, a murmur, and crackles are assessed. These parameters are monitored with every complaint of chest pain or alteration in the ECG, at the time of the peak effect of antianginal medications, at intervals during the pain episode, and upon relief of the pain.

A circadian periodicity of myocardial ischemia has been identified in recent years, in which ST depression, symptomatic and asymptomatic, occurs most often in the period between 6 a.m. and 12 p.m. (noon). Sudden cardiac death and MI follow the same pattern.[128, 129] This pattern is independent of age, sex, smoking history, and hypertension and can be altered by beta-blocking drugs. Factors responsible for this pattern appear to be related to neurohumoral changes preceding awakening and arising and for several hours afterward. An early morning rise in catecholamine secretion increases heart rate, myocardial contractility, and blood pressure. Many episodes of early morning ST depression are not accompanied by signs of increased oxygen demand, however, implicating dynamic changes in coronary perfusion such as vasospasm and increased platelet aggregation as the cause of

transient ischemia.[128, 129] Studies have shown increased coronary vasomotor reactivity in the early morning hours corresponding to increases in catecholamines.[105] Catecholamines also induce platelet hyperaggregability. In the early morning there is a simultaneous increase in aldosterone activation and blood viscosity, both of which promote thrombus formation.[129]

Interestingly, these hemodynamic responses are blunted in nonambulatory persons who do not arise after awakening.[129] Nevertheless, many of them change their body position from supine to semirecumbent and participate in activities such as washing, eating, and moving in bed. Yasue and associates[105] found that in the period between 12 a.m. (midnight) and 8 a.m. even minor activities such as shaving, straining at stool, or urination could provoke coronary vasospasm with resultant angina and ECG changes.

CLINICAL THERAPIES

The overriding objective in the management of ischemia is the preservation of ischemic and viable tissue. The therapeutic goals in meeting this objective are aimed at reducing the myocardial oxygen demand and increasing the oxygen supply. Many therapies have one or both of these benefits. Table 2–5 lists the pharmacological and nonpharmacological therapies classified according to the therapeutic goals they meet. Prevention of ischemia is an additional important goal, and modification of significant risk factors will also be discussed.

Pharmacological Therapies

Pharmacological therapies reduce oxygen demand of the heart by lowering the metabolic work due to heart rate, preload and afterload, and contractility. Agents that improve oxygen supply to the heart act by dilating coronary arteries, lysing thrombus and preventing thrombus formation, and increasing coronary perfusion time, coronary perfusion pressure, and arterial oxygen content.

The pharmacological agents and the mechanisms of their effects on the oxygen supply-demand balance of the heart are summarized in Table 2–6. The reader is referred to the

TABLE 2–5 CLINICAL THERAPIES FOR THE MANAGEMENT OF MYOCARDIAL ISCHEMIA

Goals	Pharmacological	Nonpharmacological
Reduce tissue oxygen demand	Vasodilators Calcium antagonists Beta-blocking agents Antiarrhythmics ACE inhibitors*	Rest Stress reduction Avoidance of metabolic stimulants (e.g., heat, infection, caffeine) Hypothermia Education
Increase tissue oxygen supply	Thrombolysis Vasodilators Antiplatelet agents and anticoagulants Antiarrhythmics Oxygen Red blood cell transfusion	Percutaneous transluminal coronary angioplasty Coronary artery bypass graft Exercise Education

*ACE, angiotensin-converting enzyme

references cited in the table[130–162] for a more complete discussion of each agent or class of agents. A brief review of thrombolysis and oxygen therapy will be included here.

A major advance in the nonsurgical management of thrombosis in the coronary arteries is the use of thrombolysis with several available agents: streptokinase, recombinant tissue plasminogen activator (t-PA), and anisoylated plasminogen streptokinase activator complex (APSAC).[155–158] The Second International Study of Infarct Survival[156] (ISIS-2) was a clinical trial of streptokinase or aspirin or both in 17,000 subjects suspected of acute MI. There was a significant mortality benefit at 5 weeks after thrombolysis, with the most benefit achieved in those subjects receiving streptokinase within 4 hours after the onset of symptoms. There was a decreasing but still significant mortality benefit up to 24 hours after the start of symptoms. This late benefit was most evident in persons at highest risk

TABLE 2–6 PHARMACOLOGICAL MANAGEMENT OF ISCHEMIA AND EFFECT ON MYOCARDIAL OXYGEN SUPPLY-DEMAND BALANCE

Agent	Effect on O_2 Supply and Demand	Mechanism of Effect
Vasodilators*		
Nitrates (nitroglycerin, isosorbide dinitrate, nitroprusside)	↓ O_2 demand ↑ O_2 supply	↓ Preload, ↓ afterload Coronary vasodilation
Morphine sulfate	↓ O_2 demand	↓ Preload, ↓ afterload
Calcium channel blockers(nifedipine, diltiazem, verapamil)	↑ O_2 supply ↓ O_2 demand	Coronary vasodilation, prevents vasospasm ↓ Myocardial contractility (especially with verapamil)
Beta Blockers		
(Propranolol, metoprolol, timolol)	↓ O_2 demand ↑ O_2 supply	↓ Myocardial contractility ↓ Heart rate, ↑ coronary perfusion time, controls ventricular arrhythmias
Antiarrhythmics	↓ O_2 demand ↑ O_2 supply	↓ Rapid ventricular rates ↑ Coronary perfusion, ↑ ventricular filling time ↑ ventricular volume from atrial contraction
Antiplatelets and Anticoagulants		
(Aspirin [ASA], dipyridamole, sulfinpyrazone, heparin)	↑ O_2 supply	↓ Platelet aggregation and ↓ thrombus formation Vasodilation (dipyridamole)
Thrombolytics	↑ O_2 supply	Dissolves thrombus and prevents further thrombus formation
ACE Inhibitors†*	↓ O_2 demand ↑ O_2 supply	↓ Afterload Coronary vasodilation
Oxygen	↑ O_2 supply	↑ Oxygen content of arterial blood

*Many of these agents have the secondary effect of increasing myocardial oxygen supply because the reductions in preload and afterload result in lowered intraventricular pressure, which increases the pressure gradient for coronary perfusion.
†ACE = angiotensin-converting enzyme

of death: women, the elderly, hypotensives, those with anterior MI, and those with reinfarction. ISIS-3 was conducted to compare streptokinase with t-PA. Preliminary findings[157] show that t-PA resulted in a higher rate of fatal strokes (0.7 per cent), thought to be due to cerebral hemorrhage, compared with streptokinase (0.3 per cent), although t-PA resulted in earlier recanalization of the infarct-related artery.

In order to maximize salvage of ischemic myocardium, it is critical that the nurse in the emergency department or coronary care unit be alert to patients suitable for thrombolysis and facilitate prompt administration of the drug. The feasibility of prehospital administration of thrombolytic agents as a means of providing early intervention has been demonstrated by the Seattle Myocardial Infarction, Triage, and Intervention Group.[158] This group is currently comparing the safety and efficacy of prehospital versus early emergency department administration of streptokinase.

Reperfusion of an area of the myocardium that has been ischemic for more than a few minutes may cause reperfusion injury, as evidenced by left ventricular dysfunction that may persist for several hours or days before improvement and by ventricular arrhythmias.[44, 71] Commonly used clinical indicators of successful reperfusion are abrupt cessation or diminishing chest pain, appearance of arrhythmias, return of ST segment to baseline, and an early rapid peak of creatine kinase (CK) and CK-MB enzymes. These indicators, however, are insensitive and nonspecific.[163] Further description of the indicators has been shown to have higher concordance with coronary angiographic patency,[164] and Kleven[165] has adapted them as follows for the critical care unit:

(1) ST segment normalization that is abrupt or rapidly progressive, decreases to 50% of baseline value in the most affected lead, and is associated with improvement in chest pain; (2) chest pain that ceases abruptly or progressively decreases within 30 minutes of the first noted improvement; (3) any change in heart rate or rhythm that is associated with chest pain improvement or ST segment normalization; (4) a rapid increase (2.2-fold increase or an increase of 50 U/liter/hour) in CK rise that occurs within 3 hours of administering thrombolysis. Peak serum levels of CK and CK-MB should

occur within 12 hours of beginning therapy (pp. 114–115).

Reocclusion of the vessel and worsening of the ischemia is another risk of thrombolysis. Indices of ischemia, such as angina, ST wave changes, and signs of ventricular failure, must be assessed frequently.[166]

Increasing the arterial oxygen content by increasing the fraction of inspired oxygen or by increasing hemoglobin level when necessary can be an important means of improving myocardial oxygen supply. It is common practice to give high concentrations of inspired oxygen to the patient presenting with acute ischemia and suspected MI. A number of animal and human studies[160–162] have shown, however, that high arterial oxygen tensions (PaO_2) decrease myocardial contractility; increase heart rate, blood pressure, and systemic vascular resistance; and may worsen some measures of ischemia. The issue of whether adverse effects result from administering increased levels of oxygen in the setting of acute myocardial ischemia is not clear-cut. Nevertheless, if a patient is hypoxemic or presenting with signs of ventricular failure, administration of supplemental oxygen is clearly warranted to achieve a PaO_2 sufficient to saturate hemoglobin. Higher arterial oxygen tensions would add no further advantage and could be deleterious to myocardial function. Current guidelines[167] of the American College of Cardiologists and the American Heart Association recommend high oxygen flows initially until oxygenation status can be assessed.

Nonpharmacological Therapies

Therapies to Reduce Oxygen Demand

There are nonpharmacological methods for lowering tissue oxygen demand, some of which have immediate effects (e.g., hypothermia) and others that require much longer periods to demonstrate benefits (e.g., stress reduction). Resting of the tissue or body part is probably one of the most important therapeutic interventions used to treat ischemia. The myocardium can never rest completely, but when individuals present with an ischemic event, exercise limitation becomes a necessary means of reducing MVO_2. Bed rest is initially prescribed with a program of gradually progressive exercise designed to prevent deconditioning, with early ambulation and discharge in the patient with uncomplicated MI.[168, 169] Uncomplicated MI is usually defined as the absence of angina, arrhythmias, and heart failure.[168, 170] Research indicates that rapid mobilization by day 4 after infarction in patients judged to have nearly normal ventricular function results in no deterioration of left ventricular function, extension of the MI, or expansion of the infarction scar.[171] Gradual resumption of activities within the limits of cardiac reserve may also increase the patient's confidence that full functional capacity may be regained.

Several studies by nurses and others have examined the cardiovascular responses to early exercise and various personal care activities after acute MI.[171–176] Although patient selection, activity protocols, and cardiovascular variables differed among these studies, the results consistently demonstrated that changes in position, chair sitting, toileting at the bedside, showering or tub bath, and both light and vigorous ambulation generally caused clinically insignificant changes in heart rate, rhythm, blood pressure, double product, oxygen consumption, and various measures of left ventricular function. However, a small number of patients in these studies manifested further ischemia, pointing out the need to evaluate all patients before beginning activity progression.

Patients with MI complicated by heart failure, persistent ischemia, or arrhythmias are not suitable candidates for early mobilization programs.[171, 177] The progression of activity will necessarily be delayed until ventricular function improves or, if this is not possible, will occur very slowly and with careful evaluation of the patient's responses. The presence of severe dyspnea and ECG changes in the setting of very low ejection fraction (less than 20 per cent) and maximal medical management preclude anything other than very limited activity.[177]

Low-level exercise testing has been utilized in acute MI patients prior to discharge as a means of identifying a level of activity that is safe for them to perform at home and as a means of predicting long-term outcomes.[178, 179] The patient is tested on a treadmill with a slow walking speed and low grade that requires only about 3 to 4 metabolic equivalents (METS) of energy consumption. ST changes or angina or both are highly predictive of future cardiac events.[179] This testing is also useful in determining the presence of cardiac dysfunction requiring further intervention and as a means of reassuring patients and families that a normal functional status can be achieved.

Resumption of sexual activity is of concern to many persons with angina or after MI or coronary artery bypass graft. The cardiovascular demands during peak sexual response, although increased, are transitory.[95, 180] The patient should be instructed that usual sexual activity can be gradually resumed beginning 4 to 8 weeks after the MI. Nitroglycerin should be taken if angina is experienced, and the patient and spouse are cautioned to avoid intercourse after a full meal or drinking alcoholic beverages. If palpitations, dizziness, excessive dyspnea, and chest pain unrelieved by rest or nitroglycerin occur, the patient should seek medical advice quickly.[181]

Hypothermia has been used to preserve the ischemic myocardium during the periods of circulatory arrest required to obtain a motionless operative field in cardiac surgical procedures.[2] Hypothermia prolongs the period of ischemia that can be tolerated by the heart before the point of irreversible injury occurs. Myocardial metabolism is reduced by 50 per cent for every 10° C drop in temperature, and the degree of hypothermia is determined by the estimated length of the ischemia.[182] A myocardial temperature of 20° C allows 60 minutes of ischemia without irreversible injury to mitochondrial functions.

The brain also benefits by hypothermia during these periods of circulatory arrest. Hypothermia does not totally halt metabolic activity but slows it down sufficiently to increase the period of time the brain, like the heart, can tolerate an absence of perfusion.

Psychological stress increases sympathetic nervous system activity and as a result increases arterial blood pressure, heart rate, and contractility.[183] Increased sympathetic discharge may be partly responsible for the enhanced coronary vasomotor tone seen in patients with variant angina.[105] Relaxation therapy has been shown to be beneficial in a variety of populations.[184–188] Benson and associates[184] described a progressive muscle relaxation strategy that significantly reduced the occurrence of premature ventricular contractions in patients with ischemic heart disease. This strategy helps the individual identify even mild tension and elicits the relaxation response. It is an easy technique for nurses to use and teach.

Guzzetta[185] studied patients in a coronary care unit and found a significant lowering of the apical heart rate and an increase in peripheral skin temperature after each of three sessions of relaxation or music therapy. Bohachick[186] used Benson's relaxation technique in a group of participants in a cardiac exercise program and demonstrated significant reductions in state anxiety scores and in measures of somatization, interpersonal sensitivity, anxiety, and depression as compared with a control group. A similar relaxation technique was used by a "nurse clinician"[187] in open-heart surgical patients to reduce the incidence of psychiatric reactions occurring postoperatively. The findings were in the predicted direction, but a significant relationship between relaxation and psychiatric reactions was not demonstrated.

Education of the patient and family is among the most important nursing responsibilities in the care of any patient. Patients with chronic ischemic conditions such as coronary artery disease need instruction regarding physiology and pathophysiology, medications, risk factors, and activity.[189, 190] The primary objectives in providing such instruction include not only increasing the knowledge of the patient and family but also influencing positive changes in both attitude and behavior that enhance adherence to treatment.

Studies of patient teaching methods have examined the timing of teaching, the anxiety level of the patient, and the various instructional approaches. Several reviews of the studies that have examined patient teaching in the cardiac surgical and medical populations[189, 191, 192] agreed that structured patient teaching methods resulted in better measures of recall and lowered anxiety levels. Murdaugh[189] determined from her review that timing of the teaching varied among the studies and that timing in relation to level of patient anxiety and impact on learning ability was not well delineated. Patients have indicated that learning about MI and life style changes is more effective after discharge.[190]

Therapies to Increase Oxygen Supply

Nonpharmacological interventions for improving tissue oxygen supply involve procedures for direct reperfusion: percutaneous transluminal coronary angioplasty (PTCA) and coronary artery bypass graft (CABG). The overall success of PTCA in improving clinical outcome has been approximately 85 to 95 per cent in patients with single or multivessel disease up to 2 years post-PTCA.[193] Reports have indicated significant improvements in symptoms, ventricular function, ECG signs of ischemia, exercise,[193–195] and quality of life[196] after PTCA.

Major complications of PTCA are arterial dissection, coronary embolism from atheromatous material, hemorrhage, and vasospasm. These most often occur during the procedure or within 6 hours. Repeat angioplasty is often successful but may warrant emergency coronary artery bypass graft.[195] The rate of acute occlusion is approximately 2 to 6 per cent. Late restenosis days or months after PTCA occurs invariably in almost 30 per cent of patients.[193] Persons at highest risk of restenosis are those with greater than 50 per cent stenosis post-PTCA, lesions occurring at branches or bends in the vessel, and thrombus superimposed on the lesion.[193] Observations of worsening ischemia or infarction are critical in the post-PTCA period and can be accomplished by continuous ECG monitoring with the lead corresponding to the area of myocardium subtended by the dilated vessel. Additionally, a 12-lead ECG should be obtained for complaints of chest pain.[193]

New technology being developed to prevent restenosis includes the use of laser balloon angioplasty,[197] coronary stents,[198, 199] and atherectomy.[200] A number of clinical trials investigating safety and efficacy of these technologies are currently ongoing.

Coronary artery bypass graft surgery has become a successful alternative to medical therapy for the management of coronary artery disease.[201, 202] In 1988 over 350,000 CABG procedures were performed in the United States.[5] Survival in surgically treated patients is improved compared with medically treated patients when two- or three-vessel disease and a left anterior descending artery lesion are present.[203] Survival for men and women is identical at both 5 and 10 years, although women tend to have less relief from angina at 10 years than do men. There is a gradual loss of angina relief and survival benefit over time, which accelerates after the first 6 years, probably due to the appearance of new lesions in the grafts as well as the native arteries.[203, 204] Saphenous vein grafts are prone to closure, whereas internal mammary artery grafts have an 85 to 95 per cent patency rate after 7 to 10 years.[205] CABG did not lower the rate of silent myocardial ischemia, as shown in a recent study.[206] The presence of symptomatic or nonsymptomatic ischemia in patients during exercise testing at 6 months post-CABG predicted poorer long-term survival than in those with no evidence of ischemia.

Despite improved medical outcomes after CABG, there has not been a concomitant improvement in psychological adjustment or return to work. Allen[87] summarized the results of many studies indicating that psychiatric symptoms of depression, isolation, and dependency existed up to 1 year after surgery in 20 to 30 per cent of subjects. Sexual functioning improved or stayed the same in the majority of subjects in the studies reviewed but worsened in others. Studies of return to work have been consistent in showing that many individuals, despite improved exercise performance and relief of disabling angina, do not return to work. In 15 studies reviewed[87] 80 per cent showed a decrease in employment, and 20 per cent demonstrated an increase. Preoperative unemployment or invalidism longer than 6 months predicted a 50 per cent chance of permanent inactivity after surgery. Other factors that influenced this variable included age, sex, educational level, job characteristics, and perceived advice from physicians.[87] Since over half of all CABG surgeries performed in the United States in 1988 were in those under age 65 and ·the majority of these persons were younger than age 55,[5] there may be serious psychosocial and economic consequences to the individual and society from lost wages and increased disability costs.

Coronary Risk Factor Modification

Modification of those factors that are known to increase the individual's risk of myocardial ischemia and that can be controlled is the most important step in the primary and secondary prevention of ischemia. The important risk factors for coronary artery disease are smoking, hyperlipidemia, hypertension, sedentary life style, and type A behavior pattern. Of these, smoking cessation is probably the single most effective in substantially lowering the rates of fatal reinfarction, sudden death, and total mortality.[207] The ability to modify these risk factors as part of a long-term change in life style is

influenced by a complex interaction of multiple factors: level of knowledge, attitudes, health beliefs, the relationship with the caregiver, and the cost required of the individual to adhere to a prescribed regimen in terms of time, money, effort, and social acceptance. The patient's level of knowledge is the easiest of all these factors to change, and national educational campaigns such as The National High Blood Pressure Education Program and The National Cholesterol Education Program have been vital in informing the public about ways to reduce cardiovascular disease risk. In fact, the increased public knowledge about risk factors and life style modifications are credited with having greater effects on lowering the incidence of cardiovascular diseases and related mortality than the most modern and optimal medical management.[8, 13] Knowledge may also allow individuals to improve coping skills, reduce anxiety and feelings of helplessness, and increase their confidence that life style changes will be beneficial.[207]

Much of nursing's efforts toward assisting risk factor modification have relied on educational approaches. An instructional program by itself, however, usually is insufficient to cause sustained change in behaviors and attitudes, since it addresses only some of the factors that determine life style modification and adherence.[208–210] Interventions that incorporate combinations of behavioral modification strategies,[211, 212] contracting,[210] and frequent follow-up and support[212] are needed. A considerable amount of the literature has been devoted to factors that influence adherence to treatment plans, and the reader is referred to several comprehensive reviews of the subject.[213–217]

A number of important studies have shown that risk factors can be modified significantly by behavioral changes or drugs that result in meaningful improvements in the number of subsequent cardiac events.[211, 212, 218–224] The reader is invited to review these trials for in-depth presentation of the data. Major new lines of inquiry and potentially effective interventions are discussed below.

Lowering total cholesterol and saturated fatty acids results in significant lowering of serum total cholesterol and LDL in normal children and children with familial hyperlipidemia.[225] The safety of a low-saturated fat diet and lipid-lowering drugs in children has not yet been established, but early intervention is critical. It is known that as children enter adolesence they often develop other cardiac risk factors, such as cigarette smoking, obesity, and sedentary activity, that persist into adulthood and that are associated with atherogenic lipid profiles in childhood.[225] Further research is needed to define appropriate dietary recommendations for cholesterol and fats for children and to develop lipid-lowering strategies that can be effective for families as they work with children in altering diet and activity level.

New evidence in humans has shown that dietary and drug-induced lowering of serum cholesterol and low-density lipoproteins can cause regression of coronary atherosclerosis in native and coronary bypass grafts.[226–229] It is not known why some lesions regress while others progress in the same patient. More effective methods of imaging the lesions and defining the characteristics of regression and progression are yet needed.[230]

Evidence in Alaskan Eskimos is accumulating that diets high in omega-3 fatty acids, the fish oils, are associated with significantly lower risk of coronary artery disease.[231] Early studies have shown that when omega-3 fatty acids were administered several days before[232] and for several weeks or months following PTCA[232, 233] a decreased rate of coronary restenosis occurred in comparison with controls. This effect is mediated in several possible ways: by lowering serum triglyceride levels (although this may be mitigated by a variable effect on LDL levels), by decreasing platelet aggregability and increasing bleeding time, by causing coronary vasodilation, and by inhibiting leukocyte chemotaxis and the inflammatory response. A partial mechanism for these effects is that over time the omega-3 fatty acids replace arachidonic acid as the chief fatty acid in cell membranes. The species of thromboxane produced by the metabolism of the omega-3 fatty acids has effects opposite of those of arachidonic acid thromboxane A_2, which are platelet aggregation and vasoconstriction.[231] Important risks of omega-3 oil administration are increased bleeding time and hemorrhage, fat-soluble vitamin toxicity, and environmental contamination from fish sources of the oils.

Another dietary intervention proposed for reducing the risk of coronary artery disease is the ingestion of water-soluble fiber from sources such as citrus fruits, barley, oats, dried beans, and peas. Studies of oat bran have shown a dose-response lowering of total cholesterol and triglyceride with no change in HDL. Persons with higher cholesterol and triglyceride levels had greater reductions than those with lower lipid levels.[234] When high fiber intake was combined with reduced intake of cholesterol and saturated fats, there was an even greater decrease in cholesterol.[231, 235]

Exercise as an intervention to modify a sedentary life style can be accomplished in a nonsupervised setting, such as the home or a health club, or in a supervised setting as part of a cardiac rehabilitation program. In the primary prevention of CHD, large, well-controlled studies have demonstrated that a regular program of aerobic exercise has resulted in a modest but significant reduction in the occurrence of CHD and overall mortality.[236] Results are less definitive with regard to the secondary prevention of CHD, attributable in part to design limitations and high drop-out rates. Nevertheless, a recent meta-analysis[237] of 22 randomized trials of exercise post-MI revealed a significant reduction in total and cardiovascular mortality that was evident at 1 year and was sustained for at least 3 years.

The beneficial effects of exercise training include improved skeletal muscle oxygen extraction, reduced heart rate and blood pressure response to exercise, and increased cardiac output.[207] These benefits translate into a reduction or elimination of angina.[238–240] Shephard[240] also noted the possible placebo effect of exercise in reducing angina in some patients, thus pointing out the complex psychophysiology that is part of the angina experience and the response to exercise. Other major benefits from exercise training are the increased rate of return to work following an MI or CABG,[239] subjective reports of increased activities of daily living, improved sexual function, lessened feelings of fear and depression, and a sense of well-being.[207]

Special populations such as the elderly also derive a significant benefit from exercise by increasing functional capacity, joint mobility, self-sufficiency, and alertness.[207] Patients with congestive heart failure or left ventricular dysfunction utilizing low intensity exercise achieve improved exercise capacity probably owing to improved muscle oxygen extraction.[207]

The safety of exercise training has been well established.[241–243] A recent review[244] of pooled data from 167 exercise rehabilitation programs with a total of 51,303 exercising individuals documented 21 cardiac arrests (three fatal) and eight nonfatal MIs. These events reflect a rate of occurrence of one cardiac arrest per 111,996 patient-hours of exercise and one MI per 293,990 patient-hours. This analysis revealed no relationship between the cardiac events and the size of the exercise group or the extent of ECG monitoring.

The type A behavior pattern (TABP) was first described by Friedman and Rosenman in 1959[17] and consists of a sense of time urgency and free-floating hostility. A review panel convened by the National Heart, Lung, and Blood Institute[245] concluded that TABP was an independent risk factor for CAD. The modification of TABP requires an alteration of lifetime habits and interaction patterns over several months or years.[211] Modification usually consists of the use of small group sessions combined with the use of a diary and strategies to increase client awareness of TABP and to moderate responses to everyday situations.[211] Friedman and associates[211, 220] were able to demonstrate significant and sustained reductions in TABP with an associated reduction in the recurrence of MI and the number of cardiac deaths.

ILLUSTRATIVE CASE STUDY

The following case study is presented as an example of how the phenomenon of myocardial ischemia can be manifested.

Mr. T.H. is a 63-year-old man who was admitted for percutaneous transluminal coronary angioplasty of stenoses in the saphenous vein bypass graft of his left circumflex (LCF) artery and in his native LCF artery. Mr. H.'s history of ischemic heart disease began in 1974 when he sustained two MIs. He continued to have exertional post-infarction angina and in 1976 underwent a bypass graft of his LCF and right coronary arteries. His angina was relieved by surgery; however, his left ventricular function gradually deteriorated to a point at which he was placed on afterload-reducing drugs in 1983.

In June 1984 he began complaining of both exertional and rest angina. He was placed on isosorbide dinitrate (Isordil), with relief of chest pain resulting, but began to experience increasing shortness of breath and pedal edema. In August 1984 a coronary arteriogram revealed 100 per cent stenosis of the first obtuse marginal branch of the LCF and 99 per cent occlusion of the LCF bypass graft. Left ventricular ejection fraction was 25 per cent at that time, and ventriculography revealed anteroseptal akinesia. He was not considered a candidate for another bypass graft owing to his poor left ventricular function.

In this patient the goal of PTCA was relief of his angina by maximizing perfusion through his left circumflex artery (LCF). Stenoses in the left anterior descending artery (LAD) were inoperable.

Mr. H.'s PTCA was complicated by intraoperative occlusion of the second obtuse marginal branch of the LCF. His ECG showed pseudonormalization of T waves and widened QRS waves in V_5 and V_6. He experienced no angina at the time, but auscultation of breath sounds revealed increased crackles from baseline. A Swan-Ganz catheter was inserted for close observation of his hemodynamic status. He was placed on intravenous sodium nitroprusside and nitrates to reduce preload and afterload. Diltiazem was begun to prevent vasospasm. At midnight his hemodynamic status was as follows: blood pressure of 140/70, heart rate of 70 in normal sinus rhythm, pulmonary capillary wedge (PCW) pressure elevated at 12 to 16 mm Hg, and cardiac output (CO) of 3 to 4 L/minute. A creatine phosphokinase (CPK) level drawn post-PTCA was 2530 IU/L (normal is 2 to 83 IU/L); the MB band was 628 IU/L, diagnostic of an infarct. Over the course of the next 3 days, Mr. H. experienced six spontaneous episodes of severe, crushing, substernal chest pain that did not radiate. One episode lasted 1 to 1½ hours and required high doses of intravenous (IV) nitroglycerin and 9 mg of morphine IV to relieve it. Table 2–7 illustrates the manifestations of myocardial ischemia that accompanied Mr. H.'s chest pain. As can be seen, the PCW pressure was consistently elevated with each episode, and an S_3 gallop was usually heard. Arterial blood pressure often dropped, although there was one episode of an increase, and once the blood pressure and heart rate did not change. ECG changes consisted of ST elevations or

TABLE 2–7   MANIFESTATIONS OF MYOCARDIAL ISCHEMIA IN A HEART PATIENT (MR. H.)

Date/Time	Duration of Angina	ECG	BP	HR	PCW	Heart Sounds	Lung Sounds	Other Subjective Data
10/11 4:00 a.m.	40 min.	ST ↑>3 mm T ↑	$\frac{140 \rightarrow 110}{74 \quad 70}$	72→90	15→38	+S$_3$	Crackles at bases	Nausea, dyspnea
10/12 6:00 a.m.	55 min.	ST ↑>3 mm T ↑	$\frac{140 \rightarrow 108}{64 \quad 60}$	82→104	15→45	+S$_3$	Crackles at bases	Nausea, emesis, dyspnea
10/13 4:05 p.m.	60 to 80 min.	ST ↑>3 mm T ↑	$\frac{105 \rightarrow 133}{48 \quad 60}$	85→115	28→52	+S$_3$	Diffuse crackles	Nausea, dyspnea
10/13 9:15 p.m.	30 min.	ST ↑>2 mm	$\frac{136 \rightarrow 130}{54 \quad 50}$	84→90	24→36	+S$_3$	Diffuse crackles	None
10/14 8:00 a.m.	45 min.	ST ↑>3 mm T ↑	$\frac{140 \rightarrow 90}{62 \quad 30}$	80→110	20→35	+S$_3$	Crackles at bases	Nausea, emesis, dyspnea
10/14 3:30 p.m.	30 min.	ST ↑>2 mm T ↑	$\frac{114 \rightarrow 110}{60 \quad 50}$	80→96	22→38	+S$_3$	Crackles at bases	None

ECG, electrocardiogram; BP, blood pressure; HR, heart rate; PCW, pulmonary capillary wedge pressure; ↑, elevation; ↓, depression; →, change in the value from baseline.

depressions of 2 to 3 mm and T wave elevations that were not in the area of his infarct. Rhythm changes were primarily PVCs well controlled with lidocaine. Additionally, Mr. H. reported dyspnea and nausea several times, usually accompanied by emesis.

The impression at this time was a large inferolateral MI post-PTCA with subsequent anterior ischemia secondary to vasospasm of the LAD collaterals. Isosorbide dinitrate (Isordil) was increased, and nifedipine was added to maximize coronary vasodilation and afterload reduction. Angina episodes were not alleviated, but extension of the infarction was ruled out.

Thrombolysis was performed with relief of chest pain and improved hemodynamics. Although left ventricular function remained poor, Mr. H. was able to be transferred out of the critical care unit (CCU). The remainder of his hospital stay was marked by severe depression, which improved with haloperidol (Haldol) and the support of his family. Mr. H. was discharged home 20 days after admission, having experienced no angina since thrombolysis was performed.

REVIEW OF RESEARCH FINDINGS

Findings related to potential sources of psychological and physiological stress in the hospitalized post-MI patient are reviewed in this section. This area was chosen because nursing has a major responsibility for identifying stressors and intervening to attenuate their effects on MVo$_2$.

Potential sources of physiological stress during the acute phase of an ischemic cardiac event are family visitation in the CCU[246] and interactions with caregivers.[247] Brown[246] found that 10-minute family visits had variable effects on blood pressure and heart rate compared with the values before family visits, with the mean effect being an increased systolic blood pressure. Subsequent visits (up to three visits) resulted in a higher sustained blood pressure and pulse after the visit. More research is needed to define the source of stress and its effect on the ischemic myocardium.

The simple act of having radial pulses taken and social interactions with caregivers in the CCU cause changes in heart rate, rhythm, and the incidence of ectopic beats.[247] The clinical significance of these responses is unknown. The mechanisms appear to be influenced by the central nervous system. Not all interactions with caregivers produce these changes or are harmful to patients. Bauer and Dracup[248] found that a 6-minute standardized back massage given to 25 patients with uncomplicated MI had no effect on heart rate or rhythm, systolic and diastolic blood pressures, muscle tension, skin temperature, or skin conductance. In 59 patients hospitalized for MI, CABG, or valve disease, Weiss[249] showed that four different types of touch caused a decrease in heart rate, diastolic pressure, and state anxiety and no change in systolic pressure and no arrhythmias when compared with baseline measurements. The decrease in state anxiety was found only in the men. Interestingly, two different types of verbal encounters elicited significant increases in heart rate, thought to be a result of central nervous system stimulation secondary to orienting or processing of information in the subject. The same protocol was repeated the next day, and the same responses were found, pointing out the stability of the subjects' reactions. The author speculated that the reduced arousal elicited by touch could have been because the subjects perceived the touch as caring or therapeutic rather than threatening. Their subjective responses after the experiment tended to support this view. Weiss cautioned that the data indicated only that the four touches used were not stressful to stable cardiac patients and not that touch was therapeutic. More studies are needed to clarify the effects of touch on persons of different ages, sex, cultures, and states of cardiovascular health.

Many coronary care units have policies restricting caffeine intake in acute MI patients because of the belief that caffeine increases MVO_2 and is arrhythmogenic.[250] Caffeine stimulates catecholamine secretion, causing acute increases in blood pressure in the caffeine-naive individual.[251] Over a few hours or days tolerance to catecholamines develops and attenuates this response. The data are less clear regarding the arrhythmogenic properties of caffeine, with several studies demonstrating conflicting results.[251] The weight of current evidence in normal subjects is that caffeine does not cause clinically significant arrhythmias.[252] A recent study[250] showed that caffeine increased the susceptibility to serious arrhythmias (e.g., ventricular tachycardia) in patients and normal controls in whom these arrhythmias could be induced at baseline. Several of the patients who had inducible arrhythmias after caffeine ingestion experienced cardiac symptoms after drinking coffee in their everyday lives. More study in this area is needed using electrophysiologic laboratory methods in larger samples. Also, there is a need to better differentiate the effects of caffeine from the numerous other chemicals in coffee.[251] Until more is known, it is wise to caution persons with heart disease or those who experience cardiac symptoms after drinking coffee to abstain from or minimize their caffeine intake.[251]

Another precaution practiced in many CCUs is restriction of ice water ingestion in acute MI patients, but Kirchoff and associates[253] found that only 6 of 89 post-MI subjects demonstrated clinically significant ST or T wave changes up to 25 minutes after rapidly drinking 200 or 400 ml of ice water. The functional significance of the ECG changes or whether they indicated ischemia or increased risk of arrhythmias is not known and needs further study. There were no changes in heart rate or blood pressure during the time periods studied. The authors acknowledged that a blanket policy against drinking ice water would be unduly restrictive for most patients. They recommended that the nurse monitor newly admitted patients while drinking ice water and compare their ECG with baseline values to determine who should be restricted.

IMPLICATIONS FOR FURTHER RESEARCH

Despite the accumulated literature and research efforts that have contributed to our understanding of ischemia, much remains to be learned. A number of research needs have been identified throughout this chapter, but areas that are potentially fruitful for nursing research will be highlighted here. The identification of serum markers that signify ischemic injury has occurred is critical, as it would allow for reliable determination of tissue that is salvageable and amenable to treatment. Hypoxanthine and adenosine show some promise in this regard. Measures currently in use (e.g., elevated venous lactate levels) do not necessarily correlate with the degree or area of injury and have not been shown to relate directly to tissue dysfunction.

Investigation is essential to identify the psychological, social, cultural, and spiritual responses to ischemic events. Several studies have demonstrated the complex psychodynamics that promote CHD, that come into play when the individual's life has been threatened by an ischemic event, and that influence outcomes in the recovery process. Examples of questions that need to be addressed are the following: What role does denial play in coping with CHD, recovery from an acute ischemic event, adherence to treatment, and long-term outcomes? What are the best indicators of depression, denial, and other responses that the nurse can use to predict who is at risk for adverse outcomes, and what are effective strategies for attenuating these consequences? How do women, the elderly, and different ethnic groups experience acute MI or CABG, and how do they differ from the white, middle-aged male model of CHD? How can the nurse best assess and support family functioning during the recovery process?

Another area that remains to be explored is what, if any, activity restrictions should be instituted in patients demonstrating silent ischemia. The effects of various nursing and personal care activities need to be explored in patients with unstable angina and in those who are post-PTCA or who have undergone thrombolysis. Additional studies are needed that examine the learning needs of patients and families in the critical care environment,[254] quality of life after a cardiac event, and family adaptation to the crisis of a cardiac event.[191]

In regard to prevention of myocardial ischemia much research is needed in the area of risk factor modification in children and adolescents. Also, testing of strategies for educating young people and adults about the hazards of cocaine use is needed. In secondary prevention of myocardial ischemia, large controlled trials are necessary in order to clarify the therapeutic benefits of exercise (type, amount, and frequency) in a variety of populations, such as women, the elderly, and individuals with congestive heart failure. Researchers need to explore nonpharmacological strategies for lowering blood pressure and modifying other risk factors. The potential for the relaxation response to minimize stress, lower blood pressure, and reduce arrhythmias shows promise and needs to further identify those who would benefit the most. It is vital to identify persons who are likely to have difficulty adhering to a treatment plan. Nurses need to develop behavioral strategies that influence healthy, long-term life style changes.

Recent reviews of cardiovascular[191, 255] and critical care[254] nursing research of the last decade have indicated growth in the quality and complexity of nursing research in that studies have increasingly demonstrated significantly fewer methodological problems and more correlational and intervention designs.[254] Nevertheless, additional efforts are needed to develop studies that demonstrate greater utilization of theory bases and larger samples, to limit topics having a single research study, and to conduct more meta-analyses of topics already having significant numbers of studies,[254, 255] such as cardiac patient education and measurement of cardiac output.[254]

REFERENCES

1. Trump, B.F., Berezesky, I.K., Cowley, R.A. (1982). Cellular and subcellular characteristics of acute and chronic injury with emphasis on the role of calcium. In R.A. Cowley & B.F. Trump (eds.), *The Pathophysiology of Shock, Anoxia, and Ischemia* (pp. 6–46). Baltimore: Williams and Wilkins.
2. Hearse, D., Braimbridge, M., Jynge, P. (1981). Protection of the ischemic myocardium. *Cardioplegia.* New York: Raven Press.
3. Astrup, J. (1982). Energy-requiring cell functions in the ischemic brain. J Neurosurg 56:482–497.
4. Velican, C., Velican, D. (1989). *Natural History of Coronary Atherosclerosis.* Boca Raton, FL: CRC Press.
5. American Heart Association. (1991). 1991 Heart and Stroke Facts. Dallas: American Heart Association.
6. Metropolitan Life Foundation (1989). Continued progress against cardiovascular diseases. Stat Bull Metrop Insur Co 70:16–23.
7. Metropolitan Life Foundation (1989). Progress against mortality from stroke. Stat Bull Metrop Insur Co 70:18–29.
8. McKinlay, J.B., McKinlay, S.M., Beaglehole, R. (1989). A review of the evidence concerning the impact of medical measures on recent mortality and morbidity in the United States. Int J Health Serv 19:181–208.
9. Passamani, E.R., Frommer, P.L., Levy, R.I. (1984). Coronary heart disease: An overview. In N.K. Wenger & H.K. Hellerstein (eds.), *Rehabilitation of the Coronary Patient* (2nd ed., pp. 1–15). New York: John Wiley and Sons.
10. Goodstein, R.K. (1983). Cerebrovascular accident and the hospitalized elderly: A multidimensional clinical problem. Am J Psychiatry 140:141–147.
11. Frohlich, E.D. (1990). Left ventricular hypertrophy: An independent risk factor. Cardiovasc Clin 20:85–94.
12. The health consequences of smoking: Cardiovascular disease. A report of the Surgeon General (1983). Rockville, MD: Depart of Health and Human Services.
13. Gorlin, R. (1991). Hypertension and ischemic heart disease: The challenge of the 1990s. Am Heart J 121:658–663.
14. LaRosa, J.C., Hunninghake, D., Bush, D., Criqui, M.H., Getz, G.S., Gotto, A.M., Jr., Grundy, S.M., Rakita, L., Robertson, R.M., Weisfeldt, M.L. (1990). The cholesterol facts. A summary of the evidence relating dietary fats, serum cholesterol, and coronary heart disease. A joint statement by the American Heart Association and the National Heart, Lung, and Blood Institute. The Task Force on Cholesterol Issues, American Heart Association. Circulation 81:1721–1730.
15. Grundy, S.M., Goodman, D.S., Rifkind, B.M., Cleeman, J.I. (1989). The place of HDL in cholesterol management: A perspective from the National Cholesterol Education Program. Arch Intern Med 149:505–510.
16. Paffenbarger, R.S., Wing, A.L., Hyde, R.T. (1978).

Physical activity as an index of heart attack risk in college alumni. Am J Epidemiol *108*:161–175.

17. Friedman, M., Rosenman, R.H. (1959). Association of specific overt behavior pattern with blood and cardiovascular findings. JAMA *169*:1286–1296.

18. Krantz, D.S., Contrada, R.J., Hill, D.R., Friedler, E. (1988). Environmental stress and biobehavioral antecedents of coronary heart disease. J Consult Clin Psychol *56*:333–341.

19. Eaker, E.D., Packard, B., Thom, T.J. (1989). Epidemiology and risk factors for coronary heart disease in women. Cardiovasc Clin, *19*:129–145.

20. Godsland, I.F., Wynn, V., Crook, D., Miller, N.E. (1987). Sex, plasma lipoproteins, and atherosclerosis: Prevailing assumptions and outstanding questions. Am Heart J *114*:1467–1503.

21. Stein, E.A., Steiner, P.M. (1989). Triglyceride measurement and its relationship to heart disease. Clin Lab Med *9*:169–185.

22. Betteridge, D.J. (1989). Lipids, diabetes, and vascular disease: The time to act. Diabetic Med *6*:195–218.

23. Bush, T.L., Barrett-Connor, E., Cowan, L.D., Criqui, M.H., Wallace, R.B., Suchindran, C.M., Tyroler, H.A., Rifkind, B.M. (1987). Cardiovascular mortality and non-contraceptive estrogen use in women: Results from the Lipid Research Clinics Program follow-up study. Circulation *75*:1102–1109.

24. Burkman, R.T., Robinson, J.C., Kruszson-Moran, D., Kimball, A.W., Kwitervich, A.W., Burford, R.G. (1988). Lipid and lipoprotein changes associated with oral contraceptive use: A randomized clinical trial. Obstet Gynecol *71*:33–38.

25. Miller, V.T. (1990). Dyslipoproteinemia in women. Endocrinol Metab Clin North Am *19*:381–398.

26. Frishman, W.H., Karpenos, A., Molloy, T.J. (1989). Cocaine-induced coronary artery disease: Recognition and treatment. Med Clin North Am *73*:475–486.

27. Kossowsky, W.A., Lyon, A.F., Chou, S-Y. (1989). Acute non-Q wave cocaine-related myocardial infarction. Chest *96*:617–621.

28. Klonoff, D.C., Andrews, B.T., Obana, W.G. (1989). Stroke associated with cocaine use. Arch Neurol *46*:989–993.

29. Park, Y.D., Belman, A.L., Kim, T.-S., Kure, K., Llena, J.F., Lantos, G., Bernstein, L., Dickson, D.W. (1990). Stroke in pediatric acquired immunodeficiency syndrome. Ann Neurol *28*:303–311.

30. Mizusawa, H., Hirano, A., Llena, J.F. (1988). Cerebrovascular lesions in acquired immunodeficiency syndrome (AIDS). Acta Neuropathologica (Berlin) *76*:451–457.

31. Marcus, M.L., Harrison, D.G., Chilian, W.M., Koyanagi, S., Inou, T., Tomavik, R.J., Martins, J.B., Eastham, C.L., Hiratzka, L.F. (1987). Alterations in the coronary circulation in hypertrophied ventricles. Circulation *75*(Suppl. 1):I19–I25.

32. Volpe, J.J. (1987). Hypoxic-ischemic encephalopathy: Biochemical and physiological aspects. In N.K. Volpe, *Neurology of the Newborn* (2nd ed., pp. 141–179). Philadelphia: W.B. Saunders.

33. Fenichel, G.M. (1983). Hypoxic-ischemic encephalopathy in the newborn. Arch Neurol *40*:261–266.

34. Mott, S.R., James, S.R., Sperhac, A.M. (1990). *Nursing Care of Children and Families*. Redwood City, CA: Addison-Wesley.

35. Weisfeldt, M.L., Lakatta, E.G., Gerstenblith, G. (1988). Aging and cardiac disease. In E. Braunwald (ed.), *Heart disease. A Textbook of Cardiovascular Medicine* (3rd ed., pp. 1650–1662). Philadelphia: W.B. Saunders.

36. Jansen, P.A.F., Schulte, B.P.M., Gribnau, F.W.J. (1987). Cerebral ischaemia and stroke as side effects of antihypertensive treatment; special danger in the elderly. A review of the cases reported in the literature. Neth J Med *30*:193–201.

37. Beary, J.F., Summer, W.R., Bulkley, B. (1979). Postpartum acute myocardial infarction. Am J Cardiol *43*:158–161.

38. Koniak-Griffin, D., Dodgson, J. (1987). Severe pregnancy-induced hypertension: Postpartum care of the critically ill patient. Heart Lung *16*:661–669.

39. Guyton, A.C. (1991). *Textbook of Medical Physiology* (8th ed.). Philadelphia: W.B. Saunders.

40. McCluskey, R.S. (1982). Microcirculation: Basic considerations. In R.A. Cowley & B.F. Trump (eds.), *The Pathophysiology of Shock, Anoxia, and Ischemia* (pp. 256–264). Baltimore: Williams and Wilkins.

41. Furchgott, R.F., Vanhoutte, P.M. (1989). Endothelium-derived relaxing and contracting factors. Fed Am Soc Exp Biol J *3*:2007–2018.

42. Ganong, W.F. (1991). *Review of Medical Physiology* (15th ed.). San Mateo, CA: Appleton & Lange.

43. Pasternac, A., Bourassa, M.G. (1983). Pathogenesis of chest pain in patients with cardiomyopathies and normal coronary arteries. Int J Cardiol *3*:273–280.

44. Curtis, M.J. (1991). The pathophysiological basis of arrhythmogenesis in myocardial ischemia and reperfusion: Possible target for intervention. Bratislavsli Lekarske Listy *92*:91–101.

45. Jennings, R.B. (1984). Calcium ions in ischemia. In L.H. Opie (ed.), *Calcium Antagonists and Cardiovascular Disease* (pp. 85–95). New York: Raven Press.

46. Siesjo, B.K. (1988). Historical overview: Calcium, ischemia, and death of brain cells. New York Acad Sci *522*:638–661.

47. Bonventre, J.V. (1988). Mediators of ischemic renal injury. Ann Rev Med *39*:531–544.

48. Nayler, W.G., Elz, J.S. (1986). Reperfusion injury: Laboratory artifact or clinical dilemma? Circulation *74*:215–221.

49. Forman, M.B., Puett, D.W., Virmani, R. (1989). Endothelial and myocardial injury during ischemia and reperfusion: Pathogenesis and therapeutic implications. J Am Coll Cardiol *13*:450–459.

50. Krause, G.S., White, B.C., Aust, S.D., Nayini, N.R., Kurvar, K. (1988). Brain cell death following ischemia and reperfusion: A proposed biochemical sequence. Crit Care Med *16*:714–726.

51. McCord, J.M. (1985). Oxygen-derived free radicals in postischemic tissue injury. N Engl J Med *312*:159–163.

52. Jacob, H.S. (1989). Damaging role of activated complement in myocardial infarction and shock lung: Therapeutic implications. In W.C. Shoemaker, S. Ayers, A. Grenvich, P. Holbrook, W.L. Thompson (eds.), *Textbook of Critical Care* (2nd ed., pp. 1034–1039). Philadelphia: W.B. Saunders.

53. van Echteld, C.J.A. (1988). Cardiac energy metabolism probed with nuclear magnetic resonance. In

J.W. de Jong (ed.), *Myocardial Energy Metabolism* (pp. 127–141). Boston: Martinus Nijoff Publishers.

54. Lott, J.A., Stang, J.M. (1980). Serum enzymes and isoenzymes in the diagnosis and differential diagnosis of myocardial ischemia and necrosis. Clin Chem *26*:1241–1250.

55. Allan, R.M., Horlock, P., Fox, K., Selmyn, A.P. (1981). Investigation of the mechanisms and consequences of transient myocardial ischemia. Acta Medica Scandinavica *651*(Suppl.):133–138.

56. Marmor, A., Kahana, L., Alpan, G., Grenadier, E., Keidar, S., Palant, A. (1979). Creatine kinase isoenzyme MB (CK-MB) in acute coronary ischemia. Am Heart J *97*:574–577.

57. Parmley, W., Chatterjee, K., Francis, G.S., Firth, B.G., Kloner, R.A. (1991). Congestive heart failure: New frontiers. West J Med *154*:427–441.

58. Safar, P. (1988). Resuscitation from clinical death: Pathophysiologic limits and therapeutic potentials. Crit Care Med *16*:923–941.

59. Morris, D.C., Walter, P.F., Hurst, J.W. (1990). The recognition and treatment of myocardial infarction and its complications. In J.W. Hurst, R.C. Schlant, C.E. Rachley, E.H. Sonnenblick, N.K. Wenger (eds.), *The Heart, Arteries and Veins* (7th ed., pp. 1054–1078). New York: McGraw-Hill.

60. Haljamae, J., Enger, E. (1975). Human skeletal muscle metabolism during and after complete tourniquet ischemia. Ann Surg *182*:9–14.

61. Harriman, D.G.F. (1977). Ischemia of peripheral nerve and muscle. J Clin Pathol *11*(Suppl.):94–104.

62. Modry, D.L, Chin, R.C. (1979). Pulmonary reperfusion syndrome. Ann Thorac Surg *27*:207–215.

63. Haglund, U., Bulkley, G.B., Granger, D.N. (1987). On the pathophysiology of intestinal ischemic injury. Acta Chirurgica Scandinavica *153*:321–324.

64. Hasselgren, P.O. (1987). Collective review: Prevention and treatment of ischemia of the liver. Surg Gynecol Obstet *164*:187–196.

65. Hearse, D.J. (1984). Critical distinctions in the modification of myocardial cell injury. *Calcium Antagonists and Cardiovascular Disease* (pp. 129–145). New York: Raven Press.

66. Braunwald, E., Kloner, R.A. (1985). Myocardial reperfusion: A double-edged sword? J Clin Invest *76*:1713–1719.

67. Braunwald, E., Kloner, R.A. (1982). The stunned myocardium: Prolonged, postischemic ventricular dysfunction. Circulation *66*:1146–1149.

68. Kloner, R.A., Przyklenk, K., Patel, B. (1989). Altered myocardial states: The stunned and hibernating myocardium. Am J Med *86*:14–22.

69. Babbs, C.F. (1988). Reperfusion injury of postischemic tissues. Emerg Med *17*:1148–1157.

70. Cheung, J.Y., Bonventre, J.V., Malis, C.D., Leaf, A. (1986). Calcium and ischemic injury. N Engl J Med *314*:1670–1676.

71. Ceconi, R.F., Curello, S., Cargnoni, A., Agnoletti, G., Boffa, G.M., Visioli, O. (1986). Intracellular effects of myocardial ischemia and reperfusion: Role of calcium and oxygen. Eur Heart J *7*(Suppl. A):3–12.

72. Mergner, W.J., Schaper, J. (1982). Cellular and subcellular changes in myocardial infarction. In R.A. Cowley & B.F. Trump (eds.), *Pathophysiology of Shock, Anoxia, and Ischemia* (pp. 658–681). Baltimore: Williams and Wilkins.

73. Raichle, M.E. (1983). The pathophysiology of brain ischemia. Ann Neurol *13*:2–10.

74. Sieber, F.E., Traystman, R.J. (1992). Special issues: Glucose and the brain. Crit Care Med *20*:104–114.

75. Lam, A.M., Cullen, B.F., Sundling, N. (1991). Hyperglycemia and neurological outcome in patients with head injury. J Neurosurg *75*:545–551.

76. Woo, E., Chan, Y.W., Yu, Y.L. (1988). Admission glucose level in relation to mortality and morbidity outcome in 252 stroke patients. Stroke *19*:185–191.

77. Yager, J.Y., Heitjan, D.F., Tawfighi, J., Vannucci, R.C. (1992). Effect of insulin-induced and fasting hypoglycemia on perinatal hypoxic-ischemic brain damage. Ped Res *31*:138–142.

78. Cherniack, R., Cherniack, L. (1983). *Respiration in Health and Disease* (3rd ed., p. 329). Philadelphia: W.B. Saunders.

79. Braunwald, E., Sobel, B.E. (1988). Coronary blood flow and myocardial ischemia. In E. Braunwald (ed.), *Heart Disease. A Textbook of Cardiovascular Medicine* (3rd ed., pp. 1191–1221). Philadelphia: W.B. Saunders.

80. Bagdonas, A.A., Stucky, J.H., Piera, J., Amer, N.S., Hoffman, B.F. (1961). Effects of ischemia and hypoxia on the specialized conducting system of the canine heart. Am Heart J *61*:206–218.

81. Ten Eick, R.E., Singer, D.H., Solberg, L.E. (1976). Coronary occlusion: Effect on cellular electrical activity of the heart. Med Clin North Am *60*:49–67.

82. Downar, E., Janse, M.J., Durrer, D. (1977). The effect of "ischemic" blood on transmembrane potentials of normal porcine ventricular myocardium. Circulation *55*:455–462.

83. Helgeson, V.S. (1989). The origin, development, and current state of the literature on type A behavior. J Cardiovasc Nurs *3*:59–73.

84. Eaker, E.D. (1989). Psychosocial factors in the epidemiology of coronary heart disease in women. Psychiatr Clin North Am *12*:167–173.

85. Cassem, N., Hackett, T. (1971). Psychiatric consultation in a coronary care unit. Ann Intern Med *75*:9–14.

86. Hackett, T., Cassem, N., Wishnie, H. (1968). The coronary care unit: An appraisal of its psychologic hazards. N Engl J Med *279*:1365–1370.

87. Allen, J.K. (1990). Physical and psychosocial outcomes after coronary artery bypass graft surgery. Heart Lung *19*:49–55.

88. Lowery, B.J. (1991). Psychological stress, denial and myocardial infarction outcomes. Image *23*:51–55.

89. Marsden, C., Dracup, K. (1991). Different perspectives: The effect of heart disease on patients and spouses. AACN Clin Issues Crit Care Nurs *2*:285–292.

90. Mickus, D. (1986). Activities of daily living in women after myocardial infarction. Heart Lung *15*:376–381.

91. Shanfield, S.B. (1990). Return to work after an acute myocardial infarction: A review. Heart Lung *19*:109–117.

92. Bramwell, L., Wahll, A. (1986). Effect of role clarity and empathy on support role performance and anxiety. Nurs Res *35*:282–287.

93. Gilliss, C. (1984). Reducing family stress during and after coronary artery bypass surgery. Nurs Clin North Am *19*:103–112.

94. Gilliss, C., Sparacino, P., Gortner, S., Kenneth, H. (1985). Events leading to the treatment of coronary artery disease. Implications for nursing care. Heart Lung *14*:350–356.

95. Boone, T., Kelley, R. (1990). Sexual issues and research in counseling the postmyocardial infarction patient. J Cardiovasc Nurs *4*:65–75.

96. Riegel, B. (1989). Social support and psychological adjustment to chronic coronary heart disease: Operationalization of Johnson's behavioral system model. Adv Nurs Sci *11*:74–84.

97. Parmley, W.W. (1989). Prevalence and clinical significance of silent myocardial ischemia. Circulation *80*(Suppl. IV):IV68–IV73.

98. Rashkin, M.C., Bosken, C., Baughman, R.P. (1985). Oxygen delivery in critically ill patients: Relationship to blood lactate and survival. Chest *87*:580–584.

99. Grum, C.M., Simon, R.H., Dantzker, D.R., Fox, I.H. (1985). Evidence for adenosine triphosphate degradation in critically ill patients. Chest *88*:763–767.

100. Prinzmetal, M., Kennamer, R., Merliss, R., Wada, T., Bor, N. (1959). Angina pectoris: I. A variant form of angina pectoris. Am J Med *27*:375–388.

101. Maseri, A., Severi, S., DeNes, M., L'Abbate, A., Chierchia, S., Marzilli, M., Ballestra, A.M., Parodi, O., Biagini, A., Distante, A. (1978). "Variant" angina: One aspect of a continuous spectrum of vasospastic myocardial ischemia. Am J Cardiol *42*:1019–1035.

102. Anthony, C.L., Arnon, R.G. (1983). *Pediatric Cardiology*. New York: Medical Examination Publishing Co.

103. Levene, D. (1977). *Chest Pain: An Integrated Diagnostic Approach*. Philadelphia: Lea and Febiger.

104. Basta, L.L., Raines, D., Najjar, S., Kioschos, J.M. (1975). Clinical, hemodynamic, and coronary angiographic correlates of angina pectoris in patients with severe aortic valve disease. Br Heart J *37*:150–157.

105. Yasue, H., Omote, S., Takazawa, A., Nagao, M. (1983). Coronary arterial spasm in ischemic heart disease and its pathogenesis. Circ Res *52*(Suppl.):I147–I152.

106. Fuller, C.M., Raizner, A.E., Chahine, R.A., Nahormek, P., Ishimori, T., Verani, M., Nitishin, A., Mokotoff, D., Luchi, R.J. (1980). Exercise-induced coronary arterial spasm: Angiographic demonstration of ischemia by myocardial scintigraphy and results of pharmacologic intervention. Am J Cardiol *46*:500–506.

107. Davies, A.B., Subramanian, V.B., Cashman, P.M.M., Raftery, E.B. (1983). Simultaneous recording of continuous arterial pressure, heart rate, and ST segment in ambulant patients with stable angina pectoris. Br Heart J *50*:85–91.

108. Moise, A., Theroux, P., Taeymous, Y., Descoings, B., Lesperance, J., Waters, D., Pelletier, G., Bourassa, M.G. (1983). Unstable angina and progression of coronary atherosclerosis. N Engl J Med *309*:685–689.

109. Yasue, H., Omote, S., Takazawa, A., Nagao, M., Hyon, H., Nishida, S., Horie, M. (1981). Comparison of coronary arteriographic findings during angina pectoris associated with S-T elevation or depression. Am J Cardiol *47*:539–546.

110. Berger, B., Brest, A. (1983). Exercise electrocardiography and stress thallium-201 imaging in coronary artery disease. Cardiovasc Clin *13*:253–277.

111. Picano, E. (1989). Dipyridamole-echocardiography test: Historical background and physiologic basis. Eur Heart J *10*:365–376.

112. Gotsman, M.S. (1983). Atrial pacing in the diagnosis of ischemic heart disease. Heart Lung *12*:372–382.

113. Charlap, S., Shani, J., Schulhoff, N., Herman, B., Lichstein, E. (1990). R- and S-wave amplitude changes with acute anterior transmural myocardial ischemia: Correlations with left ventricular filling pressures. Chest *97*:566–571.

114. Okin, P.M., Ameisen, O., Kligfield, P. (1987). Detection of anatomically severe coronary artery disease by the ST/HR slope. Chest *91*:582–587.

115. Osbakken, M.D. (1989). Exercise stress testing in women: Diagnostic dilemma. Cardiovasc Clin *19*:187–194.

116. Maseri, A., Chierchia, S. (1980). Coronary vasospasm in ischemic heart disease. Chest *78*(Suppl.):210–215.

117. Markham, R.V., Winniford, M.D., Firth, B., Nicod, P., Dehmer, G.J., Lewis, S.E., Willis, L.D. (1983). Symptomatic, electrocardiographic, metabolic, and hemodynamic alterations during pacing-induced myocardial ischemia. Am J Cardiol *51*:1589–1594.

118. Rock, S.M. (1991). Right ventricular myocardial infarction. J Cardiovasc Nurs *6*:44–53.

119. Beller, G.A., Gibson, R.S. (1987). Sensitivity, specificity, and prognostic significance of noninvasive testing for occult or known coronary disease. Prog Cardiovasc Dis *29*:241–270.

120. Visser, C.A., van der Wieken, R.L., Kan, G., Lie, K.I., Busemann-Sokele, E., Meltzer, R.S., Durrer, D. (1983). Comparison of two dimensional echocardiography with radionuclide angiography during dynamic exercise for the detection of coronary artery disease. Am Heart J *106*:528–534.

121. Berman, D.S., Kiat, H., Maddahi, J., Shah, P.K. (1989). Radionuclide imaging of myocardial perfusion and viability in assessment of acute myocardial infarction. Am J Cardiol *64*:9B–16B.

122. Higgins, C.B. (1990). Nuclear magnetic resonance (NMR) imaging in ischemic heart disease. Radiologica Medica *80*:164–167.

123. Johns, J.A., Leavitt, M.B., Newell, J.B., Yasuda, T., Leinbach, R.C., Gold, H.K., Finkelstein, D., Dinsmore, R.E. (1990). Quantitation of acute myocardial infarct size by nuclear magnetic resonance imaging. J Am Coll Cardiol *15*:143–149.

124. Bonow, R.O., Berman, D.S., Gibbons, R.J., Johnson, L.L., Rumberger, J.A., Schwaiger, M.R, Wackers, F.J. (1991). Cardiac position emission tomography. A report for health professionals from the Committee on Advanced Cardiac Imaging and Technology of the Council on Clinical Cardiology, American Heart Association. Circulation *84*:447–454.

125. de Jong, J.W. (1988). Diagnosis of ischemic heart disease with AMP-catabolites. In J.W. Jong (ed.), *Myocardial Energy Metabolism* (pp. 237–243). Boston: Martinus Nijoff.

126. Drew, B.J. (1991). Bedside electrocardiographic monitoring: State of the art for the 1990s. Heart Lung *20*:610–623.

127. Perchalski, D.L., Pepine, C.J. (1987). Patient with coronary artery spasm and role of the critical care nurse. Heart Lung *16*:392–402.

128. Valle, G.A., Lemberg, L. (1990). Circadian influence in cardiovascular disease (Part 1). Chest 97:1453–1457.

129. Valle, G.A., Lemberg, L. (1990). Circadian influence in cardiovascular disease (Part 2). Chest 98:216–221.

130. Conley, S.K. (1983). Administering IV nitroglycerin: Nursing implications. Dimens Crit Care Nurs 2:18–22.

131. Curfman, G.D. (1984). Intravenous nitroglycerin: Clinical use and efficacy. Int J Cardiol 5:241–244.

132. Gerber, J.G., Nies, A.S. (1990). Antihypertensive agents and the drug therapy of hypertension. In A.G. Gilman, T.W. Rale, A.S. Nies, P. Taylor (eds.), *Goodman and Gilman's Pharmacological Basis of Therapeutics* (8th ed., pp. 784–813). New York: Pergamon Press.

133. Gold, M.E. (1991). Pharmacology of the nitrovasodilators. Nurs Clin North Am 26:437–450.

134. Mueller, H.S. (1989). Management of acute myocardial infarction. In W.C. Shoemaker, S. Ayers, A. Grenvik, P.R. Holbrook, W.L. Thompson (eds.), *Textbook of Critical Care* (2nd ed., pp. 341–353). Philadelphia: W.B. Saunders.

135. Jaffe, J.H., Martin, W.R. (1990). Opioid analgesics and antagonists. In A.G. Gilman, T.W. Rale, A.S. Nies, P. Taylor (eds.), *Goodman and Gilman's Pharmacological Basis of Therapeutics* (8th ed., pp. 485–521). New York: Pergamon Press.

136. Beller, G.A. (1989). Calcium antagonists in the treatment of Prinzmetal's angina and unstable angina pectoris. Circulation 80(Suppl. IV):IV78–IV87.

137. Brodsky, S.J., Cutler, S.S., Weiner, D.A., McCabe, C.H., Ryan, T.J., Klein, M.D. (1982). Treatment of stable angina of effort with verapamil: A double-blind placebo-controlled randomized crossover study. Circulation 66:569–574.

138. The Multicenter Diltiazem Postinfarction Trial Research Group (1988). The effect of diltiazem on mortality and reinfarction after myocardial infarction. N Engl J Med 319:385–392.

139. Schlant, R.C., King, S.B. III. (1989). Usefulness of calcium entry blockers during and after percutaneous transluminal coronary artery angioplasty. Circulation 80(Suppl. IV):IV88–IV92.

140. Temkin, L.P. (1989). High-dose monotherapy and combination therapy with calcium channel blockers for angina. Am J Med 86(Suppl. 1A):23–27.

141. Urquhart, J., Patterson, R.E., Bacharach, S.L., Green, M.V., Spier, E.H., Aemodt, R., Epstein, S.E. (1984). Comparative effects of verapamil, diltiazem, and nifedipine on hemodynamics and left ventricular function during acute myocardial ischemia in dogs. Circulation 69:382–390.

142. Wei, J.Y. (1989). Use of calcium entry blockers in elderly patients. Circulation 80(Suppl. IV):IV171–IV177.

143. Beta Blocker Heart Attack Trial Research Group. (1982). A randomized trial of propranolol in patients with acute myocardial infarction. Mortality results. JAMA 247:1707–1714.

144. Lynch, P., Dargie, H., Krikler, S., Krikler, D. (1980). Objective assessment of antianginal treatment: A double-blind comparison of propranolol, nifedipine, and their combination. Br Med J 281:184–187.

145. Sadik, N.N., Tan, A., Fletcher, P.J., Morris, J., Kelly, D.T. (1982). A double-blind randomized

146. Yusof, S., Peto, R., Lewis, J., Collins, R., Sleight, P. (1985). Beta blockade during and after myocardial infarction. An overview of the randomized trials. Prog Cardiovasc Dis 17:335–371.

147. The Cardiac Arrhythmia Suppression Trial Investigators (1989). Preliminary report: Effect of encainide and flecainide on mortality in a randomized trial of arrhythmia suppression after myocardial infarction. N Engl J Med 321:406–412.

148. Keren, A., Tzivoni, D. (1990). Magnesium therapy in ventricular arrhythmias. Pacing Clin Electrophysiol 13:937–945.

149. Thielbar, S. (1984). Antiarrhythmic drug therapy: An overview. Crit Care Q 7:21–32.

150. Zheutlin, T.A., Moran, J.M., Loeb, J.M., Kehoe, R.F. (1984). Therapy of patients with malignant arrhythmias. Crit Care Q 7:35–47.

151. Mehta, J.L., Conti, C.R. (1989). Aspirin in myocardial ischemia: Why, when, and how much? Clin Cardiol 12:179–184.

152. Miller, G.J. (1989). Antithrombotic therapy in the primary prevention of acute myocardial infarction. Am J Cardiol 64:29B–32B.

153. Neri Serneri, G.G.N., Modesti, P.A., Abbate, R., Gensini, G.F. (1990). Heparin and antiaggregating therapy in unstable angina. Haemostasis 20(Suppl. 1):113–121.

154. The SCATI (Studio Sulla Calciparina Nell'Angina E Nella Trombosi Ventricolare Nell'Infarto) Group. (1989). Randomized controlled trial of subcutaneous calcium-heparin in acute myocardial infarction. Lancet 2:182–186.

155. Majerus, P.W., Broze, G.J., Miletich, J.P., Tollefson, D.M. (1990). Anticoagulant, thrombolytic, and antiplatelet drugs. In A.G. Gilman, T.W. Rale, A.S. Nies, P. Taylor (eds.), *Goodman and Gilman's Pharmacological Basis of Therapeutics* (8th ed., pp. 1311–1331). New York: Pergamon Press.

156. Second International Study of Infarct Survival Collaboration Group (1988). Randomised trial of intravenous streptokinase, oral aspirin, both, or neither among 17,187 cases of suspected acute myocardial infarction: ISIS-2. Lancet 2:349–360.

157. Lieberman, S.M. (1991). ISIS-3. J Am Coll Cardiol 18:1147–1148.

158. Kennedy, J.W., Weaver, W.D. (1989). Potential use of thrombolytic therapy before hospitalization. Am J Cardiol 64:8A–11A.

159. Linder, C., Heusch, G. (1990). ACE inhibitors for the treatment of myocardial ischemia? Cardiovasc Drugs Ther 4:1375–1384.

160. Danzig, R. (1979). Current status of oxygen therapy in acute myocardial infarction. Cardiovasc Med 4:1245–1248.

161. Ishikawa, K., Kanamosa, K., Yamakado, T., Kotori, R. (1986). The beneficial effects of 40% and 100% O_2 inhalations on acutely-induced myocardial ischemia in dogs. Tohuku J Exp Med 149:107–117.

162. Nelson, R., Tortolani, A., Hall, M., Parnell, V. (1989). Role of cardioplegia oxygen concentration in limiting myocardial reperfusion injury (abstract). Chest 96(2 Suppl.):236S.

163. Kircher, B.S., Topol, E.S., O'Neill, W.W., Pitt, B. (1987). Prediction of infarct artery recanalization after intravenous thrombolytic therapy. Am J Cardiol 59:513–515.

164. Lew, A.S., Cercek, B., Lewis, B.S., Hod, H., Shah,

P.K., Ganz, W. (1987). Efficacy of a two-hour infusion of 150 mg t-PA in acute myocardial infarction. Am J Cardiol 60:1225–1229.

165. Kleven, M.R. (1990). The critical care nurse's role in the noninvasive assessment of myocardial reperfusion. AACN Clin Issues Crit Care Nurs 1:110–118.

166. Kline, E.M. (1987). Recombinant tissue-type plasminogen activator in acute myocardial infarction: Role of the critical care nurse. Heart Lung 16:779–786.

167. American College of Cardiologists' Task Force on Assessment of Diagnostic and Therapeutic Cardiovascular Procedures (1990). American College of Cardiologists/American Heart Association Guidelines for the early management of patients with acute myocardial infarction. Circulation 82:664–707.

168. Wenger, N.K. (1984). Early ambulation physical activity: Myocardial infarction and coronary artery bypass surgery. Heart Lung 13:14–17.

169. Braun, L.T., Holm, K. (1989). Preservation of ischemic myocardium through activity management. J Cardiovasc Nurs 3:39–48.

170. Burek, K.A., Kirscht, J., Topol, E.J. (1989). Exercise capacity in patients 3 days after acute, uncomplicated myocardial infarction. Heart Lung 18:575–582.

171. Rowe, M.H., Jelinek, M.V., Liddell, N., Hugens, M. (1989). Effect of rapid mobilization on ejection fractions and ventricular volumes after acute myocardial infarction. Am J Cardiol 63:1037–1041.

172. Johnston, B.L., Watt, E.W., Fletcher, G.F. (1981). Oxygen consumption and hemodynamic and electrocardiographic responses to bathing in recent post-myocardial infarction patients. Heart Lung 10:666–671.

173. Magder, S. (1985). Assessment of myocardial stress from early ambulatory activities following myocardial infarction. Chest 87:442–447.

174. Quaglietti, S.E., Stotts, N.A., Lovejoy, N.C. (1988). The effect of selected positions on rate pressure product of the postmyocardial infarction patient. J Cardiovasc Nurs 2:77–85.

175. Winslow, E.H., Lane, L.D., Gaffney, F.A. (1984). Oxygen uptake and cardiovascular response in patients and normal adults during in-bed and out-of-bed toileting. J Cardiac Rehabilitation 4:348–354.

176. Winslow, E.H., Lane, L.D., Gaffney, F.A. (1985). Oxygen uptake and cardiovascular responses in control adults and acute myocardial infarction patients during bathing. Nurs Res 34:164–169.

177. Folta, A., Metzger, B.L. (1989). Exercise and functional capacity after myocardial infarction. J Nurs Scholar 21:215–219.

178. Sivarajan, E.S., Snydsman, A., Smith, B., Irving, J.B., Mansfield, L.W., Bruce, R.A. (1977). Low level treadmill testing of 41 patients with acute myocardial infarction prior to discharge from the hospital. Heart Lung 6:976–980.

179. Johnston, B.L. (1984). Exercise testing for patients after myocardial infarction and coronary bypass surgery: Emphasis on predischarge phase. Heart Lung 13:18–27.

180. Derogatis, L.R., King, K.M. (1981). The coital coronary: A reassessment of the concept. Arch Sex Behav 10:325–335.

181. Argondizzo, N.T. (1984). Education of the patient and family. In N.K. Wenger & H.K. Hellerstein (eds.), Rehabilitation of the Coronary Patient (2nd ed., pp. 161–178). New York: John Wiley and Sons.

182. Seifert, P.C. (1983). Protection of the myocardium during cardiac surgery. Heart Lung 12:135–142.

183. Benson, H. (1982). The relaxation response: History, physiologic basis and clinical usefulness. Acta Medica Scand 660(Suppl.):231–237.

184. Benson, H., Alexander, S., Feldman, C.L. (1975). Decreased premature ventricular contractions through use of the relaxation response in patients with stable ischemic heart disease. Lancet 2:380–382.

185. Guzzetta, C.E. (1989). Effects of relaxation and music therapy on patients in a coronary care unit with presumptive acute myocardial infarction. Heart Lung 18:609–616.

186. Bohachick, P. (1984). Progressive relaxation training in cardiac rehabilitation: Effect on psychologic variables. Nurs Res 33:283–287.

187. Aiken, L.H., Henricks, T.F. (1971). Systematic relaxation as a nursing intervention technique with open heart surgery patients. Nurs Res 20:212–217.

188. Ornish, D., Scherwitz, L.W., Doody, R.S., Kesten, D., McLanahan, S.M., Brown, S.E., DePuey, E.G., Sonnemaker, R., Haynes, C., Lester, J., McAllister, G.K., Hall, R.J., Burdine, J.A., Gotto, A.M. (1983). Effects of stress management training and dietary changes in treating ischemic heart disease. JAMA 249:54–59.

189. Murdaugh, C. (1982). Using research in practice. Focus 9:11–14.

190. Chan, V. (1990). Content areas for cardiac teaching: Patients' perceptions of the importance of teaching content after myocardial infarction. J Adv Nurs 15:1139–1145.

191. Cowan, M.J. (1990). Cardiovascular nursing research. Ann Rev Nurs Res 8:3–33.

192. Lindeman, C.A. (1989). Patient education. Ann Rev Nurs Res 7:29–45.

193. Popma, J.J., Dehmer, G.J. (1989). Care of the patient after coronary angioplasty. Ann Intern Med 110:547–559.

194. Phillips, S.J., Kongtakmorn, C., Skinner, J.R., Zeff, R.H. (1983). Emergency coronary artery reperfusion: A choice of therapy for evolving myocardial infarction. J Thorac Cardiovasc Surg 86:679–688.

195. Jones, E.L., Murphy, D.A., Crover, J.M. (1984). Comparison of coronary artery bypass surgery and percutaneous transluminal coronary angioplasty including surgery for failed angioplasty. Am Heart J 107:830–835.

196. Faris, J.A., Stotts, N.A. (1990). The effect of percutaneous transluminal coronary angioplasty on quality of life. Prog Cardiovasc Nurs 5:132–140.

197. Reis, G.J., Pomerantz, R.M., Jenkins, R.D., Kuntz, R.E., Baim, D.S., Diver, D.J., Schnitt, S.J., Safian, R.D. (1991). Laser balloon angioplasty: Clinical, angiographic and histologic results. J Am Coll Cardiol, 18:193–202.

198. Goy, J.J., Sigwart, U., Vogt, P., Stauffer, J.C., Kaufmann, U., Urban, M., Kappenberger, L. (1991). Long-term follow-up of the first 56 patients treated with intracoronary self-expanding stents (The Lausanne Experience). Am J Cardiol 67:569–572.

199. Roubin, G.S., King, S.B., Douglas, J.S., Lembo, N.J., Robinson, K.A. (1990). Intracoronary stenting during percutaneous transluminal coronary

angioplasty. Circulation *81*(Suppl. IV):IV92–IV100.

200. Safian, R.D., Gelbfish, J.S., Erny, R.E., Schnitt, S.J., Schmidt, D.A., Baim, D.S. (1990). Coronary atherectomy: Clinical, angiographic, and histologic findings and observations regarding potential mechanism. Circulation *82*:69–79.

201. Loop, F.D. (1983). Progress in surgical treatment of coronary atherosclerosis (Part 2). Chest *84*:740–755.

202. Mock, M.B., Ringquist, I., Fisher, L.D., Davis, K.B., Chaitman, B.R., Kouchoukos, N.T., Kaiser, G.C., Alderman, E., Ryan, T.J., Russell, R.O., Mullin, S., Fray, D., Killip, T., & participants in the Coronary Artery Surgery Study. (1982). Survival of medically treated patients in the Coronary Artery Surgery Study (CASS) registry. Circulation *66*:562–568.

203. Bolli, R. (1987). Bypass surgery in patients with coronary artery disease. Chest *91*:760–764.

204. Palac, R.T., Meadows, W.R., Hwang, M.H., Loeb, H.S., Pifarre, R., Gunnar, R.M. (1982). Risk factors related to progressive narrowing in aortocoronary vein grafts studied 1 and 5 years after surgery. Circulation *66*(Suppl. 1):40–44.

205. Lytle, B.W., Loop, F.D., Cosgrove, D.M., Ratliff, N.B., Easley, K., Taylor, P.C. (1985). Long-term (5 to 12 years) serial studies of internal mammary artery and saphenous vein coronary bypass grafts. J Thorac Cardiovasc Surg *89*:248–258.

206. Weiner, D.A., Ryan, T.J., Parsons, L., Fisher, L.D., Chaitman, B.R., Sheffield, L., Tristani, F.E. (1991). Prevalence and prognostic significance of silent and symptomatic ischemia after coronary bypass surgery: A report from the Coronary Artery Surgery Study (CASS) randomized population. J Am Coll Cardiol *18*:343–348.

207. Wenger, N.K. (1986). Rehabilitation of the coronary patient: Status 1986. Prog Cardiovasc Dis *29*:181–204.

208. Mills, G., Barnes, R., Rodell, D., Terry, L. (1985). An evaluation of an inpatient cardiac patient/family education program. Heart Lung *14*:400–406.

209. Sivarajan, E., Newton, K., Almes, N., Kempf, T., Mansfield, L., Bruce, R. (1983). Limited effects of outpatient teaching and counseling after myocardial infarction: A controlled study. Heart Lung *12*:65–73.

210. Swain, N., Steckel, S. (1981). Influencing adherence among hypertensives. Res Nurs Health *4*:213–222.

211. Friedman, M., Thoresen, C.E., Gill, J.J., Ulmer, D., Powell, L.H., Price, V.A., Brown, B., Thompson, L., Rabin, D.D., Breall, W.S., Bourg, E., Levy, R., Dixon, T. (1986). Alteration of type A behavior and its effect on cardiac recurrences in post myocardial infarction patients: Summary results of the Recurrent Coronary Prevention Project. Am Heart J *112*:653–665.

212. Taylor, C.B., Houston-Miller, N., Killen, J.D., DeBusk, R.F. (1990). Smoking cessation after acute myocardial infarction. Effects of a nurse-managed intervention. Ann Intern Med *113*:118–123.

213. Clark, L.T. (1991). Improving compliance and increasing control of hypertension: Needs of special hypertensive populations. Am Heart J *121*:664–669.

214. Dracup, K., Meleis, A. (1982). Compliance: An interactionist approach. Nurs Res *31*:31–36.

215. Morrow, D., Leirer, V., Sheikh, J. (1988). Adherence and medication instructions. J Am Geriatr Soc *36*:1147–1160.

216. Oldbridge, N.B. (1991). Compliance with cardiac rehabilitation services. J Cardiopul Rehab *11*:115–127.

217. Strauss, A., Glaser, B.G. (1982). *Chronic Illness and the Quality of Life*. St. Louis: C.V. Mosby.

218. Blumenthal, J.A., Emery, C.F. (1988). Rehabilitation of patients following myocardial infarction. J Consult Clin Psychol *56*:374–381.

219. Brown, W.V. (1990). Clinical trials including an update on the Helsinki Heart Study. Am J Cardiol *66*:11A–15A.

220. Friedman, M., Powell, L.H., Thoresen, C.E., Ulmer, D., Price, V., Gill, J.J., Thompson, L., Rabin, D.D., Brown, B., Breall, W.S., Levy, R., Bourg, E. (1987). Effect of discontinuance of type A behavioral counseling on type A behavior and cardiac recurrence rate of post myocardial infarction patients. Am Heart J *114*:483–490.

221. Hjermann, I., Velve Byre, K., Holme, I., Leren, P. (1981). Effect of diet and smoking intervention on the incidence of coronary heart disease, report from the Oslo Study Group of a Randomized Trial in healthy men. Lancet *2*:1303–1310.

222. The Lipid Research Clinics Program. (1984). The Lipid Research Clinics Coronary Primary Prevention Trial results. I. Reduction in incidence of coronary heart disease. JAMA *251*:351–364.

223. MacMahon, S., Peto, R., Cutler, J., Collins, R., Sortie, P., Neaton, J., Abbott, R., Godwin, J., Dyer, A., Stamler, J. (1990). Blood pressure, stroke and coronary heart disease. Part I: Effects of prolonged differences in blood pressure—evidence from 9 prospective observational studies corrected for the regression dilution bias. Lancet *335*:756–774.

224. Veterans Administration Cooperative Study Group on Antihypertensives. (1970). Effects of treatment on morbidity in hypertension: II. Results in patients with diastolic blood pressure averaging 90 through 114 mmHg. JAMA *213*:1143–1152.

225. Franklin, F.A., Brown, R.F., Franklin, C.C. (1990). Screening, diagnosis, and management of dyslipoproteinemia in children. Endocrinol Metab Clin North Am *19*:399–449.

226. Arntzenius, A.C., Kromhout, D., Barth, J.D., Reiber, J.H., Bruschke, A.V., Buis, B., VanGent, C.M., Kempen-Voogd, N., Strikwerda, S., VanDer Veide, E.A. (1985). Diet, lipoproteins, and the progression of coronary atherosclerosis: The Leiden Intervention Trial. N Engl J Med *312*:805–811.

227. Brensike, J.J., Levy, R.I., Kelsey, S.F., Passamani, E.R., Richardson, L., Loh, I.K., Stone, N.J., Aldrich, R.F., Battaglini, J.W., Moriarty, D.J., Fisher, M.R., Friedman, L., Friedwald, W., Detre, K.M., Epstein, S.E. (1984). Effects of therapy with cholystyramine on progression of coronary atherosclerosis: Results of the NHLBI Type II Coronary Intervention Study. Circulation *69*:313–324.

228. Canner, P.L., Berge, K.G., Wenger, N.K., Stamler, J., Friedman, L., Prineas, R.J., Friedwald, W. (1986). Fifteen year mortality in Coronary Drug Project patients: Long-term benefit with niacin. J Coll Cardiol *8*:1245–1255.

229. Cashin-Hemphill, L., Mack, W.J., Pogoda, J.M., Sanmarco, M.E., Azen, S.P., Blankenhorn, D.H. (1990). Beneficial effects of colestipol/niacin on coronary atherosclerosis. JAMA *264*:3013–3017.

230. Dzau, V., Braunwald, E. (1991). Resolved and

unresolved issues in the prevention and treatment of coronary artery disease: A workshop consensus statement. Am Heart J *121*:1244–1263.

231. Stone, N.J. (1990). Diet, lipids, and coronary heart disease. Endocrinol Metab Clin North Am *19*:321–344.

232. Dehmer, G.J., Popma, J.J., Van den Berg, E.K., Eichhorn, E.J., Prewitt, J.B., Campbell, W.B., Jennings, L., Willerson, J.T., Schmitz, J.M. (1988). Reduction in the rate of early restenosis after coronary angioplasty by a diet supplemented with n-3 fatty acids. N Engl J Med *319*:733–740.

233. Milner, M.R., Gallino, R.A., Leffingwell, A., Pichard, A.D., Brooks-Robinson, S., Rosenberg, J., Little, T., Lindsay, J. (1989). Usefulness of fish oil supplements in preventing clinical evidence of restenosis after percutaneous transluminal coronary angioplasty. Am J Cardiol *64*:294–299.

234. Anderson, J.W., Gustafson, N.J. (1988). Hypocholesterolemic effects of oat and bean products. Am J Clin Nutr *48*:749–753.

235. VanHorn, L.V., Liu, K., Parker, D. (1986). Serum lipid response to oat product intake with a fat modified diet. J Am Diet Assoc *86*:759–764.

236. Sadlo, H.B., Wenger, N.K. (1990). The role of exercise in the primary and secondary prevention of coronary atherosclerotic heart disease. Cardiovasc Clin *20*:177–190.

237. O'Connor, G.T., Buring, J.E., Yusuf, S., Goldhaber, S.Z., Olmstead, E.M., Paffenbarger, R.S., Hennekens, C.H. (1989). An overview of randomized trials of rehabilitation with exercise after myocardial infarction. Circulation *80*:234–244.

238. Oldbridge, N.B., LaSalle, D., Jones, N.L. (1980). Exercise rehabilitation of female patients with coronary heart disease. Am Heart J *100*:755–757.

239. Rechnitzer, P.A., Pickard, H.A., Paivia, A.U., Yurasz, M.S., Cunningham, D. (1972). Long-term follow-up study of survival and recurrence rates following myocardial infarction in exercising and control subjects. Circulation *45*:853–857.

240. Shephard, R.J. (1982). Exercise therapy in patients with angina pectoris. Adv Cardiol *31*:191–198.

241. DeBusk, R.F., Hung, J. (1982). Exercise conditioning soon after myocardial infarction: Effects on myocardial perfusion and ventricular function. Ann NY Acad Sci *382*:343–354.

242. Shaw, L.W. (1981). Effects of a prescribed supervised exercise program on mortality and cardiovascular morbidity in patients after a myocardial infarction. Am J Cardiol *48*:39–46.

243. Shephard, R.J. (1979). Recurrence of myocardial infarction in an exercising population. Br Heart J *41*:133–138.

244. VanCamp, S.P., Peterson, R.A. (1986). Cardiovascular complications of outpatient cardiac rehabilitation programs. JAMA *256*:1160–1163.

245. The Review Panel on Coronary-Prone Behavior and Coronary Heart Disease. (1981). A critical review. Circulation *63*:1199–1215.

246. Brown, A.J. (1976). Effect of family visits on the blood pressure and heart rate of patients in the coronary care unit. Heart Lung *5*:291–296.

247. Thomas, S.A., Lynch, J.J., Mills, M.E. (1975). Psychosocial influences on heart rhythm in the coronary-care unit. Heart Lung *4*:746–750.

248. Bauer, W.C., Dracup, K.A. (1987). Physiologic effects of back massage in patients with acute myocardial infarction. Focus Crit Care *14*:42–46.

249. Weiss, S.J. (1990). Effects of differential touch on nervous system arousal of patients recovering from cardiac disease. Heart Lung *19*:474–480.

250. Dobmeyer, D.J., Stine, R.A., Leier, C.V., Greenberg, R., Schaal, S.F. (1983). The arrhythmogenic effects of caffeine in human beings. N Engl J Med *308*:814–816.

251. Rosmarin, P.C. (1989). Coffee and coronary heart disease: A review. Prog Cardiovasc Dis *32*:239–245.

252. Newcombe, P.F., Renton, K.W., Rautaharju, P.M., Montague, T.J. (1988). High-dose caffeine and cardiac rate and rhythm in normal subjects. Chest *94*:90–94.

253. Kirchhoff, K.T., Holm, K., Foreman, M.D., Rebenson-Piano, M. (1990). Electrocardiographic response to ice water ingestion. Heart Lung *19*:41–48.

254. VanCott, M.L., Tittle, M.B., Moody, L.E., Wilson, M.E. (1991). Analysis of a decade of critical care nursing practice research: 1979 to 1988. Heart Lung *20*:394–397.

255. Keller, K. (1990). Cardiovascular Nursing Research Review: 1969–1988. Prog Cardiovasc Nurs *5*:26–33.

3

Cardiac Dysrhythmias

Mary Jane Sauve

Rhythmicity is inherent in all life processes whether viewed in the broader context of growth, maturation, aging, and death or in constructs such as hormone secretion. Rhythmicity is also implicit in the generation and propagation of each cardiac impulse. In the normal heart rhythmic activity results from a complex series of changes in the electrical properties of cells in the sinoatrial node, from which an impulse is generated and then is propagated in an orderly manner throughout the atria and ventricles. Dysrhythmias occur when there are changes in the electrophysiological properties of cardiac cells in one or more regions of the heart or changes in the cardiac musculature. These changes may arise from a variety of factors, including impaired oxygen and substrate transport, unequal ion and metabolic accumulation, an imbalance in autonomic innervation, aneurysms or fibrosis of the myocardium, and connective tissue disorders.[1-5]

DEFINITION

A cardiac dysrhythmia is any abnormality in the rate, regularity, initiation (formation), or conduction (transmission) of the cardiac impulse. Disturbances in cardiac rhythms can occur at any age and in a variety of clinical situations. While structural heart disease is often implicated in the genesis of dysrhythmias, they can and do occur in individuals with no evidence of heart disease or structural abnormality.

PREVALENCE AND POPULATIONS AT RISK

Cardiac dysrhythmias are ubiquitous. Changes in the rate and depth of respirations can result in wide variations in heart rate and rhythms, particularly in children. Sinus tachycardias occur with fevers, anemia, hyperthyroidism, hemorrhage, heavy exercise, or psychological or emotional stress. Slow heart rates or sinus bradycardias occur commonly in well-conditioned athletes, during sleep, in hypothyroidism, and from medications such as digitalis and beta blockers.[6]

Supraventricular tachycardia (SVT) is a common dysrhythmia in children.[2, 7, 8] In most cases the onset of SVT is paroxysmal, with rates exceeding 230 beats per minute (bpm); in infants the SVT rate is commonly 300 bpm and is often accompanied by symptoms of heart failure. SVT in youngsters is generally due to one of three major causes: Wolff-Parkinson-White syndrome, congenital heart disease, or sympathomimetic drugs such as decongestants.[8] SVT is uncommon in older individuals except as a complication of myocardial infarction. In contrast, atrial fibrillation is almost always associated with older age and structural heart disease.[9]

Atrial, junctional, and ventricular premature beats are the most common form of ectopic rhythm disturbance, tending to increase with age, whether or not structural heart disease is present.[2, 9] In normal subjects the occurrence of ventricular extrasystoles is generally benign. However, ventricular extrasystoles in patients with acute or chronic coronary artery disease, particularly if they are frequent and multifocal or paired or occur in salvos, are associated with an increased likelihood of the onset of ventricular tachyarrhythmias and sudden cardiac death (SCD).[10]

Among older individuals, the most common rhythm disturbance is bradycardia.

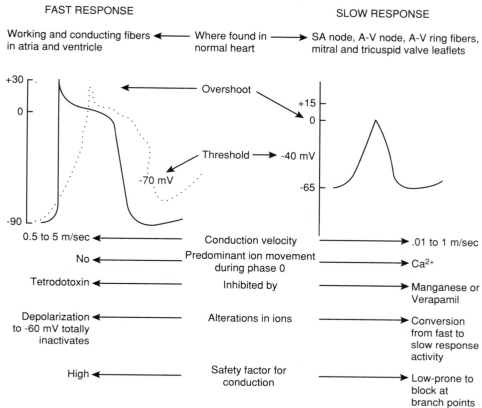

FAST RESPONSE

Working and conducting fibers ◄─── Where found in ───► SA node, A-V node, A-V ring fibers,
in atria and ventricle   normal heart   mitral and tricuspid valve leaflets

SLOW RESPONSE

Overshoot

Threshold ───► -40 mV

-70 mV

-65

0.5 to 5 m/sec ◄─────────── Conduction velocity ──────────► .01 to 1 m/sec

No ◄──────────── Predominant ion movement ──────────► Ca^{2+}
                          during phase 0

Tetrodotoxin ◄─────────── Inhibited by ──────────► Manganese or
                                                                      Verapamil

Depolarization ◄─────────── Alterations in ions ──────────► Conversion
to -60 mV totally   from fast to
inactivates   slow response
                                                                              activity

High ◄─────────── Safety factor for ──────────► Low-prone to
                          conduction   block at
                                                                              branch points

Figure 3–1. Characteristics of fast and slow action potentials. Note the different configurations of the various phases of the action potentials and the markedly disparate kinetic parameters. (From Sobel [1981]. Pract Cardiol 7:1, 31; Singh, B.H., et al. [1984]. Cellular electrophysiology of the heart. In S. Levy & M.M. Scheinmann (eds.), *Cardiac Arrhythmias: From Diagnosis to Therapy.* [p. 8]. Mount Kisco, NY: Futura Publishing Co., with permission.)

These slow heart rates are usually due to degenerative changes that cause various degrees of block in one or more areas of the cardiac conduction system, that is, sinus node disease or atrioventricular (AV) blocks. Complete heart block requiring pacemaker implantation is more likely to develop in those individuals with extensive coronary artery or valvular heart diseases.[9, 11]

MECHANISMS OF DYSRHYTHMIAS

Dysrhythmias occur because of abnormalities in the initiation and/or conduction of the cardiac impulse. Knowledge of arrhythmogenic mechanisms, as well as the salutary effects of various antiarrhythmic compounds, has been gained through the study of transmembrane potentials in various tissues of the heart under physiological and pathological conditions.[12, 13] Under physiological conditions transmembrane potentials in cardiac tissue produce two types of action potentials: (1) *slow-response* action potentials, which are found in the normal sinoatrial and AV nodes and whose phase 0 depolarization is largely calcium dependent; and (2) *fast-response* action potentials, which are characteristic of the conducting fibers in both the atria and ventricles and whose phase 0 depolarization is sodium dependent (Fig. 3–1). Knowledge of the sequential kinetics of the ionic transfers underlying depolarization (phase 0), repolarization (phases 1, 2, and 3), and spontaneous diastolic depolarization (phase 4) of the action potential in both slow- (pacemaker) and fast-response (nonpacemaker) cells is necessary in order to understand the mechanisms of arrhythmogenesis.

Phase 0 of the action potential represents rapid depolarization of the cell membrane after the resting transmembrane potential has been brought to threshold. In fast-response fibers, the onset of the action potential is mediated by two distinct inward ionic currents.[14] The first, carried by sodium ions through so-called fast channels in the cell membrane, is sudden and brief, lasting a few milliseconds. The intensity of this current is dependent upon the membrane potential from which the spike was generated, that is, the more negative the membrane potential the greater the intensity. The second inward current is carried by calcium and to a lesser extent sodium through slow channels in the cell membrane. It is a low-intensity current that contributes no more than 10 per cent to the overall depolarization phase of the action potential.[15, 16] The threshold for activation of the slow channel is -45 to -35 mV versus -70 to -65 mV for the fast channel. Inactivation of the fast inward channels is believed to be completed during phase 1 and at the latest early phase 2, while the slow channels only begin to attenuate toward the end of phase 2.[17]

The ionic current responsible for the initiation of the normal slow-response action potentials found in the sinoatrial and atrioventricular nodes closely resemble the second component of fast-response action potentials. Depolarization is dependent upon the influx of calcium and to a lesser extent sodium. Threshold potentials for slow-response fibers range from -60 to -40 mV.[15, 16]

The repolarization phases of the action potential are less well understood in terms of ionic conductance because the translocation of ions across the cell membrane varies from one cell type to another.[17] In Purkinje fibers the rapid initial repolarization seen in phase 1 is due to an outward current activated by the positive potential levels generated by depolarization and then inactivated by the ensuring equilibrium of ionic forces across the membrane. Initially, it was believed that these outward forces were due to an efflux of chloride from the cell, but it now appears that the major contributor to phase 1 repolarization is potassium.[16] Phase 2, or the plateau of the action potential, is characterized by little net current flow. The slow inward positive current secondary to calcium is balanced by the efflux of potassium. As the slow inward channels deactivate, potassium con-ductance increases, ending the plateau phase and initiating phase 3 of the action potential. This phase consists of essentially an outward current carried by potassium, which tends to increase as the membrane potential moves rapidly toward resting levels.

Phase 4 of the action potential is the interval from the completion of repolarization to the beginning of the next action potential. In pacemaker or slow-response cells phase 4 is marked by slow but steady loss of resting membrane potential due to the influx of calcium through the slow channels.[18] This characteristic diastolic depolarization of slow-response fibers, or automaticity, explains the ability of the sinoatrial node to act as the normal pacemaker of the heart. In healthy myocardial tissue only the sinoatrial node exhibits the ability to initiate action potentials without external stimulation, although cells in the atria, the AV node, and the His-Purkinje system have potential automaticity.[19] However, the sinoatrial node initiates cardiac impulses at a rate sufficiently high to overdrive or suppress any other potential automatic cell in the cardiac conduction system.

All cardiac fibers are excitable or capable of producing an action potential when stimulated sufficiently to attain threshold (Fig. 3–1). There is also an interval in each cardiac cycle during which no further impulses can be propagated; this is known as the refractory period (Fig. 3–2). During the absolute refractory period (ARP), no action potential can be induced no matter how large the stimulus. Under certain clinical conditions, such as anoxia or hyperthyroidism, the ARP is decreased because repolarization is shortened.[17] Similarly, the ARP is increased by conditions that tend to lengthen repolarization, such as hypothyroidism or drugs like quinidine and amiodarone.[17] Distinct from the absolute refractory period is the effective refractory period (ERP), which is characterized by the generation of local responses following stimulation, although a conducted impulse cannot be induced.[14, 16–18] By definition, the ERP is longer than the ARP (Fig. 3–2), but more important, it is the primary determinant of the number of impulses a specific cardiac fiber can generate per unit of time. There are two ways in which the ERP can be lengthened and thus reduce the number of sustained repetitive impulses, with one-to-one conduction, that can be generated in the fiber: (1) delay the recovery of the fast

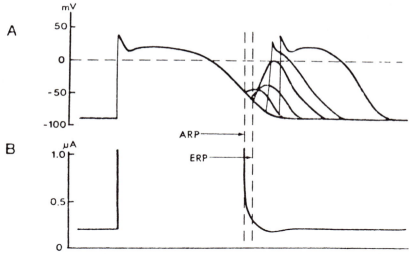

Figure 3–2. The relationship between an action potential from a fast-response cardiac fiber and the response to premature stimulation. *A,* Schematic representation of the action potential and the response elicited by an extrastimulus at various coupling intervals. *B,* This shows the change in the excitability threshold as measured by the cathodal current required for excitation during the action potential. ARP, absolute refractory period; ERP, effective refractory period. (From Singh, B.H., et al [1984]. *Cellular electrophysiology of the heart.* In S. Levy & M.M. Scheinman (eds.), *Cardiac Arrhythmias: From Diagnosis to Therapy* [p. 10]. Mount Kisco, NY: Futura Publishing Co., with permission.)

sodium channels so that an insufficient number of channels are available to support the occurrence of a propagable second spike (repolarization remains unchanged or is shortened) and (2) prolong repolarization.[17] The first of these mechanisms is an example of a time-dependent increase in ERP and is the mode of action of Class 1 antiarrhythmic agents (e.g., lidocaine). The second mechanism is an example of voltage dependent refractoriness and is the primary mode of action of Class 3 antiarrhythmics such as amiodarone. The different classes of antiarrhythmic drugs can lengthen ERP by one or both of these mechanisms (Table 3–1).

Under pathological conditions, such as ischemia, membrane potentials are altered, initiating disruptions in impulse formation or impulse conduction or in a combination of these processes.[12, 19, 20] Specific electrophysiological changes include (1) increases in rate of diastolic depolarization in Purkinje fibers, (2) decreases in membrane potentials with concomitant decreases in conduction velocity, (3) changes in either the duration or the amplitude of fast-response action potentials, and (4) increases or decreases in the duration of refractory periods.[21] These altered membrane potentials may generate ectopic activity by three different electrophysiological mechanisms: either enhanced or abnormal automaticity, triggered activity, and re-entry (Table 3–2).

Abnormal Impulse Generation

Automaticity

As noted earlier, the ionic currents responsible for phase 4 diastolic depolarization in slow-response fibers such as the sinoatrial node have been attributed to the gradual decrease in the outward ionic current carried by potassium in the presence of an inward current carried primarily by calcium.[22] The kinetics of these currents result in the accumulation of positive charges intracellularly, thereby shifting the resting transmembrane potential toward threshold potential. Catecholamine release by the sympathetic nervous system facilitates the inward currents, thus increasing the slope of phase 4 and the rate of depolarizations, while vagal activity through the action of acetylcholine depresses the slope of phase 4, thus decreasing the rate

TABLE 3–1. CLASSIFICATION OF ANTIARRHYTHMIC DRUGS

Class	Electrophysiological Action	Examples
1.	Membrane-stabilizing agents	
	a. Depress phase 0 (dv/dt) Depress conduction velocity Prolong repolarization (time-dependent ERP)	Procainamide Quinidine Disopyramide
	b. Minimal effect on phase 0 Shorten or have no effect on repolarization	Lidocaine Mexiletine Tocainide Phenytoin
	c. Depress phase 0 Markedly show conduction Differential effects on repolarization in Purkinje fibers/ventricular muscle	Flecainide Encainide Lorcainide
2.	Beta-adrenergic blocking agents Depress phase 4 depolarization Slow SA node activation Prolong AV nodel ERP	Propranolol Atenolol Sotalol* Metoprolol
3.	Agents that prolong repolarization No effect on conduction velocity Lengthen ERP by delaying voltage-dependent ERP	Amiodarone Bretylium Sotalol*
4.	Calcium channel blockers Slow SA nodal activity Prolong AV nodal conduction	Verapamil Diltiazem

*Sotalol has both Class 2 and Class 3 effects.

of depolarization in these cells (Fig. 3–3).[14, 16, 19] When the number of impulses generated by the sinoatrial node (SA) decreases because of enhanced vagal tone, SA nodal disease, or impaired impulse conduction between the SA node and atria or between atria and ventricles, a shift in pacemaker sites will normally occur.[19] In these instances the removal of overdrive suppression by the SA node allows time for the resting transmembrane potential of subsidiary pacemaker cells to decline and reach threshold prior to impulses generated from the sinus node (Fig. 3–4). However, while these latent pacemakers represent a biological safety margin, their emergence may be too slow, too fast, or too irregular to prevent significant electrical instability in the myocardium.[23]

A shift in impulse generation to an ectopic site may also occur owing to intense beta adrenergic stimulation at discrete sites in the myocardium. Such augmented subsidiary pacemakers may reach threshold prior to the SA node, thus usurping pacemaker control

of the heart. The tachyarrhythmias produced by these enhanced pacemaker cells generally take the form of accelerated junctional rhythms or idioventricular tachycardias.[24] Rosen and Reber[25] have noted that the key to recognizing enhanced automaticity from abnormal automatic mechanisms clinically is the differential response of these rhythms to overdrive pacing. Enhanced normal automaticity will be suppressed by short bursts of overdrive pacing, whereas abnormal automatic rhythms will either immediately resume their initial rate or assume the rate of the overdrive pacemaker following stimulation.

The exact ionic mechanisms responsible for the development of abnormal automaticity in Purkinje fibers and atrial and ventricular myocardial cells have not been fully elucidated. However, Bigger and colleagues[1] have shown that canine Purkinje fibers will demonstrate spontaneous diastolic depolarization when their normal resting transmembrane potentials have been shifted from -90 to -60 mV by experimentally induced ischemia. These authors have hypothesized that the most likely mechanism responsible for this change in diastolic potential was an inward current of calcium and sodium through slow-membrane channels, since the fast channels are largely[16] inoperative at -60 mV, and the outward potassium current is either depressed or inoperative at that transmembrane potential. Clinical problems that may favor the development of abnormal automaticity include hyperkalemia, acidosis, hypoxia, ischemia, and fever.[5] However, few clinical arrhythmias have been attributed to abnormal automaticity, although there is some evidence that ventricular tachycardias that develop in the late myocardial period may be generated by Purkinje fibers that demonstrate diastolic depolarization and prolonged action potentials.[26, 27]

Triggered Activity

Cranefield[28] has defined triggered activity as repetitive depolarizing currents or afterdepolarizations that shift the membrane potential in a positive direction but may or may not generate an action potential. Afterdepolarization is a term that has been used to describe the inward current of positive ions into the cell membrane during or after the final repolarization process of the action potential. The significance of afterdepolarizations rests in the fact that their occurrence is

TABLE 3–2. MECHANISMS AND CLASSIFICATIONS OF CARDIAC ARRHYTHMIAS

I. Disturbances in impulse formation
  A. Depressed sinus node automaticity
    1. Sinus bradycardia
    2. Sinus arrhythmia
    3. Wandering pacemaker
    4. Sinus pauses or arrest
  B. Enhanced automaticity
    1. Escape beats or rhythms
      a. Atrial
      b. Atrioventricular (AV) junctional
      c. Ventricular
    2. Atrial, junctional, or ventricular premature beats
    3. Ectopic supraventricular tachycardias
      a. Paroxysmal
      b. Nonparoxysmal
    4. Paroxysmal ventricular tachycardias
    5. Parasystolic rhythms
  C. Abnormal automaticity
    1. Late ischemic (postmyocardial infarction) ectopy
    2. Late ischemic tachyarrhythmias
  D. Triggered automaticity
    1. Early afterdepolarizations
      a. Ventricular ectopy
      b. Torsade de pointes
    2. Delayed afterdepolarizations
      a. Digitalis-induced ventricular dysrhythmias
      b. Exercise-induced ventricular dysrhythmias

II. Disturbances in impulse propagation
  A. Conduction blocks
    1. Sinoatrial block
    2. Intra-atrial blocks
    3. Atrioventricular (AV) blocks
      a. First-degree AV block
      b. Second-degree AV block
        (1) Mobitz type I (Wenckebach)
        (2) Mobitz type II
    4. High-degree or advanced AV block
    5. Third-degree or complete AV block
  B. Re-entry dysrhythmias
    1. Paroxysmal supraventricular tachycardias
      a. AV nodal re-entrant tachycardia
      b. Atypical AV nodal re-entrant tachycardia
      c. Orthodromic AV reciprocating tachycardia
      d. Antidromic AV reciprocating tachycardia
      e. Nodoventricular bypass tract (Mahaim)
    2. Circus movement tachycardias
      f. Atrial flutter/fibrillation
      g. Ventricular flutter/fibrillation
    3. Atrial, junctional, and ventricular extrasystoles
    4. Ventricular tachycardia

III. Mixed disturbances of impulse propagation and conduction
  E. Atrioventricular dissociation
    1. Complete
    2. Incomplete
  F. Wolff-Parkinson-White syndrome (pre-excitation)
  G. Electrical alterans
  H. Lown-Ganong-Levine syndrome

solely dependent upon the action potential that precedes them; that is, unlike abnormal pacemaker rhythms, these rhythms do not arise de novo. The development of afterdepolarizations has been experimentally associated with cardiac glycosides, hypoxia, elevated PCO_2, hypokalemia, rheumatic disease, and cardiomyopathies.[19, 25]

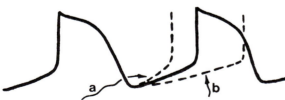

Figure 3–3. Action potential of pace-making cell. Resting phase 4 spontaneously slopes toward threshold. Increasing slope *(a)* produces acceleration; decreasing slope *(b)* produces slowing of pacemaker discharge rate. (From Mariott, H.J.L. [1988]. *Practical Electrocardiography* [8th ed., p. 112]. Baltimore: Williams & Wilkins, with permission. © 1988.)

Two types of afterdepolarizations have been described: (1) early afterdepolarizations (EADs), which occur during phase 3 of the action potential and appear to be due to a disruption in the outward flow of potassium; and (2) delayed afterdepolarizations (DADs), which occur after repolarization is complete (Fig. 3–5). DADs may result from two different mechanisms. Digitalis-induced DADs appear to result from inhibition of the sodium-potassium pump, which causes an increase in intracellular sodium, which in turn reduces the sodium-calcium exchange and subsequently results in increased intracellular calcium.[29, 30] The increase in intracellular calcium tends to load the sarcoplasmic reticulum, causing it to fluctuate in its release of calcium during systole. As a consequence, a secondary release of calcium occurs following repolarization. This secondary release of calcium creates the DAD by fostering an inward current of positive ions across the cell membrane. Those delayed afterdepolarizations not associated with digitalis appear to be due

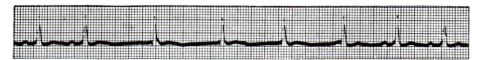

Figure 3–4. Transient sinus slowing induced by a deep breath. After the second beat, the sinus rhythm slows, and junctional escape results for four beats. The sinus node then accelerates and resumes control for the last two beats. (From Mariott, H.J.L. [1988]. *Practical Electrocardiography* [8th ed., p. 340]. Baltimore: Williams & Wilkins, with permission. © 1988.)

to an inward current carried by calcium because blockage of the slow inward current by verapamil decreases the amplitude of the DAD.[25, 28] Case studies have implicated DAD as the mechanism fostering the development of an exercise-induced ventricular tachycardia found in young people with no apparent heart disease[31–33] and ectopy following experimentally induced myocardial ischemic injury.[34] However, the significance of triggered ectopic activity due to DAD to clinically occurring dysrhythmias remains largely speculative.

Unlike DADs, which tend to occur at accelerated sinus rates,[25] early afterdepolarizations are more prominent at slower heart rates. The reason for this may be due to the

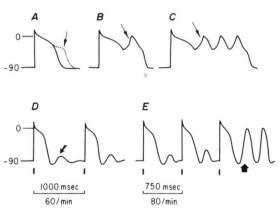

Figure 3–5. In *A*, an early afterdepolarization is indicated by the arrow. In *B*, a single triggered action potential caused by this afterdepolarization is shown, whereas in *C* a train of triggered action potentials is shown (*arrows* in *B* and *C*). In *D* and *E*, action potentials caused by propagating impulses (indicated by vertical lines) are followed by delayed afterdepolarizations (*arrow* in *D*). In *E*, triggered activity caused by the afterdepolarizations occurs at the arrow. (From Wit, A.L., & Rosen, M.R. [1981]. Cellular electrophysiology of cardiac arrhythmias: Part 2. Mod Con Cardiovasc Dis *50*:9, with permission. Copyright 1981, American Heart Association.)

fact that the repolarizing potassium currents are reduced at slower heart rates. In experimental animals blockage of the repolarizing current with cesium has been shown to initiate a torsades de pointes rhythm indistinguishable from that associated with clinical Long QT syndrome.[35, 36] Lazzara[24] speculates that EADs are responsible for the acquired Long QT syndromes that occur with use of Class 1a antiarrhythmics such as quinidine or that are seen in clinical hypokalemia (Table 3–1).

Abnormal Impulse Conduction

Re-entry

The most common mechanism believed to underlie the occurrence of clinically sustained supraventricular and ventricular arrhythmias is re-entry. The phenomena of re-entry occurs when a cardiac impulse does not die out completely after depolarizing the myocardium but instead persists and re-excites some region of the heart through which it had passed previously.[17, 24, 37] In order for re-entry to occur, there must be two anatomical or functional cardiac conduction pathways linked by a common distal pathway that have differing refractory and conduction patterns. The disparity in conduction (fast/slow) and refractory (short/long) patterns causes an area of either transient or unidirectional block to develop in the circuit.

Figure 3–6 presents the classic ring model for re-entry. In this model the normal cardiac impulse enters the proximal limb of the circuit and proceeds antegradely down the left limb and distal pathway but is blocked in the right limb. However, retrograde conduction of the impulse up the right limb of the circuit finds the area of block no longer refractory, allowing the impulse to re-enter and re-excite the tissue proximal to the block. Figures 3–7 and 3–8 present newer models of re-entry that incorporate the concept that propaga-

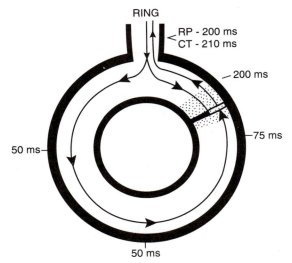

RING

RP - 200 ms
CT - 210 ms

200 ms

75 ms

50 ms

50 ms

Figure 3–6. Ring model of re-entry. Conduction times (CT) of the activation front proceeding around the ring are shown beside the ring as well as the refractory period (RP) of the entry site. A bar across the ring represents a locus of unidirectional block, and the stippled area represents a locus of slow conduction. (From Lazzara, R. [1988]. Electrophysiological mechanisms for ventricular arrhythmias. Clin Cardiol *11*:II2. Copyrighted and redrawn with the permission of Clinical Cardiology Publishing Co, Inc, and/or Foundation for Advances in Medicine and Sciences.)

tion of an impulse is really a three-dimensional process in the myocardial syncytium.[24, 38–40] In the "leading circle model" re-entry is initiated when wavefronts are blocked along a line of refractory tissue. The wavefronts circle around to the other side of the line at one end of the interface and proceed along the line of block through partially or fully recovered tissue to the other end of the interface, initiating the circuit. The circuit is maintained if the tissue along the first line of block is sufficiently recovered to allow propagation of the impulse. In the "figure eight" model re-entry is initiated when the wavefronts enter an abnormal area of the myocardium in which an arch or block is formed by sharply increased gradients of refractoriness. The wavefronts continue around both sides of the arc, returning toward the center of the arc, where they merge and cross over to the original side when the tissue near the center of the arc has recovered sufficiently for activation. The merged wavefront then divides and returns toward the ends of the arc through recovered tissue encircling the

two segments of the arc and merging between them.

In each of these models of re-entry, an area of recovered myocardium is juxtaposed against an area of refractory tissue, providing the transient or unidirectional block necessary for the establishment of the re-entry pathway. In addition, propagation of the wavefront around the block is slow enough to allow the tissue into which the wavefront is re-entering time to recover excitability,[29, 38] thus fulfilling the electrophysiological prerequisites for re-entrant excitation. Re-entrant circuits may be large or small. For example, the re-entrant circuit that produces the supraventricular tachycardia associated with pre-excitation (Wolff-Parkinson-White syndrome) involves areas in the atria, ventricles, atrioventricular node, and the accessory pathway, whereas the most common form of paroxysmal supraventricular tachycardia is associated with a re-entry circuit confined to the AV node.[7] Similarly, ventricular tachycardia can result from a large circuit, as in bundle branch re-entry, or more commonly from focal areas of ischemia in the ventricles.

The slowed conduction and unidirectional block necessary for re-entrant excitation may result from several different electrophysiological mechanisms. However, the best understood of these mechanisms has been derived from studies of ischemically injured tissue.[26, 41] As noted earlier, the size and rapidity of the depolarizing current are determined by the velocity and amplitude of phase 0 of the action potential, which in turn is the product of the resting membrane potential (normal, − 90 mV). In ischemic tissue the resting membrane potential of fast-response fibers is reduced (−60 to −70 mV), so that only a fraction of the sodium channels are available for activation. Consequently, the speed and amplitude of the upstroke (phase 0) in these fibers are decreased (depressed fast responses), and their effective refractory periods tend to outlast the action potential duration.[24, 29] The depressed upstrokes contribute to slowed conduction in the ischemic or injured area, while the prolonged refractoriness contributes to the development of conduction blocks.[17, 27, 38] Fast-response fibers in ischemic areas can also demonstrate slow-response action potentials that may contribute to the development of re-entry.[42] Although the fast inward sodium channels are inactivated at membrane potentials of − 50 mV, the slow channels are still open. Under certain conditions, such as augmented cate-

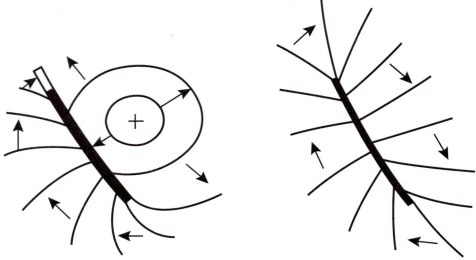

Figure 3–7. Leading circle model of re-entry. The initiation *(top)* of re-entry occurs when wavefronts that spread from the site of generation of an impulse, shown by a plus sign, encounter a line of block due to refractoriness. The wavefronts cross to the other side of the line at one extremity and proceed along the line of block through recovered tissue to cross at the other extremity and initiate the circuit. The maintenance of the circuit *(bottom)* involves wavefronts proceeding along the line of block first along one side through recovered tissue then along the other side as it recovers. (From Lazzara, R. [1988]. Electrophysiological mechanisms for ventricular arrhythmias. Clin Cardiol *11*:II2. Copyrighted and redrawn with the permission of Clinical Cardiology Publishing Co, Inc, and/or Foundation for Advances in Medicine and Science.)

cholamine release, the inward currents through the slow channel may generate an action potential. Since the inward currents are weak, the phase 0 upstroke velocity is significantly slower, giving rise to slow conduction and both unidirectional and bidirectional block.[19]

Two additional mechanisms of re-entry

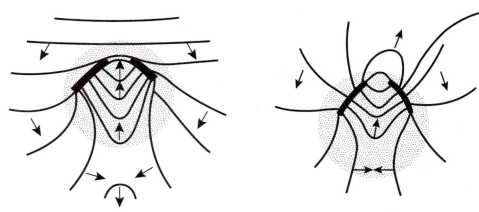

Figure 3–8. Figure eight model of re-entry. Re-entry is initiated when wavefronts of activation enter an abnormal region *(stippled)* and encounter an arc of block at a locus of sharp gradient of increasing refractoriness. The wavefronts proceed around the ends of the arc, merge near the center of the arc, and cross when refractoriness recedes. Re-entry is maintained *(bottom)* by wavefronts encircling two segments of the arc of block, merging between them. (From Lazzara, R. [1988]. Electrophysiological mechanisms for ventricular arrhythmias. Clin Cardiol *11*:II2. Copyrighted and redrawn with the permission of Clinical Cardiology Publishing Co, Inc, and/or Foundation for Advances in Medicine and Science..)

have been described: reflection and the anisotropic phenomenon.[43, 44] Reflection occurs when a propagated impulse encounters a narrow area of viable but inexcitable tissue that is connected intracellularly with excitable tissue on its distal side. Depending on the width of the gap and the intensity of the wavefront, the impulse can be passively transmitted across the gap to depolarize the distal tissue. Typically, the flow of current across the gap is very slow, so that the action potential that is generated in the distal portion can then be reflected back across the gap to re-excite the proximal tissue, producing a single extrasystole or a tachyarrhythmia.

Normal properties of atrial and ventricular muscle may also foster re-entry under certain conditions. Spach and Kootsey[44] have described the normal myocardium as an anistrophic structure, that is, one that promotes fast conduction along the length of the muscle fiber and slow conduction across the width or short axis of the fiber. Theoretically, even though membrane potentials and action potential upstrokes remain normal, these disparities in conduction patterns favor the development of re-entry. Lastly, the disparities in conduction and refractory patterns within normal sinus or atrioventricular nodal tissue can also foster re-entrant arrhythmias. For example, if a premature impulse generated by an ectopic area in the atria enters into the atrioventricular node when it is partially refractory, the impulse may be conducted slowly down nonrefractory or partially refractory tissue and blocked by refractory tissue. If the refractory tissue recovers in time to allow retrograde conduction, the re-entry circuit is established.

RELATED PHYSIOLOGICAL CONCEPTS

Other physiological phenomena related to the concept of dysrhythmia include heart rate variability, paroxysmal tachycardias, AV dissociation, and sudden cardiac death. While these phenomena share the underlying electrophysiological mechanisms resulting in the changes in rate or rhythm characteristic of all dysrhythmias, they differ in respect to their potential effects on left ventricular function, cardiac output, and perfusion of vital organ systems and as precursors of more serious rhythm disturbances. They may also differ in regard to the presence, if any, and the extent of underlying heart disease.

Heart Rate Variability

This is most pronounced in infants and children and tends to decrease with increasing age.[9, 45] Respiratory rate has a significant effect on heart rate (increasing heart rate with inspiration and decreasing it with expiration), as does the autonomic nervous system. Augmented beta-adrenergic discharge is associated with sinus tachycardias, the enhancement of subsidiary pacemakers, and abnormal automaticity. Imbalances in sympathetic tone can also cause changes in repolarization, lengthen the QT interval, and predispose the individual for a torsade type ventricular tachycardia.[36, 46, 47] Likewise, imbalances in parasympathetic or vagal tone can result in abnormally slow heart rates that can facilitate the emergence of competitive pacemakers.[6] Engel[48] has long espoused the position that the intense autonomic discharge associated with emotional arousal and psychological uncertainty can result in vasodepressor syncope in the healthy individual and sudden death in the person with a defective cardiovascular system. Singer and colleagues[49] have recently reported that there is an increased risk of recurrent sudden death in survivors of incidents of sudden cardiac death whose heart rate variability is markedly depressed. These authors believe their findings provide evidence of parasympathetic depression in patients prone to developing sudden cardiac death.

Paroxysmal Tachycardias

Paroxysmal tachycardias are usually supraventricular, although on occasion they may be ventricular, as in exercise-induced arrhythmias due to triggered activity.[7, 31, 33] These dysrhythmias are characterized by an abrupt onset and ending and rapid regular heart rates (100 to 250 bpm) and are usually initiated by an ectopic premature complex. Paroxysmal supraventricular tachycardias (PSVT) are further characterized by abnormal P waves, which may or may not be discernible; narrow QRS complexes, except in cases of a functional or underlying bundle branch block or antidromic AV reciprocating tachycardia (bypass tract conducts antegradely, and AV node conducts retro-gradely); and frequent ST-T wave depression.[50] Paroxysmal ventricular tachycardias may be sustained ($\geq$ 1 minute) or nonsustained ($\geq$ 5 beats), have right-to-left ventricular configuration, demonstrate AV dissociation, and are more often associated with underlying heart disease than are PSVTs. The most common electrophysiological mechanism believed to underlie both PSVT and paroxysmal ventricular tachycardia is reentry, although both may be caused by enhanced or an abnormal automatic foci or may be triggered as in digitalis toxicity.[7, 33]

PSVT may occur at any age, and if no heart disease is present and the rate is not excessive (> 200 bpm), the tachycardia may be well tolerated for extended periods of time.[50–52] Paroxysmal ventricular tachycardia may be equally well tolerated in young patients without discernible heart disease and in those individuals with coronary artery disease but with well-preserved ventricular function (rate generally < 200 bpm). In either case, the occurrence of symptoms is related to the rate and duration of the paroxysm as well as to the presence or absence of underlying heart disease. Individuals may therefore be completely asymptomatic or experience mild to severe palpitations, weakness, lightheadedness, shortness of breath, chest pain, or syncope, depending upon the extent of left ventricular compromise and subsequent drop in cardiac output and systemic perfusion. The prognosis for those individuals with paroxysmal tachycardias having no heart disease or with correctable clinical syndromes is generally quite good.[8]

AV Dissociation

This is defined as the independent beating of the atria and ventricles; that is, the atria and ventricles are controlled by separate pacemakers. AV dissociation is not a primary rhythm disturbance but arises from either one or a combination of four distinct mechanisms: (1) sinus bradycardia, (2) incomplete sinus node block with incomplete or complete AV block, (3) acceleration of a subsidiary pacemaker, or (4) a pause following an extrasystole or run of tachycardia.[9, 53] AV dissociation may be momentary, as occurs with a ventricular escape beat with blocked retrograde conduction; temporary, as occurs when sinus slowing facilitates the development of

an accelerated nodal rhythm; or permanent, as occurs with complete heart block.

While physiological bradycardias can develop in normal individuals (during sleep) or in athletes, with the concomitant emergence of a junctional pacemaker at or about the same rate (isorhythmic dissociation),[54] AV dissociation is usually associated with some form of cardiac disease affecting either the conduction system or ventricular myocardium.[2] Symptoms may occur in those individuals with impaired left ventricular function because the stroke volume is insufficient to maintain cardiac output. An important factor affecting stroke volume in AV dissociation is the loss of synchrony between atrial emptying and ventricular filling. In the individual with mitral stenosis, the loss of the atrial kick may be enough to precipitate symptoms of left-sided heart failure.[2] Similarly, those individuals who develop ventricular tachycardia due to an underlying structural heart disease (ischemia, valvular defects, cardiomyopathies) may also develop all of the manifestations of hemodynamic compromise due to the fast rate and lack of appropriately timed atrial contractions.[6]

Sudden Cardiac Death

Sudden cardiac death (SCD) represents the most extreme case of hemodynamic compromise due to the occurrence of a cardiac dysrhythmia. The leading cause of death in the United States, SCD is defined as a sudden arrhythmic death occurring within 1 hour of symptom onset that was neither expected by medical history nor associated with terminal heart failure, shock, or other agonal event.[55–57] Primary ventricular fibrillation is the most frequent dysrhythmia underlying this event, although some events may be preceded by organized ventricular tachycardia.[58] The individual at greatest risk for this catastrophic event is a middle-aged male with 70 per cent narrowing of at least one, but frequently two or more, coronary arteries[56, 59, 60] as well as frequent complex ventricular ectopy, ventricular wall motion abnormalities, and decreased ejection fractions.[61, 62] There is also a significant minority of patients (10 to 30 per cent) whose sudden death is not associated with coronary artery disease but with cardiomyopathies, prolonged QT syndromes (congenital or acquired), conduction abnormalities (Wolff-Parkinson-White syndrome and AV block), valvular heart disease, or no known structural dysfunction.[63]

Psychosocial factors are also believed to play a role in the genesis of SCD. Lown and colleagues[64] and Corbalan and associates[65] have developed an animal model to explain the psychophysiology of SCD and the role of the nervous system in lowering the fibrillation threshold. Several case studies have shown a relationship between specific psychosocial stressors, such as driving,[66, 67] oratory,[68] or mental arithmetic,[69–71] and the occurrence of ventricular ectopy and salvos of ventricular tachycardia. More recently, an analysis of cardiac outcomes from the Recurrent Coronary Prevention Project revealed that type A behavior was an independent predictor of sudden cardiac death but not nonsudden cardiac death or nonfatal reinfarction in post-myocardial infarction patients.[72]

RELATED PSYCHOSOCIAL CONCEPTS

Many, if not most, dysrhythmias, even potentially serious rhythm disturbances such as paroxysmal ventricular tachycardia or atrial fibrillation, can be asymptomatic for months or years and may be only brought to the attention of the individual during routine physical examination. However, if the substrate for the arrhythmia is some form of ischemic process (coronary artery disease or dilated cardiomyopathy) or if the dysrhythmia is very fast or very slow, symptoms associated with decreased cardiac output will occur. The individual's psychological response to the occurrence of cardiac dysrhythmias is determined by the severity of symptoms incurred during the dysrhythmia or from the patient's underlying heart disease and by the impact of the dysrhythmia and cardiac impairment on subsequent life style (i.e., modified work status or decreased mobility).[73, 74] The responses of individuals who have experienced sustained ventricular tachycardia or ventricular fibrillation or both illustrate this point.

Following the institution of cardiac resuscitation procedures in hospitals, several small studies of patients with myocardial infarction complicated by ventricular fibrillation were undertaken. Druss and Kornfeld[75] and Dlin and colleagues[76] reported significant short- and long-term emotional distress in these patients, including sleep disturbances, restlessness, irritability, and a strong identification with having been dead. In contrast, Dupont and colleagues[77] and Minuck and Perkins[78] found that long-term emotional disturbances were rare and that return to work among these patients was not different from that in uncomplicated myocardial infarction patients. In the most comprehensive of these early studies, Dobson and colleagues[79] reported a range of psychological responses in these patients and began to look for potential relationships. These authors found that survivors who had the greatest degree of upset in the year following their cardiac arrest also had the most frequent physical complaints (chest pain, symptoms of heart failure) and the longest delay in returning to work, while those with the least amount of or no distress had the fewest physical complaints and returned to work the earliest.

More recent studies of SCD survivors and patients with sustained ventricular tachycardia without collapse have also noted relationships among symptoms, return to work, and the occurrence of psychological distress. Haggarty and colleagues[80] noted that the psychological distress found in 51 per cent of their ventricular tachyarrhythmia patients was related to recurrences of the dysrhythmia and treatment with the then investigational drug amiodarone but not with the initial dysrhythmia, that is, nonfatal ventricular tachycardia versus ventricular fibrillation or SCD. Dunnington and colleagues[73] also found no differences in the psychological profiles of SCD and sustained ventricular tachycardia patients. Rather, the degree of psychological distress and the number of symptoms reported by their subjects were related to the presence or absence of one or more of the following factors: (1) long-term antiarrhythmic therapy, (2) forced modification of work status, and (3) more advanced cardiac impairment. In a study addressing long-term recovery in sudden death survivors, Sauve[74] found that psychological distress was related to younger age (< 52 years), symptomatology, and the severity of underlying disease.

The commonalities evident in these results, as well as data derived from interviews and group counseling of patients with ventricular tachyarrhythmias, provide the empirical basis for proposing a theoretical explanation of the psychological distress syndrome evident in this patient population.[74, 81] Two potential constructs emanate from these data: power-lessness and vulnerability. Powerlessness stems from the real or perceived losses (i.e., previous work status, role status, physical or social independence, short-term memory) experienced by these patients and their lack of control over their illness, its treatment, and its effect on their life styles. For example, one SCD survivor described his return to work and subsequent status changes thus:

> It was just hard to do things. . . . I can't visualize things sometimes the same way. . . . They tried to demote me. Well, effectively they did. I lost a lot of self-confidence.

The vulnerability experienced by these patients stems from the threat of recurrent dysrhythmia and premature death. As one young patient put it:

> I felt kind of protected in the hospital. After, when I'd be walking down the street by myself, I would just have moments . . . I'd get frightened. I could pass out right here, there'd be nobody here, I'd die right here on the spot.

For some patients, vulnerability is alleviated either by their treatment (coronary bypass, aneurysmectomy), which they consider curative, or by their ability to attribute their dysrhythmia to a specific correctable cause, such as electrolyte imbalance. In other patients vulnerability tends to wax and wane with time from the event, the effectiveness of their medical regimen, the nature and extent of their support systems, and their cognitive status alter cardiac arrest.

SITUATIONAL STRESSORS

The wide variations in clinically occurring dysrhythmias and their impact on left ventricular function, blood pressure, and cerebral, coronary, and renal perfusion, as well as patient and family responses to their occurrence, pose both a diagnostic and therapeutic challenge to physicians and nurse clinicians. The situational stressors associated with the development of serious cardiac dysrhythmias include those clinical or disease states that cause or foster changes in the electrophysiological properties of cardiac cells (e.g., ischemia, potassium imbalances) or changes in the cardiac musculature (e.g., hypertrophy, myocardial fibrosis) (Table 3–3).

Changes in Cellular Electrophysiology

The situational stressors associated with changes in the electrophysiology of cardiac cells can be divided into three main categories: ischemic heart disease, long QT syndromes, and psychosocial factors.

Ischemic Heart Disease

This is responsible for the vast majority of clinically serious dysrhythmias because of its adverse effects on cellular membrane potentials. These changes are due to a number of factors, including, but not limited to, alterations in membrane permeabilities, intracellular and extracellular ion concentrations, and disparate beta-adrenergic stimulation.[1, 3, 5, 82] The most common cause of cardiac ischemia is coronary artery disease, a disease affecting over 1 million people in the United States annually.[83] Other causes of cardiac ischemia include coronary artery spasm, congestive heart failure, atrial and ventricular hypertrophy, inflammatory processes such as myocarditis, and congenital abnormalities of the coronary circulation.[84–86]

Bigger and associates[1] note that during acute myocardial ischemia, the incidence of premature ventricular contractions ranges from 34 to 100 per cent, ventricular tachycardia from 6 to 40 per cent, and ventricular fibrillation from 1 to 11 per cent. Other arrhythmias that may complicate acute ischemic events include atrial fibrillation (7 to 29.5 per cent); supraventricular tachycardias, either atrial or junctional (1 to 27 per cent); and second and third degree heart block (2 to 10 per cent and 1.5 to 8 per cent, respectively).

After myocardial infarction, persistent ventricular ectopy, whether frequent or high grade (e.g., couplets, triplets, or salvos of ventricular tachycardia), has been shown to be a major predictor of ventricular fibrillation or sudden cardiac death independent of age, left ventricular function, or number of previous myocardial infarctions.[62, 86, 87] However, the risk of sudden cardiac death increases proportionally (up to 50 per cent in a 2-year period) when high grades of ventricular ectopy occur in association with congestive heart failure.[57] These risk factors are also applicable to those patients having dilated or congestive cardiomyopathies, hypertrophic

TABLE 3–3. SITUATIONAL STRESSORS ASSOCIATED WITH DYSRHYTHMIAS: MEDICAL DIAGNOSES AND CLINICAL STATES

I. Changes in cellular electrophysiology
  A. Myocardial ischemia
    1. Coronary artery disease
      a. Coronary artery spasm
      b. Angina pectoris
      c. Myocardial infarction
      d. Coronary thrombosis/embolism
      e. Arteritis
    2. High- or low-output heart failure
      a. Valvular heart disease
      b. Severe anemias
      c. Hemorrhagic shock
      d. Idiopathic/acquired cardiomyopathies
      e. Thyrotoxicosis
      f. Pregnancy
      g. Arteriovenous shunts
    3. Congenital abnormalities
      a. Ventricular muscle bridges
      b. Accessory bypass tracts
  B. Long QT syndromes (LQTS)
    1. Inherited
      a. Jervell and Lange-Nielsen syndrome
      b. Romano-Ward syndrome
    2. Acquired
      a. Drug induced
        (1) Antiarrhythmic drugs
        (2) Thiazide diuretics
        (3) Tricyclic antidepressants
      b. Electrolyte imbalances
        (1) Hypokalemia
        (2) Hypomagnesemia
        (3) Hypocalcemia
      c. Central nervous system dysfunctions
        (1) Subarachnoid hemorrhage
        (2) Acute traumas
      d. Severe bradyarrhythmias
      e. Mitral valve prolapse
  C. Psychosocial factors
    1. Socioenvironmental factors
      a. Life changes
      b. Social supports
      c. Educational level
      d. Socioeconomic status
      e. Physical restraint
      f. Human touch
      g. Hospital rounds
    2. Behavioral traits/coping strategies
      a. Type A coronary-prone behavior
      b. Smoking
      c. Alcohol or drug abuse
      d. Psychiatric drug side effects
      e. Manic and catatonic states
      f. REM sleep and arousal from sleep
      g. Denial/hypervigilance
    3. Emotional and cognitive states
      a. Grief and bereavement
      b. Anger/hostility
      c. Depression/anxiety
      d. Hopelessness/helplessness
II. Changes in cardiac musculature
  A. Decreased cardiac contractile units
    1. Intrinsic myocardial disease
      a. Coronary artery disease
      b. Myocarditis (viral, bacterial, mycotic)
      c. Endocarditis (viral, bacterial, mycotic)
      d. Myocardial tumors
      e. Carcinoid syndrome
    2. Primary cardiomyopathies
      a. Idiopathic
      b. Alcoholic
      c. Postpartum
    3. Secondary cardiomyopathies
      a. Infiltrative diseases
        (1) Lupus erythematosus
        (2) Sarcoidosis
        (3) Scleroderma
      b. Neuromuscular
        (1) Muscular dystrophy
        (2) Friedreich's ataxia
      c. Drug induced
        (1) Cocaine
        (2) Doxorubicin
        (3) Amphetamines
  B. Increased cardiac workload
    1. Resistance to ventricular filling/emptying
      a. Hypertension
      b. Aortic or pulmonary stenosis
      c. Hypertrophic cardiomyopathy
      d. Acute pericarditis
      e. Chronic pericardial effusion
      f. Chronic pericarditis
    2. Increased stroke volume
      a. Valvular insufficiencies
      b. Congenital right-to-left shunts
    3. Progressive hypertrophy and dilation
      a. Chronic congestive cardiomyopathy
      b. Hypertensive cardiomyopathy

cardiomyopathies, aortic or mitral value disease in association with heart failure, and ventricular ectopy.

Long QT Syndromes (LQTS)

These refer to a group of both congenital and acquired conditions that are characterized by prolongation of the QT interval and recurrent attacks of syncope and sudden death.[46, 47] The mechanism of syncope is a form of ventricular tachycardia known as torsades de pointes, or twisting of the points; that is, the apices of the QRS complexes are sometimes positive and sometimes negative.[88, 89] The rhythm is rapid and irregular with rates ranging from 160 to 280 bpm. At times the rhythm may alternate with monomorphic ventricular tachycardia or may not assume the classic features of torsades and

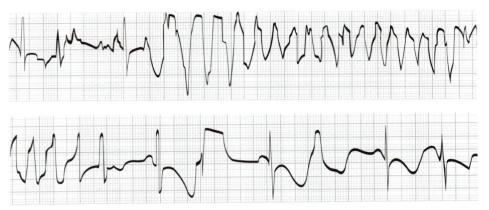

Figure 3–9. Patient 17. Electrocardiographic tracings are not continuous. *Upper tracing,* Initiation of torsades de pointes. Premature ventricular beat (2nd complex) is followed by a compensatory pause that is ended by a supraventricular beat, forming the "long" cycle length of the initiating sequence. A premature ventricular beat (4th complex) initiates torsade de pointes, forming the "short" cycle length of the initiating sequence. *Lower tracing,* Termination of a 70-second episode of torsades de pointes with progressive shortening of the QT interval and evolution of T wave changes. (From Kay, G.N., Plumb, V.J. Archiniegas, J.G., Henthorn, R.W., & Waldo, A.L. [1983]. Torsade de pointes: The long-short initiating sequence and other clinical features: Observations in 32 patients. J Am Coll Cardiol 2:813. Reprinted with permission from the American College of Cardiology.)

simply present itself as polymorphic ventricular tachycardia[46], but if it occurs in relationship with QT prolongation, it is still classified as torsades de pointes.

Congenital LQTS is an uncommon syndrome that may be inherited with or without deafness. Typically, symptoms occur in early childhood or adulthood and are characterized by attacks of presyncope and syncope precipitated by a sudden increased sympathetic tone (physical exercise, emotional arousal, or a startling noise). The risk for sudden death appears to be greater for those patients who have congenital deafness, a history of syncope, or documented ventricular tachyarrhythmias. The pathogenesis of congenital LQTS is not well understood but appears to be related to an imbalance in sympathetic innervation of the heart, with dominance of left-sided adrenergic activity as the basic defect.[47, 90]

By far the most common type of LQTS is the acquired form (Table 3–3). Antiarrhythmic agents, particularly Class 1a agents such as quinidine and disopyramide, have been commonly implicated in the prolongation of QT intervals and the occurrence of torsade.[88] Other antiarrhythmic drugs that have been associated with LQTS include encainide, flecainide, sotalol, amiodarone, and bepridil. Drug-induced torsade de pointes

usually occurs within the first 3 to 4 days of initiating drug therapy, although late onset can occur owing to dosage changes, electrolyte imbalances, or onset of bradycardia.[46] Typically, the dysrhythmia is initiated by a long-short coupling sequence (Fig. 3–9); that is, there is a pause following a late-cycle premature ventricular contraction (PVC) (the long phase), which is followed by a sinus beat whose T wave exhibits changes in shape and amplitude and whose summit is interrupted by another PVC (the short phase).[91] While controversy still exists regarding the mechanisms underlying the initiation of torsade de pointes rhythm, it is currently believed that an afterdepolarization enhanced in size by adrenergic stimuli is the basis of this dysrhythmia.[92]

Other clinical states associated with long QT and torsades-type dysrhythmias include electrolyte imbalances, particularly hypokalemia; central nervous system disorders such as subarachnoid hemorrhage; psychotrophic drug toxicity; and severe bradyarrhythmias.[46] Prolongation of the QT interval may also occur in structural heart diseases such as ischemic heart disease, but the interval change is usually due to prolongation of the QRS segment rather than a repolarization abnormality. One exception to this is mitral valve prolapse (MVP). MVP is characterized by a myxomatous degeneration of the valve (chiefly the posterior leaflet), causing it to balloon into the left atrium during systole.[93] It is a common clinical syndrome affecting 5 to 15 per cent of the general population.[94, 95] While the majority of patients with mitral value prolapse are asymptomatic, Holter monitoring studies of unselected patients with MVP have shown that ventricular arrhythmias are common.[97] However, only a small subset of these patients develops symptomatic ventricular tachycardia and sudden cardiac death.[97] High-risk patients are more likely to have mitral regurgitation,[98] prolonged QT intervals,[99] and repolarization changes on their resting electrocardiogram.[100]

Psychosocial Factors

Personality traits, defense mechanisms, emotional and cognitive states, and environmental factors such as driving and life changes have been related to the occurrence of simple dysrhythmias (atrial and ventricular extrasystoles) as well as to sudden cardiac death. Lown[10] has long espoused the position that in the presence of myocardial electrical instability (i.e., membrane potential changes due to ischemia), certain psychological and behavioral aspects may operate as acute triggers for ventricular dysrhythmias and fibrillation in predisposed individuals. The reader is referred to Binik[101] and Lynch and colleagues,[102] who have written excellent reviews and critiques of the current research related to psychosocial predictors of cardiac arrhythmias and sudden cardiac death.

Changes in the Cardiac Musculature

The pathophysiological dysfunctions associated with changes in the cardiac musculature include (1) decreased cardiac contractility due to fewer contractile units, (2) increases in cardiac work load, (3) progressive ventricular hypertrophy and dilatation, (4) interference with or restriction of ventricular filling and/or emptying, and (5) endocardial thrombus formation.[2, 57, 103] These dysfunctions most often result in low output failure due to poor myocardial contractility and increased ventricular volume and are associated with a variety of clinical dysrhythmias. For example, heart failure associated with

the large floppy heart characterizing idiopathic dilated cardiomyopathy as well as that associated with the small stiff heart found with hypertrophic cardiomyopathy is often accompanied by malignant ventricular arrhythmias.[104, 105] Atrial arrhythmias, particularly atrial fibrillation, commonly occur with mitral valve stenosis and can precipitate heart failure in these patients owing to the loss of atrial kick,[2] while aortic stenosis is more likely to cause a syncopal attack due to a ventricular tachyarrhythmia.[57]

Congenital anomalies such as muscle bridges may elicit malignant ventricular arrhythmias because they interfere with coronary blood flow during systole.[106] Accessory bypass tracts are generally associated with rapid supraventricular tachycardias, which are well tolerated.[7, 8] However, some patients with the Wolff-Parkinson-White syndrome are at risk for sudden cardiac death, most commonly from atrial fibrillation with a fast ventricular response that degenerates into ventricular fibrillation.[7, 107, 108]

Lastly, focal or diffuse fibrosis of the myocardium (scleroderma, sarcoidosis, aneurysm) or injury to the myocardial cells or vasculature due to connective tissue disorders such as lupus erythematosus results in various conduction system abnormalities as well as atrial and ventricular dysrhythmias.[2, 9]

MANIFESTATIONS OF CARDIAC DYSRHYTHMIAS

Subjective Manifestations

Palpitations, defined as a sudden or unpleasant awareness of the heart beat, are the most common manifestations of cardiac dysrhythmias. While this symptom is somewhat nonspecific because it can result from normal changes in heart rate, rhythm, or contractility, it is nevertheless the most frequent reason for initiating 24-hour ambulatory electrocardiographic (ECG) recordings through Holter monitoring.[109] When patients describe palpitations as "flip flops" or "skipped beats" or pauses followed by a "thud," extrasystoles are the most likely cause. When the rhythm is described as racing or a rapid regular heart beat that begins and stops suddenly, a ventricular, atrial, or junctional paroxysmal tachycardia may be the cause. Similarly, when the palpitation is described as a rapid irregular heart beat with an abrupt onset and termination, an atrial tachycardia or flutter with variable AV block or atrial fibrillation should be considered.[6] Factors that may be associated with the occurrence of palpitations should be investigated. These include dietary factors such as caffeinated beverages, foods containing tyramine (e.g., cheese), prescription and nonprescription drugs, and potassium-wasting reducing diets. Other factors, such as fatigue, smoking, exercise, and anxiety, can initiate a variety of benign dysrhythmias in the normal heart and life-threatening dysrhythmias in the heart already compromised by underlying coronary artery disease.[2, 9]

Slow heart rates or bradyarrhythmias may cause symptoms of fatigue, dyspnea, lethargy, and occasionally chest pain.[6] These symptoms are most often due to low cardiac output states, although symptomatology is highly dependent upon age, the mechanism underlying the bradycardia, and any concomitant cardiac, cerebral, or peripheral vascular disease. For example, compromised or diminished cerebral blood flow may cause additional symptoms of dizziness, syncope, or convulsions. Precipitous drops in heart rate (< 40 bpm) caused by transient parasympathetic discharges may also produce symptoms of presyncope and syncope.[6, 110]

Weber and colleagues[109] reported that 25 to 33 per cent of patients undergoing a 24-hour ambulatory ECG recording are suffering from symptoms of dizziness, presyncope, and syncope. In 22 to 46 per cent of these patients symptoms can be related to supraventricular tachycardias, bradyarrhythmias, or ventricular ectopy. The potential causes of these neurological symptoms may range from relatively benign vasovagal syncope to serious cardiac arrhythmias that may be prodromal of sudden cardiac death.[110] Hence, the definitive diagnosis of cardiac dysrhythmias as the cause of recurrent and unexplained syncope is essential. Since prolonged periods of ambulatory monitoring are impractical, invasive cardiac electrophysiology studies are increasingly used in this patient population to determine the presence or absence of life-threatening dysrhythmias.[111–113]

Anginal symptoms may also accompany the occurrence of cardiac dysrhythmias. In the 10 to 20 per cent of patients who complain of chest pain prior to or during ambulatory ECG, one fifth to one third of the attacks can be attributed to the occurrence of arrhythmias, while approximately one half to two thirds can be attributed to ischemia.[109] However, the majority of ischemic events recorded on Holter monitors are asymptomatic or silent.[114, 115]

Objective Manifestations

In symptomatic patients (those with palpitations, presyncope, or syncope), particularly those in whom no specific dysrhythmia has been documented, a thorough attempt should be made to identify noncardiac as well as cardiac causes of the symptomatology. Detailed physical examinations should be initiated that include an assessment of carotid hypersensitivity and postural changes in heart rate and blood pressure; laboratory analyses for electrolytes, calcium, magnesium, blood glucose, and thyroid levels; and electroencephalography for those patients with unexplained syncope.[110]

Noninvasive cardiac measures include the 12-lead ECG, ambulatory ECG, exercise stress tests, and signal-averaging techniques. While the rate and regularity of the apical and peripheral pulse can indicate the presence of a cardiac dysrhythmia, a 12-lead ECG graphically portrays many common rhythm disturbances. By a general inspection of any given ECG tracing, it can be determined whether the basic rhythm is a normal sinus rhythm or an ectopic rhythm (Table 3–1). The most common and simple dysrhythmias occur during sinus rhythm, that is, premature extrasystoles. Atrial fibrillation is the second most common rhythm disturbance followed by a less common atrial flutter.[9] Following the inspection of the ECG for rhythm, a more detailed analysis of the components of the ECG complexes is carried out (e.g., PR, QRS, QT intervals, AV synchrony). These analyses can reveal sinus pauses, various levels of AV heart block or conduction abnormalities, prolonged QT syndrome, pacemaker malfunction, and pre-excitation patterns as well as depolarization and repolarization abnormalities associated with electrolyte abnormalities and drug toxicities.[9, 116]

Continuous ambulatory ECG monitoring, including patient-activated event recorders and transtelephonic signal transmission can substantially add to the data yielded by a 12-lead ECG. A wide variety of dysrhythmias, including various tachyarrhythmias, sick sinus syndrome, intermittent high-grade AV block, alternating bilateral bundle branch block, and rate-dependent ectopies, that rarely are captured on a standard resting ECG can be detected during continuous ambulatory monitoring. Currently, ambulatory monitoring can be accomplished by two entirely different systems: conventional or Holter type systems that record each ECG complex on magnetic tape over a 24-hour period or by newer digital or "real time" recorders that encode and store data in solid state memory.[57, 115, 117] Intermittent or event recorders differ from continuous recorders in that they are capable of recording only a limited number of short data segments. These patient-activated recorders are designed to capture critical cardiac electrical events at the onset of symptoms. Some continuous and intermittent recorders are also capable of transtelephonic transmission of ECG signals directly to a centralized analysis facility. The advantage of transtelephonic systems as well as some digital systems is that they allow for immediate intervention in potentially critical situations.[118]

Clinically, ambulatory monitoring techniques are used to (1) evaluate symptoms (palpitations, dizziness, syncope, chest pain), (2) quantify known or potential dysrhythmias (atrial, ventricular arrhythmias, AV conduction defects), (3) assess the efficacy of antiarrhythmic drugs and devices such as pacemakers and implanted defibrillators, (4) evaluate ECG changes during normal occupational and recreational activities following myocardial infarction or coronary artery bypass surgery, and (5) detect silent ischemia or arrhythmias.[119]

In addition to ambulatory ECGs, another common procedure for assessing ischemic responses, arrhythmias, and cardiac performance is the *exercise stress test*.[120] In the United States, the treadmill is the preferred approach to exercise testing, and the most popular treadmill protocols are the Bruce and Naughton protocols. Each uses continuous progressive stages and differs from each other in only the rate and severity of progression at each stage. The Bruce protocol has also been modified, meaning that it has one or two very easy stages added at the beginning to give the patient a chance to warm up.[121] Whichever protocol is used, the object of the graded format is to standardize the load on the coronary circulation and to

reach an end point of 85 per cent of the age-predicted maximal heart rate.

Exercise treadmill testing (ETT) may induce virtually any disturbance in impulse formation or conduction. It can enhance or depress AV nodal and intraventricular conduction, enhance automaticity in latent automatic fibers, promote the occurrence of afterdepolarizations and arrhythmias caused by triggered activity, and facilitate the development of re-entrant dysrhythmias because of changes in depolarization, repolarization, and conduction in regional areas of ischemia.[122] However, clinically, the value of arrhythmia detection during ETT is not as important as unmasking exercise-induced myocardial ischemia. For example, frequent and high grades of ventricular ectopy in individuals who have negative ETT is generally a benign finding, but the same dysrhythmia in an individual with a positive ETT puts the individual at greater risk for subsequent cardiac events, that is myocardial infarction, cardiac arrest, and cardiac death.[57, 120, 123] Lastly, ETT may be used to assess the effectiveness of antiarrhythmic therapy, particularly in those patients with exercise-induced ventricular tachycardia.[122, 124–126]

Increasingly, *signal-averaged ECG techniques* have been employed to identify those patients following myocardial infarction or with chronic coronary artery disease and a history of complex ventricular ectopy who are at risk for sustained ventricular tachyarrhythmias or sudden cardiac death or both.[127–129] The signal-averaged ECG detects late potentials that are low-amplitude signals found in the terminal portion of the QRS complex and ST segments. These low-amplitude signals have been shown to originate from small areas of myocardium at the periphery of an infarcted area where the mixture of normal myocardial tissue and interstitial fibrosis favor anisotropic conduction and the development of re-entry dysrhythmias.[129, 130] Clinically, the ability of the signal-averaged ECG to identify patients at risk for potentially lethal ventricular arrhythmias allows for the noninvasive assessment of patients with asymptomatic high grades of ventricular ectopy, nonsustained ventricular tachycardia, unexplained syncope, and broad complex tachycardias.[57, 127–129] The presence of late potentials can alert the physician to the need for invasive serial drug testing (electrophysiological studies) in these individuals. Conversely, the absence of late potentials has a high negative predictive accuracy, identifying those patients who are at low risk for life-threatening arrhythmic events.[57, 130]

Basically, signal-averaging techniques reduce the ambient noise present in conventional electrocardiographic recordings so that late potentials, which are very low-frequency signals, can be detected. There are currently two methods for recording late potentials: temporal averaging and spatial averaging (Figs. 3–10 and 3–11).[131, 132] Temporal averaging is the most common clinical method employed because it can be done at the bedside, while spatial-averaging techniques require specialized facilities to shield the patient electrically.[130] The degree of noise reduction

achieved with temporal averaging is proportional to the number of complexes sampled. The lower the initial baseline noise, the fewer beats will be necessary for averaging. Usually 200 to 300 beats are sufficient to allow recording of a signal with baseline noise level of under 0.5 μV. Spatial averaging relies on the summation of potentials simultaneously recorded from 5 to 16 pairs of closely spaced electrodes to reduce ambient noise.[130, 132, 133] The rationale for this approach is based upon the fact that the ECG signal developed between any pair of electrodes is almost identical if the electrodes are closely spaced, whereas the noise caused by the electrode-skin interface, amplifiers, and electromyographic potentials may not be correlated ex-

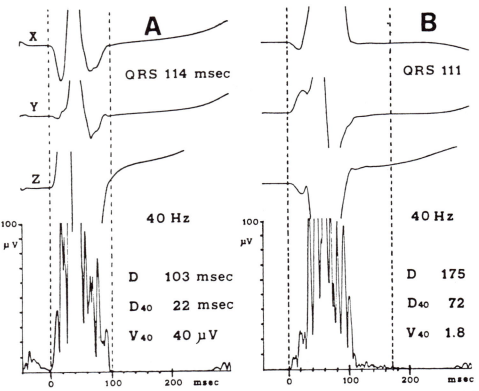

Figure 3–10. Examples of signal-averaged ECGs in two patients with prior myocardial infarction. *A,* Tracing without late potentials. *B,* Tracing with late potentials. Signal-averaged leads X, Y, Z *(top).* Filtered QRS complex *(bottom).* The quantitative analysis of the waveform includes measurement of the amplitude of the signals in the last 40 ms of the filtered QRS (V_{40}), the total duration of the filtered QRS (D), and the duration of the terminal low-amplitude signals (D_{40}). QRS = QRS complex at the standard ECG. Vertical dashed line indicates the end of the filtered QRS complex. (From Verzoni, A., Romano S., Pozzoni, L., Tarricone, D., Sangiogio, S., & Croce, L. [1989]. Prognostic significance and evolution of late ventricular potentials in the first year after myocardial infarction: A prospective study. PACE Pacing Clin Electrophysiol *12*:43, with permission.)

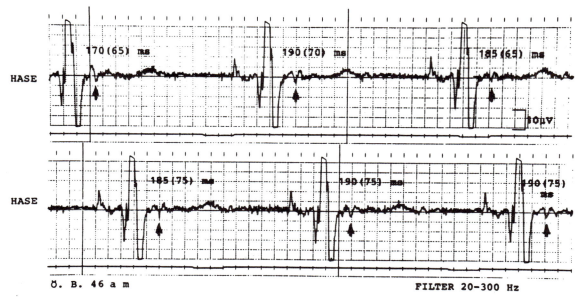

HASE

HASE

Ö. B. 46 a m   FILTER 20-300 Hz

Figure 3–11. Spatial averaging. Note the varied duration of late potentials at the end of the QRS complex. (Reproduced with permission from Int J Cardiol.) (From Kuchar, D.L., & Rosenbaum, D.S. [1989]. Noninvasive record of late potentials: Current state of the art. PACE Pacing Clin Electrophysiol *12*:1545, with permission.)

actly. In practice, however, additional techniques to decrease or to attenuate the fairly coherent electromyographic signals are necessary prior to the averaging process. The advantage of spatial averaging over temporal averaging is that it provides a beat-to-beat real time analysis of low-level signals even when the cardiac rhythm is irregular, interrupted by ectopic rhythms, or changed because of drug therapy or the onset of ischemia.[130, 132]

Lastly, objective evidence of cardiac dysrhythmias can be obtained during intracardiac electrophysiological studies (EPS). Generally carried out in a catheterization laboratory (although with portable equipment they can be performed at the bedside), EPS consist of pacing and programmed stimulation as well as intracardiac electrographic recordings from multiple sites in the heart. An electrophysiological study is indicated in those individuals who have symptomatic, recurrent, or drug-resistant supraventricular or ventricular tachyarrhythmias, especially if the tachydysrhythmia is hemodynamically compromising; in those individuals whose tachydysrhythmia occurs so infrequently that noninvasive measures are not diagnostically helpful; in those individuals with unexplained syncope; in those individuals in

whom nonpharmocological therapy such as surgery, ablation, or automatic internal cardiodefibrillator (AICD) implantation is contemplated; and lastly in those individuals in whom supraventricular tachycardia and aberrant conduction must be differentiated from ventricular tachycardia.[134]

Diagnostically, EPS are used to confirm the presence and nature of a particular dysrhythmia and to characterize, when possible, their electrophysiological mechanism. For example, the two most common forms of symptomatic PSVT in adults are re-entry arrhythmias: AV nodal re-entry tachycardia due to dual AV nodes and orthodromic tachycardia resulting from a concealed AV nodal bypass tract that only conducts retrogradely (Kent bundles).[7, 135] The tachydysrhythmia associated with AV nodal re-entry can be reproducibly initiated during EPS with the introduction of one or more programmed atrial extrastimuli during atrial pacing. The atrial premature stimuli are blocked in the fast pathway because these tissues have long refractory periods and cause conduction delays in the slow pathway, thus setting up the appropriate conditions for the initiation of the re-entry loop (Fig. 3–12). Orthodromic tachycardias can also be initiated in this manner, or they can be initiated by a pro-

TYPICAL FORM

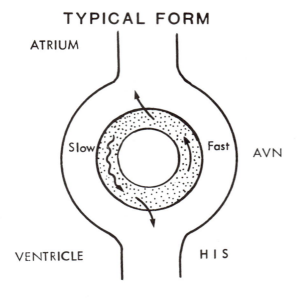

Figure 3–12. Typical form of atrioventricular nodal re-entrant tachycardia. The re-entry circuit is confined to the atrioventricular node (AVN); the slow pathway serves as the antegrade limb of the circuit and the fast pathway as the retrograde limb. Since the ventricles are depolarized via the His-Purkinje axis, the QRS complex (ECG) is narrow unless there is abnormal intraventricular conduction. Atrial and ventricular depolarizations usually occur simultaneously, thus the P waves are buried within the QRS complex and are not apparent. (From Morady, F., & Scheinmann, M.M. [1982]. Paroxysmal supraventricular tachycardia: Part 1. Diagnosis. Mod Con Cardiovasc Dis *51*:108, with permission. Copyright 1982, American Heart Association.)

grammed ventricular extrastimuli or ventricular premature depolarization (Fig. 3–13). SVTs resulting from automatic or triggered mechanisms are more difficult to elucidate during EPS. Some atrial tachydysrhythmias resulting from an automatic focus can be characterized by a gradual increase in rate (warm up phenomena) and slowing before termination, some may exhibit overdrive suppression with atrial pacing, while others cannot be reproducibly initiated or terminated with atrial extrastimuli.[19] Some investigators believe that triggered atrial tachycardias have several distinguishing characteristics, including a critical range of pacing rates and

a direct relationship between the prematurity of the initiating complex and the coupling interval of the tachydysrhythmia.[25] As with SVTs, the majority of ventricular tachydysrhythmias reproduced during EPS are reentrant arrhythmias, and only a minority can be attributed to either automatic foci or triggered mechanisms.

Therapeutically, EPS are used to assess the efficacy of antiarrhythmic drugs and surgical or ablation therapies; to gauge the risk of future arrhythmic occurrences, including sudden cardiac death; and to terminate specific dysrhythmias (Table 3–4).[135] The bedside variants of intracardiac EPS, such as, the esophageal or atrial wire electrogram (AEG) as well as the ventricular electrogram (VEG),

ATRIOVENTRICULAR BYPASS TRACT
ORTHODROMIC TACHYCARDIA

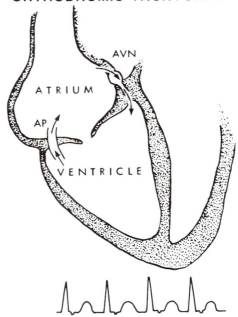

Figure 3–13. Orthodromic reciprocating tachycardia involving an atrioventricular accessory bypass tract (AP). The re-entry circuit consists of atrioventricular node (AVN), atrium, AP, and ventricle. Antegrade conduction through the AVN results in a normal pattern of ventricular depolarization; rapid retrograde conduction through the AP results in an atrial depolarization that occurs just after ventricular depolarization. The electrocardiogram (ECG) thus shows a narrow QRS complex followed closely by a P wave. (From Morady, F., & Scheinmann, M.M. [1982]. Paroxysmal supraventricular tachycardia: Part 1. Diagnosis. Mod Con Cardiovasc Dis *51*:109, with permission. Copyright 1982, American Heart Association.)

TABLE 3–4. INDICATIONS FOR INVASIVE ELECTROPHYSIOLOGICAL STUDIES

I. Diagnosis and mechanisms of dysrhythmias
  A. Sick sinus syndrome
  B. Conduction system disease
    1. Atrioventricular (AV) nodal blocks
    2. Intra-His blocks
    3. Bundle branch blocks
  C. Supraventricular tachycardias
    1. AV nodal re-entrant
      a. Typical
      b. Atypical
    2. Orthodromic
    3. Antidromic
    4. Nodoventricular (Mahaim)
    5. Intra-atrial re-entrant
    6. Automatic atrial
  D. Ventricular tachyarrhythmias
    1. Nonsustained
    2. Sustained monomorphic
    3. Ventricular flutter
    4. Ventricular fibrillation
II. Arrhythmia mapping
  A. Arrhythmic surgery (bypass tract, foci)
  B. Ablation of arrhythmic foci
III. Therapy application
  A. Termination of tachydysrhythmias
  B. Ablation therapy
    1. Catheter
    2. Radio frequency
    3. Alcohol
    4. Laser
IV. Evaluation of antiarrhythmic therapies
  A. Antiarrhythmic drugs
  B. Antitachycardia pacemakers
  C. Antiarrhythmic cardiac surgeries
    1. Coronary artery bypass graft
    2. Aneurysmectomy
    3. Excision of bypass tracts
  D. Automatic internal cardioverter defibrillators

may also be used to diagnose specific dysrhythmias or to define the mechanism underlying the dysrhythmia. For example, these electrograms can be used to differentiate an SVT with aberrancy from ventricular tachycardia or, by clarifying atrial depolarization patterns, to identify whether a narrow complex tachydysrhythmia is due to atrial flutter, AV nodal re-entry, or a concealed bypass tract.[134, 136–138] In addition, both atrial and ventricular pacing can be accomplished with these catheter electrodes so that specific dysrhythmias can be controlled or terminated.

SUGGESTED ACTIVITIES FOR PRACTICE AND RESEARCH

Research activities and the clinical care of cardiac dysrhythmia patients have been pri-marily directed toward identifying arrhythmogenic mechanisms, developing diagnostic methods and therapeutic interventions to prevent future occurrences, and evaluating medical therapies through the analysis of morbidity and mortality data. However, much remains to be learned about both the physiological and psychological factors favoring the development of dysrhythmias, the impact of life-threatening arrhythmias on the long-term psychosocial and occupational adaptation of these patients and their families, and, lastly, what nursing assessment and intervention strategies need to be developed or modified to facilitate positive patient outcomes.

More specific questions regarding the physiological factors favoring the development of dysrhythmias might center around the relationship of sleep and sleep disturbances to the occurrence of cardiac arrhythmias. For example, is there a difference in sleep patterns between patients with coronary and noncoronary artery disease? Do the sleep disruptions that occur in critical care units alter the frequency of arrhythmias? What are the effects of cardiac drugs on sleep patterns? Questions regarding the psychological factors favoring arrhythmias might address areas such as the interaction of specific emotions like depression, the type of underlying heart disease, and the arrhythmia occurrence. Additional questions might be generated about the interactions of emotional state and deleterious coping strategies such as smoking and arrhythmia frequency and complexity.

While there are some initial studies in the literature that address the psychological and occupational outcomes of survivors of sudden cardiac events, none has addressed outcomes in other life-threatening arrhythmia groups, such as patients with recurrent Wolff-Parkinson-White syndrome that degenerates into atrial fibrillation. How do factors such as age, arrhythmia recurrence, and type of therapy affect long-term outcomes? What factors increase or decrease the patient's sense of vulnerability or perceived control over the dysrhythmia? How do cognitive deficits that may be incurred following delayed or less effective cardiopulmonary resuscitation affect long-term outcomes and family dynamics? Do devices such as the Automatic Internal Cardiac Defibrillator (AICD) affect the patient's perception of quality of life? What is the relationship among extent and type of heart disease, symptomatology, psychological status, and recurrent episodes of sudden cardiac death?

Modification of current nursing assessment strategies might include assessing all patients admitted for cardiac arrhythmias for cognitive status. For example, do patients with congestive heart failure and nonsustained ventricular tachycardia have similar changes in cognition due to transient hypoxia as patients who have been resuscitated? Do patients with recurrent syncope due to either severe bradyarrhythmias or tachyarrhythmias incur temporary or permanent cognitive losses? If so, what kind of modifications in patient teaching strategies need to be considered? In the acute setting or in the telemetry unit, which ECG lead system best facilitates the bedside diagnosis of ventricular versus supraventricular tachycardia? Does heart rate variability or lack thereof predict arrhythmia occurrence in patients admitted for acute myocardial infarction, sustained ventricular tachycardia, or ventricular fibrillation? What is the effect of multiple electrophysiological studies or the use of experimental antiarrhythmic drugs and devices on the patient's perception of health and well-being? To what extent does establishing long-term therapeutic relationships with patients enhance compliance with drug regimens, recommended life style changes, and perceived control over arrhythmia recurrence?

In summary, research as well as research-based clinical nursing practice for patients with cardiac arrhythmias in both the acute care and community setting is only in its beginning stages. Relationships among factors need to be clarified and their direction documented for various dysrhythmia groups, and both nursing assessment and intervention strategies need to be documented and evaluated for their effects on short- and long-term patient and family outcomes.

REFERENCES

1. Bigger, J.T., Presdale, R.J., Heissenbuttel, R.M., Weld, F.M., & Wit, A.L. (1977). Ventricular arrhythmias in ischemic heart disease: Mechanism, prevalence, significance and management. Prog Cardiovasc Dis *19*:255–293.
2. Sokolow, M., & McIlroy, M.B. (1990). Cardiac arrhythmias. In *Clinical Cardiology* (pp. 471–517). Palo Alto: Lange Medical Publications.
3. Verrier, R.L., & Hagestad, E.L. (1985). Role of the autonomic nervous system in sudden death. Cardiovasc Clin *15*:41–63.
4. Fisch, C. (1973). Relation of electrolyte disturbances to cardiac arrhythmias. Circulation *47*:408–419.
5. Arnsdorf, M.F. (1977). Membrane factors in arrhythmogenesis: Concepts and definitions. Prog Cardiovasc Dis *19*:413–429.
6. Platia, E.V. (1987). Approach to the diagnosis of a cardiac arrhythmia. In E.V. Platia (ed.), *Management of Cardiac Arrhythmia: The Nonpharmacologic Approach* (pp. 3–8). Philadelphia: J.B. Lippincott.
7. Morady, F., & Scheinman, M.M. (1982). Paroxysmal supraventricular tachycardia: Part I. Diagnosis. Mod Con Cardiovasc Dis *51*:107–112.
8. Gaston, A., Jr. (1990). Abnormalities of cardiac rate and rhythm. In F.A. Oski, C.D. De Angelis, R.D. Feigin, & J.B. Warshaw (eds.), *Principles and Practice of Pediatrics* (pp. 1501–1505). Philadelphia: J.B. Lippincott.
9. Chung, E.K. (1989). Introduction. In *Principles of Cardiac Arrhythmia* (4th ed., pp. 1–13). Baltimore: Williams & Wilkins.
10. Lown, B. (1979). Sudden cardiac death—1978. Circulation *60*:1593–1599.
11. Peters, R.W., Scheinman, M.M., Modin, G., O'Young, J., Somelofski, C.A., & Mies, C. (1979). Prophylactic permanent pacemakers for patients with chronic bundle branch block. Am J Med *66*:978–985.
12. Hauswirth, O., & Singh, B.N. (1979). Ionic mechanisms in heart muscle in relation to the genesis and pharmacological control of cardiac arrhythmias. Pharm Review *30*:5–63.
13. Singer, D.H., Baumgarten, C.M., & Ten Eick, R.E. (1981). Cellular electrophysiology of ventricular and other dysrhythmias: Studies of diseased and ischemic heart. In E.H. Sonneblock & M. Lesch (eds.), *Sudden Cardiac Death* (pp. 13–72). New York: Grune & Stratton.
14. Fozzard, H.A. (1977). Cardiac muscle: Excitability and passive electrical properties. Prog Cardiovasc Dis *19*:343–359.
15. Zipes, D.P., Besch, H.R., & Watanabe, A.M. (1975). Role of the slow current in cardiac electrophysiology. Circulation *51*:761–766.
16. Josephson, M.E., & Seides, S.F. (1979). *Clinical Cardiac Electrophysiology*. Philadelphia: Lea & Febiger.
17. Singh, B.H., Ikeda, N., Nodemanee, K., & Hauswirth, D. (1984). Cellular electrophysiology of the heart: Basis for elucidating the origin of cardiac arrhythmias and the action of antiarrhythmic agents. In S. Levy & M.M. Scheinman (eds.), *Cardiac Arrhythmias: From Diagnosis to Therapy* (pp. 1–36). Mount Kisco, NY: Futura Publishing Co.
18. Wallace, A.G. (1990). Electrical activity of the heart. In J.W. Hurst (ed.), *The Heart* (5th ed., pp. 473–561). New York: McGraw-Hill.
19. Wit, A.L., & Rosen, M.R. (1981). Cellular electrophysiology of cardiac arrhythmias: Part 1. Arrhythmias caused by abnormal impulse generation. Mod Concepts Cardiovasc Dis *50*:7–12.
20. Cranefield, P.F., Wit, A.T., & Hoffman, B.E. (1973). Genesis of cardiac arrhythmias. Circulation *47*:190–204.
21. Mazzoleni, A. (1973). Electrophysiologic mechanisms of sudden death in patients with coronary artery disease. Heart Lung *2*:841–846.

22. Fisch, C. (1974). Electrophysiologic basis of clinical arrhythmias. Heart Lung *3*:52–56.
23. Temte, J.L. (1975). Precoronary electrophysiology. In B. Lown (ed.), *Clinician: Sudden Death* (pp. 27–35). Chicago: Searle Laboratories.
24. Lazzara, R. (1988). Electrophysiological mechanisms for ventricular arrhythmias. Clin Cardiol *11*:(Suppl.)1–15.
25. Rosen, J.R., & Reder, R.F. (1981). Does triggered activity have a role in the genesis of cardiac arrhythmias? Ann Intern Med *94*:794–801.
26. Wit, A.L., & Friedman, P.L. (1975). Basis for ventricular arrhythmias accompanying myocardial infarction: Alterations in electrical activity of ventricular muscle and Purkinje fibers after coronary artery occlusion. Ann Intern Med *135*:459–472.
27. Gough, W.B., Mehra, R., Restivo, M., Zeiler, R.H., & El Sherif, N. (1985). Re-entrant ventricular arrhythmias in the late myocardial infarction period in the dog. Circ Res *57*:432–442.
28. Cranefield, P.F. (1981). Action potentials, afterpotentials, and arrhythmias. Circ Res *41*:415–423.
29. Kass, R.S., Lederer, W.M., & Tsien, R.W. (1978). Role of calcium ions in transient inward currents and after contractions induced by strophanthidin in cardiac Purkinje fibers. J Physiol *281*:187–208.
30. Tsien, R.W., Kass, R.S., & Weingart, R. (1979). Cellular and subcellular mechanisms of cardiac pacemaker oscillations. J Exp Biol *81*:205–213.
31. Sung, R.F., Shapiro, W.A., Shen, E.N., Morady, F., & Davis, J. (1983). Effects of verapamil on ventricular tachycardias possibly caused by re-entry, automaticity, and triggered activity. J Clin Invest *72*:350–360.
32. Lin, F.C., Finley, C.D., Rahimtoola, S.H., & Wu, D. (1983). Idiopathic paroxysmal ventricular tachycardia with QRS pattern of right bundle branch block and left axis deviation: A unique clinical entity with specific properties. Am J Cardiol *52*:95–100.
33. Wu, D., Kou, H.C., & Hung, J.S. (1981). Exercise triggered paroxysmal ventricular tachycardia. Ann Intern Med *95*:410–414.
34. El Sherif, N., Goush, W.B., Zeiler, R.H., & Mehra, R. (1983). Triggered ventricular rhythms in 1-day-old myocardial infarction in the dog. Circ Res *52*:566–579.
35. Brachmann, J., Scherlag, B.J., Rosenshtraukh, L.V., & Lazzara, R. (1983). Bradycardia-dependent triggered activity: Relevance to drug-induced multiform ventricular tachycardia. Circulation *68*:846–856.
36. Schecter, E., Freeman, C., & Lazzara, R. (1984). Afterdepolarizations as a mechanism for the long QT syndrome: Electrophysiological studies of a case. J Am Coll Cardiol *3*:1556–1561.
37. Wit, A.L., & Rosen, M.R. (1981). Cellular electrophysiology of cardiac arrhythmias: Part 2. Arrhythmias caused by abnormal impulse conduction. Mod Concepts Cardiovasc Dis *50*:7–11.
38. Wit, A.L., & Rosen, M.R. (1984). Cellular electrophysiology of cardiac arrhythmias. In M.E. Josephson & H.J. Wellens (eds.), *Tachycardias-Mechanisms, Diagnosis, Treatment* (pp. 1–27). Philadelphia: Lea & Febiger.
39. Allessie, M.A., Bonke, F.I.M., & Schopman, F.J.G. (1977). Circus movement in rabbit atrial muscle as a mechanism of tachycardia. III. The "leading circle" concept: A new model of circus movement

in cardiac tissue without the involvement of an anatomical obstacle. Circ Res *41*:9–18.
40. El Sheriff, N., Mehra, R., & Gough, W.S. (1982). Ventricular activation pattern of spontaneous and induced ventricular rhythms in canine one-day-old myocardial infarction. Evidence for focal and re-entrant mechanisms. Circ Res *51*:152–166.
41. Cranefield, P.F., Klein, H.O., & Hoffman, B.F. (1971). Conduction of the cardiac impulse. I. Delay, block, and one-way block in depressed Purkinje fibers. Circ Res *28*:199–219.
42. Cranefield, P.F. (1975). *The Conduction of the Cardiac Impulse: The Slow Response and Cardiac Arrhythmias.* Mount Kisco, NY: Futura Publishing Co.
43. Antzelevitch, C., Jalife, J., & Moe, G.K. (1980). Characteristics of reflection as a mechanism of re-entrant arrhythmias and its relationship to parasystole. Circulation *61*:182–191.
44. Spach, M.S., & Kootsey, J.M. (1983). The nature of electrical propagation in cardiac muscle. Am J Physiol *244*:H3–H22.
45. Marriott, H.J.L. (1988). Incidence of arrhythmias in normal populations. In *Practical Electrocardiology* (8th ed., pp. 106–107). Baltimore: Williams & Wilkins.
46. Bhandari, A.K., & Scheinman, M.M. (1985). The long QT syndrome. Mod Concepts Cardiovasc Dis *54*:45–50.
47. Moss, A.J., Schwartz, P.J., Crampton, R.S., Locati, E., & Carleen, E. (1985). The long QT syndrome: A prospective international study. Circulation *71*:17–25.
48. Engel, G.L. (1978). Psychologic stress, vasodepressor syncope, and sudden death. Ann Intern Med *89*:403–412.
49. Singer, D.H., Martin, G.J., Magid, N., Weiss, J.S., Schaad, J.W., Kehoe, R., Zheutlin, T., Fintel, D.J., Hsieh, A.M., & Lesch, M. (1988). Low heart rate variability and sudden cardiac death. J Electrocardiol *21*:(Suppl.)S46–S55.
50. Marriott, H.J.L. (1988). Supraventricular tachycardias. In *Practical Electrophysiology* (8th ed., pp. 159–181). Baltimore: Williams & Wilkins.
51. Wu, D., Denes, P., Amat-y-Leon, F., Dhingra, R., Wyndham, C.R.C., Bowerfeind, R., Latif, P., & Rosen, K.M. (1978). Clinical, electrocardiographic and electrophysiologic observations in patients with paroxysmal supraventricular tachycardia. Am J Cardiol *41*:1045–1050.
52. Epstein, M., & Benditt, D. (1981). Long-term evaluation of persistent supraventricular tachycardia in children: Clinical and electrocardiographic features. Am Heart J *102*:80–84.
53. Marriott, H.J.L. (1988). Escape and dissociation. In *Practical Electrocardiology* (8th ed., pp. 338–351). Baltimore: Williams & Wilkins.
54. Schubart, A.F. (1958). Isorhythmic dissociation: Atrioventricular dissociation with synchronization. Am J Med *24*:209–215.
55. Kannel, W.B., Doyle, J.T., McNamara, P.M., Quickenton, P., & Gordon, T. (1975). Precursors of sudden coronary death: Factors related to the incidence of sudden death. Circulation *51*:606–613.
56. Weinberg, M. (1978). Sudden cardiac death. Yale J Biol Med. *51*:207–217.
57. Greene, H.L. (1988). Definition of patients at high risk of sudden arrhythmic cardiac death. Clin Cardiol *11*:II5–II16.

58. Nikolic, G., Bishop, R.L., & Singh, J.B. (1982). Sudden death recorded during Holter monitoring. Circulation 66:218–222.

59. Gillum, R.F. (1988). Sudden coronary death in the United States. Circulation 79:756–765.

60. Roelandt, J., & Hugenholtz, P.G. (1986). Sudden death: Prediction and prevention. Eur Heart J 7:(Suppl. A)169–180.

61. Myerburg, R.J., Conde, C.A., Sung, R.J., Mayorge-Cortes, A., Mallon, S.M., Sheps, P.S., Appel, R., & Costellanos, A. (1980). Clinical electrophysiologic and hemodynamic profile of patients resuscitated from prehospital cardiac arrest. Am J Med 68:568–576.

62. Schulze, R.A., Jr., Strauss, H.W., & Pitt, B. (1977). Sudden death in the year following myocardial infarction: Relation to ventricular premature contractions in the late hospital phase and left ventricular ejection fraction. Am J Med 62:192–199.

63. Tresh, D.D., Grove, J.R., Keelan, M.H., Seigal, R., Boncheck, L.I., Olinger, G.N., & Brooks, H.L. (1981). Long-term follow-up of survivors of prehospital sudden coronary death. Circulation 64:(Suppl. II)1–6.

64. Lown, B., Verrier, R.L., & Rabinowitz, S.H. (1977). Neural and psychologic mechanisms and the problem of sudden cardiac death. Am J Cardiol 59:890–902.

65. Corbalan, R., Verrier, R.L., & Lown, B. (1974). Psychological stress and ventricular arrhythmias during myocardial infarction in the conscious dog. Am J Cardiol 34:692–696.

66. Taggert, P., Gibbon, D., & Somerville, W. (1969). Some effects of motor car driving on the normal and abnormal heart. Br Med J 4:130–134.

67. Bellet, S., Roman, L., Kostis, J., & Slater, A. (1968). Continuous electrocardiographic monitoring during automobile driving: Studies in normal subjects and patients with coronary disease. Am J Cardiol 22:856–860.

68. Taggert, P., Carruthers, M., & Somerville, W. (1973). Electrocardiogram, plasma catecholamines and lipids, and their modification by oxprenolol when speaking before an audience. Lancet 2:341–346.

69. Lown, B., & DeSilva, R.A. (1978). Roles of psychologic stress and autonomic nervous system changes in provocation of ventricular premature complexes. Am J Cardiol 41:979–985.

70. Sime, W.E., Buell, J.C., & Eliot, R.S. (1980). Cardiovascular responses to emotional stress (quiz interview) in post-myocardial infarction patients and matched control subjects. J Hum Stress 6:39–46.

71. Tavazzi, L., Zotti, A.M., & Rondanelli, A. (1986). The role of psychologic stress in the genesis of lethal arrhythmias in patients with coronary artery disease. Eur Heart J 7:(Suppl. A)99–106.

72. Brackett, C.D., & Powell, L.H. (1988). Psychosocial and physiological predictors of sudden cardiac death after healing of acute myocardial infarction. Am J Cardiol 61:979–983.

73. Dunnington, C.S., Johnson, N.L., Finkelmeier, B.A., Lyons, J., & Keohoe, R.F. (1988). Patients with heart rhythm disturbances, variables associated with increased psychologic distress. Heart Lung 17:381–389.

74. Sauve, M.J. (1985). Survivors of sudden cardiac death: The medical and psychosocial factors related to self reports of physical status, mental health, and perceived health status. Ph.D. dissertation. Ann Arbor, MI: University Microfilms.

75. Druss, R., & Kornfeld, D. (1967). The survivors of cardiac arrest, a psychiatric study. JAMA 201:75–80.

76. Dlin, B.M., Stern, A., & Poliakoff, S.J. (1974). Survivors of cardiac arrest. Psychosomatics 15:61–67.

77. Dupont, B., Flensted-Jensen, E., & Sandoe, E. (1969). The long-term prognosis for patients resuscitated after cardiac arrest. Am Heart J 78:444–449.

78. Minuck, M., & Perkins, R. (1970). Long-term study of patients successfully resuscitated following cardiac arrest. Anesth Analg 49:115–118.

79. Dobson, M., Tattersfield, A.E., Alder, M.W., & McNicol, M.U. (1971). Attitudes and long-term adjustment of patients surviving cardiac arrest. Br Med J 3:207–212.

80. Haggarty, T.T., Burkett, M.B., & Foster, J.R. (1983). Psychological dysfunction in patients surviving ventricular tachycardia or fibrillator. Circulation (Abstracts) 68:(Suppl. III)108.

81. DeBasio, N., & Rodenhausen, N. (1984). The group experience: Meeting the psychological needs of patients with ventricular tachycardia. Heart Lung 13:597–602.

82. Opie, L.N., Nathan, D., & Lubbe, W.F. (1979). Biochemical aspects of arrhythmogenesis and ventricular fibrillation. Am J Cardiol 43:131–148.

83. Rosenman, R.H., Friedman, M., Straus, R., Wurm, M., Kositchek, R., Hahn, W., & Werthessan, N.T. (1964). A predictive study of coronary heart disease: The western collaborative group study. JAMA 89:103–110.

84. Langberg, J.J., Ports, T., Sauve, M.J., & Scheinman, M.M. (1982). Coronary artery system and aborted sudden death in patients without structural heart disease. (Abstract). Circulation 74:I1–I11.

85. Hinkle, L.E., Jr., & Thaler, H.T. (1982). Clinical classification of cardiac deaths. Circulation 65:457–464.

86. Bigger, J.T., Jr., Fleiss, J.L., Kleiger, R., Miller, J.P., & Rolmtzky, L.M. (1984). The relationship between ventricular arrhythmias, left ventricular function and mortality in the two years after myocardial infarction. Circulation 69:250–258.

87. Pfister, M., Burke, T.F., Follath, F., & Burckhardt, D. (1988). Prospective controlled randomized trial of prophylactic antiarrhythmic therapy in post-myocardial infarction patients with asymptomatic ventricular arrhythmias—study design and initial results. Clin Cardiol 11:II41–II44.

88. Marriott, H.J.L. (1988). Other tachyarrhythmias. In Practical Electrocardiography (8th ed., pp. 227–228). Baltimore: Williams & Wilkins.

89. Horowitz, L.N., Greenspan, A.M., Spielman, S.R., & Josephson, M.E. (1981). Torsades de pointes: Electrophysiologic studies in patients without pharmacologic or metabolic abnormalities. Circulation 63:1120–1128.

90. Moss, A.J., & Schwartz, P.J. (1982). Delayed repolarization (QT or QTU prolongation) and malignant ventricular arrhythmias. Mod Concepts Cardiovasc Dis 51:85–90.

91. Kay, G.N., Plumb, V.S., Arciniegas, J.G., Henthorn, R.W., & Waldo, A.L. (1983). Torsade de pointes: The long short initiating sequence and other clinical features: Observations in 32 patients. J Am Coll Cardiol 2:806–817.

92. Schechter, E., Freeman, C., & Lazzara, R. (1984). After-depolarization as a mechanism for the long QT syndrome: Electrophysiologic studies of a case. J Am Coll Cardiol 3:1556–1561.

93. Davidson, L.J., & Weaver, W.D. (1981). Mitral valve prolapse: Its recognition and nursing implications. Cardiovasc Nurs 15:7–12.

94. Savage, D.D., Levy, D., Garrison, R.J., Castelli, W.P., Kligfield, P., Devereaux, R.B., Anderson, S.J., Kannel, W.B., & Feinleib, M. (1983). Mitral valve prolapse in the general population. 3. Dysrhythmias: The Framingham Study. Am Heart J 160:582–586.

95. Procacci, P.M., Savran, S.V., Schreiter, S.L., & Bryson, A.L. (1976). Prevalence of clinical mitral-valve prolapse in 1169 young women. N Engl J Med 294:1086–1088.

96. Winkle, R.A., Lopes, M.G., Fitzgerald, J.W., Goodman, D.J., Schroeder, J.S., & Harrison, D.C. (1975). Arrhythmias in patients with mitral valve prolapse. Circulation 52:73–81.

97. Kligfield, P., Levy, D., Devereaux, R.B., & Savage, D.D. (1987). Arrhythmias and sudden death in mitral valve prolapse. Am Heart J 113:1298–1307.

98. Kligfield, P., Hochreiter, C., Kramer, H., Devereaux, R.B., Niles, N., Kramer-Fox, R., & Borer, J.S. (1985). Complex arrhythmias in mitral regurgitation with and without mitral valve prolapse: Contrast to arrhythmias in mitral valve prolapse without mitral regurgitation. Am J Cardiol 55:1545–1549.

99. Bekheit, S.G., Ali, A.A., Deslin, S.M., & Jain, W.C. (1982). Analysis of QT interval in patients with idiopathic mitral valve prolapse. Chest 81:620–625.

100. Winkle, R.A., Lopes, M.G., Popp, R.L., & Hancock, E.L. (1976). Life-threatening arrhythmias in the mitral valve prolapse syndrome. Am J Med 60:961–967.

101. Binik, Y.M. (1985). Psychosocial predictors of sudden death: A review and critique. Soc Sci Med 20:667–680.

102. Lynch, J.J., Paskewitz, D.A., Gimbel, K.S., & Thomas, S.A. (1977). Psychological aspects of cardiac arrhythmias. Am Heart J 93:645–657.

103. McKenna, W.J. (1988). Noninvasive assessment and management of the patient at high risk of sudden cardiac death. Clin Cardiol 11:II22–II25.

104. Dargie, H.J., & Cleland, J.G.F. (1988). Arrhythmias in heart failure—the role of amiodarone. Clin Cardiol 11:II26–II30.

105. Francis, G.S. (1986). Development of arrhythmias in the patient with congestive heart failure: Pathophysiology, prevalence and prognosis. Am J Cardiol 57:3B–7B.

106. Eldar, M., Sauve, M.J., & Scheinman, M.M. (1987). Aborted sudden cardiac death: Long term clinical follow-up. J Am Coll Cardiol 10:291–298.

107. Klein, G.J., Bashove, T.M., Seller, T.D., Pritchett, W.M., & Gallagher, J.J. (1979). Ventricular fibrillation in the Wolff-Parkinson-White syndrome. N Engl J Med 301:1080–1085.

108. Sharma, D.D., Yee, R., Guiraudon, G., & Klein, G.J. (1987). Sensitivity of invasive and noninvasive testing for the risk of sudden death in Wolff-Parkinson-White syndrome. J Am Coll Cardiol 10:373–381.

109. Weber, H., Schmidinger, H., Avinger, C.H., Wolfram, J., Rimpfl, T., Norman, G., & Schmid, R. (1989). Holter ECG and the evaluation of patient's symptoms. In V. Hombach, H.H. Hiler, & H.L. Kennedy (eds.), Electrocardiography and Drug Therapy (pp. 47–57). Dordrecht, the Netherlands: Kluwer Academic Publishers.

110. Garan, H., Schneller, S.J., & Ruskin, J.N. (1987). The valuation of syncope and presyncope. In E.V. Platia (ed.), Management of Cardiac Arrhythmias: The Nonpharmacologic Approach (pp. 99–110). Philadelphia: J.B. Lippincott.

111. Doherty, J.H., Pembrook-Rogers, D., Grogan, E.W., Falcone, R.A., Buxton, A.E., Marchlinski, F.E., Cassidy, D.M., Kienzie, M.G., Almendral, J.M., & Josephson, M.E. (1985). Electrophysiologic evaluation and follow-up characteristics of patients with recurrent unexplained syncope and presyncope. Am J Cardiol 55:703–712.

112. Olshansky, B., Mazuz, M., & Martins, J.B. (1985). Significance of inducible, tachycardia in patients with syncope of unknown origin: A long-term follow-up. J Am Coll Cardiol 5:216–223.

113. Hess, D.S., Morady, F., & Scheinman, M.M. (1982). Electrophysiologic testing in the evaluation of patients with syncope of undetermined origin. Am J Cardiol 50:1309–1315.

114. Stern, S., & Tzivoni, D. (1987). Silent myocardial ischemia: Diagnosis, clinical significance and management. Herz 12:318–327.

115. Levin, R.I. (1988). Quantification of transient myocardial ischemia by digital, ambulatory electrocardiography. Am J Cardiol 61:13B–17B.

116. Dubin, D. (1982). Rapid Interpretation of EKG's (3rd ed.). Tampa: Cover Publishing Co.

117. ACC/ANA Task Force (1989). Guidelines for ambulatory electrocardiography. Circulation 79:206–215.

118. Cohn, P.F. (1989). Ambulatory electrocardiography (Holter monitoring). In Silent Myocardial Ischemia and Infarction (2nd ed., pp. 103–122). New York: Marcel Dekker, Inc.

119. Bigger, J.J., Jr., Reiffel, J.A., & Coromilias, J. (1987). Ambulatory electrocardiography. In E.V. Platia (ed.), Management of Cardiac Arrhythmias (pp. 36–61). Philadelphia: J.B. Lippincott.

120. Cohn, P.F. (1989). Exercise testing. In Silent Myocardial Ischemia and Infarction (2nd ed., pp. 123–135). New York: Marcel Dekker, Inc.

121. Mark, D.B., Hlatky, M.A., & Pryor, D.B. (1988). The exercise treadmill test in patients recovering from an acute myocardial infarction. In R.M. Califf, D.B. Mark, & G.S. Wagner (eds.), Acute Coronary Care in the Thrombolytic Era (pp. 573–591). Chicago: Year Book Medical Publishers.

122. Fintel, D.J., & Platia, E.V. (1987). Exercise testing and cardiac arrhythmias. In E.V. Platia (ed.), Management of Cardiac Arrhythmias (pp. 28–36). Philadelphia: J.B. Lippincott.

123. McHenry, P.L., Morris, S.N., Kavalier, M., & Jordan, J.W. (1976). Comparative study of exercise-induced ventricular arrhythmias in normal subjects and patients with documented coronary artery disease. Am J Cardiol 37:609–616.

124. Nixon, J., Pennington, W., Ritter, W., & Shapiro, W. (1978). Efficacy of propanol in the control of exercise-induced or augmented ventricular arrhythmias. Circulation 57:115–122.

125. Woelfel, A., Foster, J., McAllister, R., Simpson, R.J., & Gettes, L.S. (1985). Efficacy of verapamil

in exercise-induced ventricular tachycardia. Am J Cardiol 56:292–297.

126. Buckingham, T.A., & Kennedy, H.L. (1985). Exercise testing and ambulatory electrocardiography in normal individuals and in patients at risk of sudden cardiac death. In J. Morganroth, & L.N. Horowitz (eds.), *Sudden Cardiac Death* (pp. 57–86). Philadelphia: Grune & Stratton.

127. Verzoni, A., Romano, S., Pozzani, L., Tarricone, D., Sangiorgio, S., & Croce, L. (1989). Prognostic significance and evolution of late ventricular potentials in the first year after myocardial infarction: A prospective study. PACE Pacing Clin Electrophysiol 12:41–51.

128. Kuchar, D.L., Thorburn, C.W., Freund, J., Yeates, M.G., & Sammel, N.L. (1989). Noninvasive predictors of cardiac events after myocardial infarction. Cardiology 76:18–31.

129. Breithardt, G., Borggrete, M., Podazeck, A., Haerten, K., & Martinez-Rubio, A. (1989). Clinical and prognostic significance of ventricular late potentials. Experience with averaging technique. In V. Hombach, H.H. Hilger, & H.L. Kennedy (eds.), *Electrocardiography and Cardiac Drug Therapy* (pp. 204–217). Dordrecht, the Netherlands: Kluwer Academic Publishers.

130. Kuchar, D.L., & Rosenbaum, D.S. (1989). Noninvasive recording of late potentials: Current state of the art. PACE Pacing Clin Electrophysiol 12:1538–1551.

131. Simpson, M.B. (1987). Signal averaging. Circulation 75:(Suppl. III)III69–III73.

132. Flowers, N.C. (1987). Signal averaging as an adjunct in detection of arrhythmias. Circulation 75:(Suppl. III)III74–III78.

133. Sederholm, M. (1988). Monitoring of acute myocardial infarction evolution by continuous spatial electrocardiography. In R.M. Califf, D.B. Mark, & G.S. Wagner (eds.), *Acute Coronary Care in the Thrombolytic Era* (pp. 444–458). Chicago: Year Book Medical Publishers.

134. Zipes, D. (1988). Genesis of cardiac arrhythmias: Elecrophysological considerations. In E. Braunwald (ed.), *Heart Disease, A Textbook of Cardiovascular Medicine* (3rd ed., pp. 581–620). Philadelphia: W.B. Saunders.

135. Platia, E.V. (1987). The electrophysiologic study. In E.V. Platia (ed.), *Management of Cardiac Arrhythmias. The Nonpharmacologic Approach* (pp. 62–98). Philadelphia: J.B. Lippincott.

136. Quaal, S.J., Phillips, B., Howery, T., & Jadvar, H. (1989). The pill electrode. Prog Cardiovasc Nurs 4:10–17.

137. Sulzbach, L.M., & Lansdowne, L.M. (1991). Temporary atrial pacing after cardiac surgery. Focus Crit Care 18:65–74.

138. Lin, D.P., DiCarlo, L.A., & Jenkins, J.M. (1988). Identification of VT using intracauity ventricular electrograms: Analysis of time and frequency domain patterns. PACE Pacing Clin Electrophysiol 11:1592–1606.

4

Circadian Rhythm Disorders

Dorothy M. Lanuza

Rhythms are ubiquitous in the world. The changes in the phases of the moon, the ebb and flow of the tide, seasonal fluctuations, and alternations of light and darkness are just a few examples of the rhythms that abound in the environment. Rhythmic variations are also found in all levels of the hierarchy of living organisms, from a single cell to a complex living organism such as a human being. The circadian, or daily, rhythm is the periodicity most often investigated in human beings. Virtually all physiological variables capable of being measured by laboratory tests have exhibited circadian rhythms. Selected variables and their acrophases and the timing of their peak values in relation to the sleep-wake cycle are shown in Figure 4–1.[1]

Circadian rhythms are believed to be adaptive mechanisms that enable individuals to adjust to the changing temporal structure of the environment.[2, 3] For example, plasma cortisol levels begin to rise shortly before or just after the time of the individual's usual awakening, as though preparing the person to meet the challenges of the day.[4] It has been suggested that in the healthy state rhythms are in synchrony[5] and that illness[6–10] and aging[11–14] may be associated with circadian rhythm disorders.

In order to understand circadian rhythm disorders, it is important to become familiar with rhythm terminology. A *rhythm* is a regularly occurring oscillating process. The maximum value of a rhythm is called the *peak*; the *acrophase* is the time when the peak value occurs, the *mesor* is the rhythm adjusted mean, the minimum value is the *trough* or *nadir*, and the difference between the mesor and the peak represents the rhythm's ampli-

tude. The *period* of a rhythm is the time occupied by one *cycle* and is measured from peak to peak or trough to trough. It is the shortest part of a rhythm that continuously repeats itself. Illustrations of these terms are shown in Figures 4–2 and 4–3. Rhythm cycles may vary in frequency from a millisecond (e.g., neuronal activity), to once approximately every 24 hours (e.g., cortisol and temperature rhythms), to monthly (e.g., women's menstrual cycle), to seasonal (e.g., testosterone and follicle-stimulating hormone circannual rhythms in males).[15]

Rhythms may be exogenous or endogenous. An *exogenous* rhythm is one that develops in response to an external periodic stimuli. The changing tide, which is a passive response to the movement of the moon, is an example. *Endogenous* rhythms originate within the organism and are self-sustaining, even in the absence of external periodic stimuli. Rhythmic fluctuations in physiological variables, such as body temperature, plasma and urinary cortisol, electrolytes, blood constituents, and urinary excretion patterns, are examples. Characteristics of endogenous circadian rhythms are listed in Table 4–1. *Entrainment* refers to the adjustment of an endogenous rhythm's phase or cycle length to the periodicity of environmental stimuli, which do not differ greatly from the rhythm's own frequency.[16] Rhythms entrained by external stimuli or time cues to the 24-hour day are called *circadian rhythms*; and the stimulus or cue, which is the dominant factor in determining the expression of a rhythm, is called a *synchronizer* or *Zeitgeber*. The light-dark cycle is the most important Zeitgeber for animals, while the alternation of rest and activity related to work and social interaction

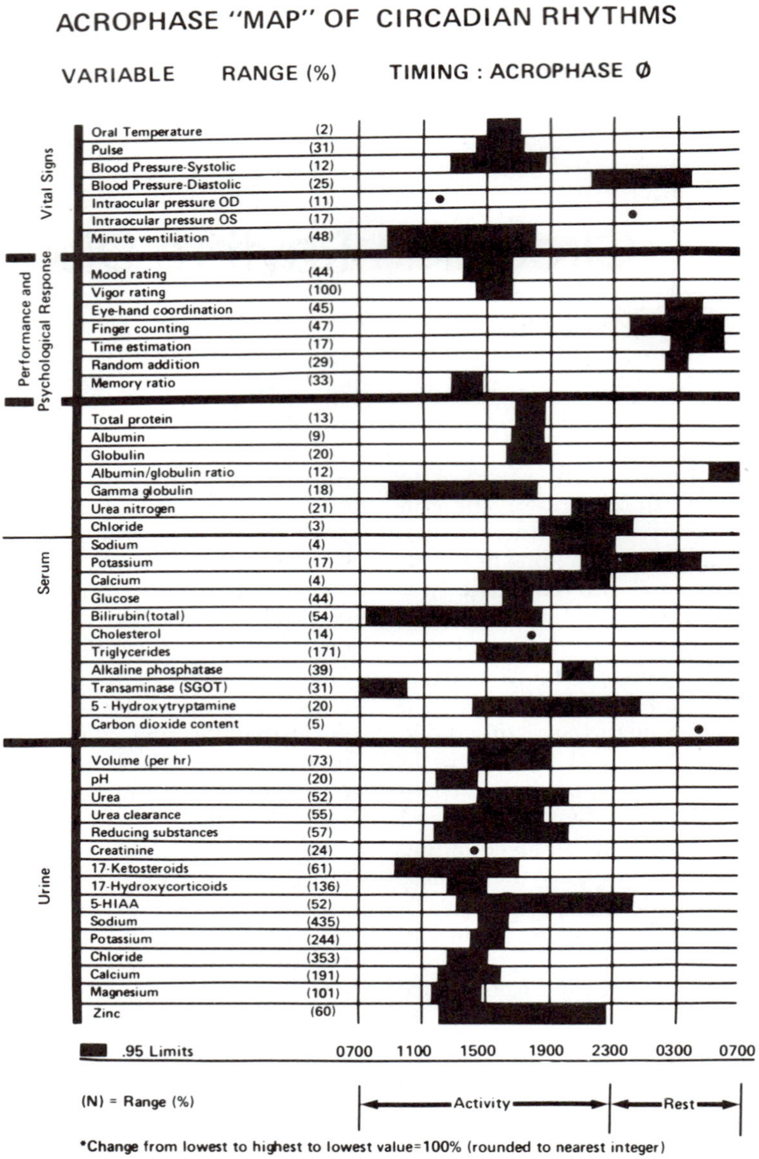

ACROPHASE "MAP" OF CIRCADIAN RHYTHMS

VARIABLE   RANGE (%)   TIMING : ACROPHASE Ø

Vital Signs

Variable	Range (%)
Oral Temperature	(2)
Pulse	(31)
Blood Pressure-Systolic	(12)
Blood Pressure-Diastolic	(25)
Intraocular pressure OD	(11)
Intraocular pressure OS	(17)
Minute ventilation	(48)

Performance and Psychological Response

Variable	Range (%)
Mood rating	(44)
Vigor rating	(100)
Eye-hand coordination	(45)
Finger counting	(47)
Time estimation	(17)
Random addition	(29)
Memory ratio	(33)

Serum

Variable	Range (%)
Total protein	(13)
Albumin	(9)
Globulin	(20)
Albumin/globulin ratio	(12)
Gamma globulin	(18)
Urea nitrogen	(21)
Chloride	(3)
Sodium	(4)
Potassium	(17)
Calcium	(4)
Glucose	(44)
Bilirubin (total)	(54)
Cholesterol	(14)
Triglycerides	(171)
Alkaline phosphatase	(39)
Transaminase (SGOT)	(31)
5 - Hydroxytryptamine	(20)
Carbon dioxide content	(5)

Urine

Variable	Range (%)
Volume (per hr)	(73)
pH	(20)
Urea	(52)
Urea clearance	(55)
Reducing substances	(57)
Creatinine	(24)
17-Ketosteroids	(61)
17-Hydroxycorticoids	(136)
5-HIAA	(52)
Sodium	(435)
Potassium	(244)
Chloride	(353)
Calcium	(191)
Magnesium	(101)
Zinc	(60)

■■■ .95 Limits   0700   1100   1500   1900   2300   0300   0700

(N) = Range (%)   ◀——Activity——▶ ◀—Rest—▶

*Change from lowest to highest to lowest value=100% (rounded to nearest integer)

Figure 4–1. A composite of circadian rhythm data adapted from Halberg (1977) and Kanabrocki and associates (1973). The darkened area represents the time when the variable's peak response (acrophase) occurs within a 95 per cent confidence interval. (From Kabat, H. F. [1981]. Circadian rhythms and drug dosing. In Walker, C. A., Winget, C. M., & Soliman, K. F. A. (eds.), *Chronopharmacology and Chronotherapeutics* [p. 10]. Tallahassee: Florida A & M University Foundation.)

is thought to be the most important Zeitgeber for humans.[17] Recent studies, however, have indicated that light is a much more important environmental synchronizer than previously thought.[18]

Rhythms are generally classified according to the frequency of their cycle into ultradian, circadian, and infradian rhythms. Rhythms with a periodicity of approximately 24 hours are called *circadian*. Rhythms that are shorter than 24 hours are classified as *ultradian* (e.g., sleep cycles), and those longer than 24 hours are classified as *infradian* (e.g., the menstrual cycle). *Free-running rhythms* are those that are no longer entrained by external time cues to the 24-hour day and thus follow their own

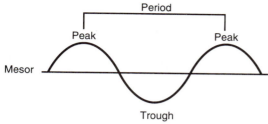

Figure 4–2. A cycle is the shortest part of the rhythm that continuously repeats itself. The period is measured from peak to peak or trough to trough. The mesor is the rhythm-adjusted mean.

TABLE 4–1 CHARACTERISTICS OF ENDOGENOUS CIRCADIAN RHYTHMS

Regularly occurring oscillating process with a periodicity of approximately 24 hours
Genetically inherited
Endogenous and self-sustaining
Role in promotion of adaptation to the temporal environment
Influenced by many factors (e.g., environmental, social)
Synchronized by a multioscillator system
Entrained to the 24-hour day by environmental time cues (Zeitgebers)
Ubiquitous, found in all living organisms
Found at all levels of organization from cells to the whole organism
Sensitive to light intensity
Objectively and subjectively measurable
Predictable

periodicity. Free-running rhythms result in desynchronization of rhythms that were temporally related.

The term *transient internal rhythm desynchronization* indicates a temporary phase shift of less than 24 hours between or among temporally related rhythms to an earlier or later time along a time axis.[19, 20] For example, shift work and transmeridian (across several time zones) jet travel can result in transient internal desynchronization. When an individual abruptly changes from the day to the night shift, the sleep-wake cycle and body temperature rhythm become temporarily desynchronized. Normally, low body temperature levels are associated with low activity and performance levels and sleep onset, while higher temperatures are associated with increased alertness, activity, and performance levels. When shift rotation occurs, the synchronization between these rhythms is disrupted.[21] Transmeridian travel to a very different time zone also requires the individual's rhythms to adapt. Temperature rhythms are considered good indicators of the adjustment of internal circadian rhythms. Similar to the adjustment that takes place in the shift worker, adjustment of the traveller's body temperature to a new schedule occurs by gradual phase shifting of the rhythm. When a *phase shift* occurs, the shape of the rhythm remains the same, but the acrophase is moved

either earlier (phase advance) or later (phase delay) along the time axis. A phase shift to an earlier schedule takes longer to adjust to than to a later schedule.[22] Characteristics of desynchronized rhythms are listed in Table 4–2.

In contrast to transient internal desynchronization, *spontaneous internal rhythm desynchronization* occurs when two or more rhythms that had similar or inverse time patterns no longer exhibit the same rhythm frequency and demonstrate a steady state of continuously changing phase relationships of more than 24 hours (i.e., 360 degrees).[19] Examples of this type of desynchronization are demonstrated in human subjects who are isolated from external time cues (temporal isolation). Initially, their body temperature and activity rhythms are in synchrony, free-running with a cycle of 25.7 hours, and maintaining a relatively fixed temporal relationship. After about 2 weeks without environmental Zeitgebers to entrain them to the 24-hour day, these rhythms undergo spontaneous desynchronization, resulting in new periodicities of 25.1 hours for temperature and 33.4 hours for activity.[23]

DEFINITIONS OF CIRCADIAN RHYTHM DISORDERS

Circadian rhythm disorders are abnormalities in the circadian time-keeping system. When malfunctioning of the circadian system occurs, rhythm disorders can be classified as (1) disorders of phase relations (timing), (2) disorders of amplitude (magnitude of

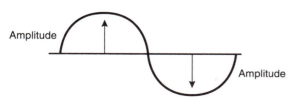

Figure 4–3. The amplitude of a rhythm is the difference between the mesor and the peak.

TABLE 4–2 CHARACTERISTICS OF TRANSIENT AND SPONTANEOUS DESYNCHRONIZED RHYTHMS

Rhythm desynchrony (i.e., a change in the phase relationships among two or more temporally related rhythms)
Change in rhythm entrainment to the 24-hour day
Multidimensional effects (i.e., physiological, cognitive, psychological, and behavioral)
Universal, could affect anyone under certain conditions; vulnerable populations at increased risk include very young, very old, neurotic individuals, people exposed for long periods of time to environments with little or no temporal cues (e.g., ICU patients), transmeridian jet travellers, shift workers, and individuals who experience injury to or alteration of their circadian pacemakers.
Possible pathophysiological and/or psychological consequences

change), and (3) disorders of entrainment (synchronization).[3] These disorders hinder the individual's ability to adapt to the external temporal environment and disturb the internal circadian sequencing of physiological and metabolic events, which may contribute to the development of disease.[3]

PREVALENCE AND POPULATIONS AT RISK

Although biological rhythms are omnipresent, the prevalence of disorders of the circadian system depends on the category of the rhythm disorder. For example, internal desynchronization is an example of a phase disorder. Internal rhythm desynchronization may be either transient or spontaneous. While transient internal desynchronization is common in transmeridian travellers, shift workers, and individuals who score high on tests of neuroticism,[24] the extent of spontaneous internal rhythm desynchronization has been reported mainly in relation to temporal isolation studies. Disturbances of the sleep-wake cycle (see Chapter 20, Impaired Sleep) are the most obvious indication of circadian system disorders and are frequently reported by individuals who experience rhythm desynchronization.

Delayed sleep phase insomnia, another example of a circadian rhythm phase relation problem, is a sleep disorder that reportedly affects approximately 10 per cent of individuals with sleeping difficulties.[25, 26] Malfunction of circadian phase relations and rhythm amplitudes has been reported to be associated with changes in the temporal patterns and quality of sleep found in the elderly[27] and in some patients with affective illness.[7, 28–30]

In addition to individuals who have circadian disorders involving alterations in phase relations and amplitudes, a small population of individuals has demonstrated rhythms that are not entrained to the 24-hour day in spite of being exposed to environmental time cues.[3]

SITUATIONAL STRESSORS

Phase relation and amplitude disorders are associated with shift work, jet lag, exposure to environments without time cues, affective disorders, illness,[31–33] head injuries,[10] and surgery.[34–36]

Clinical States and Medical Diagnoses

Phase Relations Disorders

Desynchronized rhythms are examples of phase relation disorders. The term *desynchronized rhythms* refers to a condition in which the temporal relationship between two or more rhythms is disrupted. Internal desynchronized rhythms are classified as transient or spontaneous.

Transient Internal Rhythm Desynchronization

The cause of transient rhythm desynchronization may be an abrupt change in the sleep-wake cycle due to shift work, transmeridian jet travel, or living in an environment with minimal or no external time cues.[3] Initially, the individual's internal body rhythms are in synchrony, but they are out of synchrony with the external temporal environment. While the individual's rhythms are in the process of adapting to the new 24-hour sleep-wake pattern, they become temporarily internally desynchronized.

Shift Rotation. It is estimated that 27 per cent of the male and 16 per cent of the female work force are shift workers.[37] Shift work, which causes a person suddenly to change from being active during the day and sleeping at night to being active at night and sleeping during the day, is difficult for most people to adjust to. It takes time to adapt to changes in sleep-wakefulness patterns, quality and quantity of sleep, and social activities. Until adjustment occurs, rhythms that normally varied in a temporal relationship may be out of phase with one another.

The rhythm adjustment times for different measured parameters vary. For example, nurses working during the day and sleeping at night demonstrated normal circadian rhythms for body temperature and urinary electrolytes, but after rotating from the day to the night shift, the nurses' peak body temperature and urinary measurements were phase delayed 3 to 4 hours. Following 5 days on the night shift, the nurses rotated back to the day shift. While most of the nurses' urinary measurements returned within a few days to previous day-active patterns, their body temperatures and urinary potassium patterns were still not readjusted 10 days after completion of the night shift.[38] In another study, 7 days were not sufficient for nurses' plasma cortisol, calcium, and magnesium rhythms to readjust completely to their previous day-active patterns after abruptly reversing their sleep-wake cycle to a night activity schedule for 1 week.[4]

In spite of the impact shift work has on circadian rhythms, controversy exists over its effects on workers' general health. Most shift workers are considered to be as healthy as day workers.[39] However, the incidence of morbidity associated with shift work may have been underestimated, since workers who experience the most difficulties usually select not to engage in shift work. Furthermore, the influence of workers' age and the effects of different types of shift work have not been taken into consideration when shift work morbidity has been examined.[40] Shift work is thought to be detrimental to the health of approximately 20 per cent of workers who have great difficulties adjusting to different work schedules.[39, 41] This subpopulation of individuals is unable to adapt to changing sleep-wake patterns or have medical conditions (e.g., respiratory and cardiovascular diseases and epilepsy) that are exacerbated by disruptions of their circadian system.

Shift maladaption syndrome is the term that

has been applied to the symptoms experienced by individuals who cannot successfully adjust to shift work.[40] The major consequences of shift work are alterations in the quantity and quality of sleep, persistent fatigue, behavioral changes, decreased performance, changes in response to medications, and an increased incidence of coronary artery disease and gastrointestinal disorders, such as general gastric discomfort and peptic ulcers.[40–42]

A shortening of sleep length by approximately 2 to 4 hours has been reported for night-shift workers; subsequently, their rapid eye movement (REM) and stage II sleep are also reduced.[43] Optimal waking efficiency is thought to depend more on maintenance of regular sleep-wakefulness patterns than on total number of hours slept.[44] The shift workers' changing sleep-wake patterns and conflicting environmental time cues intensify the adverse effects of sleep deficit on their performance and sense of well-being.

Although some studies have reported that sleep difficulties in shift workers increase with age,[45, 46] no age-related differences were found in oral temperature rhythms or in reports of sleepiness in 145 female nurse shift workers (age 22 to 49) when adjusting to night work.[47] Since measurement of both oral temperature and perceived alertness/sleepiness (as rated on a visual analogue scale) were scheduled every 2 hours while the individual was awake and not throughout the entire day, this would reflect diurnal, or day-night, changes rather than true 24-hour circadian changes. Furthermore, the subjects in this study were less than 50 years of age, while the age-related differences in adjusting to shift work were reported in studies involving much older individuals.[27, 48] Thus, there may be a critical age that must be reached before age-related changes are observed.

It is not surprising that reports of general fatigue are more common in those who work different schedules, particularly night shift workers.[45, 49] A study of shift workers in a paper mill demonstrated that fatigue ratings were highest and catecholamine excretion, diuresis, and self-reported performance (i.e., perceived effectiveness) ratings were lowest during the night shift.[50] Fatigue has been shown to have a circadian variation, with maximum levels occurring in the early morning.[43]

Poor tolerance to shift work is almost always associated with transient internal rhythm desynchronization; however, a desynchronized state may be present in an individual who is without symptoms or complaints. For example, 15 male subjects, 12 of whom were shift workers, were trained to measure and record every 4 hours, except during sleep, the following: (1) information about their sleep-wake cycle; (2) self-ratings of drowsiness, attention, and fatigue; (3) heart rate; (4) grip strength of both hands, and (5) their peak respiratory expiratory flow.[51] In addition, an ambulatory monitoring system was used to measure their axillary temperature and wrist movements. The investigators reported finding internal desynchronization of three to seven variables out of 10 in the shift workers. Interestingly, the self-rated variables were found to be desynchronized less often than objectively measured variables. They concluded that finding a number of desynchronized circadian rhythms in healthy shift workers was not uncommon and was not always associated with decreased performance or increased intolerance to shift work. The severity of symptoms due to shift work seemed to vary with the sensitivity of the individual to rhythm desynchronization.[51] The attitude of shift workers, their personality, and their social context are all factors that influenced their adaptation to shift work.

In addition to interest in the effects of shift work on the worker's health, there are major concerns about the effects of differing work schedules on the worker's performance and safety. Investigations of performance usually use body temperature as a marker rhythm of the individual's endogenous clock. The body temperature rhythm of day-active/night-sleep individuals is one in which the temperature is lowest at the time of usual sleep and begins to rise during the day, usually reaching a peak in late afternoon or early evening and declining to minimal levels at night. An illustration of the circadian rhythm of temperature for a day-active individual is shown in Figure 4–4.[52, 53] Several types of performance rhythms, such as serial search, verbal reasoning,[54] and vigilance patterns,[55] have been found to be temporally associated with body temperature rhythms; that is, the performance rhythm peak is associated with the body temperature rhythm peak, and the performance trough is associated with low temperature. When individuals rotate from the

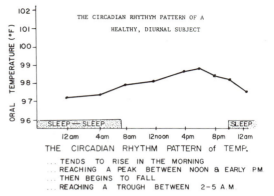

Figure 4–4. Circadian rhythm of oral temperature of a day-active individual. (From Lanuza, D.M. [1976]. Symposium on biological rhythms. Nurs Clin North Am *11*:584.)

day to the night shift, it may take days to weeks before their body temperature pattern changes to be resynchronized with their activity. Until this occurs, these individuals are active during a time when their body temperature and some of their performance rhythms are at their lowest.

The nighttime reduction in productivity and safety that has been reported in shift workers is thought to be caused by the workers' lack of adjustment to the night shift and their efforts to work when they have not received sufficient sleep and many of their performance capabilities are at a low ebb.[54] Therefore, it is not surprising that the incidence of performance errors, delays, and single-vehicle accidents is higher between 3 a.m. and 5 a.m. than at any other time of day.[56–58] In fact, it has been suggested that the shift-work schedule may have been a factor in the Three Mile Island accident,[59] the Chernobyl incident, and the Bhopal incident,[54] since all occurred between midnight and 4 a.m.

Jet Lag. Jet lag is a syndrome that occurs when a traveller rapidly crosses multiple time zones, usually four or more, and is exposed to the environmental stimuli of the new local time. The symptoms associated with jet lag are quite similar to those associated with shift rotation and are believed to be due to the fatigue associated with the flight, sleep loss, and the traveler's attempt to adapt rapidly to the new time zone with its different temporal patterns of light-dark cycle, temperature, and social activities.[60]

Reductions of subjectively assessed sleep

quality and quantity have been reported in aircrew volunteers following both eastward and westward flights across multiple time zones.[60, 61] Eastward flights, which shorten the day, result in phase advances with more variable and fragmented sleep patterns than westward flights, which lengthen the day, and result in phase delays in circadian rhythms.[61, 62] It takes several days to weeks for the transmeridian traveller's various physiological variables and functions, such as body temperature, sleep, and appetite, to adjust to the new temporal environment. Jet lag–induced psychological and behavioral alterations, however, adjust more rapidly. Since there is a great deal of interindividual differences, severity of the jet lag symptoms will vary greatly among individuals. It is estimated that approximately 30 per cent of transmeridian travelers adjust easily, while a similar percentage do not.[63]

Spontaneous Internal Rhythm Desynchronization

Absence of Time Cues. In an attempt to determine whether or not rhythms were endogenous and self-sustaining, early rhythm studies were conducted in environments as free as possible from the influences of Zeitgebers, such as light-dark alternations, atmospheric changes, and external time cues. Studies conducted on human subjects isolated from environmental time cues by living in caves or specially constructed apartments have shown that the rhythms of most physiological variables persist but, when no longer entrained by environmental Zeitgebers, would free run at frequencies slightly longer or shorter than 24 hours.[19] When free-running occurs, the rhythms of body core temperature, REM sleep, plasma cortisol, and urinary potassium excretion separate from the rhythms of rest/activity, skin temperature, slow-wave sleep, plasma growth hormone, and urinary calcium excretion (Fig. 4–5).[20, 64]

Patients in Intensive Care Units. Patients exposed over an extended period of time to an environment lacking temporal structure and environmental time cues are believed to be susceptible to developing rhythm desynchronization.[17] Intensive care units (ICUs) are examples of environments that often lack temporal structure owing to the maintenance of fairly constant lighting, activity, and noise levels throughout the 24-hour day. In addition, ICU patients might be more susceptible

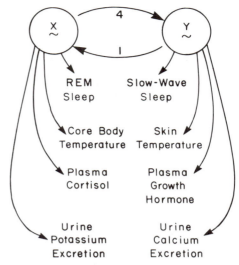

Figure 4–5. Two groups of rhythms are driven by separate pacemakers, X and Y. Pacemaker X drives REM sleep, core body temperature, plasma cortisol, and urine potassium excretion, while pacemaker Y influences slow-wave sleep, skin temperature, plasma growth hormone, and urine calcium excretion. The couping force generated by X is postulated to be approximately four times greater than that of Y on X. (From Moore-Ede, M.C. [1983]. The circadian timing system in mammals: Two pacemakers preside over many secondary oscillators. Fed Proc *42*:2803.)

to rhythm desynchronization owing to the severity of their illness as well as to the medications and treatments (e.g., continuous respiratory therapy, parenteral infusions, and surgery) that they receive.[17] For example, several studies have shown that circadian rhythms of numerous physiological variables are altered or totally suppressed in patients who had brain lesions or head injury,[10, 65, 66] who underwent surgery,[34, 35, 67–70] or who were in an ICU.[71] Sleep loss together with desynchronized rhythms may play a role in the development of the syndrome called ICU delirium, which is estimated to occur in 12 to 38 per cent of conscious patients admitted to critical care settings.[17, 72]

Would the provision of increased environmental time cues prevent or diminish the incidence of rhythm desynchrony and/or psychological disturbances in ICU patients? In a retrospective survey of 150 patients who stayed 48 hours in ICUs that had rooms with (n = 72) or without windows (n = 78), it was found that patients in ICUs with windows reported a higher recall of their stay and better time orientation than those in ICUs without windows.[73] Since ICU patients are exposed to many different and changing environmental stimuli or factors that impact on their circadian rhythms, this is indeed an area in need of further investigation.

Delayed Sleep Phase Syndrome (DSPS)

A clinical example of a phase relation disorder is DSPS insomnia, a circadian disorder of sleep timing or phase in which the individual has chronic difficulty in initiating sleep at a socially desirable time. Usually, the individual reports being unable to fall asleep until early in the morning yet has no problem remaining asleep once sleep occurs.[25, 26, 74] Since the length of the DSPS patient's normal sleep period is approximately 7 to 9 hours, having a long-delayed sleep onset makes awaking early in the morning very difficult. On the other hand, when not required to follow a strict time schedule on the weekends or when on vacation, patients with DSPS report no difficulty sleeping.[25, 74]

The cause of DSPS is not known, but it is postulated that individuals with this syndrome have a very limited ability to achieve large phase-advances of their sleep-wake cycle,[3, 25] and thus have difficulty adjusting to variations in their bedtime and awakening patterns. If they increase their awake portion of their sleep-wake cycle, they activate their phase-delay mechanism. Over a period of time, their sleep-wake pattern will demonstrate their consistent tendency to go to sleep later each night.[25] A method of treating DSPS is to reset the patients' circadian clock by sequentially phase delaying their sleep around the clock until the desired sleep-wake schedule is achieved.[74] This procedure is called chronotherapy.

Affective Disorders

Disorders of the circadian system have been implicated in the pathogenesis of affective disorders. Manic-depression (bipolar depression) and endogenous depression (unipolar depression) have been postulated to have abnormalities in circadian rhythm timing and phase control that result in (1) early morning awakening; (2) a diurnal pattern of depression, with symptoms most severe just after awakening and gradually improving throughout the day; and (3) seasonal recurrences.[7, 28–30, 75] Decreases in the amplitude of cortisol,[76, 77] melatonin,[77] thyroid-stimulating hormone[78]

sleep,[79] and temperature[80] rhythms have been demonstrated in patients with endogenous depression. Therefore, some affective disorders are examples of not only amplitude but also phase relation abnormalities, as discussed previously. Nevertheless, controversy exists over whether blunting of the temperature rhythm amplitude in affective disorders is due to the illness or a masking effect.[81, 82] The term *masking effect* refers to alterations produced in the rhythm of a variable as a result of changes in environmental conditions such as physical activity and timing of sleep.[82] The smaller or blunted temperature amplitudes that have been reported in some depressive patients may be influenced by changes in the patients' sleep-wake cycle.[79]

Three hypotheses have been proposed to explain the relationship between circadian rhythms and affective disorders: the advanced phase hypothesis, the internal desynchronization hypothesis, and the delayed phase hypothesis.[81] These hypotheses all postulate that sleep and other circadian rhythms are out of phase with each other.

The advanced phase hypothesis proposes the existence of a phase advance of circadian rhythms, which would explain the early morning awakening, the daily fluctuations in moods, and the seasonal recurrences of affective symptoms in patients with depressive conditions.[75] For example, the timing of the maximal and minimal body temperature would phase advance to an earlier time with respect to the sleep-wake cycle.[79] However, according to this hypothesis, sleep is not as phase advanced as other variables that exhibit circadian rhythms.[29]

The internal desynchronization hypothesis suggests that an affective illness episode is triggered by the interfacing of the peaks of two rhythms, one of which is free-running.[83] This hypothesis is supported by a longitudinal study of seven manic-depressive patients who demonstrated spontaneous internal desynchronization of circadian rhythms in moods, temperature, and urinary constituents.[84] Furthermore, four of these patients also exhibited phase advances of their temperature acrophases, suggesting not only that manic-depressive patients become symptomatic after their circadian rhythms uncouple from environmental Zeitgebers and begin rapid free-running but also that they are more susceptible to rhythm desynchronization and experience severe symptoms of mood disorders. Their investigations also suggest that the effectiveness of lithium, one of the drugs used to treat manic-depressive patients, is related to the drug's ability to slow down the patient's circadian oscillator once uncoupling occurs and to prevent future rhythm uncoupling.[84]

The delayed phase mood hypothesis postulates that circadian rhythms have abnormalities in their phase relationships and are phase delayed in relation to sleep.[29] Lewy suggests that future research may find that a phase delay in circadian rhythms is the major circadian abnormality of depressed patients.[29] He believes that when the sleep-wake cycle, which is influenced primarily by social cues, is disrupted, it results in disturbances of phase relationships among circadian rhythms. For example, circadian rhythms of patients with winter depression are thought to be abnormally phase delayed in relation to sleep.[29]

Several studies have not totally supported the advanced phase or internal desynchronization hypotheses.[85, 86] Yet, several investigators believe that reports of positive effects of manipulation of the sleep-wake cycle in patients with affective illness strongly links the circadian system to depression and mania.[29, 30, 87] Seasonal affective diseases are also thought to be strongly associated with circadian rhythm disorders.[88]

There is considerable interest in investigating the similarities in symptoms, such as sleep and appetite disturbances and feelings of malaise, that occur as a result of shift work, jet lag, and affective illness.[8, 28] While the intensity of the symptoms is usually greatest in individuals with affective disorders, several of the treatments for these conditions are similar. Although those who experience distress from shift work and jet lag share some similarities with people with affective disease, they differ in two major ways. First, shift workers and individuals with jet lag can correctly attribute their symptoms to a cause, while those with affective disease cannot.[8, 28] Second the circadian rhythms of shift workers and transmeridian travellers are initially internally synchronized but out of synchrony with the external environment. In contrast, the various hypotheses proposed for affective illness suggest that these individuals experience symptoms as a result of abnormal internal circadian rhythmicities. Could it be that those individuals who experience distress

from shift work and jet lag do so only after their internal rhythms develop abnormal phase relationships? Healy and Waterhouse believe that further investigation is needed of the factors and social events that contribute to vulnerability to distress from shift work, jet travel, and affective illness.[28]

Phase shifts have also been reported in the elderly.[48, 89–92] Variables such as body temperature[48] and cortisol,[90, 93] have been shown to be phase advanced in the elderly. While age-related phase shifts in circadian rhythms are believed to reflect biological changes,[90] they may also partially reflect changes in life habits and social activity.[14]

Disorders of Rhythm Amplitude

Diminutions in amplitude have been reported in the elderly[14, 90, 91] and in populations living near the Arctic Circle, who experience prolonged periods of continuous darkness or daylight.[94] Other potential causes of low-rhythm amplitudes include injury to or failure of the central biological clock or internal oscillator mechanisms or the variables that they control.[3]

Entrainment Failure

There is a small population of individuals whose endogenous circadian rhythms are not entrained to the environmental 24-hour period.[3] For example, the *hypernychthemeral syndrome* is a condition in which individuals demonstrate progressively later sleep onsets, resulting in a 24.5- to 26-hour sleep-wake cycle.[25, 95] This syndrome is an excellent example of entrainment failure.

DEVELOPMENTAL ASPECTS OF CIRCADIAN RHYTHMS

Most circadian rhythm investigations in human beings have been conducted in adults,[96] however, more recent research is examining age and gender differences in circadian patterns. Selected examples of rhythm development in the young and rhythm changes in the elderly will be addressed next.

Infants, Children, and Adolescents

The circadian rhythms of heart rate, respiratory movement, and rest and activity, which are probably driven by maternal oscillators, have been detected in the fetus.[31, 97] Since these rhythms are not observed immediately after birth, it is believed that the newborn's biological time-keeping system is not yet able to sustain them independently. During the early neonatal period, more electroencephalographic, respiratory, and heart rate ultradian than circadian rhythms have been reported.[97] While endogenous rhythmicity is hereditary, a maturation process seems necessary before most rhythms emerge as fully developed circadian rhythms.[98] In fact, it has been postulated that some circadian rhythms (e.g., cortisol) develop from the gradual lengthening of the infant's ultradian rhythms.[96, 99] An alternative suggestion is that with maturation ultradian rhythms decrease and circadian rhythms begin to dominate.[100] However, not all ultradian rhythms disappear, since both ultradian and circadian rhythms have been reported in adults for the same variable.[36, 69, 100]

Body Temperature

Since body temperature is relatively easy to measure, the development of infants' temperature circadian patterns has been studied more extensively than other variables. Yet, equivocal results have been reported regarding the presence of temperature circadian rhythms in the first weeks to months after birth. Early research reported an absence of temperature circadian rhythms in newborn infants.[100, 101] In fact, diurnal rhythms of body temperature, indicating higher values during the day than at night, were not demonstrated until infants were 4 weeks or older.[101–103] Instead of a temperature circadian rhythm, shorter ultradian cycles have been reported for infants.[104] Although infants within a month or so of birth manifested a 24-hour axillary temperature periodicity, the circadian rhythm of body temperature with respect to phase was reportedly not established until children were approximately 1 year of age. An adult-type temperature circadian rhythm with respect to phase and amplitude was not fully established until children were about 5 to 7 years of age.[101, 102]

Recent advances in monitoring technology and statistical techniques have provided more accurate and sensitive methods for detecting circadian rhythms. By measuring the infant's skin temperatures with thermistors every 3 hours for 24 hours and by using cosinor analysis, significant circadian rhythms for temperature were reported for five of six preterm infants (34 to 37 weeks' gestational age) who were 10 to 20 days postnatal.[105] However, in keeping with findings of earlier studies,[101, 102] the phase and amplitude of the temperature rhythm were found to differ from that of adults, suggesting that a maturational process is needed before the circadian rhythm is fully developed.[105]

Similarly, Mirmiran and associates[106] reported body temperature circadian rhythms in five out of nine preterm infants (24 to 34 weeks' gestational age). The infants' temperatures were measured with a rectal probe over a period of 1 to 3 days, and data were recorded approximately every 4 minutes and analyzed with a cosinor program. Although the investigators stated they could not explain why circadian rhythms were not found in four infants, a plausible explanation could be that these infants had ultradian rather than circadian rhythms.

More recently, Thomas reported ultradian temperature rhythms in preterm infants (30 to 34 weeks' gestational age).[107] Five to 10 days after birth, the temperature cycles ranged from 2 to 6 hours in three of the five preterm infants. The infants' skin temperatures were measured with thermistors, and a sampling interval of one measurement per minute was used. Data were analyzed using an autocorrelation method because previous research[104] had reported ultradian temperature rhythms in infants, and cosinor analysis is not capable of detecting cycles whose periodicity is less or more than 24 hours. It is possible that the two preterm infants who did not demonstrate an ultradian temperature pattern had longer rhythm cycles. The investigator stated that the data collection period was not adequate to determine circadian rhythmicity because the strength of autocorrelation analysis is determined partially by the number of times the cycle is repeated, and the 24-hour cycle was not repeated.[107]

The three preceding studies in preterm infants demonstrate that length of the sampling interval and data collection period as well as choice of the statistical analysis technique can influence whether or not circadian or ultradian temperature rhythms are found. For example, Thomas[107] compared her research findings with those of Updike and associates.[105] and suggested that the 3-hour sampling interval used by Updike and associates was not frequent enough to detect cycles with lengths less than 6 hours, since the ability to determine the length of a cycle is based on the length of the sampling interval multiplied by two.[107, 108] It could also be argued that data collected in periods less than or equal to 24-hour data collection periods, as used in the studies of Updike and associates[105] and Thomas,[107] were sufficient to examine ultradian rhythms but not sufficient to examine circadian rhythmicity. On the other hand, the data collection period in the study of Mirmiran and associates[106] occurred over a longer length of time (1 to 3 days) and was sufficient to determine circadian rhythmicity. As in the study of Updike and associates,[105] Mirmiran and colleagues'[106] choice of statistical technique limited the rhythm period that could be identified to a circadian cycle, and thus rhythms that were longer or shorter than 24 hours were not found.

Since light and social cues have been shown to be strong Zeitgebers for human beings, there is interest in determining what influence the 24-hour lighting, incubators, and environmental activity of an ICU may have on the developing temperature rhythms of neonates and young children.

Cortisol

Until recently, the development of circadian rhythms in hormones such as cortisol has been difficult to investigate in infants because multiple blood sampling or frequent urine collections were required. A cortisol diurnal rhythm with higher morning than evening values was initially reported in children between the ages of 1 and 3 years.[109] Several years later, serum cortisol circadian rhythms were demonstrated in infants 3 months of age[110] and in those 6 months of age or older.[111] Currently, the ability to detect cortisol in saliva has made it possible to examine more readily and noninvasively cortisol circadian rhythms in very young subjects. Similar to the serum cortisol studies, an adult-like circadian variation of salivary cortisol has been found in 3- to 6-month-old infants.[112, 113]

Animal research has shown that stimuli applied during the developmental phase of the rhythm can permanently alter the adult rhythm. For example, when young rats were given corticosteroids on their seventh to ninth or seventeenth to nineteenth day of life, their adult corticosteroid circadian rhythms and stress responses were permanently suppressed.[114, 115] These findings may have implications for infants who receive steroid therapy.

Blood Pressure

Although very little information is available on rhythmicities in children and adolescents, a few studies on circadian rhythms for systolic and diastolic blood pressure have been reported.[116–119] A study that investigated blood pressure circadian rhythms of children with hypertensive and normotensive parents reported that only 30 per cent of the children demonstrated a circadian blood pressure rhythm. No significant group differences in rhythm amplitude, acrophase, or mesor were found. Plausible explanations given by the investigator for such a small number of children exhibiting circadian rhythms were that their blood pressure rhythms were ultradian and had not yet developed into a circadian periodicity and were not entrained to the 24-hour day or that the study period of one 24-hour cycle was not long enough to detect a circadian rhythm. More rhythm research on children and adolescents is needed to elucidate the maturational process involved in the development of blood pressure rhythms.[116]

Aging and Gender

Many investigators have suggested that rhythm desynchrony occurs with aging. Thus far, animal and human research indicates that circadian rhythmicity persists in the elderly, but there are changes in certain characteristics of the rhythms, such as the amplitude, mesor, and acrophase.[14, 31, 93, 120] In human research changes in rhythm characteristics of several variables, such as body temperature[27] and sleep-wake[121] rhythms, have been reported. Although Vitello and associates[122] found no significant age differences when they examined the timing of temperature rhythms of 10 young males (m = 24 years) and eight senior males (m = 68.5 years), Weitzman and associates[27] reported that the temperature patterns of six older men (53 years and older) demonstrated a shorter period, a higher mesor, an earlier nighttime minimum temperature, and smaller rhythm amplitudes than those in six younger men (23 to 30 years). Czeisler and associates, who found associations among earlier bedtimes, earlier temperature minimal levels, and earlier waking times in elderly versus young subjects, concluded that age-related changes in temperature rhythms are associated with concurrent changes in the timing and quality of sleep.[121] Similar to the phase advance reported in temperature rhythms of elderly subjects,[27, 121] phase advances have also been reported for cortisol,[90, 91] circulating leukocytes and lymphocytes,[92] and activity.[89] In contrast, a phase delay in urinary volume excretion of older individuals has been reported, with subjects voiding a greater amount of urine during the night than during the day.[123]

Gender differences in individuals over 60 years of age have been noted in several variables, such as temperature[48, 89] and blood cortisol.[93] In general, the body temperature of older women has been shown to peak more than an hour earlier than that of men of comparable ages.[48, 89] It was postulated that shorter sleep periods and earlier awakenings reported by older females may be associated with an earlier rise in their body temperature.[48] Another gender-mediated difference has been reported for total cortisol, which is reported to be higher in elderly women than in elderly men.[93] These gender differences in temperature acrophase and cortisol mesor warrant serious consideration when evaluating circadian rhythm studies and their application to patient assessment and health care.

BIOLOGICAL RHYTHM MECHANISMS

In the last several decades there have been many efforts to elucidate the anatomy and physiology of the circadian timekeeping system in living organisms. Data from numerous studies on both human beings and lower animals support the postulate that the circadian system is a multioscillator system, that is, oscillators acting as pacemakers that drive the rhythms.[19, 64, 124, 125] The terms *oscillator* and *pacemaker* have been used interchangeably, and the term *biological clock* usually refers to two or more major oscillators. In addition, numerous investigators[19, 99, 124, 126, 127] have suggested that there are multiple secondary internal circadian oscillators, which are loosely coupled with each other but are coordinated in a hierarchial system by two or more major circadian oscillators. For example, circadian rhythmicities have been demonstrated at the cellular level of several organs, such as the adrenal gland, heart, and liver.[64] These rhythms are considered to be generated by secondary oscillators within the tissues and synchronized under the influence of a major oscillator, the clock.[64]

Under certain conditions, such as the absence of external time cues and environmental phase shifts related to shift work and transmeridian jet travel, circadian rhythms may temporarily change their phase relation to each other and become transiently internally desynchronized or even spontaneously desynchronized, uncoupled, and free-running at different frequencies. Approximately one third of human subjects who live in an environment without external Zeitgebers will exhibit internal desynchronization of their body temperature and sleep-wakefulness rhythms.[19] Rather than oscillating within the same circadian period, the temperature rhythm assumes a periodicity of about 25 hours, and the sleep-wakefulness rhythm may change to a periodicity of 33 hours,[19] indicating that these rhythms are driven by at least two major independent pacemakers. Under normal circumstances, both major pacemakers are entrained by external environmental Zeitgebers so that only circadian rhythms are manifested.

Wever developed a protocol called "fractional desynchronization" to investigate further the concept of two internal pacemakers.[128] Fractional desynchronization involves shortening or lengthening the period of a group of Zeitgebers. When the critical limit of entrainment of an oscillator to a Zeitgeber is reached, the oscillator will break away, and its periodicity will free run. Body temperature is an example of a rhythm that cannot adjust to an entrainment period of less than 23 hours or more than 27 hours.[126] Under experimental conditions that exposed subjects to days that are not within the body temperature's entrainment period, the temperature rhythm would break away and resume its free-running cycle. If more than one internal oscillator exists, then the different oscillators would separate at different Zeitgeber periods in accordance with the critical limit of their entrainment.

The pacemaker or oscillator associated with the core body temperature rhythm is postulated to be very strong, since its periodicity is maintained within a very limited entrainment range of 23 to 27 hours. The oscillator generating the temperature rhythm has been referred to as pacemaker X, whereas the oscillator associated with the sleep-wake rhythm is called pacemaker Y. The latter is hypothesized to be much weaker, since sleep-wake rhythms have a much wider range of entrainment. The coupling strength of pacemaker X is believed to be four times stronger than that of pacemaker Y.[64] Both neural and hormonal factors are believed to link the X and Y pacemaker systems.[64, 129] In addition to core body temperature, pacemaker X entrains plasma cortisol, REM sleep, and urine potassium rhythms, while pacemaker Y entrains skin temperature, plasma growth hormone, slow-wave sleep, and urinary calcium excretion (Fig. 4–5).[64] Although both the X and the Y pacemakers may influence a variable's rhythm, one pacemaker predominates. There is substantial evidence that pacemaker Y is located in the suprachiasmatic nuclei (SCN) in the anterior hypothalamus, but the exact location of pacemaker X has not been determined.[64]

A method of ascertaining the anatomic site responsible for generating endogenous circadian rhythms is to determine whether destruction or surgical isolation of a suspected site results in the elimination of or alteration in rhythmicities. Lesions made in the anterior-ventral hypothalamus of rodents were found to disrupt circadian rhythmicity in wheel running,[130] whereas specific lesions to the SCN of rats abolished several circadian rhythms, such as plasma corticosterone,[131] drinking and locomotor activity,[130, 132] and sleep/wakefulness.[133] Circadian variations in the number of adrenergic, cholinergic, dopaminergic, and benzodiazepine receptors have also been shown to be abolished following SCN ablation.[134] Thus the SCN is considered a major circadian pacemaker.

Light is a Zeitgeber that plays a very important role in entraining endogenous rhythms of living organisms to the 24-hour day.[18, 64] Light is transmitted via the retinohypothalamic afferent neural projections to the SCN, where it influences circadian rhythmicity by transmitting information from the SCN via efferent neural pathways to the receptor organs and tissues.[131] In addition to the light Zeitgeber, which entrains circadian rhythms via neural pathways, melatonin from the pineal gland can also function as a Zeitgeber to entrain circadian rhythms.[135] Thus,

circadian oscillators are influenced by both neural and hormonal input.[131, 135]

To determine how light is transmitted to the SCN, rodents were either blinded by bilateral enucleation or behaviorally blinded by bilateral destruction of their optic tracts in the area of the lateral geniculate. The enucleated animals developed free-running of their sleep-wakefulness,[133] rectal temperature, and serum corticosterone[136] rhythms, whereas the behaviorally blinded rodents maintained their circadian rhythmicity and did not free run. In the former case, no light could be transmitted to the SCN. In the latter case, the retinohypothalamic fibers were still intact and transmitting light from the retina to the SCN, thus maintaining the entrainment of the sleep-wakefulness rhythm to the environmental light-dark cycle.[133] However, there was still a question of whether the SCN generates circadian rhythms or merely serves as a relay nucleus of another pacemaker.[137] To answer this question, investigators surgically isolated the SCN by severing the neural connections from the anterior hypothalamic area of rats. Electrical rhythmicity was observed only in the area of the isolated tissue containing the SCN and not in brain areas outside the island. These findings indicate that the SCN is the site of a major circadian pacemaker. Additional support for this finding was provided by a recent study, which showed that when SCN grafts from donor animals were implanted in an arrhythmic animal whose own SCN was ablated, overt behavioral circadian rhythmicity was restored.[138] Furthermore, the restored rhythm reflected the genotypic rhythm of the donor tissue and not that of the recipient.[138]

While lesions of the SCN in rodents have been shown to eliminate activity, sleep/wakefulness, plasma corticosterone levels, and drinking behavior rhythms, temperature circadian rhythms persisted.[132, 139] Therefore, another central pacemaker other than the SCN (i.e., pacemaker Y) must be responsible for generating core body temperature rhythms. Moore-Ede has suggested that, similar to body temperature rhythms, plasma cortisol rhythms in human beings may also be controlled by the X pacemaker.[64] This hypothesis is supported by the observation that ablation of the SCN in Rhesus monkeys does not abolish the circadian variation of cerebrospinal fluid cortisol levels.[140] On the other hand, the corticosterone rhythm in nocturnal animals (e.g., rodents) is predominantly influenced by the Y oscillator in the SCN, since its destruction abolishes the corticosterone circadian rhythm.[136] Further investigations are needed to clarify the mechanisms and sites of the human circadian oscillator systems.

RELATED PHYSIOLOGICAL CONCEPTS

Sleep, insomnia, fatigue, and susceptibility rhythms are related to circadian rhythm disorders. Changes in sleep quality and quantity and concomitant experiences of increased fatigue, as discussed earlier, are commonly associated with the internal desynchronization of rhythms associated with shift work, jet travel, and affective illness. If the rhythm desynchronizations are prolonged, insomnia can develop. The following discussion will focus on the concept of susceptibility rhythms.

Susceptibility Rhythms

Susceptibility rhythm is the term used to indicate that an organism's response to stressors varies throughout the 24-hour day. The existence of susceptibility rhythms is very relevant to health. For example, many studies have shown that a circadian variation exists for susceptibility to noxious stimuli,[141] endotoxins,[142] and drugs.[143] Although this phenomenon has been studied in both human beings and animals, the reproducibility of results is especially impressive in animal studies, where the groups are kept under controlled, comparable, and standardized conditions. The morbidity and mortality in mice from physical agents, toxins, or chemicals have been shown to be several times higher at one time of day than another. If a noxious stimulus, such as noise, is applied shortly after mice awaken, the probability of convulsions occurring is much greater than if the stimulus is applied toward the end of the animals' sleep period.[141] The response of rats to injections of pneumococci also shows a circadian variation, with the greatest survival rates being associated with rats who received the injections during their highest activity span.[144]

Although susceptibility rhythms are not as well documented in human beings as in animals, research in this area is rapidly growing. In a study of the allergic response of individuals to intradermally injected histamine, the mildest skin response was seen at 11 a.m., and the most severe response was seen at 11 p.m.[145] In relation to the timing of drug administration, the time that cyproheptadine (Periactin), an antihistamine, was administered was shown to influence the duration of its effects. Cyproheptadine provided 16 hours of relief when taken at 7 a.m. and only 7 hours of relief when taken at 7 p.m.[146]

Studies have also shown that if an individual is receiving adrenal steroid therapy, the time at which the drug is administered determines whether the individual's endogenous cortisol levels are suppressed, maintained, or augmented. The plasma cortisol rhythm pattern for day-active individuals is one in which cortisol levels begin to rise in the latter part of the usual sleep period, reach a peak shortly before or just after awakening, then decline irregularly throughout the day and evening until minimal levels are reached early in the usual sleep cycle.[4, 20] Patients who receive transplanted organs are placed on lifetime steroid therapy in order to augment their endogenous cortisol levels and prevent rejection of the donor organ. Under these circumstances, the goal of treatment is to reinforce the intrinsic adrenocortical activity with negligible suppression. In order to achieve this a synthetic glucocorticoid, such as prednisone, is given after the peak secretion of endogenous cortisol in a daily or alternate day midmorning dose.[147, 148] On the other hand, if the goal is to suppress adrenocortical activity, then the synthetic steroid is given shortly before the time of the endogenous cortisol peak.[143, 147] Finally, in situations in which the goal of treatment is replacement, such as in adrenocortical insufficiency, it is recommended that the steroid be given in a way that mimics the natural endogenous rhythm; that is, the steroid would be administered in two unequal doses with approximately two thirds in the morning on awakening and one third prior to retiring in the evening.[148, 149]

Most of our knowledge concerning human susceptibility rhythms has been on subjects whose rhythms have been assumed to be in synchrony. Future research should include the examination of what occurs to susceptibility rhythms when the subjects' rhythms are desynchronized.

Chronopharmacology

Studies like those described in the previous section have led to the development of a new area of investigation, clinical chronopharmacology, which uses the information from susceptibility rhythm studies to determine methods of optimizing therapeutic interventions by manipulating the time that drugs are administered.[143] The ultimate goal of chronopharmacology is to determine the best time to administer the lowest possible dose of a drug when it would be most effective and have the fewest undesirable side effects.

Chronopathology

Knowledge of susceptibility rhythms is also used in chronopathology, the study of the time factor associated with symptoms and disease. For example, the incidence and intensity of asthmatic symptoms is reported to be greatest between 2 a.m. and 7 a.m., with few symptoms being reported during the day.[150] A diurnal study of asthmatics showed that the patients' subjective self-reports of dyspnea were greatest upon awakening around 7 a.m. and lowest around 3 p.m., while their peak expiratory flow (PEF) varied in a complimentary manner, being lowest at 7 a.m. and highest around 3 p.m.[151] These investigators suggest that (1) an increase in nighttime airway resistance, (2) an increase in pulmonary resistance, (3) an increase in bronchial reactivity to irritants, (4) a decrease in bronchodilator substances like catecholamines and cortisol, and (5) a decrease in β-adrenergic tone and an increase in vagal tone[148, 151] play a role in time-dependent susceptibility to nocturnal or early morning asthma attacks.[151] Since asthma symptoms occur mainly at night, an evening scheduling of medications, such as sustained-release theophyllines, to treat asthma has been suggested.[148]

Evidence also indicates that a population circadian rhythm exists for the occurrence of myocardial infarctions. The most extensive data (n = 8900) on the time of onset of myocardial infarction pain, published by the World Health Organization and based on information from 19 European countries, showed that the peak incidence occurred between 8 and 11 a.m.[152] These findings were recently confirmed by Muller and co-workers, who showed that the subjective report (n = 2999) of the onset of myocardial pain had a peak incidence between 6 a.m. and 12 p.m. (noon).[153] An objective method, using serial plasma cardiac creatine-kinase MB levels (n = 703) to determine the onset of myocardial infarction, showed a peak incidence occurring between 5 a.m. and 2 p.m. It is possible that the increased incidence of myocardial infarction in the morning may be associated with the shift from a resting state to an active state as well as with the rhythmic increase in plasma catecholamines, systemic arterial pressure, heart rate, and coronary vessel tone.[154] Interestingly, patients with Prinzmetal's variant angina also were found to have more angina and ST-segment elevations when they were subjected to a treadmill test between 5 and 8 a.m. than when exposed to a more strenuous and longer treadmill exercise in the afternoon.[155]

ASSOCIATED PSYCHOSOCIAL CONCEPTS

Affective Diseases

Affective diseases are related to circadian rhythm disorders, whereas seasonal affective disease (SAD) is a form of depression associated with seasonal changes in the duration and intensity of light.[156] This infradian rhythm of depression, which is manifested by marked detrimental seasonal changes in mood and energy, occurs in all races and affects people with many different occupations. SAD is more common in females than males (4:1), and while it occurs in all age groups, 20- to 40-year-olds seem most susceptible.[157] In the United States it is estimated that SAD affects about 6 per cent of the population, and an additional 14 per cent of the population have a milder form of the condition, called the winter blues.[157]

MANIFESTATIONS

Objective Manifestations

Sensitivity to desynchronized circadian rhythms varies among individuals and at different times and under different circumstances within an individual. Symptoms associated with desynchronized rhythms are sleep-arousal disorders such as wakefulness or sleep at inappropriate times, changes in sleep-wake patterns, decreases in quantity and quality of sleep, and gastrointestinal irregularity, including hunger or anorexia at inappropriate times, constipation, and peptic ulcers. Continuous monitoring of an individual's vital signs, plasma and urinary hormones, and electrolytes will indicate changes in the phase or the amplitude of the specific rhythm from reported standard patterns. This can be used to detect internal rhythm desynchronization.

Subjective Manifestations

Individuals who experience desynchronized rhythms may report feelings of fatigue, irritability, general malaise, decreased mental alertness and reaction time, and regular use of medications to induce sleep. They often report feeling inappropriately awake or sleepy, hungry or anoretic, fatigued, and irritable. They may experience general malaise and perceive a decrease in their cognitive and physical performance abilities.

SURVEILLANCE AND MEASUREMENT

Understanding normal circadian variations in the patient's physiological variables and being able to assess, predict, and eventually prevent changes indicative of impending homeostatic instability are important goals of clinical rhythm research and clinical surveillance.

In order to determine whether patients are experiencing circadian rhythm disorders, it is necessary to first assess their "normal" circadian pattern. For example, what is the usual sleep-wake and mealtime pattern? When do feelings of mental—and physical— best occur? Some of the following instruments could be used to assess circadian rhythms: Tom's[158] Tool for Assessing Circadian Patterns, Horne and Ostberg's[159] Morning-Eveningness Questionnaire, and rest/activity diaries or logs. In addition, physiological measurements of variables, such as vital signs and hormonal levels could be used to document patterns and to identify changes

that would be indicative of circadian rhythm desynchronization.

When one is designing circadian rhythm studies, it is essential to ensure that the data collection period is adequate. It should be preferably longer than one 24-hour cycle in order to capture the circadian rhythm cycle, and the sampling intervals should be frequent enough to detect changes.[160] Sampling frequency can be a problem in conducting circadian rhythm studies, especially in infants. When possible, noninvasive data collection methods should be used. It is also important to take into consideration potential masking effects.[82] For example, the change in body temperature caused by a change in the degree of physical activity may be superimposed on the temperature rhythm and thus affect the findings. When appropriate, statistical methods need to include the ability to detect 24-hour rhythms and rhythms that may be shorter or longer than 24 hours.

Methods used to measure circadian rhythms include continuous telemetry or ambulatory monitoring devices and thorough assessments of rhythmic patterns of routinely measured physiological variables (e.g., body temperature, blood pressure, urinary output) and patient logs/diaries or questionnaires that indicate patterns of sleep/wakefulness, mealtimes, activity, and mood states. While telemetry monitoring is usually used in hospital settings, there are several monitoring devices that can be used in ambulatory care and community settings to measure continuously various physiological parameters such as blood pressure, heart rate, body temperature, and activity. These instruments can be powerful tools in circadian rhythm research.

If computerized equipment is available, the data can be collected, stored, and then transmitted to a larger computer for statistical analysis. A gross estimate of a circadian rhythm can be made by a visual examination of the data plotted on graph paper. For example, if the temperature values of a patient who is active during the day and sleeps at night were plotted, do they indicate that the peak value occurs in late afternoon or early evening? Are the lowest temperature values noted during the individual's usual sleep time?

The techniques that nurses use to study the circadian rhythms of patients include the continuous cardiac, oxygen, and respiratory telemetry monitoring equipment readily available in hospitals, especially in neonatal, pediatric, labor and delivery, coronary care, medical, and surgical ICUs. When blood specimens are required for a study, often they can be obtained from an indwelling arterial or venous catheter. The volume of blood or plasma required for analysis involving hormonal or hematological parameters is low, making multiple analyses of other blood variables possible. In some cases, urine and saliva specimens are appropriate alternatives to using blood for analyzing hormone levels. Even when advanced technology is not available, circadian rhythms can be determined for variables such as temperature, heart rate, blood pressure, and urinary output with the standard equipment usually available in all hospitals, ambulatory centers, and nursing homes.

In the community setting, ambulatory temperature, blood pressure, heart rate, and activity systems have been used to study these variables in children and adults. For example, nocturnal labor onset has been reported for preterm and term deliveries.[161] Since it is possible for preterm mothers to monitor their uterine contractions with a portable tocodynamometer, the circadian rhythm of uterine contractility can be determined, and the effects of scheduling the timing of medications that suppress uterine contractility to coincide with the time of peak uterine contraction activity could be investigated.

If advanced monitoring systems are not available, patients can be taught to monitor their temperature and blood pressure and to keep logs of their activity, meals, periods of sleep, and moods. Nurses in every setting (hospital, community, nursing home) working with any type of patient (psychiatric, obstetric, medical-surgical) in any age group (neonatal to elderly) can use their knowledge of circadian rhythms to improve the care they provide. For example, a nurse specialist in geriatrics who provided health care to patients in their homes assessed the circadian rhythms of elderly patients and used that information for planning rehabilitation activities with them.[162] She reported that when she modified her usual assessment to include information about her clients' life styles and circadian rhythms, they demonstrated consistent sustained improvement in their rehabilitation. There is a need for systematic inclusion of knowledge about circadian rhythms into nursing practice and also for systematic evaluation of how practice is affected.

THERAPIES

Patients in ICU settings are often placed in situations in which time cues are minimal or absent. The unit's routines and activities may require an abrupt change in the patient's usual sleep-wake patterns and mealtimes. It is thought that these circumstances, as well as the effects of the stressors associated with the hospitalization, could lead to internal desynchronization. Measures that nurses can use to minimize circadian rhythm disorders include the prevention of sleep loss and sleep pattern irregularity and the maintenance of a regular wake-up schedule, regular eating times, and time orientation.

There are several promising new strategies being proposed or under investigation. These new treatment modalities include chronotherapy, phototherapy, diet, and medications.

Chronotherapy

Chronotherapy has been shown to be effective in treating delayed sleep phase syndrome. For example, an individual suffering from delayed sleep–onset insomnia was treated by phase shifting his rhythms. He was instructed to follow a progressive clock-hour delay of 3 hours each day until a sleep period of 11 p.m. to 7 a.m. was reached.

The adverse effects associated with shift rotation have also been found to be mitigated by the use of schedules that minimize circadian rhythm disruption. For example, rapid rotation schedules of only 1 or 2 days have been proposed, since the shift exposure to night work is insufficient to allow any rhythm change from the worker's usual sleep-activity pattern.[59] A major disadvantage of a rapid rotation schedule, however, is that people never adapt to working the night shift and that might be problematic if the work is of a critical nature. While dedicated "straight" shifts promote better adaptation to the shift-work schedule, there is an insufficient number of workers willing to work straight evening or night shifts. A more realistic chronotherapeutic method of rotating shifts would be a slow rotation (i.e., greater than 1 week but less than 5 weeks) from days to evenings to nights, resulting in a phase delay.

In addition, temporal isolation studies showed that anchor sleep (i.e., some sleep that is taken at the same time each day) was sufficient to synchronize an individual's body temperature and urinary excretion to the 24-hour day.[99] Chronotherapy could be used by nurses to try to provide a structured temporal environment for patients experiencing circadian rhythm disorders, such as patients in ICUs and patients with affective illness.

Phototherapy or Light Therapy

Phototherapy has been shown to be an effective treatment for a variety of circadian disorders. Takahashi and associates reported that the circadian pacemaker in human beings could be reset by as many as 12 hours by properly timed exposure to bright light and darkness.[163] Thus, usefulness of bright light therapy to promote adaptation in shift workers has been investigated.[164] A recent study of night workers treated for 4 days with bright light (7000 to 12,000 luxes) during the night and with darkness during the day showed that their temperature nadirs were significantly shifted to a midafternoon hour.[165] This shift was indicative of the workers' circadian adaptation to working at night and sleeping during the day. In contrast, the control group of night workers who were not exposed to light therapy continued to demonstrate temperature nadirs during the night. Light therapy is also thought to be beneficial for individuals experiencing jet lag.[166, 167]

Light therapy, alone or in combination with antidepressant medication, has been shown to be an effective treatment for seasonal affective disease.[168, 169] The exact mechanism of action of light as an antidepressant is not readily known.[170]

Diet

Ehret strongly advocates anticipatory rescheduling of rest/activity and mealtimes as time cues.[59] A schedule of meals is to be followed for 3 days prior to rotating to a new shift or travelling. The meals are planned to coincide with the new rest/activity schedule. On the first day the individual eats three large meals: breakfast and lunch are high in protein and dinner is high in carbohydrates. The next day involves fasting, with no carbohydrates allowed and other food is eaten sparingly. On the third day, the individual

again feasts on a large protein breakfast and lunch and a large carbohydrate dinner. Although this chronohygiene program has become fairly well known, more evidence is needed to support its effectiveness.

Medications

Methylxanthines such as theophylline, caffeine, and ethanol are examples of drugs known to affect the circadian clocks of lower animals by phase delays or phase advances.[59, 171] Currently, the search for pharmacological agents that can be used to reset the circadian system is in the early investigative stage.

REVIEW OF RESEARCH FINDINGS

In addition to the research cited, clinical studies are focusing on the effects of stressors such as illness, injury, and surgery on patients' circadian rhythms. For example, the circadian abnormality found in the endocrine disorder Cushing's syndrome,[172] in which the patient's cortisol levels usually do not vary but stay continuously elevated, is such a common characteristic that it is used as a diagnostic indicator.

An alteration in or lack of circadian variation in temperature has also been noted in patients with elevated brain ventricular pressure,[173] in patients with brain lesions,[65] and in head injury patients.[10, 66] For example, the temperature and heart rate rhythms of 10 patients with acute head injury were studied. Heart rate was measured every 5 minutes (288 observations per 24 hours) with a Hewlett Packard heart monitor and then transmitted to a microprocessor where it was stored for subsequent analysis. Rectal temperature was measured every 2 hours using an electronic thermometer. The data collection period ranged from 2.5 to 9 days (m = 6.5 days). The Method of Partition[174] was used to analyze the data because it was considered a rigorous test of periodicity that could handle missing data, could explain more variance within the data than the more commonly used cosinor method,[175] and did not require a prior assumption of periodicity. Only one of the 10 patients demonstrated circadian rhythms for body temperature and heart rate with peaks occurring at appropriate times. Three other patients had significant rhythms for these variables, but they were ultradian rather than circadian. No significant rhythmicity was found for the remaining six patients.[10] Limitations of this study included the inability to control for medications and treatments the patients were receiving.

Altered circadian rhythms have also been reported following different types of general surgery.[70, 176] For example, plasma cortisol rhythms were reported to be phase delayed in 10 patients undergoing general surgery. The patients were classified as undergoing minor (not requiring an abdominal incision) surgery (n = 4) and major (requiring an abdominal incision) surgery (n = 6). Two days before surgery and 2 days postoperatively blood samples were obtained every 20 minutes for 24 hours from an indwelling catheter, and patients kept logs to record stressful events during that period. Nonlinear cosinor regression analysis was used to analyze the data. The patients' cortisol circadian rhythms were found to be maintained postoperatively, but the high-trauma and low-trauma patients showed cortisol rhythm phase delays of approximately 5.5 hours and 1.5 hours, respectively.[70]

Although temperature acrophases were unchanged in 11 women who underwent abdominal surgery as compared with 10 women volunteers in the control group, phase delays were reported in their acrophases of urinary 17-ketosteroid and catecholamine metabolites.[67] Similarly, postoperative plasma cortisol circadian rhythms were also reported to be altered in 11 out of 13 coronary artery bypass graft (CABG) male patients (plasma cortisol rhythms were phase delayed in three patients and absent in eight) and in six of seven patients who underwent automatic implantable cardioverter/defibrillator (AICD) procedures (one patient exhibited a phase-delayed rhythm, and five had no cortisol circadian rhythms).[34, 35]

When the rhythms for heart rate and blood pressure were investigated in 10 cardiac transplant patients, the majority of the patients demonstrated circadian rhythms. The peak values for systolic, diastolic, and mean arterial pressures, however, were phase shifted to early morning hours, which are usually the times of low blood pressure values. In contrast, most of the patients demonstrated significant circadian heart rate rhythms with peaks occurring at the expected time of late afternoon or early evening.[36]

The influence of environmental stimuli in the ICU on the circadian rhythms of a critically ill patient on a ventilator were studied. The results showed that times of high heart rate variability were associated with times of high environmental stimuli,[69] and thus the investigators suggested that a reduction in environmental stimuli may be helpful in order to differentiate between a physiological response to external stimuli and an acute episode of physiological instability requiring treatment.

ILLUSTRATIVE CASE STUDIES

ALTERED CIRCADIAN RHYTHMS

Ms. B. F., a 55-year-old woman admitted for coronary artery bypass surgery, was anxious and unable to sleep the night before surgery. She reported getting virtually no sleep the night of surgery because of nursing interventions and very little sleep on her first 2 postoperative days. Her reports of lack of sleep were confirmed by the charting of the night nurses caring for her. Ms. B. F. reported that she was unable to sleep because of pain and that the ICU was too bright and too noisy. She also stated she has difficulty sleeping in unfamiliar surroundings. Her nurses reported that Ms. B. F. seemed reluctant to ask for pain medication. Ms. B. F. was transferred to a step-down unit on her third postoperative day. It was reported that she slept on and off that night and throughout the next day. On Ms. B. F.'s fourth postoperative day she appeared to have trouble concentrating and to be depressed. She stated she felt very tired but still had difficulty sleeping at night because of noise. She also had difficulty participating in her morning physical therapy program. In addition, her appetite was poor, and she found it even harder to eat, since the meals were served so early (i.e., 0700, 1100, and 1700 hours). She was used to eating her breakfast at 0900 hours, lunch at 1300 hours, and dinner at 1830 hours. Her participation in her morning physical therapy regimen was reported to be minimal.

Ms. B. F.'s sleep history indicated that she had been used to going to bed at 2400 hours and awakening at 0800 hours. She needs a dark, quiet room to be able to sleep and 8 hours of sleep to feel rested. When asked when she usually felt most mentally and physically alert, she specified the afternoon.

The brightness of Ms. B. F.'s room in the ICU and the noise were environmental factors that are under the control of nurses. Her early reluctance to ask for pain medication was related to her misperception that she shouldn't ask for pain medication unless her pain became unbearable. The nurses could have assessed her pain and her knowledge of the importance of requesting pain medication before her pain became severe.

Although it is unknown whether rhythm disturbances were affecting this patient's recovery, significant changes did occur in her sleep-wake pattern. Ms. B. F. was transferred to a private room on her fifth postoperative day. She reported that she had very little pain or discomfort. Plans were made so that she would not be bothered before 8 a.m. so that she could return to her regular wake-up time. The dietitian visited the patient, and a compromise was negotiated so that the timing of her meals adhered more closely to her usual schedule. Physical therapy was contacted, and Ms. B. F.'s therapy time was changed to the afternoon. Prior to discharge 3 days later, Ms. B. F. reported that she was sleeping much better, was more active, and had an improved appetite.

DELAYED SLEEP ONSET PHENOMENON

Dave, a 22-year-old college student, was in an automobile accident as a result of falling asleep at the wheel. He was admitted with a broken arm and slight concussion. During his history and physical he reported that he had a chronic problem with being unable to sleep until 3 or 4 a.m. When he had school the next day, he had difficulty waking up in time to make his 8 a.m. class. He also reported that he has felt extremely tired, fatigued, and irritable throughout the semester. In addition, he said that he had trouble concentrating on his courses and had fallen asleep during class several times. During his mid-semester break, when he worked an evening shift and didn't have to wake up early, he stated he had no

difficulty sleeping. While in the hospital, he was given a referral to the sleep disorders clinic, where he was diagnosed as having DSPS insomnia. He underwent a chronotherapeutic phase-shift regimen in which he began a progressive clock-hour delay of 3 hours per day until a sleep period of 11 p.m to 7 a.m. was reached. During the therapy, he was instructed to maintain a lights on-and-off schedule that coincided with the phase-shift program. He eventually established a regular sleep-wake schedule and no longer had difficulties falling asleep at night or waking up in the morning. His concentration improved, and he reported that he was doing well in his classes.

IMPLICATIONS FOR RESEARCH

Because nurses deliver around-the-clock care, they have many reasons and opportunities to play an important role in biological rhythm research. The number of nurses doing circadian rhythm and sleep research is increasing, but more nurse researchers are needed. Many questions need answers. Some examples of questions for future research include the following:

1. How are patient's circadian rhythms affected by illness?
2. How do stressors such as the uncertainty of diagnosis, surgery, and pain associated with hospitalization affect patient's rhythms?
3. If the patient's rhythms are desynchronized by illness or a treatment regimen, does the return to a normal pattern hasten recovery?
4. What interventions help prevent desynchronization of circadian rhythms during the patient's hospitalization, especially while in ICUs?
5. Would circadian rhythms of maternal origin for heart rate, respiratory movement, and rest/activity, which are usually detectable in the fetus, be present in situations in which the mother is drug addicted? What effects would the mother's drug use have on the baby's circadian rhythm development?
6. What circadian rhythm changes associated with aging and gender are amendable to interventions?

7. Will utilizing knowledge of the patient's performance (mental and physical) rhythms significantly affect the outcomes of education programs and physical therapy?

REFERENCES

1. Kabat, H.F. (1981). Circadian rhythms and drug dosing. In C.A. Walker, C.M. Winget, & K.F.A. Soliman (eds.), *Chronopharmacology and Chronotherapeutics* (p. 10). Tallahassee: Florida A & M University Foundation.
2. Aschoff, J. (1965). Circadian rhythms in man. Science *148*:1427–1432.
3. Moore-Ede, M.C., Czeisler, C.A., & Richardson, G.S. (1983). Circadian timekeeping in health and disease. Part II. Clinical implications of circadian rhythmicity. N Engl J Med *309*:530–536.
4. Lanuza, D.M., & Marotta, S.F. (1976). Circadian and basal interrelationships of plasma cortisol and cations in women. Aerospace Med *45*:864–868.
5. Felton, G. (1987). Human biologic rhythms. Annu Rev Nurs Res *5*:45–77.
6. Luce, C.G. (1970). *Biological Rhythms in Psychiatry* (Public Health Service Publication No. 2088). Rockville, MD: National Institute of Mental Health.
7. Wehr, T.A., Sack, D., Rosenthal, N., Duncan, W., & Gillan, J.C. (1983). Circadian rhythm disturbances in manic-depressive illness. Fed Proc *42*:2809–2814.
8. Healy, D., & Williams, J.M.G. (1988). Dysrhythmia, dysphoria, and depression: The interaction of learned helplessness and circadian dysrhythmia in the pathogenesis of depression. Psychol Bull *103*:163–178.
9. Moore-Ede, M.C., Czeisler, C.A., & Richardson, G.S. (1983). Circadian timekeeping in health and disease. Part I. Recent advances in characterizing the properties of hypothalamic circadian pacemakers. N Engl J Med *309*:469–476.
10. Lanuza, D.M., Robinson, C.A., Marotta, S.F., & Patel, M.K. (1989). Body temperature and heart rate rhythms in acutely head-injured patients. Appl Nurs Res *2*:135–139.
11. Moore-Ede, M.C. (1981). Hypothermia: A timing disorder of circadian thermoregulatory rhythms? In R.S. Posos (ed.), *The Nature and Treatment of Hypothermia*. Minneapolis: University of Minnesota Press.
12. Rosenberg, R.S. (1984). Aging and biological rhythms: Complaints of insomnia in the elderly. In E. Hans & H. Kabat (eds.), *Chronobiology 1982–1988* (pp. 345–349). Paris: S. Karger.
13. Smolensky, M.H., & D'Alonzo, G.E. (1988). Biologic rhythms and medicine. Am J Med *85*:34–36.
14. Van Gool, W.A., & Mirmiran, M. (1986). Aging and circadian rhythms. Prog Brain Res *70*:255–277.
15. Bellastella, A., Criscuolo, T., Sinisi, A.A., Iorio, S., Sinisi, A.M., Rinaldi, A., & Faggiano, M. (1986). Circannual variations of plasma testosterone, luteinizing hormone, follicle-stimulating hormone, and prolactin in Klinefelter's syndrome. Neuroendocrinology *42*:153–157.
16. Conroy, R.T.W.L., & Mills, J.N. (1970). *Human Circadian Rhythms*. London: J. & A. Churchill.
17. Campbell, I.T., Minors, D.S., & Waterhouse, J.M. (1986). Are circadian rhythms important in intensive care? Intensive Care Nurs *1*:144–150.
18. Czeisler, C.A., Kronauer, R.E., Allan, J.S., Duffy, J.F., Jewett, M.E., Brown, E.N., & Ronda, J.M. (1989). Bright light induction of strong (type O) resetting of the human circadian pacemaker. Science *244*:1328–1333.
19. Wever, R.A. (1979). *The Circadian System of Man: Results of Experiments under Temporal Isolation*. New York: Springer Verlag.
20. Moore-Ede, M.C., Sulzman, F.M., & Fuller, C.A. (1982). Circadian timing of physiological systems. In M.C. Moore-Ede, F.M. Sulzman, & C.A. Fuller (eds.), *The Clocks that Time Us* (pp. 201–317). Cambridge: Harvard University Press.
21. Wever, R.A. (1984). Toward a mathematical model of circadian rhythmicity. In M.C. Moore-Ede & C.A. Czeisler (eds.), *Mathematical Models of the Circadian Sleep-Wake Cycle* (pp. 17–79). New York: Raven Press.
22. Folkard, S., Minors, D.S., & Waterhouse, J.M. (1985). Chronobiology and shiftwork: Current issues and trends. Chronobiologia *12*:31–34.
23. Eastman, C. (1984). Are separate temperature and activity oscillators necessary to explain the phenomena of human circadian rhythms? In M.C. Moore-Ede & C.A. Czeisler (eds.), *Mathematical Models of the Circadian Sleep-Wake Cycle* (pp. 81–103). New York: Raven Press.
24. Lund, R. (1974). Personality factors and desynchronization of circadian rhythms. Psychosom Med *36*:224–228.
25. Weitzman, E.D., Czeisler, C.A., Coleman, R.M., Spielman, A.J., Zimmerman, J.C., Dement, W.C., Richardson, G.S., & Pollak, C.P. (1981). Delayed sleep phase syndrome: A chronobiologic disorder with sleep onset insomnia. Arch Gen Psychiatry *38*:737–746.
26. Anders, T.F. (1982). Biological rhythms in development. Psychosom Med *44*:61–72.
27. Weitzman, E.D., Moline, M.L., Czeisler, C.A., & Zimmerman, J.C. (1982). Chronobiology of aging: Temperature, sleep-wake rhythms and entrainment. Neurobiol Aging *3*:299–309.
28. Healy, D., & Waterhouse, J.M. (1990). The circadian system and affective disorders: Clocks or rhythms? Chronobiol Int 7:5–10.
29. Lewy, A.J. (1990). Reply to Healy, D., & Waterhouse, J.M.: The circadian system and affective disorders: Clocks or rhythms? Chronobiologic disorders, social cues and the light-dark cycle. Chronobiol Int 7:15–24.
30. Wehr, T.A. (1990). Reply to Healy, D., & Waterhouse, J.M.: The circadian system and affective disorders: Clocks or rhythms? Chronobiol Int 7:11–14.
31. Mirmiran, M., Swaab, D.F., Witting, W., Honnebier, M.B.O.M., van Gool, W.A., & Eikelenboom, P. (1989). Biological clocks in development, aging, and Alzheimer's Disease. Brain Dysfunction *2*:57–66.
32. Otsuka, A., Mikami, H., Katahira, K., Nagamoto, Y., Minamitani, K., Imaoka, M., Nishide, M., & Ogihara, T. (1990). Absence of nocturnal fall in blood pressure in elderly persons with Alzheimer-type dementia. J Am Geriatr Soc *38*:973–978.
33. Witting, W., Kwa, I.H., Eikelenboom, P., Mirmiran, M., & Swaab, D.F. (1990). Alterations in cir-

cadian rest-activity rhythm in aging and Alzheimer's disease. Biol Psychiatry 27:563–572.
34. Lanuza, D.M. (1988). Plasma cortisol changes
associated with implantation of the automatic
cardioverter/defibrillator. Circulation 78 (Suppl.
II):II-2.
35. Lanuza, D.M. (1989). The effects of two types of
cardiac surgery on plasma cortisol levels and its
circadian rhythm. Proceedings of 13th Annual
Midwest Nursing Research Society Conference—
Nursing Research: Impact on Social Issues (p. 2).
Cincinnati, Ohio.
36. Lanuza, D.M., Grady, K., Grusk, B., & Johnson,
M. (1991). Blood pressure and heart rate circadian
rhythm changes post cardiac transplantation. (Abstract). Circulation 84 (Suppl. II):II-695.
37. Danchik, K.M., Schoenborn, C.A., & Elison, J., Jr.
(1979). Basic data from Wave I of the National
Survey of Personal Health Practice and Consequences: United States (DHHS publication No.
(PHS) 81–1162). Hyattsville, MD: Public Health
Services.
38. Felton, G. (1976). Body rhythm effects on rotating
work shifts. Nurs Digest 4:29–32.
39. Thiss-Evenson, E. (1969). Shift work and health.
In A. Swensson (ed.), Proceedings of the International
Symposium on Night Shift Work (pp. 81–83). Stockholm: National Institute of Occupational Health.
40. Moore-Ede, M.C., & Richardson, G.S. (1985).
Medical implications of shiftwork. Annu Rev Med
36:607–617.
41. Bruusgaard, A. (1969). Shiftwork as an occupational health problem. In A. Swensson (ed.), Proceedings of the International Symposium on Night and
Shift Work (pp. 9–14). Stockholm: National Institute of Occupational Health.
42. Hakkinen, S. (1969). Adaptability to shift work. In
A. Swensson (ed.)., Proceedings of the International
Symposium on Night and Shift Work (pp. 68–80).
Stockholm: National Institute of Occupational
Health.
43. Akerstedt, T. (1987). Sleep/work disturbances in
working life. In E.J. Ellingson, N.M.F. Murray, &
A.M. Halliday (eds.), The London Symposia (EEG
Suppl. 39, pp. 360–363). Limerick, Ireland: Elsevier Science.
44. Taub, J.M., & Berger, R.J. (1973). Performance
and mood following variations in the length and
timing of sleep. Soc Psychophysiol Res 10:559–
570.
45. Akerstedt, T. (1985). Shifted sleep hours. Ann Clin
Res 17:273–279.
46. Kerhoff, G. (1985). Individual differences in circadian rhythms. In S. Folkard & T.H. Monk (eds.),
Hours of Work, Temporal Factors in Work-Scheduling
(pp. 29–36). New York: John Wiley.
47. Harma, M., Knauth, P., Ilmarinen, J., & Ollila, H.
(1990). The relation of age to the adjustment of
the circadian rhythms of oral temperature and
sleepiness to shift work. Chronobiol Int 7:227–
233.
48. Campbell, S.S., Gillin, J.C., Kripke, D.F., Eriksen,
P., & Clopton, P. (1989). Gender differences in the
circadian temperature rhythms of healthy elderly
subjects: Relationships to sleep quality. Sleep
12:529–536.
49. Ostberg, O. (1973). Interindividual differences in
circadian fatigue patterns of shift workers. Br J
Ind Med 30:341–351.
50. Froberg, J., Karlsson, C.-G., Levi, L., & Seeman,
K. (1969). Circadian rhythms in catecholamine
excretion, psychomotor performance, and ratings
of stress and fatigue during a 75-hour vigil. In A.
Swensson (ed.), Proceedings of the International Symposium on Night and Shift Work (pp. 64–67). Stockholm: National Institute of Occupational Health.
51. Reinberg, A., Motohashi, Y., Bourdeleau, P., Touitou, Y., Nouguier J., Nouguier, J., Levi, F., &
Nicolai, A. (1989). Internal desynchronization of
circadian rhythms and tolerance of shift work.
Chronobiologia 16:21–34.
52. Kleitman, N., & Ramsaroop, A. (1948). Periodicity
in body temperature and heart rate. Endocrinology
43:1–20.
53. Lanuza, D.M. (1976). Circadian rhythms of mental
efficiency and performance. Nurs Clin North Am
11:583–594.
54. Folkard, S. (1990). Circadian performance
rhythms: Some practical and theoretical implications. Philos Trans R Soc Lond [Biol] B327:543–
553.
55. Colquhoun, W.P. (1971). Circadian rhythms in
mental efficiency. In W.P. Colquhoun (ed.), Biological Rhythms and Human Performance (pp. 39–107).
New York: Academic Press.
56. Brown, R.C. (1949). The day and night performance of teleprinter switch board operations. Occup
Psychol 23:1–6.
57. Bjerner, B., Holm, A., & Swensson, A. (1955).
Diurnal variation in mental performance. A study
of three-shift workers. Br J Ind Med 12:103–110.
58. Harris, W. (1977). Fatigue, circadian rhythm, and
truck accidents. In R. Mackie (ed.), Vigilance Therapy, Operational Performance, and Physiological Correlates (pp. 133–146). New York: Plenum Press.
59. Ehret, C.F. (1981). New approaches to chronohygiene for the shift worker in the nuclear power
industry. In A. Reinberg, N. Vieux, & T. Andlauer
(eds.), Night- and Shift-Work. Biological and Social
Aspects (pp. 263–270). Oxford: Pergamon Press.
60. Gander, P., Myhre, G., Graeber, R.C., Andersen,
H.T., & Lauber, J.K. (1989). Adjustment of sleep
and the circadian temperature rhythm after flights
across nine time zones. Aviat Space Environ Med
60:733–743.
61. Samel, A., Wegmann, H.M., Summa, W., & Nau-
mann, M. (1991). Sleep patterns in aircrew operating on the polor route between Germany and
East Asia. Aviat Space Environ Med 62:661–669.
62. Graeber, R.C., Dement, W.C., Nicholson, A.N.,
Sasak, M., & Wegmann, H. (1986). International
cooperative study of aircrew layover sleep: Operational summary. Aviat Space Environ Med
57(Suppl.):B10–13.
63. Klein, K.E., Wegmann, H., Athanassenas, G.,
Hohlweck, H., & Kuklinski, P. (1976). Air operations and circadian performance rhythms. Aviat
Space Environ Med 47:221–230.
64. Moore-Ede, M.C. (1983). The circadian timing
system in mammals: Two pacemakers preside over
many secondary oscillators. Fed Proc 42:2801–
2808.
65. Dauch, W.A., & Bauer, S. (1990). Circadian
rhythms in the body temperatures of intensive care
patients with brain lesions. J Neurol Neurosurg
Psychiatry 53:345–347.
66. Okawa, M., Takahashi, K., & Sasaki, H. (1986).
Disturbance of circadian rhythms in severely brain-

damaged patients correlated with CT findings. J Neurol *233*:274–282.

67. Farr, L.A., Campbell-Grossman, C., & Mack, J.M. (1988). Circadian disruption and surgical recovery. Nurs Res *37*:170–175.

68. Farr, L., Keene, A., Samson, D., & Michael, A. (1984). Alterations in circadian excretion of urinary variables and physiological indicators of stress following surgery. Nurs Res *33*:140–146.

69. Felver, L., & Pike, R. (1990). Relationship of heart rate, respiratory rate, and arterial blood pressure rhythms in a mechanically ventilated patient to environmental variables in an intensive care unit. In D.K. Hayes, J.E. Pauly, & R.J. Reiter (eds.), *Chronobiology: Its role in Clinical Medicine, General Biology, and Agriculture. Part A—Progress in Clinical and Biological Research* (Vol 341A). New York: John Wiley.

70. McIntosh, T.K., Lothrop, D.A., Lee, A., Jackson, B.T., Nabseth, D., & Egdahl, R.H. (1981). Circadian rhythm of cortisol is altered in postsurgical patients. J Clin Endocrinol Metabol *53*:117–122.

71. Campbell, I.T., Bell, C.F., Minors, D.S., & Waterhouse, J.M. (1983). A preliminary study of body temperature rhythms in intensive care [Abstract]. Chronobiologia *10*:114.

72. Easton, C., & MacKenzie, F. (1988). Sensory perpetual alterations: Delirium in the intensive care unit. Heart Lung *17*:229–235.

73. Keep, P., James, J., & Inman, M. (1980). Windows in the intensive therapy unit. Anesthesia *35*:257–262.

74. Czeisler, C.A., Richardson, G.S., Coleman, R.M., Zimmerman, J.C., Moore-Ede, M.C., Dement, W.C., & Weitzman, E.D. (1981). Chronotherapy: Resetting the circadian clocks of patients with delayed sleep phase insomnia. Sleep *4*:1–21.

75. Goodwin, F.K., Wirz-Justice, A., & Wehr, T. (1982). Evidence that the pathophysiology of depression and the mechanism of action of antidepressant drugs involve alterations in circadian rhythms. Adv Biochem Pharmacol *31*:1–11.

76. Sachar, E., Hellman, L., Roffwarg, H., Halpern, F., Fukushima, D., & Gallagher, T. (1973). Disrupted 24 hour pattern of cortisol secretion in psychotic depression. Arch Gen Psychiatry *28*:19–24.

77. Beck-Friis, J., Lyungren, J.G., Thoren, M., von Rosen, D., Kjellman, B.F., & Wetter, L. (1985). Melatonin, cortisol, and ACTH in patients with manic-depressive disorder and healthy humans with special reference to the outcome of the dexamethasone suppression test. Psychoneuroendocrinology *10*:173–186.

78. Weeke, A., & Weeke, J. (1980). The 24 hour pattern of serum TSH in patients with endogenous depression. Acta Psychiatrica Scand *62*:69–74.

79. Beersma, D.G., van den Hoofdakker, R.H., & Van Berkestijn, H.W. (1983). Circadian rhythms in affective disorders: Body temperature and sleep physiology in endogenous depressives. Adv Biol Psychiatry *11*:114–117.

80. Avery, D.H., Wildschlodtz, G., & Rafaelson, O.J. (1982). Nocturnal temperature in affective disorders. J Affect Disord *4*:61–71.

81. Checkley, S. (1989). The relationship between biological rhythms and affective disorders. In J. Arendt, D.S. Minors, & J.M. Waterhouse (eds.), *Biological Rhythms in Clinical Practice* (pp. 160–183). London: Wright.

82. Wever, R.A. (1985). Internal interactions within the human circadian system: The masking effect. Experientia *41*:332–342.

83. Halberg, F. (1968). Physiological considerations underlying rhythmometry with special reference to emotional illness. In J.A. Juriaguerra (ed.), *Cycles Biologiques et Psychiatrie*. Paris: Georg, Geneve, & Masson.

84. Kripke, D.F., Mullaney, D.J., Atkinson, M., & Wolf, S. (1978). Circadian rhythm disorders in manic-depressives. Biol Psychiatry *13*:335–351.

85. Mortola, J.F., Lieu, J.H., Gillin, J.C., Rasmussen, D.D., & Yen, S.S.C. (1987). Pulsatile rhythms of adrenocorticotropin (ACTH) and cortisol in women with endogenous depression: Evidence of increased ACTH pulse frequency. J Clin Endocrinol Metab *65*:962–968.

86. Rubin, T.R., Poland, R.E., Lesser, I.M., Winston, R.A., & Blodget, A.L.N.I. (1987). Cortisol secretory dynamics in patients and matched control subjects. Arch Gen Psychiatry *44*:328–336.

87. Sack, D.A., Duncan, W., Rosenthal, N.E., Mendelson, W.B., & Wehr, T.A. (1988). The timing and duration of sleep in partial sleep deprivation theory of depression. Acta Psychiatr Scand *77*:219–224.

88. Lewy, A.J., Sack, R.L., Miller, L.S., & Hobun, T.M. (1987). Anti-depressant and circadian phase-shifting of light. Science *235*:352–354.

89. Lieberman, H., Wurtman, J.J., & Teicher, M.H. (1989). Circadian rhythms in healthy young and elderly humans. Neurobiol Aging *10*:259–265.

90. Sherman, B., Wysham, C., & Pfohl, B. (1985). Age related changes in the circadian rhythm of plasma cortisol in man. J Clin Endocrinol Metab *6*:439–443.

91. Haus, R., Nicolau, G., Lakatua, D.J., Sackett-Lundeen, L., & Petrescu, E. (1989). Circadian rhythm parameters of endocrine functions in elderly subjects during the seventh to the ninth decade of life. Chronobiologia *16*:331–352.

92. Swoyer, J., Irvine, P., Sackett-Lundeen, L., Conlin, L., LaKatua, D.J., & Haus, E. (1989). Circadian hematologic time structure in the elderly. Chronobiol Int *6*:131–137.

93. Touitou, Y., Sulon, J., Bodan, A., Touitou, C., Reinberg, A., Beck, H., Sodoyez, J-C., Demey-Ponsart, E., & Van Cauwenberge, H. (1982). Adrenal circadian system in young and elderly human subjects: A comparative study. J Endocrinol *93*:201–210.

94. Lobban, M.C. (1960). The entrainment of circadian rhythms in man. Cold Spring Harb Symp Quant Biol *25*:325–332.

95. Woolman, M., Lavie, P., & Peled, R. (1985). A hypernychthemeral sleep-wake syndrome: A treatment attempt. Chronobiol Int *2*:277–280.

96. Minors, D.S., & Waterhouse J.M. (1981). *Circadian Rhythms and the Human*. Littleton, MA: John Wright PSG.

97. Honnebier, M.B.O.M., Swaab, D.F., & Mirmiran, M. (1989). Diurnal rhythmicity during early human development. In S.M. Reppert (ed.), *Development of Circadian Rhythmicity and Photoperiodism in Mammals*. Ithaca, NY: Perinatology Press.

98. Aschoff, J. (1979). Circadian rhythms: General features and endocrinological aspects. In D.T.

Krieger (ed.), *Endocrine Rhythms* (pp. 1–61). New York: Raven Press.

99. Minors, D.S., & Waterhouse, J.M. (1981). Circadian rhythms in infancy. In J.A. Davis & J. Dobbins (eds.), *Scientific Foundations of Paediatrics* (2nd ed.) London: Heinemann.

100. Rietveld, W.M. (1990). The current control and ontogeny of circadian rhythmicity. Eur J Morphol 28:301–307.

101. Hellbrugge, T. (1960). The development of circadian rhythms in infants. Cold Spring Harb Symp Quant Biol 25:311–323.

102. Abe, K., Sasaki, H., Takebayashi, K., Fukui, S., & Nambu, H. (1978). The development of circadian rhythm of human body temperature. J Interdisciplinary Cycle Res 9:211–216.

103. Hellbrugge, T., Lange, J.E., Rutenfranz, J., & Stehr, K. (1964). Circadian periodicity of physiological functions in different stages of infancy and childhood. Ann NY Acad Sci 117:361–373.

104. Zurbruegg, R.P. (1976). Hypothalamic-pituitary-adrenocortical regulation: A contribution to its assessment, development and disorders in infancy and childhood with special reference to plasma cortisol circadian rhythm. Monogr Pediatr 17: 12–17.

105. Updike, P.A., Accurso, F.J., & Jones, R.H. (1985). Physiologic circadian rhythmicity in preterm infants. Nurs Res 34:160–163.

106. Mirmiran, M., Kok, J.H., de Kleine, M.J.K., Koppe, J.G., Overdijk, J., & Witting, W. (1990). Circadian rhythms in preterm infants: A preliminary study. Early Human Dev 32:139–146.

107. Thomas, K. (1991). The emergence of body temperature biorhythm in preterm infants. Nurs Res 40:98–102.

108. Lentz, M. (1990). Times-series-issues in sampling. West J Nurs Res 12:123–128.

109. Franks, R. (1967). Diurnal variation of plasma 17-hydroxy-corticosteroids in children. J Clin Endocrinol Metab 27:75–78.

110. Vermes, I., Dohanics, J., Toth, G., & Pongracz, J. (1980). Maturation of the circadian rhythm of the adrenocortical functions in human neonates and infants. Horm Res 12:237–244.

111. Onishi, S., Miyazawa, G., Nishimura, Y., Sugeyama, S., Yamahawa, T., Inagaki, H., Katoh, S., Itah, U., & Isobe, K. (1983). Postnatal development of circadian rhythm serum cortisol levels in children. Pediatrics 72:399–404.

112. Price, D.A., Close, G.C., & Felding, B.A. (1983). Age of appearance of circadian rhythms in salivary cortisol values in infants. Arch Dis Child 58:454–456.

113. Spangler, G. (1991). The emergence of adrenocortical function in newborns and infants and its relationship to sleep, feeding, and maternal adrenocortical activity. Early Human Dev 25:197–208.

114. Taylor, A., Lorenz, R., Turner, B., Ronneklein, O., Casady, R., & Branch, B. (1976). Factors influencing pituitary-adrenal rhythmicity: Its ontogeny and circadian variations in stress responsiveness. Psychoneuroendocrinology 1:291–301.

115. Naumenko, E.V., Markel, A.L., Laurie, S.B., & Kazin, E.M. (1985). Circadian adrenocortical periodicity changes in adult rats stimulated during early development—I. Effect of prednisolone. Chronobiol Int 2:243–251.

116. Grossman, D.G.S. (1991). Circadian rhythms in blood pressure in school-age children of normotensive and hypertensive parents. Nurs Res 40:28–34.

117. Halberg, F., Halberg, E., Halberg, J., & Halberg, F. (1984). Chronobiologic assessment of human blood pressure variation in health and disease. In M. Weber & J.I.M. Drayer (eds.), *Ambulatory Blood Pressure Monitoring* (pp. 13–156). New York: Springer Verlag.

118. Rabatin, J.S., Sothern, R.B., Brunning, R.D., Goetz, F.C., & Halberg, F. (1981). Circadian rhythms in blood and self-measured variables in ten children 9 to 14 years of age. In F. Halberg, L.W. Scheving, E.W. Powell, & D.K. Hayes (eds.), *Chronobiology, Proceedings of XIII International Conference, International Society for Chronobiology* (pp. 373–385). Milan: Il Ponte.

119. Scarpelli, P.T., Romano, S., Cagnoni, M., Livi, R., Scarpelli, L., Bigioli, F., Corti, C., Croppi, E., De Scalzi, M., Halberg, J., Halberg, E., & Halberg, F. (1985). The Florence children's blood pressure study: A chronobiologic approach by multiple measurements. Clin Exp Hypertens 1:355–359.

120. Casals, G., & deNicola, P. (1984). Circadian rhythms in the aged: A review. Arch Gerontol Geriatr 3:267–284.

121. Czeisler, C., Rios, C., & Sanchez, R. (1986). Phase advance and reduction in the amplitude of the endogenous circadian oscillator correspond with systematic changes in sleep-wake habits and daytime functioning in the elderly. Sleep 15:268.

122. Vitello, M., Smallwood, R., Avery, D., Pascualy, R., Martin, D., & Prinz, P. Circadian temperature rhythms in young adult and aged men. Neurobiol Aging 7:97–100.

123. Guite, H.F., Biss, M.R., Mainwaring-Burton, R.W., Thomas, J.M., & Drury, P.L. (1988). Hypothesis: Posture is one of the determinants of the circadian rhythm of urine flow and electrolyte excretion in elderly female patients. Age Aging 17:241–248.

124. Aschoff, J., & Wever, R. (1976). A multioscillatory system. Fed Proc 35:2326–2332.

125. Moore, R.Y. (1983). Organization and function of a central nervous system circadian oscillator: The suprachiasmatic hypothalamic nucleus. Fed Proc 42:2783–2789.

126. Wever, R. (1975). The circadian multi-oscillator system of man. Int J Chronobiol 3:19–55.

127. Moore-Ede, M.C., Schmelzer, W.S., Kass, D.A., & Herd, J.A. (1976). Internal organization of the circadian timing system in multicellular animals. Fed Proc 35:2333–2338.

128. Wever, R. (1983). Fractional desynchronization of human circadian rhythms. A method of evaluating entrainment limits and function in dependencies. Pflugers Arch 395:128–137.

129. Rusak, B., & Zucker, I. (1979). Neural regulation of circadian rhythms. Physiol Rev 59:449–527.

130. Stephan, F.K., & Zucker, I. (1972). Circadian rhythms in drinking behavior and locomotor activity of rats are eliminated by hypothalamic lesions. Proc Natl Acad Sci USA 69:1583–1586.

131. Moore, R.Y., & Eichler, V.B. (1972). Loss of circadian adrenal corticosterone rhythm following suprachiasmatic lesions in the rat. Brain Res 42:201–206.

132. Fuller, C.A., Lydic, R., Sulzman, F.M., Albers, H.E., Tepper, B., & Moore-Ede, M.C. (1981). Circadian rhythm of body temperature persists after

superchiasmatic lesions in the squirrel monkey. Am J Physiol *241*: R385–R391.

133. Ibuka, N. (1979). Suprachiasmatic nucleus and sleep-wakefulness rhythms. In M. Suda & O. Hayaishi (eds.), *Biological Rhythms and Their Central Mechanism* (pp. 325–334). Amsterdam: Elsevier-North Holland Biomedical Press.

134. Kafka, M.S., Wirz-Justice, A., Naber, D., Moore, R.Y., & Benedito, M.A. (1983). Circadian rhythms in rat brain neurotransmitter receptors. Fed Proc *42*:2796–2801.

135. Armstrong, S.M. (1989). Melatonin and circadian control in mammals. Experientia *45*:932–945.

136. Haus, E., Lakatua, D., & Halberg, F. (1967). The internal timing of several circadian rhythms in the blinded mouse. Exp Med Surg *25*:7–45.

137. Kawamura, H., & Inouye, S.T. (1979). Circadian rhythm in a hypothalamic island containing the suprachiasmatic nucleus. In M. Suda & O. Hayaishi (eds.), *Biological Rhythms and Their Central Mechanisms* (pp. 335–341). Amsterdam: Elsevier-North Holland Biomedical Press.

138. Ralph, M.R., Foster, R.G., Davis, F.C., & Menaker, M. (1990). Transplanted suprachiasmatic nucleus determines circadian period. Science *247*:975–978.

139. Nakayama, T., Arai, S., & Yamamoto, K. (1979). Body temperature and its central mechanism. In M. Suda & O. Hayaishi (eds.), *Biological Rhythms and Their Central Mechanisms* (pp. 395–403). Amsterdam: Elsevier-North Holland Biomedical Press.

140. Reppert, S.M., Perlow, M.J., Ungerleider, L.R., Mishkin, M., Tamarkin, L., Orloff, D.G., Hoffmann, H.J., & Klein, D.C. (1981). Effects of damage to the suprachiasmatic area of the anterior hypothalamus on the daily melatonin and cortisol rhythms in the rhesus monkey. J Neurosci *1*:1414–1425.

141. Halberg, F., & Howard, R.B. (1958). 24-hour periodicity and experimental medicine: Examples and interpretations. Postgrad Med *24*:349–358.

142. Halberg, F., Johnson, E., Brown, B.W., & Bittner, J.J. (1960). Susceptibility rhythm to *E. coli* endotoxin and bioassay. Proc Soc Exp Biol Med *103*:142–144.

143. Reinberg, A., Smolensky, M., Labrecque, G., & Hallek, M. (1987). Aspects of chronopharmacology and chronotherapy in children. Chronobiologia *14*:303–323.

144. Feigin, R.D., San Joaquin, V.H., Haymond, M.W., & Wyatt, R.G. (1969). Daily periodicity of the susceptibility of mice to pneumococcal infection. Nature *224*:379–380.

145. Reinberg, A., Sidi, E., & Ghata, J. (1965). Circadian reactivity rhythms of human skin to histamine or allergen and the adrenal cycle. J Allergy *36*:273–282.

146. Reinberg, A., & Sidi, E. (1966). Circadian changes in the inhibitory effects of antihistaminic drug in man. J Invest Dermatol *46*:415–419.

147. DiRaimondo, V.C., & Forsham, P.H. (1958). Pharmacologic principles in the use of corticoids and adrenocorticotropin. Metabolism *7*:5–24.

148. Smolensky, M.H., McGovern, P., Scott, P.H., & Reinberg, A. (1987). Chronobiology and asthma. II. Body-time dependent differences in the kinetics and effects of bronchodilator medications. J Asthma *24*:91–134.

149. Reinberg, A., Ghata, J., Halberg, F., Apfelbaum, M., Gervais, P., Boudon, P., Abulker, C., & Du-

pont, J. (1976). Treatment schedules modify circadian timing in human adrenocortical insufficiency. In L.E. Scheving, F. Halbert, & J.E. Pauly (eds.), *Chronobiology* (pp. 168–173). Tokyo: Igaku Shoin, Ltd.

150. Dethlefsen, U, & Repges, R. (1985). Ein neues Therapieprinzip bei nachtlichem Asthma. Med Klin *80*:44–47.

151. Reinberg, A., Guillet, P., Gervaise, P., Ghata, J., Vignaud, D., & Abulker, C. (1977). One month chronocorticotherapy (Dutimelan, 8–15 mite). Control of the asthmatic condition without adrenal suppression and circadian rhythm alteration. Chronobiologia *4*:295–312.

152. Smolensky, M.H. (1983). Aspects of human chronopathology. In A. Reinberg & M.H. Smolensky (eds.), *Biological Rhythms and Medicine* (pp. 131–209). New York: Springer-Verlag.

153. Muller, J.E., Stone, P.H., Turi, Z.G., Rutherford, J.D., Czeisler, C.A., Parker, C., Poole, W.K., Passamani, E., Roberts, R., Robertson, T., Sobel, B.E., Willerson, J.T., Braunwald, E., & the MILIS study group. (1985). Circadian variation in the frequency of onset of acute myocardial infarction. N Engl J Med *313*:1315–1322.

154. Smolensky, M.H., Tatar, S.E., Bergman, S.A., Losman, J.G., Barnard, C.N., Dacso, C.C., & Kraft, I.A. (1976). Circadian rhythmic aspects of human cardiovascular function: A review by chronobiologic statistical methods. Chronobiologia *3*:337–371.

155. Yasue, H., Omote, W., Takizawa, A., Nagao, M., Miwa K., & Tanaka, S. (1979). Circadian variation of exercise capacity in patients with Prinzmetal's variant angina: Role of exercise-induced coronary arterial spasm. Circulation *59*:938–948.

156. Rosenthal, N.E., & Wehr, T.A. (1987). Seasonal affective disorders. Psychiatr Ann *17*:670–674.

157. Rosenthal, N.E. (1989). *Seasons of the Mind*. New York: Bantam Books.

158. Tom, C.K. (1976). Nursing assessment of the biological rhythms. Nurs Clin North Am *11*:621–630.

159. Horne, J.A., & Ostberg, O. (1976). A self-assessment questionnaire to determine morningness-eveningness in human circadian rhythms. Int J Chronobiol *4*:97–110.

160. Monk, T.H., & Fookson, J.E. (1986). Circadian temperature rhythm power spectra: Is equal sampling necessary? Psychophysiology *23*:472–479.

161. Cooperstock, M., England, J.E., & Wolfe, R.A. (1987). Circadian incidence of labor onset hour in preterm birth and chlorioamnionitis. Obstet Gynecol *70*:852–855.

162. Hall, L.H. (1976). Circadian rhythms: Implications for geriatric rehabilitation. Nurs Clin North Am *11*:631–638.

163. Takahashi, J.S., DeCoursey, P.J., Bauman, L., & Menaker, M. (1984). Spectral sensitivity of a novel photoreceptive system mediating entrainment of mammalian circadian rhythms. Nature *308*:186–188.

164. Eastman, C.I. (1987). Bright light in work-sleep schedules for shiftworkers: Application of circadian rhythm principles. In L. Rensing, U. van der Heiden & M.C. Mackey (eds.), *Temporal Disorder in Human Oscillatory Systems*. Berlin: Springer-Verlag.

165. Czeisler, C.A., Johnson, M.P., Duffy, J.F., Brown, E.N., Ronda, J.M., & Kronauer, R.E. (1990). Exposure to bright light and darkness to treat physi-

ologic maladaptation to night work. N Engl J Med *322*:1253–1259.

166. Daan, S., & Lewy, A.J. (1984). Scheduled exposure to daylight: A potential strategy to reduce "jet lag" following transmeridian flight. Psychopharmacol Bull *20*:566–568.

167. Czeisler, C.A., & Allan, J.S. (1987). Acute circadian phase reversal in man via bright light exposure: Application to jet-lag sleep research. Sleep Res *16*:605.

168. Biehar, M.C., & Rosenthal, N.E. (1989). Seasonal affective disorders and phototherapy. Arch Gen Psychiatry *45*:469–474.

169. Rosenthal, N.E., Sack, D.A., Skwerer, R.G., Jacobson, F.M., & Wehr, T.A. (1988). Phototherapy for seasonal affective disorder. J Biol Rhythms *3*:101–120.

170. Terman, M. (1988). On the question of mechanism in phototherapy for seasonal affective disorder: Considerations of clinical efficacy and epidemiology. J Biol Rhythms *3*:155–172.

171. Moore-Ede, M.C., Sulzman, F.M., & Fuller, C.A. (1982). A physiological system measuring time. In M.C. Moore-Ede, F.M. Sulzman, & C.A. Fuller (eds.), *The Clocks That Time Us* (pp. 1–29). Cambridge: Harvard University Press.

172. Vagnucci, A.H. (1979). Analysis of circadian periodicity of plasma cortisol in normal man and in Cushing's syndrome. Am J Physiol *236*:R268–281.

173. Page, R.B., Galicich, J.H., & Grunt, J.A. (1973). Alteration of the circadian temperature rhythm with third ventricular obstruction. J Neurosurg *38*:308–319.

174. Patel, M.K. (1987). Estimation of periodicity by Method of Partition. Paper presented at the American Statistical Association and Biometric Society Meetings. August 17–20, San Francisco, CA.

175. Tong, Y.L. (1976). Parameter estimation in studying circadian rhythms. Biometrics *32*:85–94.

176. Farr, L.A., Gaspar, T.M., & Mann, D.F. (1984). Desynchronization with surgery. In E. Haus & H.F. Kabat (eds.), *Chronobiology* (pp. 544–547). New York: Karger.

5

Anorexia

Melissa C. Behnke
Marcia Grant

DEFINITION

The association between "good appetite" and "good health" is a well-recognized clinical phenomenon. The magnitude and the satiability of the appetite, however, are subject to a wide variety of physiological, cultural, psychosocial, and environmental influences. These influences all play a role in the selection of nutrients by the individual in order to maintain normal digestive and metabolic functioning.

Food intake is primarily controlled by an individual's desire for food. When this desire for food (a normal state) is compromised or absent, an individual is said to *experience* anorexia. Anorexia may be a transient state, unassociated with significant metabolic change. The *existence* of anorexia, or loss of appetite, on more than an occasional basis, however, is descriptive of an abnormal state.

For the purposes of this chapter, anorexia is defined as a complex, primarily subjective phenomenon in which there is a loss of appetite or lack of desire to eat resulting in a spontaneous decrease in intake. Anorexia is a phenomenon that frequently occurs throughout the life cycle in a wide variety of clinical situations and disease states.

In this chapter the phenomenon of anorexia is presented from a pathophysiological perspective. The primary focus is on those clinical states in which anorexia is a major consequence.

PREVALENCE OF ANOREXIA

Anorexia and concomitant weight loss accompany innumerable disease states (both medical and psychiatric in origin), are common side effects of drug therapy (e.g., analgesics, antibiotics, digitalis preparations, and chemotherapeutic agents), and occasionally signal drug toxicity.[1] Many systemic disorders produce significant changes in nutrient intake, absorption, and metabolism that thereby result in altered nutritional status. Increased basal metabolic rate and negative nitrogen balance are common. Alterations in taste acuity, infection, emotional stress, intestinal obstruction, endocrine dysfunction, pain, and fever may precipitate and worsen anorexia.[2] Individual allergies, food intolerances, vegetarian life styles, and diabetes may also limit the variety of intake of a diet already restricted and may contribute to nutritional deficiencies. Nonspecific gastrointestinal complaints, including anorexia, account for a high percentage of the reasons individuals seek medical care in both acute and chronic conditions. Often it is the existence of anorexia or weight loss that convinces an individual of the need to seek medical care.

The "subjectiveness" of the phenomenon and the wide variety of disorders associated with anorexia make quantitative analysis of the prevalence or frequency of occurrence extremely difficult. It is estimated that approximately 40 to 50 per cent of all general medical and surgical patients admitted to the hospital have some evidence of clinically significant protein-calorie malnutrition (PCM).[3] Of these, 5 to 10 per cent suffer from severe PCM.[4] The incidence of malnutrition appears to depend primarily on the clinical setting, the lowest incidence occurring in outpatient ambulatory settings. Among elderly hospitalized patients in the acute setting, malnutrition is reported to be between 17 and 65 per cent, while institutionalized elderly have an incidence of malnutrition ranging from 26 to 59 per cent.[5] Malnutrition in the nursing home population has reached epidemic proportions. A recent survey of nursing homes in Florida reports that 58 per cent of its residents have some degree of malnutrition.[6] The percentage of these patients who become anorexic (i.e., patients who are anorexic while in a long-term care facility) and the percentage of those who have existing anorexia (i.e., patients who are anorexic prior to admission to the facility), are unreported, but this anorexia contributes to a poor nutritional state.

Many of the patients who develop clinically significant PCM enter the hospital with a history of weight loss resulting from the anorexia and increased catabolism associated with the stress of many disease states.[3] Other patients become malnourished after admission as a consequence of the catabolic stress of surgery or sepsis. Semistarvation regimens commonly used for the critically ill (e.g., 5 per cent dextrose in water) and fasting periods imposed for diagnostic tests further compromise the patient's nutritional state.

In order to accurately identify the frequency with which anorexia and nutritional deficiencies occur in the general patient population, a thorough nutritional history/ assessment as well as measurement of other clinical parameters needs to be done for all patients admitted to a hospital, nursing home, or health care agency. A preliminary evaluation of every patient seen by a physician or nurse in a health care facility will increase the likelihood of detecting the presence of anorexia or accompanying nutritional deficiencies.

"Because anorexia is a major mechanism in the current endemic of protein-energy undernutrition in hospitals in the United States, the intake of nutrients must be measured in one of three ways: by recall, by diary (outpatient), or by observation (inpatient)."[7] Without accurate measurement and meticulous recording there is no way to estimate the number of individuals experiencing anorexia or its resulting nutritional deficiencies. While measurement of nutrient intake and meticulous and accurate recording do not measure anorexia, they do serve as a rough guide in identifying the presence of the phenomenon.

SITUATIONAL STRESSORS AND POPULATIONS AT RISK

The phenomenon of anorexia affects many patient populations. There are individuals who because of the existence of various situational or developmental stressors or their responses to these stressors have an increased predisposition to anorexia. Children between 2 and 6 years of age who present with chronic ear infections and are on prolonged antibiotic therapy often develop anorexia as a result of the therapy. Adolescents often develop erratic eating patterns, which can create significant nutritional problems. The elderly are also at risk for developing anorexia owing to numerous physical and sociocultural factors associated with aging. Several disease states also predispose individuals to anorexia.

In Table 5–1 populations at risk for developing anorexia are identified in the left column. Risk factors (stressors) that place an individual in a possible high-risk category for becoming anorexic are presented in the right column. These two categories intermesh and are not all-inclusive. Many of the high-risk factors listed affect numerous high-risk groups and vice versa. Almost any patient in any clinical setting is at potential risk for being anorexic and for developing PCM. Factors that contribute to anorexia are extremely diverse and range from a disturbance in the hunger-satiety regulatory system to taste abnormalities and to a psychological reaction to disease and treatment[8] (see Chapter 14, Hunger).

DEVELOPMENTAL DIMENSIONS

Nonspecific gastrointestinal complaints are the most frequently reported disorders in childhood.[9] It is well documented that children are particularly susceptible to the anorexigenic effects of prolonged antibiotic therapy. Antibiotic-associated gastrointestinal symptoms are common in general pediatric outpatients and can account for a significant percentage of the nutritional deficiencies and diminished food intake reported in this population.[10]

Perhaps the most frequent association made by the general public with regard to anorexia is the disease anorexia nervosa. This disorder primarily affects previously healthy adolescent females in whom loss of appetite

TABLE 5–1 POPULATIONS AT HIGH RISK FOR ANOREXIA

High-Risk Populations	Stressors
Patients over 65 years	Dental/masticatory problems
	Diminished olfaction
	Unpalatable institutional diets (hospitals, nursing homes)
	Institutionalization
	Inadequate income
	Social isolation/depression
Cerebrovascular accident (CVA, or stroke)	Immobilization/bed rest
	Paresis/paralysis
	± Difficulty chewing or swallowing
Trauma/burn	Hypermetabolic state or increased basal metabolic rate (BMR)
	Decreased intake and utilization of nutrients
Septic shock	Fever, infectious processes
Cancer	Pain
Head and neck	Altered taste/odor perception
Gastrointestinal	Chemotherapy
Colorectal	Radiation therapy
Pancreatic	Social isolation
Kaposi's sarcoma (HIV-positive status)	Fatigue
	Anxiety/depression
Postoperative patients	Prolonged IV therapy
	Anesthesia
	Major surgery
Chronic disease states	
Diabetes mellitus	Insulin dependency/diet restrictions
Chronic obstructive pulmonary disease (COPD)	Dyspnea, fatigue
Renal failure	Nausea, dyspepsia
	"Bad" taste or ammonia taste in mouth
Rheumatoid arthritis	Pain
	Decreased mobility
	General malaise
	Drug side effects
	Depression
Heart disease	
Congestive heart failure (CHF)	Prolonged drug therapy (digoxin, antihistamines, diuretic agents)
Coronary artery disease (CAD)	Venous congestion and tissue edema in the gastrointestinal tract
Psychogenic disturbance	Anxiety
	Depression
	Job stress
Anorexia nervosa	Marital changes
Anorexia bulimia	Academic stress
Senile dementia	Hospitalization/change in familiar surroundings
	Illness/unknown diagnosis
	Death and fears of isolation, diagnosis, pain
Alcoholism/cirrhosis	Excessive alcohol ingestion
Advanced liver disease	Inadequate intake of proper nutrients
	Electrolyte imbalances
	Ascites
	Metabolic abnormalities
Nutritional deficiencies	Magnesium deficiency
	Copper deficiency
Alcohol/drug dependency	Zinc deficiency
	Thiamine deficiency
Hepatitis	Jaundice/increased bilirubin
Addison's disease	Underdosage of maintenance corticosteroids
Adrenal deficiencies	Hyponatremia
	Hypercalcemia

Abbreviation: HIV, human immunodeficiency virus.

or refusal to eat may lead to self-starvation and an emaciated appearance. Both physiological and psychological mechanisms are thought to play a role in the development of the disease. The onset of anorexia nervosa most commonly occurs between the ages of 13 and 25 years, and those affected are usually white females from middle-class to upper-class backgrounds (although there is evidence that the disease is increasing in men and in the elderly).[5, 11, 12] Although extreme weight loss and loss of appetite in young women lead physicians or health care workers to suspect anorexia nervosa, a wide variety of gastrointestinal tract disorders or primary intestinal diseases may mimic or accompany anorexia nervosa. Anatomical and developmental obstructions, such as intestinal malrotation and achalasia and esophageal, gastric, or duodenal webs and diaphragms, as well as ulcers, tumors, tuberculosis, and gastritis can also cause vague abdominal pain, resulting in a loss of appetite, avoidance of food, and subsequent weight loss.[13]

Suspected anorexic patients should be carefully screened for malabsorption syndromes such as celiac disease and inflammatory bowel syndrome or early Crohn's disease, as these disease processes may be very similar to anorexia nervosa. In a study by Gryboski and colleagues, three out of ten adolescent girls with anorexia and weight loss that clinically resembled anorexia nervosa proved to have Crohn's enteritis.[11] Upper gastrointestinal, small bowel, and colonic radiographs assist in making a differential diagnosis of anorexia.[14]

In addition to bowel disease, endocrine disorders must be differentiated from anorexia nervosa. Hypopituitarism, or adrenocortical insufficiency, is a possible diagnosis in young women with anorexia, weight loss, or amenorrhea.[15] The presenting complaint is usually one other than "loss of appetite." Anorectic patients show a decrease in appetite with subsequent weight loss but have little if any disturbance in body image or fear of obesity, which often accompanies the patient with anorexia nervosa.[5] Thus, assessment should include an intake evaluation as well as a thorough review of symptoms, including menstrual information to help formulate differential diagnoses and rule out physical illness.

Aging is characterized by a gradual deterioration of physiological function, which adversely affects the appetite and may result in anorexia. Numerous oral-gustatory factors hinder the elderly person's desire or ability to ingest an adequate diet. Taste buds diminish in sensitivity with advancing age, and the elderly patient may derive less pleasure from eating. Often dental problems increase with age and interfere with mastication. Ill-fitting dentures, fewer teeth, gum atrophy or disease, or inadequate salivary secretion may narrow food choices and dietary intake and result in a change in normal eating patterns. Many of the most nutritional and necessary foods, such as lean and organ meat (high in protein and iron), become difficult to chew and are eliminated from the diet and replaced with a diet high in carbohydrates, which are not only economical and easily masticated but also lead to increased gastric distention and early satiety or a sensation of fullness.[16]

The aging process also affects the physiological parameters of gastrointestinal secretion, absorption, and mobility.[17] The stomach appears to be particularly subject to structural changes due to aging. Histological abnormalities occur, resulting in a decrease in mucosal thickness and consequent atrophy.[18] There is an increasing incidence of achlorhydria, with a decline in the total volume of acid secretion in both men and women. Atrophic changes in the secreting glands of the stomach that hinder hydrochloric acid and pepsin secretion occur in approximately 80 per cent of all individuals older than 50 years of age. Diminished cellular renewal of the stomach epithelium, which normally occurs every 5 days, has also been shown.[17] Motor activity is also altered, with diminution in hunger contractions and delayed gastric emptying.[18] Presbyesophagus, delayed emptying of the esophagus, and chronic atrophic gastritis are common age-related changes that affect the desire or ability of the elderly to consume adequate calories for nutritional maintenance.[19]

Morphologically, aging of the small intestine is reflected in gut weight reduction and muscle fiber atrophy. Lipids are absorbed more slowly, and the pancreatic enzymes occur in smaller amounts, thereby affecting the absorption of amino acids and sugars.[17] Additional structural and physiological information regarding age-specific changes in the small and large intestine is scant.

Because of a diet of marginal adequacy secondary to economic or other factors, the elderly are susceptible to the negative effects of drug therapy and reduced rates of drug inactivation and excretion.[13] A careful history of temporal relationships to initiation of drug therapy is needed.

Many elderly patients report that despite maintaining usual dietary intake and exercise patterns, their weight gradually decreases. Frequently, the exact time of onset is unclear. Patients report complaints such as: "I just don't feel like eating," "My appetite seems smaller," "Food doesn't taste good," and "I have a bad taste in my mouth all the time."[13]

Possibly, decreasing mobility, visual acuity, and mental alertness may also affect dietary intake negatively. A hearing impairment can result in reluctance to converse with mealtime companions, feelings of isolation, and reduced enjoyment and intake of food.[19] Restricted financial income also limits the amount and types of food purchased. Money may be spent instead on medications, many of which adversely affect the appetite.[5]

The impact of emotional and behavioral patterns on the gastrointestinal tract is profound, frequently constituting the sole source of an individual's complaint.[18] Depression, cognitive impairment (dementia), and social isolation (feelings of alienation) are frequent causes of anorexia in the aged. In elderly depressed patients, food may lose some of its symbolism (i.e., warmth, acceptance, caring) or may be used as a weapon manifested by a subintentional death wish by refusing to eat.[6, 20] In persons aged 65 and older the incidence of significant clinical depression is 8 to 15 per cent in the general population and up to 50 per cent in nursing home populations.[21] Depression over loss of health and vigor, spouse, family, friends, and role as well as concern over changing self-image contributes to anorexia and inadequate nutrition.

It is estimated that 5 to 6 million Americans will suffer some form of dementia by the year 2000 and that currently the prevalence of dementia is 2 to 3 per cent between the ages of 65 and 79 and 20 per cent in individuals over age 80.[6, 22, 23] Many institutionalized patients are dependent on others for providing dietary intake, and often, because of a lack of time, these needs are not met.

Other contributing factors to anorexia in the aged include various disease processes, especially diabetes, heart disease, and chronic obstructive pulmonary disease (COPD). The ingestion of a variety of medications, both over-the-counter and prescribed, in addition to vitamin and mineral supplements may ultimately impair appetite and absorption, storage, and utilization of nutrients while giving a false sense of "adequate nutrition." Zinc deficiency has been shown to decrease food consumption either through abnormal regulation of appetite or through learned aversion to the deficient diet.[5]

Specific Situational Stressors

Anorexia in Patients with Liver Disease

Cirrhotic or alcoholic anorexia and weight loss are possibly a result of alterations in carbohydrate, protein, fat, and vitamin metabolism. The signs and symptoms are related to the occurrence of hepatocellular necrosis (similar to acute hepatitis) or to the complications of cirrhosis primarily as a result of the rise in intrahepatic vascular resistance leading to portal hypertension, ascites, and esophageal varices. These in turn produce jaundice, anorexia, nausea and vomiting, a sense of fullness, early satiety, and general discomfort.[24] A profound degree of anorexia usually precedes the more overt clinical manifestations in viral hepatitis. It is thought that changes in the stomach or bowel as a result of hepatitis can produce anorexia. For instance, it is possible that visceral reflexes reduce peristalsis, and anorexia, nausea, and vomiting result. The anorexia invariably subsides with morphological and biochemical evidence of hepatic improvement.[13]

Numerous mechanisms of anorexia in liver disease have been postulated. These mechanisms, as outlined by DeWys,[25] include the following: (1) a nonspecific alarm reaction to sickness may influence the central nervous system (CNS) to reduce appetite; (2) postprandial hyperglycemia associated with liver disease may signal the CNS glucostat in such a way as to reduce appetite; (3) hepatic glucoreceptors, which fire the vagus nerve in response to glucose perfusion in the liver, may be involved in anorexia; (4) liver disease may produce hypersensitivity of these hepatic glucoreceptors, and thus inappropriate messages may reach the central appetite control center and lead to anorexia; and (5) liver disease may result in amino acid imbalance in plasma, which may also lead to anorexia. In patients with cirrhosis and chronic active hepatitis, elevated levels of the amino acid tyrosine may be observed.

Anorexia in Cancer Patients

Both physiological and psychosocial factors responsible for the decline of food intake in cancer patients have been postulated (Fig. 5–1). A large number of these factors have been proposed to account for the anorexia occurring in this population.

Abnormalities in taste sensation may play a significant role in the cancer patient's reduced oral intake, or the "anorexia of malignancy." Reported abnormalities of taste sensation correlate with reduced caloric intake in cancer patients. DeWys and Walters found the detection and recognition threshold for sweet (sucrose) greater in tumor patients than in a normal control group; the symptom of meat aversion in this same group correlated with a lowered taste threshold for bitter (urea).[26–28] This lowered threshold for bitter may be related to the amino acid polypeptide and the purine content of meat, which in pure form have a bitter taste.[27] Investigators propose that elevated thresholds for salt recognition occur, particularly in colon cancer patients who undergo resection of the bowel and subsequent 5-fluorouracil therapy.[29, 30] Williams and Cohen's work,[31] in contrast to DeWys' and Walters' studies, reported that lung cancer patients experienced borderline significant reductions in taste acuity for sourness. Other taste parameters did not prove to differ significantly from normal.

The mechanism behind these taste abnormalities in cancer patients is still poorly understood. Nutritional deficiencies may play a role. Zinc, copper, nickel, niacin, and vitamin A have all been implicated in altered taste sensations.[32] Zinc deficiency has been researched most widely. Henkin and associates studied cancer patients exhibiting anorexia and hypogeusia (decreased taste acuity).[33] Of those patients studied (n = 7), all had significantly lowered serum zinc. Treatment with zinc sulfate restored normal taste.

In addition to the above factors, anorexia can be attributed to abnormalities in the metabolism of glucose and triglycerides, to the imbalance of specific plasma amino acids, to decreased insulin sensitivity, and to delayed digestion.[34]

Tumors of the head and neck (oral cavity, pharynx, esophagus) impair food intake by mechanical means. Sometimes the problem is compounded by both surgical resection and irradiation, which may further interfere with mastication and swallowing or cause xerostomia, stomatitis, pharyngitis, and esophagitis.[35]

Gastrointestinal malignancies and associated mechanical problems impair ingestion, digestion, and absorption of foodstuffs. Nutrient assimilation is markedly diminished in patients with gastrointestinal tumors and may be the result of inadequate pancreatic enzymes and bile salts owing to neoplastic obstruction, fistulous bypass of the small bowel, infiltration of the bowel by cancer cells, blind loop syndrome secondary to partial obstruction, and intestinal mucosal cell changes sec-

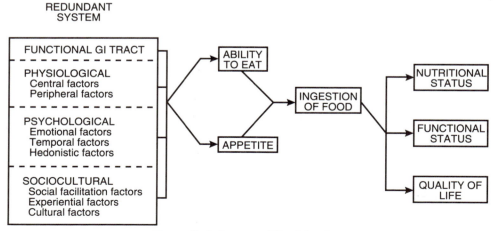

Figure 5–1. Impact of food intake.

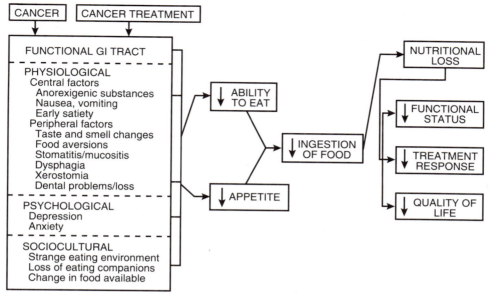

Figure 5–2. Changes in food intake during cancer and cancer treatment.

ondary to malnutrition.[35] Mucosal atrophy and destruction of villi of the small intestine result in disruption in absorptive capacity of the epithelial lining of the intestines. The microvilli of the lining must be present if absorption of nutrients is to occur.[36] A gastric malignancy may present with the sole nonspecific symptom of anorexia before the development of other complaints such as bloating, a feeling of fullness, or dyspepsia. The cause of anorexia in gastric cancer is not known, but later in the course of the disease it is attributed to diminution of gastric tone and peristalsis secondary to neoplastic infiltration. The decreased desire for food reduces the total caloric intake, and progressive weight loss results. Inadequate diet may lead to vitamin deficiencies and malnutrition. Severe dyspnea results from diffuse pulmonary lymphatic spread of gastric cancer and also interferes with intake.[37]

In addition to altered taste perceptions, conditioned food aversions, especially in children receiving radiation and chemotherapy, play an important role in cancer anorexia. Studies indicate that learned aversions to foods consumed shortly before chemotherapy arise in both adults and children and result in specific foods being associated with nausea, vomiting, and malaise.[38] Odors of foods are partially responsible for the food aversions experienced by cancer patients.[39]

Tumor growth alone can also produce se-vere anorexia.[40] The severity of the anorexia correlates with the extent of disease (or tumor) but not with histological type of tumor. A decline in food intake may be a result of psychological distress occurring at various times during the patient's clinical course.[41] Fears of death, isolation, and pain can negatively influence a patient's intake. Psychological and physical deterioration often intensify the problem of inadequate intake and are compounded by the side effects of surgery, chemotherapy, and radiation therapy. Thus, the situational stressors of "the unknown," in addition to many of the conventional therapies used in cancer treatment, pose extra stresses for the cancer patient (Figs. 5–2 and 5–3).

Anorexia in HIV Infection and AIDS

The severe malnutrition that accompanies acquired immunodeficiency syndrome (AIDS), as with other chronic disease states, increases morbidity and mortality. Maintaining weight, strength, and level of functioning is important for self-image and overall quality of life.

Anorexia in human immunodeficiency virus (HIV) infection and AIDS is associated with multiple factors. Any infection and inflammatory or neoplastic disease associated with HIV infection or AIDS may produce side effects in the oral cavity, pharynx, esoph-

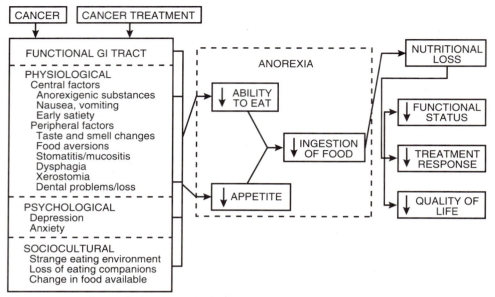

Figure 5–3. Anorexia during cancer and cancer treatment.

agus, and central nervous system. Such side effects interfere with normal appetite clues and may produce mechanical changes in food intake. Other physiological factors include general metabolic abnormalities leading to vitamin deficiencies and poor eating habits. The devastating psychological and psychosocial impact of HIV infection may include increased anxiety and depression, which may in turn decrease appetite. Adequate nutritional intake may improve response to treatment, help to prevent complications, and minimize further impairment of immune function.[42] The multiple pharmacological agents commonly used in the treatment of AIDS may also cause significant loss of appetite.[43]

Anorexia in Cardiac Disease, Congestive Heart Failure and End-Stage COPD

Individuals suffering from congestive heart failure (CHF) experience hypoxia (a "malnutrition") of the tissues that occurs as a result of decreased cardiac output and venous congestion of the gastrointestinal tract secondary to severe edema. These patients may appear overweight until successful diuretic therapy is initiated.[44] The congestion of intestinal veins may cause some impairment of intestinal absorption, which in turn may also contribute to anorexia.

Anorexia in cardiac disease is usually accompanied by nausea and bloating or abdominal fullness, which also has a negative effect on appetite because of central causes, congestion, or the resulting hepatomegaly. These symptoms may also result from digoxin toxicity. Gastrointestinal symptoms arise from the effects of digoxin on the chemoreceptor trigger zone in the medulla rather than as a result of direct stimulation of the gastrointestinal system.[24] Anorexia is present prior to the onset of cardiac rhythm changes in only 50 per cent of cases.[24]

With severe CHF and COPD, the anorexia may be a result, in part, from the extra work performed by the respiratory muscles, the increase in oxygen consumption by the hypertrophied heart, and the general discomfort or fatigue of the patient. These factors increase the basal metabolic rate (BMR) and the caloric requirements of the individual.[45] Rarely, severe right-sided heart failure, a protein-losing enteropathy, may significantly alter the synthesis of protein and contribute to anorexia and a protein-calorie malnutrition. The combination of reduced caloric intake and increased caloric expenditure results in a reduction of tissue mass and, in severe cases, cardiac cachexia, which resembles the cachexia seen in cancer patients with disseminated disease.[46]

In less severe disease states, chronic bronchitis can also interfere with food intake. The swallowing of expectorated sputum can lead to continual gastric upset and nausea, interfering with appetite and food ingestion.[19] As food intake diminishes, PCM progresses, with catabolism of body proteins for fuel. Organ dysfunction then occurs: Cardiac contractility and output are diminished, and respiratory muscles atrophy with destruction of alveolar tissue.[36] Vital capacity and tidal volume are depressed, mucociliary clearance is abnormal, and the cough becomes ineffective.

Anorexia in Chronic Renal Disease (Uremic Syndrome)

Anorexia is one of the earliest manifestations of uremia and significantly contributes to the PCM often seen in patients with this disease. During the dialysis process, most patients experience prolonged and marked anorexia as well as nausea and vomiting. The anorexia improves following dialysis, and therefore it is possible that dialyzable factors, such as cyanates, amino acids, and small polypeptides, may be possible causative factors in the anorexia.[25] Another cause of anorexia in patients with chronic renal disease may be food aversions. These are common and are probably related to the ammonia taste that develops in the mouth as urea in the saliva breaks down to ammonia. The "uremic fetor," a uriniferous odor of the breath, is often associated with unpleasant taste sensations and reduction in intake.

Dialysis patients experience an appreciable amount of chronic blood loss due to the dialysis process as well as a decreased absorption of iron across the gut wall. These two factors plus decreased erythropoietin production contribute to a significant and irreversible anemia.[47] Reduced energy level, lack of activity, apathy, anorexia, and disinterest in food can result from this anemia. Anorexia accompanies depression (thoughts of suicide and frequent death wishes), which is common in patients with this chronic disease.

MECHANISMS

Anorexia occurs in response to abnormalities in the hunger-satiety regulatory system. The integration of many neural, chemical, and hormonal influences makes comprehensive study of the regulation of food intake extremely complex. It is known that physiological mechanisms and conditioning, as a result of complex social, cultural, and emotional events, control our eating.

Physiological Mechanisms

See Chapter 14, Hunger, for a more detailed discussion of the central mechanisms of appetite regulation. The theories of hormonal and psychological influences most pertinent to an understanding of the phenomenon of anorexia are discussed next.

Thermostatic Theory

The thermostatic theory suggests that body temperature and the heat released from the metabolism of food are regulators of food intake. It has been observed in mammals that feeding adjustments are made in response to environmental temperature; that is, mammals eat more in the cold and less in the heat. It is unclear whether eating responses to changing temperature are related to changes in core or peripheral temperature sensors.[48] Clinically, the febrile or hypermetabolic patient is often anorectic. Alternately, a patient who has lost considerable weight may become hypothermic on exposure to cold temperature. In PCM states, patients may be basally somewhat hypothermic.

Aminostatic Theory

In the aminostatic theory, the concentration and pattern of amino acids in the blood and extracellular fluids are important signals for food intake regulation. Excesses and deficiencies of plasma amino acids play a role in the initiation or inhibition of food intake. It has been found that amino acid–imbalanced diets decrease the appetite as measured by decreased food intake. Many brain neurotransmitters are affected by the supply of amino acids in the blood and from the diet. It is possible that feeding behavior may also be influenced by these amino acids.[48, 49]

In recent years, dopamine receptors have been found in various parts of the brain and there has been an increasing recognition of the function of norepinephrine, dopamine, and serotonin as neurotransmitters.[50] In addition, research findings suggest the participation of monoamine systems in the regulation of food intake. For example, interruption of monoamine pathways or depletion of dietary monoamine content affects food intake. Serotonin (the serotoninergic system) may play a role in regulating normal feeding behavior, and derangements in the system may explain the pathogenesis of some of the anorexia that occurs in cancer patients.[50, 51] Data also suggest that cholinergic neurons and the neurotransmitter acetylcholine may have a role in receiving and transmitting information for the regulation of feeding.

Hormonal Influences

Research indicates that numerous hormones affect appetite, including insulin, glucagon, epinephrine, enterogastrone, cholecystokinin, and others.[52] Increased serum insulin possibly stimulates appetite, whereas decreased insulin production or decreased sensitivity to insulin (as in the cancer patient) results in a decreased stimulation of appetite. Glucagon reduces food intake indirectly through its effect of raising peripheral blood glucose levels.[53] Epinephrine antagonizes the insulin effect, alters gastrointestinal motility, and results in breakdown of glycogen in the liver. Insulin secretion is inhibited, and appetite is curtailed. The release of enterogastrone and cholecystokinin into the blood after food intake may also inhibit consumption by registering a satiety signal.

Data on other hormones in anorectic patients are scant, and DeWys suggests that a study of hormone levels in anorexia is a worthwhile approach.[48] Many metabolic and physiological factors influence food intake and regulation, but additional research is needed in this area to clarify these relationships.

Psychological Influences

The psychological influences on anorexia are as numerous as the physiological ones. Anxiety, whether in reaction to hospitalization, uncertainty of disease and its diagnosis, or change or loss in job status, increases the basal metabolic rate and demands a concomitant increase in food intake if nutritional status is to be maintained. Factors that often accompany illness, such as stress, depression, fear of isolation, or fear of pain, all decrease the desire to eat. In addition to anxiety, the patient may exhibit mood swings, difficulty in concentrating, anorexia, and insomnia.[41]

Feelings of hopelessness or the feeling that "nothing can be done" produces the emotionally oriented response of inactivity.[54] This is a natural reaction, especially in cancer patients who may associate cancer with death. These reactions may result not only in a decrease in appetite but also in a decrease in absorption of what is eaten and a decrease in the metabolism and utilization of what is absorbed. Anecdotal clinical evidence indicates that if feelings of hopelessness persist for any length of time, there will be a loss of appetite (anorexia), malaise, and weight loss even in physically healthy individuals.[41]

Patients who are allowed to participate in their treatment and their recovery may feel more highly motivated and independent. These factors may override other factors that reduce intake. The psychological significance of emphasizing the eating of a high-calorie diet as important therapy for the cancer patient needs further study. Hammill studied 18 head and neck cancer patients who received radiation therapy for their tumors. Half were randomized to the experimental group, which consisted of pretreatment with nutritional counseling, including an unspecified amount of protein and high-calorie liquid supplement. Results showed the experimental group had a more stable dietary intake and lost less weight than the control subjects during treatment.[55]

Anorexia cannot be explained by physiological alterations alone. Psychological factors do contribute to the presence of anorexia and weight loss in many patient populations, although the instruments for studying these factors are still in the developmental stage.

Pathological Consequences

There are numerous potentially detrimental consequences or outcomes associated with prolonged anorexia. If anorexia results in progressive and concomitant weight loss, a cycle of physical deterioration begins (Fig. 5–4).

The presence of malnutrition has been shown to significantly affect the hospital course of patients and directly increases the morbidity and mortality. There is evidence that severe protein loss not only reduces resistance to infection but impedes tissue repair and interferes with the synthesis of enzymes and plasma proteins. A threefold to tenfold increase in morbidity and related mortality can exist from undiagnosed and untreated malnutrition.[7]

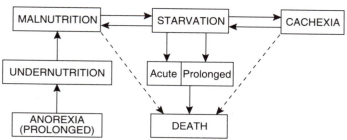

Figure 5–4. Cycle of physical deterioration in prolonged anorexia. Undernutrition, inadequate dietary intake and inability to metabolize nutrients normally (McBrydes); malnutrition, insufficient consumption of protein and calories resulting in the progressive loss of lean body mass and adipose tissue; starvation, a clinical state/condition in which the body is deprived of essential nutrients, a manifestation of malnutrition; cachexia, systemic metabolic derangement resulting in progressive wasting. (See *MacBrydes Signs and Symptoms*, 6th ed.)

If anorexia is prolonged and nitrogen balance is not restored or disease is not controlled, progressive nutritional deterioration of the individual results in a downhill spiral of malnutrition, cachexia, and death. Thus, the combined effects of inadequate intake, possibly altered metabolism, and loss of protein reserves due to prolonged anorexia may result in the most extreme form of protein-calorie malnutrition, cachexia. If this state is not reversed, the physiological derangements continue and death results.[56]

RELATED PATHOPHYSIOLOGICAL CONCEPTS

The concept of anorexia, although having a unique set of characteristics, must be differentiated from other similar and related concepts. Astute observation and skilled history taking and recording are valuable tools used by the clinician in differentiating characteristics of closely related concepts.

A pathophysiological concept closely related to anorexia is nausea, a very disagreeable feeling experienced in the back of the throat, the epigastrium, and generaly accompanied by vomiting. The same stimuli that cause an individual to be anorectic can also cause an individual to be nauseated. Anorexia and nausea, similarly, are ineffective responses associated with a variety of psychophysiological and organic disorders. Psychic stimuli (strong odors) can trigger anorexia, nausea, or vomiting. Stimulation of the hypothalamus can also trigger anorexia, nausea, or vomiting.[57]

Similarly, the stimuli that cause anorexia and nausea are extremely varied and include such clinical states as pregnancy, diabetic ketoacidosis, vascular shock, cardiac diseases, Ménière's disease, and many others. If either anorexia or nausea continues for a prolonged period of time, malnutrition and weight loss result.

Nausea, like anorexia, may arise from visceral discomfort, treatments, or medications used in illness or therapy; it may also arise from various psychological reactions (pain, fear, emotional stress). Nausea, like anorexia, is a subjective sensation; however, it creates discomfort in both the throat and abdomen. Unlike anorexia, nausea is described as an uncomfortable "tight" feeling in the throat during which an individual feels like vomiting. The feeling is accompanied by a decrease in gastric contractions and spasms of the duodenum.[1]

Anorexia appears to be a factor associated with the circumstances of all episodes of nausea. When nausea is accompanied by anorexia, the motivation to eat is completely extinguished.[45] Any individual who is nauseated has no desire for food.[58] In nausea, thoughts of food and eating are repulsive and may even worsen the existing nausea, which may then be followed by vomiting. In anorexia, the desire to eat is absent and there is a general disinterest in food, but the individual may nonetheless still experience the physiological sensation of hunger.

ASSOCIATED PSYCHOSOCIAL CONCEPTS

The psychosocial concept identified as occurring most frequently in association with anorexia is depression. It is well documented that depression can cause a decrease in appetite with subsequent weight loss. The anorectic patient often complains of feeling "weak" and "tired" (fatigued), appears apathetic and exhausted, and expresses a lack of interest in activities of daily living. These same manifestations may also describe a clinically depressed patient.[59] The crucial element in differentiating depression from anorexia is skilled and accurate nursing assessment and history taking. An assessment of feelings of diminished self-worth or self-esteem is useful, since these are indicators of depression and not likely to be present with anorexia alone. The nurse clinician must learn to identify and treat the causes rather than the symptoms of these related concepts and must be "cued-in" to patient responses in order to make the task of differentiating closely related concepts easier. In addition, a psychiatric consultation/evaluation should be considered early so that chemotherapy can be carefully monitored and appropriately maintained (or changed, if necessary).

Depression in patients with cancer exacerbates other symptoms (e.g., pain, anorexia). Sadness and a depressed mood, as well as anorexia, are common occurrences in cancer patients and are normal responses to the disease; these symptoms are frequently nonresponsive to pharmacological measures. The diagnosis of morbid depression, which will be amenable to pharmacological intervention, is extremely difficult in these patients because the somatic symptoms that usually provide the indicators of depressive illness are also common symptoms of cancer itself.[60] Sleep disturbances, anorexia, weight loss, and loss of libido are all common in both depressed patients and cancer patients. A trial of antidepressants is often indicated when a diagnosis is in doubt and to help combat the devastating effects severe emotional depression has on appetite.[60, 61] Improvement in mood with a trial of antidepressants may help the clinician differentiate between depressive illness and anorexia.

Depression resulting in anorexia may be due to changes in physical attractiveness or altered body state, self-worth, or wholeness.[61] Overwhelming disinterest in all aspects of life is the hallmark of profound depression, while a disinterest in food may be the only clue that the patient is anorectic. Research indicates that the presence of anorexia in a cancer patient with less advanced disease is more likely due to a reactive depression than to the disease itself.

A second psychosocial concept, sitophobia, which is defined as "the fear of eating because of subsequent or associated discomfort,"[1] must also be differentiated from anorexia. This particular state frequently occurs in patients with regional enteritis (especially those with partial obstruction) or in patients with a gastric ulcer following either partial or total gastric resection.[45] Sitophobia is also a common occurrence in patients with end-stage pulmonary disease. In this group of patients, the increase in both mucus production and respiratory effort that accompanies eating may increase or create dyspnea and shortness of breath. The memory of the discomfort and the physical inability to tolerate the concomitant disturbance in oxygenation may discourage the patient from eating. Thus, sitophobia is an actual fear of eating because of the pain or discomfort associated with food. Anorexia, however, is not a fear of eating but a loss of interest in eating. Unlike sitophobia, anorexia is infrequently associated with painful eating; however, pain, discomfort, or fear of something related to illness can result in an anorectic state.

In sitophobia, unlike anorexia, appetite usually persists and the patient continues to experience feelings of hunger; however, the ingestion of food is nonetheless curtailed. Anorectic individuals will complain that even though the appetite is extinguished, they may experience feelings of hunger until they begin to eat. As soon as they begin to ingest food, the feelings of hunger disappear.

MANIFESTATIONS

Anorexia is primarily a subjective phenomenon; however, a number of objective manifestations are used to identify the presence of anorexia.

Objective manifestations of anorexia include, first, a decreased food intake recorded over time. This implies that intake is consistently low for a period of time and that the pattern has somehow been documented. Second, a significant decrease in food and fluid intake with an associated weight loss is observed. If the anorexia is progressive or continues for an extended period of time, laboratory data, anthropometric measurements, and other clinical parameters are valuable in identifying the extent of nutritional deficiency resulting from the anorexia.

It is of primary importance that those individuals caring for the anorectic patient be aware that some patients may not report a change in appetite or eating patterns and yet actually have a significant decrease in caloric intake, which signifies an unrecognized anorexia.[62] In one study of 303 elderly patients, 83 per cent rated their intake as good or excellent; controlled observation, however, showed that only 60 per cent actually had good intake.[19] A meticulous and strict calorie count and diet history are vital in identifying this group of patients.

Subjective manifestations of anorexia are extremely variable, and one must listen carefully to patients' "verbal cues" in order to recognize those complaints that pertain to a loss of appetite. For example, often patients, upon questioning, report their old clothes "don't fit anymore" or that "they are much too large." Any patient data regarding normal or adequate intake are based on recollection. Changes in appetite may be gradual, and the patient may underestimate the magnitude of the change. Subjective manifestations frequently encountered in clinical practice are listed in Table 5–2.

SURVEILLANCE AND MEASUREMENT

Numerous clinical parameters are used to monitor anorexia over time. In both the acute and chronic phases, however, the importance of a nursing data base cannot be overemphasized. This data base incorporates a diet history and assists the clinician in assessing the current nutritional status of the individual as well as in monitoring the patient's progress throughout the intervention process. An evaluation of all physiological as well as psychological factors contributing to the development and progression of anorexia must be included.[63]

History

A routine baseline nutritional screening is needed in all hospitalized patients in order to identify those individuals at high risk for development of significant problems. Table 5–3 lists the parameters for a patient at high risk for PCM.[64, 65] The presence of any one of these parameters increases the risk for malnutrition as compared with the normal population. Patients with cancer often experience two or more of these parameters and are the most likely patient population to suffer from some form of PCM at the time of hospitalization.

The history of an anorectic patient should include the following data: (1) frequency and intensity with which anorexia occurs; (2) duration of the anorexia; (3) specificity of the complaint; (4) what foods, if any, aggravate or relieve the feeling (i.e., anorexia for all or special foods); and (5) drug history (especially laxative use and digitalis, hypertensive, and hydrochlorothiazide or antihistamine therapy). When assessing a patient for the presence or absence of anorexia, one must determine the frequency and intensity of the anorexia. The anorexia should be described according to a standard scale. The use of a

TABLE 5–2 SUBJECTIVE MANIFESTATIONS OF ANOREXIA

Patient Complaints (Physiological)	Subjective Reports (Behavioral)
Pain	"I've lost my appetite."
Nausea/vomiting	"I just don't feel like eating."
Alterations in odor or taste perception	"I've lost my taste for food." "Food just doesn't taste good anymore."
Early satiety	"I feel so full after just a few bites."
Tiredness, weakness, listlessness, apathy	"I don't enjoy food like I used to."
Fever	"Can't seem to put weight on and I'm eating like I always did."
Drug therapy side effects	"I'm not hungry."
• Stomatitis	"The thought of food nauseates me."
• Diarrhea	"Food is so bland, tasteless."
Dysphagia	"Food all tastes the same and I used to really enjoy eating."
Malaise/fatigue	

TABLE 5–3 PARAMETERS FOR A PATIENT AT HIGH RISK* FOR PROTEIN-CALORIE MALNUTRITION[64, 65]

1. A recent 7 to 10 per cent weight loss or an unintentional weight loss of more than 2.2 pounds (1 kilogram) per week.
2. Major surgery within the past 6 months.
3. Treatment with radiation therapy or chemotherapy within the past 6 months.
4. Any illness that has lasted more than 3 weeks within the last 6 months.

*A patient is at high risk for protein-calorie malnutrition if one or more of the above parameters is present.

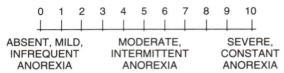

Figure 5–5. Example of a scale for assessing frequency and intensity of anorexia. (From Donoghue, M., Nunnally, C., & Yasko, J. [1982]. *Nutritional Aspects of Cancer Care* [pp 83–145]. Reston, VA: Reston Publishing.)

simple likert-type scale is suggested. This type of scale is quickly and easily administered while providing accurate subjective data which can be used over time for evaluation and comparison of interventions.[65] (Fig. 5–5).

An anorexia instrument developed by Grant and associates for head and neck cancer patients consists of 22 items formatted as 100-mm linear analogue scales.[66] Seven subscales are represented in the instrument: appetite, ability to eat, appetite-hunger factors, oral-gustatory factors, general symptoms, psychological factors, and sociocultural factors. The one item for appetite consisting of a 100-mm linear scale anchored with the words "no appetite" and "large appetite" could be used clinically to monitor appetite changes in patients suffering from anorexia. Use of this instrument in cancer patients reflects changes that occur in a predictable pattern as patients are undergoing radiation treatments wherein appetite changes are expected.[67] Clinicians should use these tools not only to assess the presence and severity of the anorexia but also to evaluate the distress associated with it. Refining our assessments in clinical practice will better direct the supportive approaches to the individual client.

Dietary and weight information, any recent changes in appetite, difficulty swallowing or chewing, nausea or vomiting, food allergies or intolerances, change in bowel habits or presence of constipation or diarrhea, and usual daily diet patterns (time, place, amounts) should be included in an initial nutritional screening. Tables 5–4 and 5–5 summarize evaluation areas of patients at risk for malnutrition. Consultation with a clinical dietitian regarding the results of the nutritional screening will assist in formulation of an appropriate diet for the patient.

Additional facets of the medical history that may affect nutritional status and influence anorexia are as follows: type, duration, and location of tumor (if cancer is the diagnosis); medications (nutrient-drug interactions, length of time drugs are taken, laxative and glucocorticoid usage); previous surgery that might affect nutrient intake (e.g., head and neck, gastrointestinal procedures); current treatment; pre-existing acute or chronic processes (e.g., infections, diabetes mellitus, coronary artery disease, liver disease, hypertension); and psychological or socioeconomic factors that may affect food intake (e.g., income, outside assistance with food preparation, facilities for food preparation, persons in the home).

Medical audits reveal that height, weight, serum albumin, and total lymphocyte counts are not routinely measured,[68] and many other areas affecting nutritional status are

TABLE 5–4 INFORMATION FOR EVALUATING PATIENTS AT RISK FOR MALNUTRITION AS A RESULT OF PROLONGED ANOREXIA*

Criterion	Present (+)	Absent (−)
Recent weight less than 10 per cent of usual body weight		
Serum albumin less than 3.0 per cent		
Total lymphocyte count less than 1500/mm³		
Patient NPO for 5 days or maintained on D_5W or clear liquid diet for more than 5 days		
Presence of decubitus ulcers		
Elevated metabolic requirements (fever, infection, burns, trauma)		
External losses (draining fistula, wounds, abscesses)[33]		

Adapted from Mueller, K., Buzby, G., & Mullen, J. (1982). Therapeutic nutritional practices for the cancer patient. Penn Med, 2:59–63.

*If one or more of the above criteria is observed, a detailed nutritional assessment is indicated.

Abbreviation: NPO, nothing by mouth.

TABLE 5–5 AREAS TO INCLUDE IN NUTRITIONAL ASSESSMENT USING MNEMONIC DEVICE ABCDE

A	=	Anthropometric measurements
B	=	Biochemical or laboratory data
		Hemoglobin and hematocrit
		White blood cell count with differential
C	=	Clinical observation
D	=	Diet recall/food frequency questionnaire
E	=	Everything else (includes socioeconomic and psychological factors that interfere with food intake)

TABLE 5–6 ANTHROPOMETRIC MEASUREMENTS TO ESTIMATE THE DEGREE OF MUSCLE AND FAT DEPLETION*

Measurement	Comments
Triceps skinfold thickness (TSF)	A gross measurement of the fat reserves in the body
Midarm circumference (MAC)	A gross measurement of the body's muscle stores using the nondominant arm
Creatine height index (CHI)	An estimate of total muscle mass via excretion rates of creatinine

*Parameters must be compared with normal standards.

TABLE 5–7 VALUES OF SERUM ALBUMIN AND DEGREE OF DEPLETION

Value	Degree of Depletion
4.5 to 3.8 g/dl	Normal level
3.7 to 3.0 g/dl	Mild protein depletion
2.9 to 2.5 g/dl	Moderate protein depletion
2.5 g/dl or less	Severe protein depletion

Adapted from Donoghue M, Nunally C, Yasko J. (1982). *Nutrition Aspects of Cancer Care* (pp. 83–145). Reston, VA: Reston Publications.

omitted from medical records. To provide optimal nutritional care for patients, the nutritional assessment data base must be accurate and complete.

The major areas to be included in a detailed nutritional assessment data base are presented next.

Assessment of Somatic Protein Compartment

Depletion of the somatic protein compartment is evidenced by fat and muscle wasting. The parameters used to evaluate the somatic protein compartment are height and weight index, or the weight of the patient in proportion to his or her height. In order to minimize error, the same scale should be used each time; the patient needs to be weighed at the same time each day, in the same clothing, and with an empty bladder to ensure an accurate baseline. Anthropometric measurements (Table 5–6) should also be made. The above parameters provide an estimate of the degree of muscle and fat depletion when compared with normal standards for each.

Assessment of Visceral Protein Compartment

Visceral proteins circulate in the blood stream. Depletion of the visceral protein stores is evidenced by decreased blood protein levels and affects the ability of the patient to repair normal cells and heal wounds. Visceral protein measurement includes serum albumin, which falls rapidly with protein malnutrition; total lymphocyte count (TLC), which reflects the status of the immune system; and prealbumin measurement, which can be used to assess the individual's visceral protein status on a short-term basis. Albumin has a half-life of 18 to 20 days, and any changes in nutritional status will often take this long to be reflected in albumin levels. Albumin levels remain one of the major indicators of nutritional status, and have been valuable in predicting morbidity and mortality. Both serum albumin and TLC are evaluated by comparison with a table of standard values. Cell-mediated immunity, measured by delayed hypersensitivity skin testing, and transferrin or total iron-binding capacity (TIBC) are assessed when more accurate and detailed laboratory data measurements are needed.[64, 65] Several factors limit the overall usefulness of skin testing in assessing nutritional status and may be reduced in only severe malnutrition. Standard values of serum albumin and lymphocyte depletion are listed in Tables 5–7 and 5–8.

Physical Assessment

In addition to an assessment of the somatic and visceral protein compartments, a physical assessment is essential to determine the nutritional status of the anorectic patient. Table

TABLE 5–8 VALUES OF LYMPHOCYTE DEPLETION

Value	Degree of Depletion
1800/mm³ or greater	Normal
1800 to 1500/mm³	Mild depletion
1500 to 1200/mm³	Moderate depletion
1200/mm³ or less	Severe depletion

Adapted from Donoghue M, Nunally C, Yasko J. (1982). *Nutrition Aspects of Cancer Care* (pp. 83–145). Reston, VA: Reston Publications.

5–9 summarizes the areas in the physical examination pertinent to nutritional status.[69]

Nutrient Requirement and Diet Recall

Another area included in a nutritional assessment is the determination of nutrient requirement and diet recall. This area includes a written record of all food or fluids consumed in a 3-day period and a record of calorie and protein needs for the patient. Intake is then compared with the amount of calories and protein needed as predicted from the calculated basal energy expenditure (BEE). The BEE is calculated using the Harris-Benedict equation:

In men
$$\text{Kcal/day} = 66 + (13.7 \times \text{wt}) + (5 \times \text{Ht}) - (6.8 \times \text{age})$$

In women
$$\text{Kcal/day} = 655 + (9.6 \times \text{wt}) + (1.7 \times \text{Ht}) - (4.7 \times \text{age})$$

Wt is the actual weight in kilograms; Ht is the height in cm. The BEE then can be multiplied by a factor reflecting additional calories needed for activity level or stress of surgery.

Diet recall must be used cautiously, as patients, especially those who are outpatients, may report or record intake inaccurately and thus information may not reflect a patient's true dietary intake. With the confused or memory-impaired person, observation and documentation of meal intake by the health care provider are generally required.

Dietary Composition

Once caloric needs are established, the composition of the diet and the best method of providing essential nutrients must be determined. Because there is no protein reserve for energy in the body, the goal of nutritional therapy is to protect or restore the body's protein. Nitrogen balance is a measure of the protein balance in the body. Positive nitrogen balance implies intact body protein, whereas negative nitrogen balance implies protein depletion. To maintain a positive nitrogen balance, at least 7 to 8 per cent of the total calories must be provided by protein. For the hypermetabolic individual, protein requirements will double and should be 15 to 20 per cent of the total calories; patients with liver or renal impairment may need protein intake to be limited.[32]

THERAPIES AND THERAPEUTIC GOALS

The primary goal of management for the anorectic patient is to maintain or restore optimal nutritional status and positive nitrogen balance. To achieve this goal, the major objectives include (1) providing adequate oral intake to prevent malnutrition, (2) minimizing factors (environmental and others) that contribute to patient anorexia, and (3) monitoring nutritional status parameters, such as body weight. The planning, implementing, and evaluating of individual patient needs, while providing opportunity for maximum

TABLE 5–9   NUTRITIONAL ASSESSMENT BY A PHYSICAL EXAMINATION

Physical Examination	Comments
Skeletal muscles	Check for presence or absence of muscle wasting (especially of supraclavicular and interosseous muscles),[66] hemorrhages into muscles, calf tenderness, and weakness.
Subcutaneous fat	Check for presence or absence of subcutaneous fat (especially abdomen, arms)
Skin and mucous membrane	Observe for condition, color, and tone. Observe condition of scrotal and rectal areas as well as dorsum of feet for dry, scaling skin, or petechiae.
Mouth, tongue, and gums	Observe for beefy red or scarlet tongue (glossitis), presence of dry red fissures at angles of lips (cheilosis), and spongy, pale, receding gums (gingivitis).
Edema	Observe sacral area and feet for pitting edema.
Vital signs	Check to assess hydration status of patient and also check for elevated blood pressure, arrhythmias, increased or decreased heart rate, and decreased pulse amplitude.
Masticating/swallowing	Observe for effectiveness[59] and identify and record difficulties.
Hair, nails, and eyes	Check for any appearance of dry, brittle, sparse/thin hair; Bitot's spots in eyes; and brittle, rigid nail.[66]

patient contribution, are vital to fulfilling the goals of therapy successfully.

Current trends in health care systems focus on the need for outpatient ambulatory management whenever possible. This trend places additional demands on the nurse to prepare patients for greater participation in self-care and management/prevention techniques related to the side effects of treatment. Teaching patients about their disease, treatments, and what to expect reduces fear, increases self-confidence, and may improve compliance and enhance participation in treatment.[70]

The side effects of the treatment or disease process are an important dimension in determining the quality of life for the patient. Quality of life is defined according to the individual patient's perception of current level of functioning compared with a possible or ideal level. In a study by Coates and associates, patients were asked to rank the severity of chemotherapy-induced side effects.[71] Most of the patients ranked the side effects that affected them on a day-to-day basis as the most severe, including anorexia, nausea and vomiting, loss of hair (alopecia), fatigue, weight loss, oral ulcerations, taste changes, and diarrhea. These complaints are often viewed by the health care providers as relatively minor, with infection and bleeding viewed as the most serious side effects. To the patient these serious side effects do not occur as frequently, nor do they cause discomfort on a daily basis. It is vital to deal with those problems that the patient views as troublesome and to establish with the patient and family the goal of therapy and how it will affect quality of life.

Numerous techniques or clinical therapies may be used to nourish the patient with an intact gastrointestinal system. Initially, an assessment of the patient's eating environment needs to be determined to identify the presence of noxious stimuli that might contribute to anorexia. Consultation with a dietitian and family members is essential in helping to create a pleasant atmosphere for meals. Certain odors (from dressings, food, other patients) can trigger and increase anorexia; these need to be eliminated from the environment, or the patient should be moved whenever possible. Attention needs to be directed toward the appearance, aroma, texture, and temperature of food as well. Favor-

ite or familiar foods can be brought from home and frozen for future use. The dietitian takes patient food preferences into consideration when planning meals and allows the patient as much freedom in choice and selection of foods as possible.[72]

External as well as internal factors may cause or aggravate anorexia. Lack of social interaction and unfamiliar hospital environment as well as limited selection and often unpalatable hospital food can contribute to and increase anorexia. Restrictive or unpalatable diets may also result in a loss of interest in food. Making food readily available and providing a relaxed atmosphere for group dining by ambulatory inpatients improve intake and patient morale.[30] It is suggested that access to "kitchen galleys" where adults are allowed to prepare their own snacks and meals encourages increased consumption.[30] The monotony of the hospital food service can be relieved by allowing ambulatory patients to select their own meals in the hospital cafeteria or coffee shops or at vending machines or local restaurants, when appropriate.[30]

Prior to discharge, the nurse explores possibilities for enrolling the patient in a free meal-delivery program, especially if the patient lives alone. If the patient returns to a family residential setting, efforts can be made by the patient to help others deal with social situations, which may contribute to nutritional compromise and diminished quality of life. The nurse encourages patients to join support groups (especially patients with HIV infection who experience a great deal of social isolation due to their disease), where problems can be shared and often creatively solved by other group members. Learning how others cope with similar issues is a valuable approach to the anorectic client.[73]

For pediatric patients, especially those with cancer or prolonged hospitalizations, pizza parties, banana split days, and picnics are some examples of activities that can be planned to improve appetite and food consumption. Children undergoing therapy prefer the same foods that most children prefer: pizza, hot dogs, hamburgers, potato chips, french fries, and popsicles.[30] These should be provided or served when possible. For adults, social atmosphere and the setting are improved by the serving of wine and the addition of soft music to stimulate appetite and increase social interaction. Family members are encouraged to eat with the patient if this is preferred. Patients should be encouraged to sit on the side of the bed or up in a chair, since eating in bed may encourage the "sick role." Silverware from home, cloth instead of paper napkins, and glasses in place of paper cups may improve acceptance and oral intake.

Many anorectic patients find cold protein foods more palatable than hot ones,[68] and the odor from hot food is often more offensive. Cold protein items (salad plates of fruit, cheese), cold snacks high in protein, and fresh fruit in protein-containing desserts should be made available, when possible.[29] The anorectic nonambulatory patient needs support in trying a variety of foods, as the monotony of a simple diet further aggravates the existing anorexia.[74] Sandwiches (cold meat or peanut butter), milkshakes, popsicles, cottage cheese and fruit, and vegetable salads are suggested if the patient prefers cold foods.

Patients should avoid drinking fluids with meals, as this can stimulate the volume receptors in the stomach and intestines and produce a feeling of fullness. Instead, the patient should take frequent small sips and cups of fluids throughout the day to minimize the development of a feeling of fullness. Patients are advised to eat the largest meal early in the day when the appetite is best.

DeWys and Pascucci-Amino recommend that foods of high nutritional density be encouraged, especially for cancer patients, those receiving chemotherapy or radiation therapy, or anyone with PCM.[74] The use of double-strength milk (1 cup dried skim milk added to 1 quart whole milk) or half-and-half flavored with strawberry, raspberry, or maple syrups; vanilla extract; molasses; and fruit purees or juices is suggested. The use of double-strength milk in the preparation of cream soups and creamed foods, puddings, custards, baked goods, and any food to which milk is ordinarily added is also recommended.[8] Although expensive, shakes and puddings are also commercially available with increased caloric content in a variety of flavors. Cream-style chicken soup and instant oats or bran oatmeal are available commercially from Forta. Calorie and protein content in these products is doubled.

Caution is exercised in recommending the use of milk to patients, since clinically symptomatic lactose intolerance is frequently observed in the adult. Lactase deficiency in the American adult population may be as high as 16 per cent in caucasians and 70 per cent in blacks.[75] In addition, the cancer patient may be at a greater risk for development of a related lactose intolerance because of possible gastrointestinal mucosal damage from the malignancy, chemotherapy, radiotherapy, or pre-existing malnutrition. The use of a gluten-free, lactose-free, low-residue diet in children receiving radiation therapy has resulted in complete prevention of acute and chronic radiation enteritis in one study.[32] If milk is contraindicated or the patient has a history of lactose intolerance, the use of any lactose-free commercial diet supplement (Citrotein, Osmolite, Isocal) needs to be explored for use in adding calories to the diet. DeWys and Herbst reported that a panel of 25 cancer patients rated Ensure, a lactose-free supplement, the most acceptable (with regard to taste) in a group of seven other supplements.[76] The addition of sauces, butter, or sour cream to foods, if tolerated, adds calories and helps to minimize weight loss. When needed, Polycose R, a tasteless glucose polymer (32 calories/teaspoon), can also be added to foods and beverages to increase calories.[64]

Canned liquid supplements frequently exacerbate the metallic taste some patients experience. Therefore, liquid supplements, packaged in waxed cartons, are desirable.[73]

Oral elemental, chemically defined formulas and standard supplements are important ways to add nutrients, calories, and protein to the diet of an anorectic patient. These nutritionally balanced liquid supplements augment the basic diet, but individual taste should dominate which product is selected.[72] Supplements are especially useful with patients who develop malnutrition secondary to malabsorption states, draining fistulas, decreased intake after colon surgery, and radiation- and chemotherapy-induced intestinal changes.[61] Availability and cost to the patient are also factors to consider in choosing a supplement because many preparations are not covered by standard medical insurance policies.[77] For both the lactose-tolerant and lactose-intolerant patient, appropriate additions, such as ice cream, whipped cream or a nondairy topping, rum, crème de menthe, or amaretto, according to the likes and dislikes of the individual can enhance the flavor of many of the supplements.[74] The addition of fresh fruits (strawberries, blueberries, peaches), vanilla extract, or nutmeg enhances vanilla supplements, and other flavors can be frozen to resemble frozen dairy desserts.[64] The wide variety of fresh fruits and vegetables now available to individuals (e.g., kiwi fruit, papaya, pear-apples, snow peas) allows them to diversify and add variety to their diets in order to increase their intake.[78] Usually, the chemically defined products are more acceptable to patients if served as a slush or ice or used in a recipe.[77]

Most patients prefer supplements chilled and served in a glass. Supplements are best tolerated in small quantities of 2 to 4 ounces and at frequent intervals.[63] A "taste test" tray with approximately 1 ounce of five different supplements may be brought to the patient for selection of the preferred supplement. The client is advised to sip the supplement slowly, preferably between meals, and to report the occurrence of any unusual side effects, such as gastric distention, abdominal cramping, nausea, or diarrhea. As a result of the high osmolality of most supplements, diarrhea frequently occurs.[64] If diarrhea does occur, advise the patient to sip 8 ounces of the supplement over an 8-hour period or to dilute the supplement. A lactose-free supplement may be necessary for persistent diarrhea. For temporary lactose deficiency due to anorexia, LactAid can be prescribed to convert lactose to lactic acid and permit the use of milk.[77]

In dietary planning, consideration of a patient's ethnic and religious background is also vital for improving food intake (kosher, vegetarian). Clinical experience brings to mind the case of a Chinese woman 3 days postcholecystectomy who, from nurses' and physicians' reports, was progressing well except for unexplained "anorexia"—not touching any of the liquids on her tray. The patient did not speak English and was unable to communicate the fact that many Chinese people do not drink fluids until they sit at room temperature for a period of time. Her tray of fluids was taken away before she had a chance to drink them. Finally, with the help of a Chinese nursing student, this fact was discovered and the "anorexia" subsided. Additionally, most adult blacks, Asians, and Mediterranean southern Europeans do not tolerate milk well.[78] Facts such as these are most helpful to those individuals involved in dietary planning for the anorectic patient. Cultural food preferences do influence the acceptance of standard hospital menus and nutritional intake.[30]

Many anorectic cancer patients (because of early satiety) find that small frequent feedings (every 2 to 4 hours) increase food tolerance. Decreasing the quantity and size of portions served often is more appealing to the anorectic patient. Gradually increasing the amount of food served at each meal is recommended, as a full plate is often overwhelming to the anorectic patient.

Oral hygiene to reduce "taste fatigue"[79] as well as offering a warm washcloth for cleansing hands and face prior to meals is also helpful in stimulating the appetite. Normal saline irrigations of the oral cavity, half-strength mouth wash, lemon drops, or chewing gum may also help freshen the mouth and stimulate the production of saliva.

Some drugs demonstrate specific appetite-stimulating effects. Data suggest that cyproheptadine (Periactin), an antihistamine/antiserotonin agent, is useful in promoting weight gain in geriatric patients, adults with essential anorexia, and adolescents with anorexia nervosa. A study using 4-mg doses of cyproheptadine three times a day in adults with anorexia showed the cyproheptadine to be more effective than placebo in improving appetite and affecting significant weight gain.[41, 80] Research indicates that dronabinol (delta 9-tetrahydrocannabinol, THC—the active ingredient in marijuana), promotes weight gain and produces mild mood elevation in cancer and geriatric patients.[41, 47, 81] Regelson and colleagues reported that dronabinol at a dose of 15 mg/day caused cancer patients significantly to improve appetite and gain weight as compared with controls taking a placebo.[81] The patients, however, developed serious side effects (including sedation, orthostatic hypotension, ataxia, and dizziness). Current studies are underway to determine whether lower doses of dronabinol can achieve the same positive appetite stimulation.[82]

The use of insulin and hormonal therapy (corticosteroids/androgens) to increase well-being and appetite and enhance weight gain is widely documented, but the long-term effects are virtually unknown, and side effects, even on a short-term basis, are significant.[41, 47] Reports indicate that prednisone enhances appetite in anorectic patients with lupus erythematosus and in patients receiving renal transplants. Nandrolone decanoate (Deca-durabolin) enhances appetite in anorectic patients with anemia.[47] In a double-blind, cross-over trial, prednisolone (5 mg three times daily for 2 weeks and then reduced for the third week) proved significantly more effective than placebo (p < 0.001) in improving the appetite of 41 cancer patients on a short-term basis. No weight change was reported in either the placebo or prednisolone group, thus demonstrating that no appreciable water retention developed with the prednisolone therapy at study dosage. A major placebo effect (50 per cent) indicates that there is a possible psychological basis for anorexia in some patients.[83] The patients in the above study had a variety of solid tumors, with gastrointestinal tumors the most common. All of the patients showed a similar pattern of response to treatment.

In studies by Shinshanker and associates[84] and Kris and associates,[85] metoclopramide was found to improve gastric emptying in patients with impaired gastric motility and the feeling of abdominal fullness. Using a radionucleotide scan, Shinshanker and associates studied a group of patients with gastrointestinal malignancy and no mechanical explanation for the delayed emptying and early satiety.[84] They found symptoms were reversed by metoclopramide. Kris and associates, using a similar scan, found corresponding gastric paresis in a group of patients with advanced lung cancer.[85] They confirmed the beneficial response to metoclopramide.

In addition to these therapies, megestrol acetate, a progestational agent that stimulates the appetite to improve food intake and enhances cellular metabolism while contributing to weight gain, is currently being evaluated for use. Tchekmedyian and associates used high-dose megestrol (480 to 1600 mg/day) therapy with 33 patients with advanced breast cancer.[86] Several patients reported marked increase in appetite while receiving megestrol therapy; 27 of 28 completing the study reported weight gain. The use of megestrol acetate, especially in high doses, induces weight gain in patients with advanced cancer regardless of response to therapy or extent of disease.[87] Loprinzi and colleagues[88] designed a randomized, double-blind placebo-controlled study of adult patients with advanced incurable cancer (other than breast and endometrial) to determine whether megestrol acetate offers a significant benefit in terms of weight gain (15 pounds and over). Studies are currently under way to determine the role of megestrol acetate in appetite increase, weight gain, and improvement of symptomatic care.[89]

The use of hydrazine sulfate, an inhibitor of gluconeogenesis, also has been demonstrated to have a positive effect on appetite. In a randomized study by Chlebowski and associates,[90] 61 cancer patients who had lost 10 per cent of their body weight received hydrazine sulfate (60 mg three times a day), and 40 patients received a placebo.[90] After 1 month, appetite improved and there was an increase in caloric intake and subsequent weight gain in the patients receiving hydrazine. A significant improvement toward normalization was noted in glucose tolerance as well. Research by Chlebowski and associates with non–small cell lung cancer patients supports the above finding and also reports improved nutritional parameters and increased median survival.[91]

Certain metals, especially zinc and copper, may play an important role in maintaining normal sensory functions. Some disorders of taste can be corrected with the administration of oral zinc sulfate.[8] These results, however, have not been supported by controlled clinical trials. Recent work suggests that abnormalities in endogenous opiate regulation of appetite may play a role in the anorexia of zinc deficiency.[92]

Interventions for Sensory Compensation

Anorexia resulting from chemosensory disorders (changes in taste and smell) significantly impact on nutritional status and food habits. Individuals who are able to adjust their appreciation for food and their habits to compensate for the missing sensation are at less risk for negatively affecting their nutritional status. One method of compensation is to vary the texture as well as the temperature of foods to add to mealtime enjoyment. Foods with homogeneous texture (e.g., sherbet and pudding) were given lower preference ratings by patients in a study by Doty.[93]

For selected patients, food enjoyment is improved by including condiments that stimulate the trigeminal nerve and add a spicy or hot quality (e.g., horseradish, peppers, fresh mint).[94] Citrus fruits and drinks and pickled and acidic foods, if tolerated, stimulate taste buds. The use of carbonated water as a mouth rinse may also help "clear" the taste buds. A Mexican meal (tacos, burritos) includes hot spicy sauces complemented by cold sour cream or guacamole and a crisp, crunchy tortilla. This type of meal can stimulate the patient visually and through a variety of textures and temperatures.[82] As a result of taste or smell changes, the degree of anorexia will vary from individual to individual. For some patients, the smell of food may be pleasant; for others it may be perceived as foul and interfere with intake. It is important that the clinician take individual preferences into account.

Pain and nausea contribute greatly to anorexia; therefore, the judicious use of appropriate drugs approximately 30 minutes prior to meals in order to control the pain and nausea may also help to enhance appetite.[95] Haloperidol (Haldol), prochlorperazine (Compazine), and chlorpromazine (Thorazine) are more effective antiemetics than promethazine (Phenergan), trimethobenzamine (Tigan), or diphenhydramine (Benadryl) in controlling nausea.[41, 95] Research from Johns Hopkins Oncology Center suggests that for patients receiving chemotherapy dexamethasone (Hexadrol) is a more effective antiemetic than prochlorperazine (Compazine).[96] Effective dosage as well as an ongoing evaluation of the effectiveness of prescribed medications to control distressing symptoms may help to improve oral intake.

Numerous drugs and drug interactions have been demonstrated to decrease dietary intake by causing anorexia, nausea, and vomiting and by altering the sense of taste.[47] These need to be evaluated carefully in the anorexic patient. Drug substitutions should be considered if appetite is altered.[97, 98] Anorexia and weight loss in a digitalized patient who is elderly or taking diuretics suggest digitalis toxicity, and careful follow-up of these patients is crucial. The clinician must be aware of the possibility of drug interactions as a possible source of altered food consumption. Careful recording on the patient's medical record of any comments made about change in appetite supports the team effort for maintaining dietary intake.

Many of the pharmacological therapies used in the supportive care of patients may contribute to the anorectic syndrome. The use of narcotic analgesics is known to depress appetite and decrease gastric motility, thus resulting in constipation. Constipation can also interfere with appetite and intake by creating a feeling of fullness and a bloated sensation. High-fiber diets and bran supplements should be recommended with caution, as they may reduce available nutrients and minerals and depress appetite for other foods.[82] Patients are advised to try mature fruits and prune juice, which produce a natural laxative effect while adding calories without causing untoward side effects.

Tricyclic antidepressants are frequently used in conjunction with narcotic analgesics for their synergistic and sedative effects. The side effects of this class of drugs include dry mouth, delayed gastric time, and constipation—all symptoms that can interfere with food intake. Doxepin, desipramine, and trazodone are reported to have fewer anticholinergic effects and should be considered or substituted for patients who are taking prescribed antidepressants.[42]

Fluoxetine (Prozac), a widely prescribed antidepressant that blocks the reuptake of the neurotransmitter serotonin, is used with increasing frequency for hospital (reactive) depression because of the report of limited side effects. A known weight loss of 6 to 10 pounds in a small percentage of patients has been reported and, consequently, fluoxetine should be used judiciously in patients with anorexia and weight loss due to an advanced disease process.

Nonsteroidal anti-inflammatory drugs (NSAIDs), including aspirin, are also frequently used as adjuncts to pain management. They are known to increase gastric acidity, resulting in indigestion, reflux, or ulceration as well as nausea, vomiting, diarrhea, and constipation, which can also negatively affect food intake.[82] The use of an enteric-coated tablet or one of the more recently developed NSAIDs, e.g., Lodine, has been shown to have fewer gastrointestinal side effects than ASA.

Chronic antibiotic therapy can cause structural changes in the gastrointestinal tract, resulting in ulceration or colitis that can lead to malabsorption, diarrhea, anorexia, and other gastrointestinal disorders, especially in patients with AIDS.[99] Tetracycline is perhaps the most potentially damaging, and substitutions should be considered if possible. Other drugs known to have anorexigenic effects include corticosteroids, antihistamines, antihypertensives, antacids, dopaminergic agents, antihyperlipidemics, antineoplastics, laxatives, and digitalis.

A large percentage of advanced cancer patients with anorexia or nausea develop "dumping syndrome." These patients have responded favorably to the use of cimetidine to alleviate symptoms and improve appetite.

Research supports the fact that behavioral modification techniques, especially the use of self-hypnosis in children, are valuable techniques for controlling anorexia in order to improve food intake.[41, 95] Hypnosis, progressive muscle relaxation, guided imagery, systematic desensitization, and cognitive distraction are some of the symptom control techniques found to be most successful or effective in blocking cancer treatment—related distress and in controlling anticipatory side effects of chemotherapy.[100] Further exploration of these techniques, primarily utilizing group participation in both children and adult populations, may prove useful.

The nutritional interventions are individualized according to the cause of nutritional compromise. Many problems of the anorectic client are interrelated and mandate creative solutions.[73]

Interventions for Dietary Compensation

For anorexic patients unable to ingest adequate amounts of food voluntarily, enteral nutrition (tube feeding using nasogastric, nasoduodenal, esophagostomy, gastrostomy, or jejunostomy tubes) offers an alternative to oral feeding. Total parenteral nutrition (TPN) is the next alternative when feeding via the gastrointestinal tract is contraindicated.

Krause and associates proposed that therapeutic manipulation of plasma-free tryptophan levels by the administration of hypertonic dextrose might paradoxically increase appetite, while the administration of oral branched-chain amino acids might also produce the same result. If this theory is hypothetically correct, the treatment of anorexia by pharmacological manipulation of plasma tryptophan is a distinct possibility.[101] Additional research in this area, however, is needed.

Educational and Counseling Interventions

An educational approach with dietary counseling and written or videotaped materials may be a valuable intervention for the anorectic patient. Improved food intake results if the patient is actively involved in the planning and selection of nutrients when possible.[67] In a quasiexperimental study of 41 cancer patients undergoing radiation therapy for head and neck cancer, subjects were randomized to a control group that received the usual supportive care during radiation therapy or to an experimental group that received a structured nutritional counseling program.[67] The structured program included (1) an audiovisual program illustrating common nutritional problems occurring during radiation therapy and self-care measures for each (e.g., sore mouth and related care), (2) written directions given to each patient on the content of the program, (3) a copy of the book *Eating Hints*[99] available from the National Cancer Institute, and (4) feedback on the weekly analysis of dietary intake compared with recommended and individualized calorie and protein intake. Anorexia was measured on the anorexia scale developed by Grant and associates.[66] Objective measurement of anorexia was calculated as actual calorie and protein intake and percentage of the recommended amounts of each. The analysis revealed that the experimental group was composed of a group of patients highly susceptible to anorexia related to a history of greater weight loss prior to treatment. Both groups lost a significant amount of weight during therapy. The experimental group maintained dietary intake at levels higher than the control group despite greater losses of appetite and the ability to eat. These results point to the possibility that coaching and counseling patients on needed dietary intake during a period of nutritional vulnerability can override the anorexia present and provide some impact on food intake. The book *Eating Hints*,[99] a valuable resource for the anorectic patient, was written from material derived from interviews with cancer patients and includes many useful and easily prepared meals.

The health care provider must avoid handing out printed materials and instructions without communicating verbally with the patient or a family member. Material needs to

TABLE 5–10 SUMMARY OF SELECTED PARAMETERS IN A PATIENT WITH ANOREXIA

Date	Weight*	Digoxin Level†	Dose	Serum Albumin	Total Lymphocytes
1/15	(admission) 135 pounds	Elevated	0.25 mg q.d.	2.8 g/dl	1350 mm³
1/20	136 pounds	Elevated	0.125 mg q.d.	3.5 g/dl	1425 mm³
2/1	139 pounds	WNL	0.125 mg q.d.	4.0 g/dl	1600 mm³
2/21	142 pounds	WNL	0.125 mg q.d.	4.2 g/dl	1700 mm³

*Ideal weight: 150 pounds
†Elevated, > 2.0 mm³
WNL, within normal limits; q.d., every day

be reviewed to ensure that it is understood. Ideally, teaching should occur during the absence of negative symptoms and before the problem occurs.

Distraction is a valuable technique to focus attention away from the annoying symptom of anorexia and to improve intake. A favorite television program, enjoyable music, or talking about a favorite subject can be valuable in improving intake. Adolescents enjoy rock music videos, and adult patients may enjoy classical, country, or religious radio channels. These must be individualized to the likes and dislikes of each patient.

Hospitalized patients are encouraged to take an increasingly active role in evaluating their own illnesses, monitoring their symptoms, and developing treatment plans. Providing the patient with a hospital diary is one useful method for reinforcing this type of behavior.[102] Patients are encouraged to keep a written record of any questions they may have regarding their treatment, diet, exercise plans, medications, or illness in general. The diary functions as an important link between patient and health care workers and encourages continued involvement of the patient in his or her own care.[103]

Nursing intervention with the anorectic patient is challenging. Continual assessment and evaluation—reassessment and re-evaluation—are needed in order to manage the problem successfully.

CASE STUDIES

The following two case studies illustrate some of the manifestations of anorexia, particularly if prolonged.

CASE STUDY NO. 1

Mr. J. W., a 76-year-old white male, was admitted to the medical floor of a large metropolitan hospital from a convalescent nursing home with the diagnosis of "progressive weight loss" and "loss of appetite." The patient stated that he couldn't keep weight on because "I just don't feel like eating." Mr. W. reported being initially bedridden in the nursing home for the past 6 months since suffering a stroke, which left him with a residual left-sided paralysis. He does not go to the dining hall and dislikes eating alone. He picks at the food on his tray, frequently eating only the dessert and drinking the coffee. The patient is a widower (2 years) with no immediate family in the area except for a 78-year-old brother who is unable to drive owing to failing eyesight; he lives 30 miles from the hospital. Mr. W. is left-handed, and this creates additional difficulty with his eating. The patient also complains that his dentures no longer fit and that he has difficulty chewing many of the foods he likes the best (especially meats and caramel candy). Mr. W. reports no nausea or vomiting, no food allergies, and no diarrhea.

The patient has taken digoxin, 0.25 mg daily, and hydrochlorothiazide, 50 mg daily for 10 years, and reports taking over-the-counter laxatives (Ex-Lax) daily for the past 3 years to "keep his bowels regular." The patient has maintained a regular daily pattern of elimination despite his bedridden status.

On admission the patient weighed 135 pounds in a hospital gown, and his height was recorded as 5 feet 9½ inches without shoes. He reported his usual weight as about 150 pounds, "give or take a few pounds." Initial orders included digoxin levels, calorie counts, daily weights, and dietary consultation. Serial serum albumin, total lymphocyte counts, and anthropometric measurements were also ordered (see Table 5–10 for a summary of results). The patient was placed on a high-protein, high-calorie diet served in six small feedings. A physical therapy program was initiated.

Following reduction of the digoxin dose from 0.25 mg/day to 0.125 mg/day, Mr. W.'s appetite steadily improved, and the anorexia subsided. The patient was placed on docusate (Colace) and psyllium hydrophilic mucilloid (Metamucil) daily to soften and add bulk to his stool. The over-the-counter laxative preparation used prior to admission was eliminated from his routine. The patient was placed in a community home near his older brother who was able to come daily to assist Mr. W. with his meal preparation and eating. The social interaction and medication change greatly increased Mr. W.'s appetite. Mr. W. was fitted with new dentures and is now able to adequately chew many of the foods he had been unable to chew before, with a few modifications. Preparing his own meals with the assistance of his brother has made mealtimes much more enjoyable. Mr. W. was last seen in the outpatient clinic 2 months after discharge and was steadily gaining weight. There was no evidence of any appetite disorder, and the anorexia had completely subsided.

CASE STUDY NO. 2

In November Ms. F. M., a 53-year-old woman, was admitted via the emergency room with complaints of "loss of appetite and nausea" as well as a 15-pound weight loss over the past 2 months with no reported decrease in amount of food consumed: "I've been eating the way I always do but I'm still losing weight." The patient reported that for the 2 weeks prior to admission her urine had appeared darker in color and she felt excessively fatigued. "I'm always tired out and I have no energy even after a good 10 hour night's sleep." Ms. M. also complained of midsternal pressure on swallowing and a feeling of fullness after meals. "I take a few bites and I feel like there is a weight on my chest right between my breasts." On physical examination, sclera and skin appeared jaundiced and there was midepigastric tenderness. The liver edge was palpated 2 cm below the right costal margin. Past history revealed a right radical mastectomy was performed for intraductal

carcinoma of the breast 2 years previously, and there was evidence of possible "ulcer disease" for 3 years. The patient states, "I'm afraid I might have cancer again."

Barium swallow, performed on the third hospital day, revealed a mass in the upper third of the stomach; gastroscopy with biopsy revealed adenocarcinoma of the stomach. Exploratory laparotomy on the fifth hospital day revealed a large unresectable midepigastric tumor involving lymph nodes, liver, and other major blood vessels and organs. Palliative abdominal radiation and chemotherapy with 5-fluorouracil (12 mg/kg) was initiated 10 days postsurgery in order to allow for healing of the surgical incision.

Combination radiation and chemotherapy increased the patient's chances of developing gastrointestinal tract complications due to destruction of gastric enzymes. Anorexia markedly increased toward all foods, and the patient stated "nothing tastes good; the thought of food nauseates me." Diarrhea (of up to 20 stools per day) developed during therapy. In addition, the patient acquired moniliasis, a frequent side effect of chemotherapy, and gingival sores, which further complicated an already compromised nutritional state. Ms. M.'s laboratory values are shown in Table 5–11.

Immediately after her course of radiation and chemotherapy Ms. M.'s anorexia improved, and she was able to tolerate a soft diet in six small feedings in addition to a liquid supplement. Two weeks later, however, the anorexia markedly worsened and the patient was readmitted to the hospital, unable to tolerate solid foods and complaining of a total loss of appetite for all foods. Ms. M. appeared dehydrated with evidence of dry cracked lips and tenting of subcutaneous tissue on the upper extremities, and 4+ pitting edema of the lower extremities. Intravenous therapy with 5 per cent dextrose in water, nasal oxygen at 2 L/minute, and morphine sulfate 10 mg every 2 hours was initiated. A massive pulmonary edema developed 36 hours after readmission, and the patient succumbed to her disease.

These case studies illustrate the multiple complexities of anorexia. It is a clinical phe-

TABLE 5–11   CHANGES IN SELECTED PARAMETERS IN A PATIENT WITH ANOREXIA

	Date	Hct.*	Hgb.†	Albumin‡	Weight§
Admission	11/21	35 per cent	11 g/100 ml	3.5 g/dl	115 pounds
After surgery	11/25	28 per cent	8 g/100 ml	3.0 g/dl	112 pounds
Prior to radiation therapy and chemotherapy	12/4	32 per cent	10 g/100 ml	3.7 g/dl	117 pounds
After chemotherapy complete	1/13	24 per cent	6 g/100 ml	2.8 g/dl	105 pounds
One week postchemotherapy	1/20	30 per cent	8 g/100 ml	2.9 g/dl	107 pounds
Two weeks after chemotherapy and second admission	1/27	22 per cent	6 g/100 ml	2.4 g/dl	99 pounds

*Normal Hct. = 38 to 41 per cent
†Normal Hgb. = 12 to 16 g/100 ml
‡Normal albumin = 4.5 to 3.8 g/dl
§Usual weight = 130 pounds (height = 5 feet, 4 inches)
Hct., hematocrit; Hgb., hemoglobin

nomenon that occurs frequently as a human response to many varied conditions.

REVIEW OF RESEARCH FINDINGS

Little nursing research has been reported about anorexia, and clinical (empirical) research on anorexia involving human subjects is rare. Multiple variables influence the clinical picture and make the study of anorexia extremely difficult. The premorbid nutritional status of the individual and variable responses to illness are two of the host variables that are extremely difficult to measure. The measurement of anorexia and the incidence, degree, and timing of its occurrence create further difficulty for the researcher.

Although recognition of the problem of anorexia is documented in both medical and nursing literature and suggestions for improving appetite of the anorectic patient are made, these are essentially unsupported with reliable research or accurate statistical data. A majority of the existing research on anorexia is presented in relationship to cancer and the cancer population and to the effects of nutritional therapy (TPN and elemental diets) on the cancer population, especially during treatments (chemotherapy, radiation therapy) that result in anorexia. A small number of studies have also been done on anorexia as a side effect of drug therapy. Selected studies are discussed below.

Research on Anorexia and Cancer

Anorexia and concomitant weight loss occur frequently in cancer patients. Weight loss has recently been recognized as one of the major determinants of survival, a fact that makes the understanding of its pathogenesis of prime clinical relevance. Many factors are involved in the pathogenesis of this weight loss, but few scientific studies document the interrelationships. Anorexia is probably a prime pathway. Spontaneous consumption of food decreases in some patients more than in others. In many patients, complete nutritional depletion occurs and death ensues.[104]

In a study by Costa and associates, food consumption was estimated in 199 ambulatory cancer patients and in 205 normal subjects (matched control group).[104] Nutrition interviews, including medical and weight histories, height, anthropometric parameters, and estimates of food intake by 24-hour recall, made up the data. The data showed that male cancer patients ate significantly less than the healthy controls (1894 kcal/day versus 2358 kcal/day, p < .005), while female cancer patients maintained their food consumption near the level of their normal counterparts (1556 kcal/day versus 1612 kcal/day). In a subset of male lung cancer patients with well-documented weight history, anorexia could not explain weight loss. The inability of anorexia to explain weight loss leads one to believe that weight loss is possibly a consequence of altered host metabolism.

In a preliminary report of results from a multi-institutional study evaluating anorexia in cancer patients, the conclusion that decreased caloric intake is important in the weight loss of cancer patients was supported.[105] The caloric intake of 89 cancer patients (varying sites and stages) was estimated from 3-day diet diaries using a computerized nutrient analysis system. Symptoms that might be related to food intake were elicited by semistructured interview. Basal energy expenditure was calculated by computer. The results show that 22 patients (25 per cent) had calorie intake below BEE. In an interview, patients were requested to report symptoms that might be interfering with eating. Symptoms referable to the oronasal area were most frequent and were reported in one form or another by 67 (75 per cent) patients. The most frequently reported symptom was altered taste sensation, noted by 53 (60 per cent) patients. Thirty-five patients (39 per cent) related symptoms referable to the gastrointestinal tract, with the most frequent being a sense of filling up quickly (22 patients). These results provided clues to the pathophysiological mechanisms of decreased caloric intake.[105]

From a preliminary study using an assay performed on the urine of anorectic cancer patients, the investigators reported the presence of substances in the urine that strongly suppress the level of activity, thirst, and appetite.[106] These substances have not been purified, but evidence from earlier studies indicates that they may be peptides. Injection of peptides experimentally into animals with cancer allows researchers to study the effect on food intake and promotes a better understanding of the pathogenesis of anorexia in cancer.[50]

In a report by Hall and associates, 31 patients attending a surgical oncology outpatient clinic after primary resection of a gastrointestinal tumor were studied.[107] The purpose of the study was to identify those factors that best reflect protein-calorie malnutrition in this population. Outcome measure included daily protein and caloric intake, three plasma protein estimations, two upper limb anthropometric measurements, and estimated weight loss. The patients were divided into three groups depending on (1) the absence of clinically detectable tumor (9 patients), (2) the presence of clinically detectable tumor with survival over the ensuing 4-month period (10 patients), and (3) clinically detectable tumor without survival over the ensuing 4-month period (12 patients). The variables least able to reflect malnutrition in this sample were dietary intake data and estimates of weight loss, which failed to differentiate between groups of patients and to interrelate with other measures of malnutrition in a cross-correlation matrix.

The failure of dietary intake data to mirror

the anorexia so commonly admitted by patients with advanced gastrointestinal cancer is revealing. The inaccuracy of dietary measurement, combined with the wide variation in the quantity of food consumed by patients, makes demonstration of differences in trials of fixed sample size extremely difficult. Recruitment of a large number of patients potentially alleviates this problem. Alternatively, anorexia can be investigated in small numbers of patients using longitudinal studies in which the interpatient variation is excluded by each patient acting as his or her own control. Such studies will remain negative unless real changes in dietary intake exceed errors of measurement. This may be one of the primary reasons the anorexia of cancer escapes detailed study.

Studies of head and neck cancer patients reveal the presence of anorexia and its exacerbation during periods of therapy. Several studies have documented that as many as 40 per cent of patients with cancer of the head and neck area are at nutritional risk at the time of diagnosis, having experienced anorexia and weight loss prior to seeking medical help.[108, 109] This vulnerable population demonstrates persistent nutritional problems during radiation therapy, with anorexia and weight loss occurring commonly.[67, 110] Several studies have examined the effects of counseling and coaching on maintaining adequate intake and decreasing weight loss despite persistent and frequently increasing anorexia.[67, 111, 112]

Results of Grant's study have been discussed previously and point to the potential value of coaching or counseling patients to maintain adequate oral intake.[67] In Daly and associates' study oral intake was compared with enteral nutrition in head and neck cancer patients undergoing radiation therapy.[111] Results revealed that the tube-fed group had better maintenance of weight during radiation therapy when compared with the oral intake group. No differences in either response to radiation therapy or patient survival occurred in either group. In the study by Foltz and colleagues 180 patients with advanced colorectal or non–small cell lung cancer were randomized to three levels of nutritional support: control (no nutritional counseling and ad lib diet), standard (nutritional counseling to achieve a target weight), and augmented (nutritional counseling for a target caloric intake with 25 per cent of total calories derived from protein sources).[112] After 4 weeks, nutritional counseling produced a significant increase in caloric intake. These studies indicate a beginning understanding of the value of coaching or counseling patients in an effort to overcome anorexia and maintain adequate nutritional intake.

Research on Drug Therapy and Anorexia

Because the nutritional complications of drug usage are subtle and seemingly nonspecific and protracted in cause, research on drug therapy and anorexia is practically nonexistent. Virtually any pharmacological agent may produce anorexia and subsequent undernutrition by a wide variety of other mechanisms, including interference with intestinal absorption, binding to plasma proteins, decreased transport across cell membranes, peripheral utilization, transformations intracellularly, storage, turnover, elimination, and excretion.[13] Anorexia is such a common phenomenon in clinical settings that clinicians often fail to search for underlying mechanisms. Drugs may cause undernutrition (inadequate dietary intake and inability to metabolize nutrients normally) by reducing food intake. This commonly occurs when the drug being taken produces anorexia. Two drugs especially implicated in appetite suppression are levodopa (Dopar and Larodopa) and digitalis (digoxin).[19]

Digoxin is a well-known cause of chronic anorexia and insidious weight loss. Yet, it is often forgotten that patients can lose so much weight from this that a malignancy may be suspected.[81, 82] Smith and Habere found that of six patients interviewed only two admitted to anorexia with hindsight and the other four had only intermittent symptoms.[98] Digoxin, because of the anorexia it produces, should be considered as a potential cause of insidious weight loss.[82]

Research shows that in addition to digoxin, certain categories of drugs, such as the thiazide diuretics, over-the-counter appetite suppressants, laxatives, narcotic and non-narcotic analgesics (especially aspirin), non-steroidal anti-inflammatory drugs, and antidepressants, are particularly likely to cause anorexia and drug-induced nutritional deficiencies. It has also been shown that antibiotics are a notorious cause of anorexia and

delayed digestion of food. Ferrous sulfate (Feosol) and phosphate binders commonly cause anorexia, nausea, and vomiting. Many anesthetic agents and chemotherapeutic agents (e.g., 5-fluorouracil, vincristine), alter taste sensitivity and contribute to anorexia, although research in this area is scant.

Chemotherapeutic agents are known to cause severe prolonged anorexia. Food intake may be limited owing to a reduction or loss of taste or smell acuity.[13] An example of this phenomenon is the agent penicillamine, which has been shown to cause a loss of taste acuity by binding to zinc and removing it from the body.[113] Active laboratory research is currently underway to explore this important area.[13]

When food seems tasteless or "bland," there is little impetus to eat. Drugs may also cause loss of interest in eating by a central mechanism when the patient becomes anxious, depressed, or withdrawn or when a more severe psychiatric disorder develops.[114]

IMPLICATIONS FOR RESEARCH

Many areas of study need to be explored in order to understand more fully the phenomenon of anorexia. Perhaps the greatest need for research on anorexia is for a comprehensive study in a uniform population in order to develop specific patterns that characterize the anorectic patient. This is beginning to happen in the studies describing anorexia in head and neck cancer patients. Other areas for further nursing investigation and evaluation are (1) factors to be included in an initial as well as long-term nutritional assessment of the anorexic patient and the most practical and reliable method for establishing nutritional needs of anorexic patients, (2) the effectiveness of various nursing interventions in alleviating anorexia and in improving food acceptance in specific populations and of most benefit to specific patient groups, (3) nutritional preparations and drug therapies that are most beneficial to patients with anorexia and those that need to be developed and field tested in clinical trials, and (4) assessment parameters that can most accurately measure response to nutritional therapy.[115] In addition to identifying and evaluating therapies for the anorectic client and establishing whether patient survival is improved, there are many questions and topics germane to nursing that need to be investigated. For example, how can anorexia be measured? What parameters can be used to measure the magnitude and extent of anorexia? Since eating behavior is controlled by numerous cues or control mechanisms, future research should be directed at delineating a hierarchical ranking of these food intake cues.[48] Definitive studies of the energy expenditure of cancer patients are needed, since weight loss is not always due to anorexia and decreased caloric intake. Clinical trials of nutritional and metabolic intervention in patients should include an evaluation of the effects on appetite and anorexia.[48]

Comprehensive and effective nursing management of the challenging and complex problem of anorexia depends on our knowledge of populations at risk, our assessment skills, and our expertise in designing nursing interventions based on empirically tested research that will ultimately improve care given to the anorectic client.

REFERENCES

1. Jones, D., Dunbar, C., & Jirovic, M. (1978). *Medical-Surgical Nursing: A Conceptual Approach* (p. 557). New York: McGraw-Hill.
2. Nutritional status of cancer patients. (1980). Nutr Rev *21*:378.
3. Blackburn, G.L., & Harvey, K.B. (1982). Nutritional assessment as a routine in clinical medicine. Postgrad Med *71*:46–63.
4. Salmond, S. (1980). How to assess the nutritional status of acutely ill patients. Am J Nurs 80:922–924.
5. Morley, J.E., Mooradian, A.D., Silver, A.J., Heber, D., & Alfin-Slater, R.B. (1988). Nutrition in the elderly. Ann Intern Med *109*:890–904.
6. Morley, J., & Silver, A. (1988). Anorexia in the elderly. Neurobiol Aging *9*:9–16.
7. Rudman, D. (1980). Syndromes of undernutrition: Assessment of nutritional status. In K. Isselbacher, et al. (eds.), *Harrison's Principles of Internal Medicine* (9th ed., p. 405). New York: McGraw-Hill.
8. Johnson, J. (1979). Anorexia in the cancer patient. In J. Wollard (ed.), *Nutritional Management of the Cancer Patient* (pp. 83–95). New York: Raven Press.
9. Woods, C.G., Rylance, M.E., Cullen, R.E., & Rylance, G.W. (1987). Adverse reactions to drugs in children. Br Med J *294*:869–870.
10. Bruppacher, R., Gyr, M., & Fisch, T. (1988). Abdominal pain, indigestion, anorexia, nausea and vomiting. Baillières Clinical Gastroenterol 2:275–292.
11. Gryboski, J., Katz, J., Sangrie, H., & Herskovic, T. (1968). Eleven adolescent girls with severe anorexia. Clin Pediatr 7:684.
12. Akridge, K. (1989). Anorexia nervosa. J Obstetr Gynecol Neonatal Nurs 18(1):25–30.
13. Blacklow, R. (1983). Anorexia. *MacBrydes Signs and Symptoms: Applied Pathologic Physiology and Clinical Interpretation* (6th ed., pp. 62–65). Philadelphia: J.B. Lippincott.
14. Wyllie, R. (1984). Differential diagnosis of anorexia: A challenge. Consult *3*:8–9.
15. Sleisenger, M.H., & Fordtram, J.S. (1983). *G.I. Disease: Pathophysiology, Diagnosis and Management* (3rd ed., vol. 1, p. 138). Philadelphia: W.B. Saunders.
16. Claggert, M. (1980). Managing anorexia in the elderly. Home Health Rev *3*:12–15.
17. Tichy, A.M., & Malasanos, L.T. (1979). Physiological parameters of aging, Part II. J Gerontol Nurs *5*:38–41.
18. Sklar, M. (1983). G.I. diseases in the aged. In W. Reichel (ed.), *Clinical Aspects of Aging* (2nd ed., p. 205). Baltimore: Williams and Wilkins.
19. Olson-Noel, C., & Bosworth, M. (1989). Anorexia and weight loss in the elderly. Postgrad Med *85*:140–144.
20. Kaplan, S., & Tuckman, T.B. (1986). Considerations for those providing nutritional care to the elderly. J Nutr Elderly *5*:53–58.
21. Garetz, F. (1976). Breaking the dangerous cycle of depression and faulty nutrition. Geriatrics *31*:73–75.
22. Winegrad, C.H., & Jarvik, L. (1986). Physician management of the demented patient. J Am Geriatr Soc *34*:295–308.
23. Gurland, B., & Goss, P. (1982). Epidemiology of psychopathology in old age: Some implications for clinical services. Psychiatr Clin North Am *5*:110–126.
24. Wyngaarden, J., & Smith, L. (1988). *Cecil's Textbook of Medicine* (18th ed., p. 843). Philadelphia: W.B. Saunders.
25. DeWys, W.D. (1970). Working conference on anorexia and cachexia of neoplastic disease. Cancer Res *30*:2816–2818.
26. DeWys, W.D. (1974). Abnormalities of taste as a remote effect of a neoplasm. Ann NY Acad Sci *230*:427–434.
27. DeWys, W.D., & Walters, K. (1975). Abnormalities of taste sensation in cancer patients. Cancer *36*:1888–1896.
28. DeWys, W.D. (1977). Taste and feeding behavior in patients with cancer. In M. Winick (ed.), *Current Concepts in Nutrition* (vol. 6). New York: John Wiley.
29. Carson, J.S., & Gormician, A. (1977). Taste acuity and food attitudes of selected patients with cancer. J Am Diet Assoc *70*:361.
30. Gormican, A. (1980). Influencing food acceptance in anorexic cancer patients. Postgrad Med *68*:145–152.
31. Williams, L., & Cohen, M. (1978). Altered taste thresholds in lung cancer. Am J Clin Nutr *31*:122–125.
32. Szeulga, D., Groenwald, S., & Sullivan, D. (1990). Nutritional disturbances. In S. Groenwald, M. Frogge, M. Goodman, & C. Yarbro (eds.), *Cancer Nursing: Principles and Practice* (2nd ed., pp. 495–519). Boston: Jones and Bartlett.
33. Henkin, R., Schechter, P., & Hoye, R. (1971). Idiopathic hypogeusia with dysgeusia, hyposmia, and dysosmia: A new syndrome. JAMA *217*:434–440.
34. Henkin, R.I. (1977). New aspects in the control of food intake and appetite. Ann NY Acad Sci *300*:321–334.
35. Mueller, K., Buzby, G., & Mullen, J. (1982). Ther-

apeutic nutritional practices for the cancer patient. Penn Med February:59–63.

36. Schroeder, S. (ed.) (1989). *Current Medical Diagnosis and Treatment*. Norwalk, CT: Appleton & Lange.

37. Sodeman, W. (ed.) (1985). *Sodeman's Pathologic Physiology—Mechanisms of Disease* (7th ed.). Philadelphia: W. B. Saunders.

38. Bernstein, I., & Bernstein, I. (1981). Learned food aversions and cancer aversions and cancer anorexia. Cancer Treat Reports *65*(Suppl. 5):43–47.

39. Nielsen, S., Theologides, A., & Vickers, Z. (1980). Influence of food odors on food aversions and preferences in patients with cancer. Am J Clin Nutr *33*:2253-2261.

40. Morrison, S.D. (1978). Origins of anorexia in neoplastic disease. Am J Clin Nutr *33*:1104.

41. Holland, J., Rowland, J., & Plumb, M. (1977). Psychological aspects of anorexia in cancer patients. Cancer Res *37*:2425–2428.

42. Keithley, J. (1990). Management of nutritional problems in patients with AIDS. Oncol Nurs Forum *17*:23–27.

43. Greene, J. (1988). Clinical approach to weight loss in the patient with HIV infection. Gastroenterol Clin North Am *17*:573–586.

44. Luckman, L., & Sorenson, K. (1980). *Medical Surgical Nursing: A Psychophysiologic Approach*. Philadelphia: W.B. Saunders.

45. Isselbacher, K. (1980). *Harrison's Principles of Internal Medicine* (9th ed., p. 197). New York: McGraw-Hill.

46. Braunwald, E. (ed.) (1988). *Heart Disease* (3rd ed.). Philadelphia: W.B. Saunders.

47. Kensit, M. (1978). Appetite disturbances in dialysis patients. JAMA *6*:194–199.

48. DeWys, W.D. (1977). Anorexia in cancer patients. Cancer Res *37*:2354–2358.

49. Morley, J., & Levine, A. (1983). The central control of appetite. Lancet *1*:398–401.

50. Theologides, A. (1981). Anorexia in cancer: Another speculation on its pathogenesis. Nutr Cancer *2*:133–135.

51. Krause, R., Greep, J., & Fische, A. (1979). Central mechanism for anorexia in cancer: Role of the neurotransmitter serotonin (abstract). Br J Surg *66*:885–886.

52. Novin, D., Wywicks, W., & Bray, G. (eds.) (1976). *Hunger: Basic Mechanisms and Clinical Implications*. New York: Raven Press.

53. Krause, M., & Mahan, L. (1981). *Food, Nutrition, and Diet Therapy* (6th ed., pp. 553–556). Philadelphia: W.B. Saunders.

54. Schmale, A. (1979). Psychological aspects of anorexia. Cancer *3*(Suppl. 2):2087–2092.

55. Hammill, P. (1978). Nutritional assessment and intervention to improve the nutritional status of cancer patients. M.A. thesis. University of Rochester School of Nursing.

56. Van Eys, J. (1982). Nutrition and neoplasia. Nutr Rev *40*:353–356.

57. Roy, C., Sister, & Roberts, S.L. (1981). *Theory Construction in Nursing: An Adaptation Model* (pp. 102–104). Englewood Cliffs, NJ: Prentice-Hall.

58. Norris, C. (1982). Nausea and vomiting. In C. Norris (ed.), *Concept Clarification in Nursing* (pp. 81–110). Rockville, MD: Aspen Publications.

59. Renneker, M., & Leib, S. (1979). *Understanding Cancer* (2nd ed., p. 242). Palo Alto, CA: Bull Publishing.

60. Hanks, G.W. (1984). Psychotropic drugs. Clin Oncol *3*:135–151.

61. Donovan, M., & Peirce, S. (1976). *Cancer Care Nursing*. New York: Appleton-Century-Crofts.

62. DeWys, W.D. (1979). Anorexia as a general effect of cancer. Cancer *43*:2013–2019.

63. Donoghue, M. (1981). Nursing interventions: Anorexia in nursing care of the cancer patient with nutritional problems. *Ross Roundtable on Oncology Nursing* (session III, pp. 27–34). Columbus, OH: Ross Laboratories.

64. Donoghue, M., Nunnally, C., & Yasko, J. (1983). Anorexia (protein calorie malnutrition). In J. Yasko (ed.), *Guidelines for Cancer Care: Symptom Management* (pp. 159–183). Reston, VA: Reston Publishing.

65. Donoghue, M., Nunnally, C., & Yasko, J. (1982). *Nutritional Aspects of Cancer Care* (pp. 83–145). Reston, VA: Reston Publishing.

66. Grant, M., Padilla, G., & Rhiner, M. (1991). Patterns of anorexia in cancer patients. Proceeding of the First National Nursing Research Conference. Atlanta: American Cancer Society. Publication Number 71-25M-3332-03 PE

67. Grant, M. (1987). Effects of a structured teaching program for cancer patients undergoing head and neck radiation therapy on anorexia, nutritional status, functional status, treatment response, and quality of life. Ph.D. dissertation. University of California, San Francisco.

68. Thiele, V. (1980). *Clinical Nutrition* (2nd ed.). St. Louis: C.V. Mosby.

69. Donoghue, M. (1986). Nutritional aspects of cancer and chemotherapy in the elderly. In D. Welch-McCaffrey (ed.), *Nursing Considerations in Geriatric Oncology* (pp. 23–26). Philadelphia: Adria Laboratories.

70. Frank-Stromborg, M. (1986). The role of the nurse in cancer detection and screening. Semin Oncol Nurs *2*:191–199.

71. Coates, A., Abraham, S., & Kaye, S. B. (1983). On the receiving end—Patient perception of the side effects of chemotherapy. Eur J Clin Oncol *19*:203–208.

72. Schein, P., MacDonald, J., Waters, C., & Haidak, D. (1979). Nutritional complications of cancer and its treatment. In L. Kruse, et al. (eds.), *Cancer: Pathophysiology, Etiology, and Management* (pp. 364–377). St Louis: C.V. Mosby.

73. Weaver, K. (1991). Reversible malnutrition in AIDS. Am J Nurs AJN *91*:25–31.

74. DeWys, W., & Pascucci-Amino, M. (1978). Anorexia, taste changes and diet in cancer. Compr Ther *4*:7–12.

75. Zamcheck, N., & Broitman, S.A. (1973). Nutrition in diseases of the intestines. In R. Goodhart & M. Shils (eds.), *Modern Nutrition in Health and Disease*. Philadelphia: Lea and Febiger.

76. DeWys, W.D., & Herbst, S.H. (1977). Oral feeding in the nutritional management of the cancer patient. Cancer Res *37*:109–111.

77. Drasin, H., Rosenbaum, E.H., Stitt, C.A., & Rosenbaum, I.R. (1979). The challenge of nutritional maintenance in cancer patients. West J Med *130*:145–152.

78. Dairy Council Digest. (1988). National Dairy Council, *59*:5.

79. Mitchell, P., & Lousteau, A. (1981). *Concepts Basic to Nursing* (3rd ed.) New York: McGraw-Hill.

80. Pawlowski, G.J. (1975). Cyproheptadine: Weight gain and appetite stimulation in essential anorexic adults. Curr Ther Res 18:673–678.

81. Regelson, W., Regelson, W., Butler, J. R., & Schultz, J. (1976). Delta-9-tetrahydrocannabinol as an effective antidepressant and appetite-stimulating agent in advanced cancer patients. In N. Braude & S. Szara (eds.), *The Pharmacology of Marijuana*. New York: Raven Press.

82. Spaulding, M. (1989). Recent studies of anorexia and appetite stimulation in the cancer patient. Oncology (Suppl.) 3:17–23.

83. Willox, J., Corr, J., Shaw, J., Richardson, M., Calman, K.C. & Drennan, M. (1984). Prednisolone as an appetite stimulant in patients with cancer. Br Med J 288:27.

84. Shinshanker, K., Bennett, R., & Haynie, T.P. (1983). Tumor-associated gastroparesis: Correction with metoclopramide. Am J Surg 145:221–225.

85. Kris, M.G., Yeh, S.D., Gralla, R.J., & Young, C.W. (1985). Symptomatic gastroparesis in cancer patients. A possible cause of cancer associated anorexia that can be improved with oral metoclopramide (Abstract). Proc Am Soc Clin Oncol 4:267.

86. Tchekmedyian, N.S., Tait, N., Moody, M., Greco, F.A., & Aisner, J. (1986). Appetite stimulation with megestrol acetate in cachectic cancer patients. Semin Oncol 13(Suppl. 4):37–43.

87. Schacter, L., Rozencweig, M., Canetta, R., Kelley, S., Nicaise, C., & Smaldone, L. (1989). Megestrol acetate: Clinical experience. Cancer Treat Rev 16:49–63.

88. Loprinzi, C.L., Ellison, N.M., Schaid, D.J., Krook, J.E., Athmann, L.M., Dose, A.M., Mailliard, J.A., Johnson, P.S., Ebbert, L.P., & Geeraerts, L.H. (1990). Controlled trial of megestrol acetate for the treatment of cancer anorexia and cachexia. J Natl Cancer Inst 82:1127–1132.

89. Tait, N., & Aisner, J. (1989). Nutritional concerns in cancer patients. Semin Oncol Nurs 5:58–62.

90. Chlebowski, R.T., Bulcavage, L., Grosvenor, M., Tsunoki, R., Block, J.B., Heber, D., Scrooc, M., Chlebowski, J.S., Chi, J., & Oktay, E., et al. (1987). Hydrazine sulfate in cancer patients with weight loss. Cancer 59:406–410.

91. Chlebowski, L., Bulcavage, L., Grosvenor, M., Oktay, E., Block, J.B., Chlebowski, J.S., Ali, I., & Elashoff, R. (1990). Hydrazine sulfate: Influence on nutritional status and survival in non-small cell lung cancer. J Clin Oncol 8:9–15.

92. Theologides, A. (1988). Appetite in anorexia of cancer. Curr Concepts Nutr 16:101–124.

93. Doty, R.L. (1977). Food preference rating of congenitally anosmic humans. In M. Kare & O. Maller (eds.), *Chemical Senses and Nutrition II*. New York: Academic Press.

94. Duffy, V., & Ferris, A.M. (1989). Nutritional management of patients with chemosensory disturbances. Ear, Nose Throat J. 68:395–397.

95. Costa, G., & Donaldson, S. (1980). The nutritional effects of cancer and its therapy. Nutr Cancer 2:22–29.

96. Markman, M., Sheidler, V., Ettinger, D.S., Quaskey, S.A., & Mellits, E.D. (1984). Antiemetic efficacy of dexamethasone. N Engl J Med 311:549–552.

97. Banks, T., & Ali, N. (1974). Digitalis cachexia (letter to the editor). N Engl J Med 290:746–747.

98. Smith, T., & Habere, E. (1973). Digitalis. N Engl J Med 289:1010, 1115, 1063.

99. *Eating Hints*. (1987). NCI Publication No. 87–2079. Washington, DC: US Dept of Health and Human Services.

100. McCabe, M. (1991). Psychological support for the patient on chemotherapy. Oncology 5:91–99.

101. Krause, R., Humphrey, C., von Mayenfeldt, M., James, H., & Fischer, J. (1981). A central mechanism for anorexia in cancer: A hypothesis. Cancer Treat Rep 65(Suppl. 5):15–20.

102. Bedell, S.E., Cleary, P.D., & Delbanco, T.L. (1984). The kindly stress of hospitalization. JAMA 77:592–596.

103. Vebrugge, L. (1980). Health diaries. Med Care 18:73–95.

104. Costa, G., Bewley, P., Aragon, M., & Siebold, J. (1981). Anorexia and weight-loss in cancer patients. Cancer Treat Rep 65(Suppl. 5):3–7.

105. DeWys, W.D., Costa, G., & Henkin, R. (1981). Clinical parameters related to anorexia. Cancer Treat Rep 65(Suppl. 5):49–53.

106. Barai, B., & DeWys, W. (1980). Assay for presence of anorectic substance in urine of cancer patients (abstract). Proc Am Soc Cancer Res 21:378.

107. Hall, J.C., Lawton, J., Appleton, N., Stocks, H., & Giles, G.R. (1980). The assessment of protein-calorie malnutrition in patients with gastrointestinal cancer. Aust NZ J Surg 50:289–292.

108. Bassett, M.R., & Dobie, R.A. (1983). Patterns of nutritional deficiency in head and neck cancer. Head Neck Surg 91:119–125.

109. Flyan, M.B., & Leighty, F. (1987). Postoperative outpatient nutritional support of patients with squamous cancer of the upper aerodigestive track (abstract). Joint Annual Meeting of the Association of Head and Neck Oncologists of Great Britain, British Association of Surgical Oncology, Society of Head and Neck Surgeons, and Society of Surgical Oncology, April 25–30.

110. Johnston, C.A., Kease, J., & Prudo, S.M. (1982). Weight loss in patients receiving radical radiation therapy for head and neck cancer: A prospective study. J Parenter Enteral Nutr 6:399–402.

111. Daly, J.M., Hearne, B., Dunaj, J., LePorte, B., Vikram, B., Strong, E., Green, M., Muggio, F., Groshen, S., & DeCosse, J.J. (1984). Nutritional rehabilitation in patients with advanced head and neck cancer receiving radiation therapy. Am J Surg 148:514–520.

112. Foltz, A. (1987). Effectiveness of nutritional counseling on calorie intake, weight change, and percent protein intake in patients with advanced colorectal and lung cancer. Nutrition 3:263–271.

113. MacFarland, M.D. (1974). Penicillamine and zinc. Lancet 2:962.

114. Aiach, J.M. (1980). Effects of diet on the absorption of drugs. Pharm Ada Hebr 55:210.

115. Valencius, J. (1979). Nutritional support of the cancer patient. In C. Kellog & B. Sullivan (eds.), *Current Perspectives in Oncologic Nursing* (vol. 2, pp. 45–55). St. Louis: C.V. Mosby.

6

Cancer Cachexia

Ada M. Lindsey

DEFINITION

Cachexia, as a debilitating wasting syndrome, may be seen in conditions other than cancer; for example, wasting occurs with prolonged infection, severe traumatic injuries, some cardiac or pulmonary conditions, and other chronic illnesses such as liver disease. Cachexia may occur as a consequence of anorexia, infection, ulceration, loss through drainage, or a number of other attendant debilitating conditions. Wasting is the distinguishing characteristic of cachexia. However, because of the complexity of the phenomenon, the frequency with which it is observed, and the morbidity and mortality associated with it in cancer patients, the focus of this chapter is the cachexia of malignancy. It occurs more commonly with some malignancies, such as lung cancer, and less frequently with other malignancies, such as breast cancer. There is accumulating evidence to begin to elucidate at least a few of the specific mechanisms involved in this wasting phenomenon associated with some types of cancer and in patients with infection or trauma. The monokine cachectin/tumor necrosis factor–alpha (TNF) has been proposed as one endogenous mediator resulting in the cachetic syndrome. The primary distinguishing features of cancer cachexia define the phenomenon; it is a syndrome of progressive wasting associated with alterations in host metabolism.

PREVALENCE AND POPULATIONS AT RISK

Prior to the effectiveness of the current cancer therapies, cachexia was the leading cause of death in cancer patients.[1] With the increased survival rates and lengthened disease-free intervals resulting from current therapies, cancer is now considered to be a chronic disease. Thus, it is anticipated that more cancer patients will experience cachexia. With exacerbations of the disease, people are treated more aggressively and are kept alive longer. With better health care and greater accessibility to services, more people will be diagnosed with cancer. As the age of the population increases (i.e., more older people), the incidence of cancer is projected to increase. All of these circumstances contribute to the potential increase in the number of cancer patients who will experience cachexia at some time in the course of the disease and the treatment regimen.

Figures on the exact incidence of cachexia are unknown. It is estimated that one half to two thirds of cancer patients with varying tumor types experience cachexia and that two thirds of those who succumb to cancer are cachectic at death.[1, 2] In a large study by the Eastern Cooperative Oncology Group, more than 50 per cent of 3000 cancer patients had lost weight.[3] Weight loss for patients with some types of cancer such as breast cancer and sarcoma was not significant, but for others with lung cancer or cancer of visceral organs the weight loss was significant. Others have reported cachexia or evidence of protein-calorie malnutrition (PCM) in 50 to 80 per cent of cancer patients.[4, 5] These data suggest that 50 per cent or more of patients with cancer will have clinically detectable cachexia. Considering the magnitude of the incidence of cancer as a major health problem, the prevalence of cancer cachexia is great. Because cachexia contributes significantly to the morbidity and mortality of cancer patients, it is a substantial clinical problem.

Elderly individuals, children, and adolescents are more vulnerable to the development of cachexia. Cancer patients, regardless of age or tumor type, who experience prolonged episodes of anorexia (a loss of appetite resulting in a decline in spontaneous food intake) are at greater risk for the occurrence of progressive wasting, particularly when the intake over time does not meet the metabolic needs of the host.

Patients whose malignancies are in sites that cause interference with the ingestion, digestion, and/or absorption of nutrients are more likely to experience cachexia. Those who receive radiation therapy to sites involved in the ingestion, digestion, and absorption processes also are at greater risk for the development or progression of cachexia. Cancer patients who have other concomitant debilitating conditions, such as infection or open draining wounds, are at obvious risk for cachexia, if the food intake is insufficient for the altered metabolic state. Although not well documented with empirical evidence, clinical observations suggest that cachexia occurs more frequently in certain tumor types, for example, small cell lung cancer. Given the complexity of the phenomenon and the number of contributing etiological stressors, all cancer patients need to be assessed periodically for their potential risk for the development or progression of cachexia.

SITUATIONAL STRESSORS

Major stressors that may influence the development of cachexia include the side effects of chemotherapy and radiation therapy, the location and type of cancer, and the extent of the tumor burden. Side effects of treatment frequently include nausea and vomiting, stomatitis, mucositis, and anorexia, all of which act to diminish intake. Some individuals develop learned food aversions in response to therapy. The presence of infection or an open draining wound is also a stressor that has an impact on development of cachexia.

Clinical State

In all the cancer and nutrition literature, there is no one simple set of parameters that definitively identifies when an individual is recognized or diagnosed as having cancer cachexia. Nutritional assessment data are those most frequently used in studies to determine metabolic status, and normative values of these parameters are available for comparisons.[6–9] In addition to weight loss and objective loss of protein and fat, cachectic individuals may have hyperglycemia and hyperlipidemia. Less easily accessible parameters, such as resting metabolic rate, degree of insulin resistance, whole body nitrogen, and total body potassium, are also used in clinical studies conducted to assess the metabolic alterations occurring in cancer patients. From a more simple and practical perspective, the following indicators are suggested for use by the nurse in determining when cachexia is present. If a cancer patient has a greater than 10 per cent weight loss within a 6-month period, an intake less than a calculated basal energy expenditure (BEE) times a factor of 1.5 for more than 1 month, a triceps skinfold measurement and a mid-arm muscle circumference determination that fall 10 per cent below the reference standard, or a 10 per cent change in those measures from the individual's baseline values, the clinical evidence would strongly suggest cachexia.

DEVELOPMENTAL DIMENSIONS

The elderly cancer population is at increased risk for the development of cachexia because the digestive and absorptive functions may already be compromised by the aging process and because there is increased incidence of cancer with advancing age. Children and adolescents who are at critical growth periods and who are being treated aggressively with chemotherapy are also vulnerable to development of cachexia. Development and maintenance of body mass at any age require an energy balance wherein the intake and metabolic processes are sufficient to meet the requirements imposed by energy expenditure.

MECHANISMS

One explanatory mechanism for the development and progression of cancer cachexia is prolonged anorexia in which the intake is not adequate for the metabolic needs of the individual. However, this explanation does not account for all the observed cases of cachexia. There are examples in which neither the quality nor quantity of nutritional intake can account for the degree of wasting observed. There is considerable variation in food intake among individuals. Food intake in healthy individuals is thought to be regulated by both short-term and long-term feedback systems (see Chapter 14, Hunger). Examples of substances participating in short-term feedback affecting feeding include blood glucose, amino acid concentrations, circulating free fatty acids, and a host of hormones, such as insulin, glucagon, and bombesin. In cancer patients, alterations in glucose, lipid, and amino acid kinetics have been reported. The extent to which these or other alterations influence the regulatory mechanisms involved in feeding and result in anorexia is not clear. Even when other factors, such as fever and drainage, are considered, there are still examples of cachexia that remain unexplained by alterations in intake. Anorexia more recently has been associated with TNF production.

The tumor mass observed at autopsy usually accounts for less than 5 per cent of the body weight.[10] The quantity of malignant tissue, that is, the tumor burden, in comparison to total body weight is an impressively small figure when one considers the degree of wasting observed. Overt cachexia has been observed when tumors are less than 0.01 per cent of body weight.[2] A number of theories about the pathogenesis of cancer cachexia have been proposed and are reviewed in more detail elsewhere[11–31] (Table 6–1). Several of these theories are described here to explain the variety of mechanisms that could contribute to or account for cancer cachexia.

Tumors have a higher rate of anaerobic glycolysis, resulting in an increased lactate

TABLE 6–1 CANCER CACHEXIA: PROPOSED EXPLANATORY MECHANISMS

Anorexia
Increased gluconeogenesis
Decreased sensitivity to insulin
Increased metabolic rate
Tumor versus host competition for nutrients
Mobilization of lipids
Failure of compensatory mechanisms to increase food intake
Paraneoplastic phenomenon, abnormal synthesis of peptides by tumor
Cachectin/tumor necrosis factor–alpha and other cytokines

production.[13, 32, 33] The metabolic pathways involved in converting glucose to lactate and recycling (Cori cycle) to glucose, that is, the use of lactate for the synthesis of glucose (gluconeogenesis), require energy. This energy-requiring process has been proposed as one of the theories of pathogenesis.[34–38] Other investigators estimate that the energy drain from the increased Cori cycle activity may contribute to cachexia but that it could not solely account for a sufficient expenditure of energy (particularly in view of the tumor mass versus host mass) to explain the weight loss observed.[10, 13, 32, 33, 39] However, the highest Cori cycle activity in cancer patients was found in those with the greatest energy expenditure.[32]

Patients with advanced cancer also have an abnormal glucose tolerance curve similar to that seen in diabetics.[35, 37, 40, 41] There is a resistance or decreased sensitivity to insulin, and the disappearance rate of glucose is decreased in the cachectic individual.[40–42] The observed alterations in carbohydrate metabolism in individuals with cancer are plausible contributory factors in the genesis of cachexia but are not adequate as the sole explanation for the phenomenon of wasting.

Clinical observations confirm that there is increased growth of tumor tissue while wasting of nontumor host tissue occurs. In some cancer patients, the wasting is observed before a decline in intake is identified, or wasting may occur without a decline in intake. One hypothesis is that the metabolic rate of cancer patients is higher than normal, and several investigators have reported an increased metabolic rate in patients with advanced cancer.[13, 39, 43] Other investigators have reported contradictory findings; in some cases the rate is hypometabolic or within a normal range, and for others it is hypermetabolic.[35, 44–49] In some cases, the metabolic rate is increased while there is a decrease in intake.[10, 39] Another theory for the accelerated energy utilization is that malignant cell growth proceeds continuously in contrast to the diurnal periodicity of the metabolic activity observed for normal cells; thus, the metabolism of the malignant cells results in greater energy expenditure.[7, 34, 35] However, this theory alone also does not provide a sufficient explanation, since the metabolic energy expenditure of the tumor is relatively low when compared with the apparent total increase in energy loss in some cases.[50]

Other theories proposed to explain the development of cachexia suggest that the tumor growth and host wasting can be attributed to tumor-versus-host competition for selected nutrients.[43, 51–56] There is experimental evidence of nitrogen trapping by tumor tissue, but again considering the proportion of tumor mass to host mass, the increased uptake of nitrogen (amino acids) is also insufficient to account for the total extent of wasting observed. Cancer patients provided with a diet adequate in calories and protein content were shown to have decreased protein synthesis, and an increased metabolism of some amino acids has been found in cancer patients who have lost weight.[57, 58] There are two mechanisms involved. There is a redistribution of selected elements from host to tumor tissue. When nutrients are removed selectively by malignant cells, host cells are forced to use less efficient metabolic pathways, resulting in greater energy expenditure.[35, 38, 59]

Wasting of muscle mass in cachectic individuals is clinically evident. Studies have produced contradictory findings on whether the loss of muscle is due to increased degradation or to decreased protein synthesis.[56, 60] Current findings suggest net loss in protein is due to decreased synthesis, and in a recent study cancer patients had increased rates of whole body protein turnover.[55, 56, 61] TNF also has been implicated in the aberrations observed in protein metabolism, but the findings are controversial.[62–65]

Alterations in lipid metabolism have also been observed in some types of cancers. Mobilization of lipids, as free fatty acids, was the predominant finding. Lipid-mobilizing properties or responses have been observed in laboratory studies using the serum and urine from tumor-bearing animals and from some humans with cancer.[1, 2] There is also clinical evidence of the progressive depletion of fat reserves in individuals with advancing cancer. In some individuals with cancer, there is evidence that lipid sources are used as a predominant energy source.[13, 52, 54] TNF may play a role in promoting cachexia as a consequence of its inhibiting action on a key enzyme in lipid synthesis, lipoprotein lipase (LPL). TNF has been shown to suppress LPL activity in vitro and in vivo; also LPL is one of several enzymes that has been found to be depressed in cancer patients.[66–72]

In humans and animals, a number of integrated and interrelated mechanisms are involved in the control of food intake[2, 73] (see Chapter 14, Hunger). When intake falls below required levels, the usual adaptive response is to increase intake. In cachectic cancer patients, there is a failure in this compensatory mechanism.[2, 74] Which food intake control mechanisms are involved in this process and how they are implicated are being studied.

For some individuals with cancer, alterations in host metabolism distinct from nutritional intake are involved in the development and progression of cachexia. It has been proposed that in some cases cachexia may be another consequence of paraneoplastic phenomena.[75, 76] It is known that some malignant tumors abnormally synthesize biochemical substances that produce systemic metabolic effects; that is, these molecules affect host cells distant from the tumor site. These effects result in severe metabolic alterations and are characterized by the absence of the effective, normal physiological feedback control mechanisms. An example is ectopic hormone production by tumors of nonendocrine cell origin.[77, 78] One theory about the pathogenesis of cancer cachexia is based on this model; that is, some malignant cells may produce peptides that could alter normal enzyme functions.

All cells contain the same genetic components. As cells normally differentiate and become specialized, different genes are repressed in different cell types; as a result, normal cells derive their specific functional capacities. It has been postulated that some malignant tumor cells have lost or have impairment of this selective gene repression phenomenon, which could result in the synthesis of abnormal molecules.[77] Evidence to support the postulated existence of such a paraneoplastic phenomenon is the frequent finding of embryonic antigens in specific malignant tissues and the documented paraneoplastic ectopic hormone syndromes.[77, 78] There now is some evidence that malignant cells may produce TNF.[23, 79, 80]

The most significant new work has been the identification of cachetin/tumor necrosis factor-alpha and the studies that have been conducted to determine its role in the many aberrations associated with cancer cachexia and in infection, sepsis, and trauma.[20, 24, 25, 28, 69, 70, 81–94] Brennan, in an early comparison of cancer cachexia and starvation, observed that some of the metabolic abnormalities that occur with trauma and sepsis are similar to those that have been documented in individuals with cancer cachexia.[95] Subsequently, some of these effects have been found to be associated with the production of the peptide cytokines TNF and interleukin-1 (IL-1) by activated monocytes and macrophages in response to injury and infection. These cytokines have an effect on adipose tissue and skeletal muscle and are associated with anorexia.[19, 62, 69]

It is suggested that the release of these mediators in the inflammatory response may be the factor that contributes to the wasting phenomenon that is seen not only with cancer but also with injury, trauma, and possibly other diseases. These findings lead to a new hypothesis for explanation of some of the metabolic alterations that are characteristic of cancer cachexia.[20, 22, 27] The abnormalities may be a result of the production of the mediating cytokines.

Moldawer and colleagues put forth the hypothesis that the increased production of monokines such as TNF-alpha and IL-1, which occurs during active tumor growth, are the metabolic inducers of the complex host response that results in cancer cachexia.[22] They acknowledge, however, that this host-response model may not be appropriate for persons with breast cancer or sarcoma, as cachexia rarely occurs with those cancer types. In fact, at death some people with cancer are not cachetic. Kern and Norton also suggest that cancer cachexia is the result of a host response to the tumor; the tumor stimulates a host defense immune response resulting in the production of cytokines.[27] Although they propose that this immunological response is ineffective with rapidly growing tumors, the secretion of the cytokines continues, and the secondary effects of these active peptides result in the nutritional and metabolic abnormalities associated with the development and progression of cachexia. The question of how this proposed immune response can be explanatory for noncachectic cancer patients remains to be answered.

The initial metabolic response to infection and trauma is similar to that which occurs with some types of cancer. Loss of skeletal muscle mass, increase in hepatic protein synthesis, hyperglycemia and hypertriglyceremia, and anorexia are examples. With infection or trauma these changes occur quickly, and when treated they revert to normal.

However, with cancer, the metabolic changes initially occur more slowly, and with actively growing tumor the aberrations become more devastating, resulting in the cancer cachexia syndrome. With the resolution of infection or trauma the stimuli for the production of the blood monocyte and tissue macrophage products (IL-1 and TNF) are removed. This is in contrast to the host response that continues the production of these cytokines in the presence of tumor. With the successful removal or regression of the tumor, cancer cachexia is also reversed.

TNF production is induced by endotoxins, viruses, and mitogens; it can also be stimulated by cytokines (IL-1, IFN-2) and colony-stimulating factors.[18] While evidence suggests that TNF production may have a role in the host defense system, there is also evidence of a deleterious role of TNF in infectious diseases, for example, endotoxic shock, acute phase responses to infection, and malaria.[60, 96–98]

Current evidence suggests that cachectin (TNF) serves a protective function when small amounts are produced; when production is chronic, anorexia and a wasting syndrome occur. When large amounts are produced, the resulting state of shock can be lethal.[30, 96]

Like other cytokines, TNF participates in a range of cell regulatory, immune, and inflammatory processes and has an inhibitory or enhancing action on other cytokines.[18] TNF, as part of the cytokine network, is also stimulated by other cytokines. TNF exerts these regulatory activities through interaction with specific receptors on cell surfaces. Receptors for cachectin are present on liver, muscle, adipose, and most tissues, including normal and malignant cells.[69, 96, 99] When TNF binds to its specific receptors, intracellular protein synthesis is altered, thus cell functions are affected. One form of TNF is membrane bound and has properties similar to transmembrane proteins. Although through cleavage a form of TNF becomes an extracellular molecule, it has been suggested that membrane-bound TNF is the active molecule in macrophage-mediated cytotoxicity.[100]

Whether or not cachectin/TNF is detectable in the serum of cancer patients with cachexia is controversial.[29, 63, 64, 80, 86, 101] Twenty-three weight-losing cancer patients were included in a study to determine the plasma concentration and in vitro production of TNF and IL-1.[86] None of the 23 had detectable plasma levels of bioactive TNF; however, in vitro TNF production by their blood monocytes remained normal. The investigators concluded that biologically active TNF in the plasma is not critical to the development of cancer cachexia. Other investigators also have not found detectable levels of TNF in serum samples from weight-losing cancer patients.[101] There has been some evidence that blood monocytes from cancer patients with actively growing tumors spontaneously produce TNF and produce more TNF in vitro when stimulated than do blood monocytes in noncancer patients.[80] It is possible that the sensitivity of the current assay techniques is insufficient to detect circulating levels of TNF. Another consideration is that the half-life of TNF in plasma is reported to be very short in animals and in humans, from 6 to 20 minutes.[102]

A cachectic animal model has now been developed.[103] This model should be helpful in determining the mechanisms in progressive cancer cachexia. While the causes of cancer cachexia still remain incompletely understood, the current plausible explanation, for at least some forms of cancer, implicates TNF and IL-1 as the metabolic inducers of the phenomenon. These peptides may be produced by activated monocytes and macrophages as a host response to actively growing tumor. With their continued production over time, their secondary effects result in the progressive wasting of the cancer cachexia phenomenon. Studies have shown that TNF has a role in many actions, including hemorrhagic necrosis in tumors, suppression of the enzyme lipoprotein lipase, activation of neutrophils and neutrophil adherence to endothelial cells (suggesting a role in the inflammatory process), stimulation of angiogenesis and mitogenicity, induction of osteoclastic bone resorption and inhibition of bone collagen synthesis, acceleration of growth of normal fibroblasts, and induction of collagenase, prostaglandin E_2, IL-1, and granulocyte macrophage colony-stimulating factor production.[18, 83, 91, 104–115] It is possible that TNF may facilitate tumor spread through its lytic effect on bone and tumor growth via its stimulatory effects on angiogenesis and mitogenicity. There are conflicting theories and data about the role of TNF

in promoting cancer and cachexia and its role in effecting hemorrhagic tumor necrosis. Additional research is required before all the actions and interactions of TNF can be elucidated in some logical pattern of function.

The contribution that decreased intake, alterations in metabolism in the tumor tissue, alterations in the metabolism in nontumor host tissue (as a result of systemic humoral effects), and other factors make to the development and progression of cancer cachexia remains a complex, not completely elucidated phenomenon. Probably the contribution of each of these components to the cachectic state is variable according to type, stage, and grade of the tumor. It is plausible that no single theory will explain all the observed cases of cachexia. If this is the case, therapies for preventing or reducing cachexia will also be different. Progress has been made in understanding the underlying mechanisms, but additional research is required to find effective anticachexia therapies for individuals, particularly when cancer therapy is not curative.

PATHOLOGICAL CONSEQUENCES

With cancer cachexia, there are alterations in host metabolism and in composition of the body tissues and there is progressive wasting. The cachectic syndrome is physiologically and psychologically catastrophic. Even minor weight loss has been shown to be prognostic of shortened survival time.[3, 116] Despite food intake, cancer cachexia can be lethal.[21]

Cachexia may limit the extent to which anticancer therapies can be undertaken. There may be less rapid "rebound" or recovery between drug administration cycles or between the fractionated delivery of radiation therapy. This less rapid recovery may necessitate delays or interruptions in therapy, a decrease in dose, or in some cases cessation of therapy. All of these may compromise the effectiveness of the therapeutic regimen.

Cachectic individuals are prone to infection and to impaired wound healing. Impaired immune function is observed in cachectic individuals. Whether this immunoincompetence is a result of the nutritional status, the therapy, the tumor, or the cachexia is unclear.[117–122] (For a more extensive review of immune system dysfunction, see Chapter 17, Immunosuppression.)

The cachectic individual appears physically

ill as progressive asthenia and emaciation occur. Weakness, decreased effort tolerance, pale and atrophic skin, and muscle wasting have been noted. The muscle wasting eventually results in weakness of the respiratory muscles, with the resultant tendency for atelectasis, pulmonary infection, and deterioration of the individual's respiratory capacity.

Behavioral indicators of cachexia may include changes in appetite or in eating patterns, a progressive decline in motor activity and functional performance, or other evidence of fatigue. Terminally, the associated behavioral component is recognized as apathy, flatness of affect, detachment, and, for some individuals a reported longing for annihilation. The attendant pathological consequences of cancer cachexia are of considerable scope and magnitude[17]; the presence and progression of cachexia impact quality of life and survival. The clinical significance of this complex phenomenon requires further research to elucidate the underlying mechanisms and to develop effective anti-cachexia therapies. If cachexia is not reversed, death occurs.

RELATED PATHOPHYSIOLOGICAL CONCEPTS

Cardiac cachexia and pulmonary cachexia may be viewed as related physiological concepts. Regardless of underlying pathology, when energy expenditure exceeds energy supply, wasting will occur. There is a different temporal dimension to the occurrence of cachexia resulting from this kind of energy imbalance. For some, wasting occurs early in the illness; for others, it progresses more slowly.

Anorexia and starvation are two pathophysiological concepts that have characteristics both similar and dissimilar to those of cachexia. Anorexia, if defined as a loss of appetite resulting in spontaneous decline in intake or an intake that is inadequate for host needs, is one factor that may contribute significantly to the development and progression of cachexia.[123–132] Anorexia may be antecedent to or occur concomitantly with the progression of cachexia; however, a number of other factors may also contribute to the occurrence of cachexia—thus the two concepts are not mutually inclusive. A number of studies about the influence of taste changes

on anorexia in cancer patients have been conducted.[133–139] Studies about food preferences and food aversions in cancer patients have also been reported.[140–143] Whereas anorexia is conceptually bound to dimensions of appetite and intake, cachexia is conceptualized to include nutritional status data, host metabolism alterations, and redistribution of body composition components. Cancer cachexia is a clinical syndrome involving a broader constellation of distinguishing characteristics than anorexia. (For a more inclusive overview of anorexia, see Chapter 5, Anorexia.)

Over time, with a decline in intake that is inadequate for the metabolic needs of the host, starvation will occur. Although some aspects of the PCM occurring with starvation are observed in individuals with cancer, cachexia resulting from a malignant tumor appears to be mediated by different mechanisms than those that regulate the metabolic alterations occurring with starvation.[95] Feedback mechanisms that act to preserve life in starvation appear to be impaired in patients with uncontrolled malignant tumor growth. When starvation occurs in individuals without cancer, a number of adaptive, compensatory mechanisms result. However, in the individual with cancer cachexia, these adaptive mechanisms are not observed to occur. The resting metabolic rate is increased in some individuals with cancer cachexia, whereas in prolonged PCM the resting metabolic rate decreases; thus, resting energy expenditure is greater for some cachectic individuals with advanced cancer.[42, 43, 95, 144–146]

Other physiological alterations are reported to occur with cancer cachexia and not with starvation. Nausea, dysphagia, anorexia, and early satiety are common phenomena in cancer cachexia, and these subjective sensations may be so severe as to depress food intake completely.[123, 133] In addition, altered taste sensation and food aversions may be experienced by cachectic cancer patients.[133–139, 143]

Thus, the syndrome of cancer cachexia can be distinguished from that of starvation. The metabolic alterations that occur in starvation are adaptive and compensatory, while those alterations that occur in cachexia may contribute to the progressive wasting. Starvation results from inadequate intake, while cancer cachexia has been observed when the quality and quantity of food intake could not alone account for the wasting. There are differences in the causes.

ASSOCIATED PSYCHOSOCIAL CONCEPTS

Two psychosocial phenomena that may occur as a result of an individual's experiencing cancer, cancer therapy, and cancer cachexia are depression and alterations in self-concept, particularly body image. It is difficult, if not impossible, to ferret out the extent to which having cancer versus experiencing the progressive wasting associated with cachexia contribute to expressions of depression and changes in body image perceptions. Alternatively, depression may influence the progression of cachexia, expecially if the depression results in decreased activity and decreased intake. For some, altered body image perceptions result from the physical changes that occur; these changes may be very devastating and may become part of the "cancer experience." It is apparent that there are relationships between these physiological and psychosocial concepts, and they are complex.

MANIFESTATIONS

Objective Manifestations

Cancer cachexia is a syndrome characterized by progressive physical deterioration. The most obvious clinical manifestation is loss of weight. For some individuals with cancer, weight loss is the initial symptom; for others, weight loss occurs with progression of the malignancy.

Because cachexia is a syndrome in which a wide range of metabolic alterations may be involved, it is necessary for the nurse to use multiple objective parameters to identify and describe the magnitude of the phenomenon (Table 6–2). Anthropometric measures used for assessment of nutritional status are parameters to be considered in identifying cachexia. In addition to weight change, there is evidence of loss of body fat and muscle mass. Serum albumin and serum transferrin values (which can be measured directly or calculated from total iron-binding capacity) are indicators of visceral protein status. There is contradictory evidence about serum albumin values in patients with advanced cancer who are cachectic; some studies show a decrease while others show normal to increased values. Differences can be related to

TABLE 6–2 OBJECTIVE MANIFESTATIONS OF CANCER CACHEXIA

Progressive physical wasting
    Weight loss
    Loss of fat
    Loss of muscle mass
Impaired immune function
    Anergy (decreased response to skin test antigens)
    Decreased lymphocyte count
Energy imbalance
    Decreased intake
    Negative nitrogen balance
    Energy expenditure exceeding energy intake
Behavioral changes
    Decreased tolerance for activity
    Increased weakness, fatigue with usual activities
    Decreased enthusiasm for enjoyable activities
    Expressions of apathy

state of hydration. Calculations of mid-arm muscle circumference and creatinine height index are used to estimate somatic protein status, that is, lean body mass. Additional measures, such as total body water and total body potassium, provide more definitive data but also require more sophisticated techniques and personnel for measurement. Changes in fat reserves are estimated from triceps skinfold thickness measurements. Lymphocyte count as a percentage of white blood cells and sensitivity to skin testing with recall antigens, such as *Candida*, mumps, and purified protein derivative (PPD), are indicators of the state of immunocompetence.[117–122] These measures are well described in the nutritional assessment literature.[6–9] Weight change, caloric intake, nitrogen balance, and caloric intake as a percentage of calculated BEE are indicators of the individual's metabolic status, that is, anabolism versus catabolism. The extent of the excursion seen for each of these parameters from the normal range of values will be dependent somewhat on the magnitude of the cachectic state and the time period over which the cachexia has developed. Examples are given in the illustrative case history.

Behavioral manifestations of cachexia are more subtle, but deterioration of activity and tolerance for activity are the significant observations. The nurse needs to be astute in chronicling these changes. For example, less energy is exerted in the individual's physical movements and conversation. Increasing weakness becomes apparent as individuals use their hands and arms to lift themselves out of a chair or use a stair railing to assist their ascent of the steps. Difficulty in lifting or carrying objects signifies increasing weakness. Even eating becomes a "chore" and tires the cachectic individual. General decline in all motor activities is observed. There are noticeable changes in the individual's affect as well. Usual enthusiasm for going places or doing things wanes.

As the cachexia progresses, the individual may become apathetic and express acknowledgment about their terminal state. The wasting of cancer cachexia is recognized by the individual and is perceived to signal impending death.

Subjective Manifestations

Cachectic individuals classically express a sensation of tiredness, lack of energy, and abject fatigue. Some express experiencing appetite-related sensations such as feeling bloated after eating a small quantity of food, some report developing aversions to certain foods, and some discuss experiencing taste changes. Feeling nauseated is a fairly common experience. Again, the perceived changes or the expression of the changes in sensations will occur over time and they may be subtle. The professional nurse should be sensitive to these expressions as they are revealed in the progression of cachexia. The cachectic individual may also discuss the more obvious physiological and behavioral manifestations described above, such as the feeling of general weakness, fatigue, and the decline in motor activity. Spouses and partners or family members describe vividly the increasing frequency of the resting and withdrawal behaviors with comments such as "stayed on the couch all day," "naps most of the day," or "didn't want to go play cards with our friends." It is the astute professional nurse who recognizes these subjective expressions as signaling the development or progression of cachexia.

Cachexia is reversible, and improvement in all of the described manifestations does occur. Cachexia is reversed when cancer therapy (surgery, chemotherapy, or radiation) is effective in eliminating the tumor or in achieving tumor regression.

SURVEILLANCE AND MEASUREMENT

The professional nurse has responsibility for monitoring the physiological parameters and changes in behavior already cited as well as for identifying the changes that occur over time; this is important in determining the development, progression, or remission of cancer cachexia. Specific surveillance parameters include weight, triceps skinfold thickness, midarm circumference, and mid-arm muscle determinations. Reference standards for these measurements are published; in addition to the normal range, values for mild, moderate, and severe deficits are also given.[6–9] Thus, it is possible for the nurse not only to determine changes over time from the individual's baseline measurements but also to compare the individual's measurements with normative standards.

Data for other objective parameters can be obtained by calculating the creatinine height index, nitrogen balance, caloric intake, and caloric intake as a percentage of the calculated BEE.[147] Serum albumin, serum transferrin, and lymphocyte count should also be monitored over time. Behavioral and metabolic indicators of cachexia may precede other signs of neoplastic growth. Early recognition of the behavioral, physiological and metabolic indicators of cancer cachexia is imperative if attempts to reduce the attendant morbidity are to be successful. Because studies to date involving cachectic subjects have included multiple types of cancer, the incidence, development, and progression of cachexia in specific types of cancer is unknown.

Additional data about the nutritional, metabolic, and behavioral components of the phenomenon of cancer cachexia occurring with specific malignant tumors are needed. The current knowledge, however, does provide direction for clinical practice. The role of the nurse involves assessment and continued surveillance based on information about the clinical indicators of cachexia.

After an individual is identified as being at risk for cachexia, surveillance of specific parameters should be done periodically, at least once every 6 weeks. These parameters are anthropometric measurements, including changes in weight and adipose tissue and muscle mass; food intake patterns; appearance of tissue and skin; changes in strength and endurance; and selected biochemical measures as previously specified. The important component of surveillance is that data collected serially over time are compared over time to determine response to therapy or disease progression.

CLINICAL THERAPIES

Primarily, therapies are directed to remove or eliminate the tumor or to induce tumor regression, as reversion of cachexia appears to be dependent on the effectiveness of the cancer therapy. Currently, there are no standard therapies specific for treating cachexia. If specific pathogenic mechanisms are found to be responsible for the development and progression of cachexia, it will become possible to create therapies specific for cachexia. There are, however, therapies that are associated in some way with cachexia; for example, treatment of an infection that may be compounding the wasting and administration of fluids, blood, or blood products for dehydration from decreased intake or from loss through drainage or replacement of elements lost through removal of effusions. The professional nurse shares responsibility for instituting these therapies, explaining the rationale for their use as well as the procedures employed and monitoring the responses to the therapies.

The investigational drug hydrazine sulfate is being used as an anticachexia agent in trials with advanced cancer patients.[37, 38, 148, 149] Hydrazine sulfate is a specific enzyme-blocking agent that interrupts the conversion of lactate to glucose (Cori cycle, gluconeogenesis); the intent is to decrease energy expenditure from this process. There is some objective and subjective evidence of the effectiveness of this investigational drug in decreasing the progression of cachexia in some patients; however, additional study is required.

Another agent, megestrol acetate, has also been proposed as a possible treatment for cancer cachexia, as high doses of megestrol acetate in clinical trials for women with stage IV estrogen-receptor positive breast cancer resulted in a weight gain for 81 per cent of the patients and an increased appetite for 53 per cent.[150–152] Megestrol acetate results in increased anabolic enzymes; this may account partially for the observed weight gain.[151] How megestrol acetate influences the cachexia syndrome and the mechanisms involved in weight gain remain to be studied.

TNF has also been used in phase I and II clinical trials as an anticancer agent because of its demonstrated cytotoxic or cytostatic action for in vitro human cancer cell lines and its tumor necrotizing effects.[81] However, in these TNF trials minimal antitumor effects have been observed.[102, 153–160] Toxicities commonly associated with clinical trials of TNF were fever, chills, local pain, and inflammation. Additional manifestations of toxicity occurred in some of the trials. In a phase I trial, TNF was administered by 24-hour continuous infusion to 15 patients with advanced metastatic adenocarcinoma; while 11 patients had tumor progression, one showed a minor response, and in three others there was no tumor progression during the 2 months of TNF therapy.[102] Indomethacin was used to decrease the side effects; however, the dose-limiting systemic toxicities included chills, fever, myalgias, headache, and thrombocytopenia. These are similar to the side effects observed with use of other lymphokines.

In a phase II study of 25 patients with advanced disease (melanoma and renal cancer) who were given escalating doses of TNF intramuscularly, there was progression of disease in 22 while in three the disease remained stable.[155] It has been suggested that using TNF with other agents or following administration of other agents may enhance its antitumor effectiveness.

If TNF or other products are continuously released in patients with some types of cancer and if these products are the mediators of the complex cachetic phenomena, it should be possible to design drugs to interfere with their interactions. Thus, the development of agents that block or compete for the TNF or IL-1 receptors may become useful therapeutically for cancer cachexia.

Progressive tumor growth is associated with nutritional problems.[5, 132, 161–171] Despite successes reported in earlier nonrandomized clinical studies, nutritional support in more recent randomized clinical trials has not been effective in increasing response to therapy or in increasing survival.[21, 169, 170] Bozzetti summarized the findings on the effects of TPN for cachectic cancer patients.[172] In the studies reviewed TPN was used for relatively short periods, and during the administration, no nutritional variable worsened.[172] In some studies body weight and fat mass increased. Opinions and findings about the use of parenteral feedings as nutritional support for cancer patients remain controversial, and thus the ability of nutritional support to influence clinical outcomes is not clearly established.[44, 55, 56, 168–179]

Because there is controversy about whether use of nutritional interventions produces increased tumor growth, the current recommendation is that interventions be implemented while the cancer patient is concurrently undergoing active anticancer therapy. Increasing tumor growth (cell division) in this way may in fact enhance cell kill by the chemotherapeutic agents or radiation therapy. The precise nutritional needs of the cancer patient have not been determined; thus, one possible explanation is that the effects of nutritional support have not been optimal because the supplementation does not meet specific nutritional needs. Preoperative TPN, however, has been shown to reduce operative mortality and previous post-surgical complications.[171, 172] While nutritional support may not ameliorate cachexia or lengthen survival, it may have other beneficial effects, such as reduction of complications.

The professional nurse must be involved in explaining and administering the nutritional intervention as well as monitoring over time the response to the therapy. Education of the patient and family about preventive and promotive behaviors to decrease risk for infection and to maintain an adequate nutritional intake (such as small frequent feedings that are high in calories and protein) is an important responsibility of the professional nurse.[180] Recommendations for managing the nutrition-related problems observed in cancer patients, such as anorexia, stomatitis, food aversions, nausea, and vomiting, and for improving their intake are reviewed by others.[143, 174, 181–183] Use of relaxation or other therapies to diminish nausea and vomiting, organization of activities to decrease energy expenditure, and engaging in enjoyable, fun activities are other examples of preventive and promotive behaviors that may have some therapeutic advantages.

Clinical responsibilities of the professional nurse include early recognition of behavioral and metabolic indicators of impending or progressing cachexia; patient and family education about aspects of preventive, curative, or palliative therapies; and contributions to the care of the individual receiving aggressive nutritional support and cancer therapies.

REVIEW OF RESEARCH FINDINGS

Historically, there have been reports of spontaneous regression of cancer associated with a prior infection. Subsequently, the monokine secreted by macrophages in response to bacterial stimulation was discovered and eventually was named TNF. The first evidence that TNF was produced by host cells (monocytes and macrophages) was reported in 1975, and by the early 1980s the TNF gene had been cloned and expressed.[81, 85, 87, 89] It now has been shown that TNF production is induced by endotoxin; this explains the spontaneous tumor regression that historically was reported following bacterial infections.[184, 185] Using blood from a cachectic animal model, a humoral mediator of cachexia was identified and called cachectin.[20, 25, 82] In an animal model this polypeptide acts to inhibit an enzyme (lipoprotein lipase) important in the synthesis of lipids. There is also evidence that TNF is produced by human tumor cell lines.[186] Cachectin now has been shown to be closely related or identical to TNF.[18, 19, 84, 90] Human TNF has been purified and characterized as a polypeptide chain of 157 amino acids. The gene that codes for human TNF has been isolated and cloned, and TNF is available as a purified recombinant product.[87, 88] The gene is located in the same region as the major histocompatibility complex.[187] It is also near the gene that codes for the cytokine lymphotoxin, which is believed to be associated with lymphocyte-mediated killing.

It has been shown that mice inoculated with tumor cells that secrete TNF become cachectic.[23] This and other animal studies suggest an association between TNF and cancer cachexia; however, studies with humans have produced conflicting findings.[101] The research on the identification of TNF and the studies to determine its actions have been very significant in deriving some insight into the many metabolic aberrations associated with cancer cachexia. The research has also been important in proposing that TNF and possibly other cytokines are the common mediators in the consequences observed with infection, trauma, and septic shock.

The study by Vlassara and colleagues is illustrative; they reported a 35 per cent decrease in lipoprotein lipase activity in a group of 28 cancer patients.[68] The decrease in the enzyme activity was correlated with the percentage of weight loss and was related to tumor type. For example, lung cancer patients showed the greatest weight loss and the lowest enzyme activity and breast cancer patients had minimal weight loss and normal lipoprotein lipase activity.

Cachexia is acknowledged as a significant debilitating manifestation of progressive malignancy; yet systematic studies of the development and progression of cachexia, when specifically defined as a systemic derangement of host metabolism, are lacking. The findings reported are fragmentary and sometimes contradictory. Observations frequently have been collected on a one-time basis or for only a short time period and in subjects with markedly varying tumors and time since diagnosis and undergoing various therapies. Thus, these studies have not provided adequate information to determine whether or not different tumors have different or predominant patterns of metabolic alterations resulting in cachexia. A variety of studies that address variables associated with cachexia have been reported; some of these are reviewed below.

In one study of the resting energy expenditure of 200 cancer patients with varying tumor types and time since diagnosis, 26 per cent were found to be hypermetabolic and time since diagnosis was significantly longer for those subjects.[146] Thirty-three per cent of the subjects, however, were reported to be hypometabolic. Thus, findings do not support the hypothesis of a consistent increase in energy expenditure for all cancer patients.

Findings from a retrospective study of 1000 patients with various types of malignancy showed that a significant weight loss occurred in approximately one half the subjects.[76] In a large study, weight loss was associated with a shorter survival time; cancer patients with no weight loss lived longer.[3] Nielsen and colleagues documented significantly greater weight loss in lung cancer patients than in patients with other tumor types.[140] A loss of greater than 6 per cent of the pre-illness weight was observed in approximately 50 per cent of 316 patients with limited or extensive non–oat cell carcinoma of the lung.[161] In another study, Costa and colleagues found that weight loss occurred prior to diagnosis in most patients with carcinoma of the lung and that after diagnosis, weight loss continued and did not correlate with the observed extent of the malignancy; weight was a predictor of death.[162] For 50 surgically treated lung cancer patients, Costa and Donaldson found that in 16 patients (25 per cent of the subjects) weight loss was evident months before a relapse was documented.[76]

From a chart review of 479 lung cancer patients and diet intakes for 205 voluntary normal subjects and 198 cancer patients, Costa and colleagues concluded that survival was influenced significantly by an initial weight loss (within 2 months) of 5 per cent or greater and that anorexia could not solely account for the observed weight loss.[163, 164] Other investigators concluded from an initial dietary assessment of 22 cancer patients (with different tumor types, varying duration of cancer, and undergoing different therapies) that in those who lost weight, the protein and caloric intakes were "markedly below normal."[144]

Burke and associates also reported a decline in protein and caloric intake in those cancer patients who lost weight.[165] In a longitudinal prospective study in which 10 male small cell lung cancer patients were followed, it was suggested that the spontaneous decline in intake could be the significant factor contributing to the observed loss in weight that occurred during a 5-month period following diagnosis.[132] The investigators concluded that the intake was less than adequate for any activity beyond a basal state.

In a study in which the effects of intravenous hyperalimentation were examined, a better outcome was reported for subjects with adenocarcinoma of the lung who at the time of diagnosis had less than a 4 per cent weight loss and a greater than 74 per cent triceps skinfold thickness.[167] Copeland and colleagues reported finding a positive correlation between adequate nutritional status and response to chemotherapy in 175 patients for whom intravenous hyperalimentation was administered in addition to the chemotherapy regimen.[177] For 100 surgical patients receiving intravenous hyperalimentation preoperatively and postoperatively, fewer complications occurred and there were no deaths. In another study of cancer patients with a variety of tumors, survival time for those receiving chemotherapy and intravenous hyperalimentation was not greater than for those receiving food.[188] Findings were reported from a study of the nutritional status of eight allogeneic bone marrow recipients followed for a 3-month period.[178] In the immediate post-transplant period the subjects received supplemental TPN. All eight subjects had some alteration in nutritional status; four of these experienced greater declines in nutritional status and had many complications that led to longer hospitalizations or to death. TPN had a varying positive effect but was not sufficient (in amounts given) to prevent the decline in nutritional status observed in four of the eight subjects.

With depletion of protein, loss of immunocompetence has been observed. Delayed or impaired sensitivity to skin test antigens was examined in a study of nutritional assessment and cancer patient outcome during therapy. One hundred per cent mortality was observed in patients who remained anergic.[179] Increased survival for cancer patients has been correlated positively with immunocompetence before and during therapy.[177, 179] A response to chemotherapy was observed only in those who had a positive skin test. These findings provide evidence that cell-mediated immunity can be restored, at least initially, with adequate nutritional support and that immunological competence is influenced by nutritional status.[177]

Numerous other studies can be cited. The ones included here have been selected as representative of those that have more immediate clinical relevance for the professional nurse.

ILLUSTRATIVE CASE STUDY

Cachexia may develop insidiously, and changes in the values for a variety of the parameters may go unnoted if the values are not routinely obtained serially and compared over time. Data for a patient diagnosed with small cell lung carcinoma are used as an example to illustrate the development of cachexia.

Mr. P. was a 53-year-old white unmarried man who lived alone. Initially, he noticed that the nature of his cough changed and his shortness of breath with activity and fatigue increased. He also experienced hemoptysis. These changes triggered his seeking medical assistance. Following biopsy, the diagnosis of small cell lung cancer was confirmed. He estimated his usual (6 month pre-illness) weight to be 165 pounds; his weight recorded at the time of diagnosis was 152 pounds. Although he had sustained a weight loss of greater than 10 pounds in a few months before diagnosis, for his height and build his ideal weight is considered to be 151 pounds. Clinically, for some parameters it is probably more important to use the

subject's own baseline data for comparison of changes over time and to use normative data to estimate when the patient deviates significantly from the norm. Obviously, there are parameters for which normal values must be used for comparison (e.g., serum albumin and blood glucose).

Mr. P. had been well all his life with no other significant health problems reported. He had a long smoking history and stated that his appetite was good at the time of diagnosis except that for several weeks before diagnosis he noticed a "witch hazel taste" associated with drinking vodka.

Mr. P. was started on an aggressive chemotherapy protocol and received prophylactic cranial radiation approximately 10 weeks following initiation of therapy. The chemotherapy regimen required that he return every 3 to 6 weeks for drug administration, and he was hospitalized periodically for administration of cisplatin.

The diagnosis was confirmed in mid-November; despite aggressive therapy, however, by mid-April progression of the malignancy to the mediastinum was shown on radiographs. He commented that he ate well in the mornings but did not consume much thereafter. When encouraged to use food supplements (and samples were provided), Mr. P. refused to eat them, commenting that they made him "nauseated." Before and after the diagnosis, he ate most of his meals at a small cafe near his apartment. Weight changes, mean caloric intake, and caloric intake as a percentage of calculated BEE over time for Mr. P. are given in Table 6–3, which shows that his intake progressively declined over time. He did not consume sufficient calories to meet even BEE needs, and a decline in weight occurred. Values obtained over time for his mid-arm muscle circumference, triceps skinfold thickness, and other selected parameters are shown in Table 6–4.

Mr. P. also began to express thoughts about the outcome of his disease: "I'm not thinking about only one year to live." In May he reported episodes of spontaneous vomiting not preceded by nausea. His voice was hoarse and weak; Mr. P. was a quiet man, and over time his voice demonstrated a lack of vitality and energy.

TABLE 6–3 CHANGES IN WEIGHT AND INTAKE OVER TIME SINCE CANCER DIAGNOSIS IN A PATIENT (MR. P.) WITH CACHEXIA

Time from Diagnosis	Weight (kg)	Caloric Intake (kcal)	Caloric Intake as Percentage of BEE*	Caloric Intake as Percentage of BEE* × 1.5†
Diagnosis	69.1	1929	127	85
2 months	71.6	2018	133	89
4 months	69.1	1491	99	66
6 months	65.4	1202	79	53
8 months	62.2	827	55	36
10 months	53.0	0	0	0

*BEE for males = 66 + (13.7 × weight in kg) + (5 × height in cm) − (6.8 × age in years) (Blackburn et al, 1977); caloric intake as percentage of BEE calculated using weight at time of diagnosis (BEE = 1513 kcal).
†BEE multiplied by a factor of 1.5 to account for moderate activity (BEE × 1.5 = 2270 kcal).

It seemed to require much effort for him to talk. In June, left vocal cord paralysis was observed and there was persistent mediastinal adenopathy. Radiation therapy to the mediastinum was initiated, and partial response of the tumor was noted.

Mr. P. gradually showed less energy and less quickness in his movements and less enthusiasm in his expressions, but he maintained a keen mental ability throughout the course of his illness. In mid-August, he was too weak to return to the clinic for follow-up; he remained at home in bed for a few days and experienced severe nausea and vomiting (with virtually no intake). He was admitted to the hospital, and feeding via a nasogastric tube was initiated. Persistent narrowing of the distal esophagus due to extension of disease was confirmed by radiographs. Within 2 weeks, he was discharged home and readmitted in several days for dehydration and then again within 2 weeks for "no

intake at all." He stated "I can't eat anything, everything I swallow, I gag, I am very unsteady and fall; my situation has gotten worse." After a week of hospitalization, he was discharged to the care of his sister, who came from out of town to be with him (he had continued to live alone throughout this period of time). Two days later, he underwent emergency thoracentesis and died 1 day later. The course of his entire illness had occurred in less than 1 year (10½ months) from the time of diagnosis. Cachexia, indeed, had occurred and progressed.

Although this patient example clearly demonstrates fairly rapid progression, there are other examples in which the effectiveness of therapy is apparent and the values for the parameters being monitored serially show return to a normal range. The professional nurse needs to be sensitive to both the obvious changes and to the more subtle changes in energy level, motor function, intake, and other

TABLE 6–4 CHANGES OVER TIME SINCE CANCER DIAGNOSIS IN SELECTED PARAMETERS IN A PATIENT WITH CACHEXIA

Time from Diagnosis	Midarm Muscle Circumference* (Percentage of Standard†)	Triceps Skinfold Thickness* (Percentage of Standard†)	Serum Albumin (g/dl)	Serum Transferrin (mg/dl)
Diagnosis	98	93	3.3	196
2 months	106	94	4.4	220
4 months	93	93	4.3	202
6 months	91	90	4.0	194
8 months	89	87	3.2	184
10 months	86	84	2.5	170

*Left arm.
†See Blackburn et al., 1977.

behavioral characteristics that herald either remission or progression of the phenomenon. Assisting the individual through the course of the illness and concomitant cachexia when there is such rapid compromise of the individual's health status is critical and challenging for the professional nurse.

IMPLICATIONS FOR FURTHER RESEARCH

The relative contribution of any of the selected parameters or combination of parameters to the development and progression of cachexia in a specified type of cancer remains unknown. The studies in which parameters indicative of cachexia have been investigated and reported primarily have been measured during periods of hospitalization, have rarely included serial measurements of the nutritional and metabolic status parameters over time, and have rarely examined the relationships of these parameters in patients with a similar tumor type treated by a similar therapeutic regimen. The study of the incidence and temporal occurrence of the cachexia of malignancy is difficult because of the requisite longitudinal nature of data collection and to the inherent subjective components of the phenomenon. It is difficult, if not impossible, to separate the contributions of the malignancy itself to the occurrence of cachexia from the effects of the treatment regimen on the development of cachexia.

Because cachexia may influence the patient's tolerance and response to treatment and because evidence that heralds the development and progression of cachexia may precede other more specific signs of neoplastic growth or recurrence, it is imperative that a more complete and definitive description of the phenomenon be developed for use in nursing practice. That is, knowledge about the signs and symptoms of cachexia and their temporal relationships to the existence and progression of the cancer may conceivably (1) influence the timing of medical treatment, (2) provide the basis for preventing or easing the morbidity of the disease, (3) provide the basis for therapies that would enhance the effectiveness of the prescribed medical treatment of the disease, (4) facilitate the early diagnosis of cancer or its recurrence, and (5) serve as indicators of tumor activity.

Cancer cachexia is a frequent and substantial clinical problem; it is an observable phenomenon with behavioral and biochemical components that influence cancer morbidity and therapy. Accumulating evidence suggests that the real devastation produced by some malignant neoplasms is not the direct effect of invasion of adjacent normal cells but rather is the abnormal synthesis and elaboration of biochemical substances that produce altered metabolic effects at sites distant to the tumor.

It is important to determine whether for some tumor types cachexia results from TNF production, selective nutrient utilization by the tumor, increased metabolic rate, decreased intake, alterations in anatomic structures that result in interference with digestive or absorptive processes, treatment regimen, some combination of these factors, or some other plausible explanation. Another question to be answered is whether there are differences in the pathogenesis of cachexia in the various tumor types. It is apparent that there are numerous areas requiring considerable work before the answers become the knowledge base to direct nursing practice.

REFERENCES

1. Theologides, A. (1977). Cancer cachexia. Curr Concepts Nutr 6:75–94.
2. Morrison, S. D. (1976). Control of food intake in cancer cachexia: A challenge and a tool. Physiol Behav 17:705–714.
3. DeWys, W. D., Begg, D., Lavin, P. T., Brand, P. R., Bennett, J. M., Bertino, J. R., Cohen, M. H., Douglas, H. O., Engstrom, P. F., Ezdinli, E. Z., Horton, J., Johnson, G. J., Moertel, C. G., Oken, M. M., Perlia, C., Rosenbaum, C., Silversteen, M. N., Skeel, R. T., Sponzo, R. W., & Tormay, D. C. (1980). Prognostic effect of weight loss prior to chemotherapy in cancer patients. Am J Med, 69:491–497.
4. Buzby, G. P., Mullen, J. F., Mathews, D. C., Hobbs, C. L., & Rosato, E. F. (1980). Prognostic nutritional index in gastrointestinal surgery. Am J Surg, 139:160–167.
5. Nixon, D. W., Heymsfield, S. B., Cohen, A. E., Kutner, M. H., Ansley, J., Lawson, D. M., & Rudman, D. (1980). Protein-calorie undernutrition in hospitalized cancer patients. Am J Med, 68:683–690.
6. Blackburn, G. L., Bistrian, B. R., Maini, B. S., Schlamm, H. T., & Smith, M. F. (1977). Nutritional and metabolic assessment of the hospitalized patient. J Parenter Enter Nutr, 1:11–22.
7. Butterworth, C. E., & Blackburn, G. L. (1975). Hospital malnutrition. Nutr Today 10:8–18.

8. Frisancho, A. R. (1981) New norms of upper limb fat and muscle areas for assessment of nutritional status. Am J Clin Nutr *34*:2540–2545.

9. Metropolitan Life Insurance Company. (1983). *Tables of Ideal Weights*.

10. Waterhouse, C. (1974). How tumors affect host metabolism. Ann NY Acad Sci *230*:86–93.

11. Theologides, A. (1972). Pathogenesis of cachexia in cancer. Cancer *29*:484–488.

12. Costa, G. (1977). Cachexia, the metabolic component of neoplastic diseases. Cancer Res *37*:2327–2335.

13. Young, V. R. (1977). Energy metabolism and requirements in the cancer patient. Cancer Res, *37*:2336–2347.

14. Strain, A. J. (1979). Cancer cachexia in man: A review. Invest Cell Pathol *2*:181–193.

15. Theologides, A. (1982). Pathogenesis of anorexia and cachexia in cancer. Cancer Bull, *34*:140–149.

16. Lawson, D. H., Richmond, A., Nixon, D. W., & Rudman, D. (1982). Metabolic approaches to cancer cachexia. Annu Rev Nutr, *2*:277–301.

17. Lindsey, A. M. (1982). The phenomenon of cancer cachexia: A review. Oncol Nurs Forum *9*:38–42.

18. Balkwill, F. R.: Tumor necrosis factor. Br Med Bull *45*:389–400.

19. Beutler, B., Greenwald, D., Hulmes, J. D., Charg, M., Pan, Y. C., Mathison, J., Ulevitch, R., & Cerami, A. (1985). Identity of tumor necrosis factor and the macrophage-secreted factor cachectin. Nature *316*:552–554.

20. Beutler, B., & Cerami, A. (1986). Cachectin and tumor necrosis factor as two sides of the same biological coin. Nature *320*:584–598.

21. Fearon, K. C., & Carter, D. C. (1988). Cancer cachexia. Ann Surg *208*:1–5.

22. Moldawer, L. L., Georgieff, M., & Lundholm, K. (1987). Interleukin-1, tumor necrosis factor alpha (cachectin) and the pathogenesis of cancer cachexia. Clin Physiol *7*:263–274.

23. Oliff, A., DeFeo-Jones, D., Boyer, M., Martinez, D., Kiefer, D., Vuocolo, G., Wolfe, A., & Socher, S. H. (1987). Tumors secreting human TNF/cachectin induce cachexia in mice. Cell *50*:555–563.

24. Tracey, K. J., Lowry, S. F., & Cerami, A. (1988). Cachectin: A hormone that triggers acute shock and chronic cachexia. J Infect Dis *157*:413–420.

25. Beutler, B., & Cerami, A. (1988). Cachectin, cachexia, and shock. Annu Rev Med *39*:75–83.

26. Norton, J. A., Peacock, J. L., & Morrison, S. D. (1987). Cancer cachexia. Crit Rev Oncol Hematol *7*:289–327.

27. Kern, K. A., & Norton, J. A. (1988). Cancer cachexia. J Parent Enter Nutr *12*:286–298.

28. Beutler, B., & Cerami, A. (1988). Tumor necrosis, cachexia, shock, and inflammation: A common mediator. Annu Rev Biochem *57*:505–518.

29. Balkwill, F., Osborne, R., Burke, F., Naylor, S., Talbot, D., Durbin, H., Tavernier, J., & Fiers, W. (1987). Evidence for tumor necrosis factor/cachectin production in cancer. Lancet *2*:1229–1232.

30. Beutler, B. (1988). Cachexia: A fundamental mechanism. Nutr Rev *46*:369–373.

31. Oliff, A. (1988). The role of tumor necrosis factor (cachectin) in cachexia. Cell *54*:141–142.

32. Holroyde, C. P., Gabuzda, T. G., Putnam, R. C., Paul, P., & Reichard, G. A. (1975). Altered glucose metabolism in metastatic carcinoma. Cancer Res *35*:3710–3714.

33. Holroyde, C. P., & Reichard, G. A. (1981). Carbohydrate metabolism in cancer cachexia. Cancer Treat Rep *65*(Suppl. 5):55–59.

34. Gold, J. (1974). Cancer cachexia and gluconeogenesis. Ann NY Acad Sci *230*:103–110.

35. Chlebowski, R. T., & Heber, D. (1986). Metabolic abnormalities in cancer patients: Carbohydrate metabolism. Surg Clin North Am *66*:957–968.

36. Hughes, T. K., Cadet, P., & Larned, C. S. (1989). Modulation of tumor necrosis factor activities by a potential anticachexia compound, hydrazine sulfate. Int J Immunopharmacol *11*:501–507.

37. Chlebowski, R. T., Bulcavage, L., Grosvenor, M., Tsunokai, R., Block, J. B., Heber, D., Scrooc, M., Chlebowski, J. S., Chi, J., Oktay, E., Akman, S., & Ali, I. (1987). Hydrazine sulfate in cancer patients with weight loss: A placebo-controlled clinical experience. Cancer *59*:406–410.

38. Gold, J. (1987). Hydrazine sulfate: A current perspective. Nutr Cancer *9*:59–66.

39. Waterhouse, C. (1974). Lactate metabolism in patients with cancer. Cancer *33*:66–71.

40. Schein, P. S., Kisner, D., Haller, D., Belcher, M., & Hamosh, M. (1979). Cachexia of malignancy: Potential role of insulin in nutritional management. Cancer *43*:2070–2076.

41. Smith, F. P., Kisner, D., & Schein, P. S. (1980). Nutrition and cancer: Prospects for clinical research. Nutr Cancer *2*:34–39.

42. Waterhouse, C., & Kemperman, J. H. (1971). Carbohydrate metabolism in subjects with cancer. Cancer Res *3*:1273–1278.

43. Warnold, L., Lundholm, K., & Scherstén, T. (1978). Energy balance and body composition in cancer patients. Cancer Res *38*:1801–1807.

44. Souba, W. W., & Copeland, E. M. (1988). Parenteral nutrition and metabolic observations in cancer. Nutr Clin Pract *3*:183–190.

45. Dempsy, D. T., Feurer, I. D., Knox, L. S., Crosby, L. O., Buzby, G. P., & Mullen, J. L. (1984). Energy expenditure in malnourished gastrointestinal cancer patients. Cancer *53*:1265–1273.

46. Knox, L. S., Crosby, L. O., Feurer, I. D. Buzby, G. P., Miller, C. L., & Mullen, J. L. (1983). Energy expenditure in malnourished cancer patients. Ann Surg *197*:152–162.

47. Hansell, D. T., Davies, J. W. L., & Burns, H. J. G. (1986). The relationship between resting energy expenditure and weight loss in benign and malignant disease. Ann Surg *203*:240–245.

48. Lindmark, L., Bennegård, K., Edén, E., Ekman, L., Scherstén, T., Svaninger, G., & Lundholm, K. (1984). Resting energy expenditure in malnourished patients with and without cancer. Gastroenterology *87*:402–408.

49. Macfie, J., Burkinshaw, L., Oxby, C., Holmfield, J. H. M., & Hill, G. L. (1982). The effect of gastrointestinal malignancy on resting metabolic expenditure. Br J Surg *69*:443–446.

50. Blackburn, G. L., & Bothe, A. (1978). Assessment of malnutrition in cancer patients. Cancer Bull, *30*:88–93.

51. Van Eys, J. (1982). Tumor-host competition for nutrients. Cancer Bull, *34*:136–140.

52. Waterhouse, C. (1981). Oxidation and metabolic interconversion in malignant cachexia. Cancer Treat Rep, *65*(Suppl. 5):61–66.

53. Brennan, M., & Burt, M. E. (1981). Nitrogen metabolism in cancer patients. Cancer Treat Rep 65(Suppl. 5):67–78.

54. Lundholm, K., Edstrom, S., Ekman, L., Karberg, I., & Scherstén, T. (1981). Metabolism in peripheral tissues in cancer patients. Cancer Treat Rep 65(Suppl. 5):79–83.

55. Jeevanandam, M., Legaspi, A., Lowry, S. F., Horowitz, G. D., & Brennan, M. F. (1988). Effect of total parenteral nutrition on whole body protein kinetics in cachectic patients with benign or malignant disease. J Parenter Enter Nutr 12:229–236.

56. Kurzer, M., & Meguid, M. M. (1986). Cancer and protein metabolism. Surg Clin North Am 66:969–1001.

57. Stein, T. P., Oram-Smith, J. C., Leskiw, M. J., Wallace, H. W., & Miller, E. E. (1976). Tumor-caused changes in host protein synthesis under different dietary situations. Cancer Res 36:3926–3940.

58. Waterhouse, C., & Mason, J. (1981). Leucine metabolism in patients with malignant disease. Cancer 48:939–944.

59. Theologides, A.: (1979). Cancer cachexia. Cancer 43:2004–2012.

60. Mortensen, R. F., Shapiro, J., Lin, B. F., Douches, S., & Neta, N. (1988). Interaction of recombinant IL-1 and recombinant tumor necrosis factor in induction of mouse acute phase proteins. J Immunol 140:2260–2266.

61. Jeevanandam, M., Lowry, S. F., Horowitz, G. D., & Brennan, M. F. (1984). Cancer cachexia and protein metabolism. Lancet 1:1423–1426.

62. Baracos, V., Rodeman, H. P., Dinarello, C. A., & Goldberg, A. L. (1983). Stimulation of muscle protein degradation and prostaglandin E_2 release by leukocytic pyrogen: A mechanism for the increased degradation of muscle proteins during fever. N Engl J Med 308:553–558.

63. Mitchell, L. A., & Norton, L. W. (1989). Effect of cancer plasma on skeletal muscle metabolism. J Surg Res 47:423–426.

64. Moldawer, L. L., Svaninger, G., Gelin, J., & Lundholm, K. G. (1987). Interleukin-1 and tumor necrosis factor do not regulate protein balance in skeletal muscle. Am J Physiol 253:C766.

65. Flores, E. A., Bistrian, B. R., Pomposelli, J. J., Dinarello, C. A., Blackburn, G. L., & Istfan, N. W. (1989). Infusion of tumor necrosis factor/cachectin promotes muscle catabolism in the rat. J Clin Invest 83:1614–1622.

66. Kawakami, M., & Cerami, A. (1981). Studies of endotoxin-induced decrease in lipoprotein lipase activity. J Exp Med 154:631–639.

67. Semb, H., Peterson, J., Tavernier, J., & Olivecrona, T. (1987). Multiple effects of tumor necrosis factor on lipoprotein lipase in vivo. J Biol Chem 262:8390–8394.

68. Vlassara, H., Spiegel, R. J., Doval, D. S., & Cerami, R. (1986). Reduced plasma lipoprotein lipase activity in patients with malignancy-associated weight loss. Horm Metab Res 18:698–703.

69. Beutler, B., Mahoney, J., Le Trang, N., Pekala, P., & Cerami, A. (1985). Purification of cachectin, a lipoprotein lipase suppressing hormone secreted by endotoxin-induced RAW 264.7 cells. J Exp Med 161:984–995.

70. Tracey, K. J., Lowry, S. F., & Cerami, A. (1988). The pathophysiologic role of cachectin/TNF in septic shock and cachexia. Ann Inst Pasteur Immunol 139:311–317.

71. Porat, O. (1989). The effect of tumor necrosis factor alpha on the activity of lipoprotein lipase in adipose tissue. Lymphokine Res 8:459–469.

72. Fried, S., & Zechner, R. (1989). Cachectin/tumor necrosis factor decreases human adipose tissue lipoprotein lipase mRNA levels, synthesis, and activity. J Lipid Res 30:1917–1923.

73. Hall, R. J. C. (1975). Progress report: Normal and abnormal food intake. Gut 16:744–752.

74. Morrison, S. D. (1978). Origins of anorexia in neoplastic disease. Am J Clin Nutr 31:1104–1107.

75. Costa, G. (1980). Cachexia, the metabolic component of neoplastic diseases. Cancer Res 37:2327–2335.

76. Costa, G., & Donaldson, S. (1980). The nutritional effects of cancer and its therapy. Nutr Cancer 2:22–29.

77. Cox, R. P., & Ghosh, N. K. (1978). Current concepts in the ectopic production of fetal proteins and hormones by neoplastic cells. Am J Med Sci 275:232–248.

78. Lindsey, A. M., Piper, B. F., & Carrieri, V. L. (1981). Malignant cells and ectopic hormone production. Oncol Nurs Forum 8:13–15.

79. Fine, R. M. (1988). Evidence of tumor necrosis factor/cachectin production in cancer. Int J Dermatol 27:379–380.

80. Aderka, D., Fisher, S., Levo, Y., Holtmann, H., Hahn, T., & Wallach, D. (1985). Cachectin/tumour necrosis factor production by cancer patients. Lancet 2:1190.

81. Carswell, E. A., Old, L. J., Kassel, R. L., Green, S., Fiore, N., & Williamson, B. (1975). An endotoxin-induced serum factor that causes necrosis of tumors. Proc Natl Acad Sci USA 72:3666–3670.

82. Beutler, B., & Cerami, A. (1987). Cachectin: More than a tumor necrosis factor. N Engl J Med 316:379–385.

83. Dinarello, C. A., Cannon, J. G., Wolff, S. M., Bernheim, H. A., Beutler, B., Cerami, A., Figari, I. S., Palladino, M. A., Jr., & O'Connor, J. V. (1986). Tumor necrosis factor (cachectin) is an endogenous pyrogen and induces production of interleukin-1. J Exp Med 163:1433–1450.

84. Liang, C. M., Liang, S. M., Jost, T., Sand, A., Dougas, I., & Allet, B. (1986). Production and characterization of monoclonal antibodies against recombinant human tumor necrosis factor/cachectin. Biochem Biophys Res Commun 137:847–854.

85. Mannel, D. N., Moore, R. N., & Mergenhagen, S. E. (1980). Macrophages as a source of tumoricidal activity (tumor-necrotizing factor). Infec Immun 30:523–530.

86. Moldawer, L. L., Drott, C., & Lundholm, K. (1988). Monocytic production and plasma bioactivities of interleukin-1 and tumor necrosis factor in human cancer. Eur J Clin Invest 18:486–492.

87. Pennica, D., Nedwin, G. E., Hayflick, J. S., Seeburg, P. H., Derynck, R., Palladino, M. A., Kohr, W. J., Aggarwal, B. B., & Goeddel, D. V. (1984). Human tumor necrosis factor: Precursor structure, expression and homology to lymphotoxin. Nature 312:724–729.

88. Shirai, T., Yamaguchi, H., Ito, H., Todd, C. W., & Wallace, R. B. (1985). Cloning and expression

of the gene for human tumor necrosis factor. Nature *313*:803–806.

89. Tisch, H., & Gifford, B. E. (1983). In vitro production of rabbit macrophages tumor cell cytotoxin. Int J Cancer *32*:105–112.

90. Wanebo, H. J. (1989). Tumor necrosis factor. Semin Surg Oncol *5*:402–413.

91. Ziegler-Heitbrock, H. W., Möller, A., Linke, R. P., Haas, J. G., Rieber, E. P., & Riethmüller, G. (1986). Tumor necrosis factor as an effector molecule in monocyte mediated cytotoxicity. Cancer Res *46*:5947–5952.

92. Tracey, K. J., Vlassara, H., & Cerami, A. (1989). Cachectin/tumor necrosis factor. Lancet *1*:1122–1126.

93. Aderka, D., Holtman, H., Toker, L., Hahn, T., & Wallach, D. (1986). Tumor necrosis factor induction by Sendai virus. J Immunol *136*:2938–2942.

94. Starnes, H. F., Warren, R. S., Jeevanandam, M., Gabrilove, J. L., Larchian, W., Oettgen, H. F., & Brennan, M. (1988). Tumor necrosis factor and the acute metabolic response to tissue injury in man. J Clin Invest *82*:1321–1325.

95. Brennan, M. F., (1977). Uncomplicated starvation versus cancer cachexia. Cancer Res *37*:2359–2364.

96. Beutler, B., & Cerami, A. (1988). Cachectin (tumor necrosis factor): A macrophage hormone governing cellular metabolism and inflammatory response. Endocr Rev *9*:57–66.

97. Waage, A., Halstensen, A., & Espevik, T. (1987). Association between tumor necrosis factor in serum and fatal outcome in patients with meningococcal disease. Lancet *1*:355–357.

98. Grau, G. E., Fajardo, L. F., Piguet, P. F., Allet, B., Lambert, P. H., & Vassalli, P. (1987). Tumor necrosis factor (cachectin) as an essential mediator in murine cerebral malaria. Science *237*:1210–1212.

99. Aggarwal, B. B., Eessalu, T. E., & Hass, P. E. (1985). Characterization of receptors for human tumor necrosis factor and their regulation by gamma interferon. Nature *318*:665–667.

100. Kriegler, M., Perez, C., DeFay, K., Albert, I., & Lu, S. D. (1988). A novel form of TNF/cachectin is a cell surface cytotoxic transmembrane protein: Ramifications for the complex physiology of TNF. Cell *53*:43–53.

101. Socher, S. H., Martinez, D., Craig, J. B., Kuhn, J. G., & Oliff, A. (1988). Tumor necrosis factor not detectable in patients with clinical cachexia. J Natl Cancer Inst *80*:595–598.

102. Wiedenmann, B., Reichardt, P., Rath, U., Theilmann, L., Schule, B., Ho, A. D., Schlick, E., Kempeni, J., Hunstein, W., & Kommerell, B. (1989). Phase I trial of intravenous continuous infusion of tumor necrosis factor in advanced metastatic carcinoma. J Cancer Res Clin Oncol *115*:189–192.

103. Bibby, M. C., Double, J. A., Ali, S. A., Fearon, K. C., Brennan, R. A., & Tisdale, M. J. (1987). Characterization of a cachectic transplantable adenocarcinoma of the mouse colon. J Nat Cancer Inst *78*:539–545.

104. Feinman, R., Henriksen-DeStefano, D., Tsujimoto, M., & Vilcek, J. (1987). Tumor necrosis factor is an important mediator of tumor cell killing by human monocytes. J Immunol *138*:635–640.

105. Shalaby, M. R., Aggarwal, B. B., Rinderknecht, E., Svedersky, L. P., Finkle, B. S., & Palladino, M. A. (1985). Activation of human polymorphonuclear

neutrophil formations by interferon-gamma and tumor necrosis factors. J Immunol *135*:2069–2073.

106. Gamble, J. R., Harlan, J. M., Klebanoff, W. J., & Vadas, M. A. (1985). Stimulation of the adherence of neutrophils to umbilical vein endothelium by human recombinant tumor necrosis factor. Proc Natl Acad Sci USA *82*:8667–8671.

107. Sugarman, B. J., Aggarwal, B. B., Hass, P. E., Figari, I. S., Palladino, M. A., Jr., & Shepard, H. M. (1985). Recombinant human tumor necrosis factor-alpha: Effects on proliferation of normal and transformed cells in vitro. Science *230*:943–945.

108. Dayer, J. M., Beutler, B., & Cerami, A. (1985). Cachetin/tumor necrosis factor stimulates collagenase and prostaglandin E_2 production by human synovial cells and dermal fibroblasts. J Exp Med *162*:2163–2168.

109. Bertolini, D. R., Nedwin, G. E., Bringman, T. S., Smith, D. D., & Mundy, G. R. (1986). Stimulation of bone resorption and inhibition of bone formation in vitro by human tumor necrosis factors. Nature *319*:516–518.

110. Broudy, V. C., Kauschansky, K., Segal, G. M., Harlan, J. M., & Adamson, J. W. (1986). Tumor necrosis factor type alpha stimulates human endothelial cells to produce granulocyte/macrophage colony-stimulating factor. Proc Natl Acad Sci USA *83*:7467–7471.

111. Vilcek, J., Palombella, V. J., Zhang, Y., Lin, J. X., Feinman, R., Reis, L. F. L., & Le, J. (1988). Mechanisms and significance of the mitogenic and antiviral actions of TNF. Ann Inst Pasteur Immunol *139*:307–311.

112. Vilcek, J., Palombella, V. J., Henriksen-DeStefano, D., Swenson, C., Feinman, R., Hirai, M., & Tsujimoto, M. (1986). Fibroblast growth enhancing activity of tumor necrosis factor and its relationship to other polypeptide growth factors. J Exp Med *163*:632–634.

113. Leibovich, S. J., Polverini, P. J., Shepard, H. M., Wiseman, D. M., Shively, V., & Nuseir, N. (1987). Macrophage-induced angiogenesis is mediated by tumor necrosis factor alpha. Nature *329*:630–632.

114. Cerami, A., & Beutler, B. (1988). The role of cachectin/TNF in endotoxic shock and cachexia. Immunol Today *9*:28–31.

115. Stovroff, M. C., Fraker, D. L., Travis, W. D., & Norton, J. A. (1989). Altered macrophage activity and tumor necrosis factor: Tumor necrosis and host cachexia. J Surg Res *46*:462–469.

116. DeWys, W. D. (1986). Weight loss and nutritional abnormalities in cancer patients: Incidence, severity and significance. In K. C. Calman & K. C. Fearon (eds.), *Nutritional Support for the Cancer Patient* (pp. 251–261). Philadelphia: W. B. Saunders.

117. Eilber, F. R., & Morton, D. L. (1970). Impaired immunologic reactivity and recurrence following cancer surgery. Cancer *25*:362–367.

118. Anthony, H. M., Templeman, G. H., Madsen, K. E., & Mason, M. K. (1974). The prognostic significance of DHS skin tests in patients with carcinoma of bronchus. Cancer *34*:1901–1906.

119. Dominioni, L., Dionigi, R., Dionigi, P., Nazari, S., Fossati, G., Prati, U., Tibaldeschi, C., & Pavesi, F. (1981). Evaluation of possible causes of delayed hypersensitivity impairment in cancer patients. J Parenter Enter Nutr *5*:300–306.

120. Bistrian, B. R., Blackburn, G. L., Scrimshaw, N. S., & Flatt, J. P. (1975). Cellular immunity in semi-starved states in hospitalized adults. Am J Clin Nutr 28:1148–1155.

121. Cunningham-Rundles, S. (1982). Effects of nutritional status on immunological function. Am J Clin Nutr 35:1202–1210.

122. Twomey, P., Ziegler, D., & Rombeau, J. (1982). Utility of skin testing in nutritional assessment: A critical review. J Parenter Enter Nutr 6:50–58.

123. DeWys, W. (1977). Anorexia in cancer patients. Cancer Res 37:2354–2358.

124. Holland, J. C., Rowland, J., & Plumb, M. (1977). Psychological aspects of anorexia in cancer patients. Cancer Res 37:2425–2428.

125. DeWys, W. D. (1979). Anorexia as a general effect of cancer. Cancer 43:2013–2019.

126. Schmale, A. H. (1979). Psychological aspects of anorexia. Cancer 43:2087–2092.

127. Garattini, S., Bizzi, A., Donelli, M. G., Guaitari, A., Samanin, R., & Spreafico, F. (1980). Anorexia and cancer in animals and man. Cancer Treat Rev 7:115–140.

128. Krause, R., Humphrey, C., von Meyenfeldt, M., James, H., & Fischer, J. (1981). A central mechanism for anorexia in cancer: A hypothesis. Cancer Treat Rep 65(Suppl. 5):15–21.

129. Theologides, A. (1981). Anorexia in cancer: Another speculation on its pathogenesis. Nutr Cancer 2:133–135.

130. DeWys, W. D., Costa, G., & Henkin, R. (1981). Clinical parameters related to anorexia. Cancer Treat Rep 65(Suppl. 5):49–52.

131. Bernstein, I. L. (1982). Physiological and psychological mechanisms of cancer anorexia. Cancer Res 42(Suppl.):715–720.

132. Lindsey, A. M., & Piper, B. F. (1985). Anorexia and weight loss: Indicators of cachexia in small cell lung cancer. Nutr Cancer 7:65–76.

133. DeWys, W. (1974). Abnormalities of taste as a remote effect of a neoplasm. Ann NY Acad Sci 230:427–434.

134. Mossman, K. L., & Henkin, R. I. (1978). Radiation-induced changes in taste acuity in cancer patients. Int J Radiat Oncol Biol Phys 4:663–670.

135. Williams, L. R., & Cohen, M. H. (1978). Altered taste thresholds in lung cancer. Am J Clin Nutr 31:122–125.

136. Mossman, K., Schatzman, A., & Chencharick, J. (1982). Long-term effects of radiotherapy on taste and salivary function in man. Int J Radiat Oncol Biol Phys 8:991–997.

137. Bolze, M. S., Fosmire, G. J., Stryker, J. A., Chung, C. K., & Flipse, B. G. (1982). Taste acuity, plasma zinc levels, and weight loss during radiotherapy: A study of relationships. Radiobiology 144:163–169.

138. Trant, A. S., Serin, J., & Douglass, H. O. (1982). Is taste related to anorexia in cancer patients? Am J Clin Nutr 36:45–58.

139. Strohl, R. A. (1983). Nursing management of the patient with cancer experiencing taste changes. Cancer Nurs 6:353–359.

140. Nielsen, S. S., Theologides, A., & Vickers, Z. M. (1980). Influence of food odors on food aversions and preferences in patients with cancer. Am J Clin Nutr 33:2253–2261.

141. Bernstein, I. L., & Bernstein, I. D. (1981). Learned food aversions and cancer anorexia. Cancer Treat Rep 65(Suppl. 5):43–47.

142. Smith, J. C., & Blumsack, J. T. (1981). Learned taste aversion as a factor in cancer therapy. Cancer Treat Rep 65(Suppl. 5):37–42.

143. Padilla, G. V. (1986). Psychological aspects of nutrition and cancer. Surg Clin North Am 66:1121–1135.

144. Cohn, S. H., Gartenhaus, W., Vartsky, D., Sawitsky, A., Zanzi, I., Vaswani, A., Yasumura, S., Rai, K., Cortes, E., & Ellis, K. J. (1981). Body composition and dietary intake in neoplastic disease. Am J Clin Nutr 34:1997–2004.

145. Long, C. L., Merrick, H. W., Dennis, R. S., Holme, D. S., & Geiger, J. W. (1982). Energy requirements for cancer patients. Am Bull 34:155–162.

146. Knox, L. S., Crosby, L. O., Feurer, I. D., Buzby, G. P., Miller, C. L., & Mullen, J. S. (1983). Energy expenditure in malnourished cancer patients. Ann Surg 197:152–162.

147. Blackburn, G. L., Maini, B. S., Bistrian, R. R., & McDermott, W. V., Jr. (1977). The effect of cancer on nitrogen, electrolyte and mineral metabolism. Cancer Res 37:2348–2353.

148. Gold, J. (1979). Hydrazine sulfate and cancer cachexia. Nutr Cancer 1:4–9.

149. Chlebowski, R. T., Heber, D., Richardson, B., & Block, J. B. (1984). Influence of hydrazine sulfate on abnormal carbohydrate metabolism in cancer patients with weight loss. Cancer Res 44:857–861.

150. Aisner, J., Tchekmedyian, N. S., Tait N., Parnes, H., & Novak, M. (1988). Studies of high-dose megestrol acetate: Potential applications in cachexia. Semin Oncol 15(Suppl. 1):68–75.

151. Hamburger, A., Parnes, H., Gordon, G. B., Shantz, L. M., O'Donnell, K. A., & Aisner, J. (1988). Megestrol acetate-induced differentiation of 3T3-LI adipocytes in vitro. Semin Oncol 15(Suppl. 1):76–78.

152. Tchekmedyian, N. S., Tait, N., Moody, M., & Aisner, J. (1987). High-dose megestrol acetate: A possible treatment for cancer cachexia. JAMA 257:1195–1198.

153. Blick, M., Sherwin, S. A., Rosenblum, M., & Gutterman, J. (1987). Phase I study of recombinant tumor necrosis factor in cancer patients. Cancer Res 47:2986–2989.

154. Feinberg, B., Kurzrock, R., Talpaz, M., Blick, M., Saks, S., & Gutterman, J. U. (1988). A phase I trial of intravenously-administered recombinant tumor necrosis factor-alpha in cancer patients. J Clin Oncol 6:1328–1334.

155. Figlin, R., de Kernion, J., & Sarna, G. (1988). Phase II study of recombinant tumor necrosis factor (rTNF) in patients with metastatic renal cell carcinoma (RCCa) and malignant melanoma (MM). Proc Am Soc Clin Oncol 7:652.

156. Zamkoff, K. W., Newman, N. B., Rudolph, A. R., Young, J., & Poiesz, B. J. (1989). A Phase I trial of subcutaneously administered recombinant tumor necrosis factor to patients with advanced malignancy. J Biol Response Mod 8:539–552.

157. Jakubowski, A. A., Casper, E. S., Gabrilove, J. L., Templeton, M. A., Sherwin, S. A., & Oettgen, H. F. (1989). Phase I trial of intramuscularly administered tumor necrosis factor in patients with advanced cancer. J Clin Oncol 7:298–303.

158. Warren, R. S., Starnes, H. F., Gabrilove, J. L., Oettgen, H. F., & Brennan, M. F. (1987). The acute metabolic effects of tumor necrosis factor

administration in humans. Arch Surg *122*:1396–1400.

159. Lenk, H., Tenneberger, S. T., Muller, V., Ebert, J., & Shiga, T. (1989). Phase II clinical trial of high-dose recombinant human tumor necrosis factor. Cancer Chemother Pharmacol *24*:391–392.

160. Sherman, M. L., Spriggs, D. R., Arthur, K. A., Imamura, K., Frei, E. III., & Kufe, D. W. (1988). Recombinant human tumor necrosis factor administered as a five-day continuous infusion in cancer patients. Phase I toxicity and effects on lipid metabolism. J Clin Oncol *6*:344–350.

161. Lanzotti, V., Thomas, D., & Boyle, L. (1977). Survival with inoperable lung cancer. Cancer Res *39*:303–313.

162. Costa, G., Vincent, R., & Aragon, M. (1979). Weight loss and cachexia in lung cancer. Cancer Res *20*:387.

163. Costa, G., Lane, W. W., Vincent, R. G., Siebold, J. A., Aragon, M., & Bewley, P. T. (1981). Weight loss and cachexia in lung cancer. Nutr Cancer *2*:98–103.

164. Costa, G., Bewley, P., Aragon, M., & Siebold, J. (1981). Anorexia and weight loss in cancer patients. Cancer Treat Rep *65*(Suppl. 5):3–7.

165. Burke, M., Bryson, E. I., & Kark, A. E. (1980). Dietary intakes, resting metabolic ratio, and body composition in benign and malignant gastrointestinal disease. Br Med J *26*:211–215.

166. Theologides, A., Ehlert, J., & Kennedy, B. J. (1976). The calorie intake of patients with advanced cancer. Minnesota Med *50*:526–529.

167. Freeman, M., Frankmann, C., Beck, R. D., & Valdivieso, M. (1982). Prognostic nutrition factors in lung cancer patients. J Parenter Enter Nutr *6*:122–127.

168. Lindsey, A. M. (1986). Cancer cachexia: Effects of the disease and its treatment. Semin Oncol Nurs *2*:19–29.

169. Lanzotti, W. J., Copeland, E. M., George, S. L., et al. (1985). Cancer chemotherapeutic response and intravenous hyperalimentation. Cancer Chemother Rep *59*:437–439.

170. Chlebowski, R. T. (1986). Effect of nutritional support on the outcome of anti-neoplastic therapy. In K. C. Calman & K. C. Fearon (eds.), *Nutritional Support for the Cancer Patient* (pp. 365–379). Philadelphia: W. B. Saunders.

171. Klein, S., Simes, J., & Blackburn, G. L. (1986). Total parenteral nutrition and cancer clinical trials. Cancer *58*:1378–1386.

172. Bozzetti, F. (1989). Effects of artificial nutrition on the nutritional status of cancer patients. J Parenter Enter Nutr *13*:406–420.

173. Balducci, L., & Hardy, C. (1987). Cancer and nutrition: A review. Compr Ther *13*:60–69.

174. Tait, N., & Aisner, J. (1989). Nutritional concerns in cancer patients. Semin Oncol Nurs *5*(Suppl. 1):58–62.

175. Koretz, R. L. (1984). Parenteral nutrition: Is it oncologically logical? J Clin Oncol *2*:534–538.

176. Kokal, W. A. (1985). The impact of anti-tumor therapy on nutrition. Cancer *55*:273–278.

177. Copeland, E. M., III, Daly, J. M., & Dudrick, S. J. (1977). Nutrition as an adjunct to cancer treatment in the adult. Cancer Res *37*:2451–2456.

178. Layton, P. B., Gallucci, B. B., & Aker, S. N. (1981). Nutritional assessment of allogeneic bone marrow recipients. Cancer Nurs *4*:127–135.

179. Harvey, K., Bothe, A., & Blackburn, G. L. (1979). Nutritional assessment and patient outcome during oncological therapy. Cancer *43*(Suppl.):2065–2069.

180. Butler, J. H. (1980). Nutrition and cancer: A review of the literature. Cancer Nurs *3*:131–136.

181. Grant, M. M. (1986). Nutritional interventions: Increasing oral intake. Semin Oncol Nurs *2*:36–43.

182. D'Agostino, N. S. (1989). Managing nutrition problems in advanced cancer. Am J Nurs *89*:50–56.

183. Hardy, C., Wallace, C., Khansur, T., Vance, R. B., Thigpen, J. T., & Balducci, L. (1986). Nutrition, cancer and aging: An annotated review: II. cancer cachexia and aging. J Am Geriatr Soc *34*:219–228.

184. Coley, N. H., Fowler, G. A., & Bogatko, F. H. (1952). A review of the influence of bacterial infection and of bacterial products (Coley's toxins) on malignant tumors in man. Acta Med Scand (Suppl.) *276*:29–97.

185. Shear, M. F., & Perrault, A. (1944). Chemical treatment of tumors. IX. Reactions of mice with primary subcutaneous tumors to injection of a hemorrhage-producing bacterial polysaccharide. J Natl Cancer Inst *44*:461–476.

186. Spriggs, D., Imamura, K., Rodriguez, C., Horiguchi, J., & Kufe, D. W. (1987). Induction of tumor necrosis factor expression and resistance in a human breast tumor cell line. Proc Natl Acad Sci USA *84*:6563–6566.

187. Spies, T., Morton, C. C., Nedospasov, S. A., Fiers, W., Pious, D., & Strominger, J. L. (1986). Genes for the tumor necrosis factors alpha and beta are linked to the human major histocompatibility complex. Proc Natl Acad Sci USA *83*:8699–8702.

188. Lawson, D. H., Nixon, D., & Rudman, D. (1981). Effects of tumors on mineral and electrolyte metabolism (Abstract). Mol Inter Nutr Cancer 15–16.

189. Beutler, B. (1988). The presence of cachectin/tumor necrosis factor in human disease states. Am J Med *85*:287–288.

7

Hypothermia

Rebecca Phillips

DEFINITION

Hypothermia is a core body temperature less than 35° C.[1–8] The core zone is composed of organ structures located within the body cavity and head.[9] Temperature monitoring sites for evaluating the core zone are the tympanic membrane, esophagus, pulmonary artery, urinary bladder, and rectal ampulla.[4, 6, 10–12] Levels of hypothermic severity have been historically delineated into ranges moving from mild to profound[13, 14] (Table 7–1). Neurophysiologists generally agree that the location for temperature regulation is either the anterior or the lateral hypothalamus.[4, 6, 9, 15] Survival following hypothermia appears dependent upon the severity and duration of the episode.[2, 6, 16, 17]

PREVALENCE AND POPULATIONS AT RISK

There are no definitive prevalence statistics for hypothermia. The rate of occurrence of hypothermia from accidental outdoor exposure is unknown. It can be assumed that persons with mild cases do not seek medical attention. Exposure events occur more frequently in cold climates than in tropical climates.[18] However, episodes have been recorded in the sunbelt of the United States.[7, 19] Accidental hypothermia from immersion and near drowning carries a mortality rate of 2.5 deaths per 100,000 occurrences.[20–27] In demographic studies the usual age for fatality is 10 to 19 years.[22] Hypothermia in the neonate is due to an immature thermoregulatory mechanism.[28]

Incidence in this population depends upon low gestational age or low birth weight.

Hypothermia exists in the patient who has experienced pharmaceutical overdose because of the effects on the hypothalamus. Monoamine oxidase (MAO) inhibitors, tricyclic antidepressants, and narcotics reduce temperature by hypothalamic suppression.[29] The prevalence of this type of hypothermia appears to be higher during the holidays.

Physically traumatized individuals can experience hypothermia.[30, 31] Those who do not have significant neurological involvement but do have volume-deficit injuries experience central core cooling from rapid fluid resuscitation.[30] With an estimated 60 million cases of trauma annually in the United States, there is significant potential for hypothermia. The incidence of hypothermia in this setting is dependent upon the frequency of trauma and is seen more often in regional trauma centers.[32]

Danzel and associates worked with the Hypothermia Study Group to develop an outcome scoring system for victims of hypothermia.[33] Their work shows that the key survival indicator for hypothermia is the extent of end-organ damage.

Induction of hypothermia is performed in patients undergoing certain types of surgical

TABLE 7–1 HYPOTHERMIA LEVELS

Levels	Temperature (°C)
Normal	36.6–37.5
Mild	34.0–36.5
Moderate	28.0–33.5
Deep	17.0–27.5
Profound	04.0–16.5

From Phillips, R. & Skov, P. (1988). Rewarming and cardiac surgery: A review. Heart Lung *17*:511–520.

intervention. Coronary artery bypass grafting utilizes hypothermia and cardioplegia to provide myocardial cell protection and end-organ protection by reduction of oxygen demand.[34–38]

Hypothermia is used to lower total body oxygen demand and protect end organs during the major vascular repair of an ascending or aortic arch aneurysm[39, 40] or when a major neurovascular surgical reconstruction procedure is performed.[41–44] Tertiary care centers will provide these services more frequently than small community district hospitals because of their referral base.

SITUATIONAL STRESSORS AND DEVELOPMENTAL DIMENSIONS

Individuals can be exposed to situational stressors that will cause hypothermia. Accidental hypothermia occurs when there is unintentional exposure to low environmental temperature.[1, 6, 7, 17, 20, 21, 45] Deliberate induction of low core temperature is seen in the surgical procedures noted above.[4, 34, 46–48]

Developmental stressors for hypothermia occur at both ends of the life cycle, placing the individual at risk because of age or developmental status. Specific stressors and populations at risk are discussed next.

Clinical States

Hypothermia affects both sexes of all age groups through various developmental stressors. The fetus becomes hypothermic when the mother does, and a bradycardic heart rate develops as an indicator of a decrease in its core temperature.[49] Maternal hypothermia deliberately induced for emergency neurological[50] or cardiovascular surgical procedures requiring cardiopulmonary bypass can be disastrous to the fetus. Besides developing bradycardia while the mother is undergoing a bypass procedure, the fetus can be macerated at the time of a premature but viable birth because of the hypothermia.[51] The fetus may also be spontaneously aborted because of hypothermic effects at a time of nonviability.[52] However, the mother can deliver a healthy term or a viable preterm infant, even after a hypothermic episode.[53–55]

Neonates become hypothermic immediately after birth as a result of heat evaporation from their wet skin into the environment of the delivery room.[56, 57] This heat loss can be as significant as 4.5° C over the first minute of life if the neonate is left uncovered in the cold delivery room. The heat is lost by evaporation, radiation, and convection. The neonate's large surface area to mass ratio, in light of its small volume of subcutaneous tissue, makes possible this heat loss over the first minute of life.[58]

Newborns can remain hypothermic for the first 3 days of life without concern for the presence of a severely dysfunctional state.[59] Newborns should be closely monitored for hypoglycemia if they are having difficulty regulating temperature. The hypoglycemia is due to rapid utilization of brown fat to speed up metabolism and raise core temperature.[28, 60] After 3 days of life, if hypoglycemia is not occurring, the hypothermia should be investigated, as it could indicate a breakdown of the normal physiological response to sepsis.[59]

Hypothermia can occur from submersion. This happens throughout the life span[20–22] and is a two-edged sword. The submersion in extremely cold water (2 to 12° C) for a prolonged time may result in biological and clinical death. Biological death occurs because of the deleterious effects of hypothermia on the cardiovascular system.[21, 26] The clinical death from hypothermia is seen as a slowing of metabolism. This metabolic reduction has a protective effect on brain tissue. It also modulates metabolic acidosis by decreasing lactate production. Warm water submersion accident victims rarely survive in a fully intact neurological state because of the lack of hypothermic protection.[22, 23]

Severe hypothermia can also be caused by submersion in icy snow. The Mt. Hood climbing expedition disaster is an example of the devastating effects of severe hypothermia. Nine of 11 healthy athletic climbers froze to death. They were found in profoundly hypothermic states on the south side of the mount. Rewarming techniques were successful for only two of the victims.[16]

In the aged population, there is an impaired ability to thermoregulate.[61, 62] The main reason seems to be a reduction in metabolic and vasomotor responses.[63, 64] This is due to loss of lean body muscle mass as well as a reduction in thermogenic nutrients in the diet.[65] There is also a decreased ability to generate heat from a reduced capability to activate the shivering mechanism.[66] This increases the potential for accidental hypothermia in the elderly.[67, 68] Because of the reduction of thermogenic nutrients in daily dietary intake, the aged individual shows evidence of malnutrition and this more readily allows for the development of infectious processes. A febrile response may not be seen, and hypothermic septic states may ensue.[69] These episodes are more severe if metabolic-endocrine disorders are present. Thyroid dysfunction, particularly hypothyroid conditions, aids in the continuation of hypothermia. This is related to reduced thyroid-stimulating hormone (TSH) levels. TSH helps set metabolic rate. Diabetes mellitus may also cause hypothermia because intracellular glucopenia in the hypothalamic tissue causes an alteration in neurohormonal control of temperature.[70–72] Hypoglycemia-induced hypothermia can also be related to excessive alcohol ingestion.[73–76] This alcohol-induced hypothermia results in acute circulatory failure.[77] The alcoholic population is at added risk for the development of hypothermia from the vasodilating effects of alcohol at the skin surface, thus, increasing blood flow and reducing body heat by convection. The alcohol also anesthetizes the brain, reducing the individual's sensation of cold and the appropriate response to it.[78]

Every patient entering the operating room is at risk for hypothermia. If the patient is placed in an operating room where ambient temperature is less than 21° C (69.8° F), core temperature will consistently drop at a mean rate of 0.3° C per hour.[79] This holds true for open cavity and non–open cavity procedures.[80] Anesthesia aids the development of hypothermia by blocking activation of the shivering mechanism and the body's generation of heat.[81] This occurs while there is an increase in the body's heat loss through the cutaneous vasodilative effects of anesthesia.[82] The use of nitrous oxide as an anesthetic agent further compounds the temperature losses by its suppression of the thermostatic set point in the hypothalamus.[83] Comparison of anesthesia techniques, with strong controls on all other heat loss variables, revealed that the anesthetic agents themselves rapidly decreased the core temperature by 0.6° C immediately after induction.[84]

Narcotics affect temperature regulation by direct interference with the anterior hypothalamus.[85, 86] They cause vasodilatation in resistance and capacitance vascular beds, allowing for redistribution of blood away from skeletal muscle and reducing heat generation while increasing losses through the skin.[87, 88]

Specific surgical procedures utilize therapeutic hypothermia as a preservation technique for the organ system. Neurosurgeons utilize hypothermic circulatory arrest in the repair of cerebral artery aneurysms.[41–43, 89–91] However, incidental hypothermia during neurosurgical procedures not utilizing deliberate temperature reduction is of concern because of the related slow return to wakefulness and the increasing intracranial pressure caused by shivering.[92]

Various surgical procedures may benefit from the application of induced hypothermia. These procedures include (1) the repair of juxtahepatic vascular injury;[93] (2) the repair or reconstruction of a kidney;[94–98] (3) major thoracic aortic procedures, so that spinal cord function is preserved after the necessary cross clamping needed to effect repairs;[99–103] and (4) all cardiac surgical procedures, allowing for reduction in metabolic demands[104–106] and preservation of myocardial cell energetics after the required period of anoxic arrest.[107–111]

Neurologists use induced hypothermia in combination with barbiturate coma to treat refractory status epilepticus.[112] This technique is also used to treat severe Reye's syndrome.[113, 114] Cerebral anoxia and ischemia have been treated using hypothermia with or without barbiturate coma.[115–118] Current approaches to neurological salvage do not include the use of hypothermia.[119]

MECHANISMS

Physiology of Thermoregulation

To understand the pathophysiology of hypothermia, it is necessary to first examine the physiology of temperature regulation. Houdas and Ring discuss Liebermeister's 1875 work, in which he postulated that the body had a reference temperature point to which it naturally gravitated.[120] If there is a variance from this set-point, the body then activates appropriate mechanisms to return to this established temperature point.[9] This reference, or set-point, is known as the thermoneutral zone.[120] The limits of the total temperature range are set by the fragility the cell demonstrates to dehydration and ice crystal formation on the low side and by the speed of the denaturation of vital cell proteins on the high side.[13]

Each organ system has its own regulatory range. The heart and brain have very narrow temperature variance points.[120] The maintenance of temperature within this range is accomplished by adjustments in how thermal loads are sensed and processed for correction. This is temperature regulation.[13]

Homeothermy is maintained by a balance between heat lost to the environment and heat gained by production.[9, 13, 121, 122] This is controlled by positive and negative feedback system responses for both physical and chemical mechanisms. Physical mechanisms are regulated by the nervous system, which functions as a message center to send and receive thermal change requirements. The endocrine system is responsible for chemical mechanism changes. Thyroid-stimulating hormone (TSH) and adrenocorticotrophic hormone (ACTH) regulate the body's metabolic rate and speed of gluconeogenesis. Both of these mechanisms are involved in the process of regulating temperature variation from set-point.[9, 13]

Neurophysiologists have been looking for the temperature control center in the brain since 1884, when Ott made lesions in the base of the dog brain and saw a hyperthermic response.[123] Hall and associates determined that possibly there are special temperature sensors in the preoptic region.[124] Bazett and Penfield found that when there was total decerebration, there was a lack of ability to regulate temperature.[125] If unilateral decerebration occurred, there was regulatory ability, and this ability was better seen when the decerebration left the optic chiasm intact. From their studies Bazett and associates concluded that the temperature control center was found in the hypothalamic region.[125–127]

Frazier and associates noted that large lesions placed dorsal to the optic chiasm and ventral to the anterior commissure would seriously impair temperature regulation to heat, without much effect on regulation to cold.[128] However, bilateral lesions in the caudal part of the hypothalamus impaired regulatory ability to either heat or cold. Other investigators also found the same response to lesion placement.[129, 130] These studies supported the conclusion that tissue in the hypothalamic region is the center for temperature regulation.

The body handles heat loads by varying surface blood flow through deep and cutaneous vessel dilation and inducing autonomic motor outflow tracts to produce sweat.[9] This allows for heat from the core to move to the surface by means of convective transfer and countercurrent exchange.[131, 132] Evaporation of sweat also helps to cool the body and reduce heat.[133] There is a heat threshold for activation of sweating, and this varies between sexes, with the female threshold set higher than the male.[134–137]

The body handles cold loads by increasing metabolic rate, causing vasoconstriction and activation of the shivering mechanism. Metabolic heat is generated from the carbohydrates, fats, and proteins ingested in the diet. Ingested carbohydrate initiates the anaerobic glycolysis process via the Embden-Meyerhof pathway. This process oxidizes glucose, by ATP phosphorylation, into pyruvate. Pyruvate is then oxidized into acetylcoenzyme A, which enters the Krebs cycle as tricarboxylic acid.[138] The breakdown products of fats are ketoacids that also enter the Krebs cycle.[139] Proteins convert to amino acids that are deaminated to enter the energy pathway. The energy produced by these pathways elevates metabolic activities, which reflect metabolic rate and result in an increase in core temperature. These metabolic activities are regulated by TSH-released thyroxine. Low thyroxine levels reduce the efficiency of these pathways and hamper the body's ability to handle cold loads.[140] When the increase in metabolic rate is insufficient to elevate core temperature or if the skin's cutaneous cold receptors are stimulated, vasoconstriction of the superficial capillary bed occurs. The vasoconstriction shunts blood from the peripheral vascular bed to the core in an attempt to retain body heat. If this is ineffective or if there is a decrease in local blood or tissue temperature at the level of the hypothalamus, the shivering mechanism is activated.[141] Shivering in response to vasoconstriction comes from skeletal muscle tone heightened in response to impulses transmitted from myelinated nerve fibers in the cutaneous bed. These impulses then transfer to the dorsal root of the spinal column before they ascend to the central thermogenic center within the hypothalamus. Shivering is centrally activated when the hypothalamus identifies a blood temperature as being below the thermal set-point.[142] Once this center is stimulated, signals are sent from the brain stem to the spinal cord and out to the anterior motor neurons via the somatic motor outflow tracts. The motor neurons increase the tone of the skeletal muscle. This heightened tone causes oscillations that result in muscular contraction of an involuntary nature.[13, 143]

Pflug and colleagues found that shivering increased oxygen consumption by 500 per cent over the resting state.[144] This increase in consumption is attributed to increased cardiac workload, as seen by an elevation of the rate pressure product value (heart rate × systolic blood pressure). Increased consumption reduces both mixed venous and arterial oxygen (PO_2) levels, increasing cardiac and respiratory work loads.[144-148] Rodriguez and associates[147] corroborated Pflug's[144] data and demonstrated an increase in carbon dioxide (PCO_2) production during shivering episodes. This elevation in PCO_2 alters the body's acid-base balance, further taxing the cardiopulmonary system. When hypothermia occurs, the metabolic rate is increased, vasoconstriction shunts blood to the core, and the skeletal muscle shivering mechanism is activated to improve heat load to the body and increase core temperature.

Pathophysiology of Hypothermia

Hypothermia develops when heat is lost from the body. Heat can be lost by the mechanisms of convection, conduction, radiation, or evaporation[16] (Table 7–2). Convection removes heat by utilizing the circulating blood cells. Body heat is given off when the subcutaneous tissue is cooler than the temperature of the blood. When this happens, the blood cells provide heat to the tissue. Convection is also the physical mechanism by which heat is lost in cold wind or during cold water immersion. The skin gives

TABLE 7–2 HEAT TRANSFER TECHNIQUES

Mechanism	How Heat Transfer Is Effected
Convection	Uses circulating red blood cells to adjust temperature of the skin to the blood circulating in the core.
Conduction	Moves heat from one object to another by physical contact.
Radiation	Dissipates heat into the environment.
Evaporation	Reduces temperature by use of a water molecule as it changes into vapor and carries heat away.

off heat in an attempt to warm the wind or the water. Conductive transfer removes heat by shifting it to anything that comes in contact with the heated object. An example would be skin-to-clothing transfer of body heat. Radiation of heat occurs between the skin and the environment. Body heat is generated and dissipated into a cooler surrounding environment. Evaporation requires damp skin in order to reduce body heat. The fluid on the skin converts to vapor, and the vapor reduces body temperature.[149]

The effects of hypothermia can be observed on all organ systems. Some of these effects are extremely beneficial to the system functioning less than optimally. Others create life-threatening problems for the individual and a challenge to health care professionals.

The Neurological System

The pathophysiological effects of hypothermia on the neurological system vary from confusion to apparent neurological death. As the core temperature falls to levels of hypothermia, mental confusion and reduced capability to perform a mental task become apparent. This state fades to lethargy and finally coma as the temperature continues to fall.[150] This reduction in level of consciousness is related to a drop in cerebral blood flow (CBF). Each degree drop in core temperature causes a 6 to 7 per cent reduction in the CBF. At 30° C the pupils will dilate.[151, 152] As core temperature reaches 22° C, the pupils will become fixed. If hypoxia is also present, this can occur at 27° C.[153]

With these neurological signs of catastrophe present an electroencephalogram (EEG) may be performed. A core temperature below 36° C may be the cause of reduced electrical activity and electrical cerebral silence.[152-154] Evoked-potential (EP) examinations are used to assess the brain's ability to respond to external electrical stimuli. Visual, auditory, and somatic divisions can be checked for their viability.[155] These EP examinations are extremely sensitive to a decrease in core temperature. Auditory brain stem EP examinations exhibit continued, consistently reduced functioning as the temperature falls.[156, 157] Hypothermia slows axonal conduction and depresses neurotransmitter release, reducing sympathetic transmission. This causes a 7 per cent increase in the interpeak latency of the waves on the EP recording for every 1° C the temperature falls. The latency length will double to 14 per cent of normal around the 26° C mark. The latency period will totally disappear, and a flat line on the EP tracing will be present at 20° C.[40, 157] Much care must be exercised when interpreting any neurological sign if any level of hypothermia is present.

Reduced core temperature alters functioning of the sympathetic limb of the autonomic nervous system. This is demonstrated by a reduction in beta-receptor response. These receptors are located within the myocardial tissue and other sites. Activation of these sites causes increased cardiac contractility, which is a major determinant of blood pressure. This reduced beta-site response stimulates an increase in release of the neurotransmitter norepinephrine. Norepinephrine is a catecholamine that increases systemic vascular resistance (SVR) by stimulation of alpha receptors. The increase in SVR raises blood pressure, improving CBF. Therefore, elevated norepinephrine levels act as a neurologically mediated vascular attempt to protect cerebral function.[158, 159]

The Cardiovascular System

The cardiovascular system has a pathophysiological response to the presence of hypothermic conditions. As the core temperature drops, mean arterial pressure (MAP) initially increases in a compensatory metabolic attempt to increase blood flow from core to periphery.[160-162] As thermal stress increases by a further drop in core temperature, MAP falls in response to a decrease in circulating volume.[161-163] The reduction in circulating volume is attributed to fluid loss to the extravascular tissue, shunting of the blood to the smaller peripheral vessels, and fluid loss through diuresis occurring from lack of renal response to antidiuretic hormone (ADH).[164, 165] The drop in volume increases SVR two or three times above baseline in an attempt to improve blood pressure. This high SVR severely reduces preload to the left ventricle, which reduces stroke volume output from the left ventricle to the periphery. The reduced circulating volume decreases ventricular filling. A reduction in filling lowers pressure in accordance with the Starling phenomenon. Since ventricular contractility is related to filling pressure, when pressure is reduced, contractility is decreased, reducing beta-receptor site activity. This helps to further decrease ventricular

contractility.[158, 159] The hemodynamic response to a decrease in ventricular contractility is a fall in cardiac output, resulting in reduced blood pressure. At a core temperature of 31° C, peripheral blood pressure may be unrecordable.[166]

A reduction in core temperature also initiates a reduction in heart rate. This occurs from conduction defects at the atrioventricular (AV) node and bundle of His. These defects are seen on the electrocardiogram (ECG) as AV blocks, bundle branch blocks (BBB), and prolongation of the PR and QT intervals.[167] The QT interval is prolonged in response to the slowed heart rate. Since this slowing in heart rate is not from vagal stimulation, atropine is ineffective in increasing it.[161] As the temperature drops to 32° C or lower, the atrial-to-bundle of His (AH) interval is prolonged until there is a 2:1 Wenckebach pattern, showing a loss of AV node conduction rate. This occurs from freezing of the AV node.[168] As the rate continues to slow and the AV, QT, and AH intervals are progressively prolonged, the hypothermic heart demonstrates myocardial irritability. As circulatory function is depressed, anaerobic metabolism increases. This is seen as an increase in lactate production with a resultant fall in total body pH. This heightens myocardial irritability and the likelihood of episodes of atrial or ventricular fibrillation as the temperature reaches 30° C. Asystole follows as the temperature further drops to 15° C.[169]

Of the core organs, cardiac muscle is the most oxygen-consuming. Because of this, Bigelow and associates began to study the mechanism by which oxygen consumption could be reduced.[170] The results of his study demonstrated that core cooling lowers total body oxygen demands and therefore consumption. There is a near direct relationship between consumption and temperature, with a known 50 per cent fall in myocardial oxygen consumption at a temperature of 28° C.[4]

The Pulmonary System

As the core temperature drops from its set-point, respiratory rate initially increases to adjust for a falling body pH owing to impaired circulatory function.[149] Respiratory effort then falls in response to the cerebral medullary reflex response to cold. This further decreases body pH as carbon dioxide levels increase from reduced ventilation. The reduction in respiratory effort allows atelectasis to develop, creating an intrapulmonary shunt. Shunting reduces PO_2 to a hypoxic level.[171, 172] To further compound the oxygenation problem, hypothermia causes a shift of the oxyhemoglobin curve to the left, reflecting an increased oxygen affinity for hemoglobin and therefore decreased tissue oxygen uptake and utilization.[173, 174]

Another result of the cold is the attenuation of the cough reflex and the occurrence of bronchorrhea. These can result in the pooling of bronchial secretions, placing a hypothermic individual at risk for the development of pneumonia, from aspiration of bronchial secretions, and hypoxemia. Cessation of respiratory effort does not occur until core body temperature is reduced to 24° C.

The Gastrointestinal System

Ulcerations and hemorrhages in the gastric mucosa are classic indications of the occurrence of hypothermia.[175] Once core temperature falls below 34° C, gastric motility is absent. This can be seen as air and fluid lines on radiographs.[167] Pancreatitis from reduced circulatory flow may develop and is most notably seen in fatal hypothermic episodes.[176]

The Renal System

The hypothermia-induced decrease in the cardiac output causes a reduction in renal blood flow (RBF) and glomerular filtration rate (GFR).[177] Hypothermia inhibits the tubular reabsorption of sodium and water and decreases tubular response to ADH and ACTH (see the Endocrine System section). Therefore, no inhibition is placed on diuresis, and the circulating volume will not be maintained.[178, 179] This further reduces RBF and GFR while activating the cardiovascular response to falling central venous pressure.

Serum potassium (K^+) levels shift with changes in temperature. As cardiac output falls and lactate builds up, K^+ is released into the blood.[180] Based on retrospective data collected from the Mt. Hood disaster,[19] prolonged hypothermia resulted in cell lysis. This occurrence is indicated by K^+ levels in excess of 10 mEq/L. Serum K^+ levels in excess of 7 mEq/L were a grave prognostic indicator in this group of hypothermia victims. If hypothermia is controlled and not severe or prolonged, then serum levels will fall as K^+ is shifted back into the cell.[181] When diuresis occurs during hypothermia, serum K^+ can be reduced because the tubule does not reabsorb it.[182]

The Endocrine System

Hypothermia affects the endocrine system by inhibiting beta cell function in the pancreas. This causes a decrease in insulin output at a time of increased requirements as the stress response increases glucose level.[149, 183, 184]

Adrenocorticotropic hormone appears lower than normal in the animal anesthetized in a hypothermic condition. The ACTH level is regulated by corticotropin-releasing factor (CRF), which responds to oxytocin (OT) and arginine vasopressin (AVP), two peptides released by the hypothalamus. During hypothermia, AVP and OT levels are significantly reduced from normal core temperature levels. Lower AVP and OT levels reduce pituitary release of CRF, which in turn decreases ACTH levels in the circulating serum of hypothermic anesthetized animals.[185] Findings in humans have correlated well with the animal findings for all hormonal levels.[186] The renal effects of ACTH are tubular reabsorption of sodium and water and excretion of potassium. In the face of hypothermia, ACTH levels will be reduced, allowing for sodium and water losses as well as K^+ losses by the hypothermic kidneys. If there is a preexisting renal dysfunction, hypothermia worsens the effects.[182]

The Hematological System

Hypothermic conditions alter the hematological presentation of an individual and the clotting mechanism. Hematocrit levels will be elevated because of the fluid losses associated with hypothermia.[187, 188] Leukocytes are found sequestered within the liver, spleen, and splenic beds when the core temperature is reduced below 33° C. This lowers peripheral white blood cell counts and reduces the phagocytic response.[4, 189] This leaves the individual at risk for the development of an overwhelming infectious state that will not be identifiable until normothermia is re-established.

Clotting is slowed as a result of the hypothermic effects on the coagulation cascade, fibrinolytic activity, and platelet function. The series of reactions constituting the coagulation cascade slow with reduction in metabolic rate that occurs with core temperature drop, as do all enzymatic reactions in the body.[190] Fibrinolytic activity increases and is thought to be attributable to the release of a heparin-like factor that inhibits Factor X. This causes a bleeding coagulopathy that resembles disseminated intravascular coagulation. The cause of this syndrome is multifactorial and dependent on the initiating event of the hypothermia.[191]

The effect of the hypothermic state on platelets is twofold. There is sequestration of platelets in the spleen and liver.[192] Hessel and associates tagged platelets with chromium and found the majority of sequestration occurred in the liver.[193] Sequestration reduces peripheral platelets available to respond to bleeding episodes. Valeri and associates examined thromboxane B_2 levels in normothermic and hypothermic baboons.[194] (Thromboxane B_2 is the substance responsible for allowing platelets to aggregate.) The authors found that the cooler the body temperature, the lower the thromboxane B_2 level ($P < .05$), probably because the thromboxane B_2 level derives from the enzymatic breakdown of thromboxane A_2. As previously indicated, all enzyme reactions slow with the reduction of core temperature. The level of thromboxane B_2 was restored with return to normothermia.[185, 186]

The Enzyme System

The enzymes that regulate the Krebs cycle accumulate when the core temperature falls. This allows for more rapid phosphorylation of nutritional elements needed for heat generation. At the same time, the glucose-6-phosphate dehydrogenase activity, responsible for activating a competing metabolic pathway, decreases in its level of functioning. This helps to save heat-producing energy.[195]

Creatine kinase (CK) is an enzyme that is located within the brain (CK1), the heart (CK2), and the skeletal muscle mass (CK3). The presence of hypothermia ensures that total serum CK will be elevated.[196] Since CK is released when muscle damage occurs, isoenzyme levels help determine the origin of CK release and the damaged organ. (For a review of systemic effects of hypothermia, see Table 7–3.)

MANIFESTATIONS

The manifestation of hypothermia is primarily a decrease in core temperature below 35° C.[1–8] The presence of shivering may indicate that central temperature has been reduced below the physiological set-point. Abbey has done an extensive review of the literature available on the initiation of the shivering mechanism.[197] This review resulted in the development of a five-point shivering scale that can be used as a clinical assessment tool. The scale is keyed to the palpation of selected muscle groups identified as routinely involved in shivering. It allows for clinical delineation of the degree to which the individual's shivering mechanism has been activated.[197] The levels of the scale are given below:

0 = No muscle evidence of shivering.
1 = Masseter muscle groups have increased tone on palpation.
2 = Pectoralis muscle groups have increased tone on palpation.
3 = Generalized obvious shivering without teeth chattering.
4 = Teeth chattering with obvious shivering.

Care must be taken to ensure that core temperature is below the usual physiological set-point to verify that shivering is related to hypothermia.

The presence of the Osborn J on the 12-lead ECG is diagnostic for a less than normal core temperature.[4] This J wave is seen most frequently in the left chest leads. It presents as an upward deflection off of the S wave prior to the onset of the ST segment (Figure 7–1).[198] The interval lengths measured on the ECG will prolong as the sinus and AV nodes demonstrate cold response. Eventually, the sinus node will lose its ability to control the rhythm, and arrhythmias will develop.[166] Care must be exercised to avoid making a diagnosis of hypothermia on the basis of arrhythmia development. The blocks associated with hypothermia and loss of sinus node activity can occur during the evolution of an inferior wall infarct.[199] Therefore, the only true manifestation of a hypothermic episode is the recording of a core temperature less than 35° C.

SURVEILLANCE AND MEASUREMENT

Surveillance of hypothermic states is achieved by frequent monitoring of temperature values from core sites. This is usually done by continuous digital display of the

TABLE 7–3   SYSTEMIC EFFECTS OF HYPOTHERMIA

System/ Mechanisms	Temperature Range (° C)	Effects
Neurological	< 36	EEG unreliable
	< 36	Each ° C depresses neurotransmitter release.
	34	7% decrease in CBF
	30	Pupils dilate
	26	EP latency length 14% longer than normal
	22	Fixed pupils
	20	Flat line on EP
Cardiovascular	32	Prolonged AH interval
	31	BP not recordable
	30	Irritability
	28	50% decrease in MVO_2
	15	Asystole
Pulmonary	< 36	Decreased respiratory effort, atelectasis, shunting, left shift of oxyheme curve
	24	Cessation of respiratory effort
Gastrointestinal	< 34	No motility
Renal	< 36	Decreased RBF, decreased GFR, inhibited tubular response to Na and H_2O, decreased response to ADH, ACTH, and potassium
Endocrine	< 36	Inhibited B-cell function, decreased AVP, CRF, and ACTH
Hematological	< 33	Sequestered leukocytes in the liver, spleen, and splenic beds; sequestered platelets in spleen and liver; decreased thromboxane B_2 level
Enzymatic	< 35	Increased total CK, increased phosphorylation of nutritional elements for heat generation
Shivering		O_2 consumption increases 500% over resting state; increased rate-pressure product

Abbreviations: EEG, electroencephalogram; CBF, cerebral blood flow; EP, evoked potential; AH, atrial-His bundle; MVO_2, myocardial oxygen demand; PCO_2, carbon dioxide; PO_2, oxygen; RBF, renal blood flow; GFR, glomerular filtration rate; ADH, antidiuretic hormone; ACTH, adrenocorticotropic hormone; AVP, arginine vasopressin; CRF, corticotropin-releasing factor; CK, creatine kinase.

temperature values. If this type of monitoring is not available, low reading glass thermometers should be utilized. The sites usually identified as "core sites" are the tympanic membrane, esophagus, pulmonary artery and urinary bladder.[4, 6, 10–12] Although the rectal ampulla is frequently identified as being part of the core, during hypothermic events it more accurately reflects peripheral temperature. Because of this varying response, rectal temperature more approximately fits the "transitional" temperature zone. This is an area in which temperature "zone" is classified as to how the site responds to cold stress.[200, 201] When compared with the defined core temperatures, changes in rectal temperature lag behind all others during hypothermia.[202]

Mravinac and associates compared rectal, pulmonary artery, and urinary bladder temperatures in 55 adult patients who had experienced hypothermic cardiac surgery.[203]

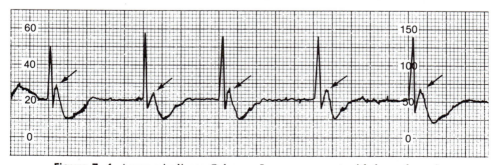

Figure 7–1. Arrows indicate Osborne J waves present with hypothermia.

Results showed a strong correlation between urinary bladder and pulmonary artery temperatures. Rectal temperature did not show a strong correlation with urinary bladder or pulmonary artery temperature. (See Research Review for a full discussion of the studies.)

The use of rectal temperature in the neonate is not considered a safe technique because of the potential for rectal perforation[204] or thermometer breakage.[205] Axillary temperatures may be falsely elevated by the high volume of brown adipose tissue at this site. Bliss-Holtz found that use of inguinal temperatures in the normal full-term neonate may be quite appropriate, as these temperatures have an extremely high correlation with rectal temperatures.[206] There is less brown adipose tissue in this area, which accounts for its correlation with rectally obtained values. Use of rectal temperature to measure hypothermia requires acknowledgment that the values lag behind more centrally located sites.

Surveillance of shivering on a continuous basis is necessary to protect patients from significant increases in oxygen consumption. Use of Abbey's scale is encouraged for documentation of the presence and severity of shivering.[197] Nurses are encouraged to monitor for shivering because it is approximately 11 per cent efficient in producing an increase in total body heat.[207] It leads, however, to a loss in core temperature, as the mechanism continues for protracted periods of time. This occurs from the vasodilation of the skeletal muscle mass as shivering progresses.[197] Hemingway indicated that shivering resembles light exercise to the muscles.[142] This exercise state requires an increase in oxygen consumption at the cost of increased cardiac and respiratory work.

THERAPIES

The major goal of initiating therapeutic measures for hypothermia is to return temperature to normothermia. The core needs to be rewarmed before the periphery in order to prevent circulatory collapse. Rewarming in this manner stops rapid dilation of the peripheral vascular bed when circulatory volume may not be sufficient to maintain blood pressure. A second major goal is the prevention of compromise to the cardiovascular and pulmonary systems during rewarming from hypothermia. As this rewarming process occurs, observation for afterdrop of core temperature must be initiated. "Afterdrop" refers to the continued falling core temperature after the initiation of rewarming techniques. It was initially thought that this reduced temperature was associated with the return of cold blood from the periphery to the core. The cold blood returns as the warming techniques dilate the vascular bed.[208] This concept has been re-evaluated, and it is now thought that afterdrop occurs because of the way that heat flows through body tissues. The occurrence is limited in its magnitude and force by convection from the circulating blood.[209] This discussion reviews both internal and external methods aimed at correcting the hypothermia (Table 7–4).

External Methods

Rewarming the individual who suffers from hypothermia can be most readily accomplished by use of an internal approach. However, external methods can be applied so that there is attenuation of further heat loss. External methods to avoid further heat loss can be active or passive. An example of a passive external technique is removal of the individual from the cold exposure (i.e., taking the person out of the cold water or out of the snow) and providing warm, dry coverings.[210] This avoids further loss of body heat to evaporation.[149] The individual undergoing surgery is relieved from the cold stress by removal from the operating room. Use of

TABLE 7–4   REWARMING TECHNIQUES

External
Passive
Warm environment
Minimal drafts
Blankets
Head covering
Active
Fluid-circulating blankets
Radiant lights
Internal
Inhalation of warmed gases
Warmed gases during surgery
Warmed IV fluids and blood
Hemodialysis
Peritoneal dialysis
Nasogastric irrigation
Colonic irrigation
Mediastinal irrigation
Cardiopulmonary bypass

reflective blankets while in the operating suite as well as appropriate head covering helps to protect the patient from heat losses to the cold environment.[211] Heat loss through the scalp can be major, particularly in the individual with limited hair covering.[13] Newborns are dried at birth and wrapped in warmed blankets prior to removal from the cold delivery room. A key aid to attenuation of this heat loss is an increase in ambient temperature.[212]

For individuals suffering from hypothermia, active external rewarming may be attempted by the use of warm fluid-filled blankets. Studies have shown, however, that these actively help only in avoidance of further heat loss when used in a warm room.[79–80, 212] Miles and Thompson showed that the fluid-filled bead bed was effective in correcting a case of hypothermia by minimizing heat loss from the core to the environment.[213] Care must be taken when using this bed to avoid hypovolemia. Insensible fluid losses will be increased in the individual resting on the warmed bed, particularly as core temperature returns to normothermia. Additional fluids must be infused to ensure that the anticipated dehydration effects from the warmed bed will not further jeopardize the survival of the individual. Newborns are routinely cared for in radiant warmer beds to keep their exposed skin surfaces warm and reduce further core temperature drops.[214]

Internal Methods

Use of internal warming methods are aimed at returning the core to normothermia before the periphery. By doing this, the periphery is aided in warming by the circulation of warm core blood. If the periphery were to return to normothermia before the core, the victim would experience "rewarm shock," a period of vasodilation with a significant decrease in systemic vascular resistance.[215] As the vascular resistance falls, an extreme state of hypovolemia would be seen. Rapid fluid resuscitation using warm fluids would be necessary in this case to maintain circulation. Therefore, the core should be rewarmed before the periphery. Internal, invasive methods of rewarming will accomplish this. Probably the most active and invasive technique is the use of cardiopulmonary bypass (CPB). In this situation, CPB can be most readily instituted by percutaneous placement

of bypass catheters into the femoral vein and artery. This allows for rapid institution of circulatory support for core rewarming.[216, 217] Use of this method in rewarming a hypothermic trauma patient is inadvisable because of the necessity for heparinization.

Barr and associates suggested using continuous warmed pleural cavity perfusion in place of full CPB.[218] In their experimental model, two chest tubes were placed into the pleural space. One tube was used for inlet of warmed fluid, the other was used to drain the pleural space. Inflow was controlled by a bypass pump that ran at a flow rate of 850 ml/minute. The technique was successful in rewarming the model from 28° C to 32° C in 56 minutes. It is a technique that might be utilized for core rewarming but has not yet been studied in humans.

Several other invasive techniques can be utilized to reverse hypothermia. Warmed nasogastric instillation has been suggested by Bar as a means of elevating core temperature.[219] Minimal electrolyte shifts occurred if solutions were warmed, instilled, drained, rewarmed, and reinstilled. Instillate warming temperature should be between 38° and 40° C. Electrolyte depletion did not occur until after six exchanges.

Peritoneal dialysis involving a warmed dialysate solution is also suggested as a means of applying direct heat to a core cavity. This is a usable technique in postoperative hypothermic patients, particularly those who have renal failure. The electrolyte imbalance of this patient group may require immediate dialysis in the postoperative period. Although warming the dialysate is not always necessary, it should be used in the hypothermic patient.[13, 220, 221] This form of dialysis is difficult to utilize in the traumatized patient population experiencing hypothermia because of the possibility of abdominal injury. Until the integrity of the abdominal contents can be assured, full use of the peritoneal space should not be attempted.

Hemodialysis also is a possible way of correcting a low temperature state, but care must be exercised when this technique is utilized because of the volume shifts that occur with dialyzer use. Volume loading of a significant quantity must be performed in a timely fashion. This is particularly important while the patient is undergoing rewarming because of the vasodilation created.[220, 221]

A less aggressive but still invasive method

for rewarming from hypothermia involves the use of warming intravenous fluids. This includes crystalloid solutions and blood and blood products. Core temperature can be reduced with each liter of cold fluid administered. The use of various blood-warming devices helps to reduce the internal temperature loss from fluid administration.[13, 220, 222, 223]

Pflug and associates evaluated the effectiveness of warmed inhalation gases on improving the temperature of a hypothermic core.[144] They were able to show that heat transferred across the mediastinum and the bronchial mucosa from the mainstem bronchus. Ventilator cascades are capable of humidifying and warming oxygen delivered to the trachea as high as 46° C without creating thermal injury. The hypothermic individual does not have to be intubated to receive heated humidified oxygen; it can be provided by any oxygen delivery system that accommodates humidification. This technique can be used to help rewarm hypothermic patients requiring mechanical ventilation.

Rewarming techniques involve active and passive external techniques as well as invasive internal methods. A combination of these techniques is usually used to help reverse a hypothermic state. The external techniques are usually the easiest methods to employ. Although they probably do not actively improve the core temperature, these interventions attenuate any further loss of body heat. Use of the invasive, internal methods actively increases core temperature. While these techniques are being utilized, supportive techniques for the cardiovascular system may be necessary. Recall that left ventricular contractility is reduced during periods of hypothermia. This reduces cardiac output and blood pressure. A beta-agonist agent should be infused intravenously to improve left ventricular stroke work. If this does not provide adequate blood pressure to improve end-organ perfusion, the addition of an alpha-agonist agent should be considered.[224]

REVIEW OF RESEARCH FINDINGS

The topic of recovery from hypothermia is not widely covered in the nursing literature. The subtopic most frequently studied is the selection of site for core temperature monitoring. This part of the chapter reviews the major studies available on the topic of core monitoring site selection.

Surveillance for hypothermia is dependent upon the reliability of temperature monitoring devices and their placement location. These devices can be placed on the tympanic membrane and in the esophagus, the pulmonary artery, urinary bladder, or rectum. Pulmonary artery, rectum, and now urinary bladder are the most common monitoring sites in the critical care environment for core monitoring. The purpose of monitoring the core temperature is to allow the clinician to determine the level of metabolic activity occurring within the individual undergoing surveillance. Shellock and Rubin demonstrated the use of pulmonary artery blood temperature as an accurate reflection of the core in their study on core temperature measurements.[10] Their results are referenced by others as the standard method for core temperature monitoring.

Evaluation of the use of urinary bladder temperature began to appear in the literature in the early 1980s. Lilly and associates compared urinary bladder temperature with rectal, esophageal, and pulmonary artery values to determine its effectiveness in reflecting core values.[11] Thirty-one adults undergoing lengthy major surgical procedures were monitored by urinary bladder temperature and at least one other temperature monitoring site. Temperature values from all sites monitored were recorded every 15 minutes from anesthesia induction through initial intensive care unit (ICU) recovery. The study does not indicate how long the temperature recordings were made at the 15-minute time interval after ICU arrival. The temperature values recorded ranged from 26.8 to 38.4° C. Values from all sites were almost identical across the recorded range during periods of unassisted circulation. This allowed high correlation coefficients and F values ($P < .001$) across the temperature range investigated. The sample regression slopes all approached unity. In those patients requiring extracorporeal circulation, temperature values recorded from urinary bladder and pulmonary artery sites during rapid rewarming sequences showed almost overlapping values. Temperatures recorded by esophageal and rectal monitors showed slower increases when compared with the urinary bladder and pulmonary artery temperatures. This was felt to be associated with a lack of fluid flow at these monitoring sites. The researchers concluded that urinary bladder temperature can be reliably used to reflect the temperature of the core.

Moorthy and associates studied urinary bladder temperature monitoring in patients experiencing the rapid changes associated with cardiopulmonary bypass and then while they were in a steady state level in the ICU.[12] The sample consisted of 12 patients undergoing cardiac surgery. Temperature monitoring sites were the nasopharynx, esophagus, rectum, urinary bladder, and skin. Thermistors were placed after anesthesia induction. Pulmonary artery temperature was not monitored intraoperatively because of the potential for error with the change in blood flow created by use of the cardiopulmonary bypass pump. It was, however, monitored continuously in the ICU.

Temperatures were recorded every 15 minutes during surgery and every hour for 6 hours postoperatively. Thereafter, values were recorded every 2 hours for 10 hours. Results intraoperatively showed that when mean esophageal and nasopharyngeal temperatures were down between 23 and 25° C, rectal and bladder temperatures were recorded at 28 and 29° C, respectively. During rapid rewarming in the operating room, rectal and bladder temperatures again lagged, while esophageal and nasopharyngeal temperatures showed return from hypothermia.[12]

Postoperatively, the rectal, urinary bladder, and pulmonary artery temperatures were all within 0.5 to 1.0° C of each other, with rectal temperature 1.0° C lower than pulmonary artery temperature. This lag in rectal temperature would be clinically significant if blankets are removed (to reduce overshoot of temperature above normothermia) based on its value. They would be removed 1° C too late if attempting to avoid overshoot of temperature in the postoperative cardiac surgery patient population.[225] There was, however, a significant difference between core and skin temperature, a questionable problem of perfusion rather than hypothermia. The research team recommended use of urinary bladder temperature as a reflection of core temperature in a steady state (one not actively being effected by cardiopulmonary bypass temperature changes).

Davis and associates evaluated tympanic membrane temperature for its usefulness as a core monitoring site.[226] Their initial study

was conducted on an animal model, comparing tympanic temperature with direct measurement of regional cerebral temperature during periods of profound hypothermia. These values were compared to nasopharyngeal, esophageal, and rectal temperatures, representing accepted core monitoring sites. The study results indicated that the tympanic membrane was reliable for evaluating cerebral temperature. Though the research report offered no statistical analysis, the results suggested that the tympanic membrane values were more closely aligned in value to the direct cerebral temperature than the other three sites.

This research team modified the animal model protocol for use in human subjects. The direct cerebral monitoring was eliminated for human subjects. Study results showed that temperature recorded at the tympanic membrane site fell more rapidly than the temperature recorded at the nasopharyngeal site during hypothermia. Tympanic membrane temperature also had less variability with respect to the esophageal temperature.

The integrity of the external auditory canal must be ascertained by otoscopic examination prior to insertion of the ear probe. An example of loss of canal integrity would be membrane rupture with deep diving and more commonly skull fracture.[227] Research results in several studies have demonstrated trauma to the tympanic membrane and the canal with use of the ear probe.[226, 228] In response to these complications, a new infrared tympanic thermometer has been developed. Clinical trials have found that the device is accurate for recording core temperature without tympanic membrane trauma.[229]

Because the tympanic membrane is used to monitor brain core temperature, it is useful in surgical procedures necessitating circulatory arrest, as it allows for monitoring of the metabolic state of the brain. This is extremely important during episodes of accidental hypothermia severe enough to mimic cerebral silence. Clinical application of tympanic membrane monitoring will assist in determining brain temperature for EEG monitoring, since cerebral silence tracings require normothermia for the brain.

CASE STUDY

An 86-year-old woman was admitted to the critical care center. She had been picked up at her home by paramedics after having not been seen by neighbors for 48 hours. Upon arrival, the paramedics found her on the floor, unresponsive to verbal or tactile stimulation. Pupils were dilated bilaterally, blood pressure was unobtainable, heart rate was 32 with an idioventricular rhythm, respiratory rate was 6 and shallow, and extremities were cold without palpable pulses. Oxygen was established by face mask at 10 L/minute. After several attempts, an intravenous line was placed in the left antecubital vein. Normal saline (NS) (1000 ml) was rapidly infused at a wide open rate. Atropine (1 mg) was given IV push without effect on the heart rate. An isoproterenol (Isuprel) drip (1 mg in 250 ml NS) was added and titrated to 2 mcg/minute to obtain a heart rate of 50 per minute. With this rate and volume, she was transported by air rescue to the hospital's emergency department with a palpable blood pressure of 40 mm Hg.

On arrival in the emergency department, a rectal temperature of 94° F was recorded, systolic blood pressure was 40 by palpation, heart rate was 52 with isoproterenol, and respiratory rate had dropped to 4 breaths per minute. A more severe hypothermic state was suspected, and a low reading thermometer was utilized. It verified a hypothermic state, with rectal temperature recorded at 30° C. Isoproterenol was continued, and a second large peripheral intravenous line was started. A dopamine infusion was begun for blood pressure support. When the dopamine infusion reached 15 mcg/kg/minute, the systolic blood pressure exceeded 100 mm Hg. The heart rate was now 60 beats per minute, so the isoproterenol infusion was discontinued. The results of various tests verified the effects of hypothermia; that is, white blood cell count was subnormal, hemoglobin was 15.6 g/dl, arterial blood gas results showed hypercarbia, the chest radiograph demonstrated bilateral infiltrates, and the ECG revealed a nodal rhythm with Osborne J waves.

At this point, the patient was transferred from the emergency department to the critical care center. On arrival, she was placed between two fluid blankets set at 40° C. A rectal probe was placed to allow for continuous temperature recording. Normal saline was continued at 200 ml/hour, and dopamine was infused to maintain a blood pressure in excess of 90 mm Hg. A Foley catheter was placed to allow for closer monitoring of urinary volume. Vital signs were obtained and showed a rectal temperature of 30° C, heart rate of 54, respiratory rate of 6, urine volume of 10 ml. One hour later the temperature had increased to 32° C.

Four hours after admission, the rectal temperature had risen to 34° C, and arterial blood gases showed hypoxemia and persistent hypercarbia. A No. 7 endotracheal tube was inserted without incident, and mechanical ventilation was begun. Supplemental oxygen was increased to 100 per cent to improve Po_2. Po_2 increased to a maximum of 68 mm Hg. Because of hypotension, positive end-expiratory pressure (PEEP) was not added. To aid in reducing heat loss, the temperature of the ventilator humidifier was increased to 39° C.

Volume repletion continued with the addition of 25 per cent albumin solution to the normal saline infusion (100 ml 25 per cent albumin for every 1.5 L of NS). A central venous introducer was placed in the right neck for pulmonary artery line insertion if volume repletion became difficult to manage. As volume status stabilized, urine output improved to 50 ml hour.

Subsequent laboratory studies showed a reduced hemoglobin from the initial value with the white blood cell count increased from baseline. The serum potassium level was 5.2 mEq, and cardiac and liver enzyme values exceeded normal levels. Renal function values indicated dehydration, and biochemical values showed poor nutritional status (decreased fat and protein levels below normal). Hyperalimentation was begun with the addition of intralipids.

Twenty-four hours after admission, rectal temperature could not be maintained at a level of 35° C. Blood pressure remained 70 to 80 mm Hg systolic, in spite of volume repletion and dopamine infusion. Heart rate remained less than 60 with varying rhythms (sinus-nodal—2:1 block). With an inspired oxygen concentration of 100 per cent, arterial Po_2 was 52 mm Hg. Arterial pH was 7.21 with PCO_2 of 24, bicarbonate (HCO_3) of 11, and base excess of minus 15. A single dose of 44 mEq $NaHCO_3$ was given to correct metabolic acidosis. PEEP of 5 cm H_2O was added to improve oxygenation without success, and a drop in blood pressure occurred. A norepinephrine (Levophed) (8 mg/250 ml D_5W) infusion was begun to increase blood pressure. Because of persistent metabolic acidosis, the serum lactate level was determined. Results showed a level of 9.2, usually a level difficult to correct (normal value is 2.5.). Because of this continuing situation, the family was approached to discuss resuscitation status. After a conference with physicians, the clinical nurse specialist, and social services, the family decided to place the patient on "do not resuscitate" status. Twenty-eight hours after admission with continued volume, pressor, and respiratory support, she died. The patient never fully recovered from the initial hypothermic state. Active internal rewarming was never attempted because of physician concern that the patient would not return to a functional neurological status. The hypotensive episode had been prolonged for over 36 hours.

IMPLICATIONS FOR FURTHER RESEARCH

In reviews of the literature on hypothermia, little is found to address the trajectory of core temperature in the accidental hypothermia victim. Information detailing the anticipated trajectory in recovery is available on deliberate hypothermia, but detailed information is necessary on the accidental hypothermia to aid in anticipating patients' responses.

Nursing has contributed very little by way of controlled research to the investigation of hypothermia, which is an important problem. Most of the available literature, both medical and nursing, is reported in case study or review format. Isolated studies have been reported on the subtopics of the metabolic effects and the pathophysiology of hypothermia, the shivering mechanism, rewarming techniques, and the studies on core temperature measurements. These topics are usually covered in the literature on cardiopulmonary bypass.

Hypothermic patients require nursing interventions to help them avoid further heat loss, but nursing has not aggressively investigated the interventions appropriate to achieve that goal. One such intervention that is poorly investigated is the use of blankets. Although used in most settings, warmed and fluid-filled blankets have not demonstrated change in low body temperature states. Since nursing practice utilizes these methods with the belief that they will elevate core temperature from moderate levels of hypothermia (see Table 7–1), nurses need to design well-controlled studies to demonstrate the effectiveness of the interventions. Suggested interventions to be studied include (1) increased ambient temperature; (2) warmed bath blankets; (3) lying on fluid-filled heated blankets; (4) covering by fluid-filled heated blankets; (5) "sandwiching" in fluid-filled heated blankets; (6) use of warmed air blown over the individual; (7) warmed fluids given intravenously, orally, nasogastrically, or rectally; or (8) a combination of all of these. These interventions should not be used in the presence of severe or profound hypothermia (see Table 7–1). For these levels of hypothermia, more aggressive and invasive methods must be utilized to ensure that core rewarming occurs first. The above list is not meant to be inclusive but a beginning from which to search for the best interventions to treat mild to moderate hypothermia.

REFERENCES

1. Carden, D., Doan, L., Sweeney, P., & Nowak, R. (1982). Hypothermia. Ann Emerg Med *11*:497–503.
2. White, J. (1982). Hypothermia: The Bellevue experience. Ann Emerg Med *11*:417–424.
3. Harnett, R., Pruitt, J., & Sias, F. (1983). A review of the literature concerning resuscitation from hypothermia: Part I—the problem and general approaches. Aviat Space Environ Med *54*:425–434.
4. Reuler, J. (1978). Hypothermia: Pathophysiology, clinical settings, and management. Ann Intern Med *89*:519–527.
5. Smith, D. (1983). Living death: Don't let hypothermia fool you into a fatal mistake. RN *46*:49–51.
6. Miller, J., Danzl, D., & Thomas, D. (1980). Urban accidental hypothermia: 135 cases. Ann Emerg Med *9*:456–461.
7. Thomas, D. (1988). Accidental hypothermia in the sunbelt. J Gen Intern Med *3*:552–554.
8. Yates, D., & Little, R. (1979). Accidental hypothermia. Resuscitation *7*:59–67.
9. Elder, P. (1989). Accidental hypothermia. In W.

Shoemaker, W.S. Ayres, A. Grenvik, P. Holbrook, & W. Thompson (eds.), *Textbook of Critical Care* (2nd ed., pp. 101–109). Philadelphia: W.B. Saunders.

10. Shellock, F., & Rubin, S. (1982). Simplified and highly accurate core temperature measurements. Med Prog Tech *8*:187–188.

11. Lilly, J., Boland, J., & Zekan, S. (1980). Urinary bladder temperature monitoring: A new index of body core temperature. Crit Care Med *8*:742–744.

12. Moorthy, S., Winn, B., Jallard, M., Edwards, K., & Smith, N. (1985). Monitoring urinary bladder temperature. Heart Lung *14*:90–93.

13. Biddle, C. (1985). Hypothermia: Implications for the critical care nurse. Crit Care Nurse *5*:34–38.

14. Clochesy, J. (1984). Profound hypothermia. Focus Crit Care *11*:19–21.

15. Hardy, J. (1961). Physiology of temperature regulation. Physiol Review *41*:521–606.

16. Hauty, M., Esrig, B., Hill, J., & Long, W. (1987). Prognostic factors in severe accidental hypothermia: Experience from the Mt. Hood tragedy. J Trauma *27*:1107–1112.

17. Weidin, B., Vanggaard, L., & Hirvonen J. (1979). "Paradoxical undressing" in fatal hypothermia. J Forensic Sci *24*:543–553.

18. DeLapp, T. (1983). Accidental hypothermia. Am J Nurs *83*:63–67.

19. Altus, P. (1980). Hypothermia in the sunny south. South Med J *73*:1491–1492.

20. McGee, M. (1989). An unusual case of accidental hypothermia due to cold water immersion. Am J Forensic Med Path *10*:152–155.

21. Clarke, E., & Niggemann, E. (1975). Near-drowning. Heart Lung *4*:946–962.

22. Spyker, D. (1985). Submersion injury: Epidemiology, prevention, and management. Pediatr Clin North Am *32*:113–125.

23. Wolf, D. (1980). Near drowning. Crit Care Update *7*:31–36.

24. Bennett, R. (1976). Drowning and near-drowning: Etiology and pathophysiology. Am J Nurs *76*:919–923.

25. Samuelson, T., Doolittle, W., Hayward, J., Mills, W., & Membroff M: Hypothermia and cold water near drowning: Treatment guidelines. Alaska Med *24*:106–111.

26. Harnett, R., O'Brien, E., Sias, F., & Pruitt, J. (1980). Initial treatment of profound accidental hypothermia. Aviat Space Environ Med *51*:680–687.

27. Hayward, J., & Eckerson, J. (1984). Physiological responses and survival time prediction for humans in ice-water. Aviat Space Environ Med *55*:206–212.

28. Kattwinkel, J., Cook, L., Hurt, H., Nowacek, G., & Short, J. (1989). Controlling temperatures of sick and at risk infants. In J. Kattwinkel (ed.), *Newborn Care: Concepts and Procedures, Book II.* Charlottesville, VA: Department of Pediatrics, University of Virginia Medical Center.

29. Wong, K. (1983). Physiology and pharmacology of hypothermia. West J Med *138*:227–232.

30. Jurkovich, G., Greiser, W., Luterman, A., & Curreri, W. (1987). Hypothermia in trauma victims: An ominous predictor of survival. J Trauma *27*:1019–1024.

31. Luna, G., Maier, R., Pavlin, E., Anardi, D., Copass, M., & Oreskovich, M. (1987). Incidence and effect of hypothermia in seriously injured patients. J Trauma *27*:1014–1018.

32. Veise-Berry, S. (1988). Evolution of the trauma cycle. In V. Cardona, P. Hevin, P. Mason, A. Scanlon-Schilpp & S. Veise-Berry (eds.), *Trauma Nursing from Resuscitation through Rehabilitation* (pp. 3–15). Philadelphia: W. B. Saunders.

33. Danzel, D., Hedges, J., & Pozos, R. (1989). Hypothermia outcome score: Development and implications. Crit Care Med *17*:227–231.

34. Galbut, D., Traad, E., & Dorman, M. (1985). Twelve-year experience with bilateral internal mammary artery grafts. Ann Thorac Surg *40*:264–269.

35. Reitz, B., & Ream, A. (1982). Use of hypothermia in cardiovascular surgery. In A. Ream & R. Fogdall (eds.), *Acute Cardiovascular Management: Anesthesia and Intensive Care* (pp. 830–851). Philadelphia: J.B. Lippincott.

36. Hearse, D., Braimbridge, M., & Jynge, P. (1981) *Protection of the Ischemic Myocardium: Cardioplegia* (pp. 167–208). New York: Raven Press.

37. Shanks, C., Wade, L., Meyer, R., & Wilkinson, C. (1985). Changes of body temperature and heat in cardiac surgical patients. Anaesth Intens Care *13*:12–17.

38. Sealy, W. (1989). Hypothermia: Its possible role in cardiac surgery. Ann Thorac Surg *47*:788–791.

39. Mahfood, S., Qazi, A., Garcia, J., Mispireta, L., Corso, P., & Smyth N. (1985). Management of aortic arch aneurysm using profound hypothermia and circulatory arrest. Ann Thorac Surg *39*:412–417.

40. Crepps, J., Allmendinger, P., Ellison, L., Humphrey, C., Preissler, P., & Low, H. (1987). Hypothermic circulatory arrest in the treatment of thoracic aortic lesions. Ann Thorac Surg *43*:644–647.

41. Spetzler, R., Hadley, M., Rigamonti, D., Carter, L., Raudzens, P., Shedd, S., & Wilkinson, E. (1988). Aneurysms of the basilar artery treated with circulatory arrest, hypothermia, and barbiturate cerebral protection. J Neurosurg *68*:868–879.

42. Baumgartner, W., Silverberg, G., & Ream, A. (1983). Reappraisal of cardiopulmonary bypass with deep hypothermia and circulatory arrest for complex neurosurgical operations. Surgery *94*:242–249.

43. Drake, C., Barr, H., & Coles, J. (1964). The use of extracorporeal circulation and profound hypothermia in the treatment of ruptured intracranial aneurysm. J Neurosurg *21*:575–581.

44. Gardner, T. (1982). Hypothermia—basic concepts. In R. Engelman & S. Levitsky (eds.), *Textbook of Clinical Cardioplegia.* Mt. Kisco, New York: Futura Publishing.

45. Vaagenes, P., & Holme, J. (1982). Accidental deep hypothermia due to exposure. Anaesthesia *37*:819–824.

46. Marta, M. (1985). Intraoperative hypothermia. AORN J *42*:240–242.

47. Shanks, C., Wade, L., Meyer, R., & Wilkinson, C. (1984). Changes of body temperature and heat in cardiac surgical patients. Anaesth Intens Care *13*:12–17.

48. Rittenhouse, E., Mohri, H., Dillard, D., & Merendino, K.A. (1974). Deep hypothermia in cardiovascular surgery. Ann Thorac Surg *17*:63–98.

49. Jadhon, M., & Main, E. (1988). Fetal bradycardia

associated with maternal hypothermia. Obstet Gynecol 72:496–497.

50. Stange, K., & Halldin, M. (1983). Hypothermia in pregnancy. Anesthesiology 58:460–461.

51. Levy, D., Warriner, R., & Burgess, G. (1980). Fetal response to cardiopulmonary bypass. Obstet Gynecol 56:112–115.

52. Boba, A. (1962). Hypothermia: Appraisal of risk in 110 consecutive patients. J Neurosurg 19:924–933.

53. Rowbotham, G., Bell, K., Akenhead, J., & Caern, A. (1957). A serious head injury in a pregnant woman treated by hypothermia. Lancet 1:1016–1019.

54. Boatman, K., & Bradford, V. (1958). Excision of an internal carotid aneurysm during pregnancy employing hypothermia and a vascular shunt. Ann Surg 148:271–275.

55. Zitnik, R., Brandenburg, R., & Shelden, R. (1969). Pregnancy and open heart surgery. Circulation 39(Suppl):257–262.

56. Ziegel, E., & Van Blarcom, C. (1972). Characteristics and nursing care of the newborn. In E. Ziegel & C. Van Blarcom (eds.), Obstetric Nursing (6th ed., pp. 535–610). New York: Macmillan.

57. Smales, C., & Kim, R. (1978). Thermoregulation in babies immediately after birth. Arch Dis Child 53:58–61.

58. Darnall, R. (1987). The thermophysiology of the newborn infant. Med Instrum 21:16–22.

59. El-Radhi, A., Jawad, M., Manson, N., Jamel, I., & Ibrahim, M. (1983). Sepsis and hypothermia in the newborn infant: Value of gastric aspirate examination. J Pediatr 103:300–302.

60. Hey, E., & Katz, G. (1969). Temporary loss of metabolic response to cold stress in infants of LBW. Arch Dis Child 44:323.

61. Kolanowski, A., & Gunter, L. (1983) Thermal stress and the aged. J Gerontol Nurs 9:13–15.

62. Robbins, A. (1989). Hypothermia and heat stroke: Protecting the elderly patient. Geriatrics 44:73–80.

63. Kramer, M., Vandik, J., & Rosin, A. (1989). Mortality in elderly patients with thermoregulatory failure. Arch Intern Med 149:1521–1523.

64. Wagner, J., Robinson, S., & Marino, R. (1974). Age and temperature regulation of humans in neural and cold regulation. J Appl Physiol 37:562–566.

65. Emslie-Smith, D. (1981). Hypothermia in the elderly. Br J Hosp Med 11:442–452.

66. Collins, K., Easton, J., & Exton-Smith, A. (1985). Shivering thermogenesis and vasomotor responses with convective cooling in elderly. MMWR 34:753–754.

67. Fox, R., Woodward, P., Exton-Smith, A., Green, F., Donnison, D., & Wicks, M. (1973). Body temperature in the elderly: A national study of physiological, social and environmental conditions. Br Med J 1:200–206.

68. Collins, K., Exton-Smith, A., Fox, R., Macdonald, I., & Woodward, M. (1977). Accidental hypothermia and impaired temperature hemostasis in the elderly. Br Med J 1:353–356.

69. Lewin, S., Brettman, L., & Holtzman, B. (1981). Infection in hypothermic patients. Arch Intern Med 141:920–925.

70. Maclean, D., Murison, J., & Griffiths, P. (1973). Acute pancreatitis and diabetic ketoacidosis in accidental hypothermia and hypothermic myxoedema. Br Med J 4:757–761.

71. Fitzgerald, F., & Jessop, C. (1982). Accidental hypothermia: A report of 22 cases and review of the literature. Adv Intern Med 27:127–150.

72. Freinkel, N., Metzger, B., & Harris, E. (1972). The hypothermia of hypoglycemia. N Engl J Med 287:841–845.

73. Freinkel, N., Singer, D., & Arky, R. (1963). Alcohol hypoglycemia—I. carbohydrate metabolism of patients with clinical alcohol hypoglycemia and the experimental reproduction of the syndrome with pure ethanol. J Clin Invest 42:1112–1133.

74. O'Keefe, S., & Marks, V. (1977). Lunchtime gin and tonic, a cause of reactive hypoglycemia. Lancet 1:1286–1288.

75. Tucker, H.S.G., & Porter, W.B. (1942). Hypoglycemia following alcoholic intoxication. Am J Med Sci 204:559–566.

76. Fitzgerald, F. (1980). Hypoglycemia and accidental hypothermia in an alcoholic population. West J Med 133:105–107.

77. Raheja, R., Pure, V., & Schaffer, R. (1981). Shock due to profound hypothermia and alcohol ingestion. Crit Care Med 9:644–646.

78. Weyman, E., Greenbaum, M., & Grace, J. (1974). Accidental hypothermia in an alcoholic population. Am J Med 56:13–21.

79. Morris, R., & Wilkey, B. (1970). The effects of ambient temperature on patient temperature during surgery not involving body cavities. Anesthesiology 32:102–107.

80. Morris, R. (1971). Influence of ambient temperature on patient temperature during intra-abdominal surgery. Ann Surg 173:230–233.

81. Flacke, W. (1963). Temperature regulation and anesthesia. Int Anesthesiol Clin 2:43–54.

82. Pertwee, R., Marshall, N., & MacDonald, A. (1986). The effect of subanaesthetic partial pressures of nitrous oxide and nitrogen on behavioral thermoregulation in mice. In K. Cooper, P. Lomax, E. Schonbaum, & W. Veale (eds.), Homeostasis and Thermal Stress: Experimental and Therapeutic Advances (pp. 19–21). Farmington, CT: Karger.

83. Sessler, D., Rubinstein, E., & Eger, E. (1987). Core temperature changes during N_2O/fentanyl and halothane/O_2 anesthesia. Anesthesiology 67:137–139.

84. Sessler, D., Olofsson, C., Rubinstein, E., & Beebe, J. (1988). The thermoregulatory threshold in humans during halothane anesthesia. Anesthesiology 68:836–842.

85. Lotti, V., Lomax, P., & George, R. (1966). Heat production and heat loss in the rat following intracerebral and systemic administration of morphine. Int J Neuropharmacol 5:75–83.

86. Rosow, C., Miller, J., Pelikan, E., & Cochin, J. (1980). Opiates and thermoregulation in mice. I. Agonists. J Pharmacol Exp Ther 213:273–283.

87. Miller, R., Forsyth, R., & Melmon, K. (1972). Morphine-induced redistribution of cardiac output in the unanesthetized monkey. Pharmacology 7:138–148.

88. Nieminen, M., Rosow, C., Triantafillou, A., Schneider, R., Lowenstein, E., & Philbin, D. (1983). Temperature gradients in cardiac surgical patients—a comparison of halothane and fentanyl. Anesth Analg 62:1002–1005.

89. Silverberg, G., Reitz, B., & Ream, A. (1981). Hypothermia and cardiac arrest in the treatment of

giant aneurysms of the cerebral circulation and hemangioblastoma of the medulla. J Neurosurg *55*:337–346.

90. Silverberg, G., Reitz, B., & Ream, A. (1980). Operative treatment of a giant cerebral artery aneurysm by hypothermia and circulatory arrest: Report of a case. Neurosurgery *6*:301–305.

91. Houston, C. (1984). Hypothermia and cardiac arrest in the treatment of giant aneurysms. J Neurosurg Nurs *16*:15–22.

92. Goldblat, A., & Miller, R. (1972). Prevention of incidental hypothermia in neurosurgical patients. Anesth Analg *51*:536–543.

93. Launois, B., De Chateaubriant, P., Rosat, P., & Keroff, G. (1989). Repair of suprahepatic caval lesions under extracorporeal circulation in major liver trauma. J Trauma *29*:127–128.

94. McCoy, G., & Barry, J. (1989). Transplant techniques applied to general urology. Urology *33*:110–115.

95. Wickham, J., Hanley, H., & Joekes, A. (1967). Regional renal hypothermia. Br J Urol *39*:727.

96. Hanley, H., Joekes, A., & Wickham, J. (1968). Renal hypothermia in complicated nephrolithotomy. J Urol *99*:517.

97. Stubbs, A., Resnick, M., & Boyce, W. (1978). Anatrophic nephrolithotomy in the solitary kidney. J Urol *119*:457.

98. Hulme, B. (1972). Kidney preservation by surface cooling: Analysis of 130 transplants. Br Med J *4*:139.

99. Colon, R., Frazier, O., Cooley, D., & McAllister, H. (1987). Hypothermic regional perfusion for the protection of the spinal cord during periods of ischemia. Ann Thorac Surg *43*:639–643.

100. Katz, N., Blackstone, E., Kirklin, J., & Karp, R. (1981). Incremental risk factors for spinal cord injury following operation for acute traumatic aortic transection. J Thorac Cardiovasc Surg *81*:669.

101. Pontius, R., Brockman, H., & Hardy, E. (1954). The use of hypothermia in the prevention of paraplegia following temporary aortic occlusion: Experimental observations. Surgery *36*:33.

102. DeBakey, M., Cooley, D., & Creech, O. (1955). Resection of the aorta for aneurysms and occlusive disease with particular reference to the use of hypothermia: Analysis of 240 cases. Surgery *5*:153.

103. Cooley, D., Oh, D., Frazier, O., & Walker, W. (1981). Surgical treatment of aneurysms of the transverse aortic arch: Experience with 25 patients using hypothermic techniques. Ann Thorac Surg *32*:260.

104. Blair, E. (1968). *Clinical Hypothermia.* New York: McGraw-Hill.

105. Berne, R. (1965). Myocardial function in severe hypothermia. Circ Res *2*:90–95.

106. Kirklin, J., & Barratt-Boyes, B. (1986). Hypothermia, circulatory arrest, and cardiopulmonary bypass. In J. Kirklin & B. Barratt-Boyes (eds.), *Cardiac Surgery* (pp. 29–82). New York: John Wiley.

107. Fuhrman, G., Fuhrman, F., & Field, J. (1950). Metabolism of rat heart slices, with special reference to effects of temperature and anoxia. Am J Physiol *163*:62.

108. Griepp, R., Stinson, E., & Shumway, N. (1973). Profound local hypothermia for myocardial protection during open heart surgery. J Thorac Cardiovas Surg *66*:731–741.

109. Heineman, F., MacGregor, D., Wilson, G., & Nenomuja J. (1981). Regional and transmural myocardial temperature distribution in cold chemical cardioplegia. J Thorac Cardiovasc Surg *81*:851–859.

110. Stiles, Q., Hughes, R., & Lindesmith, G. (1977). The effectiveness of topical cardiac hypothermia. J Thorac Cardiovasc Surg *73*:176–180.

111. Tyers, G., Williams, E., Hughes, H., & Waldhausen, J. (1976). Optimal myocardial hypothermia at 10 degrees to 15 degrees centigrade. Surg Forum *27*:233–234.

112. Orlowski, J., Erenberg, G., Lueders, H., & Cruse R. (1984). Hypothermia and barbiturate coma for refractory status epilepticus. Crit Care Med *12*:367–372.

113. Frewen, T., Swedlow, D., Watcha, M., Raphally, R., Godinez, R., Heiser, M., Kettreck, R., & Bruce, D. (1982). Outcome in severe Reye syndrome with early pentobarbital coma and hypothermia. J Pediatr *110*:663–665.

114. Boutros, A., Hoyt, J., & Menezes, A. (1977). Management of Reye's syndrome. Crit Care Med *5*:234.

115. Safar, P. (1978). Introduction: on the evolution of brain resuscitation. Crit Care Med *6*:119.

116. Safar, P., Bleyaert, A., & Nemoto, E. (1978). Resuscitation after global brain ischemia–anoxia. Crit Care Med *6*:215.

117. Breivik, H., Safar, P., & Sands, P. (1978). Clinical feasibility trials of barbiturate therapy after cardiac arrest. Crit Care Med *6*:28.

118. Brennan, R. (1978). Resuscitation from metabolic coma and encephalitis. Crit Care Med *6*:277.

119. Walleck, C. (1989). Controversies in the management of the head-injured patient. Crit Care Nurs Clin North Am *1*:67–74.

120. Houdas, Y., & Ring, E. (1987). Temperature regulation. In Y. Houdas, & E. Ring (eds.), *Human Body Temperature: Its Measurement and Regulation* (pp. 135–141). New York: Plenum Press.

121. Abels, L. (1986). Thermoregulation. In Abels L. (ed.), *Critical Care Nursing: A Physiologic Approach* (pp. 548–587). St. Louis: C.V. Mosby.

122. Cabanac, M., & Massonnet, B. (1977). Thermoregulatory responses as a function of core temperature in humans. J Physiol *265*:587–596.

123. Ott, I. (1987). Heat center in the brain. J Nerv Ment Dis *14*:152.

124. Hall, J., Polte, J., Kelley, R., & Edwards, J. (1954). Skin and extremity cooling of clothed humans in cold water immersion. J Appl Physiol *7*:188.

125. Bazett, H., & Penfield, W. (1922). A study of the Shevington decerebate animal in the chronic as well as the acute condition. Brain *45*:185.

126. Bazett, H., McGlone, B., & Brocklehurst, R. (1930). The temperatures in the tissues which accompany temperature sensations. J Physiol *49*:88.

127. Bazett, H., Alpers, J., & Erb, H. (1933). Hypothalamus and temperature control. Arch Neurol Psychiatr *30*:728.

128. Frazier, C., Alpers, B., & Lewy, F. (1936). The anatomical localization of the hypothalamic centre for the regulation of temperature. Brain *59*:1222.

129. Clark, G., Magoun, W., & Ranson, S. (1939). Hypothalamic regulation of body temperature. J Neurophysiol *2*:202.

130. Ranson, S. (1940). Regulation of body temperature. Association for Research in Nervous & Mental Diseases Proceedings *20*:342–399.

131. Roddie, I., Shepherd, J., & Whelan, R. (1956). The effect of heating the legs and of posture of the

blood flow through the muscle and skin of the human forearm. J Physiol *132*:47P.

132. Roddie, I., Shepherd, J., & Whelan, R. (1958). Evidence from venous oxygen saturation measurements that the increase in forearm blood flow during body heating is confined to the skin. J Physiol *134*:444.

133. Adolph, E. (1946). The initiation of sweating in response to heat. Am J Physiol *145*:710.

134. Hardy, J., & Soderstrom, G. (1938). Heat loss from the nude body and peripheral blood flow at temperatures of 22 degrees centigrade to 35 degrees centigrade. J Nutr *161*:493.

135. Gagge, A. (1937). A new physiological variable associated with sensible and insensible perspiration. Am J Physiol *120*:277.

136. Hardy, J., Milhorat, A., & DuBoise, E. (1941). Basal metabolism and heat loss of young women at temperatures from 22 degrees centigrade to 35 degrees centigrade. J Nutr *21*:383.

137. Gibson, T., & Shelley, W. (1948). Sexual and racial differences in the response of sweat glands to acetylcholine and pilocarpine. J Invest Dermatol *11*:137.

138. Brobeck, J. (1980). Energy balance and food intake. In V. Mountcastle (ed.), *Medical Physiology* (14th ed.). St. Louis: C.V. Mosby.

139. Brobeck, J., & DuBoise, A. (1980). Energy exchange. In V. Mountcastle (ed.), *Medical Physiology* (14th ed.). St. Louis: C.V. Mosby.

140. Gale, C. (1973). Neuroendocrine aspects of thermoregulation. Annu Rev Physiol *35*:391.

141. Bruck, K. (1978). Thermoregulation: Control mechanisms and neural processes. In J. Sinclair (ed.), *Temperature Regulation and Energy Metabolism in the Newborn*. Philadelphia: Grune & Stratton.

142. Hemingway, A. (1963). Shivering. Physiol Rev *43*:397.

143. Holtzclaw, B. (1990). Shivering: A clinical nursing problem. Nurs Clin North Am *25*:977–986.

144. Pflug, A., Iasheim, G., Foster, C., & Martin, R. (1978). Prevention of post anaesthesia shivering. Can Anaesth Soc J *25*:43–49.

145. Bay, J., Nunn, J., & Prys-Roberts, C. (1968). Factors influencing arterial pO₂ during recovery from anaesthesia. Br J Anaesth *40*:398.

146. Prys-Roberts, C. (1968). Post-anesthesia shivering. In J. Artusio (ed.), *Clinical Anesthesia* (p. 358). Philadelphia: F.A. Davis.

147. Rodriguez, J., Weissman, C., Damask, M., Askanazi, J., Hyman, A., & Kinney, J. (1983). Physiologic requirements during rewarming: Suppression of the shivering response. Crit Care Med *11*:490–497.

148. Michanfelder, J., Whlen, A., & Daw, F. (1965). Moderate hypothermia in man: Hemodynamic and metabolic effects. Br J Anaesth *37*:738.

149. Bligh, I. (1985). Regulation of body temperature in man and other animals. In A. Shetzer, & R. Eberhart (eds.), *Applications* (vol. 1, pp. 26–28). New York: Plenum Press.

150. Coleshaw, S., Van Somern, R., Wolff, A., Davis, H., & Keatinge, W. (1983). Impaired memory registration and speed of reasoning caused by low body temperature. J Appl Physiol *55*:27–31.

151. Dugui, H., Simpson, R., & Stowers, J. (1961). Accidental hypothermia. Lancet *2*:1213–1219.

152. Huet, R., Karliczek, G., & Coad, N. (1989). Pupil size and light reactivity in hypothermic infants and adults. Intensive Care Med *15*:216–217.

153. Quasha, A., Tinker, J., & Sharbrough, F. (1981). Hypothermia plus thiopental: Prolonged electroencephalographic suppression. Anesthesiology *55*:636–640.

154. Levy, W. (1984). Quantitative analysis of EEG changes during hypothermia. Anesthesiology *60*:291–297.

155. Giubilato, R., & Metcalf, J. (1984). Evoked potentials: Nursing perspectives. J Neurosurg Nurs *16*:241–247.

156. Kileny, P., Dobson, D., & Gelfand, E. (1983). Middle-latency auditory evoked responses during open heart surgery with hypothermia. Electroencephalogr Clin Neurophysiol *55*:268–276.

157. Markand, O., Lee, B., Warren, C., Stoelting, R., King, R., Brown, J., & Mahomed, Y. (1987). Effects of hypothermia on brainstem auditory evoked potentials in humans. Ann Neurol *22*:507–513.

158. Bergh, U., Hartley, H., Landsberg, L., & Ekblom, B. (1979). Plasma norepinephrine concentration during submaximal and maximal exercise at lowered skin and core temperature. Acta Physiol Scand *106*:383–384.

159. Johnson, D., Hayward, J., Jacobs, T., Collis, M., Eckerson, J., & Williams, R. (1977). Plasma norepinephrine responses of man in cold water. J Appl Physiol *43*:216–220.

160. Hayward, J., Eckerson, J., & Kemna, D. (1984). Thermal and cardiovascular changes during three methods of resuscitation from mild hypothermia. Resuscitation *11*:21–33.

161. Kolodzik, P., Mullin, M., Krohmer, J., & McCabe, J. (1986). The effects of antishock trouser inflation during hypothermic cardiovascular depression in the canine model. Am J Emerg Med *6*:584–590.

162. Anzai, T., Turner, M., & Gibson, W. (1978). Blood flow distribution in dogs during hypothermia and post hypothermia. Am J Physiol *234*:706–710.

163. Fedor, E., & Fisher, B. (1959). Simultaneous determination of blood volume with Cr51 and T-1824 during hypothermia and rewarming. Am J Physiol *199*:703–705.

164. D'Amato, H., & Hagnauer, A. (1953). Blood volume in the hypothermic dog. Am J Physiol *173*:100–102.

165. Morray, J., & Pavlin, E. (1985). Hemodynamic effects of acute and prolonged hypothermia in the dog. Anesthesiology *63*:278.

166. Harari, A., Regnier, B., & Rapier, M. (1975). Hemodynamic study of prolonged deep accidental hypothermia. J Intens Care Med *1*:65–70.

167. Duguid, H., Simpson, R., & Stowers, J. (1961). Accidental hypothermia. Lancet *2*:1213–1219.

168. Jacob, A., Lichstein, E., & Ulano, S. (1978). A-V block in accidental hypothermia. J Electrocardiol *11*:399–402.

169. O'Keefe, K. (1977). Accidental hypothermia: A review of 62 cases. JACEP *6*:491–496.

170. Bigelow, W., Lindsay, W., Harrison, R., Gordon, R., & Greenwood, W. (1950). Oxygen transport and utilization in dogs at low body temperature. Am J Physiol *160*:125.

171. Bangs, C. (1984). Hypothermia and frost bite. Emerg Med Clin North Am *2*:475–487.

172. Stine, R. (1977). Accidental hypothermia. JACEP *6*:413–416.

173. Fahey, P. (1983). Overall clinical assessment of the

role of continuous SVO₂ measurement in hemo-dynamic monitoring in the ICU. In I. Schweiss (ed.), *Continuous Measurement of Blood Oxygen Saturation in the High Risk Patient* (vol. I, pp. 113–122). San Diego: Beach International.

174. Welton, D., Mattox, K., & Miller, R. (1978) Treatment of profound hypothermia. JAMA *240*:2291–2292.

175. Hirvonen, I. (1976). Necropsy findings in fatal hypothermia cases. Forensic Sci *8*:155–164.

176. Read, A., Emslie-Smith, D., Gough, K., & Holmes, R. (1961). Pancreatitis and accidental hypothermia. Lancet *2*:1219–1221.

177. Vander, A. (1980). *Renal Physiology* (2nd ed.). New York: McGraw-Hill.

178. Zatzman, M. (1984). Renal and cardiovascular effects of hybernation and hypothermia. Cryobiology *21*:593–614.

179. Boylan, J., & Hong, S. (1966). Regulation of renal function in hypothermia. Am J Physiol *211*:1371–1378.

180. Rosenfeld, J. (1963). Acid-base and electrolyte disturbances in hypothermia. Am J Cardiol *18*:678–682.

181. Koht, A., Cane, R., & Cerullo, L. (1983). Serum potassium levels during prolonged hypothermia. Intensive Care Med *9*:275–277.

182. Tepperman, J. (1980). *Metabolic and Endocrine Physiology* (pp. 169–194). Chicago: Year Book Medical Publishers.

183. Bickford, A., & Mottram, F. (1960). Glucose metabolism during induced hypothermia in rabbits. Clin Sci *19*:345.

184. Kuroshima, A., Doi, K., & Ohno, T. (1978). Role of glucagon in metabolic acclimation to cold and heat. Life Sci *23*:1405.

185. Gibbs, D. (1985). Inhibition of corticotropin release during hypothermia: The role of corticotropin-releasing factor, vasopressin, and oxytocin. Endocrinology *116*:723–727.

186. Egdahl, R., Nelson, D., & Hume, D. (1957). Effect of hypothermia on 17 hydroxycorticosteroid secretion in adrenal venous blood in the dog. Science *121*:506.

187. Corbett, J. (1982). Hematology tests. In J. Corbett (ed.), *Laboratory Tests in Nursing Practice* (pp. 25–54). Norwalk, CT: Appleton-Century-Crofts.

188. Kee, J. (1987). Laboratory tests. In J. Kee (ed.), *Laboratory and Diagnostic Tests with Nursing Implications* (pp. 187–189). Norwalk, CT: Appleton and Lange.

189. Finlayson, D., & Kaplan, J. (1979). Cardiopulmonary bypass. In J. Kaplan (ed.), *Cardiac Anesthesia* (pp. 415–418). Philadelphia: Grune & Stratton.

190. Niemezura, R., & DePalma, R. (1979). Optimum compress temperature for wound hemostasis. Surg Res *26*:570–573.

191. Mahajan, S., Myer, T., & Baldini, M. (1981). Disseminated intravascular coagulation during rewarming following hypothermia. JAMA *245*:2517–2581.

192. Vellalobos, T., Addson, E., & Riley, P., et al. (1958). A cause of the thrombocytopenia and leukopenia that occur in dogs during deep hypothermia. J Clin Invest *37*:1–7.

193. Hessell, E., Schner, G., & Dillard, D. (1980). Platelet kinetics during hypothermia. J Surg Res *28*:23–34.

194. Valeri, C., Cassidy, G., & Khuri, S., et al. (1987).

Hypothermia-induced reversible platelet dysfunction. Ann Surg *205*:175–181.

195. Torlinska, T., Paluszak, J., Kozlik, J., Kruk, D., Gryczka, A., & Krauss, H. (1982). Activity of certain enzymes in the mitochondrial and cytoplasmic fractions of liver cells, myocardium and skeletal muscle of the rat during short-lasting hypothermia. Acta Physiol Pol *33*:545–550.

196. McDaniel, R., & Devine, J. (1980). Elevations of creatine kinase isoenzyme CK in patients with exposure induced hypothermia. Ann Clin Lab Sci *10*:155–159.

197. Abbey, J. (1982). Shivering and surface cooling. In C. Norris (ed.), *Concept Clarification in Nursing* (pp. 223–242). Rockville, MD: Aspen Systems.

198. Best, R., Syverud, S., & Nowak, R. (1985). Trauma and hypothermia. Am J Emerg Med *3*:48–55.

199. Harper, R., Gold, H., & Leinbach, R. (1980). Acute myocardial infarction. In R. Johnson, E. Haber, & W. Austen (eds.), *The Practice of Cardiology* (pp. 310–338). Boston: Little, Brown and Company.

200. Davis, F., Paremelazshagan, K., & Harris, E. (1977). Thermal balance during cardiopulmonary bypass with moderate hypothermia in man. Br J Anaesth *49*:1127–1132.

201. Sladen, R. (1982). Management of the acute cardiac patient in the ICU. In A. Ream & R. Fogdall (eds.), *Acute Cardiovascular Management: Anesthesia and Intensive Care* (pp. 405–541). Philadelphia: J.B. Lippincott.

202. Molnar, G., & Read, R. (1974). Studies during open-heart surgery on the special characteristics of rectal temperature. J Appl Physiol *36*:333–336.

203. Mravinac, C., Dracup, K., & Clochesy, J. (1989). Urinary bladder and rectal temperature monitoring during clinical hypothermia. Nurs Res *38*:73–76.

204. Fonkalsrud, E., & Clatworthy, H. (1965). Accidental perforation of the colon and rectum in newborn infants. N Engl J Med *272*:1097–1100.

205. Lau, J., & Ong, G. (1981). Broken and retained rectal thermometers in infants and young children. Aust Pediatr J *17*:93–94.

206. Bliss-Holtz, J. (1989). Comparison of rectal, axillary and inguinal temperatures in full-term newborn infants. Nurs Res *38*:85–87.

207. Horvath, S., Spurr, G., Hutt, B., & Hamilton, L. (1956). Metabolic cost of shivering. J Appl Physiol *8*:595–602.

208. Webb, P. (1986). Afterdrop of body temperature during rewarming: An alternative explanation. J Appl Physiol *60*:385–390.

209. Iampietro, P., Vaughn, J., Goldman, R., Kreider, M., Masucci, F., & Bass, D. (1960). Heat production from shivering. J Appl Physiol *15*:632–633.

210. Mills, W. (1983). Summary of treatment of the cold injured patient, hypothermia. Alaska Med *25*:29–31.

211. Bourke, D., Wurm, H., Rosenberg, M., & Russell, J. (1984). Intraoperative heat conservation using a reflective blanket. Anesthesiology *60*:151–154.

212. Roizem, M., Sohn, Y., L'Hommedieu, C., Wiley, E., & Ota, M. (1980). Operating room temperature prior to surgical draping: Effect on patient temperatures in recovery room. Anesth Analg *59*:852–855.

213. Miles, J., & Thompson, G. (1987). Treatment of severe accidental hypothermia using the clinitron bed. Anaesthesia *42*:415–418.

214. Baumgart, S. (1987). Current concepts and clinical strategies for managing low-birth-weight infants under radiant warmers. Med Instrum *21*:23.

215. Reitz, B., & Ream, A. (1982). Use of hypothermia in cardiovascular surgery. In A. Ream & R. Fogdall (eds.), *Acute Cardiovascular Management: Anesthesia and Intensive Care* (pp. 830–851). Philadelphia: J.B. Lippincott.

216. Laub, G., Baraszak, D., Kupferschmid, J., Magovern, G., & Young, J. (1989). Percutaneous cardiopulmonary bypass for the treatment of hypothermic circulatory collapse. Ann Thorac Surg *47*:608–611.

217. Seuffert, G. (1984). An Alaskan experience with cardiopulmonary bypass in resuscitating patients with profound hypothermia and cardiac arrest. Alaska Med *26*:31–33.

218. Barr, G., Halvorsen, L., & Donovan, A. (1988). Correction of hypothermia by continuous pleural perfusion. Surgery *103*:553–557.

219. Bar, Z. (1984). Central heating for intraoperative hypothermia. Crit Care Med *12*:1082.

220. Goel, I., Mundth, E. (1981). Cardiac surgery in chronic renal failure. In D. Lowenthal, R. Pennock, W. Likoff, G. Onesti (eds.), *Management of the Cardiac Patient with Renal Failure* (pp. 191–198). Philadelphia: F.A. Davis.

221. Lazarus, J., Morgan, A., & Tilney, N. (1982). Patients with chronic renal failure: General management and acute surgical illness. In N. Tilney & J. Lazarus (eds.), *Surgical Care of the Patient with Renal Failure* (pp. 14–15). Philadelphia: W.B. Saunders.

222. Smith, J., & Snider, M. (1989). An improved technique for rapid infusion of warmed fluid using a level 1 fluid warmer. Surg Gynecol Obstet *168*:273–274.

223. Flancbaum, L., Trooskin, S., & Pedersen, H. (1989). Evaluation of blood-warming devices with the apparent thermal clearance. Ann Emerg Med *18*:355–359.

224. Frame, S., Timberlake, G., & McSwain, N. (1987). Trauma rounds. Problem: Iatrogenic hypothermia in the trauma patient. Emerg Med *19*:99–100, 103.

225. Rafalowski, M. (1987). Relationship of core temperature at time of blanket removal to subsequent core temperature in patients immediately after coronary artery bypass. Heart Lung *16*:9–13.

226. Davis, F., Barnes, P., & Bailey, J. (1981). Aural thermometry during profound hypothermia. Anaesth. Intensive Care *9*:124–128.

227. Farmer, J. (1990). Ear and sinus problems in diving. In A. Bove & J. Davis (eds.), *Diving Medicine* (pp. 200–222). Philadelphia: W.B. Saunders.

228. Rawson, R.O., & Hammel, H.T. (1963). Hypothalamic and tympanic membrane temperatures in rhesus monkeys. Fed Proc *22*:283.

229. Shinozaki, T., Deane, R., & Perkins, F. (1988). Infrared tympanic thermometer: Evaluation of a new clinical thermometer. Crit Care Med *16*:148–150.

8

Apnea

Helen L. Dulock

Apnea is a respiratory pattern abnormality and is a manifestation of a deficit in the control of breathing. Apnea occurs across age groups but has been described primarily in premature newborns, older infants, and adults with obstructive sleep apnea syndromes (see Chapter 20, Impaired Sleep). This chapter is devoted to an exploration of the phenomenon of apnea in premature newborns.

The breathing pattern of newborns may be categorized as regular, irregular, periodic, or apneic. These four breathing patterns reflect the underlying coordination, integration, and maturation of the central and peripheral nervous systems, chest wall stability, lung compliance, sleep state, and chemical control of respiration. The full-term newborn normally will have achieved a degree of maturation that permits coordination and integration of these systems. This will be reflected in a breathing pattern that consists of regular respiration (equal breath-to-breath intervals) interspersed with irregular respirations (unequal breath-to-breath intervals). Apnea in a full-term newborn is a serious symptom requiring investigation. The premature newborn (less than 37 weeks' gestation) will not have achieved as high a degree of maturation, coordination, or integration of these systems. This will be reflected in a breathing pattern that consists of irregular respiration interspersed with periodic breathing or apneic episodes or both.

DEFINITION

A variety of definitions of periodic breathing and apnea may be found in both the research and clinical literature. Apnea is cessation of respiratory airflow, whether the cause is due to lack of respiratory effort (central apnea) or to upper airway obstruction (obstructive apnea) or to a combination of these two events (mixed apnea). Periodic breathing consists of three or more respiratory pauses of greater than 3 seconds' duration with less than 20 seconds of respiration between pauses. Definitions of periodic breathing and types of apnea are presented in Box 8–1.[1]

BOX 8–1

Definitions: Periodic Breathing and Apnea

Periodic breathing is a breathing pattern in which there are three or more respiratory pauses of greater than 3 seconds' duration with less than 20 seconds of respiration between pauses. Periodic breathing can be a normal event.

Apnea is cessation of respiratory air flow. The respiratory pause may be central or diaphragmatic (i.e., no respiratory effort), obstructive (usually due to upper airway obstruction), or mixed. Short (15 seconds) central apnea can be normal at all ages.

Pathological apnea is an abnormal respiratory pause, one that is prolonged (20 or more seconds) or associated with cyanosis, abrupt marked pallor, hypotonia, or bradycardia.

Apnea of prematurity (AOP) is periodic breathing with pathological apnea in a premature infant. Apnea of prematurity usually ceases by 37 weeks' gestation (menstrual dating) but occasionally persists for several weeks past term.

Periodic breathing and apnea have many common characteristics (Box 8–2).[2] Periodic breathing is a common breathing pattern in premature newborns that is usually not of pathological significance. It has often been stated that apnea of prematurity is associated with periodic breathing and that neither periodic breathing nor apnea generally occur in the first 36 to 48 hours of postnatal life. However, it has been suggested that periodic breathing does not precede apnea in premature newborns.[3] Additionally, it has been demonstrated by multichannel recordings of respiratory variables during the first 12 hours of life that significant apnea, but not periodic breathing, is a frequent occurrence before 36 hours of age.[3] Significant apnea was defined in this study as cessation of nasal airflow for 15 seconds or more if associated with a fall

---

BOX 8–3

Types of Apnea

Central apnea is the absence of respiratory efforts (or diaphragmatic activity) and is manifest by absence of both respiratory effort and airflow at the nares.

Obstructive apnea is due to obstruction of the airway, usually at the pharyngeal level, and is manifest by the presence of respiratory efforts and the absence of airflow at the nares.

Mixed apnea is characterized by having a component of both central and obstructive apnea. Most mixed apneas begin as central apnea followed by an obstructive event.

---

in heart rate of at least 20 per cent from the previous baseline or a decrease in oxygen saturation of at least 10 per cent.

Apnea is classified according to origin into three types: central, obstructive, or mixed (Box 8–3). Traditionally, central apnea has been thought to be the major type of apnea in premature infants. However, the majority of cases of apnea in premature infants appear to be noncentral in origin; that is, the combination of mixed and obstructive apneas is greater than the occurrence of central apneas.[4, 5]

Apnea in premature infants also needs to be differentiated according to its cause. Apnea occurs in association with or secondary to many specific pathophysiological conditions, such as respiratory distress syndrome, sepsis, or patent ductus arteriosus (discussed under the text on Clinical States). However, the most common type of apnea is not associated with underlying pathophysiological conditions and is thought to be due to developmental immaturity of central respiratory control mechanisms. This type of apnea is referred to as "apnea of prematurity" or as "idiopathic" apnea.[6] Apnea of prematurity is a diagnosis of exclusion; that is, it is a diagnosis made only after clinical conditions associated with apnea in premature infants have been ruled out. The diagnosis of apnea of prematurity should not be made if the neonate is more than 38 weeks postconceptual age.[7]

PREVALENCE AND POPULATIONS AT RISK

Those most at risk for development of periodic breathing and apnea are premature

---

BOX 8–2

Characteristics of Periodic Breathing and Apnea

Common Characteristics
Occurrence inversely related to gestational age.
Rarely occurs after 36 weeks' gestational age.
Frequency may increase during first weeks of life, depending on degree of immaturity.
May be initiated by conditions that reduce functional residual capacity or that produce hypoxemia.
May be abolished by increasing functional residual capacity or by maintaining normal arterial oxygenation.
Once occurs, tends to reoccur.
Tends to occur more frequently in association with active (REM) sleep.
Differentiating Characteristics
Periodic Breathing:
Cessation of respiration for greater than 3 seconds, with less than 20 seconds of respiration between pauses.
Not generally associated with changes in heart rate, arterial oxygenation, or cyanosis.
A common respiratory pattern, especially in infants less than 1500 g.
Apnea:
Cessation of respiration for 10 to 20 seconds or longer.
Usually accompanied by bradycardia, fall in blood pressure, hypoxemia, cyanosis, pallor, or hypotonia.
Occurrence of repeated episodes of hypoxemia may result in CNS damage.

infants, especially those born earlier than 34 weeks' gestation or those weighing less than 1500 g.

The incidence of apnea varies inversely with gestational age and with postnatal age. There is also great variability in incidence among different premature infants of the same gestational age. Studies vary in their definitions of apnea and in the use of either gestational age or birth weight as the criterion for sample inclusion. For these reasons, it is difficult to make comparisons among different studies. A large prospective study of 25,152 live births reported the incidence of recurrent apnea (three or more episodes of apnea greater than 20 seconds) as 78 per cent at 26 to 27 weeks' gestation and 75 per cent at 28 to 29 weeks' gestation.[8] At 30 to 31 weeks' gestation the incidence was 54 per cent and had decreased to 7 per cent by 34 to 35 weeks' gestation. This inverse relationship between age and incidence suggests that immaturity is a major underlying factor. With the increased survival of premature neonates of lower gestational ages, apnea has become a major clinical problem in intensive and intermediate care nurseries. Apnea is also a common occurrence for very-low-birth-weight neonates treated with surfactant replacement therapy for respiratory distress syndrome. In these neonates, weaning from mechanical ventilation may be accomplished earlier than was possible before surfactant replacement therapy became widely used. Thus, these premature newborns may have mature lungs, but are still immature neurologically, which may be manifest as apnea. Current trends are for premature infants to be discharged home or to be transferred to smaller hospitals at earlier ages. Thus, questions regarding what constitutes a normal breathing pattern, that is, how much periodic breathing or what amount and duration of apnea is normal for premature infants at the time of hospital discharge, take on added significance.

SITUATIONAL STRESSORS

Apnea may be precipitated in some premature infants by situational stressors present in the environment in which care is provided, such as thermal stimuli. Hypothermia (less than 36° C skin temperature or less than 36.2° C rectal or axillary temperature) is associated with an increase in oxygen consumption and metabolic rate, which may result in apnea. Similarly, hyperthermia (greater than 37° C skin temperature or rectal or axillary temperature greater than 37.5° C) also increases oxygen consumption and metabolic rate and may precipitate apneic episodes.[9]

Perlstein and associates found that apneic episodes were more frequently preceded by rising ambient air temperature in incubators than by constant or decreasing air temperatures.[10] For example, when the temperature servo control probe became detached from the skin, the incubator temperature turned on, and the resulting rise in air temperature was associated with the onset of apnea. Later, when the temperature set-point was changed from 36.0 to 36.6° C, resulting in an increase in incubator air temperature, this was again associated with an onset of apnea. A significant increase in the incidence of apnea in premature infants was also observed by Daily and colleagues when the skin temperature was maintained at 36.8° C, rather than at 36° C.[11]

Thus, there seems to be a susceptible group of premature infants in whom apneic episodes can be induced by thermal stimuli; however, the exact mechanisms by which this occurs is not known. The heating unit of an isolette or of a radiant heat warmer is turned on or off, depending on the neonate's skin temperature. When servo control is used, it is important to document the skin temperature of the neonate and the ambient temperature inside the isolette. A rise in incubator temperature might reflect hypothermia in the neonate. The neonate should be maintained in a neutral thermal environment (NTE). An NTE provides conditions that permit maintenance of normal core temperature while simultaneously maintaining metabolic rate and oxygen consumption at minimal levels.

DEVELOPMENTAL DIMENSIONS AND MECHANISMS

The fetus who is born prematurely has several interrelated developmental and physiological characteristics that place it at increased risk for periodic breathing and apnea. The premature infant has a greater oxygen consumption than the adult (4 to 6 ml/kg/minute versus 3 to 4 ml/kg/minute) and a relatively smaller lung volume and oxygen stores. Therefore, the premature infant requires greater alveolar ventilation to maintain a normal arterial oxygenation and pH. Adequate ventilation in the premature infant requires relatively more work than in the term newborn or adult because of smaller airways, lack of surfactant, and less efficient respiratory muscles. Several physiological and developmental characteristics that influence the stability of the respiratory pattern of the premature infant are discussed below.

Neuronal Development

Premature infants have incomplete myelination of most neurons and have sparse dendritic development. Unmyelinated neurons propagate impulses more slowly and therefore make it more difficult to achieve temporal summation. Temporal summation occurs when repeated afferent stimuli cause new excitatory postsynaptic potentials (EPSP) before previous EPSP have decayed. Sparse dendritic development makes it more difficult to achieve spatial summation. Spatial summation occurs when activity is present in more than one synaptic knob at the same time. These factors decrease the ability of the premature neonate to achieve the alternating excitation and inhibition of impulses that are necessary for the establishment of a rhythmic breathing pattern.[12] As a result, any presynaptic or postsynaptic inhibitory activity, whether it is chemical, electrical, or ionic, has a greater inhibitory effect in premature infants than in mature persons later in life. The preponderance of inhibitory activity makes the respiratory control system of premature infants more unstable. Factors that impair nerve cell metabolism, such as hypoxia, brain stem edema, hyperbilirubinemia, hypoglycemia, hypocalcemia, or sepsis, can interfere with the rhythmic activity of respiratory neurons and cause periodic breathing and apnea.[13]

Properties of Chest Wall Muscles and Lungs

One stimulus to respiration is the neural drive. The response to this stimulus is an inspiratory-expiratory cycle. However, between the stimulus and the response are the respiratory muscles and the lungs. Normal functioning of these structures is necessary if ventilation is to be adequate. An unstable chest wall or a reduction in the lung's compliance reduces ventilation and contributes to periodic breathing and apnea.[13]

The chest wall of the premature is unstable (not fixed) and highly compliant. As the diaphragm descends during inspiration, the chest wall retracts, therefore limiting the ability to generate the negative intrathoracic pressure that is required to inflate the relatively stiff lungs. This reduces inspiratory volume. At end-expiration, the compliant chest wall makes it more difficult to maintain a negative intrapleural pressure. This increases the natural tendency of the lungs to collapse toward residual volume. The result may be atelectasis and hypoxemia, which are thought to contribute to developing periodic breathing and apnea. Once atelectasis occurs, the compliant chest wall makes it more difficult to develop a transpulmonary pressure that is sufficient to re-expand the lungs.

The respiratory muscles, like other muscles, are subject to fatigue. The diaphragm is the principal muscle of respiration. In the premature infant it is thought that the diaphragm is less able to sustain high work loads for long periods of time. Muscle resistance to fatigue is related to the percentage of type 1 high oxidative fibers in the muscles. The adult diaphragm has about 50 per cent of these type of fibers, the full-term newborn has about 25 per cent, and the premature infant has less than 10 per cent.[12] Fatigue slows the respiratory rate, decreases tidal volume, and may produce periodic breathing and apneic episodes.[12] The work of breathing is increased in premature infants owing to the small size of the airways, the presence of lung disease, and rapid eye movement (REM) sleep. Premature infants may also have decreased surfactant. A deficiency of surfactant decreases lung compliance and increases the amount of transpulmonary pressure needed for lung inflation. Thus, even an adequate neural drive and muscular effort are less efficient in producing an adequate ventilatory response in premature infants.

Chemoreceptors

The chemical drive to ventilation is mediated through the peripheral and central chemoreceptors. The peripheral chemoreceptors (carotid and aortic bodies) respond primarily to hypoxemia. In the adult, when the arterial oxygenation falls below about 60 torr, the carotid bodies are stimulated and ventilation increases. However, in both full-term and premature newborns, the initial response to induced hypoxemia is a slight increase in minute ventilation followed by a 10 to 20 per cent decrease of minute ventilation below control values by the third minute of hypoxemia.[14] This biphasic ventilatory response to hypoxemia is not affected by gestational age but is affected by postnatal age. Full-term newborns show this biphasic response for approximately 10 days, and premature infants, for approximately 18 days after birth. Thereafter, the response to hypoxemia in both groups is one of sustained ventilation.[14] Clinically, this means that in premature newborns hypoxemia depresses their ventilation for about the first 3 weeks of life. This response may play a role in inducing periodic breathing and apnea in premature infants. It is believed that hypoxemia causes a central depressing effect on ventilation that overrides the peripheral stimulation of the carotid bodies.[15] In studies with fetal animals, hypoxemia causes cessation of fetal breathing movements. Both hypoxemia and hyperoxemia can produce irregular respiratory patterns. In many premature infants, a rapid increase in FIO_2 from 21 to 100 per cent results in intermittent respiratory pauses followed by a regular respiratory pattern in a few minutes.

The medullary chemoreceptors are primarily responsive to changes in hydrogen ion concentration. An increase in carbon dioxide increases the arterial hydrogen ion concentration, which increases ventilation. During normoxia, this ventilatory response to carbon dioxide is essentially the same in term newborns as in adults.[16] Hypoxemia makes the premature neonate less responsive to increased levels of carbon dioxide. In premature infants, the higher the inspired oxygen concentration, the steeper the response to carbon dioxide; the lower the inspired oxygen concentration, the flatter the response to carbon dioxide.[15] Hypercarbia with hypoxemia in premature infants tends to create a cycle in which ventilation remains depressed. Thus, hypoxemia not only may cause premature infants to hypoventilate but also decrease their ability to increase ventilation in response to hypercarbia. Interventions aimed at reducing hypercarbia and hypoxemia are important if an adequate ventilatory drive is to be maintained. Preterm neonates with apnea, compared with a matched group without apnea, also show a decreased ventilatory response to carbon dioxide;[17] this suggests that abnormal ventilatory control may contribute to the development of apnea.

Sleep States

Sleeping and breathing are interrelated biological events. Sleep affects respiratory rate, depth, and control of breathing. Any difficulty with breathing is likely to increase during sleep and may therefore lead to sleep disturbances. There are three identifiable sleep states in the newborn period: (1) active or rapid eye movement (REM), (2) quiet or non–rapid eye movement (NREM), and (3) indeterminate (Box 8–4).

The predominant sleep state of the premature infant is active sleep. During active sleep, breathing is less responsive to metabolic influences and is more driven by the behavioral system, thus variability in ventilatory patterns and responses are more common.[18] Premature infants spend a greater proportion of the 24 hours asleep than term newborns, and 65 to 80 per cent of total sleep time is spent in active sleep.[19, 20] During active sleep, the respiratory rate and depth are irregular, and the frequency and duration of respiratory pauses are increased. Apneic episodes occur more frequently during active sleep. Gabriel and coworkers examined 493 apneic episodes occurring in eight healthy premature infants.[20] Seventy-nine per cent of the episodes occurred during active sleep,

---

BOX 8–4

Definitions of Sleep States

   Active or rapid eye movement (REM) sleep is characterized by rapid eye movements despite closed eye lids; frequent limb, body, or facial movements; and irregular respiratory and heart rates.

   Quiet or non–rapid eye movement (NREM) sleep is characterized by absence of eye or body movements, presence of startles, and regular respiratory and heart rates.

   Indeterminate or undifferentiated sleep states are those that do not meet the criteria for either REM or NREM sleep.

even though active sleep made up only 65 per cent of the total sleep time. Fifteen per cent of the apneic episodes occurred during indeterminate sleep states. Only 6 per cent of the apneic episodes occurred during quiet sleep, which accounted for 18 per cent of the total sleep time.

Hypoxemia has been proposed as a possible initiating event for apnea in premature infants.[14] Gabriel and associates measured transcutaneous oxygen ($tcPO_2$) levels during different sleep states in seven healthy prematures of 32 to 34 weeks' conceptual age.[21] The lowest and most variable $tcPO_2$ values were found during active sleep, and the highest $tcPO_2$ values were found during quiet sleep. Although apneic episodes occurred predominantly (86 per cent of 149) during active sleep, the incidence of apnea did not correlate with the decreased $tcPO_2$.

One reason that periodic breathing and apneic episodes occur more frequently during active sleep may be related to chest wall instability and decreased functional residual capacity. The intercostal muscles are inhibited during active sleep.[22] This inhibition causes the rib cage to move inward when the diaphragm contracts and the abdomen moves outward (chest distortion). To achieve the same tidal volume, the diaphragmatic contraction has to increase, since part of its work is being used to move the ribs inward, not to move environmental gases.[23] The work of breathing in active sleep is therefore higher than in other sleep states. In addition, the functional residual capacity (FRC) has been shown to be reduced approximately 30 per cent in active sleep as a result of the inhibition of the intercostal muscles.[24] Because of this, local areas of atelectasis may develop, leading to a decrease in ventilation/perfusion ratios, lower arterial oxygenation, and unstable breathing patterns.

CLINICAL STATES AND MEDICAL DIAGNOSES

Apnea occurs in conjunction with a wide variety of clinical conditions (Box 8–5). These conditions should be considered as possible causes for the apnea within the context of intrapartum events and the neonatal course preceding the onset of apnea. Appropriate diagnostic tests should be performed in an attempt to determine, if possible, the

---

BOX 8–5

Conditions Associated with Apnea in Premature Infants

Central Nervous System
  Intracranial bleeding
  Seizures (apnea may be the manifestation of seizure activity)
  Myelomenigocele
  Bilirubin encephalopathy
Respiratory System
  Respiratory distress syndrome
  Pneumonia
  Pulmonary edema
Cardiovascular System
  Patent ductus arteriosus with congestive heart failure
  Anemia
  Polycythemia
Metabolic System
  Hypoglycemia
  Hypocalcemia
  Hypernatremia
Environmental Factors
  Temperatures in upper zone of neutral thermal environment
  Rewarming hypothermic newborn too rapidly
Infections
  Sepsis
  Meningitis
  Necrotizing enterocolitis
Other
  Reflex stimulation of suction or feeding catheters
  Refluxed gastric contents
  Uncoordinated sucking, swallowing, and breathing during feeding

---

cause of the apnea. Treatment is then directed simultaneously toward both the underlying primary condition and the resultant apneic episodes.

Periventricular intracerebral (intraventricular) hemorrhage is commonly associated with apnea in premature infants, especially in those with a history of an anoxic episode at the time of delivery.[25]

Apnea may be a manifestation of subtle seizures. In this situation, apnea is almost always accompanied or preceded by sustained eye opening with ocular fixation or eye deviation or both.[26] In premature infants, however, apneic episodes are more likely to be due to mechanisms other than seizure activity.

Respiratory distress syndrome (RDS) is the clinical expression of an immature lung, with small respiratory units that inflate with diffi-culty and do not remain inflated between respirations. This feature is due in part to decreased pulmonary surfactant. Without surfactant, the surface tension at the inter-face of gas and alveolar wall is high and the lung becomes progressively atelectatic. RDS is often associated with apnea. Decreased lung compliance, chest wall instability, hypox-emia, and hypercarbia, combined with in-creased respiratory work and muscle fatigue, are all factors that contribute to exhaustion of the respiratory drive in premature infants with RDS. During the recovery phase from RDS, apnea may occur in conjunction with a large left-to-right shunt due to patent ductus arteriosus and the subsequent development of pulmonary edema and left ventricular failure.

Pneumonia may contribute to apnea by increasing vagal reflexes and by causing hy-poxemia.[25, 27] Neonatal infection should al-ways be considered when apnea occurs, as it is usually fatal if untreated. Apnea may be the only or the major presenting symptom of sepsis. Group B streptococcus is the most common cause of sepsis in premature infants. Apnea during the first 24 hours of life should always be considered secondary to sepsis until proven otherwise. After the second week of life, apnea in hospitalized premature infants may be due to nosocomial infections.

Apnea and periodic breathing may be as-sociated with anemia (hematocrit ≤ 30 to 40 per cent) due to decreased oxygen-carrying capacity of the blood. However, the effect of transfusing packed red blood cells (PRBCs) on the incidence of apnea or periodic breath-ing is unclear. Some studies have shown no effect of transfusion of PRBCs on the inci-dence of either apnea or bradycardia,[28, 29] but other studies have shown a decrease in the number of apneic episodes, duration of pe-riodic breathing, and bradycardia.[30] Apneic episodes may be one of the manifestations seen in the early postnatal period in neonates with polycythemia.[31]

Premature newborns who undergo surgery and anesthesia around the time of discharge (i.e., for repair of inguinal hernia) frequently experience episodes of periodic breathing and apnea postoperatively. These infants should have surgery performed in hospitals that can provide ventilatory support, if needed, and should have respiratory rate, heart rate, and pulse oximetry monitoring for at least 24 hours postoperatively.[32]

Periodic breathing is thought to be a be-nign condition, especially if it is not inter-mixed with recurrent apneas that require assisted ventilation to prevent or treat hypox-emia. However, apnea with repeated epi-sodes of hypoxemia may result in neurolog-ical sequelae;[33] the highest incidence of sequelae has been noted in neonates of lowest gestational age. More recently, it has been shown that when apneic episodes are accom-panied by moderate bradycardia (heart rate > 80 or < 100 beats per minute) or severe bradycardia (heart rate < 80 beats per min-ute), systemic blood pressure decreases, ac-companied by a decrease in cerebral blood flow velocity. Thus, repeated episodes of ap-nea with moderate to severe bradycardia may potentially contribute to causing or exacer-bating hypoxic-ischemic brain injury.[34]

RELATED PATHOPHYSIOLOGICAL CONCEPTS

Apnea is a phenomenon that occurs not only in premature infants, but also during early infancy in association with a variety of clinical conditions and in adults with obstruc-tive sleep apnea syndromes (see Chapter 20, Impaired Sleep). Three conditions in early infancy in which apnea is either hypothesized or known to play a role are discussed below. Definitions of these conditions are given in Box 8–6.

Sudden Infant Death Syndrome

Currently, sudden infant death syndrome (SIDS) is the leading cause of postnatal (be-tween 28 days of age and the end of the first year of life) death in the United States. Two definitions of SIDS are given in Box 8–6; the first has been the definition used for more than two decades; the second is a new defi-nition developed by an expert panel con-vened by the National Institute of Child Health Development.[35] The incidence of SIDS is approximately 1 to 2 per cent per 1000 live births, or 6000 to 7000 infants each year. The incidence has not changed in the past 2 decades despite decreases in other causes of infant mortality.[1] An increased risk for SIDS occurs among infants born prema-turely, infants with low birth weight for ges-tational age, infants of young multiparous women with short intergestational intervals, infants of low socioeconomic status, and black infants. An increased incidence of SIDS has been noted in methadone- and cocaine-exposed infants[36, 37]; however, this has not been a consistent finding in other studies of in utero exposure to cocaine.[38] Both maternal cocaine use and SIDS have overlapping risk factors, such as low socioeconomic status; therefore, the relationship between the two may vary in different populations.

A relationship between apnea and SIDS has been postulated since 1972, when Steinschneider reported two of five infants with prolonged sleep apnea subsequently dying of SIDS.[39] However, the role of apnea as a factor in SIDS continues to be an area of controversy and the focus of intense scientific investigations. Apnea and SIDS are not synonymous terms (see Box 8-6 for definitions). The apnea hypothesis is only one of several proposed hypotheses for SIDS, which include cardiac arrhythmias and abnormal brain stem control mechanisms.

The National Institute of Child Health and Human Development SIDS Cooperative Epidemiologic Study found that apnea during the neonatal period was not a specific risk factor for SIDS.[40] Apnea of prematurity is not an additional risk factor for SIDS (i.e., it does not add to the risk already imposed by premature birth). Overall, 18 per cent of infants with SIDS were born prematurely.[41] The percentage of cases of SIDS with a previously reported history of postneonatal apnea (episode of turning blue or stopped breathing) is reported to be 7 per cent.[41]

Apparent Life-Threatening Event

An apparent life-threatening event (ALTE) describes a general clinical syndrome. The classic description involves a presumed healthy infant who is unexpectedly found by the parent or caretaker to be not breathing, blue, and limp. The infant is revived with stimulation, mouth-to-mouth resuscitation, or cardiopulmonary resuscitation. Terminology used in the past for this event, such as "near-miss SIDS" or "aborted crib death," has been abandoned because of the potentially misleading association between this type of event and SIDS.[1] Infants presenting with a history of an ALTE need a complete workup to identify a possible cause. The clinical diagnoses of infants presenting with an ALTE from one study are shown in Table 8-1.[42] In this study, in 61 per cent of the cases that presented as ALTE, a specific clinical diagnosis could be made. The incidence of ALTE in the general population is estimated to be 2 to 3 per cent.[43] The incidence of SIDS is increased in infants who have had repeat ALTE episodes, especially a small subgroup who have experienced sleep apnea that required vigorous stimulation or resuscitation.[44] However, most infants who die of SIDS do not come from the group that has previously experienced an ALTE.

Apnea of Infancy

Apnea of infancy (AOI) refers to infants who are more than 37 weeks postconceptual age at the onset of pathological apnea and for whom no specific cause of ALTE can be identified (idiopathic ALTE).[1]

ASSOCIATED PSYCHOSOCIAL CONCEPTS

Parents' responses to the birth of a premature newborn have been well documented.

TABLE 8–1   CLINICAL DIAGNOSES OF INFANTS ADMITTED WITH ALTE (N = 2779)

	Number	Percentage
Known Origin	1695	61
Digestive (e.g., gastroesophageal reflux, pyloric stenosis aspiration, infection)	733	46
Neurological (e.g., epilepsy, brain tumor, infection)	509	30
Respiratory (e.g., infection, airway abnormality, congenital alveolar hypoventilation)	289	10.4
Metabolic and endocrine (e.g., hypocalcemia, hypoglycemia, hypothyroidism)	41	2.4
Cardiovascular (e.g., cardiomyopathy, arrhythmia, infection)	34	2
Miscellaneous (e.g., smothering, drug effect, sepsis)	49	2.8
No Known Origin		
Apparently minor incident	695	25
Apparently severe incident	389	14

From Kahn, A., Rebuffat, E., Sottiaux, M., & Blum, D. (1988). Problems in management of infants with an apparent life threatening event. Ann NY Acad Sci *533*:78–88.

However, less well documented are parents' responses to the specific and sequential nature of medical complications such as respiratory distress syndrome, patent ductus arteriosus, sepsis, or hyperbilirubinemia as they arise, often one on top of the other, during the neonatal course of illness. Apnea usually occurs during the first 1 to 2 weeks of life, when the premature infant is no longer receiving ventilatory support and may be thought to be in a more stable physiological state. The impact of apnea as "one more thing happening to my baby" is described below by the mother of a premature infant born at 28 weeks' gestation and weighing 2 pounds and 10 ounces.[45]

> He was requiring only a small amount of oxygen and seemed to be doing well. While we chatted and watched, Andrew stopped breathing, which sent his monitor into a noisy tail spin. The nurse calmly reached over and gave his mattress a thump, bump, and he started breathing again. She explained that apnea is very common and should be expected in a baby born so early.

It was still very frightening. We left a bit later, still shaken by the experience. This was my first true moment of reality since his birth. I had been so high all day phoning friends and relatives. My world was okay as long as I didn't have to deal with too much of the reality at a time.

> During the next few weeks we would have good news one day and bad news the next. It was described by one of the doctors as a "roller coaster ride" during the first few weeks in a premature baby's life. . . . When Andrew was two and a half weeks old we got the phone call that all parents of hospitalized babies dread. Andrew was having more apnea than usual and they didn't know what was causing it. They were doing blood cultures, and a spinal tap was necessary to rule out meningitis. . . . We were on the roller coaster again and could not deal with the pain he must be enduring. That, for me, was the hardest part of the whole ordeal. It just didn't seem fair. . . . When they phoned us in the night, we had already fallen asleep from sheer exhaustion. When Tom answered the phone, I couldn't bear to hear, so I put my hands over my ears like a little child and prayed one last time. Good news— it wasn't meningitis. His hemoglobin was low and that seemed to be causing the increase in apnea. He was given blood and by the next day, he was doing well.

This mother's story reminds us that although apnea may be a common occurrence in premature infants, it is not seen as a common event by the parents. Their interpretation of and response to this event in their premature infant's life depend upon our explanation of apnea. This can best be done in the context of the premature infants' gestational age, postconceptual age, and concurrent medical conditions. Telling the parents the premature infant "forgot to breathe" is probably not helpful and raises more questions than it answers.

MANIFESTATIONS

Apneic episodes may result in physiological changes, primarily decreases in oxygenation and heart rate and alterations in hemodynamics. Factors that may influence the degree of oxygen desaturation are the duration of apnea and the arterial oxygenation prior to the onset of apnea.[5] Because of the smaller FRC in premature infants, it could be expected that the arterial oxygenation prior to the onset of apnea would influence both the rate of fall of oxygenation and the lowest oxygenation reached during an apneic episode. The type of apnea (central, obstructive, or mixed) has not been found to be significantly related to the degree of oxygen desaturation in premature infants.[5, 46] In adults, however, oxygen desaturation occurs more rapidly with obstructive apnea.[47] An early hypothesis that hypoxemia occurring before the onset of apnea was the primary event in triggering apnea has not been supported.[48]

The cardiovascular response to apnea occurs after the onset of apnea and varies with the duration of apnea. Bradycardia (heart rate < 100 beats per minute) frequently occurs after the onset of apnea. The heart rate generally does not increase until after resumption of breathing. Peripheral vasoconstriction occurs, and blood pressure may increase initially but decreases with continuation of the apnea.[49, 50] Blood pressure measurements made directly (intra-arterially) during episodes of apnea and bradycardia showed that decreases in blood pressure are consistently related to the degree of bradycardia.[51] With mild and moderate decreases in heart rate (< 120 and < 100 or > 80 beats per minute, respectively) diastolic blood pressure decreases. With severe bradycardia (heart rate < 80 beats per minute), decreases occur in both diastolic and systolic blood pressure. The changes in systemic hemodynamics during apnea and bradycardia are reflected by similar changes in cerebral hemodynamics; that is, cerebral blood flow velocity consistently decreased as a reflection of decreases in systemic blood pressure and heart rate. Thus, repeated episodes of apnea with associated hypoxemia and severe bradycardia may contribute to hypoxic-ischemic brain injury.[51]

SURVEILLANCE

Apnea Monitors

Premature infants of low birth weight (≤ 1800 g) and low gestational age, especially those less than 34 weeks, should be monitored for heart rate and respiratory rate continuously in the first weeks of life. This is important to detect apnea and bradycardia and thus prevent episodes of hypoxemia.

Historically, the eyes of the nurse have been the apnea monitor. Mechanical apnea monitors were introduced in intensive care nurseries in the late 1960s. Apnea monitors are of three major types: motion or pressure-sensitive monitors, thoracic impedance monitors, and airflow detection monitors.

Motion or Pressure-Sensitive Monitors

The apnea mattress monitor detects pressure changes in an air-filled mattress caused by breathing movements. These monitors also have an alarm that can be set to sound after a predetermined period of time during which there is no respiration. With this type of apnea monitor any movement, such as seizure or vibration from equipment, may register as respiration, and therefore the monitor may fail to detect a true apneic episode. If upper airway obstruction occurs, respiratory movements may continue and severe hypoxemia may develop before the alarm is activated.[52]

Thoracic Impedance Monitoring

This is the most commonly used method of respiratory monitoring. The technique of measuring respiratory efforts by means of changes in electrical resistance across the chest is called impedance plethysmography or impedance pneumography. It is based on the principle that volume changes within a given electrical field during breathing are accompanied by changes in electrical resistance. The magnitude of transthoracic impedance is influenced by the relative nonconductive (air) and conductive (blood and interstitial fluid) volumes in the thorax. With breathing, the impedance fluctuates as the air-fluid ratio changes and the fluctuations produce a voltage change. A change of voltage above a given level is registered as a breath. The alarms of these apnea monitors can be set to sound after a predetermined time period, during which no breath has been registered. This type of apnea monitor has been widely used since 1969. One advantage of this type of respiratory monitoring device is the ability to detect heart rate with the same electrodes.

The nurse should be aware of several characteristics of this type of apnea monitor. Transthoracic impedance monitors detect respiratory efforts; therefore, they do not detect obstructive apnea, which is characterized by respiratory efforts but no airflow. Similarly, a disorganized breathing pattern consists of respiratory efforts that may be ineffective for ventilation, and both obstructive apnea and a disorganized breathing pattern may cause hypoxemia.[53, 54] Mixed and obstructive types of apnea have been documented to occur more frequently than central apnea in premature infants.[5]

Nurses rely on apnea monitors to alert them to the premature infant's respiratory status and to document apneic episodes. However, thoracic impedance apnea monitors in newborn nurseries have failed to detect many apneic episodes.[55, 56] Monitoring for heart rate should accompany monitoring for apnea. Therefore, if the impedance monitor fails to detect apnea, the heart rate monitor, with a low heart rate alarm, will detect bradycardia.

Southall and associates noted that when apnea is accompanied by bradycardia, stroke volume has to increase if cardiac output is to be maintained.[57] Thus, with an increase in stroke volume there are greater changes in the volume of blood in the ventricles between systole and diastole and therefore greater differences in electrical impedance. The impedance changes between systole and diastole may be interpreted as a respiratory signal by impedance apnea monitors. This imitation of a respiratory signal by a cardiac signal during an apneic episode accompanied by bradycardia may account for some of the failures of impedance monitors to detect apnea.

Thoracic impedance monitors have to be able to respond to respiratory signals from infants of varying weights and to varying strength of signals. Therefore, the sensitivity setting on the apnea monitor is a critical variable. Setting the manual sensitivity control determines how weak a signal the monitor will detect as a breath.[58] If the sensitivity is set too high, heart beats, vibrations from nearby equipment, or other artifacts may be recorded as respiratory movements even though respiration has stopped. This could lead to undetected apnea. If the sensitivity is set too low, the alarm is triggered "falsely" and may therefore tend to be ignored or turned off. At lower sensitivity settings, it is more likely that only respiration will be detected.[58] Observing the respiratory pattern while adjusting the monitor to the lowest possible setting that can detect most breaths should provide the proper sensitivity. Shallow respirations may produce signals that are below the detection capability of the monitor. This is a common cause of false alarms.

Respiratory signals of low amplitude may also be due to electrode placement, loose electrode belt, or limited chest excursions. In addition to setting the sensitivity, one can also set the lower limit for the respiratory rate. If respiration falls below this rate, the alarm will be activated. The appropriate lower limit should be checked and documented at the beginning of each shift. Most, if not all, apnea monitors used for home monitoring have an automatic sensitivity control setting only.

One report addresses the current state of the art in the design and clinical application of apnea monitoring by transthoracic impedance.[59] Selected infant home apnea monitors have been evaluated for their reliability and safety.[60]

Airflow Monitors

This type of monitor detects the presence or absence of airflow at the nares and includes the pneumotachygraph and measurements of end-tidal (expired) carbon dioxide. These techniques are mainly restricted to short-term research use, however, owing to the expense and size of the apparatus.

The acoustic monitor detects breath sounds at the nose through a microphone at the end of a small catheter.[52] The signal from the microphone is amplified and filtered. In a comparison of the acoustic monitor and thoracic impedance monitors on a small group of premature infants for a short time, the impedance monitor detected only seven out of 26 apneic episodes (less than or equal to 15 seconds in duration) that were detected by the acoustic monitor. The techniques available to monitor respiratory airflow in neonates have been reviewed.[61]

Current generations of apnea monitors or "event recorders" have the capability of storing data surrounding a respiratory event, interfacing with pulse oximeters to record not only respiratory effort and heart rate but also oxygen saturation, and recording the time the monitor was in actual use. Thus, these recorders are helpful in distinguishing between true and false alarms and in documenting the compliance of the caregiver. In a study evaluating the performance of event recorders in the home, 92 per cent of more than 14,000 alarms did not reflect true apnea or bradycardia.[62] Most of the false alarms (69 per cent) were due to movement-loose leads. Conversely, true events may be documented by event recorders that otherwise might be missed, such as apneas that do not activate the alarm but that do cause oxygen desaturation. Compliance of the caregiver in using the monitor at home can now be readily assessed. Noncompliance or undercompliance may need to be addressed by education of the caregiver, discontinuation of home monitoring, or, if the condition warrants, rehospitalization of the infant.

The cost of event recordings may preclude their routine use; however, this issue requires further study. Event recordings increase the cost of monitoring because of the equipment, and the analysis of the data collected; however, with event recorders, the total length of monitoring time may be decreased. Event recording is recommended for documentation of frequent alarms in a symptomless infant; recording type, frequency, and duration of events in infants with ALTE; and for assistance in decision making by parents who have concerns regarding weaning from monitoring.[63]

THERAPIES

Therapeutic Goals

The therapeutic goal is to reduce the frequency and duration of apneic episodes and to restore a regular breathing pattern. Treatment of apnea begins with determination of the cause. Apnea associated with an underlying clinical condition is resolved by treating the underlying condition; however, therapy for the apneic episode also needs to be simultaneously instituted. The same therapies will be utilized for apnea of prematurity, which is thought to be due to developmental immaturity and not associated with an underlying clinical condition. The following clinical therapies are discussed according to their degree of invasiveness and risks. The most noninvasive therapies should be considered first, and one or more of them should be employed simultaneously.

Increase in Afferent Stimuli

Respiratory afferents require a certain level of afferent impulses coming into the respiratory center in order to maintain breathing. Thus, increasing afferent input increases afferent activity. This is the theoretical basis for cutaneous stimulation, vestib-

ular stimulation, and ambient temperature maintenance in the lower zone of the neutral thermal environment.

Cutaneous stimulation has long been used to resolve apneic attacks but is usually effective only if employed early in the apneic episode.[11] If the infant is apneic for many seconds or if the incidence of apneic episodes is high, cutaneous stimulation is seldom effective. Prophylactic cutaneous stimulation (rubbing an extremity for 5 out of 15 minutes) reduced the frequency of apneic episodes by 35 per cent over the control period.[8] The effect persisted for several minutes after the stimulation had been discontinued. There is not always agreement on which cutaneous areas of the premature infant should be stimulated, but the greatest density of tactile receptors is in the palms of the hands and the soles of the feet. These areas are most sensitive to tactile stimulation throughout life.[64]

In utero, vestibular-proprioceptive stimulation occurs as the fetus floats in the amniotic fluid. The vestibular system begins myelination at 4 months' gestation and is fully mature at term. The early maturity of the vestibular system may make it one of the most potent avenues for providing developmentally relevant stimulation to premature infants. Oscillating waterbeds have been used to simulate vestibular stimulation in utero. Their use was reported to be effective in significantly reducing the frequency of apneic episodes.[65, 66] However, a randomized clinical trial with an oscillating air mattress showed no benefit in reducing apnea or in enhancing growth and development.[67]

Maintaining ambient temperatures in the lower zone of the neutral thermal environment is supported by the observation that premature infants have an increased incidence of apnea when the environmental temperatures are near the upper limit of the thermoneutral zone or when there is a sudden rate of increase in the incubator environmental temperature.[10, 11] Fluctuations in environmental temperatures, especially intermittent blasts of warm air, may also increase the incidence of apnea. Minimizing fluctuations can be done by entering the microenvironment of the infant as little as possible and by constructing incubators that do not allow warm air currents to flow directly over the infant. Rewarming a hypothermic infant too rapidly may also induce apneic episodes.

Maintenance of Normoxia

Hypoxemia is one of the consequences of apnea. In general, the longer hypoxemia is present, the longer it will take to resolve once therapy is initiated. For some premature infants, increasing the inspired oxygen concentration from 21 to 23 per cent may be sufficient to alleviate recurring apneic episodes. Maintaining the arterial oxygen concentration between 60 and 80 torr, or the oxygen saturation about 90 per cent, may alleviate apneic episodes that occur at lower arterial oxygen levels. Monitoring oxygenation is best done by a pulse oximeter (oxygen saturation) or a skin surface (transcutaneous) oxygen monitor. Arterial oxygenation can rise abruptly with slight changes in FIO_2 and can vary greatly with changes in infant state. The hematocrit value should be checked to ensure that it is 40 per cent or above. A transfusion of packed red blood cells to increase the hematocrit to greater than 40 per cent may be therapeutic. The frequency of apnea and periodic breathing in growing premature infants has been shown to be reduced following transfusion of packed red blood cells.[68, 69] However, this is controversial, and the risks of transfusion therapy should be weighed against the possible benefits to the infant.

Ventilation with Bag and Mask

If the apneic episode is not resolved quickly, ventilation with a bag and mask will be necessary to restore breathing. The inspired oxygen concentration delivered via bag and mask should not routinely be increased, as frequently the premature infant will become hyperoxic. Hyperoxia often induces an irregular breathing pattern. Repeated episodes of hyperoxia may increase the risk of retinopathy of prematurity. As spontaneous breathing is restored, the bag and mask ventilation should be gradually reduced and hyperventilation should be avoided, as respiratory alkalosis abolishes or decreases the ventilatory drive. It is also useful to produce a positive end-expiratory pressure of 2 to 4 cm H_2O during bag and mask ventilation and to maintain this pressure for a couple of minutes after the re-establishment of a breathing pattern.

Continuous Positive Airway Pressure

Continuous positive airway pressure (CPAP) increases functional residual capacity and alveolar size by increasing transpulmonary pressure. In addition, CPAP prevents airway closure, maintains alveolar distention at end-expiration, and causes distention of the pulmonary stretch receptors. The resultant increase in lung volume increases lung compliance, improves oxygenation, and reduces the work of breathing. Low levels of CPAP are effective in decreasing the frequency of apneic attacks in premature infants with and without primary pulmonary disease.[70, 71] In one report, CPAP reduced the incidence of mixed and obstructive apnea but had no effect on central apnea.[72]

Central Respiratory Stimulation: Theophylline and Caffeine

Kuzemko and Paala were the first to report that aminophylline (75 to 80 per cent theophylline) was effective in decreasing the frequency of apneic episodes in premature infants.[73] Since their report was published, other studies have confirmed their findings.[74–77] Theophylline and caffeine both increase the sensitivity of the respiratory center to carbon dioxide (CO_2). The slope of the CO_2 response curve is increased and shifted to the left; therefore, the ventilatory response to CO_2 is more vigorous and occurs at a lower PCO_2.[78] Other effects of these drugs that may relate to the reduction of apneic episodes include (1) increased transmission of neural impulses, (2) improved skeletal muscle contraction, and (3) improved oxygenation secondary to increased cardiac output.[79] Lopes and associates showed that theophylline given to premature infants with apnea improved diaphragmatic contractility and reduced the number of severe apneic episodes caused by fatigue.[80] Thus, the efficacy of theophylline in premature infants may be related to both a central and peripheral effect.

Theophylline regularizes the breathing pattern, stabilizes arterial oxygenation, and decreases the number of hypoxic episodes.[81] Theophylline does not increase respiratory frequency[58] but does increase tidal volume.[78] Caffeine increases respiratory frequency with minimal effects on tidal volume. Theophylline has more potent cardiovascular and diuretic effects, with intermediate effects on the central nervous system. Caffeine has the most effect on the central nervous, muscular, and respiratory systems.[82] Giving theophylline or aminophylline to premature infants with apnea has been associated with a decrease in the number of apneic episodes of greater than or equal to 20 seconds and of bradycardias of 80 beats per minute or less.[83] Monitoring only heart rate when neonates are receiving theophylline would fail to detect some episodes of apnea.

The side effects of theophylline are tachycardia, jitteriness, abdominal distention, feeding intolerance, and vomiting. These effects are dose-related and reversible with discontinuation of the drug. Caffeine does not appear to produce these side effects, even at high plasma levels, but it does increase metabolic rate and has the potential to cause poor weight gain in premature infants.[79] Both drugs have much longer half-lives and decreased clearance in premature infants compared with adults.[84, 85] A minimum of four biological half-lives must elapse before a steady state serum level can be achieved with any drug. Therefore, a loading dose is usually given followed by a maintenance dose. A loading dose of 5.5 to 6 mg/kg has been recommended.[84, 85] The recommended maintenance dose/rate is about 1 mg/8 hours or 2 mg/12 hours, with the dosage adjusted to maintain a serum level of 10 mg/L (range of 6 to 13 mg/L).[79] These recommendations are for intravenous administration. Oral theophylline is 80 per cent absorbed, so the dose should be multiplied by 1.25 if oral theophylline or aminophylline is used.[77] The monitoring of serum levels of theophylline may be done 2 hours after a dose and just prior to another dose to determine the peak and trough levels, respectively. Because significant amounts of theophylline are metabolized to caffeine in premature infants, the theophylline level may not reflect the total xanthine load; therefore, the plasma caffeine levels should be monitored also.[86]

The multisystem effects of these drugs in premature infants are not known and may pose long-term risks. In adults, methylxanthines decrease cerebral blood flow secondary to increased cerebral vascular resistance.[87] There has been no reported difference in growth or in neurological or ophthalmological examinations in children at 18 to 40 months of age who were treated with caffeine as neonates.[88] The use of any therapeutic intervention requires a proper evaluation for the possible causes of the apneic episodes and of the consequences of the intervention.

Some healthy premature infants may be ready for hospital discharge but continue to have apneic episodes. Another group of premature infants are those that had apnea during their neonatal course that resolved by the time of their discharge. A third group consists of those who may have never had apnea during hospitalization but who experience apnea or an apparent life-threatening event during early infancy. Guidelines for evaluation of these three different groups of infants are shown in Table 8–2.[89]

ILLUSTRATIVE CASE STUDY

The following case study exemplifies the typical prenatal history and postnatal events prior to the onset of apnea in a premature newborn. It also demonstrates the diagnostic work-up related to apnea and the utilization of one clinical therapy for apnea.

Baby Z. was an 1130-g male born at 30 weeks' gestation to a 29-year-old para I gravida III. The baby was delivered via cesarean section because of prolonged ruptured membranes and breech presentation. The mother received two doses of betamethasone prior to delivery. The Apgar scores were 7 and 7, respectively. Baby Z. was intubated and initially received an FIO_2 of 25 per cent at ventilator pressures of 20/4 at a rate of 60 per minute. On the third day of life, he was extubated and received 23 per cent oxygen via hood for the next 2 days before being weaned to room air. During the first week of life, Baby Z. developed symptoms of patent ductus arteriosus. This was treated with indomethacin, with resolution of the murmur and hemodynamic changes. On the fourth day of life, phototherapy was started because of a total bilirubin of 9.8 with a direct bilirubin of 0.8 mg. The hematocrit level was maintained above 40 per cent via transfusions of packed red blood cells.

Toward the end of the first week of life, progressive episodes of apnea (> 15 seconds) and bradycardia (< 100 beats per minute) began to develop. A septic work-up was done, and Baby Z. was started on antibiotics. When the cultures came back negative, the antibiotics were discontinued. The glucose and calcium levels were normal. An ultrasound examination of the head showed no

TABLE 8–2   **APNEA PROBLEMS IN THREE GROUPS OF INTENSIVE CARE NURSERY GRADUATES**

Symptomatic		Asymptomatic	
a. Inpatient: apnea never resolves b. Outpatient: apnea a new problem		a. Never had apnea b. Had symptomatic apnea that resolved	
Has Apnea	*Never Had Apnea*	*Had Symptomatic Apnea That Resolved*	
RECOMMENDATION FOR EVALUATION			
1. Observation, including apnea-cardiac monitoring in hospital. 2. Trained medical staff available for CPR. 3. Medical evaluation directed by history and physical examination. 4. Appropriate clinical polygraphic study directed by clinical question and possible therapy.	1. Consider appropriate polygraphic studies in infants with significant residual neurological, cardiac, pulmonary, or other clinical problems that may contribute to apnea problems such as (a) infant with BPD, (b) anemia (Hct < 30). 2. Home apnea-cardiac monitoring to observe for apnea problems in a high-risk patient such as infant born to a narcotic addict or surviving twin of SIDS infant.	1. None, if no symptomatic apnea for 2 weeks prior to discharge during which time infant has not had methylxanthine or other respiratory stimulant treatment. 2. History of apnea should be noted in record, since anemia (Hct < 30) or effects of general anesthesia may increase risk for apnea.	
ETIOLOGY			
Disease related or idiopathic.	High-risk group; residual dysfunction.	None.	
TREATMENT			
1. Treatment of disease alone may be sufficient if apnea resolves. 2. In those infants who continue to have apnea in the hospital, a trial of methylxanthines is worthwhile. 3. Home apnea-cardiac monitoring, particularly in those infants in whom apnea does not resolve.	1. Clinical observation only. 2. Therapy to support residual problem, for example supplemental O_2 in BPD infant with suboptimal ($Po_2 < 50$) oxygenation (home apnea-cardiac monitoring may be helpful in selected cases). 3. Home apnea-cardiac monitoring in selected cases. 4. Parents trained in CPR; document observations of monitor alarms and interventions daily and review with physician on a regular basis.	None.	

Modified from Ballard, R.A. (1988). *Pediatric Care of the ICN Graduate* (p. 269). Philadelphia: W.B. Saunders.
BPD, bronchopulmonary dysplasia; CPR, cardiopulmonary resuscitation; Hct, hematocrit; SIDS, sudden infant death syndrome.

indications of intraventricular bleeding. Theophylline was started, and within 24 to 36 hours episodes of apnea and bradycardia had ceased.

The serum theophylline level was 9 µg/ml on the third day after the medication was started. Chest radiographs during this time demonstrated intermittent atelectasis. The infant was continuously monitored on a heart rate and respiratory monitor and was breathing room air. Transcutaneous oxygen monitoring indicated $tcPo_2$ readings between 58 and 80 torr.

At 3 weeks' postnatal age, Baby Z. was transferred to a community hospital closer to his home and was continued on theophylline, heart rate monitoring, and respiratory monitoring. The theophylline was discontinued at 6 weeks' postnatal age, but heart and respiratory rates continued to be monitored. There were no further episodes of apnea or bradycardia, and Baby Z. was discharged home at 8 weeks' postnatal age.

REVIEW OF RESEARCH FINDINGS

The following research articles have been selected for review because of their relevance to nursing practice and because each study represents a major contribution toward isolating and describing factors associated with the phenomenon of apnea or the efficacy of thoracic impedance monitoring devices in the detection of apnea.

Daily and colleagues' classic study in 1969 was one of the first in which thoracic impedance monitoring was used to follow the respiratory pattern and heart rate changes in a group of premature infants known to be at risk for apnea.[11] Twenty-two premature infants (birth weight range of 765 to 2552 g) were continuously monitored for 7 to 16 days during the first 16 days of life. Seven of the premature infants were recovering from mild respiratory distress syndrome, and one had aspiration pneumonia. The remaining 14 were clinically well. An attempt was made to maintain the environmental temperature in the thermoneutral zone at all times. Throughout the study, the apnea monitor alarm was set to activate 20 seconds after the onset of apnea. The accuracy of the alarm was verified by observation. No stimulation of respiration was used between the twentieth and thirtieth second after the onset of apnea. From the thirtieth to forty-fifth second, diffuse cutaneous stimulation was applied. After 45 seconds, bag and mask resuscitation with 96 per cent oxygen was instituted. All apneic episodes of 20 seconds or greater were tabulated from the recordings and correlated with the stimulus required to reinitiate respiration. The appearance of the infant during apnea was observed. The relationship between environmental temperature and apnea was assessed in six additional infants. In this group, the skin temperature was alternately maintained at 36 and 36.8° C every 12 hours by an abdominal skin temperature probe.

A total of 540 apneic episodes of 20 or more seconds were observed in 13 of the 22 infants monitored (nine of the premature infants had no apneic episodes longer than 20 seconds). Of the 540 episodes, 79 per cent (428/540) exceeded 30 seconds in duration. All episodes of 30 or more seconds' duration were tabulated to estimate the incidence of apnea. The incidence was expressed as a per cent of infants studied on a given day who were having apneic episodes of greater than 30 seconds' duration. On the basis of this criterion, the incidence was calculated to be approximately 25 per cent of the infants studied in the first 10 days of life.

Clinical observation of the premature infants during apnea revealed that for the first 20 to 30 seconds they usually remained pink and appeared to have good tone but rapidly became limp, pale, cyanotic, and unresponsive after that time. The smaller premature infants tended to become cyanotic and to experience bradycardia, hypotonia, and cyanosis more rapidly. Between the thirtieth and forty-fifth second, cyanosis, pallor, loss of muscle tone, and failure to respond to cutaneous stimulation became more apparent.

Respiration began spontaneously in 37 per cent of the 540 apneic episodes and in association with cutaneous stimulation in another 55 per cent. Bag and mask ventilation was required in 8 per cent of the episodes, even though cutaneous stimulation was initiated at 30 seconds. All apneic episodes were noted to begin in expiration during periodic breathing.

The mean heart rates at the onset of apnea were not significantly different. In apneic episodes of more than 45 seconds 65 per cent were associated with bradycardia (heart rate < 100 beats per minute) occurring within 15 seconds. In apneic episodes of shorter duration, the bradycardia was often preceded by a short period of tachycardia, which implies the tachycardia is reflexive in origin. Regardless of the ultimate duration of apnea, bradycardia was always present by 30 seconds.

On the basis of these observations, these researchers suggested that apnea be defined as the nonbreathing interval that a given infant cannot tolerate without bradycardia and cyanosis; for large premature infants this may be about 20 seconds, but for smaller infants this may be as short as 5 seconds.

In the six different subjects with periodic breathing and apnea in whom skin temperature varied from 36.0 to 36.8° C every 12 hours, apnea was more frequent at the higher skin temperature. This suggests some apneic episodes may be initiated by thermally induced changes.

In this study, periodic breathing and apnea

also occurred within 15 minutes of feeding in 49 per cent (21/43) of feeding intervals that could be documented.

This classic study in apnea research exemplifies beginning research efforts in describing and defining a clinical phenomenon (apnea), in documenting the changes in variables (heart rate, color, muscle tone) associated with the onset and duration of the phenomenon, and in describing the contextual or environmental factors (temperature, feeding) that influence the occurrence of the phenomenon. This beginning research effort was greatly enhanced by the simultaneous and continuous electronic monitoring of the respiratory pattern and heart rate combined with documentation of clinically observable events temporally associated with apnea and the effects of different levels of interventions.

From this study, the incidence of apneic episodes greater than 30 seconds' duration was determined to be approximately 25 per cent in infants studied in the first 10 days of life. The incidence has been determined to be much higher (see Prevalence and Populations at Risk earlier in the chapter). However, the incidence is certainly influenced by the higher survival rate of lower gestational age premature infants (now compared with the survival rate in 1969) and by the fact that in this study the incidence of apnea was based on apneic episodes greater than 30 seconds' duration, whereas most current studies are based on apneic episodes of 20 seconds' duration or shorter.

The observation that apnea is not preceded by changes in heart rate but that bradycardia and associated cardiovascular changes frequently follow apneic episodes has been confirmed by others.[90, 91] Previous observations and reports by others regarding temperature as a variable possibly related to apnea influenced Daily and colleagues to study the association between apnea frequency and skin temperature.[11] Their finding that apnea was more frequent at higher skin temperatures and Perlstein and colleagues'[10] later observation that onset of apnea was often preceded by rising air temperature in incubators (see the section Situational Stressors) have contributed to our understanding of variables that need to be controlled not only in research but also in practice.

In another study, the detection of apnea by conventional thoracic impedance monitoring was compared with apnea detection by a continuous computer data acquisition system.[5] In clinical practice, the conventional method for detecting apnea in premature infants consists of thoracic impedance apnea monitors with alarms for absence of respiratory effort and low heart rate to alert the nursing staff. It is known that this type of apnea monitor does not detect mixed or obstructive types of apnea and that in nurseries many episodes of apnea are missed. A total of 1266 apneic episodes were documented from 27 infants studied between 1 and 21 days of postnatal life. All were experiencing clinical apnea at the time of the study. Apnea was defined as an episode of 15 seconds or greater with an associated decrease in heart rate and oxygenation. Selected findings from this study are summarized in Table 8–3. Findings were as follows: (1) obstructive and mixed apneas were a more common occurrence than central apneas, (2) thoracic impedance monitoring was less reliable in documenting mixed and obstructive apneas, and (3) mixed apneas were associated with a longer mean duration. Apnea duration was positively correlated with both a decrease in heart rate and oxygen saturation. Also, of all apneic episodes, 75 per cent were associated with a decrease in heart rate to less than 100 beats per minute and subjects receiving theophylline therapy did not demonstrate a significant decrease in heart rate with central and mixed apnea but did with obstructive apnea.

This study reinforces the inadequacy of thoracic impedance apnea monitoring in detecting the occurrence of apnea, especially mixed and obstructive types, in nurseries. Previous studies have also documented this problem.[92] There continues to be a need to

TABLE 8–3 TYPE, DETECTION, AND DURATION OF APNEA

	Central (%)	Mixed (%)	Obstructive (%)
Type of apnea	46	44	10
Detection by thoracic impedance	64	50	31
Duration			
< 20 seconds	32	22	40
20–30 seconds	48	48	45
30–50 seconds	18	26	13
> 50 seconds	2	4	2

From Muttitt, S.C., Finer, N.N., Tierney, A.J., & Rossman, J. (1988). Neonatal apnea: Diagnosis by nurse versus computer. Pediatrics *82*:113–720. Reproduced with permission, © 1988.

develop apnea monitoring equipment that is more reliable and has greater sensitivity and specificity.

IMPLICATIONS FOR RESEARCH

Although there are multiple developmental and physiological factors known to be related to the propensity of the premature infant to develop apnea, it is also clear that environmental factors can increase the risk and frequency of apneic episodes. Environment has been identified as one of the central phenomenon of the discipline of nursing.[93, 94] Based on Roy's adaptation model, adaptation is viewed as a process of responding positively to environmental changes.[95, 96] Adaptative responses are those that promote the integrity of the person in terms of the goals of survival, growth, reproduction, and self-mastery. Ineffective responses are those that do not contribute to those goals. In Roy's model the goal of nursing is to promote adaptation. Based on Roy's adaptation model, a framework (Fig. 8–1) is proposed for nursing research in apnea in premature infants.

The focal stimuli (the stimuli immediately confronting the individual and the one to which an adaptative response must be made) are uncoordinated neural impulse generation, transmission, and integration. The nervous system is the source of the neural drive, and the activity of brain stem respiratory neurons must be maintained through continuous postsynaptic excitation. This neural drive is often unstable in premature infants owing to neuronal immaturity. Even if there is an adequate neural drive, properties of the respiratory muscles (fatigue) or of the lungs (decreased compliance) or sleep state (REM sleep) may reduce or modify ventilatory output. The premature infant has limited ability to regulate autonomic functions such as heart rate and respiratory rate. The ventilatory pattern may become unstable and result in periodic breathing or apnea.

The residual stimuli, according to Roy's model, include those factors that may be relevant in the current situation but whose effects cannot be measured or validated. In the proposed framework, the residual stimuli are conceptualized as factors related to the intrauterine environment that might influence the control of breathing, such as episodes of fetal hypoxia, maternal cigarette smoking, and alcohol intake, and as events related to or causing the premature delivery.

The background or contextual stimuli are all other stimuli in the situation. Contextual stimuli in this situation would include gestational age, since the occurrence of apnea is inversely related to gestational age, and the presence or absence of concurrent illnesses, since there are several clinical conditions known to be associated with apnea. Other contextual stimuli are environmental factors such as thermal, tactile, or vestibular stimuli, which have been shown to affect apnea through changes in afferent input to the respiratory center.

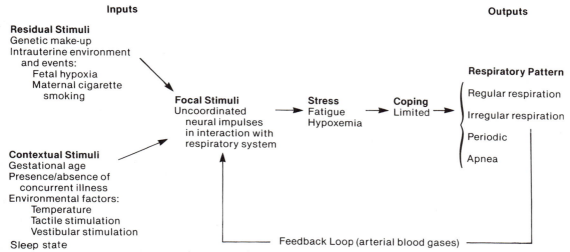

Figure 8–1. Adaptation model and apnea in premature infants.

The context in which apneic episodes occur deserves close scrutiny in order to identify clusters of factors that may exist in the environment, including caregiver activities, to result in apnea. For example, a physical examination, a chest radiograph, and then a bolus gavage feeding may be followed by an apneic episode. Frequently, it is only the nurse who has observed this entire sequence of events and the subsequent impact on the premature infant.

Overwhelming stimuli from the environment may initiate apnea in some premature infants.[97] The documentation of the clustering or sequencing of environmental events that may be related to apnea should include the entire 24-hour cycle to take into account various levels of environmental stimuli and the developing circadian rhythm of the premature infant. The timing and sequencing of interventions may be just as important as the effects of the interventions themselves.

On another level of investigation, nursing research needs to focus on considering what contextual stimuli might be important in augmenting respiratory center output and thus promoting a more regular respiratory pattern. The converse also needs to be considered: What contextual stimuli might be minimized or reduced that contribute to an unstable respiratory pattern? For example, would continuous gavage feedings rather than intermittent bolus feedings reduce the frequency of postfeeding apnea?

Variables such as vestibular stimulation, tactile stimulation, and maintaining the skin temperature in the lower range of the neutral thermal environment have all been shown to be effective in reducing the frequency of apnea. Perhaps the incidence of apnea in a given nursery might be reduced by systematically incorporating into practice interventions based on the variables shown to affect the incidence of apnea.

Sleep in premature infants is characterized by frequent sleep state transitions, and the respiratory system may be most unstable during these transition periods. In the premature infant of less than 30 weeks' gestation, these transitions between the poorly organized sleep states may also correlate with periods of oscillating rhythmicity in respiration.

Many premature newborns are discharged home wearing apnea monitors. The impact of this technology on the family and on their interactions and relationships requires further investigation.

REFERENCES

1. *Consensus Development Conference: Infantile Apnea and Home Monitoring* (1986). (NIH Publication No. 87-2905). Bethesda, MD: National Institutes of Health.
2. Dulock, H. (1981). Apnea and periodic breathing. J Calif Perinat Assoc *1*:27–33.
3. Barrington, K.J., & Finer, N.N. (1990). Periodic breathing and apnea in preterm infants. Pediatr Res *27*:118–121.
4. Dransfield, D., Spitzer, A.R., & Fox, W.W. (1983). Episodic airway obstruction in premature infants. Am J Dis Child *137*:441–443.
5. Muttitt, S.C., Finer, N.N., Tierney, A.J., & Rossmann, J. (1988). Neonatal apnea: Diagnosis by nurse versus computer. Pediatrics *82*:113–720.
6. Kattwinkel, J.B., Nearman, H.S., Fanaroff, A.A., Katona, P.G., & Klaus, H.K. (1975). Apnea of prematurity: Comparative therapeutic effects of cutaneous stimulation and nasal continuous positive airway pressure. J Pediatr *86*:588.
7. Brooks, J.G. (1984). Relationship of apnea of infancy to SIDS. Perinatol Neonatol *8*:15–18.
8. Henderson-Smart, D.J. (1981). The effect of gestational age on the incidence and duration of recurrent apnea in newborn babies. Aust Pediatr J *17*:273–276.
9. Lemons, J.A., & Kisling, J.A. (1982). Thermoregulation. In R. Schreiner & J.A. Kisling (eds), *Practical Neonatal Respiratory Care*. New York: Grune & Stratton.
10. Perlstein, P., Edwards, N., & Sutherland, J. (1970). Apnea in premature infants and incubator–air temperature change. N Engl J Med *282*:461.
11. Daily, W., Jr., Klaus, M., & Meyer, H.B.F. (1969). Apnea in premature infants: Monitoring, incidence, heart rate changes, and effects of environmental temperatures. Pediatrics *43*:510.
12. Bryan, A.C., & Bryan, M.H. (1978). Control of respiration in the newborn. Clin Perinatol *5*:269–281.
13. Schulte, F.J. (1977). Apnea. Clin Perinatol *4*:165.
14. Rigatto, H., & Brady, J.P. (1972). Periodic breathing and apnea in preterm infants: Hypoxia as a primary event. Pediatrics *50*:219–228.
15. Rigatto, H., de la Torre Verduzco, R., & Cates, D.B. (1975). Effects of O_2 on the ventilatory response to CO_2 in preterm infants. J Appl Physiol *39*:896–899.
16. Rigatto, H. (1977). Ventilatory response to hypercapnia. Semin Perinatol *1*:363–367.
17. Gerhardt, T., & Bancalavi, E. (1984). Apnea of prematurity: I. Lung function and regulation of breathing. Pediatrics *74*:58–62.
18. Phillipson, E.A., Murphy, E., & Kozer, L.F. (1976). Regulation of respiration in sleeping dogs. J Appl Physiol *40*:688–694.
19. Parmelee, A., Wenner, W., Akiyama, Y., Schultz, M., & Stern, E. (1967). Sleep states in premature infants. Dev Med Child Neurol *9*:70–77.
20. Gabriel, M., Albani, M., & Schulte, F.J. (1976). Apneic spells and sleep states in preterm infants. Pediatrics *57*:142–147.
21. Gabriel, M., Helmin, U., & Albani, M. (1980). Sleep induced Po_2 changes in pre-term infants. Eur J Pediatr *134*:153–154.
22. Hagan, R., Bryan, A.C., Bryan, M.H., & Gulston, G. (1976). The effects of sleep state on intercostal muscle activity and rib cage motion. Physiologist *93*:214–218.

23. Krill, R., Andrew, S.W., Bryan, A.C., & Bryan, M.H. (1976). Respiratory load compensation in infants. J Appl Physiol *40*:357–361.

24. Henderson-Smart, D.J., & Read, D.J. (1978). Depression of intercostal and abdominal muscle activity and vulnerability to asphyxia during active sleep in the newborn. In C. Guilleminault & W. Dement (eds.), *Sleep Apnea Syndromes.* New York: Alan R. Liss.

25. Rigatto, H. (1977). Apnea and periodic breathing. Semin Perinatol *1*:375–381.

26. Volpe, J.J. (1987). Neonatal seizures. In J.J. Volpe (ed.), *Neurology of the Newborn* (2nd ed.). Philadelphia: W.B. Saunders.

27. Kattwinkel, J. (1977). Neonatal apnea: Pathogenesis and therapy. J Pediatr *90*:342–247.

28. Keyes, W.B., Donohue, P.K., Spivak, J.L., Jones, M.D., & Oski, F.A. (1989). Assessing the need for transfusion of premature infants and role of hematocrit, clinical signs and erythropoietin level. Pediatrics *84*:412–417.

29. Blank, J.P., Sheagren, T.G., & Vajaria, J. (1984). The role of RBC transfusion in the premature infant. Am J Dis Child *138*:831–833.

30. Joshi, A., Gerhardt, T., & Shandloff, P. (1987). Blood transfusion effect on the respiratory pattern of preterm infants. Pediatrics *80*:79–84.

31. Phibbs, R.H. (1987). Neonatal polycythemia. In A.M. Rudolph (ed.), *Pediatrics* (18th ed.). Norwalk, CT: Appleton and Lange.

32. Liu, L.M.P., Cote, C.J., & Goudsouzian, N.G. (1983). Life threatening apnea in infants recovering from anesthesia. Anesthesiology *59*:506–508.

33. Naeye, R. (1979). Neonatal apnea: Underlying disorders. Pediatrics *63*:8–12.

34. Perlman, J.M., & Volpe, J.J. (1985). Episodes of apnea and bradycardia in the preterm newborn: Impact on cerebral circulation. Pediatrics *76*:333–338.

35. Willinger, M., James, L.S., & Catz, C. (1991). Defining the sudden infant death syndrome (SIDS): Deliberations of an expert panel convened by the National Institute of Child Health Development. Pediatr Pathol *11*:617–684.

36. Chavez, C.J., Ostrea, E.M., Stryker, J.C., & Smialek, Z. (1979). Sudden infant death syndrome among infants of drug-dependent mothers. J Pediatr *95*:407–409.

37. Chasnoff, I.J., Burns, K., & Burns, W.J. (1987). Cocaine use in pregnancy: Perinatal morbidity and mortality. Neurotoxicol Teratol *9*:291–293.

38. Hadeed, A.J., & Siegel, S.R. (1989). Maternal cocaine use during pregnancy: Effect on the newborn infant. Pediatrics *84*:205–210.

39. Steinschneider, A. (1972). Prolonged apnea and the sudden infant death syndrome: Clinical and laboratory observations. Pediatrics *50*:646–654.

40. Hoffman, H.J., Damus, K., Hillman, L., & Krongrad, E. (1988). Risk factors for SIDS. In P.J. Schwartz, D.P. Southall, M. Valdes-Dapena (eds.), *The Sudden Infant Death Syndrome: Cardiac and Respiratory Mechanisms and Interventions.* Ann NY Acad Sci *533*:13–30.

41. Hoffman, H.J., Damus, K., Krongrad, E., & Hillman, L. (1986). Apnea, birth weight and SIDS: Results of the NICHD Co-operative Epidemiological Study of Sudden Infant Death Syndrome (SIDS) Risk Factors. In Consensus Report, *Infantile Apnea and Home Monitoring.* Rockville, MD: National Institutes of Health.

42. Kahn, A., Rebuffat, E., Sottiaux, M., & Blum, D. (1988). Problems in management of infants with an apparent life-threatening event. Ann NY Acad Sci *533*:78–88.

43. Brooks, J.G. (1990). Apparent life-threatening events. In *Current Therapy in Perinatal-Neonatal Medicine* (vol. 2.). Philadelphia: B.C. Decker p. 514–518.

44. Oren, J., Kelly, D., & Shannon, D.C. (1986). Identification of a high risk group for Sudden Infant Death Syndrome among infants who were resuscitated for sleep apnea. Pediatrics *77*:495–499.

45. Redmon, L. (1983) Born too soon: One family's story. Genesis *5*:18–21.

46. Dulock, H.L. (1989). Arousal Response to Respiratory Events in Premature Newborns. Ph.D. dissertation. University of California, San Francisco, School of Nursing.

47. Tilkian, A.G., Guilleminault, C., Schroeder, J.S., Lehrman, K.L., Simmons, F.B., & Dement, W.C. (1976). Sleep induced apnea syndrome: Hemodynamic studies during wakefulness and sleep. Ann Intern Med *85*:714–719.

48. Hiatt, M.I., Hegyi, T., Indyk, L., Dangman, B.C., & James, L.S. (1981). Continuous monitoring of PO_2 during apnea of prematurity. J Pediatr *98*:288–291.

49. Storrs, C.N. (1977). Cardiovascular effects of apnea in preterm infants. Arch Dis Child *52*:534–540.

50. Girling, D.J. (1972). Changes in heart rate, blood pressure, and pulse pressure during apneic attacks in newborn babies. Arch Dis Child *47*:405–410.

51. Perlman, J.M., & Volpe, J.J. (1985). Episodes of apnea and bradycardia in the preterm newborn: Impact on cerebral circulation. Pediatrics *76*:333–338.

52. Stark, A. (1982). Apnea monitors—1982. Med Instrument *6*:160–162.

53. Warburton, D., Stark, A., & Taeusch, H.W. (1977). Apnea monitor failure in infants with upper airway obstruction. Pediatrics *60*:742–744.

54. Peabody, J., Gregory, G., Willis, M., Alistar, G.S., Lucey, P., & Lucey, J. (1979). Failure of conventional monitoring to detect apnea resulting in hypoxemia. In A. Huch, R. Huch, & J.F. Lucey (eds.), *Hypoxemia, Continuous Transcutaneous Blood Gas Monitoring.* The National Foundation–March of Dimes Birth Defects (vol. 15, no. 4). New York: Alan R. Liss.

55. Stein, I., & Shannon, D.C. (1975). The pediatric pneumogram: A new method for detecting and quantifying apneas in infants. Pediatrics *55*:599–603.

56. Shannon, D. (1975). Prevention of apnea and bradycardia in low birth weight infants. Pediatrics *55*:589–594.

57. Southall, D.P., Richards, J.M., Lau, K.C., & Shinebourne, E.A. (1980). An explanation for failure of impedance apnea alarm systems. Arch Dis Child *55*:64–65.

58. Emergency Care Research Institute (1980). Infant apnea monitors. Health Devices *9*:247–283.

59. Technical Information Report (1989). *Apnea Monitoring by Means of Thoracic Impedance Pneumography.* Arlington, VA: Association for the Advancement of Medical Instrumentation.

60. Emergency Care Research Institute (1987). Infant home apnea monitors. Health Devices *16*:79–109.

61. Dransfield, D.A., & Philip, A.G.S. (1985). Respira-

tory airflow measurement in the neonate. Clin Perinatol *12*:21–30.

62. Weese-Mayer, D.E., Brouillette, R.T., Morrow, A.S., Conway, L.P., Klemka-Walden, L.M., & Hunt, C.E. (1989). Assessing validity of infant monitor alarms with event recording. Pediatrics *115*:702–708.

63. Bush, L. (1989). Cardiorespiratory monitoring. Medical Electronics *2*:1–4.

64. Humphrey, T. (1978). Function of the nervous system during prenatal life. In S. Uwe (ed.), *Perinatal Physiology* (pp. 651–683). New York: Plenum Medical Book.

65. Körner, A.F., Kraemer, H.C., Haffner, M.E., & Cosper, L.M. (1975). Effects of waterbed floatation on premature infants: A pilot study. Pediatrics *56*:361.

66. Körner, A.F., Guilleminault, C., Van den Hoed, J., & Baldwin, R.B. (1978). Reduction of sleep apnea and bradycardia in preterm infants on oscillating waterbeds: A controlled polygraphic study. Pediatrics *61*:528–533.

67. Saigal, S., Watts, J., & Campbell, D. (1986). Randomized clinical trial of an oscillating air mattress in preterm infants: Effect on apnea, growth and development. J Pediatr *109*:857–860.

68. DeMaio, J.G., Harris, M.C., Deuber, C., & Spitzer, A.R. (1989). Effect of blood transfusion on apnea frequency in growing premature infants. J Pediatr *114*:1039–1041.

69. Joshi, A., Gerhardt, T., Shandloff, P., & Bancalari, E. (1987). Blood transfusion effect on the respiratory pattern of preterm infants. Pediatrics *80*:79–84.

70. Gregory, G., & Tooley, W.H. (1971). Blood gas changes during bag and mask ventilation. Clin Res *19*:220.

71. Boros, S.J., & Reynolds, J.W. (1976). Prolonged apnea of prematurity. Clin Pediatr *15*:123.

72. Miller, M.J., Carlo, W.A., & Martin, R.J. (1985). Continuous positive airway pressure selectively reduces obstructive apnea in preterm infants. J Pediatr *106*:91–95.

73. Kuzemko, J.A., & Paala, J. (1973). Apneic attacks in the newborn treated with aminophylline. Arch Dis Child *48*:404.

74. Aranda, J.V., Gorman, W., Bergsteinsson, H., & Gunn, T. (1977). Efficacy of caffeine in treatment of apnea in low birth weight infant. J Pediatr *90*:467–472.

75. Myers, T., Milsap, R.L., Krauss, A.N., Auld, P.A.M., & Reidenberg, M.M. (1980). Low dose theophylline therapy in idiopathic apnea of prematurity. J Pediatr *96*:99–103.

76. Peabody, J.L., Gregory, G.A., Willis, M.M., & Tooley, W.H. (1978). Transcutaneous monitoring in aminophylline treated apneic infants. Pediatrics *62*:698–701.

77. Uvay, R., Shapiro, D.L., Smith, B., & Warshaw, J.B. (1975). Treatment of severe apnea: Apnea in prematures with orally administered theophylline. Pediatrics *55*:595–598.

78. Davi, M.J., Simmons, K.F., & Seshia, M.M. (1978). Physiological changes induced by theophylline in treatment of apnea in preterm infants. J Pediatr *92*:91–95.

79. Aranda, J., & Turner, T. (1979). Methylxanthines in apnea of prematurity. Clin Perinatol *6*:87–108.

80. Lopes, J.M., LeSouy, P.N., Bryan, M.H., & Bryan, A.C. (1982). The effects of theophylline on diaphragmatic fatigue in the newborn. (Abstract) Pediatr Res *16*:355.

81. Peabody, J. (1979). Transcutaneous oxygen measurement to evaluate drug effects. Clin Perinatol *6*:109–121.

82. Ritchie, J.M. (1975). Central nervous system stimulants: The xanthines. In L.S. Goodman & A. Gilman (eds.), *The Pharmacological Basis of Therapeutics* (5th ed.) New York: MacMillan.

83. Southall, D.P., Levitt, G.A., Richards, J.M., Jones, R.A.K., Kong, C., Farndon, P.A., Alexander, J.R., & Wilson, A.J. (1983). Undetected episodes of prolonged apnea and severe bradycardia in preterm infants. Pediatrics *72*:541–551.

84. Aranda, J., Sitar, D.S., Parson, W., Loushnan, P.M., & Neims, A.H. (1976). Pharmocokinetic aspects of theophylline in premature newborns. N Engl J Med *295*:413–417.

85. Giacoia, G., Jusko, W.J., Menke, J., & Koup, S.R. (1976). Theophylline pharmacokinetics in premature infants with apnea. J Pediatr *89*:829–835.

86. Bory, C., Baltassat, P., Porthault, M., Bethenod, M., Frederich, A., & Aranda, J.V. (1979). Metabolism of theophylline to caffeine in premature newborn infants. J Pediatr *94*:988–993.

87. Wechsler, R.L., Kleiss, L.M., & Kety, S.S. (1952). The effect of intravenous administered aminophylline on cerebral circulation and metabolism in man. J Clin Invest *29*:28–30.

88. Gunn, T.R., Metrakos, K., Riley, P., Willis, D., & Aranda, J.V. (1979). Sequelae of caffeine treatment in preterm infants with apnea. J Pediatr *94*:106–109.

89. Ariagno, R.L. (1988). Management of apnea in the ICN graduate. In R.A. Ballard (ed.), *Pediatric Care of the ICN Graduate*. Philadelphia: W.B. Saunders.

90. Peabody, J., Gregory, G., Willis, M., Alistar, G.S., Lucey, P., & Lucey, J. (1979). Failure of conventional monitoring to detect apnea resulting in hypoxemia. In A. Huch, R. Huch, & J.F. Lucey (eds.), *Continuous Transcutaneous Blood Gas Monitoring*. The National Foundation–March of Dimes Birth Defects (Vol. 15, No. 4). New York, Alan R. Liss.

91. Stein, I., & Shannon, D.C. (1975). The pediatric pneumogram: A new method for detecting and quantifying apneas in infants. Pediatrics *55*:599–603.

92. Shannon, D., Gotay, F., Stein, I.M., Rogers, M.C., Todres, I.D., & Moylan, F.M.B. (1975). Prevention of apnea and bradycardia in low birth weight infants. Pediatrics *55*:589–594.

93. Fawcett, J. (1978). The what of theory development. In Theory development: What, Why and How. New York: National League for Nursing.

94. Fawcett, J. (1983). Hallmarks of success in nursing theory development. In P Chinn (ed.), *Advances in Nursing Theory Development*. Rockville, MD: Aspen Systems.

95. Roy, C. (1976). Introduction to Nursing: An Adaptation Model. Englewood Cliffs, NJ: Prentice-Hall.

96. Roy, C., & Roberts, S. (1981). *Theory Construction in Nursing: An Adaptation Model*. Englewood Cliffs, NJ: Prentice Hall.

97. Gorski, P.A., Davison, M.F., & Brazelton, T.B. (1979). Stages of behavioral organization in the high risk neonate: Theoretical and clinical considerations. Semin Perinatol *3*:61–72.

9

Alterations in Consciousness

Marylou Muwaswes

DEFINITION OF "CONSCIOUSNESS"

In 1980 the American Nurses Association (ANA) issued a definition of nursing that reflects the past function of nursing and the present influence of nursing theory on the discipline. It states: "Nursing is the diagnosis and treatment of human responses to actual or potential health problems"[1] (p. 9). Nursing is concerned with alterations of consciousness because these are changes in human behavior that impair the individual's ability to interact. Nursing has acknowledged its responsibility to assist the individual to adapt to these changes, and inherent in this responsibility is acquisition of knowledge. The knowledge that nurses seek regarding alterations of consciousness relates to the physiological, psychological, and anatomical theories of conscious behavior, methods to evaluate these behaviors, knowledge of etiological factors, and intervention strategies to assist the individual to adapt.

"Consciousness" is a word used continually, but it is difficult to define precisely because the operational properties and physiological mechanisms of conscious behavior are largely unknown.[2] Plum and Posner in their classic text, *The Diagnosis of Stupor and Coma,* define consciousness as the

> state of awareness of self and the environment . . . the content of consciousness represents the sum of the cognitive and affective mental functions. Arousal is the other aspect of consciousness and . . . behaviorally is closely linked to the appearance of wakefulness[3] (p. 3).

This definition conceptualizes consciousness into two aspects related to the behavioral function of the brain: content and arousal.

Cortical and subcortical areas of the brain interact to produce conscious behaviors. These behaviors are expressed as the ability to be aroused and the multiple complex behaviors of an individual, such as memory, thinking, and reasoning. This definition is useful, for it emphasizes the importance of utilizing behavioral descriptions to define the wide spectrum of states that represent consciousness. Consciousness cannot be observed or measured directly. Rather, observation and measurement of the behavior of an individual are done at one moment or over a given period of time. The collections of behavioral observations that are acquired about an individual then become the description of that individual's consciousness—the observed behaviors—the phenomenon of consciousness.

Using the ANA's definition of nursing as the organizing principle for the multiple levels of nursing function, alterations in consciousness can be defined as changes in the individual's behavior that impairs his or her ability to interact with the internal and external environment and to respond to change. In this chapter conscious behavior is described within the context of two clinical syndromes that commonly produce an alteration in consciousness: delirium and dementia. These two syndromes are chosen because they represent dissimilar etiological events, initial presentation, temporal patterns of signs and symptoms, and management strategies.

Although the precipitating pathophysiological events may not always be of neurological origin, the syndromes of delirium and dementia represent an abnormal state of neurological function. These syndromes are the consequence, expressed in behaviorally defined observations, of a wide variety of diseases and etiological factors. Lipowski conceptualizes each as representative of global disorders of cognitive function and identifies the primary defects in both syndromes as deficits in memory, judgment, directed thinking, and intellectual performance.[4, 5] For each of these syndromes, a definition is presented, manifestations described, and classification methods outlined.

DEMENTIA

Definition

The word "dementia" means a loss of acquired intellectual function. This is a broad term that requires further definition and description to understand its application, but even operational definitions have limitations.[6–10] Joynt and Shoulson, in a paper on dementia, state that the term means "an unusual loss of intellectual function . . . as opposed to mental retardation in which the intellect was never normal"[8] (p. 475). In addition, these authors make several pertinent points regarding the use of the term dementia: (1) the term does not imply gradual loss of intellectual function, (2) dementia is a symptom of many diseases and not a diagnostic entity, and finally, (3) dementia may be reversible. Attention directed to these points is based on the growth in knowledge in the last two decades in the fields of neurology and neuroscience and the need to clarify outdated perspectives, in particular, that dementia is not a normal consequence of the aging process but rather a consequence of specific pathophysiological disease states.[9, 10]

Prevalence and Populations at Risk

Four to 5 per cent of the United States population who are older than age 65 suffer from severe dementia. Another 10 per cent of the population older than age 65 are affected by mild to moderate dementia.[10] Jorm and associates reviewed 47 studies from 1945 to 1985 to determine the prevalence of dementia and found that the occurrence of all dementias increases with age, with rates doubling every 5.1 years.[6] Data from the Framington Study[11] and other studies confirmed this finding.[12–14] In addition to age, the prevalence of dementia varies with specific disease states. Unequivocal statistics are difficult to ascertain because of several factors: (1) the differences in diagnostic criteria used to confirm dementia vary across studies and (2) geographical and population differences are not accounted for in studies.[14]

An extensive number of diseases may cause dementia. The list provided in Table 9–1 was developed by Haase and includes more than 50 diseases.[15] Two other disorders—sarcoidosis[1] and acquired immunodeficiency syndrome (AIDS), which may produce AIDS dementia complex[16]—have been added to the list. The diffuse parenchymatous diseases and other degenerative diseases listed produce dementia by direct interference with cellular metabolism. These primary disorders are progressive, and the mental changes are irreversible.

Other etiological factors, such as space-occupying lesions, anoxia, and endocrine, cardiovascular, and metabolic disorders, secondarily may produce degenerative changes in the brain to cause the syndrome of dementia, either transiently or, if the cellular damage is severe, permanently. In addition, these factors may predispose an individual to the development of dementia if he or she is threatened by subsequent cerebral insult. The reversible causes of dementia are noted in Table 9–2.[17]

In the United States, the most common cause of severe dementia is Alzheimer's disease, which accounts for 50 to 60 per cent of all reported cases.[10] Cerebrovascular disease, which produces multi-infarct dementia, is believed to account for approximately 20 to 22 per cent of the cases of dementia. Treatable causes of dementia are estimated to account for approximately 15 per cent of cases.[10, 12] Alzheimer's disease and cerebrovascular disease dementia are known to coexist.[12] Within each category of etiological factors that may produce dementia, a relative risk may be estimated or calculated. For instance, the prevalence of dementia among patients with Parkinson's disease is between 22 and 40 per cent.[18] The most consistent complication after head injury is the development of mental symptoms.[19] Kase reviewed the epidemiology of dementia and found that multi-infarct dementia occurred more predominantly in

TABLE 9–1   DISEASES CAUSING DEMENTIA

Diffuse parenchymatous
 diseases of the central
 nervous system
So-called presenile
 dementias
 Alzheimer's disease
 Pick's disease
 Kraepelin's disease
 Parkinson-dementia
  complex of Guam
 Huntington's chorea
Senile dementia
Other degenerative
 diseases
 Hallervorden-Spatz
  syndrome
 Spinocerebellar
  degenerations
 Progressive myoclonus
  epilepsy
 Progressive
  supranuclear palsy
 Parkinson's disease
Metabolic disorders
 Myxedema
 Disorders of the
  parathyroid glands
 Wilson's disease
 Liver disease
 Hypoglycemia
 Remote effects of
  carcinoma
 Cushing's syndrome
 Hypopituitarism
 Uremia
 Dialysis dementia
 Metachromatic
  leukodystrophy
Vascular disorders
 Arteriosclerosis
 Inflammatory disease
  of blood vessels
 Disseminated lupus
  erythematosus
 Thromboangiitis
  obliterans
 Arteriovenous
  malformation
 Binswanger's disease
 Arteriovenous
  malformations
Normal pressure
 hydrocephalus
Hypoxia and anoxia

Deficiency diseases
 Wernicke-Korsakoff
  syndrome
 Pellagra
 Marchiafava-Bignami
  disease
 Vitamin B_2 and folate
  deficiency
Toxins and drugs
 Metals
 Organic compounds
 Carbon monoxide
 Drugs
Brain tumors
Trauma
 Open and closed head
  injuries
 Punch-drunk syndrome
 Subdural hematoma
 Heat stroke
Infections
 Brain abscess
 Bacterial meningitis
 Fungal meningitis
 Encephalitis
 Subacute sclerosing
  panencephalitis
 Progressive multifocal
  leukoencephalopathy
 Creutzfeldt-Jakob
  disease
 Kuru
 Behçet's syndrome
 Lues
Other diseases
 Multiple sclerosis
 Muscular dystrophy
 Whipple's disease
 Concentration-camp
  hypoxia and anoxia
  syndrome
 Kufs's disease
 Familial calcification of
  basal ganglia

From Haase, G. R. (1977). Diseases presenting as dementia. In C. E. Well (ed.), *Dementia* (pp. 27–28). Philadelphia: F. A. Davis.

men whereas Alzheimer's disease occurred more frequently in women.[12]

Prospective research reviews to determine the nature and course of Alzheimer's disease have described a familial pattern of occurrence. The estimated risk of Alzheimer's dis-

ease is 1 in 4 by age 90 for those who have first-degree relatives with the disease.[20] The pattern of incidence is not clear, and the precise genetic abnormality is uncertain. It has been found that the neuropathological features of Alzheimer's disease dementia often develop in adults with Down syndrome.[21-24] The relationship between these disorders and their genetic similarities is being investigated.

Clinical States

Dementia is a constellation of signs and symptoms that may be associated with a variety of clinical states that affect brain metabolism and function. For that reason, the methods used to classify dementia are presented. Dementia may be classified according to the age of onset, such as early-onset (before age 65) and late-onset (after age 65) primary degenerative dementia of the Alzheimer's type. Dementia is also classified ac-

TABLE 9–2   REVERSIBLE CAUSES OF DEMENTIA

Depression ("pseudodementia")
Intoxication
 Therapeutic drugs
 Alcohol
 Other substances (heavy metals, carbon monoxide)
Metabolic-endocrine derangements
 Renal failure
 Hyponatremia
 Volume depletion
 Hypoglycemia
 Hepatic failure
 Hypothyroidism
 Hyperthyroidism
 Hypercalcemia
 Cushing's syndrome
 Hypopituitarism
Brain disorders
 Stroke
 Subdural hematoma
 Infection (meningitis, neurosyphilis, abscess)
 Tumors (primary or metastatic)
 Normal pressure hydrocephalus
Cardiopulmonary disorders (congestive heart failure, arrhythmias, chronic obstructive pulmonary disease)
Generalized infection (those causing deficiencies of vitamin B_{12}, folate, and niacin)
Miscellaneous causes
 Sensory deprivation (blindness, deafness)
 Hospitalization (from isolation or anesthesia)
 Fecal impaction
 Anemia
 Remote effects of cancer

From UCLA Conference (1982). Dementia in the elderly: the silent epidemic. *Ann Intern Med, 97*:235. Reprinted with permission.

cording to etiology, which attempts to define specific characteristics of disease and differentiate the presentation of manifestations.[25] A method to classify dementia on the basis of associated clinical signs and symptoms and laboratory data is outlined in Table 9–3.[26] In addition, classification can be etiologically based on whether the dementia is reversible or irreversible (see Table 9–2).

Developmental Dimensions

The prevalence of severe dementia changes from less than 1 per cent at ages 65

TABLE 9–3   CLASSIFICATION OF DEMENTIAS

Diseases in which dementia is usually associated with clinical and laboratory signs of other medical disease
Hypothyroidism
Cushing's syndrome
Nutritional deficiency states such as pellagra, the Wernicke-Korsakoff syndrome, and subacute combined degeneration of spinal cord and brain (vitamin B_{12} deficiency)
Chronic meningoencephalitis, general paresis, meningovascular syphilis, cryptococcosis
Hepatolenticular degeneration (familial and acquired)
Brominism, chronic barbiturate intoxication

Diseases in which dementia is associated with other neurological signs but not with other obvious medical diseases
Huntington's chorea (choreoathetosis)
Schilder's disease and related demyelinative diseases (spastic weakness, pseudobulbar palsy, blindness, deafness)
Parkinson's disease
Amaurotic familial idiocy and other lipid-storage diseases (myoclonic seizures, blindness, spasticity, cerebellar ataxia)
Myoclonus epilepsy (diffuse myoclonus, generalized seizures, cerebellar ataxia)
Creutzfeldt-Jakob disease (diffuse myoclonus)
Cerebrocerebellar degeneration (cerebellar ataxia)
Cerebral-basal ganglion degeneration (apraxia-rigidity)
Dementia with spastic paraplegia (spastic legs)
Thrombotic or embolic cerebral infarction (multi-infarct)
Brain tumor (primary or metastatic, abscess)
Brain trauma, such as cerebral contusion, midbrain hemorrhage, chronic subdural hematoma
Marchiafava-Bignami disease (often with apraxia and other frontal lobe signs)
Communicating (low pressure) or obstructive hydrocephalus (often with ataxia of gait)

Diseases in which dementia is usually the only evidence of neurological or medical disease
Alzheimer's disease and senile dementia
Pick's disease

Adapted from Adams, R. A., & Victor, M. (1985). *Principles of Neurology* (p. 316). New York: McGraw-Hill.

to 70 to over 15 per cent by age 85.[10] The popular science writer Lewis Thomas has characterized Alzheimer's disease as the "disease of the century."[27] Terry and Katzman explain this characterization and speculate on the future impact that dementia may have on society.[28] If the incidence of death from heart disease, cancer, and stroke continue to decline, life expectancy rates would increase. Within this context of an increasingly aging population, dementia would become "the number one health problem"[10] (p. 498).

In summary, the syndrome of dementia may result from multiple processes that may or may not be reversible. The key issue in the search for a diagnostic entity and treatable problem represents initially the attempt to prevent further deterioration in mental function. Whatever the etiological events, the changes in mental function in dementia are somewhat stereotypical. Little is known about the precise biochemical abnormalities of each disorder or the exact anatomical correlates associated with the various types of dementia.

Mechanisms

Since the early 1970s, the number of morphological and biochemical changes described as occurring with dementia has increased.[29–34] The uncharted areas that need further exploration involve (1) knowledge of the precise relationship or causal relationship between these changes and the cognitive changes that occur with dementia and (2) the increased incidence of dementia with certain neurological diseases, such as Parkinson's disease.[35] This portion of the chapter describes the cellular changes and hypotheses of the relationship of these changes to cognitive function observed in individuals with dementia. In the text on Manifestations, the functional testing of individuals with dementia is described.

Morphological Changes

The morphological changes that occur in the brain of a person with Alzheimer's disease are also found, to a lesser degree and with a different distribution, in nondemented aged brains.[36] The gross changes in the anatomy of the brain in dementia include decreased brain weight and thinning of the sulci, suggestive of atrophy.[14] Cortical and central atrophy is common in all types of dementia.

Often the functional neurological deficits are greater than these gross changes indicate, which suggests that the cellular abnormalities are at a more microscopic level.

The cellular degeneration found in the brains of individuals with Alzheimer's disease is characterized by the presence and number of neurofibrillary tangles and the presence of neuritic or amyloid plaques found in the hippocampus and widely distributed in the cerebral cortex.[10, 14, 37, 38] In addition, granulovascular changes have been found in the Hirano bodies in the hippocampus.[28, 39] Evidence suggests a specific pattern of cellular pathology that involves the major projection neurons of the hippocampal formation, which in effect isolates the association cortices, basal forebrain, thalamus, and hypothalamus from the hippocampus.[30, 38]

Since the initial work of Tomlinson and associates,[40] which correlated the degree and severity of the morphological changes (neurofibrillary tangles and neuritic plaques) with the occurrence of dementia, the severity and degree of clinical presentation of dementia in Alzheimer's disease are believed to be correlated positively with the extent of neuroanatomical abnormalities, specifically the number of amyloid plaques.[41, 42]

Neurofibrillary tangles are also found at post-mortem examination in brains of individuals with Down syndrome,[10] Parkinson's dementia,[43] and postencephalitic parkinsonism.[36] The histological pattern of lesions described as occurring in Alzheimer's disease represents the most common pattern found in demented individuals. With multi-infarct dementia, which commonly is caused by cerebrovascular disease or hypertension, multiple areas of cellular infarction characterized by cellular degeneration typical of ischemia occur. The areas involved in multi-infarct dementia are primarily cortical, with white matter degeneration. The infarcts may be large or small, cortical and subcortical, or lacunar, with widespread white matter ischemic changes.[44]

Biochemical Changes

A reduced concentration of the enzyme choline acetyltransferase (ChAT) in the neocortex and hippocampus is the biochemical abnormality confirmed most often in brain tissue of individuals affected by Alzheimer's disease.[32] This enzyme catalyzes the acetylation of choline to the neurotransmitter acetylcholine and is present in small quantities in cholinergic cells.[39] Muscarinic cholinergic receptors are present in normal amounts in the brain tissue.[10] The reduction of ChAT, and therefore acetylcholine, in the cortex may be related to the decreasing numbers of neurons in the basal forebrain nuclei. The relationship of these cellular abnormalities to the clinical manifestations of Alzheimer's disease is based on the finding that the neuroanatomical pathways involved with maintenance of memory are cholinergic pathways and that cells of the hippocampus involved with memory are innervated by cholinergic pathways.[30] In fact, the degree of reduction of ChAT has been correlated positively with the density of neurofibrillary tangles, senile plaques, and the degree of dementia.[23] The cholinergic deficiencies found in Alzheimer's disease, although the severest, may be only one of many interacting biochemical abnormalities of synaptic transmission.[45] A recent promising avenue of research has identified specific gene mutations of DNA in persons with Alzheimer's disease.[41]

Pathological Consequences

The treatable dementias outlined in Table 9–2 represent a form of dementia in which the cognitive impairment may be reversible if treated early and with success. The primary dementias, such as Alzheimer's disease, Creutzfeldt-Jakob disease, and Pick's disease, represent forms of dementia in which there is a progressive decline in cognitive function. The inevitable outcome of this decline results in the inability to perform self-care activities and progressive and continued social, physical, and intellectual isolation.[46]

The pathophysiological alterations, measured by morphological and biochemical changes in cellular brain function, vary according to the underlying causes of the dementia.

Related Pathophysiological Concepts

Alterations in consciousness (dementia) are related to other pathophysiological concepts in either a causative or an outcome relationship. Ischemia and hypoxia are two states that can cause an alteration in consciousness through their pathological effects on cellular metabolism in the brain. Sleep is a concept that is considered to be a "normal" variation in consciousness, that is, not caused by illness or pathology but a variation nonetheless. Because of the dysfunction in cognition that affects an individual's ability to care for oneself, those with dementia may at any point in their course experience alterations in other physiological phenomena. For instance, sleep patterns are often disturbed in individuals with Alzheimer's and Parkinson's diseases. Alterations in mobility, infection, and appetite may result from the inability to care for oneself.

In normal aging, morphological changes occur, as previously mentioned, that differ in severity, extent, and location as compared with the changes that occur in dementia.[36] The similarity of these changes to those observed in dementia has encouraged some investigators to speculate on whether a certain type of dementia associated with aging (Alzheimer's disease) may represent an accelerated aging process in the brain.[20]

Associated Psychological Concepts

Benign senescent forgetfulness may resemble dementia.[47] As the nervous system ages, some functional changes in complex neuronal circuits occur as a result of a slowdown in reaction time. These cellular changes may be manifested functionally as an inability to remember and recall names and details rapidly or as problems in responding to novel situations.[48, 49] These changes are called benign because they do not interfere with maintaining an independent life style; they do not progress, as in dementia; and life expectancy is not shortened. The range and severity of intellectual dysfunction seen in dementia are not apparent in careful testing of benign senescent forgetfulness.

Dementia and depression may resemble each other, especially early in the course of dementia, when memory impairment may be the only prominent feature.[7] The manifestation common to both depression and dementia is the subjective reporting of some type of memory impairment. The subjective memory complaints must be followed up with formal testing. Subjective, rather than objective, memory impairment is more common

in depressive illness. Memory lapse that is severe enough to interfere with intellectual function, as measured objectively through the mental status examination, is termed "pseudodementia." Sufficient overlap may occur between the results of mental status function in a demented individual and one with depression. Complicating the differentiation of depression from dementia is the fact that depression can coexist with dementia.[50–52]

Manifestations

Objective Manifestations

Consciousness cannot be measured directly. Dementia and delirium represent syndromes that delineate specific observable behaviors related to conscious behavior. The physiological measurements described here represent attempts to visualize brain structures and measure brain function. None of these measurements is diagnostic for delirium or dementia but provides information that aids in the differential diagnosis of the etiological factors that may cause cognitive impairment.

Electroencephalographic (EEG) findings in Alzheimer's disease with moderate or severe dementia show symmetrical, usually diffuse slowing from the normal pattern of waveform. There is a high degree of correlation between slowing of the EEG and the presence and degree of cognitive impairment.[10, 53] The EEG slowing is not diagnostic for Alzheimer's disease, since it occurs in other diseases that involve cognitive impairment, such as multi-infarct dementia, and forms of delirium other than delirium tremens.[4] The value of the EEG lies in its ability to help differentiate whether the etiological process underlying the cognitive changes is focal or diffuse.[28] For example, the EEG of multi-infarct dementia shows more frequent paroxysmal activity and focal abnormalities.

Computed tomography (CT) and magnetic resonance imaging (MRI) are techniques used to visualize the structural components of the brain. The CT scan is a more widely used and less expensive procedure. Like MRI, it can detect brain atrophy and structural lesions and is helpful in the differential diagnosis of dementia. MRI is superior to CT scan in the differential diagnosis of multi-infarct dementia versus Alzheimer's disease.

MRI provides greater resolution of brain structures, and therefore detection of small subcortical infarcts and white matter changes is possible.[54-57]

Global cerebral blood flow is reduced in both multi-infarct dementia and Alzheimer's disease, the amplitude of the reduction often depending on the severity of the dementia. Cerebrovascular disease may produce dementia by causing infarction of large and small vessels, and the reduction in global cerebral blood flow is often bilateral. These processes then interfere with cognitive function. The precise relationship between specific vessel disease and the development of cognitive impairment is not known.[44]

Several investigative groups have described the pattern of lesion distribution in cases of ischemic stroke with and without dementia. Dementia associated with ischemic stroke occurred more frequently, with bilateral and dominant hemisphere lesions often in the temporoparietal lobe.[57] Infarcts associated with dementia were also found in the thalamus and basal ganglia, although not exclusively in these regions.[54, 56]

Particular patterns were noted on the positron emission tomographic (PET) scan of individuals with Alzheimer's disease. This imaging technique studies brain function in vivo, not brain structure, as do CT scans and MRI. Researchers found that although oxygen extraction is normal[28] (unlike that in an ischemic event), glucose metabolism and blood flow oxygen metabolism were reduced in the temporal and parietal lobes.[58] Progression of dementia severity often leads to involvement of decreasing cortical metabolism.

The phrase "intellectual function" covers a wide variety of complex mental operations—what Plum and Posner describe as the content of consciousness.[2] Operations such as memory, thinking, abstraction, and reasoning are impaired. Plum and Posner also suggest that the decline in cognitive function observed in dementia is not necessarily accompanied by a reduction in the arousal aspect of consciousness. Other brain functions may also be affected in dementia, but usually defects in these functions are not described specifically as dementia[5] and may be related to the specific diseases that cause dementia.

The *Diagnostic and Statistical Manual of Mental Disorders* (DSM-III-R)[7] presents criteria that define the critical aspects of the syndrome of dementia. Application of these criteria in the clinical setting (Table 9–4) does not delineate etiological factors but those behaviors specific to dementia and distinct from delirium. Although dementia is described as a change in behavior, the use of dementia as a diagnostic entity is meaningless unless the results of the clinical examination, formal testing, and patient history are placed within the context of a clear chronological history of cognitive impairment and the findings from a complete medical examination to determine the causative factor.

With progressive degenerative dementia, such as Alzheimer's disease, the memory loss initially may be so mild that it goes unnoticed. The loss of intellectual function eventually becomes evident in those behaviors of daily living that require intellectual ability rather than physical ability. In cases of primary degenerative dementia, loss of intellectual function leads to loss of physical function. Distinction is made between global decline in intellectual function that can be evaluated by the mental status examination and tested through questions of memory, orientation, and the individual's history and a specific loss of intellectual function, as represented by aphasia, apraxia, and agnosia.[46, 47]

The central features in the clinical presentation of Alzheimer's disease are impairment of recent memory and subsequent progressive decline in cognitive function.[10] Other salient features, perhaps resulting from these primary impairments, include changes in personality and manifestations of affective disturbances.[46] The clinical course of an individual with Alzheimer's disease subsequent to the initial memory loss may demonstrate individual differences and patterns of progression. Other neurological findings in Alzheimer's disease that occur later in the course include aphasia, agnosia, and apraxia. The inevitable effect of Alzheimer's disease on the individual is progressive, irreversible loss of functional ability to a state of total dependence.[14, 59] The diagnosis of Alzheimer's disease during life is based on clinical criteria for the presence of dementia, medical testing to rule out other clinical conditions that may resemble the dementia of Alzheimer's disease, and pathological confirmation post mortem to identify specific neuroanatomical abnormalities found with Alzheimer's disease. Because there is presently no definitive clinical marker for Alzheimer's disease, a diagnosis made on the basis of clinical find-

TABLE 9–4   DIAGNOSTIC CRITERIA FOR DELIRIUM AND DEMENTIA

Dementia (At Least Three of the Following Must Be Present)
A. Demonstrable evidence of impairment in short-term and long-term memory. Impairment in short-term memory (inability to learn new information) may be indicated by inability to remember three objects after 5 minutes. Long-term memory impairment (inability to remember information that was known in the past) may be indicated by inability to remember past personal information (e.g., what happened yesterday, birthplace, occupation) or facts of common knowledge (e.g., past presidents, well-known dates).
B. At least one of the following:
   (1) Impairment in abstract thinking, as indicated by inability to find similarities and differences between related words, difficulty in defining words and concepts, and other similar tasks.
   (2) Impaired judgment, as indicated by inability to make reasonable plans to deal with interpersonal, family, and job-related problems and issues.
   (3) Other disturbances of higher cortical function, such as aphasia (disorder of language), apraxia (inability to carry out motor activities despite intact comprehension and motor function), agnosia (failure to recognize or identify objects despite intact sensory function), and "constructional difficulty" (e.g., inability to copy three-dimensional figures, assemble blocks, or arrange sticks in specific designs).
   (4) Personality change (i.e., alteration or accentuation of premorbid traits).
C. The disturbance in A and B significantly interferes with work or usual social activities or relationships with others.
D. Not occurring exclusively during the course of delirium.
E. Either (1) or (2):
   (1) There is evidence from the history, physical examination, or laboratory tests of a specific organic factor (or factors) judged to be etiologically related to the disturbance.
   (2) In the absence of such evidence, an etiological organic factor can be presumed if the disturbance cannot be accounted for by any nonorganic mental disorder (e.g., major depression accounting for cognitive impairment).

Criteria for Severity of Dementia
Mild: Although work or social activities are significantly impaired, the capacity for independent living remains, with adequate personal hygiene and relatively intact judgment.
Moderate: Independent living is hazardous, and some degree of supervision is necessary.
Severe: Activities of daily living are so impaired that continual supervision is required (e.g., unable to maintain minimal personal hygiene, largely incoherent or mute).

Delirium (At Least Three of the Following Must Be Present)
A. Reduced ability to maintain attention to external stimuli (e.g., questions must be repeated because attention wanders) and to appropriately shift attention to new external stimuli (e.g., perseverates answer to a previous question).
B. Disorganized thinking, as indicated by rambling, irrelevant, or incoherent speech.
C. At least two of the following:
   (1) Reduced level of consciousness (e.g., difficulty keeping awake during examination).
   (2) Perceptual disturbances: misinterpretations, illusions, or hallucinations.
   (3) Disturbance of sleep-wake cycle with insomnia or daytime sleepiness.
   (4) Increased or decreased psychomotor activity.
   (5) Disorientation to time, place, or person.
   (6) Memory impairment (e.g., inability to learn new material, such as the names of several unrelated objects after 5 minutes, or to remember past events, such as history of current episode of illness).
D. Clinical features develop over a short period of time (usually hours to days) and tend to fluctuate over the course of a day.
E. Either (1) or (2):
   (1) Evidence from the history, physical examination, or laboratory tests of a specific organic factor (or factors) judged to be etiologically related to the disturbance.
   (2) In the absence of such evidence, an etiological organic factor can be presumed if the disturbance cannot be accounted for by any nonorganic mental disorder (e.g., manic episode accounting for agitation and sleep disturbance).

From *Diagnostic and Statistical Manual of Mental Disorders III-Revised.* (1987). Washington, D.C.: American Psychiatric Association.

ings alone may be erroneous, particularly early in the disease.[14]

During the early course of dementia due to multiple infarcts, the picture of cognitive impairment may resemble that of Alzheimer's disease, and differentiation between these two entities poses a problem. The Hachinski Ischemic Score, a clinical tool developed by Hachinski and associates,[60] has been used with some success to differentiate Alzheimer's disease from multi-infarct dementia.[60] Table 9–5 presents the items scored during the examination and emphasizes, in particular, that a higher score, indicating greater risk of ischemic dementia, is based on a past history of cardiac disease, the presence of associated focal neurological findings, and an abrupt onset and fluctuating course of mental symptoms.[61, 62] Other investigators have pointed out that the temporal relation-

TABLE 9–5 HACHINSKI ISCHEMIC SCORE

Instructions: Record the presence or absence of the clinical features of dementia listed below and add the point values assigned each feature (value in parentheses) whenever "present" is checked. Summation of points produces an ischemic score. A score of 4 indicates a patient with pure Alzheimer's type of dementia (ATD); a score of 7 indicates a patient with multi-infarction dementia (MID) or mixed ATD and MID.

Feature	Point Value	Absent	Present
Abrupt onset	(2)		
Stepwise deterioration	(1)		
Fluctuating course	(2)		
Nocturnal confusion	(1)		
Relative preservation of personality	(1)		
Depression	(1)		
Somatic complaints	(1)		
Emotional incontinence	(1)		
History of hypertension	(1)		
History of strokes	(2)		
Evidence of associated atherosclerosis	(1)		
Focal neurological symptoms	(2)		
Focal neurological signs	(1)		
TOTAL ISCHEMIC SCORE:			

Modified from Hachinski, V. C., Iliff, L. D., Zilkha, E., DuBoulay, G. H., McAllister, V. L., Marshall, J., Russell, R. W. R., & Symon, L. (1975). Cerebral blood flow in dementia. Arch Neurol 32:632–637. Copyright 1975, American Medical Association.

ship between the evidence of brain ischemia and dementia is another important clinical factor in differentiating multi-infarct dementia from Alzheimer's disease.[44]

DELIRIUM

Definition

Delirium is defined as "a transient mental disorder reflecting acute brain failure due to widespread derangement of cerebral metabolism."[4, 5] Delirium is characterized by disorders of cognition, wakefulness, and psychomotor behavioral disturbances.

Prevalence and Populations at Risk

The prevalence of delirium is difficult to know directly because, like dementia, it is not a diagnostic entity and precise epidemiological studies do not exist.[64] Engel and Romano estimated that between 10 and 15 per cent of individuals in acute medical and surgical units have some form of delirium.[63] Morse and Litin, retrospectively, identified 60 postoperative patients with delirium over a 6-month period.[65] This group represented 54 per cent of the postoperative patients for this period, exclusive of those undergoing surgical procedures that could alter sensory intake. Dubin and associates, in a retrospective literature review, found that between 1967 and 1977 the reported incidence of postcardiotomy delirium changed from 13 to 67 per cent.[66] In another study, 20 per cent of elderly patients admitted to an acute care hospital experienced delirium during their hospital stay. The following factors were associated with the appearance of delirium: abnormal sodium levels, severe illness, chronic pre-existing cognitive dysfunction, hypothermia or hyperthermia, use of psychoactive drugs, and azotemia.[67]

As with dementia, the etiological factors that may cause delirium are extensive. In fact, because of its complex organization, the brain is particularly vulnerable to any adverse change in its internal environment. The wide range of processes and diseases that potentially may produce delirium reflect this principle, and the development of delirium is often multifactorial.

Plum and Posner noted that of all the metabolic etiological factors that may alter consciousness (Table 9–6) and produce the syndrome of delirium, the most commonly encountered in an acute care setting are ischemia, hypoxia, hypoglycemia, drug intoxications, and postsurgical or intensive care unit psychosis.[2] These investigators have identified a group of disorders that can cause delirium but do not cause stupor and coma and that are generally self-limited but can be fatal if not treated properly and adequately. These include withdrawal from sedative drugs and alcohol; acute intoxication with drugs such as propranolol, cimetidine, and digitalis; and intoxications with a wide range of psychotropic drugs.[68] In elderly individuals or people with systemic disease that interferes with drug metabolism, delirium from drug ingestion can appear at lower than expected drug dosages. In drug intoxication, although the agent can often be identified, the biochemical abnormality is uncertain, and

TABLE 9–6   CAUSES OF STUPOR AND COMA

I. **Deprivation of oxygen, substrate, or metabolic cofactors**
   *A. Hypoxia (interference with oxygen supply to the entire brain, cerebral blood flow [CBF] normal)
      1. Decreased Po_2 and O_2 content: pulmonary disease, alveolar hypoventilation, decreased atmospheric oxygen tension
      2. Decreased blood O_2 content, Po_2 normal—"anemic anoxia": anemia, carbon monoxide poisoning, methemoglobinemia
   *B. Ischemia (diffuse or widespread multifocal interference with blood supply to brain)
      1. Decreased CBF resulting from decreased cardiac output: Stokes-Adams syndrome, cardiac arrest, cardiac arrhythmias, myocardial infarction, congestive heart failure, aortic stenosis, pulmonary embolus
      2. Decreased CBF resulting from decreased peripheral resistance in systemic circulation: syncope, carotid sinus hypersensitivity, low blood volume
      3. Decreased CBF flow associated with generalized or multifocal increase in cerebrovascular resistance: hyperventilation syndrome, increased blood viscosity (polycythemia, cryoglobulinemia and macroglobulinemia, sickle cell anemia), subarachnoid hemorrhage, bacterial meningitis, hypertensive encephalopathy
      4. Decreased local CBF owing to widespread small vessel occlusion: disseminated intravascular coagulation, systemic lupus erythematosus, subacute bacterial endocarditis, cardiopulmonary bypass, fat embolism, cerebral malaria
   *C. Hypoglycemia: from exogenous insulin, spontaneous (endogenous insulin, liver disease)
   D. Cofactor deficiency: thiamin (Wernicke's encephalopathy), niacin, pyridoxine, folic acid, cyanocobalamin

II. **Diseases of organs other than brain**
   *A. Diseases of nonendocrine organs: liver, hepatic coma; kidney, uremic coma; lung, CO_2 narcosis
   B. Hyperfunction or hypofunction of endocrine organs: pituitary, thyroid (myxedema-thyrotoxicosis), parathyroid (hyperparathyroidism and hypoparathyroidism), adrenal gland (Addison's disease, Cushing's disease, pheochromocytoma), pancreas (diabetes, hypoglycemia)
   C. Other systemic diseases: diabetes mellitus, cancer, porphyria, sepsis, fever

III. **Exogenous poisons**
   *A. Sedative drugs: barbiturates, tranquilizers, bromides, ethanol, opiates
   B. Acid poisons or poisons with acidic breakdown products: paraldehyde, methyl alcohol, ethylene glycol, ammonium
   C. Psychotropic drugs: tricyclic antidepressants and anticholinergic drugs, amphetamines, lithium, phenothiazides, lysergic acid diethylamide (LSD)-mescaline, monoamine oxidase inhibitors
   D. Others: penicillin, anticonvulsants, steroids, cardiac glycosides, salicylates, heavy metals, cimetidine, organic phosphates

IV. **Abnormalities of fluid, ionic or acid-base environment of CNS:** hyponatremia, hypoosmolality and hyperosmolality, acidosis (metabolic and respiratory), alkalosis (metabolic and respiratory); magnesium (hypermagnesemia and hypomagnesemia), calcium (hypercalcemic and hypocalcemia) phosphorus (hypophosphatemia) disorders

V. **Disordered temperature regulation:** hypothermia, heat stroke, fever

VI. **Infections or inflammation of the central nervous system:** leptomeningitis, encephalitis, acute encephalopathy, cerebral vasculitis, subarachnoid hemorrhage

VII. **Miscellaneous diseases of unknown cause:** seizures and postictal states, concussion, acute delirious states* (sedative drug withdrawal, postoperative delirium, intensive care unit delirium, drug intoxication)

From Plum, F., & Posner, J. B. (1980). *The Diagnosis of Stupor and Coma* (3rd ed., pp. 178–180). Philadelphia: F. A. Davis.
*Alone or in combination, the most common causes of delirium seen on medical or surgical wards.

in such disorders as postoperative delirium, neither the agent nor the abnormality is well known.[69, 70]

Psychotropic drugs with anticholinergic properties can induce delirium. Other drugs, although they may not directly affect brain cholinergic systems, can, if used in conjunction with anticholinergics, potentiate the action of these drugs through synergistic action; clonidine is an example.[71] The tricyclic antidepressants can cause delirium in the elderly.[72] The least potent antipsychotic drugs, such as chlorpromazine and thioridazine, also have the most potent anticholinergic effects[72, 73] (Table 9–7.)

Situational Stressors

There appear to be individual differences in susceptibility to delirium in response to any specific etiological factor. The nature of this susceptibility has remained elusive. Several etiological factors have been defined that are by no means conclusive or inclusive. Lipowski lists these as follows: (1) age 50 years or older, (2) addiction to alcohol or drugs, and (3) cerebral damage due to any cause and sustained at any age[4] (p. 244). Additional factors, such as prolonged immobilization, sleep deprivation, and situations that alter

TABLE 9–7   PSYCHOTROPIC DRUGS, POTENCIES, AND SIDE EFFECTS

Agent	Relative Potency	Predominant Side Effects	Usual Initial Daily Dose for the Elderly
Chlorpromazine	100	Sedating, anticholinergic	10–25 mg b.i.d. or t.i.d. times a day
Thioridazine	95–100	Sedating, anticholinergic	10–25 mg b.i.d. or t.i.d. times a day
Thiothixene	5	Extrapyramidal	2–3 mg
Haloperidol	2	Extrapyramidal	0.5–2 mg
Fluphenazine	2	Extrapyramidal	0.5–2 mg

From Thompson, T.L., Moran, M.G., & Nies, A.S. (1983). Psychotropic drug use in the elderly. Pt II. Reprinted by permission of The New England Journal of Medicine. *308*:194–199.

the quality and quantity of sensory input, may also facilitate the onset of delirium or increase its severity or duration.

Clinical States

Another difficulty with estimating incidence of delirium is that the terminology used by various disciplines—medicine and psychiatry, for example—is not consistent in describing the behavioral manifestations that occur with this syndrome. For example, metabolic encephalopathy is a term used in medicine to describe any number of behavioral changes that result from disruption of metabolism of the brain. Plum further defines this state on the basis of the initial presenting metabolic defect.[68] Primary, or endogenous, encephalopathy results when there is intrinsic failure of neuronal or glial metabolism. Secondary, or exogenous, encephalopathy is a disruption of brain metabolism owing to extracerebral causes. The clinical pattern of presentation of behavioral symptoms may resemble either dementia or delirium. The conditions mentioned previously that place the individual at risk for delirium—ischemia, hypoxia, and hypoglycemia—are also the clinical states associated with the syndrome of delirium.

Mechanisms

Delirium can be viewed as a widespread and generalized impairment of cerebral function that accompanies diffuse metabolic and multifocal cerebral disease.[4, 70] The precise pathophysiological mechanism responsible for producing the signs and symptoms of delirium depends on the etiological event. Whatever the event (or more likely, events), it involves primary or secondary disruption in systemic systems that influence cerebral cellular respiration: energy supply, delivery

of adequate substrate to meet metabolic needs, and requirements to remove metabolic waste products. Delirium is manifested by an alteration in cognitive function as well as an alteration in arousal.[2, 69] The observation that the symptoms and signs of delirium reflect global brain dysfunction suggests that the impairment in cellular function is also global and widespread. The alteration in behavior produced by any illness or disease that causes delirium is quantitatively related to the degree of loss of cortical cellular function.[74]

Delirium may occur in the pathophysiological states of hypoxia and hypoglycemia, in which availability of the substrates oxygen and glucose is diminished. The clinical appearance of delirium usually accompanies oxygen uptakes below 2.5 ml per 100 g of brain tissue per minute; when the uptake falls below 2.0 ml per 100 g of brain tissue per minute, most patients are unconscious.[74] The appearance of clinical symptoms that occur with hypoxia depends not only on the absolute arterial oxygen levels—levels below 50 mm Hg cause delirium, and those below 25 mm Hg cause coma—but also on the hemoglobin concentration, cerebral blood flow, and serum pH. The appearance of clinical signs and symptoms with hypoglycemia may vary from individual to individual. Posner suggests, in general, that glucose levels below 30 mg/dl cause confusion.[74]

The neuroanatomical appearance of the brain in some individuals who have been delirious during life is normal at post-mortem examination.[74] In other instances, identifiable pathological cerebral changes can be seen, most commonly those observed after anoxia, ischemia, or hypoglycemia. These changes consist of the appearance of microscopic microvacuoles in the cytoplasm of the neurons of the cortex and hippocampus that represent swollen mitochondria. As the insult becomes more severe, Nissl granules appear and there is generalized pallor. With prolonged insult, neurons in the cerebral cortex may disappear and the third layer of the cortex may disintegrate. Anoxic changes may affect the basal ganglia, and there may be diffuse demyelination of subcortical gray matter.[74] A pathological finding in individuals who have died of uremia, hypoxemia, diabetic coma, or carbon dioxide narcosis is cerebral swelling.[74]

In many cases of metabolic encephalopathy that cause delirium, the cerebral oxygen uptake declines in approximate proportion to the degree of brain dysfunction observed through the clinical examination—unlike the findings in Alzheimer's disease. The most severe consequence is that if delirium is left untreated, a potentially reversible process becomes irreversible.

Several authorities suggest that the clinical presentation in many of the above disorders is similar.[74, 75] The variation of presentation seen in individuals, as outlined previously, may be the result of the severity of the metabolic derangement rather than of the specific etiological factor. This is difficult to confirm, partly because of the problems in administering a mental status examination to a delirious individual, but it is certainly an interesting question to address.

Related Pathophysiological Concepts

As with dementia, the physiological concepts related to delirium are the etiological factors. These are presented in Table 9–6. In clinical situations in which the causative factor can be clearly identified, such as drug-induced delirium or hypoxia-induced delirium, the underlying mechanism is related to the pathophysiological events specific to that condition. In other clinical situations, such as intensive care unit psychosis or postsurgical delirium, the pathophysiological events are unclear. Whether or not there is a common biochemical abnormality present in all the clinical states that produce delirium is open to speculation. The commonality of behavioral manifestations has encouraged some investigators to hypothesize that cholinergic pathways[48] or central monoamine pathways may be altered with metabolic encephalopathies.

Stupor, coma, confusion, and obtundation are other terms used to define clinical conditions or states. These states are related to

delirium because of an overlap of certain manifestations of each. In stupor, coma, and obtundation, the similarity to delirium is related to the observations that these states represent and are manifested by a defect in arousal, which makes evaluation of the content of consciousness impossible. In confusion, which is an imprecise term, the content and arousal aspects of consciousness may be altered.[3] Delirium may precede stupor and coma in specific clinical disorders but does not always progress to stupor and coma.

Related Psychological Concepts

Delirium is classified by the DSM III-R[7] under the category of organic brain syndromes as one of seven descriptive psychopathological syndromes, as is dementia. The other syndromes that delirium must be distinguished from are hallucinosis, the amnestic syndrome, organic personality syndrome, organic affective syndrome, and organic delusional syndrome. The distinguishing characteristics are presented for each of these syndromes (Table 9–8). The classification of these last two syndromes remains controversial because they lack the traditional characteristics that allow categorization of these behaviors as organic and because they overlap with disorders regarded as functional.[4, 31]

Manifestations

Objective Manifestations

Both global and focal brain functional abnormalities can be produced by disruptions of cerebral metabolism either directly or indirectly. The global symptoms include alterations in the level of alertness, attention, comprehension, and cognitive synthesis.[74] Focal abnormalities include defects in recent memory storage and recall, language recognition and synthesis, and perhaps hallucinations.

The clinical manifestations of delirium may vary from individual to individual. The onset, which may be rapid or gradual, is characterized as acute or subacute and is a transient phenomenon. Although it is difficult to quantify delirium relative to the observed mental status changes, Lipowski outlines a pattern of severity that is helpful as a basis for organ-

TABLE 9–8   DIAGNOSTIC CRITERIA FOR ORGANIC BRAIN SYNDROMES OTHER THAN DELIRIUM AND DEMENTIA

Disorder	Criterion
Organic hallucinosis	A. Prominent, persistent or recurrent hallucinations. B. Evidence from the history, physical examination, or laboratory tests of a specific organic factor (or factors) judged to be etiologically related to the disturbance. C. Not occurring exclusively during the course of delirium.
Amnestic syndrome	A. Demonstrable evidence of impairment in both short-term and long-term memory; with regard to long-term memory, very remote events are remembered better than more recent events. Impairment in short-term memory (inability to learn new information) may be indicated by inability to remember three objects after 5 minutes. Long-term memory impairment may be indicated by inability to remember past personal information. B. Not occurring exclusively during the course of delirium and does not meet the criteria for dementia. C. There is evidence from the history, physical examination, or laboratory tests of a specific organic factor (or factors) judged to be etiologically related to the disturbance.
Organic delusional syndrome	A. Prominent delusions. B. There is evidence from the history, physical examination, or laboratory tests of a specific organic factor (or factors) judged to be etiologically related to the disturbance. C. Not occurring exclusively during the course of delirium.
Organic mood syndrome	A. Prominent and persistent depressed, elevated, or expansive mood. B. There is evidence from the history, physical examination, or laboratory tests of a specific organic factor (or factors) judged to be etiologically related to the disturbance. C. Not occurring exclusively during the course of delirium. Specify manic, depressed, or mixed.
Organic anxiety syndrome	A. Prominent, recurrent, panic attacks or generalized anxiety. B. There is evidence from the history, physical examination, or laboratory tests of a specific organic factor (or factors) judged to be etiologically related to the disturbance. C. Not occurring exclusively during the course of delirium.
Organic personality syndrome	A. A persistent personality disturbance, either lifelong or representing a change or accentuation of a previously characteristic trait, involving at least one of the following: (1) affective instability (e.g., marked shifts from normal mood to depression, irritability, or anxiety) (2) recurrent outbursts of aggression or rage that are grossly out of proportion to any precipitating psychosocial stressors (3) markedly impaired social judgment (e.g., sexual indiscretions) (4) marked apathy and indifference (5) suspiciousness or paranoid ideation. B. There is evidence from the history, physical examination, or laboratory tests of a specific organic factor (or factors) judged to be etiologically related to the disturbance. C. This diagnosis is not given to a child or adolescent if the clinical picture is limited to the features that characterize attention-deficit hyperactivity disorder. D. Not occurring exclusively during the course of delirium and does not meet the criteria for dementia. Specify explosive type if outbursts of aggression or rage are the predominant feature.

Compiled from *Diagnostic and Statistical Manual of Mental Disorders III-Revised.* (1987). Washington, D.C.: American Psychiatric Association.

izing the clinical features of this syndrome.[5] In the early stages, the symptoms may reflect changes in mentation and awareness. These changes may be transient and fluctuate throughout the day. Sleep disturbances are common during the early stages of delirium and may first appear as vivid dreams or nightmares. In fact, Lipowski states that delirium may be characterized as a disturbance of the sleep-wake cycle.[4, 5] It is not uncommon for this cycle to be reversed or for the sleep to be frequently interrupted. The seemingly mild initial changes in mental status that characterize delirium in fact herald potentially severe consequences. Although some individuals may never progress beyond these mild changes, these changes may precede a more intense phase of delirium.

Lipowski points out that during the early phases of delirium the individual may recognize the change in cognitive function and may develop coping behaviors to manage the adverse behaviors.[4, 5] These coping behaviors may present as depression, anxiety, anger, guilt, shame, withdrawal, and denial. The depressed individual may remain quiet, and therefore the cognitive changes will not be recognized unless specific testing is performed to ascertain them.

If the delirium progresses, the milder features may give way to more severe manifestations that reflect increased brain tissue involvement. The misperceptions of the early phase may progress to hallucinations worsened by sleep disturbances. The manifestations of this more severe phase characterize not only the increased disorganization of cognitive function but also the unique variability of each affected individual's behavior. One individual may react with wild fear and become combative and agitated, whereas another may become withdrawn and develop an apathetic demeanor and may be interested only in picking at the bedsheets in a seemingly purposeless manner. During this phase, the abnormal behavior observed may again fluctuate between normal and abnormal, with brief intervals when the individual is lucid.

Lipowski emphasizes that individuals with delirium may appear either quiet or hyperalert. He succinctly describes this: "Thinking may be slow, labored and impoverished or the contrary—speeded up and rich with disturbed imagery"[76] (p. 191). In either case, recall for the period the memory disturbance occurred may be lost; when recovery occurs, the individual is amnestic for this period. In individuals who can recall their misperceptions, it is not known whether this may reflect a less severe form of delirium.

Posner and Plum offer a helpful organization to evaluate the wide array of behavioral changes that occur with delirium.[2] The defects observed in delirium can be evaluated in terms of attention, alertness, orientation, grasp, memory, affect, and perception. In the early phases of delirium, mental status testing can be helpful. But once the point of stupor is reached, the examination becomes difficult to use and inaccurate to apply. Strub

and Black highlight this latter point in their text, *The Mental Status Exam,* noting that when the individual loses the ability to attend or pay attention to the environment, use of the question-answer format of the mental status examination becomes difficult to administer and interpret.[77] The phrase they use to emphasize this concern is "attention presupposes alertness but alertness does not imply attention."[77]

EEG waves were always slowed in delirium, reflective of the widespread derangement.[63] Obrecht and Sachdev and their associates indicated that the value of the EEG in acute confusional states is based on the finding that specific focal abnormalities can be demonstrated suggestive of focal intracranial pathology, as opposed to the general slowing seen with metabolic encephalopathy.[78, 79] Others have disagreed with this finding, citing the example of delirium tremens.[2, 76] More extensive studies of brain metabolism during delirium are lacking because of the problem inherent in testing individuals during such an acute phase of illness.

Subjective Manifestations

Individuals may not notice the mental changes that occur with delirium, or they may complain of a wide variety of mental changes related to concentration, memory, disturbance of the sleep-wake cycle, and misperceptions. Complaints may be expressed about the vividness of dreams or the presence of hallucinations.[2] There may be indications that the individual has difficulty focusing and sustaining attention on tasks that require concentrated mental efforts. In some cases of a mild disorder, the individual may awake confused and disoriented and have problems recognizing the surroundings if they are unfamiliar. In such instances, the individual can be assisted by reorientation. Reports of awareness of disorientation and hallucinations appeared in the literature related to postcardiotomy delirium.[80] Because the nature and severity of the delirium was not well described, it is difficult to evaluate the meaning of these reports. The disorientation and difficulty with memory commonly are unrecognized by the individual, and on recovery there is no recall of the delirious period.

SURVEILLANCE AND MEASUREMENT OF DELIRIUM AND DEMENTIA

The clinical measurement of the behavioral manifestations of the syndromes of delirium and dementia follows a systematic and organized format that includes observation, history taking, and specific testing techniques based on a hierarchical system of stimulus and response. Because mental status and cognitive function in particular may be elusive phenomena to test clinically, various methods of evaluation and measurement have been proposed.

When one is evaluating any tool or format that assesses mental status, three considerations should be kept in mind: (1) know the purpose of the tool and why it was developed, (2) determine the accuracy of the tool in its ability to detect and evaluate mental changes, and (3) realize that medical diagnosis of the etiological events that produce the syndromes of delirium and dementia is based on differential evaluation of multiple diagnostic and clinical examinations, not solely on the mental status examination. A nursing diagnosis also incorporates the findings of several evaluation processes. A thorough history that includes the chronology of mental status changes is critical. In addition, adequate screening must be done prior to the administration of the mental status examination to ascertain the visual, auditory, and language function of the individual. Nursing care of individuals with either of these syndromes involves the trained use of accurate, consistent assessment techniques to establish the presence of mental changes and to follow these changes over time. It also involves evaluation of the impact that mental changes have on the individual's ability to interact with the environment.

A number of tools for testing mental status have been developed and reported.[77, 81–84] The instruments described here have been chosen because of the universal nature of their use and because they serve as prototypes for discussion.

The DSM-III-R,[7] used by psychiatrists to standardize diagnostic entities, sets forth criteria of evaluation to determine the presence of delirium and dementia. These criteria are used for initial screening and are also followed over time to evaluate change.

The traditional mental status examination is part of the more complete neurological examination. Although every individual who presents with change in mental status should have a complete neurological examination, the outline presented in Table 9–9 is the mental status examination specifically. The

TABLE 9–9 FORMAT OF MENTAL STATUS EXAMINATION

Level of consciousness
Behavioral observations
   Psychomotor behavior
   Mood and affect
   Physical appearance
Attention
Memory
Language
Constructional ability
Higher cognitive functions
Related cortical functions

methods to evaluate each item, including questions, have been well described.

Indications of changes may be detected initially through incidental observations.[82] This means that the nurse must be alert continually to the behavior of the individual. Cohen stresses the importance of distinguishing between observations and inferences; conclusions that are derived from observations must be based upon formal and informal testing methods that validate the observation.[82] The mental status examination provides a framework to validate observations. Evaluation of the individual over time is established by testing and retesting with the mental status examination.

The Mini-Mental State Examination (MMSE) is a tool developed by Folstein and associates to detect cognitive impairment.[83] One of the purposes in developing this tool was to provide clinicians with a brief and accurate method to evaluate cognitive functions. The MMSE tests cognitive function in several specific areas. It assesses orientation to time and place, instantaneous recall, short-term memory, and abilities to perform serial subtractions or reverse spelling. The MMSE also measures constructional capabilities and the use of language (Table 9–10). The results of each section are added together for a total score ranging from 0 to 30, with 0 indicating the lowest score. The term "mini" is used because it is not a complete mental status examination, as it does not include evaluation of mood, abnormal mental experiences, and thought processes.[83] The advantages cited with the use of the MMSE are that inter-rater reliability is high,[83, 85] training individuals to administer the examination takes little time,[83, 86] and the time to administer it is short, an estimated 5 to 10 minutes. The MMSE has been advocated as a reliable screening tool for individuals who have men-

TABLE 9–10 MINI-MENTAL STATE EXAMINATION

Orientation

Maximum Score	Score	
5	( )	What is the (year) (season) (date) (day) (month)?
5	( )	Where are we (state) (county) (town) (hospital) (floor)?

Registration

3	( )	Name 3 objects: 1 second to say each. Then ask the patient all 3 after you have said them. Give 1 point for each correct answer. Then repeat them until he learns all 3. Count trials and record. Trials _____

Attention and Calculation

5	( )	Serial 7's. 1 point for each correct. Stop after 5 answers. Alternatively spell "world" backwards.

Recall

3	( )	Ask for the 3 objects repeated above. Give 1 point for each correct.

Language

9	( )	Name a pencil and watch (2 points). Repeat the following "No ifs, ands, or buts" (1 point). Follow a 3-stage command: "Take a paper in your right hand, fold it in half, and put it on the floor" (3 points). Read and obey the following: Close your eyes (1 point), write a sentence (1 point), copy a design (1 point).
_____		Total Score Assess level of consciousness along a continuum

Alert   Drowsy   Stupor   Coma

Modified from Folstein, M. F., Folstein, S. E., & McHugh, P. R. (1975). Mini-mental state—a practical method for grading the cognitive state of patients for the clinicians. Reprinted from J Psychiatr Res *12:*189–198. With permission from Pergamon Press Ltd, Oxford.

tal status changes accompanied by an inability to concentrate for long periods of time. Unlike the traditional mental status examination, which includes testing of behaviors associated with focal brain function (such as constructional ability), the MMSE reliably determines the presence of more diffuse changes only.[85]

Researchers have found one of the inherent pitfalls of the MMSE to be a high false-positive rate for the finding of cognitive impairment.[86] The error has been attributed to the tool's lack of sensitivity in accounting for a low educational level. This is consistent with the problems of mental status evaluation in general when educational level, the effects of social isolation, and cultural factors are difficult to delineate and define.

In nursing practice, the purposes of surveillance with the syndromes of delirium and dementia are to monitor behavior to (1) continue to evaluate these syndromes, (2) evaluate the effects of therapy, (3) evaluate the underlying condition, and (4) evaluate the need for additional therapy. The mental status examination currently provides the best method to evaluate behavior over time. Evaluation of the effects of therapy and the underlying condition involves use of the mental status examination, the physical examination, and other diagnostic procedures specific to determination of a causative factor. A more extensive review of the diagnosis of delirium and dementia is presented in a number of other works.[3, 10, 69]

CLINICAL THERAPIES FOR DEMENTIA AND DELIRIUM

Principles of Management and Therapeutic Goals

When the treatment of the syndromes of dementia and delirium is considered, it is important to distinguish the type of care possible and the management principle applied. The first principle for both of these syndromes is treatment of the underlying disorder. The inherent notion involved is that of brain resuscitation. This includes not only treatment of a specific disorder that may be the causative factor in the production of delirium and dementia but also supportive therapies to facilitate restoration of normal physiological function of the brain and prevent deterioration of systemic function. For example, treatment of the memory loss associated with Korsakoff's syndrome is replacement of the B vitamin complex. With a barbiturate-addicted individual who is delirious from abrupt withdrawal of this drug, reinstitution of the drug is started and a program of gradual withdrawal begun. For these types of disorders, clinical therapies are specific.

The second principle of management is focused not on reversal of a pathological process but on treatment of particular symptoms, for instance, lack of sleep or combative behavior. Clinical pharmacological therapies have been used to improve the memory loss associated with Alzheimer's disease, and several investigative drugs are being tested. Pharmacological therapies also are available to manage some of the more striking behavioral symptoms, such as the agitated, combative behavior that may occur with delirium.

The third principle of management can be conceptualized as aimed toward prevention or amelioration of environmental factors that may precipitate mental status changes. Reality orientation is a treatment strategy that illustrates this management principle. Another way to describe this form of management is environmental manipulation.

The following text describes some common behavioral dysfunctions associated with the syndromes of delirium and dementia and reviews the pertinent literature regarding their management.

Pharmacological Research on Treatment of Memory Loss

The observations that cholinergic pathways, particularly in the hippocampus, may be involved in the functional deficits of memory loss in individuals with Alzheimer's disease sparked researchers to investigate the use of cholinergic agonists to ameliorate these deficits. The hypothesis that the synthesis of acetylcholine is decreased because of a reduction in ChAT (the acetylcholine synthesizing enzyme) has encouraged the attempt to treat memory loss through facilitation of the cholinergic system. Pharmacological research has focused on two categories of drug action: (1) improving or maintaining cognitive function and (2) improving behavior.

Terry and Katzman conceptualized the pharmacological studies directed to the cholinergic hypothesis as following four avenues of investigation[10]: (1) direct replacement of acetylcholine with dietary choline, which crosses the blood-brain barrier, or lecithin, a biosynthetic precursor to acetylcholine; (2) inhibition of the normal hydrolysis of acetylcholine with esterase blockers, such as physostigmine; (3) use of an analogue of acetylcholine, such as arecholine; and (4) increasing the sensitivity of the muscarinic receptors to facilitate the action of the smaller quantities of acetylcholine that may be present. The numerous clinical trials based on these principles of therapy have not demonstrated any consistent or lasting improvements in memory function.[87]

Cooper reviewed the other major areas of pharmacological research for drugs used in Alzheimer's disease.[88] The use of nootropics (drugs used to increase neuron metabolic activity) is one line of current research. Nootropics are postulated to improve memory dysfunction by producing protein synthesis and phospholipid metabolism and by facilitating cholinergic neurotransmission.

The ergoloid mesylates are compounds that decrease vascular resistance, thereby increasing cerebral blood flow.[89] Lasting improvement in memory has not been demonstrated, although improvement in the level of alertness has been reported. Other drugs have been investigated that attempt to improve other central neurotransmitter systems (besides acetylcholine) through replacement therapy or that attempt to improve cerebral cellular integrity through vascular mechanisms.[90-92]

Pharmacological Treatment of Behavioral Disturbances

A number of affective and behavioral changes have been described in association with dementia distinct from the cognitive impairments that occur. These include problems such as sleep disturbances characterized by insomnia with night wandering, mild to severe agitation, combativeness, emotional lability, and suspiciousness. No behavior or pattern of presentation has been noted consistently for all dementias, although mania appears less common in Alzheimer's disease. The spectrum of severity of these behavioral manifestations may range from mild to severe. Another way to grade the intensity of these manifestations is to determine to what degree they are a problem to the management and care of the demented individual. The mental status changes that occur in an individual with delirium, such as agitated confusion, may jeopardize treatment and may place the individual at risk for injury; therefore, immediate attention is vital.

The neuroleptics are antipsychotic agents that, when used in low doses, may be helpful in managing agitation in individuals with delirium and dementia.[72, 73, 93] Table 9–7 is a list of the more common agents used in this class, the relative potency of each agent compared with chlorpromazine (arbitrarily assigned the potency of 100), and the predominant side effects of each. A preferred drug in management of agitation is haloperidol (a nonphenothiazine antipsychotic), which is administered in low doses and increased in small increments to achieve therapeutic effects.[64, 93, 94] The advantages of this agent are that it is a relatively potent antipsychotic and the sedative and anticholinergic effects are lower than those of chlorpromazine and thioridazine. Haloperidol does have the highest incidence of side effects manifesting as extrapyramidal symptoms, which include tremors, dystonias, pseudoparkinsonism, and akinesthesias.[72]

The benzodiazepines are a class of sedative drugs often prescribed for mild anxiety or agitation. They are less efficient than neuroleptics for severe agitation but do not produce extrapyramidal signs. Use of these drugs in elderly individuals with agitated delirium or in a demented individual may be hazardous because of the tendency of the elderly to experience paradoxical excitement with usage and because these drugs may exacerbate symptoms of dementia. In addition, the benzodiazepines have been found to suppress rapid eye movement (REM) sleep and produce rebound nightmares in the elderly.[64, 72]

Use of barbiturates for sleep disturbances associated with delirium and dementia is not advised.[94] The potent sedative effects of this class of drugs may blur an already clouded mental picture and make further clinical evaluations difficult. In addition, the risk of cardiopulmonary depression and an increased tendency to falls complicate the mental state of already compromised individuals. Mild sleep-inducing agents that are metabolized and excreted rapidly are recommended.

Pharmacological treatment of the affective and behavioral disturbances of the demented or delirious individual should be instituted only after thoughtful consideration of the nature of the problem, with confidence that the benefits outweigh the risks of treatment and in conjunction with psychological intervention strategies. The behavioral disturbances associated with dementia may be the result of physical, social, or environmental dysfunction and as such can be managed with therapies to adjust these dysfunctions without the use of drugs. The behavioral disturbances associated with delirium may be the result of perceptual illusions or hallucinations, and psychological intervention should be directed toward management of these. If drug therapy is used, it should be specific to the identified problem and judiciously administered to prevent untoward mental changes or physical reactions. Because most demented individuals are elderly, this group is particularly vulnerable to the untoward effects of drug therapy owing to the altered sensitivity of organs and altered ability to metabolize and excrete drug products.

Environmental Therapies

Reality orientation (RO) is an intervention strategy that was first used with confused individuals. It was developed by Folsom to reduce disorientation in elderly people.[95] The techniques of RO, as first developed, are composed of two forms of treatment. Class RO involves rehearsal with individuals of everyday events, such as noting the time or weather or the events of the day, for a specified period each day. Within this structure are three levels of function based on the degree of disorientation. The other form is 24-hour RO. In this form, confused individuals are presented with information throughout the day about the time, place, and the events of the day. Information about these orientation markers are structured into every interaction that the staff may have with the confused individual. In 24-hour RO, the environment is structured with signs and cues to help the individual remain aware of the surroundings.

Systematic studies done to evaluate reality orientation have focused on elderly populations. Difficulties encountered in interpreting the findings are related to (1) the different study groups used, (2) different measurement techniques used to evaluate outcome, and (3) the difficulty in ascertaining the effects of RO on all aspects of functional behavior.[95] In spite of these methodological problems, utilization of 24-hour reality orientation techniques is recommended as part of the care of institutionalized elderly individuals.[96, 97]

Psychological Support Measures

Psychological support measures are part of the management of the individual with delirium, and their use has been outlined and described utilizing various formats. The principles of psychotherapeutic measures emphasized by those who work with individuals with postcardiotomy delirium include establishment of a relationship, reassurance, environmental support, consultative relationships with the staff, and allowance of ventilation of feelings.[65]

Boss conceptualizes nursing management of the individual with delirium under two main categories of interventions. Those interventions that (1) minimize the need for impaired functions and (2) those interventions that maintain and maximize utilization of intact cortical functions.[98] Using the principles of RO, Boss lists nursing care activities within each main category of interventions. Examples of the activities that would be utilized by the nurse to minimize the need for impaired functions include placing written cues in the environment to serve as signals and establishing and maintaining a constant environment. Nursing care activities that maintain and maximize the use of an individual's intact cortical functions include continual interpersonal orientation with contact and face-to-face contact during interactions.[99]

ILLUSTRATIVE CASE STUDIES

CASE STUDY NO. 1

An 80-year-old retired surgeon was admitted to the hospital with a 2-week history of left upper quadrant pain, described as sharp, intermittent, and radiating toward the midline and back. The patient complained of occasional diarrhea for the past week, with no melena, and of loss of appetite and a 15-pound (6.8 kg) weight loss over the past month. He had been taking meperidine (100 mg) orally every 4 to 6 hours for the past 2 weeks for pain.

His past medical history was positive for type II diabetes (non—insulin-dependent) controlled by diet and for mild congestive heart failure. He had a 40-pack-year history of smoking and did not drink alcohol. He was myopic and was

experiencing a bilateral hearing loss, for which he wore a hearing aid.

Initial laboratory data, including glucose, were normal. Physical examination was unremarkable except for the cardiac examination, which revealed a 2/6 systolic ejection murmur; no clicks, rubs, or gallops were auscultated. Blood pressure was 150/98 mm Hg. A CT scan of the abdomen was negative. Ultrasonography of the abdomen revealed a splenic mass. The neurological examination performed on admission described the patient as alert and oriented to time, place, and person without evidence of focal neurological deficits.

Two days after admission, surgery was performed using general anesthesia. An abdominal laparotomy revealed pancreatic cancer, and resection of the pancreatic tail was done at this time. Five units of packed red blood cells were transfused during surgery.

The first postoperative night was uneventful. The patient received fluid replacement with 5 per cent dextrose in 0.5 normal saline with 20 mEq of potassium at 125 ml per hour, a Jackson-Pratt (JP) tube was in place to drain the peritoneum, and a nasogastric tube (NG) was inserted to drain the stomach. Vital signs were stable except for a temperature elevation to 38.8 C° rectally. Meperidine (75 mg) was ordered for pain every 4 to 6 hours as needed.

The next morning the nurse found the patient agitated, mumbling to himself, attempting to remove the Foley catheter, JP drain, and NG tube. The patient stated that he was at home and needed to go to work; and that the year was 1956. He was oriented to person. The nurse was able to comfort and quiet him with gentle persuasion. He was medicated for pain once again. During the course of the day, he became increasingly more restless and agitated. He did not recognize his family when they visited and became more insistent that he was at home. His hands were restrained because he continued to pull at his intravenous line and tubes. The patient's record was reviewed and postoperative course evaluated to determine the etiological events that may have led to his disoriented, agitated state.

Laboratory data from the morning showed the following values: sodium, 126 mEq/L; potassium, 3.5 mEq/L; chloride, 98 mEq/L; hematocrit, 30 ml/dl; hemoglobin, 8 g/100 ml; blood urea nitrogen, 17 mg/100 ml; creatinine, 2 mg/100 ml; osmolality, 293 mOsm/Kg; and glucose, 300 mg/100 ml. The blood gases were PaO_2, 54 mm Hg; HCO_3, 22 mEq/L; $PaCO_2$, 45 mm Hg; pH, 7.33; and base excess, +3 mEq/L.

Over a 12-hour period fluid intake was 1500 ml, urine output was 1000 to 1200 ml, and NG tube output was 500 to 800 ml. The urine specific gravity was 1.025.

The physical examination revealed temperature, 38.8° C; blood pressure 100/82 mm Hg; pulse, 110 bpm; respiratory rate, 18. The jugular veins were not visible at 45 degrees. A systolic ejection murmur of 2/6 was heard best at the third left intercostal space; no rubs, clicks, or gallops were auscultated. The point of maximal impulse was 2 cm lateral to the midclavicular line at the fifth intercostal space. No chest pain was reported.

Another neurological examination was performed. (The outline for the mental status examination can be reviewed in Table 9–9.) The patient was agitated, mumbling to himself, picking at the sheets, and fumbling with his tubes and abdominal dressing. He was alert, easily distracted by noise, and thought that the nurse was his daughter. He had difficulty focusing on the questions asked, and often the initial response was unrelated to the question. He was disoriented to time, place, and situation. He stated his birthdate accurately but was unable to state his present address, name the current president, or remember and repeat digits presented to him. Abstraction of proverb interpretation was difficult, and he became increasingly agitated as the examination progressed. His speech was clear, without aphasia. The motor, sensory, and cranial nerve examination revealed no focal deficits, which would indicate the presence of a structural lesion.

Because the changes in his mental status were believed to be the result of postoperative metabolic abnormalities, his age, and a change in his sensory environment, he was started on haloperidol (1 mg) to manage these acute behavioral symptoms. Medical treatment also included oxygen therapy and fluid replacement, with correction of the sodium imbalance. Nursing management included

a nursing order for 24-hour one-to-one care, using the family to assist with reorientation, and re-evaluation of the patient as requiring total nursing care.

This case study describes a patient at high risk for delirium. The factors that may have contributed to his delirium are age (80); acute pain and possibly inadequate pain relief or inability to handle medication; hearing loss and myopia, which alter sensory intake; a major surgical procedure; physical changes such as dehydration, hyponatremia, hypoxia, and blood loss; and an unfamiliar environment.

The neurological examination was performed to rule out the possibility of any other acute pathological process as the cause for his mental changes, such as stroke. In addition, since a detailed neurological examination was not done on admission, the examination and findings at this point served as a baseline. As evaluation continues, it would be important to interview the family to gather information about his mental status that could be added to the baseline data.

CASE STUDY NO. 2

The patient, a 55-year-old man, was in good health until 6 months ago, when he began to complain of severe bifrontal headaches. His wife noted that he had difficulty remembering appointments and that he was no longer able to balance their checkbook. On admission to the hospital, he appeared thin, in good health, and in mild discomfort from his headache. The mental status examination revealed impaired short-term and immediate memory; he was oriented to the year and his name but unable to state the day or the month. His speech was fluent, without aphasia. He was alert and attentive during the examination and seemed unconcerned about his physical health and uninformed about the reason for admission to the hospital.

The neurological examination revealed no focal motor or sensory deficits. Papilledema was seen on examination of the optic discs. The physical examination revealed no deficits or abnormalities.

A CT scan of the head revealed a left parasagittal mass extending past the midline, with surrounding brain edema. Three days after admission to the hospital, a craniotomy was performed and the tumor mass removed.

Thirteen months after discharge from the hospital, this patient returned to work as an electrician.

This case illustrates an example of a patient with mental status changes suggestive of dementia. The clinical presentation of the development of memory loss over a period of 6 months is the marker that points to this. The accompanying physical symptom of severe headache occurring simultaneously with the mental changes suggests a structural etiological process as the causative factor in producing the picture seen here.

REVIEW OF RESEARCH FINDINGS

Most of the text on management has de-scribed the individual with the syndromes of delirium and dementia from a primary care perspective. Concern has been expressed that total care of the individual involve consider-ation of the individual within the family unit. This is important, particularly when the di-agnosis of dementia is presumed to represent a stressful experience for family members, and requires the creation of a new role—that of caregiver—within the family network. For these reasons, this review focuses on studies related to the role of the family caregiver.

Recognition of the role of the family in the care of a dependent individual was expressed keenly by Sanford, who stated, "the sup-porter is the hub around which the future of the patient revolves"[100] (p. 472). The impor-tance of including family members in the care of the individual with dementia is re-peatedly emphasized in the literature by au-thors who manage these individuals.[101, 102] Eisdorfer and Cohen provide a helpful out-line for those who work with families and individuals with dementia[103] (Table 9–11).

Severity of illness (of the care recipient) has been implicated as an important predic-tive variable of caregiver well-being.[104, 105] Several indicators that measure severity of illness have been used alone or in combina-tion to describe the extent and intensity of Alzheimer's disease. Measures of dementia and functional and physical ability and be-havioral descriptions of the symptoms asso-

TABLE 9–11   TWELVE-ITEM CHECKLIST FOR MANAGING DEMENTIA SYNDROMES

1. Provide the family with specific information about the nature of dementing illnesses. Be certain to emphasize that resources exist to help the family cope with the illness.
2. Give both medical and psychiatric care to maximize level of functioning for both patient and family. This includes a thorough medical assessment to rule out treatable causes of dementia. Supportive psychotherapy, various group approaches, and concerned citizen groups have all been found to be useful.
3. Refer families to appropriate medical specialists, even when a relative has a profound dementia. This maximizes the patient's "level of functioning."
4. Refer to appropriate community and social services. This includes home repair and chore services, home health aids, visiting nurses, adult day care programs, transportation services, laundry services, physical and occupational therapy, and respite care.
5. Help families in decisions regarding institutionalization.
6. Refer families for appropriate legal and financial counseling. Although not the true province of the physician, financial planning, power of attorney, and legal guardianship are frequently overlooked and may, at a later stage, become much more complicated.
7. Refer families, when appropriate, for psychotherapeutic intervention.
8. Obtain an evaluation of the home setting, to identify specific problems that should be discussed with the family.
9. Periodically reassess the patient's intellectual capacities. This identifies new problems that should be discussed with the family.
10. Work with the caregivers to develop a comprehensive strategy that addresses the needs of the patient and family.
11. Refer the patient and family to community self-help groups (e.g., Alzheimer's Disease Association); this allows the sharing of ideas and management strategies.
12. Provide appropriate medication as necessary. Drugs designed to improve behavioral manifestations often oversedate the patient unless carefully titrated.

Data from Eisdorfer, C., & Cohen, D. (1981). Management of the patient and family coping with dementing illness. J Fam Pract *12*:832. Reprinted from Appleton & Lange, Inc.

ciated with the disease are examples of the factors used to estimate the variable severity of illness.[106, 107]

Assumption of the caregiver role was shown to have a number of negative effects on caregiver health and perceived psycholog-ical status,[108–112] although other studies have noted no negative consequences or have found that the effects were related to individ-ual factors not captured by the measurement methods.[113–117]

In an attempt to capture the impact and consequences that caregiving has on the caregiver, the concept of burden was used as an outcome variable in studies of caregivers. "Burden" has been defined as the cost to the caregiver demanded by assuming the caregiver role and responsibilities.[104] An important distinction was further developed that conceptualized burden into objective and subjective categories for the purposes of providing clarity to the concept and for instrument development.[117, 118] "Subjective burden" is defined as a measure of the perceptions or feelings of the caregiver. "Objective burden" is defined as changes in the caregivers' lives that can be quantified.[105]

The relationship between severity of illness and caregiver burden was assumed to be positive, with the more severe the illness, the greater the caregiver burden. Studies over the past several years yielded inconclusive results to support this hypothesis.[105, 119] Zarit and associates found that as the length of caregiving increased, caregivers developed greater tolerance for memory and behavioral problems; this tolerance was negatively correlated with burden.[114] Montgomery suggested that burden is perceived as greater by caregivers when their freedom was limited rather than when the severity of illness was considered.[117]

Several authors proposed that burden may be influenced by a number of confounding variables, in addition to severity of illness measures.[105, 120, 121] These were identified as (1) caregiver involvement with the care recipient, (2) the caregiver's tolerance to the impairments of the care recipient, (3) the caregiver's perception of lack of freedom, and (4) caregiver characteristics, such as the kinship relationship, sex, and the quality of the prior relationship.

In addition to these factors, Vitaliano and associates[105] and Barer and colleagues[120] identified several methodological issues related to the study of the concept of burden over the past 10 years. These were summarized as including problems with diverse definitions and conceptual models, the use of varied measurement approaches, the application of nonspecific burden measures to nonhomogeneous populations, and the lack of consideration of the changes that may develop over time in the caregiving situations[105] (p. 68).

Future research should consider the preceding methodological issues as well as en-sure that instrument development considers measures to test for construct and content validity, analysis of the relationship of the caregiver to the care recipient, objective and subjective burden as separate phenomena, and caregiving circumstances.[105, 121]

IMPLICATIONS FOR FURTHER RESEARCH

Several areas specific to nursing management of individuals with delirium and dementia deserve attention in regard to future research. One is related to the methods that nurses use to identify mental changes. Nursing-generated studies need to address the discrepancy of terminology, definitions, and evaluative methods used to collect data. The model of risk factor identification applied to various institutional populations might be incorporated into educational and research literature. With proper identification of high-risk individuals and early detection of mental changes, some of the untoward reactions associated with disorientation and perceptual problems might be avoided. Williams and colleagues describe this type of nursing activity as preventive.[122] Wolanin and Phillips have written a book that incorporates the nursing process with patient outcome criteria for nursing interventions related to the client who is confused.[123] The instructional method recommended in this text for assessment of the client is a unique approach that warrants recognition and testing in the clinical area.

More study in the use of environmental manipulation techniques should be encouraged. This includes such diverse topics as use and management of staff, use of family members to assist with care, and exploration and research on how the setting influences management of an individual and how the environment affects behavior. Although the techniques of reality orientation are used, these methods were developed for use in controlled environments with elderly individuals. The results of the application of these techniques to other populations in different settings are unknown.

The ANA definition of nursing[1] could be utilized to begin to define human responses that result from complex interactive variables that may cause delirium and dementia. In addition, the human response model could be used as an organizing system for developing ways to measure outcomes of various intervention techniques.

REFERENCES

1. American Nurses' Association. (1980). *Nursing: A Social Policy Statement.* Kansas City, MO: American Nurses' Association.
2. Gazzaniga, M. S., & Le Doux, J. E. (1978). *The Integrated Mind.* New York: Plenum Press.
3. Plum, F., & Posner, J. B. (1980). *The Diagnosis of Stupor and Coma* (3rd ed.). Philadelphia: F. A. Davis.
4. Lipowski, Z. J. (1980). A new look at organic brain syndromes. Psychiatry *137*:674–678.
5. Lipowski, Z. J. (1990). *Delirium: Acute Confusional States.* New York: Oxford University Press.
6. Jorm, A. F., Korten, A. E., & Henderson, A. S. (1987). The prevalence of dementia: A quantitative integration of the literature. Acta Psychiatr Scand *76*:465–479.
7. American Psychiatric Association (1987). *Diagnostic and Statistical Manual of Mental Disorders III Revised.* Washington, D. C.: American Psychiatric Association.
8. Joynt, R. J., & Shouldson, I. (1979). Dementia. In K. M. Heilman & E. Valenstein (eds.), *Clinical Neuropsychology.* New York: Oxford University Press.
9. National Institutes of Health Consensus Development Conference Statement (1988). Differential diagnosis of dementing diseases. Alzheimer Dis Assoc Disord *2*:4–15.
10. Terry, R., & Katzman, R. (1983). Senile dementia of the Alzheimer's type: Defining a disease. In R. Katzman & R. Terry (eds.), *The Neurology of Aging* (pp. 51–84). Philadelphia: F. A. Davis.
11. Kase, C. S., Wolf, P. A., Bachman, D. L., Linn, R. T., & Cupples, L. A. (1989). Dementia and stroke: The Framington Study. In M. D. Ginsberg & W. D. Deitrich (eds.), *Cerebrovascular Diseases, Sixteenth Research Conference* (pp. 193–197). New York: Raven Press.
12. Kase, C. S. (1991). Epidemiology of multi-infarct dementia. Alzheimer Dis Assoc Disord *5*:71–76.
13. Evans, D. A., Funkenstein, H. H., Albert, M. S., Scherr, P. A., Cook, N. R., Chown, M. J., Hebert, L. F., Hennekens, C. H., & Taylor, J. O. (1989). Prevalence of Alzheimer's disease in a community population of older persons. Higher than previously reported. JAMA *262*:2551–2556.
14. Byrne, E. J., Smith, C. W., & Arie, T. (1991). The diagnosis of dementia. I. Clinical and pathological criteria: A review of the literature. Int J Geriatr Psychiatry *6*:199–208.
15. Haase, G. R. (1977). Diseases presenting as dementia. In C. E. Well (ed.), *Dementia* (pp. 27–67). Philadelphia: F. A. Davis.
16. Derix, M. M. A., deGans, J., & Portegies, P. (1990). Mental changes in patients with AIDS. Clin Neurol Neurosurg *92*:215–222.
17. UCLA Conference. (1982). Dementia in the elderly: The silent epidemic. Ann Intern Med *97*:231–241.
18. Liberman, A., Dziatolowski, M., Kupersmith, M., Serby, M., Goodgold, A., Korein, J., & Goldstein, M. (1979). Dementia in Parkinson disease. Ann Neurol *6*:355–359.
19. Jennett, B., & Teasdale, G. (1981). *The Management of Head Injury.* Philadelphia: F. A. Davis.
20. Davies, P. (1991). Alzheimer's disease: Progress toward diagnosis in vivo. Geriatrics *46*:79–81.
21. Evenhuis, H. M. (1990). The natural history of dementia in Down's syndrome. Arch Neurol *47*:263–267.
22. Kosik, K. S. (1991). Alzheimer, plaques and tangles: Advances on both fronts. Trends Neurosci *14*:218–219.
23. Haxby, J. V. (1985). Clinical and neuropsychological studies of dementia in Down's syndrome. Ann Intern Med *103*:572–574.
24. Dalton, A. J., Crapper, R. M., & McLachlan, D. R. (1986). Clinical expression of Alzheimer's disease in Down's syndrome. Psychiatr Clin North Am *4*:659–670.
25. Andreoli, T. E., Carpenter, C. C. J., Plum, F., & Smith, L. T. T. (1990). Pathological alterations of consciousness. In T. E. Andreoli, C. C. J. Carpenter, F. Plum, & L. T. T. Smith (eds.), *Essentials of Medicine* (2nd ed., pp. 667–689) Philadelphia: W. B. Saunders.
26. Adams, R. A., & Victor, M. (1990). *Principles of Neurology.* New York: McGraw-Hill.
27. Thomas, L. (1981). On the problems of dementia. Discover, August, pp. 34–36.
28. Terry, R. D., & Katzman, R. (1983). Senile dementia of the Alzheimer type. Ann Neurol *14*:497–506.
29. Pedley, T. A., & Miller, J. A. (1983). Clinical neurophysiology of aging and dementia. In R. Mayeux & W. G. Rosen (eds.), *The Dementias* (pp. 31–49). New York: Raven Press.
30. Hyman, B. T., van Hoesen, G. W., Damasio, A. N., & Barnes, C. L. (1984). Alzheimer's disease: Cell specific pathology isolates the hippocampal formation. Science *25*:1160–1170.
31. Prusnier, S. B. (1984). Prions. Sci Am *251*:50–59.
32. Fibiger, H. C. (1991). Cholinergic mechanisms in learning, memory and dementia: A review of recent evidence. Trends Neurosci *14*:220–223.
33. Haan, J., & Roos, R. A. C. (1990). Amyloid in central nervous system disease. Clin Neurol Neurosurg *92*:305–310.
34. Blass, J. P., Baker, A. C., Ko, L., & Black, R. S. (1990). Induction of Alzheimer antigen by an uncoupler of oxidative phosphorylation. Arch Neurol *47*:864–869.
35. Ruberg, M., Ploska, A., Javoy-Agid, F., & Agid, Y. (1982). Muscarinic binding and choline acetyltransferase activity in Parkinsonian subjects with reference to dementia. Brain Res *Z32*:129–139.
36. Cote, L. (1981). Aging of the brain and dementia. In R. W. Kandel, & J. H. Schwartz (eds.), *Principles of Neural Science* (pp. 574–575). New York: Elsevier.
37. Gorelick, P. B., & Bozzola, F. G. (1991). Alzheimer's disease—clues to the cause. Post Med *89*:231–232, 237–238, 240.
38. Muller-Hill, B., & Beyreuther, K. (1989). Molecular biology of Alzheimer's disease. Ann Rev Biochem *58*:287–307.
39. Coyle, J. T., Price, D. L., & DeLong, M. R. (1983). Alzheimer's disease: A disorder of cortical cholinergic innervation. Science *219*:1184–1189.
40. Tomlinson, B. E., Blessed, G., & Roth, M. (1970) Observations on the brains of demented old people. J Neurol Sci *11*:205–242.

41. Selkoe, D. J. (1992). Aging brain, aging mind. Sci Am 267:135–142.

42. Perry, E. K., Tomlinson, B. E., Blessed, G., Bergman, K., Gibson, P. H., & Perry, R. H. (1978). Correlation of cholinergic abnormalities with senile plaques and mental test scores in senile dementia. Br Med J 2:1457–1459.

43. Whitehouse, P. J., Hedreen, J. C., White, C. L., III, & Price, D. L. (1983). Basal forebrain neurons in the dementia of Parkinson disease. Ann Neurol 13:243–248.

44. Erkinjuntti, T., & Sulkava, R. (1991). Diagnosis of multi-infarct dementia. Alzheimer Dis Assoc Disord 5:112–121.

45. McGeer, E. G. (1981). Neurotransmitter systems in aging and senile dementia. Prog Neuropsychopharmacol 5: 435–445.

46. McKhann, G., Drachman, D., Folstein, M., Katzman, R., Price, D., & Stadlan, E. M. (1984). Clinical diagnosis of Alzheimer's disease: Report of the NINCDS-ADRDA Work Group under the auspices of the Department of Health and Human Services Task Force on Alzheimer's disease. Neurology 34:939–944.

47. Gurland, B., & Toner, J. (1977). Differentiating dementia and non-dementing conditions. In C. E. Well (ed.), Dementia (pp. 1–17) Philadelphia: F. A. Davis.

48. Blass, J. P., & Plum, F. (1983). Metabolic encephalopathies in older adults. In R. Katzman & R. Terry (eds.), The Neurology of Aging. Philadelphia: F. A. Davis.

49. La Rue, A. (1982). Memory loss and aging. Psychiatr Clin North Am 5:89–103.

50. Greenwald, B., Ginsberg, E., Marin, D., Laitma, L., Hermann, K., Moms, R., & Davies, K. (1989). Dementia with co-existing major depression. Am J Psychiatry 146:1472–1478.

51. Wragg, R., & Jester, D. (1989). Overview of depression and psychosis in Alzheimer's disease. Am J Psychiatry 146:577–587.

52. Merriam, A., Aronson, N. Gaston, P., Wey, S., & Katz, R. (1988). The psychiatric symptoms of Alzheimer's disease. J Am Geriatr Soc 36:7–12.

53. Albert, M. S., Duffy, F. H., & McAnulty, G. B. (1990). Electrophysiologic comparisons between two groups of patients with Alzheimer's disease. Arch Neurol 47:857–863.

54. Jagust, W. J., & Eberling, J. L. (1991). MRI, CT, SPECT, PET: Their use in diagnosing dementia. Geriatrics 46:28–35.

55. Kertesz, A., Polk, M., & Carr, T. (1990). Cognition and white matter changes on magnetic resonance imaging in dementia. Arch Neurol 47:387–391.

56. Brown, W. D., & Frackowiak, R. S. J. (1991). Cerebral blood flow and metabolism studies in multi-infarct dementia. Alzheimer Dis Assoc Disord 5:131–143.

57. Ladurner, G., Iliff, L. D., & Lechner, H. (1982). Clinical factors associated with dementia in ischemic stroke. J Neurol Neurosurg Psychiatry 45:97–101.

58. Jagust, W. J., Reed, B. R., Seab, J. P., & Budinger, T. F. (1990). Alzheimer's disease. Age at onset and single-photon emission computed tomographic patterns of regional cerebral blood flow. Arch Neurol 47:628–633.

59. McLean, S. (1987). Assessing dementia: I. Difficulties, definitions and differential diagnosis. Aust NZ J Psychiatry 21:142–174.

60. Hachinski, V. C., Lassen, N. A., & Marshall, J. (1974). Multi-infarct dementia. A cause of mental deterioration in the elderly. Lancet 2:207–210.

61. Hachinski, V. C. (1983). Multi-infarct dementia. Neurol Clin 1:27–36.

62. Hachinski, V. C. (1991). Multi-infarct dementia: A reappraisal. Alzheimer Dis Assoc Disord 5:64–68.

63. Engel, G. L., & Romano, J. (1959). Delirium: A syndrome of cerebral insufficiency. J Chron Dis 9:260–277.

64. Fish, D. N. (1991). Treatment of delirium in the critically ill patient. Clin Pharm 10:456–466.

65. Morse, R. M., & Litin, E. M. (1969). Postoperative delirium—a study of etiologic factors. Am J Psychiatry 126:388–395.

66. Dubin, W. R., Field, H. L., & Gastfriend, D. R. (1979). Postcardiotomy delirium: A critical review. J Thorac Cardiovasc Surg 77:586–594.

67. Francis, J., & Kapoor, W. N. (1990). Delirium in hospitalized elderly. JAMA 263:1097–1101.

68. Plum, F. (1979). Consciousness and its disturbances. In P. B. Beeson, W. McDermott, & J. B. Wyngaarden (eds.), Cecil's Textbook of Medicine (pp. 639–643). Philadelphia: W. B. Saunders.

69. Lipowski, Z. J. (1987). Delirium (acute confusional states). JAMA 258:1789–1792.

70. Lipowski, Z. J. (1967). Delirium, clouding of consciousness and confusion. J Nerv Ment Dis 145:227–254.

71. Summers, W. K. (1978). A clinical method of estimating risk of drug induced delirium. Life Sci 22:1511–1516.

72. Thompson, T. L., Moran, M. G., & Nies, A. S. (1983). Psychotropic drug use in the elderly. Part I. N Engl J Med 308:134–138.

73. Thompson, T. L., Moran, M. G., & Nies, A. S. (1983). Psychotropic drug use in the elderly. Part II. N Engl J Med 308:194–199.

74. Posner, J. B. (1979). Delirium and exogenous metabolic brain disease. In P. B. Beeson, McDermott, W., & Wyngaarden, J. B. (eds.), Cecil's Textbook of Medicine (pp. 644–651). Philadelphia: W. B. Saunders.

75. Aring, C. D. (1982). Metabolic encephalopathy: Neurologic and psychiatric considerations. Heart Lung 11:516–521, 1982.

76. Lipowski, Z. J. (1980). Delirium. Springfield, Illinois: Charles C Thomas.

77. Strub, R. L., & Black, F. W. (1981). The Mental Status Examination in Neurology. Philadelphia: F. A. Davis.

78. Obrecht, R., Okhomina, F. O. A., & Scott, D. F. (1979). Value of EEG in acute confusional states. J Neurol Neurosurg Psychiatry 42:75–77.

79. Sachdev, N. S., Carter, C. C., Swank, R. L., & Blachly, P. H. (1967). Relationship between postcardiotomy delirium, clinical neurological changes and EEG abnormalities. J Thorac Cardiovasc Surg 54:557–563.

80. Owens, J. F., & Hutelmyer, C. M. (1982). The effect of preoperative intervention on delirium in cardiac surgical patients. Nurs Res 31:60–62.

81. Filskov, S. B., & Leli, D. A. (1981). Assessment of the individual in neuropsychological practice. In S. B. Filskov, & T. J. Boll (eds.), Handbook of Clinical Neuropsychology. New York: John Wiley.

82. Cohen, S. (1981). Mental status assessment. Am J Nurs *81*:1493–1518.

83. Folstein, M. F., Folstein, S. E., & McHugh, P. R. (1975). "Mini-mental state" a practical method for grading the cognitive state of patients for the clinician. J Psychiatr Res *12*:189–198.

84. Weintraub, S., & Mesulam, M. M. (1985). Mental status assessment of young and elderly adults in behavioral neurology. In M. M. Mesulam (ed.), *Principles of Behavioral Neurology.* Philadelphia: F. A. Davis.

85. Anthony, J. C., LeResche, L., Niaz, U., VonKorff, M. R., & Folstein, M. (1982). Limits of the "mini-mental state" as a screening test for dementia and delirium among hospital patients. Psychol Med *12*:397–408.

86. Dick, J. P. R., Guiloff, R. J., Stewart, A., Blackstock, J., Bielawska, C., Paul, E. A., & Marsden, C. D. (1984). Mini-mental state examination in neurological patients. J Neurol Neurosurg Psychiatry *47*:496–499.

87. Volger, B. W. (1991). Alternatives in the treatment of memory loss in patients with Alzheimer's disease. Clin Pharm *10*:447–456.

88. Cooper, J. K. (1991). Drug treatment of Alzheimer's disease. Arch Intern Med *151*:245–249.

89. Hollister, L. (1984). Ergoloid mesyltates for senile dementias: Unanswered questions. Ann Intern Med *100*:894–898.

90. Harris, R. J., Branston, N. M., Symon, L., Bayhan, M., & Watson, A. (1982). Effects of the calcium antagonist, nimodipine, upon psychological responses of the cerebral vasculature and its possible influence upon focal cerebral ischemia. Stroke *13*:759–765.

91. Hollander, E., Mohs, R. C., & Davis, K. L. (1986). Cholinergic approaches to the treatment of Alzheimer's disease. Br Med Bull *42*:97–100.

92. Tariot, P. N., Sunderland, T., Cohen, R. N., Newhouse, P. A., Mueller, E. A., & Murphy, E. L. (1988). Tramylcypromine compared with L-deprenyl in Alzheimer's disease. J Clin Psychopharmacol *8*:23–37.

93. Shneider, L. S., Pollock, V. E., & Lyness, S. A. (1990). A meta-analysis of controlled trials of neuroleptic treatment in dementia. J Geriatr Soc *38*:553–563.

94. Wragg, R. E., & Jeste, D. V. (1988). Neuroleptics and alternative treatment. Psychatr Clin North Am *11*:195–213.

95. Folsom, J. C. (1968). Reality orientation for the elderly mental patient. J Geriatr Psychiatry *1*:291–307.

96. Burton, M. (1982). Reality orientation for the elderly: A critique. J Adv Nurs *7*:427–433.

97. Hogstel, M. O. (1979). Use of reality orientation with aging confused patients. Nurs Res *28*:161–165.

98. Boss, B. (1982). Acute mood and behavioral disturbances of neurological origin: Acute confusional states. J Neurosurg Nurs *14*:61–68.

99. Cammermeyer, M. (1988). Assessment of cognition. In P. H. Mitchell, L. C. Hodges, M. Muwaswes, & C. A. Walleck (eds.), *AANN'S Neuroscience Nursing: Phenomena and Practice* (pp. 155–165). Norwalk, CT: Appleton and Lange.

100. Sanford, R. A. (1975). Tolerance of debility in elderly dependent on supporters at home: Its significance for hospital practice. Br Med J *3*:471–473.

101. Gwyther, L. P. (1985). *Care of the Alzheimer's patients*: A Manual for Nursing Home Staff. Chicago: American Health Care Association and ADRDA.

102. Zarit, S. H., Orr, N. K., & Zarit, J. M. (1985). *The Hidden Victims of Alzheimer's Disease: Families Under Stress.* New York: New York University Press.

103. Eisdorfer, C., & Cohen, D. (1981). Management of the patient and family coping with dementing illness. J Fam Pract *12*:831–887.

104. Wilder, D. E., Teresi, J. A., & Bennett, R. C. (1983). Family burden and dementia. In R. Mayeux & W. G. Rosen (eds.), *The Dementia's* (pp. 239–251). New York: Raven Press.

105. Vitaliano, P. P., Young, H. M., & Russo, I. (1991). Burden: a review of measures used among caregivers of individuals with dementia. Gerontologist *31*:67–73.

106. Teunisse, S., Derix, M. M. A., & vanCrevel, H. (1991). Assessing severity of dementia. Arch Neurol *48*:274–277.

107. George, L. K., & Gwyther, L. P. (1986). Caregiver well being: A multi-dimensional examination of family caregivers of demented adults. Gerontologist *26*:253–259.

108. Miller, B. (1987). Gender and control among spouses of the cognitively impaired: A research note. Gerontologist *27*:447–453.

109. Nygaard, H. A. (1988). Strain on caregivers of demented elderly people living at home. Scand J Prim Health Care *6*:33–37.

110. Pearson, T., Verns, S., & Nellett, C. (1988). Elderly psychiatric patient status, and caregiver perceptions as predictors of caregiver burden. Gerontologist *28*:79–83.

111. Poulshock, S. W., & Deimling, G. T. (1984). Families caring for elderly in residence: Issues in measurement of burden. J Gerontol *39*:230–239.

112. Cohen, D., & Eisdorfer, C. (1988). Depression in family members caring for a relative with Alzheimer's disease. J Am Geriatr Soc *36*:885–889.

113. Hirschfeld, M. (1983). Homecare versus institutionalization: Family caregiving and senile brain disease. Int J Nurs Sci *20*:23–32.

114. Zarit, S. H., Reever, K. E., & Bach-Peterson, J. (1980). Relatives of the impaired elderly: Correlates of feelings of burden. Gerontologist *20*:649–655.

115. Teunisse, S., Derix, M. M. A., & vanCrevel, H. (1991). Assessing severity of dementia. Arch Neurol *48*:274–277.

116. Townsend, N., Noelber, L., Deimling, G., & Bass, D. (1989). Longitudinal impact of interhousehold caregiving on adult children's mental health. Psychol Aging *4*:393–401.

117. Montgomery, R. J. V., Gonyea, J. G., & Hooyman, N. R. (1985). Caregiving and the experience of subjective and objective burden. Fam Relations *34*:19–26.

118. Thompson, E. H., & Doll, W. (1982). The burden of families coping with the mentally ill: Invisible crisis. Fam Relations *31*:379–388.

119. Novak, M., & Guest, C. (1989). Caregiver response to Alzheimer's disease. Int J Aging Hum Dev *28*:67–69.

120. Barer, B. M., & Johnson, C. L. (1990). A critique of the caregiving literature. Gerontologist *30*:26–29.

121. Fitting, M., Rabins, P., Lucas, M. J., & Eastham, J. (1986). Caregiver for dementia patients: A comparison of husbands and wives. Gerontologist 26:248–252.

122. Williams, M. A., Holloway, J. R., Winn, M. C., Wolanin M. O., Lawler, M. L., Westwick, C. R., & Chin, M. H. (1981). Nursing activities and acute confusional states in elderly hip fractures. Nurs Res 28:25–35.

123. Wolanin, M. O., & Phillips, L. R. F. (1981). *Confusion: Prevention and Care*. St. Louis: C. V. Mosby.

10

Urinary Incontinence

Mary H. Palmer

DEFINITION

Urinary incontinence is a disruption in the storage and emptying mechanism of the bladder, "a condition in which involuntary loss of urine is a social or hygienic problem and is objectively demonstrable."[1] Several types of urinary incontinence have been defined. These types are stress, urge, overflow, reflex, and functional urinary incontinence.

As can be seen in Table 10–1, functional incontinence is a unique type of incontinence: The lower urinary tract is normal but environmental, physical, cognitive, or communication problems create barriers to using the toilet. Unlike in functional and urge incontinence, an individual with reflex incontinence is unaware of the need to void. The interruption of nerve transmissions to the brain due to trauma, tumor, or lesion prevents the occurrence of the conscious need to void. Bladder emptying is controlled at the spinal cord level. In overflow incontinence, urinary retention due to an obstruction at the bladder outlet or to peripheral neuropathies results in absent or ineffective contraction of the bladder's smooth muscle, the detrusor.

Uninhibited contractions of the detrusor that occur at any time during bladder filling and urine storage characterize urge incontinence. A large amount of urine loss is common. In contrast, the detrusor does not contract during stress incontinence. The pressure in the bladder overcomes the pressure in the urethra, usually during a cough or sneeze or with exercise and changes in position. Stress incontinence rarely occurs at night in bed and usually involves a small amount of urine loss.

A taxonomy for alterations in urinary elimination has been developed for nurses.[3] Urinary incontinence is conceptualized as expulsive, retentive, and mixed. Nursing diagnoses for expulsive incontinence include stress, urge, and stress-urge incontinence. The unifying characteristic is urine expulsion occurring through bladder contraction. Nursing diagnoses for retentive incontinence include acute retention and chronic retention. The common characteristic is the retention of urine and potential overflow incontinence. Nursing diagnoses for mixed incontinence include functional, reflex, and total incontinence; mixed incontinence is a combination of expulsive and retentive properties. For example, there may be voluntary retention but involuntary expulsion of urine as often seen in functional incontinence. The reader is referred to a complete discussion of the development of this taxonomy in journal articles.[3, 4]

Definitions used by older persons often differ from those used by health care professionals. In one study noninstitutionalized older adults did not use the same terminology or criteria for incontinence as the researchers.[5] For example, loss of urine, regardless of the amount, in the privacy of one's home or bathroom was not considered incontinence, but overt wetting of clothing in public places was deemed by the older adults as incontinence.

PREVALENCE AND POPULATIONS AT RISK

The prevalence of urinary incontinence refers to the degree to which the disruption is present in a given population at a specific

221

TABLE 10–1 DEFINITIONS OF URINARY INCONTINENCE

Stress	Involuntary loss of urine when intravesical pressure exceeds intraurethral pressure in the absence of detrusor activity*
Urge	Involuntary loss of urine associated with a strong urge to void*
Reflex	Involuntary loss of urine caused by abnormal reflex activity in the spinal cord in the absence of sensation usually associated with the desire to micturate*
Overflow	Involuntary loss of urine when the intravesical pressure exceeds the maximum urethral pressure associated with bladder distention but in the absence of detrusor activity*
Functional	Urinary leakage associated with the inability (because of impairments of cognitive or physical functioning, psychological unwillingness, or environmental barriers) to use toilets†

*See the International Continence Society (1980). The standardization of terminology of lower urinary tract function. Scand J Urol Nephrol Suppl *114*:5–19.[1]
†See P. Katz & E. Calkins (1989). Principles and Practice of Nursing Home Care (pp. 247–274). New York: Springer.[2]

point of time. The prevalence gives one a sense of the magnitude of the problem. It has been estimated that 10 million adult Americans, regardless of the setting, are incontinent.[6]

The incidence of urinary incontinence refers to the rate of new cases developing in a group at risk for becoming incontinent during a specific period of time. This rate gives the probability of a member of a vulnerable group becoming incontinent. Table 10–2 exhibits select studies of the prevalence of urinary incontinence in the acute care, long-term care, and community settings.

It is difficult to evaluate the prevalence of urinary incontinence in the acute care setting. There have been few studies with large samples of hospital patients in the United States. However, Sullivan and Lindsay stated that 19 per cent of the admissions of patients age 65 years and older during a 6-week period to a 730-bed teaching hospital were incontinent of urine.[7] Sier and associates reported an overall prevalence of 35 per cent during a 14-week period for 363 admissions of patients age 65 years and older to five general medical-surgical units of a university hospital.[8] Using hospital discharge information from part A of the Medicare form, the annual age-standardized prevalence for women

is calculated to be 16.6 per 10,000 and 10.1 per 10,000 for men.[9]

Lack of documentation in the medical record may lead to under-reporting of the magnitude of the problem. Also, urinary incontinence in the acute care setting may be transient in nature; incontinence appears with the acute medical condition that led to the hospitalization and resolves as the medical condition of the patient improves. The use of chemical and physical restraints may also induce incontinence owing to the lack of mobility and the increased dependency on others to perform elimination. Acute changes in mental status from elevated temperature, electrolyte imbalances, and other physiological changes can cause transient incontinence. A standardized definition of incontinence, criteria to define a case, and sensitive screening tools are necessary to record episodes of incontinence objectively throughout the course of the hospital stay.

The prevalence of urinary incontinence in nursing home residents in the United States is estimated to be approximately 50 per cent, although it has been noted that data regarding prevalence rates have not been consistently maintained.[15] Nursing home residents are vulnerable to urinary incontinence owing to physical and mental morbidity. Few longitudinal studies have been conducted to determine the incidence of incontinence in the long-term care setting. As seen in Table 10–2, a national sample of nursing home residents found that 10.7 per cent had difficulty with bladder continence alone, and 32.5 per cent had difficulty with fecal and bladder continence.

Sole reliance on medical record documentation to determine the prevalence of urinary incontinence may lead to underestimates, as was also indicated in the acute care setting.[7] Palmer and associates found inconsistent documentation of incontinence among several nursing and medical forms in the records of nursing home residents.[16] Inadequate awareness that incontinence is a disruption, not a normal process of aging, may account for the lack of documentation. Also, poor communication between the nursing and medical staffs about new cases or worsening of the existing cases of incontinence affects whether incontinence is detected, documented, and appropriately assessed.

Reports of the prevalence of incontinence in the community vary. For example, in one

TABLE 10–2   **PREVALENCE OF URINARY INCONTINENCE**

Study	Population Sample	Definition of Incontinence	Prevalence
Setting: Acute Care			
Sullivan & Lindsay (1984)[7]	315 patients (65+ years) admitted over a 6-week period	Any inappropriate loss of urine, regardless of amount or frequency (included use of external catheter, excluded indwelling catheter)	19%
Sier, Ouslander, & Orzeck (1987)[8]	363 patients (65+ years) admitted over a 14-week period.	One or more episodes of incontinence documented on incontinence monitoring record while hospitalized	Age: 65–74 = 24% 75+ = 48%
Massachusetts Medical Society (1991)[9]	41.4 million hospital discharge records (Medicare A)	First mention of incontinence in discharge records	Women: 16.6* Men: 10.1*
Setting: Long-Term Care			
Ouslander, Kane, & Abrass (1982)[10]	842 patients (65+ years) from seven nursing homes	Any uncontrolled leakage of urine regardless of amount or frequency.	50%
Ouslander & Fowler (1985)[11]	7853 VA patients in 90 nursing home facilities	Any uncontrolled leakage regardless of amount or frequency.	41%
Hing & Sekscenski (1986)[12]	1.4 million (included patients 55+ years)	Difficulty controlling bladder	10.7% bladder only; 32.5% bladder and bowel
Setting: Community			
Diokno, Brock, Brown, & Herzog (1986)[13]	1955 adults (60+ years)	Any uncontrolled urine loss in the prior 12 months without regard to severity	30% (males = 18.9%; females = 37.7%)
Harris (1986)[14]	5637 adults (65+ years) who answered questions regarding urinary problems on the National Health Interview Survey	Includes those with any degree of difficulty controlling urination as well as those with catheters	9%

*Per 10,000 population.

study the prevalence of urinary incontinence is reported to be approximately 9 per cent in a national sample of older adults dwelling in communities in the United States.[14] However, a higher prevalence rate, 30 per cent, is reported in the Michigan Medical, Epidemiological, and Social Aspects of Aging sample.[9]

Adults in the community have varying degrees of health and functional status; therefore, subgroups may have a higher prevalence of urinary incontinence than the general population. For example, Noekler found that 53 per cent of 299 impaired older adults living at home with a family caregiver were incontinent of urine.[17] Mitteness found 31 per cent of 140 elderly residents of a subsidized housing unit to be incontinent of urine at least once a week.[5] Deliberate efforts were made to contain and hide incontinence from others.

Unless the same definitions and sampling criteria are used in studies using self-reported data, the prevalence rate obtained may be underreported and may not accurately reflect the actual loss of urine control.

Several populations are at risk for becoming and remaining incontinent of urine, including individuals with a disruption in bladder filling, urine storage, or emptying of urine. Interaction between situational stressors, factors that are extrinsic to an individual such as accessibility of toilets, and developmental factors intrinsic to the individual, such as gender or age, may increase an individual's vulnerability to incontinence.

Adults aged 65 years and older have many

of the neurological and functional conditions that may lead to incontinence. For example, Parkinson's disease is the leading cause of neurological disability in older adults.[18] It has been estimated that approximately 70 per cent of older adults with Parkinson's disease are incontinent of urine.[19] However, incontinence is not caused by age and not all older adults with neurological disorders will be incontinent of urine.

Chronic illnesses and conditions that affect functional ability are prevalent among older adults. Arthritis is a prevalent geriatric problem that often limits or impedes mobility.[20] Individuals with mobility impairments resulting from arthritis, poorly fitting shoes, and muscular atrophy are at risk of becoming incontinent, especially in environments where personal assistance and toilets are inaccessible.

Concomitant illnesses or conditions that compromise awareness of the need to void also increase the risk for incontinence. Older adults with communication disorders resulting from dementia, cerebral vascular accidents, or other neurological and functional disorders are an especially threatened group. The inability to articulate the need to void or to translate neural information from the micturition center in the brain into meaningful patterns of behavior creates a vulnerability unless caregivers are scrupulous in detecting voiding behaviors and in offering toilet facilities regularly.

Therefore, functionally or cognitively impaired individuals in environments that do not promote continence by having easily and readily accessible help to use the toilet or bathrooms are at risk. However, other stressors increase susceptibility to incontinence in various groups of individuals.

SITUATIONAL STRESSORS

Situational stressors can lead to established patterns of alterations in urinary elimination as well as transient or acute episodes of incontinence in normally continent adults. This section presents situational stressors for transient incontinence. A discussion of antecedents for established types of incontinence are discussed under Clinical States.

Stressors such as changes in cognitive functioning and level of mobility, presence of inflammatory processes, and ingestion of pharmacological agents may cause incontinence. Ouslander identified the mnemonic DRIP (Delirium, Restricted mobility and retention, Infection, inflammation, impaction, and Polyuria and pharmaceuticals) to use in identifying and remembering factors that may precipitate acute incontinence.[21]

Delirium, often the first sign of an infection in the elderly, can cause incontinence as a result of a diminished ability to perceive and interpret signals from the micturition center in the cortex. Behaviors exhibited while delirious, confused, disoriented, or restless may lead caregivers to chemically or physically restrain the individual, thus limiting access to toilet facilities.

As with functional incontinence, transient incontinence can be caused by impaired mobility. The stress of a sudden change in mobility such as sprain or fracture of a lower extremity can lead a normally continent and independent adult to be incontinent until the previous level of functioning is resumed. Imposed bedrest also contributes to incomplete emptying of the bladder unless a normal voiding position is assumed.

Acute urinary tract infections, including pyuria, sometimes cause urgency and a sense of precipitation. Bacteriuria is a common finding in older adults, and its relationship to the development of urinary incontinence is not clearly understood. Asymptomatic bacteriuria is often transient in nature and generally is not treated.[22, 23] However, bacteriuria with symptoms of frequency, urgency, and dysuria is treated with appropriate antimicrobials.

Medications and medical conditions that increase the volume of urine production may also precipitate incontinence. Fast-acting diuretics can overload the bladder and shorten the time between onset of sensation of the need to void and actual voiding. Ingestion of alcohol has a diuretic effect; in sufficient amounts it clouds the consciousness of the individual, thus impairing the ability to perceive and act on the need to micturate. Anticholinergic medications have a urinary retentive effect; acute onset of overflow incontinence may result, especially in vulnerable individuals such as men with benign prostatic hypertrophy (BPH). A side effect of alpha-adrenergic agonists, beta-adrenergic agonists, and calcium channel blockers is urinary retention. Medical conditions such as hyperglycemia and hypercalcemia may induce polyuria, which in turn can create transient incontinence.

Clinical States

Urinary incontinence is not a disease but a condition or a symptom.[1] As can be seen in Table 10–3, several clinical states can result in incontinence.

Changes in the position of the female pelvic structures, such as prolapse of the bladder into the vagina, uterine prolapse into the vagina, and bulging of the rectum into the vagina, cause an anatomical deviation in the position of the bladder neck and proximal urethra that can result in stress incontinence. In postmenopausal women, atrophic vaginitis and weakening of vaginal tissues as a result of estrogen deficiency are suggested causes of stress incontinence by decreasing outlet resistance.[24] Because contraction of the pelvic musculature aids in the lengthening, support, and compression of the urethra,[25] weak or lax pelvic muscles, it is believed, would contract less efficiently and thus have a weaker effect on compressing the urethra.

Diseases and conditions such as Parkinson's disease, multiple sclerosis, dementia, neoplasms, and cerebral vascular accidents that affect the frontal lobe may result in detrusor hyperreflexia (uninhibited contractions arising from a neurological defect). If the ability to inhibit micturition sufficiently is diminished, urge incontinence results.

Suprasacral lesions, tumors, or trauma may lead to the loss of the conscious need to void and to the loss of inhibitory control of micturition by the cerebral cortex. Bladder emptying, then, is controlled by the sacral micturition center. Reflex incontinence occurs as frequent uncontrolled voiding.

Men with benign prostatic hypertrophy may experience overflow incontinence. In some cases, the prostate, which surrounds the bladder neck and proximal urethra, enlarges to the point of occluding the outlet. Men with benign prostatic hypertrophy who ingest prescribed or over-the-counter medications with side effects of urinary retention are at risk of developing acute urinary retention and overflow incontinence.

Other common bladder outlet obstructions are urethral stricture and fecal impaction. Peripheral neuropathy that disrupts afferent input to the brain stem and cortical center of control (i.e., tabes dorsalis, diabetic neuropathy) leads to diminished conscious control of micturition. Neuropathy that damages efferent motor pathways to the bladder also results in large flaccid bladders. Alcoholic neuropathy and peripheral neuropathy secondary to diabetes mellitus and lumbar disk herniation are common causes of overflow incontinence. Bladder dysfunction has been found to be related to the severity of the underlying disease process.[18]

As previously mentioned, any medical condition that impedes an individual's ability to reach a toilet or communicate the need to use the toilet can lead to functional incontinence. Also, mixed types of incontinence occur owing to various factors. For example, women who have stress incontinence, chronic cystitis, or urinary tract infections with associated sensations of urgency may have a combination of stress and urge incontinence.

TABLE 10–3 CAUSES OF URINARY INCONTINENCE

Stress	Incompetent urethra, weak pelvic floor musculature
Urge	Lower urinary tract: urinary tract infection, cystitis, bladder tumor, bladder stones Central nervous system: cerebral vascular accident, dementia, Parkinson's disease, normal pressure hydrocephalus, multiple sclerosis
Reflex	Spinal cord tumor/lesion
Overflow	Outlet obstruction: prostatic hypertrophy, fecal impaction Chronic myogenic decompensation: peripheral neuropathy
Functional	Impaired mobility, severe dementia, communication difficulties, depression, hostility, caregiver or toilets or toilet substitutes unavailable

DEVELOPMENTAL DIMENSIONS

Comparisons of old people and children with urinary incontinence have abounded for years. In 1749 a physician wrote, "children and old people often piss-a-bed in their sleep, but these come not to the physician to be cured."[26] However, the comparison ends there; an important distinction between the two groups is the current societal expectation that children eventually grow into continence and old people slip inexorably into decline.

Age-related changes occur in the bladder that include decreased bladder capacity and delayed onset of the sensation to void. The consequence of these changes is a possible frequency in voiding and a decrease in time between conscious desire to void and actual voiding. An increase in the amount of residual urine and an increase in the number of involuntary detrusor contractions are also considered changes of aging. These changes are not of such a magnitude as to cause incontinence directly; rather, they enhance the risk of incontinence if the balance between the factors that maintain continence is disrupted. Research clearly shows, however, that age alone does not cause incontinence.[27] Incontinence in older persons can often be effectively treated with remedial and restorative interventions.

Symptoms of bladder outlet obstruction due to prostatic hypertrophy include nocturia, pain during micturition, frequency, urgency, and small volumes of urine. Symptoms of obstruction of the bladder neck include hesitancy, decrease in force of stream, sensation of incomplete emptying, and prolonged voiding time.[28] Urge incontinence is more frequently seen in men and older adults.[24] About half of the men with benign prostatic hypertrophy causing obstruction of the bladder outlet also have detrusor instability and urgency.[29] Treatment includes surgical resection of the prostate.

The role of menopause in the development of incontinence in women is unclear.[6] Postmenopausal women experience thinning of the vaginal wall and increased vascular frailty. The vaginal wall is vulnerable to infection or trauma without estrogen replacement.[30] The urethra and bladder neck are also estrogen sensitive, becoming less efficient in closure and achieving a water tight seal. An associated symptom of atrophic vaginitis, in which the vulva appears dry, inflamed, and reddened, is stress incontinence.[31] Once atrophic vaginitis is treated with estrogen, incontinence is often eliminated.[18]

MECHANISMS

A review of the normal physiology of micturition and continence is necessary to understand disruptions in bladder filling and urine storage and emptying. This mechanism is mediated by intraindividual psychosocial factors, environmental influences, and societal norms. The process of socially acceptable urinary elimination involves a complex interaction between the anatomical structures of the lower urinary tract (bladder and urethra)

and the central and peripheral nervous systems.

The bladder acts as a reservoir for urine until voluntary emptying occurs. The body of the bladder passively stretches and fills with urine until stretch receptors located in the bladder wall send impulses along afferent nerve pathways to the sacral micturition center (S2–4), illustrated in Figure 10–1. The sacral micturition center, in turn, relays signals via a somatic nerve, the pudendal nerve, to sustain and increase the tone of the pelvic muscle.[24] This striated muscle surrounds the external urethral opening and is one component of what in older textbooks was referred to as the external urethral sphincter mechanism.

The other component consists of striated muscle that surrounds the urethra above the pelvic muscle and extends to the bladder neck, forming a significant portion of the outer muscular wall of the urethra as shown in Figure 10–2. There are gender differences in the smooth muscle that constitutes the bladder neck. In the female urethra this smooth muscle follows a longitudinal path in the urethral wall; in contrast, a well-defined circular collar of smooth muscle surrounds

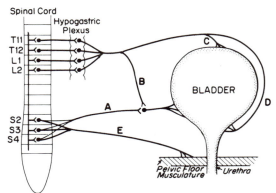

TYPE OF NERVE	FUNCTION
A PARASYMPATHETIC CHOLINERGIC (Nervi Erigentes)	Bladder contraction
B SYMPATHETIC	Bladder relaxation (by inhibition of parasympathetic tone)
C SYMPATHETIC	Bladder relaxation (β adrenergic)
D SYMPATHETIC	Bladder neck and urethral contraction (α adrenergic)
E SOMATIC (Pudendal nerve)	Contraction of pelvic floor musculature

Figure 10–1. Peripheral nerves involved in micturition. (From Ouslander, J. [1989]. Incontinence. In R. Kane, J. Ouslander, & I. Abrass [eds.], *Essentials of Geriatric Medicine* [2nd ed., p. 143]. New York: McGraw-Hill, with permission.)

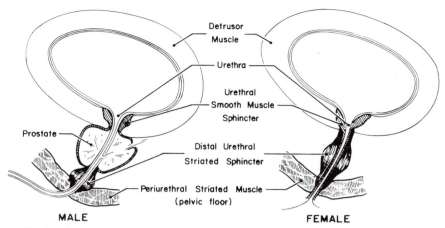

Figure 10–2. Diagram of anatomy of the lower urinary tract. (Adapted from Gosling, J. [1979]. The structure of the bladder and urethra in relation to function. Urol Clin North Am *6:*31.) (Reproduced from Wyman, J. [1988] Nursing assessment of the incontinent geriatric outpatient population. Nurs Clin North Am *23:*170, with permission.)

the male bladder neck and proximal urethra. Gosling suggested that other factors such as elastic tissue, striated muscle, and a vascular component aid in the provision of a functional watertight sphincter in women.[32]

The hypogastric plexus provides efferent sympathetic activity and relaxes the detrusor through inhibition of parasympathetic ganglionic transmission. Increases in urethral contraction occur through stimulation of adrenergic receptors in the smooth muscle sphincter located at the base of the bladder and proximal urethra.[33] In older textbooks, the smooth muscle sphincter was called the internal sphincter mechanism.

Higher neurological levels of bladder function control are alerted by the sacral micturition center. The micturition center in the brain stem, pontine-mesencephalic gray matter, comprises a common pathway to the motor neurons of the bladder.[33] This center synchronizes the relaxation of the urethral sphincter and the contraction of the bladder to facilitate voiding. The highest levels of control are located in the frontal lobe of the cerebral cortex and the basal ganglia.[34] They serve primarily to inhibit or delay voiding.[24]

As shown in Figure 10–3, initially there is little increase in intravesical pressure as the bladder fills. However, as the bladder dis-

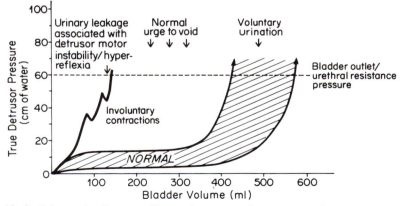

Figure 10–3. Schematic diagram illustrating normal pressure-volume relationships in the bladder and the urodynamic phenomenon of uninhibited or involuntary bladder contractions—also referred to as detrusor-motor instability or detrusor hyperreflexia. (From Ouslander, J. [1989]. Incontinence. In R. Kane, J. Ouslander, & I. Abrass [eds.], *Essentials of Geriatric Medicine* [2nd ed., p. 144]. New York: McGraw-Hill, with permission.)

tends and the pressure within the bladder increases, the conscious desire to empty the bladder increases. To maintain continence, the intraurethral pressure must exceed the intravesical pressure.[24] However, when voluntary micturition occurs, there is inhibition of somatic and sympathetic nerve activity.[21] As the resistance of the outlet at the base of the bladder decreases, the bladder neck and proximal urethra assume a funnel-like configuration, and coordinated contraction of the bladder occurs. Because the detrusor consists of interwoven bundles of smooth muscles that are woven into a complex mesh, it functions in a coordinated contraction to empty urine when stimulated. Dysfunction occurs in one or both phases of micturition (i.e., bladder filling and urine storage) and bladder emptying.[33]

Mechanism of Stress Incontinence

Individuals who involuntarily lose urine in the absence of contraction of the detrusor experience stress incontinence. Usually, a small volume of urine is lost with a sudden increase in intra-abdominal pressure that occurs, for example, in sneezing, coughing, and active exercises such as jumping jacks. The underlying cause is usually an incompetent urethra.[35] The incompetency may arise from a change in location of the bladder neck and proximal urethra during abdominal straining. Normally, the bladder neck and proximal urethra lay above the pelvic muscle within the abdominal cavity, and there occurs uninterrupted transmission of increases in intra-abdominal pressure with a corresponding increase in intraurethral pressure. When the bladder neck and proximal urethra are not supported in a position in which transmission of pressure increases is able to take place, and the intraurethral pressure is exceeded, urine leakage will occur. After a prostatectomy, men sometimes have stress incontinence due to sphincter insufficiency as a postoperative complication.[36]

Mechanism of Urge Incontinence

In contrast to stress incontinence, in which a small amount of urine is lost, urge incontinence usually involves a larger quantity of urine loss.[25, 37] Figure 10–3 demonstrates normal filling of the bladder; involuntary

contractions of the detrusor are absent or suppressed. However, when there are contractions of a sufficient magnitude that are not inhibited early in the filling cycle, incontinence may occur. Uninhibited contractions are caused by central factors such as disorders or injuries of the central nervous system control of micturition and by localized factors such as cystitis, bladder tumors, or lesions.

An underlying mechanism of uninhibited detrusor contraction is disruption in the central nervous system micturition center. An individual experiences frequency and urgency when the parasympathetic response in the spinal micturition center to infection or inflammation exceeds the inhibitory effect of the cortical micturition center. Uninhibited detrusor contractions may also result from deconditioned voiding reflexes.[38] For example, some people resort to frequent voiding and maintaining chronic low bladder volume to avoid incontinent episodes. This practice, however, reduces bladder capacity, and with time the bladder wall thickens, aggravating the condition of decreased tone and increased instability.[38] Incontinence due to uninhibited detrusor contractions in the absence of a neurological disorder is also referred to as detrusor motor instability.

Women who have stress incontinence or chronic cystitis or urinary tract infections with associated sensations of urgency may develop a habit of frequent voiding to prevent an "accident" and in turn develop a deconditioned micturition reflex.

Mechanism of Reflex Incontinence

Individuals with lesions or tumors located in the spinal cord above the sacral reflex but below the brain stem micturition center often have no conscious sensation of the need to void. This is due to an interruption in the transmission of information to the higher centers of micturition control. Also, detrusor sphincter dyssynergia—the lack of relaxation of pelvic musculature during bladder contraction—may also result from a suprasacral pathology. The result of both of these conditions is frequent voiding of moderate volume.[39]

Mechanism of Overflow Incontinence

Overflow incontinence often results from two pathological mechanisms. The first involves a bladder with normal contractibility function but which is obstructed at the outlet; this results in overdistention of the bladder. Once the intravesical pressure exceeds intraurethral pressure, urine will dribble out in a continuous fashion. The underlying mechanism of overflow incontinence caused by fecal impaction is unclear. It is thought that the distended bowel may occlude or obstruct the bladder outlet.[2] The second mechanism, chronic myogenic decompensation, often leads to overflow incontinence. The result is a large flaccid acontractile bladder.

Mechanism of Functional Incontinence

Functional incontinence occurs in individuals with an intact urinary tract. Normal bladder capacity ranges from 300 to 600 ml,[21] and it is difficult for a person to keep urine from escaping from the bladder once capacity has been achieved. Therefore, for individuals whose bladder capacity has been reached but find the distance to the bathroom or environmental barriers preventing timely access to a toilet, incontinence results. Sprecht reported that if the time taken to reach a toilet exceeds the interval between acknowledging the need to void and actual voiding, incontinence will occur.[40]

Psychological processes, such as depression and anxiety, have been implicated in the development of incontinence. Depression has been viewed as an antecedent to urinary incontinence as well as a consequence. Newman postulated that emotional breakdown through emotional isolation in older adults, similar to the experiences of prisoners of war, was a cause of incontinence.[41] A state of hopelessness evolves and hygienic behaviors sharply deteriorate. Williams and Pannill stated that institutionalized older adults are subjected to adverse stimuli to normal voiding, such as a lack of privacy during toileting.[38] They postulated that the subsequent feelings of humiliation could lead to a loss of the incentive to be continent. Motivation is thought to play an important, yet undetermined role in continence. Hadley and colleagues reported that motivation to be continent was a requirement for continence.[42]

Some older adults have a combination of the different types of incontinence previously discussed. For instance, women often report

mixed symptoms of stress and urge incontinence.[13, 43] Therefore, identification of underlying mechanisms of incontinence is necessary for appropriate interventions to be instituted.

RELATED PATHOPHYSIOLOGICAL CONCEPTS

A pathophysiological concept related to urinary incontinence is alteration in skin integrity, especially in individuals unable or unwilling to perform personal hygiene. Adults with concurrent conditions that affect the integrity of the skin, such as malnutrition, peripheral vascular disorders, dependent edema secondary to inactivity and circulatory disorders, and diabetes mellitus, may be at increased risk for pressure sores. Also, fecal incontinence, which is associated with urinary incontinence, places an individual at risk for pressure sores.[44] Fecal incontinence in the absence of urinary incontinence is uncommon. The prevalence of fecal incontinence without urinary incontinence in nursing home residents is estimated to be 1.8 per cent. However, the prevalence of double incontinence (bowel and bladder) is estimated to be 32.5 per cent.[12] Therefore, although pressure sores may not be a direct result of urinary incontinence alone, fecal and urinary incontinence are prevalent conditions found in impaired populations.

The signal to void is a full bladder; therefore, hydration is a related physiological concept. Many times, older persons limit their fluid intake in the mistaken belief that it helps to reduce incontinent episodes.[5]

ASSOCIATED PSYCHOLOGICAL CONCEPTS

Because the physiological process of storing and expelling urine is shaped by social rules for acceptable times and places for elimination, urinary incontinence represents a deviation from societal norms. Children are expected to have bladder control by age 5 or by the time they start school. School-aged children, especially boys who have difficulty with urine control at night, can be stigmatized by unsympathetic peers and adults.

Adults are expected to maintain continence to remain in the social world. Traditionally, incontinence was rarely reported to one's physician; there was, and sometimes still is, a sense of futility in finding a remedy to the problem. Ingrained social stereotypes that compare older adults to babies persist. Even though the manufacturers of adult disposable underclothing used to contain urine insist on calling them "adult briefs," the common term, diaper, is used by caregivers and sometimes the older adults themselves. The loss of continence has been interpreted as a loss of social and personal competence. Incontinence is often cited as a reason for nursing home placement.[45]

Related psychosocial concepts to urinary incontinence include stigma, shame, self-esteem, and dependency. A dictionary definition of incontinence is "lack of restraint of the passions or appetites, free or uncontrolled indulgences of the passions or appetites; especially of the sexual appetite."[46] The stigma of lack of self-control can be and often is applied to incontinent adults. Goffman discussed a stigmatized individual as one who is different and less desirable than others.[47] This person is discounted and viewed as less than whole by the normal members of society. Willington noted that incontinence has "all the stigmata of failure"[48] (p. 3). The individual reacts to the stigma of incontinence in a variety of psychological ways, such as expressing feelings of shame, denying the existence of the disruption by using cognitive strategies of defining the problem (i.e., "I'm not incontinent if I only wet my nightgown but not the bed linens"), or accepting incontinence as inevitable.

Community-dwelling women reported restricting social activities, feelings of embarrassment, and having sexual difficulties.[49] Wyman and associates used a 26-item questionnaire, The Incontinence Impact Questionnaire, and found that active women dwelling in the community who participated in outings that involved long-distance travel and unfamiliar places were most affected by incontinence.[50] The women also reported fear of embarrassment from an incontinent episode. However, Simons reported that women living in the community felt that incontinence was inevitable with advancing age and experienced no difference in self-esteem than continent women.[51] The cumulative effect on mental health of restricting interpersonal and social activities and the fear of potentially stigmatizing situations has not been determined, yet is assumed to have far-

reaching effects. Isolation reduces social support and access to health care systems and may have a negative impact on the physical and mental health of the individual.

Yu found that most incontinent nursing home residents felt that they were outcasts and were ashamed of being incontinent.[52] Yu and associates did not find their questionnaire useful in measuring the psychological stress associated with incontinence with cognitively impaired residents of nursing homes because of the severity of the cognitive impairment.[53] Therefore, the psychological impact of urinary incontinence on severely cognitively impaired adults is not known.

Another psychosocial concept related to incontinence, especially in the nursing home setting, is dependency. Miller suggested that rather than patient dependency driving nursing care, just the opposite occurs. Deterioration in functioning of patients in geriatric hospitals "is not an antecedent event which is followed by dependency, but a consequent event preceded by detrimental ward environments"[54] (p. 482). Patients who were exposed to individualized nursing care had lower dependency needs (bathing, dressing, toileting) than patients with similar baseline dependency needs who received traditional task-oriented care.[55]

As an essential part of the nursing home environment, the nursing staff acts as a powerful influence on the residents. When interactions between the staff and patients were examined, staff members were found to support dependent behaviors and to ignore independent behaviors exhibited by the residents.[56] Although independent behaviors of personal maintenance (self-care behaviors of toileting, dressing, eating) were not supported by the nursing staff, residents maintained these behaviors through a yet unexplained mechanism of chaining behaviors in clusters.[57] (In behavioral terms, behaviors to be maintained are often clustered in chains, which are series of behaviors that are linked or joined together by reinforcers.) Because the direction of the relationship between dependency and incontinence is not clear, more research is needed in a variety of settings in which incontinent adults reside.

MANIFESTATIONS

Subjective Manifestations

Table 10–4 lists some subjective and objective manifestations of each type of urinary

TABLE 10–4   MANIFESTATIONS OF URINARY INCONTINENCE

	Subjective	Objective
Stress	Report of small amount of urine loss with a cough, sneeze, laugh, change of position; sensation of heaviness in pelvic area	Leaking of urine with standing and/or lying stress test; hypermobility of urethra during voiding cystometrogram; evidence of weak vaginal tone, cystocele, atrophic vaginitis, or sphincter incompetence during pelvic exam
Urge	Report of need to void comes on too fast to get to toilet; loss of large amount of urine; frequent voiding; loss of urine at sound of water running or when waiting for access to a public toilet	Evidence of urinary tract infection, inflammation of bladder wall; uninhibited bladder contractions on cystometrogram; evidence of neurological lesion in cerebral cortex; deconditioned micturition reflex during physical exam
Overflow	Report of incomplete emptying of the bladder; dribbling of urine; painful abdomen; unaware of urine loss	Palpable bladder during abdominal exam; large amount of urine in bladder after voiding; evidence of outlet obstruction (i.e., enlarged prostate palpated during rectal exam)
Functional	Report of unable to get to bathroom on time; unable to position for toileting without assistance; lack of convenient access to toilet	No incontinence when access to toilet or assistance to toilet is available; evidence of impaired mobility, manual dexterity, communication, or cognitive skills; normal functioning of urinary tract during urodynamic testing

incontinence. It has been reported that older adults often do not report incontinence to their physician or other health care professionals out of a belief that there is nothing to be done or because of the sensitive nature of the subject.[24, 58, 59] There is little correlation between self-report of severity of incontinence and amount of urine collected in perineal pads. Warwick and Brown found that a self-report of improvement in incontinence after treatment often does not match the results of clinical testing.[60] Some women overestimated the amount of improvement despite leakage of urine during objective evaluation. Sutherst and associates used the weight of perineal pads worn by incontinent women to measure the severity of the condition.[61] The authors noted a poor correlation between quantified loss and the self-report of urine loss. Parkin and Davis reported that women with detrusor instability indicated worse symptoms when using a visual analogue scale for severity of urinary loss than did women with stress incontinence.[62] However, Frazer and coworkers found no significant relationship between the self-report of urine loss as measured by a visual analogue scale and objective measure using 2-hour perineal pad weight.[63] A detailed history and thorough physical examination is essential for diagnosis and appropriate treatment.

Objective Manifestations

Besides those listed in Table 10–4, objective manifestations of incontinence include visibly wet clothing, furniture, flooring, and bed linens. Urine odor on the person and in the living environment is usually a sign that problems with urine control exist. The amount of urine loss can be objectively determined by weighing perineal pads.[61]

SURVEILLANCE AND MEASUREMENT

Assessment includes making the distinction between transient or acute onset and established incontinence. When there is acute onset incontinence, the common causes require investigation. If the incontinence is persistent, antecedent factors and patterns of episodes should be explored. A careful history and physical examination are essential to identify underlying causes of incontinence and to determine the need for urodynamic testing.

The history of any individual with incontinence should include current medications, medical and psychiatric conditions, and a description of urinary symptoms and incontinent episodes. Information about antecedent factors and behaviors is also important: Was a diuretic ingested? How much fluid was consumed? Did the person attempt to delay voiding? Did the person make an effort to get to a toilet? What environmental factors might have hindered or enhanced access to the toilet?

The effects of incontinence on everyday life and the quality of life must be explored: Does the individual avoid social interactions or limit social outings? Are intimate relationships affected by incontinence? The methods of management should be elicited as well as the person's motivation for improving continence status. In institutionalized older adults, the level and quality of interaction between the incontinent older adult and the nursing staff should be assessed.

A written record of incontinent episodes is important in the assessment of the frequency and severity of incontinence.[64] There are several voiding diaries or bladder charts reported in the literature; only a few are referenced.[24, 29, 31, 65-67] A chart to record information regarding voiding usually includes the following information: date, time of continent voiding, time of leakage or large amount of urine loss, activities engaged in at the time of the incontinent episode, and fluids ingested throughout the day. For literate, cognitively intact, community-dwelling individuals, space on the chart for comments about factors that influence or potentially cause the incontinent episode is necessary.

The reader is also referred to select algorithms that have been developed for evaluating incontinence.[21, 68] Figure 10–4 illustrates an algorithm that is used by a nurse practitioner. Medical, physical, and environmental factors that are easily treated or modified are assessed first. Furthermore, the algorithm is also useful in identifying individuals who require consultation with a urologist and more extensive urodynamic tests. Careful history taking and physical examination are the cornerstones of this algorithm.

A thorough examination of the neurological and genitourinary systems is a necessary component of the physical examination. The abdomen should be palpated for masses and tenderness. A rectal examination should be performed to determine impaction and masses, the size of the prostate in men, and the level of sphincter tone and perineal sensation.[29] Assessment of the level of mobility and manual dexterity and mental status, especially of impaired older adults, is also necessary.

The urine should be examined for hematuria and evidence of infection. A postvoiding residual (PVR) provides information regarding the emptying capacity of the bladder; a residual volume exceeding 100 ml may indicate an obstruction at the bladder outlet or weak detrusor contraction. Blood chemistry analysis includes the determination of urea nitrogen, creatinine, and glucose levels to detect renal disease or diabetes mellitus.

Ouslander described bedside diagnostic tests to evaluate incontinence in older adults.[29] For example, the individual is requested to void to determine the amount and the volume at which the desire to void occurs. A PVR is then obtained via catheter. With the catheter in place the bladder is filled with sterile water or saline to determine bladder filling capacity and whether uninhibited detrusor contractions occur. The individual is asked to cough in the supine and sometimes in the standing position after the catheter is removed to observe for urinary leakage. Ouslander reported that these tests had a 75 per cent sensitivity and 95 per cent specificity.[29]

Urodynamic tests are also performed to determine underlying pathology. The use of urodynamic tests to evaluate all incontinent adults has been questioned.[24] However, urodynamic studies are indicated when neurological abnormalities are identified, incomplete bladder emptying occurs with overflow incontinence, and stress incontinence is associated with urethral dysfunction.[18]

Cystometrograms determine the filling and storage capacity of the bladder. Uninhibited bladder contractions are detected by transducers used to monitor intravesical pressure and intra-abdominal pressure once the bladder is filled. To evaluate bladder emptying, a noninvasive test, uroflowmetry, is employed. The rate of urine flow is measured by a strip chart recorder as the person voids into a special apparatus. This test is used to diagnose urethral obstruction.[24]

A voiding cystourethrogram evaluates pelvic relaxation in women, postprostatectomy incontinence in men, and urinary retention after abdominal-perineal resection.[18] The presence of spinal abnormalities, cystocele, urethral diverticulum, and intraurethral abnormalities as well as abnormal movement of the urethra during voiding can be detected using this procedure. There are other diagnostic urodynamic tests used to detect abnormalities in voiding and pathologic disorders in the urinary tract.

There is no system to classify severity of symptoms objectively for each type of incontinence. However, attempts have been made to classify the severity of incontinence by the quantity of urine lost. The measurement of the severity of incontinence may need to include psychological factors in addition to a quantified amount and pattern of urine loss.

In an attempt to measure the psychological stress associated with incontinence objectively, Yu and colleagues developed an Incontinence Stress Questionnaire for Patients (ISQ-P).[53] There are two versions of this instrument: one has 20 items and the other has 36 items. This tool is used to detect depressive symptoms, aesthetic and bodily concerns, and feelings of shame. The tool was of limited use with cognitively impaired adults, although some of the cognitively impaired participants in one study were able to respond to the questionnaire.

THERAPIES

Several clinical therapies are available to treat urinary incontinence. Surgical procedures to treat stress incontinence in women, to relieve bladder outlet obstruction secondary to an enlarged prostate in men, to implant artificial sphincters, and to induce denervation of the bladder at the central or peripheral level are reviewed elsewhere.[6, 36, 60]

Devices used to collect urine include external and indwelling catheters and absorbent pads and garments. An ideal external collection device for women has not been perfected, although there are several designs.[69] Indwelling catheters should be considered as a last resort for incontinence management because of the associated morbidity, that is, bacteriuria and increased risk of septicemia. However, indwelling catheters are appropriate to monitor output accurately as necessary, to maintain skin integrity and wound cleanliness, and to provide comfort for terminally ill persons and those with intractable incontinence.[70]

Absorbent pads and undergarments are useful as the sole management strategy for incontinence or used as adjuncts to other therapies, such as pelvic floor exercises.[71] Absorbent products include disposable and reusable briefs, pads, panty liners, and shields. A multitude of incontinence products are available. For example, there are products designed specifically for men who leak a small amount of urine as well as adult underpants with a superabsorbent polymer that contain large volumes of urine for hours. No single product will be appropriate for all incontinent individuals who need or desire to use these products.[72] Therefore, assessment of level of functioning and personal preferences play a part in the determination of the product best suited for the individual.

A variety of resources provide descriptions of available continence products.[15, 69, 73, 74] These products ought to be used only after careful assessment of the incontinent individual and as a last resort to promote the quality of life. These products must not be used solely for the convenience of the staff or as a substitute for human intervention.

Pharmacological Therapy

Pharmacological treatment may be used alone or in conjunction with behavioral therapies. Medications are used to improve bladder emptying, to inhibit bladder contraction, and to strengthen the bladder outlet (Table 10–5).

A cholinergic agonist, bethanechol, may be used parenterally to increase intravesical pressure to maximize bladder emptying.[75] However, because of cholinergic side effects, bethanechol may be contraindicated for use in older adults. Drugs used to treat urge incontinence by inhibiting bladder contractions include imipramine, oxybutynin, propantheline, and flavoxate. Oxybutynin and flavoxate may have a relaxant effect on the detrusor as well as anticholinergic properties. Because of the potential anticholinergic side effects of these drugs, such as blurred vision, changes in mental status, and constipation, they must be used cautiously in the older adult population.

Stress incontinence can be treated with drugs that increase bladder outlet resistance. These include alpha-adrenergic agonists, pseudoephedrine, phenylpropanolamine, imipramine, and topically applied estrogens. Alpha-adrenergic agonists are contraindicated for individuals with hypertension, hyperthyroidism, and cardiovascular disease. Estrogens are contraindicated in women with a history of carcinoma of the breast and thrombophlebotic disease.

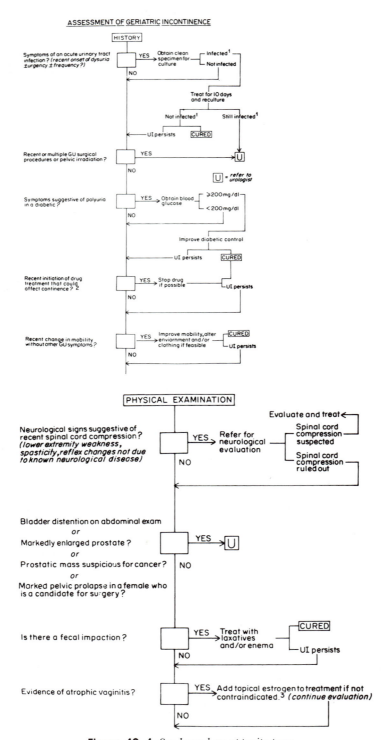

Figure 10–4. *See legend on opposite page*

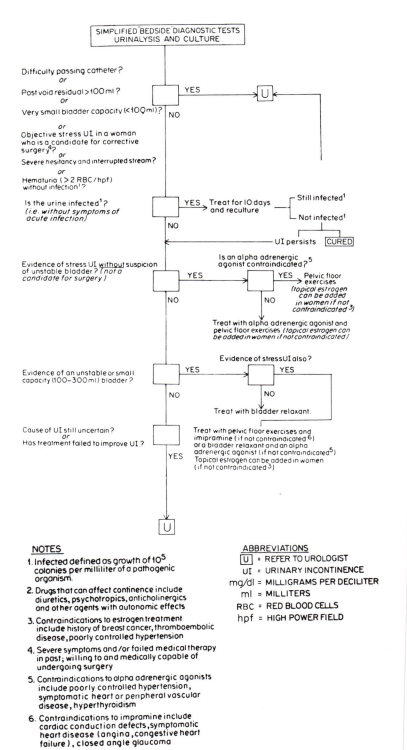

Figure 10–4. Algorithm for assessing geriatric incontinence. (From Ouslander, J. [1986]. Diagnostic evaluation of geriatric incontinence. Clin Geriatr Med *2:*726–727, with permission.)

TABLE 10–5   DRUGS USED TO TREAT URINARY INCONTINENCE

Drug	Mechanism	Uses	Nursing Implications
Anticholinergics/ spasmodics (propantheline, imipramine, oxybutynin, flavoxate, dicyclomine)	Increases bladder capacity; diminishes bladder contractions	Urge incontinence associated with bladder instability	Assess for mental status changes, urinary retention, vision changes, difficulty swallowing or eating, and constipation. Monitor blood pressure.
Alpha-adrenergic agonists (pseudoephedrine, imipramine, phenylpropanolamine)	Contracts the urethral smooth muscle	Stress incontinence associated with sphincter weakness	Assess for mental status changes, weakness, dizziness, difficulty swallowing or eating. Monitor blood pressure.
Conjugated estrogens (oral, topical)	Increases periurethral blood flow; strengthens periurethral tissues	Stress incontinence associated with sphincter weakness	Assess for vaginal bleeding, genitourinary or abdominal pain, hemorrhagic skin eruptions, and changes in sexual function. Monitor blood pressure and weight.
Cholinergic agonists (bethanechol)	Promotes bladder contraction	Overflow incontinence associated with atonic bladder	Assess for abdominal discomfort, difficulty swallowing, nausea, vomiting, and bowel pattern changes. Monitor intake and output (I&O) and blood pressure.
Antibiotics (general classification)	Treats bladder infections	Urinary tract infections	General nursing implications for all antibiotics.
Oral penicillin	Antibacterial	Urinary tract infections	Read and follow specific information for each medication.
Oral cephalosporins	Bactericidal or bacteriostatic	Urinary tract infections	Assess patients' allergies/ hypersensitivities to antibiotics.
Oral tetracyclines	Antibacterial	Urinary tract infections	Obtain a culture and sensitivity before first dose.
Oral sulfonamides	Inhibit bacterial growth	Urinary tract infections	Determine patient's weight. Monitor laboratory values. Assess for allergic reaction. Assess for overgrowth of nonsensitive organisms. Assess vital signs. Assess appetite. Assess for dizziness. Assess bowel pattern. Monitor I&O. Assess mental status for changes. Assess patient's sleep/wake patterns. Assess oral hygiene. Assess patient's ability to ambulate/ transfer safely. Assess renal and hepatic function. Teach patient to avoid sunlight. Store medication properly. Check expiration date for medication.

From McCormick, K., Scheve, A., & Leahy, E. (1988). Nurs Clin North Am 23:238–239.
Data in the first three columns are from Ouslander, J.G. (1986). Drug therapy for geriatric incontinence. Clin Geriatr Med 2:790.
Data on antibiotics are from Gever, L., Robinson, J., Rome, A., et al. (1980). *Nurse's Guide to Drugs.* Horsham, PA: Intermed Communications.

Behavioral Therapies

Behavioral therapies for incontinence in adults include scheduled toileting, bladder retraining, contingency management, biofeedback, and pelvic muscle exercises with components of other behavioral therapies. In the institutional long-term care setting, staff management techniques have been used with success to improve the continence status of elderly residents.

Scheduled toileting, also called habit training,

involves a fixed schedule, usually every 2 to 4 hours, for bladder emptying. A bladder chart is kept and is modified after the individualized pattern of continent and incontinent voiding is identified. Continence depends on the diligence of caregivers to adhere to the schedule of toileting patients. This is a frequently used intervention in institutionalized settings with cognitively impaired adults with functional or urge incontinence.[76]

Bladder retraining, also known as bladder drill or bladder training, involves a variable schedule of voiding. This intervention is suitable for an individual who is motivated and able to understand and interpret body sensations. This person keeps a bladder chart and is encouraged to expand the length of time between voidings. This intervention is used to treat urge incontinence.[77] By increasing the time between voidings, one can increase bladder capacity and urgency will eventually lessen. Drug therapy is used at times in conjunction with this intervention.[78]

Contingency management, also referred to as behavioral modification, is a consistent and systematic approach of rewarding continent voiding through verbal praise and discouraging incontinence with verbal disapproval.[37] An example of social disapproval is, "I don't understand why you wet on yourself and didn't ask for help. I come around every hour, or you can call me by pressing the buzzer."[79] Contingency management is sometimes combined with the scheduled voiding intervention. This method is used in both outpatient and inpatient settings and with cognitively impaired adults.

Biofeedback has been used for stress and urge incontinence and bladder-sphincter dyssynergia. An individual must be cognitively intact and motivated to understand visual or auditory biofeedback of various physiological parameters of urine control. Usually during a cystometric procedure, the individual watches tracings of bladder and abdominal pressure, bladder contraction, and sphincter and pelvic muscle activity. Physiological responses are changed through a process of operant conditioning in which the individual learns by observing the results of the voluntary efforts made to control bladder and sphincter activity.[80]

Pelvic muscle exercises, also called Kegel exercises, are most commonly used to treat female stress incontinence.[81] Women who are comfortable in using this technique learn how to contract the pelvic muscle without performing a Valsalva maneuver, which increases intra-abdominal pressure. Contraction of the muscle for 10 seconds and relaxation for 10 seconds, repeated for 50 to 60 contractions, are performed three times a day.[82] A device called a *perineometer* can be inserted into the vagina to provide feedback about the strength of the contraction.[83] Because the individual must comply with the exercise regimen daily, motivation is an integral part of the therapy. Pelvic muscle exercises may be used in conjunction with biofeedback, scheduled voiding, or bladder retraining.

Staff management in the institutional setting involves several components. An adequate number of primary nursing staff to care for incontinent patients is a fundamental requirement. A formula to determine the required staffing level is available.[84] Instructions for the staff to change their own behavior from cleaning up after an incontinent episode to proactive actions such as toileting patients are crucial. The staff behavior must be monitored and evaluated, with feedback given to individual staff members in the form of verbal or written praise about performance.[84]

REVIEW OF RESEARCH FINDINGS

There was little nursing research in the United States on urinary incontinence in adults, especially older adults, prior to the 1970s. Few nursing studies using case-control research designs are available. Reports in the literature are descriptive studies or clinical trials with small samples. However, there is encouraging evidence in the recent literature that nurses are becoming interested in conducting research related to incontinence and that nursing interventions are successful in the management of incontinence.

Research activities have focused on two general practice settings: long-term care and ambulatory care.

Long-term Care Setting

In the long-term care setting, anecdotal reports abound that environmental modifications such as encouraging self-toileting behavior, making toilets accessible, and positive staff attitudes improve continence status.[85–90] The characteristics of incontinent patients in nursing homes have been reported.[10, 91] Incontinent residents generally exhibit a higher level of mobility and cognitive impairment than continent residents.[92]

Behavioral therapies have long been used by clinicians to manage incontinence in various groups in institutional settings.[93] Interventions focus on modifying the antecedents or the consequences of incontinence.[37] Also Burgio and Burgio noted that behavioral therapies differ in administration.[76] Some therapies may be self-managed by the individual, such as biofeedback; other therapies are staff-managed, especially for cognitively and mobility impaired individuals.

As an example of the latter, Schnelle and colleagues described a study in which 126 residents in a long-term care facility were assigned to immediate and delayed prompted voiding therapy groups after baseline data were collected.[94] The majority of the subjects were cognitively impaired and incapable of independent voiding. Urodynamic tests at the bedside were performed by a urologist, and the level of wetness was measured throughout the day (7 a.m. to 7 p.m.). Prompted voiding treatment consisted of hourly checks of the subjects and asking if they were wet or dry. The subjects were checked for accuracy and if dry, were given social approval. If the resident was wet, clothing was changed and corrective feedback was given by telling the resident that assistance should have been requested. Socialization with the resident was minimized. Residents were also toileted and given additional social reinforcement when they expressed willingness to attempt to void. A significant predictor for success of this treatment was the first day's response—low wetness and high appropriate toileting behaviors were predictive of high continence levels. The authors suggested that residents were not learning new continence skills but were responding to increased opportunities in the environment to be continent. They also suggested that nurse managers use first-day baseline and first-day treatment responses as prognostic criteria to identify residents who would best respond to this therapy.

Creason and associates had similar results with prompted voiding therapy in 85 female residents of a long-term care facility.[95] The majority of the subjects had severe cognitive and functional impairments. Prompted voiding was an effective technique in reducing wet episodes over a 5-week period. Immediate response to treatment was not measured in this study, as it was in the study by Schnelle and colleagues, but by 5 weeks a significant reduction in incontinent episodes occurred.

Hu and colleagues used a randomized controlled experimental design to investigate the effectiveness of prompted voiding with female residents of a long-term care facility.[96] After baseline measures were obtained, 71 women were assigned to a control group and 72 women were assigned to the treatment group. The treatment period lasted 13 weeks, and follow-up data were collected at 2, 4, and 6 months after treatment. There were significant reductions in wet episodes immediately after treatment and throughout the follow-up period. The authors suggested that the treatment group continued to improve because the subjects learned to make self-initiated requests to use the toilet. It was also found that those with more severe incontinence improved more than those with less severe incontinence. The probability of improvement was greater for subjects with higher scores on the Mini-Mental State Examination,[97] and subjects who had normal bladder function responded well to training. There was an increase in labor costs over and above the savings in laundry costs. This finding supports other research showing that behavioral therapies are labor-intensive and increase costs at least initially to the facility.[98] Incentives such as financial rewards to staff who toilet patients and save money on supplies have been suggested. Also, the identification of individuals who would benefit from behavioral therapies is necessary for efficient management strategies to be implemented.

Engel and colleagues described a 3-year study that augmented a prompted voiding therapy with a staff management component.[99] Individual staff members received feedback from their supervisors regarding their performance on completing assigned toileting. Bar graphs depicting the percentage of completed toileting were shared at biweekly meetings. Letters praising performance or encouraging increased performance were given to the staff member. A 6-month summary letter signed by the director of nursing was placed in the personnel file. Behavioral therapy was effective in increasing continence, and individualized feedback was more effective than group feedback.

Ambulatory Care Setting

Mitteness, an anthropologist, provided valuable information about the cognitive organization of incontinence by older adults dwelling in the community.[5, 59] She found that elaborate plans were made to avoid detection by peers and others and that there was little effort to seek medical help. The terminology used by lay persons to discuss or describe urinary functioning differs from that of health care professionals; without this awareness poor communication and inaccurate data collection occur. Knowledge about the characteristics of incontinent adults in the community is growing.

Wells and associates reported clinical characteristics of 200 women who reported being incontinent.[100] Before treatment protocols were instituted, diagnoses were formed according to clinical criteria. A combination of urge and stress incontinence was present in 27 per cent of the sample. Pure stress incontinence was present in the majority (66 per cent) of the sample, and more than one third of the sample had atrophic vaginitis. In the community setting, women with stress incontinence have been treated on an outpatient basis with biofeedback and pelvic muscle exercises.

Baigis-Smith and associates found significant improvement in continence by using biofeedback techniques, habit training, and relaxation techniques in adults dwelling in the community.[101] Fifty-four cognitively intact older persons who were motivated to learn pelvic muscle exercises were recruited into the sample. There was a significant decrease in the number of wet episodes after pelvic muscle exercises and biofeedback. This decrease continued for 6-months to the follow-up visit. Age was not a significant factor in improvement in this study.

For frail elderly in the community, Morishita described a geriatric day hospital at which incontinent participants were evaluated and treated.[102] Nurses or nurse practitioners administer mental and functional status examinations. A nurse practitioner performs bedside diagnostic procedures described earlier in this chapter and works with a geriatrician in evaluating laboratory results and clinical findings to determine the diagnosis and treatment plan.

In treating incontinence with behavioral therapies, nurses have devised sophisticated methods of assessing pelvic muscle strength. Brink and associates evaluated the inter-rater reliability of a digital pelvic muscle rating scale.[103] This scale was tested with 338 women between the ages of 55 and 90 years who reported urinary incontinence. The scale ranged from 0, indicating no contraction of the pelvic muscle when the woman was instructed to contract the muscle during digital examination, to a score of 4, indicating a strong contraction lasting several seconds. These authors noted a positive relationship between pelvic muscle strength and ability to control urine stream and age. A three-dimensional scale to measure pressure, duration of the contraction, and displacement of the vertical plane was proposed. This scale is similar to the one devised by Worth and colleagues.[104] These authors tested a scale to measure four components of the circumvaginal muscle—pressure, duration, muscle ribbing, and position of the examiner's finger during the examination. This scale has been tested with 30 healthy young women with high inter-rater reliability ($rho = .6, P = .04$).

ILLUSTRATIVE CASE STUDIES

The following are illustrative case studies of two frequent types of incontinence in adults.

CASE STUDY NO. 1

C.L. visited a gynecologist at her daughter's insistence. She is a 66-year-old widow who lives alone in her home where she has lived for 40 years. She is active in volunteer work at the local community hospital and enjoys spending time with her three grandchildren. Ever since the birth of her last child 30 years ago, Mrs. L. experienced a small amount of urine leakage without warning when she laughed forcefully, sneezed, or coughed. She never mentioned this condition to her physician. She had not been examined by a gynecologist for 14 years, since the onset of menopause. Recently, Mrs. L. has had trouble getting to the bathroom in time. She has just started using commercially available undergarments for bladder control, limits her fluid intake during the day, and tries to go to the bathroom every hour whether or not the sensation to void is present. During a recent shopping trip with her daughter, she wet all her undergarments while attempting to get to the public restroom after lunch.

On examination, Mrs. L.'s abdomen was soft and nondistended and there were no scars. Two children had been vaginally delivered when she was 30 and 36 years old, respectively. During the pelvic examination, there was no evidence of a cystocele or uterine prolapse. While Mrs. L. was in the lying position, there was a small leakage of urine when she was instructed to cough. Further examination revealed that the vaginal walls looked pale and that there was a white discharge, indicating atrophic vaginitis. Muscle tone was weak when she was instructed to contract her vaginal muscles during the manual examination of the vagina. The rectal examination was negative for fecal impaction or rectal mass. A postvoiding residual urine was less than 50 ml.

Laboratory tests revealed serum glucose, urea nitrogen, and creatinine levels to be within normal limits. A urine culture was negative for infection.

Mrs. L. was instructed to keep a bladder diary for 14 days and to keep a record of her fluid intake. It was recommended that she attempt to drink six to eight glasses of water a day. Conjugated estrogen was prescribed intravaginally to treat atrophic vaginitis, and she was instructed to perform pelvic muscle exercises three times a day with at least 15 to 20 exercises during each session. An instruction sheet was given to remind her (1) not to tense her abdomen, buttocks, or thigh muscles during the exercises; (2) that each contraction should last 10 seconds, with 10 seconds of relaxation; (3) that the exercises should be practiced in the lying, sitting, and standing positions; and (4) to check if the correct muscle is being exercised by inserting a finger into the vagina and contracting the muscle.

After 2 weeks of regularly performing the exercises, Mrs. L. noticed a decrease in the number of incontinent episodes. She also found a pattern to some occurrences of urine loss; urine was lost when she moved from a sitting to standing position. She was instructed to use her exercises prior to changing positions. Also, a bladder-retraining schedule was instituted, initially set at every 2 hours with the anticipation of increasing the interval to 3 or 4 hours to decrease urgency symptoms. After another 6 weeks, Mrs. L. continued to be highly motivated to follow the regimen and was so pleased with the reduction in wetness that she stopped wearing bladder control undergarments.

CASE STUDY NO. 2

J.R. is a 79-year-old widowed resident of a small rural nursing home. She ambulates with great difficulty. Her feet are deformed from years of neglect and poorly fitting shoes. She is unable to walk unless she wears shoes with special supports. Mrs. R. is cognitively impaired; her score on the Mini-Mental State Examination is 15.[97] The staff must frequently reorient her to time and place. She recognizes familiar faces but does not retain names. Mrs. R. is incontinent of urine at least twice a day and once during the night. Each episode of incontinence occurs as she attempts to get to the bathroom. Mrs. R. voids in large amounts and is very distressed over being incontinent.

Her history is negative for cystocele, pelvic or rectal surgeries, or childbirth. A urine culture was negative for bacteria. Her fasting blood sugar was 100 mg/100 ml, serum creatinine was 1.5 mg/100 ml, and blood urea nitrogen was 12 mg/100 ml.

The nursing staff drew up a care plan that included a bladder chart and scheduled voiding. After 10 days, a pattern of incontinent episodes emerged and the bladder chart was refined to offer Mrs. R. assistance to the toilet immediately upon arising, before retiring at night, and every 3 hours during the day. Environmental modifications included a bedside commode at night and a second pair of shoes that offered support but were easy to slip on without assistance. The nursing staff consistently verbally praised her continent behavior and attempts at self-toileting. Incontinent episodes diminished to less than twice a week.

IMPLICATIONS FOR FURTHER RESEARCH

Although it is clear that age does not cause incontinence, there continues to be a need for research to develop a clear understanding of the natural history and development of urinary incontinence in adults. Developmental aspects must be considered in longitudinal prospective studies. It is important to learn whether incontinence that appears in active community-dwelling adults places them on a trajectory of increased impairment and disability in old age. Also, it is not clear whether results from studies of institutionalized elderly should be generalized to impaired adults in home care. Nurses need to replicate and extend research studies to other practice settings. Incontinence may present differently among various subgroups in the population, indicating that subclinical pathological processes need to be identified.

Primary health promotion strategies to maintain continence across the life span have yet to be developed.[105] Educational strategies are needed for health care professionals and lay persons to understand the normal changes in the functioning of the urinary system with age and how to access existing treatment modalities for incontinence. Through educational programs and factual information, lay and health care misconceptions that incontinence is an inevitable process with age will be changed.[106] There is little information regarding the developmental aspects of adult urinary incontinence. For example, the possible relationship between childhood enuresis and development of incontinence in later life has not been thoroughly investigated. However, Berrios reported that there was a significant association between the history of childhood enuresis and incontinence in adult psychotic patients admitted to a psychiatric ward.[107]

The relationship between personal regard for hygiene and incidence of incontinence, especially functional incontinence, has not been determined. Intra-individual factors, such as valuation of personal hygiene throughout childhood and adult life, is another underinvestigated area. Societal beliefs about aging and myths of the inevitability of decline may contribute to the development of incontinence and the reluctance to seek help on the part of many older adults.

Little is known about the effect of the social interaction between the staff and residents on the presence of urinary incontinence in the nursing home setting. The effect of adjustment to nursing homes and the presence of affective disorders in older adults, such as depression, remains to be investigated. Also the social impact of incontinence on adults in highly structured settings such as nursing homes and boarding homes has not been systematically investigated.

Concurrent with the increasing awareness of the different types of incontinence and the clinical criteria for diagnosis is the need for sensitive and specific assessment tools in the clinical setting. Development of tools to assess pelvic floor strength are underway. Reliable bladder records and diaries have been developed. Yet, there continues to be a need for practical clinical tests to assess actual urine loss in different settings. These tools will aid the nurse researcher and clinician in the identification of individuals who will most likely benefit from the array of restorative, rehabilitative, and comfort intervention strategies that are currently available.

Research has shown that nurses play a significant role in the assessment and treatment of urinary incontinence. Nurses have devised assessment methodologies that have been tested on relatively small samples. While there is a better understanding of the causes of incontinence and multiple interventions, more research, especially interdisciplinary research with large samples, is needed. Identification of individuals at risk for becoming and remaining incontinent is imperative. Palliative measures must be used as a last resort. Evaluation of current interventions employed in the clinical setting and the community is necessary. There continues to be a need for the development of new techniques and products to meet the hygienic and social needs of incontinent adults at different stages of their life.

Incontinence is a significant problem for adults, especially for those with functional and cognitive impairments. There is increased interest by nurses and health care professionals to better understand this complex phenomenon. Resources for nurses are readily available in the form of various treatments, information and education, and supplies and equipment. Considerable evidence exists that incontinence is responsive to treatment once it is detected and properly diagnosed.

REFERENCES

1. International Continence Society (1988). The standardization of terminology of lower urinary tract function. Scand J Urol Nephrol Suppl *114*:5–19.
2. Ouslander, J. (1989). Assessment and treatment of

incontinence in the nursing home. In P. Katz & E. Calkins (eds.), *Principles and Practice of Nursing Home Care* (pp. 247–274). New York: Springer Publishing.

3. Voith, A. (1988). Alterations in urinary elimination: Concepts, research, and practice. Rehab Nurs *13*:122–131.

4. Voith, A., & Smith, D. (1985) Validation of the nursing diagnosis of urinary retention. Nurs Clin North Am *20*:723–729.

5. Mitteness, L. (1987). The management of urinary incontinence by community-living elderly. Gerontology *27*:185–193.

6. Agency for Health Care Policy and Research (1992). *Urinary Incontinence in Adults: Clinical Practice Guidelines* (AHCPR Pub. No. 0038). Rockville, MD: Department of Health and Human Services.

7. Sullivan, D., & Lindsay, R. (1984). Urinary incontinence in the geriatric population of an acute care hospital. J Am Geriatr Soc *31*:694–697.

8. Sier, H., Ouslander, J., & Orzeck, S. (1987). Urinary incontinence among geriatric patients in an acute care hospital. JAMA *257*:1767–1771.

9. Massachusetts Medical Society (1991). Urinary incontinence among hospitalized persons aged 65 years and older—United States, 1984–1987. MMWR *40*:433–436.

10. Ouslander, J., Kane, R., & Abrass, I. (1982). Urinary incontinence in elderly nursing home patients. AMA *248*:1194–1198.

11. Ouslander, J., & Fowler, E. (1985). Management of urinary incontinence in Veterans Administration nursing homes. J Am Geriatr Soc *33*:33–40.

12. Hing, E., & Seksceenski, E. (1986). Use of health care-nursing home care. NCHS Anal Epidemiol Series 3 *25*:71–75.

13. Diokno, A., Brock, B., Brown, M., & Herzog, R. (1986). Prevalence of urinary incontinence and other urological symptoms in the noninstitutionalized elderly. J Urol *136*:1022–1025.

14. Harris, T. (1986). Aging in the eighties. Prevalence and impact of urinary problems in individuals age 65 years and over. NCHS Ad Data, August 27.

15. Ouslander, J., Kane, R., Vollmer, S., & Menezes, M. (1985). *Technologies for Managing Urinary Incontinence. (Health Technology Case Study 33)* (OTA-HSC-33). Washington, D. C.: Congressional Office of Technology Assessment.

16. Palmer, M., McCormick, K., & Langford, A. (1989). Do nurses consistently document incontinence? J Gerontol Nurs *15*:11–16.

17. Noekler, L. (1987). Incontinence in the elderly—care by the family. Gerontologist *27*:194–200.

18. Leach, G., & Yip, C. (1986). Urologic and urodynamic evaluation of the elderly population. Clin Geriatr Med *2*:731–755.

19. Khan, Z. (1987). Loss of bladder control in females. National Parkinson Foundation *6*:1–2.

20. White, L., Cartwright, W., Cornonu-Huntley, J., & Brock, D. (1986). Geriatric epidemiology. Annu Rev Gerontol Geriatr *6*:215–311.

21. Ouslander, J. (1989). Incontinence. In R. Kane, J. Ouslander, & I. Abrass (eds.), *Essentials of Clinical Geriatrics* (pp. 139–189). New York: McGraw-Hill.

22. Boscia, J., Kobasa, W., Knight, R., Abrutyn, E., Levison, M., & Kaye, D. (1986). Epidemiology of bacteriuria in an elderly population. Am J Med *80*:208–214.

23. Whippo, C., & Creason, N. (1989). Bacteriuria and urinary incontinence in aged female nursing home residents. J Adv Nurs *14*:217–225.

24. Wyman, J. (1988). Nursing assessment of the incontinent geriatric outpatient population. Nurs Clin North Am *23*:169–187.

25. McGuire, E. (1979). Urethral sphincter mechanisms. Urol Clin North Am *6*:39–49.

26. Kirshen, A., & Cape, R. (1984). A history of urinary incontinence. J Am Geriatr Soc *32*:686–688.

27. National Institutes of Health (1989). Urinary incontinence in adults. Conn Med *53*:27–33.

28. Staskin, D. (1986). Age-related physiologic and pathologic changes affecting lower urinary tract function. Clin Geriatr Med *2*:701–710.

29. Ouslander, J. (1986). Diagnostic evaluation of geriatric urinary incontinence. Clin Geriatr Med *2*:715–730.

30. Glowacki, G. (1983). Geriatric gynecology. In W. Reichel (ed.), *Clinical Aspects of Aging* (2nd ed., pp. 319–328). Baltimore: Williams and Wilkins.

31. Norton, C. (1986). *Nursing for Continence* (pp. 141–161). Beaconsfield: Beaconsfield Publishing.

32. Gosling, J. (1979). The structure of the bladder and urethra in relation to function. Urol Clin North Am *6*:31–38.

33. Wein, A. (1986). Physiology of micturition. Clin Geriatr Med *2*:689–699.

34. Wells, T., & Diokno, A. (1989). Urinary incontinence in the elderly. Semin Neurol *9*:60–67.

35. Schmidbauer, C., Chang, H., & Raz, S. (1986). Surgical treatment: female geriatric incontinence. Clin Geriatr Med *2*:759–776.

36. Blaivas, J., & Berger, Y. (1986). Surgical treatment for male geriatric incontinence. Clin Geriatr Med *2*:777–787.

37. Burgio, K., & Engel, B. (1987). Urinary incontinence. Behavioral assessment and treatment. In L. Carstensen & B. Edelstein (eds.), *Handbook of Clinical Gerontology* (pp. 252–266). New York: Pergamon Press.

38. Williams, M., & Pannill, F. (1982). Urinary incontinence in the elderly. Ann Intern Med *97*:895–907.

39. Resnick, N., & Yalla, S. (1985). Management of urinary incontinence in the elderly. N Engl J Med *313*:800–805.

40. Specht, J. (1986). Genitourinary problems. In D. Carnevali & M. Patrick (eds.), *Nursing Management for the Elderly* (2nd ed., pp. 447–466). Philadelphia: J. B. Lippincott.

41. Newman, J. (1962). Old folks in wet beds. Br Med J *1*:1824–1827.

42. Hadley, E., Abbey, J., Awad, S., Burgio, K., Craighead, E., Diokno, A., Engel, B., Fantl, A., Jarvis, G., Mitteness, L., Ory, M., Ouslander, J., Resnick, N., Rooney, V., Schneider, E., Schucker, B., Wells, T., Williams, M., & Willington. F. L. (1983, April). Bladder training and related therapies for urinary incontinence: Prospects and problems for clinical trials in the elderly. Prepared for the National Institute on Aging Workshop on Bladder Training. Bethesda, MD.

43. Herzog, A., Diokno, A., Brown, M., Normolle, D., & Brock, B. (1990). Two year incidence, remission, and change patterns of urinary incontinence in noninstitutionalized older adults. J Gerontol *45*:M67–74.

44. Spector, W., Kapp, M., Tucker, R., & Sternberg, J. (1988). Factors associated with presence of de-

cubitus ulcers at admission to nursing homes. Gerontologist *28*:830–834.

45. Ouslander, J. (1990). Urinary incontinence in nursing homes. J Am Geriatr Soc *38*:289–291.
46. *Webster's New Twentieth Century Unabridged Dictionary* (1977). (2nd ed., p. 925). San Francisco: Collins, World.
47. Goffman, E. (1963). *Stigma*. Engelwood Cliffs, NJ: Prentice-Hall.
48. Willington, F. L. (1976). *Incontinence in the Elderly* (p. 3). New York: Academic Press.
49. Norton, C. (1982). The effects of urinary incontinence in women. Int Rehab Med *4*:9–14.
50. Wyman, J., Harkins, S., Choi, S., Taylor, J., & Fantl, A. (1987). Psychosocial impact of urinary incontinence in women. Obstet Gynecol *70*:378–381.
51. Simons, J. (1985). Does incontinence affect your client's self-concept? J Gerontol Nurs *11*:37–40.
52. Yu, L. (1987). Incontinence stress index: Measuring psychological impact. J Gerontol Nurs *13*:18–25.
53. Yu, L., Kaltreider, L., Hu, T., Igou, J, & Craighead, W. (1989). The ISQ-P tool measuring stress associated with incontinence. J Gerontol Nurs *15*:9–15.
54. Miller, A. (1984). Nurse/patient dependency—a review of different approaches with particular reference to studies of the dependency of elderly patients. J Adv Nurs *9*:479–486.
55. Miller, A. (1985). A study of the dependency of elderly patients in wards using different methods of nursing care. Age Aging *14*:132–138.
56. Barton, E., Baltes, M., & Orzech, M. (1980). Etiology of dependency in older nursing home residents during morning care: The role of staff behavior. J Pers Soc Psychol *38*:423–431.
57. Baltes, M., Honn, S., Barton, E., Orzech, M., & Lago, D. (1983). On the social ecology of dependence and independence in elderly nursing home residents: A replication and extension. J Gerontol *38*:556–564.
58. Schwartz, D. (1977). Personal point of view—A report of seventeen elderly patients with a persistent problem of urinary incontinence. Health Bull *35*:197–204.
59. Mitteness, L. (1987). So what do you expect when you're 85? In J. Roth & P. Conrad (eds.), *Research in the Sociology of Health Care* (vol. 6, pp. 177–219). Greenwich, CT: JAI Press.
60. Warwick, R., & Brown, A. (1979). A urodynamic evaluation of urinary incontinence in the female and its treatment. Urol Clin North Am *6*:203–216.
61. Sutherst, J., Brown, M., & Shawer, M. (1981). Assessing the severity of urinary incontinence in women by weighing perineal pads. Lancet *1*:1128–1131.
62. Parkin, D., & Davis, J. (1986). Use of a visual analogue scale in the diagnosis of urinary incontinence. Br Med J *293*:365–366.
63. Frazer, M., Haylen, B., & Sutherst, J. (1989). The severity of urinary incontinence in women. Br J Urol *63*:14–15, 1989.
64. Wyman, J., Choi, S., Harkins, S., Wilson, M., & Fantl, J. (1988). The urinary diary in evaluation of incontinent women: A test-retest analysis. Obstet Gynecol *71*:812–817.
65. Ouslander, J., Urman, H., & Uman, G. (1986).

Development and testing of an incontinence monitoring record. J Am Geriatr Soc *34*:83–90.
66. Duffin, H., & Castleden, C. (1986). The continence nurse adviser's role in the British health care system. Clin Geriatr Med *2*:841–855.
67. Smith, D. (1988). Continence restoration in the homebound patient. Nurs Clin North Am *23*:207–218.
68. Hilton, P., & Stanton, S. (1981). Algorithmic method for assessing urinary incontinence in elderly women. Br Med J *282*:940–942.
69. Pieper, B., Cleland, V., Johnson, D., & O'Reilly, J. (1989). Inventing urine incontinence devices for women. Image *21*:205–209.
70. Constantino, G. (1990). Catheterization. In K. Jeter, N. Faller, & C. Norton (eds.), *Nursing for Continence* (pp. 241–265). Philadelphia: W. B. Saunders.
71. Brink, C. (1990). Absorbent pads, garments, and management strategies. J Am Geriatr Soc *38*:368–373.
72. Jeter, K. (1990). The use of incontinence products. In K. Jeter, N. Faller, & C. Norton (eds.), *Nursing for Continence* (pp. 209–222). Philadelphia: W. B. Saunders.
73. Verdall, L., & Bouda, J. (1988). *Resource Guide of Continence Products and Services* (3rd ed.). Union, SC: Help for Incontinent People.
74. Snow, T. (1988). Equipment for prevention, treatment, and management of urinary incontinence. Top Geriatr Rehab *3*:58–77.
75. Ouslander, J., & Sier, H. (1986). Drug therapy for geriatric incontinence. Clin Geriatr Med *2*:789–807.
76. Burgio, K., & Burgio, L. (1986). Behavioral therapies for urinary incontinence in the elderly. Clin Geriatr Med *2*:809–827.
77. Wells, T. (1988). Additional therapies for urinary incontinence. Top Geriatr Rehab *3*:48–57.
78. Hadley, E. (1986). Bladder training and related therapies for urinary incontinence in older people. JAMA *256*:372–379.
79. Petrilli, C., Traughber, B., & Schnelle, J. (1988). Behavioral management in the inpatient geriatric population. Nurs Clin North Am *23*:265–277.
80. Burgio, K., Whitehead, W., & Engel, B. (1985). Urinary incontinence in the elderly. Ann Intern Med *103*:507–515.
81. Kegel, A. (1948). Progressive resistance exercises in the functional restoration of the perineal muscles. Am J Obstet Gynecol *56*:238–248.
82. Palmer, M., & McCormick, K. (1991). Alterations in elimination: urinary incontinence. In E. Baines (ed.), *Perspectives in Gerontological Nursing*. Newbury Park: Sage.
83. McCormick, K., & Burgio, K. (1984). Incontinence. An update on nursing care measures. J Gerontol Nurs *10*:16–23.
84. McCormick, K., Scheve, A., & Leahy, E. (1988). Nursing management of urinary incontinence in geriatric inpatients. Nurs Clin North Am *23*:231–264.
85. Spiro, L. (1978). Bladder training for the incontinent patient. J Gerontol Nurs *4*:28–35.
86. King, M. (1980). Treatment of incontinence. Nurs Times *76*:1006–1010.
87. McDonnell, P. (1980). Promoting continence in psychogeriatric patients. Nurs Times *76*:1014–1016.
88. Bolwell, J. (1982). Dignity at all times. *Nurs Mirror* *154*:50–54.

89. Busby, J. (1983). Strategies for effective management of incontinence. Geriatr Consult July/August, pp. 24–28.

90. Jirovec, M., Brink, C., & Wells, T. (1988). Nursing assessments in the inpatient geriatric population. Nurs Clin North Am 23:219–230.

91. Burgio, L., Jones, L., & Engel, B. (1988). Studying incontinence in an urban nursing home. J Gerontol Nurs 14:40–45.

92. Ouslander, J., Morishita, L., Blaustein, J., Orzeck, S., Dunn, S., & Sayre, J. (1987). Clinical, functional, and psychosocial characteristics of an incontinent nursing home population. J Gerontol 42:631–637.

93. Wilson, T. (1948). Incontinence of urine in the aged. Lancet 2:374–377.

94. Schnelle, J., Traughber, B., Sowell, V., Newman, D., Petrilli, C., & Ory, M. (1989). Prompted voiding treatment of urinary incontinence in nursing home patients. J Am Geriatr Soc 37:1051–1057.

95. Creason, N., Grybowski, J., Burgener, S., Whippo, C., Yeo, S., & Richardson, B. (1989). Prompted voiding therapy for urinary incontinence in aged female nursing home residents. J Adv Nurs 14:120–126.

96. Hu, T., Igou, J., Kaltreider, L., Yu, L., Rohner, T., Dennis, P., Craighead, E., Hadley, E., & Ory, M. (1989). A clinical trial of a behavioral therapy to reduce urinary incontinence in nursing homes. JAMA 261:2656–2662.

97. Folstein, M., Folstein, S., & McHugh, P. (1975). Mini-mental state. A practical method for grading the cognitive state of patients for clinicians. J Psychiatr Res 12:189–198.

98. Sowell, V. (1987). A cost comparison of five methods of managing urinary incontinence. Qual Rev Bull 13:411–414.

99. Engel, B., Burgio, L., McCormick, K., Hawkins, A., Scheve, A., & Leahy, E. (1990). Behavioral treatment of incontinence in the long-term care setting. J Am Geriatr Soc 38:361–363.

100. Wells, T., Brink, C., & Diokno, A. (1987). Urinary incontinence in elderly women: Clinical findings. J Am Geriatr Soc 35:933–939.

101. Baigis-Smith, J., Smith, D., Rose, M., & Newman, D. (1989). Managing urinary incontinence in community-residing elderly persons. Gerontologist 29:229–233.

102. Morishita, L. (1988). Nursing evaluation and treatment of geriatric outpatients with urinary incontinence. Nurs Clin North Am 23:189–206.

103. Brink, C., Sampselle, C., Wells, T., Diokno, A., & Gillis, G. (1989). A digital test for pelvic floor muscle strength in older women with urinary incontinence. Nurs Res 38:196–199.

104. Worth, A., Dougherty, M., & McKey, P. (1986). Development and testing of the circumvaginal muscles rating scale. Nurs Res 35:166–168.

105. Palmer, M. (1990). Urinary incontinence. Nurs Clin North Am 25:919–934.

106. Collings, J. (1988). Educating nurses to care for the incontinent patient. Nurs Clin North Am 23:279–289.

107. Berrios, G. (1986). Temporary urinary incontinence in the acute psychiatric patient without delirium or dementia. Br J Psychiatry 149:224–227.

ALTERATIONS IN SENSATION

A sensation is defined as a perception or feeling associated with stimulation of sensory receptors or sense organs. Sensations are subjective and necessarily are modulated by the individual's experience and perceptual processes.

Examples of sensations include taste, touch, vision, hearing, and smell. Sensations may also be synonymous with symptoms such as dyspnea and pain; these symptoms are signs of pathological processes. All sensations may become symptoms when alterations in structure or function occur. Symptoms can vary from nausea, hearing difficulty, and itching to dizziness, watery eyes, and a racing heart. Numerous symptoms or sensations are assessed frequently by nurses and, as such, fall within the domain of nursing practice and research. In fact, if nursing functions are defined as the diagnosis and treatment of human responses to actual or potential health problems, a major component of nursing practice is symptom management.

This section describes sensations that are symptoms representing pathological states, including dyspnea, fatigue, pain, hunger, and nausea, vomiting, and retching. These altered sensations are human responses to illness that are assessed and managed regularly by nurses and are repeatedly seen across a wide range of diseases in a variety of chronic and acute clinical settings. Dyspnea reflects alterations in the sensation of breathing as a result of a variety of chemical, neural, and muscular stimuli integrated in the cortex. Fatigue occurs with several diseases, including cancer and cardiac, renal, and pulmonary disorders. Fatigue is a distressing sensation that is experienced normally in day-to-day living, sometimes with disease or clinical therapies and often with exercise. Pain may result from a variety of noxious stimuli. The kind and extent of the pain are shaped by the stimuli and the individual's perception, which is affected by personal, situational, and physiological variables. Hunger can result from a variety of alterations in food intake. Attention to this phenomenon usually occurs when it is publicized as an international problem. In this section, however, the focus of hunger is its occurrence in the hospitalized population. Frequently used therapies, including hyperalimentation, intravenous infusions, and enteral feedings may in fact be accompanied by hunger in the critically ill patient if adequate volume and nutrients are not provided. The chapter on nausea, vomiting, and retching is an example of a sensation, nausea, which is followed by the observable behaviors of vomiting and retching.

All of these sensations involve complex interrelationships and processes; multiple theories relating to causation and the effects of moderator variables are hypothesized. With the possible exception of pain, the scientific community is just beginning to appreciate the individual variation in perception and behavior and how other variables covary with these sensations. These physical sensations are influenced by numerous physiological and psychosocial processes. Adequate study of the sensations requires consideration of multiple theoretical perspectives, including information processing theories, physiological mechanisms, psychological factors, sociocultural determinants, and developmental stages.

Scientists would agree that theoretically pain is at the highest level of development. Pain as a symptom has been studied extensively with most of the related moderator variables being well known and scientifically investigated. In contrast, dyspnea, until now, has been studied from a pathophysiological perspective with little emphasis on relevant psychosocial variables or the meaning of the symptom to the person. Most of research on fatigue has been focused on the measure of work fatigue. This pervasive symptom is only now being recognized and studied in the context of health and illness. Hunger and appetite have been confused conceptually in the literature. The hunger felt by acutely ill patients and those variables that may influence the frequency and intensity of this hunger are addressed in this section. Nurse researchers have described and studied conceptual models and cognitive-behavioral therapies for the treatment of nausea and vomiting. This chapter includes a discussion of this development in nursing knowledge relevant to nausea and vomiting and the associated physiological responses.

The probability that these symptoms will be reported by the individual may vary as a function of demographic variables such as age, gender, occupation, residential status, and culture. Self-reports of sensations such as shortness of breath or fatigue differ widely depending on the personal perception and the meaning and definition that the symptom has to the person. In addition, physical impairment does not always correlate with the reporting of frequency or severity of these sensations, indicating the importance of considering a multifactorial model that includes demographic, personal, psychosocial, and cultural variables.

With knowledge of the mechanisms, manifestations, and clinical therapies relevant to these sensations, the professional nurse is able to monitor accurately the human response over time and plan appropriate interventions. The following chapters provide theoretical and experiential knowledge that is useful for the valid assessment and plan of care necessary in professional nursing practice.

11

Dyspnea

Virginia Carrieri-Kohlman
Susan Janson-Bjerklie

DEFINITION

Dyspnea is defined as the subjective sensation of difficult, uncomfortable breathing and includes both the perception of labored breathing by the patient and the reaction to that sensation.[1] Authors have proposed various definitions that emphasize the awareness of increased effort needed to breathe,[2] the uncomfortable and unpleasant feeling of inability to breathe,[3] the conscious awareness of increased commands to the inspiratory muscles,[4] or the "pathological" nature of the breathlessness.[5]

The lack of a precise definition of dyspnea may in part be attributable to the nature of the varied respiratory sensations.[6] Guz reported different respiratory sensations resulting from breath-holding, irritation, obstruction, and inability to obtain enough air.[7] More recently, Simon and colleagues suggested that the term "breathlessness" may encompass multiple sensations.[8, 9] When presented with different stimuli, such as breath-holding, carbon dioxide (CO_2) inhalation, exercise, and resistive loads, normal volunteers were able to distinguish between different sensations of breathlessness depending on the stimulus. Extending these findings, this group of investigators found that different clusters of descriptors were chosen by subjects with different pulmonary conditions, including pulmonary vascular disease, neuromuscular and chest wall diseases, chronic obstructive pulmonary disease (COPD), pregnancy, and interstitial lung disease. In addition, there was an association between clusters of descriptors and specific conditions. Descriptions of sensations were clustered into the categories of rapid exhalation, shallow, work, suffocating, hunger, tight, and heavy.

Another group of researchers have continued this exploration of verbal descriptors for breathlessness used by cardiopulmonary patients.[10] A list of 45 descriptors of breathing discomfort related to exertion was administered to 208 patients on two different occasions; 169 patients were considered reliable. The descriptors clustered into 12 groups that seemed to describe different aspects of breathing discomfort. Patients with various diseases did seem to identify different aspects of breathing discomfort. Patients with COPD chose distress more often, patients with asthma tended to indicate wheeziness, patients with restrictive disorders reported rapid breathing, and patients with cardiac disease described a need to sigh more often. Other investigators have found that during exercise, patients breathing added resistive loads could distinguish between the sensations of breathlessness, effort, and tension.[11]

Phrases used by patients with various pulmonary diseases to describe dyspnea have included the following. "I feel short of breath", "hard to breathe," "It's hard to move air," "I can't get enough air," and "I feel chest tightness."[12] Children use words such as "It's hard to breathe," "can only get a little in," and "tightness, lungs feel shut" to describe their shortness of breath.[13] Most authors agree that dyspnea encompasses more than simply the sensation of the intensity of the effort of breathing. One researcher suggested that the word dyspnea should be replaced by breathlessness or shortness of breath, the words commonly used by patients with uncomfortable respiratory sensations.[14]

Dyspnea, like pain, has an important affective dimension of distress and is clearly affected by cognitive and contextual factors; the threshold for perception of the sensation varies widely.[15] The stimulus intensity of "just noticeable difference" may be the same among patients with similar lung pathology, but the distress of dyspnea, the affective component, may vary greatly. The affective component is hypothesized to be modulated by personal, health status, and situational variables, much like other symptoms are.[16] Normal subjects exercising in the laboratory have been able to differentiate the distress of dyspnea from the intensity of the sensation.[17]

Dyspnea should be distinguished from other changes in breathing pattern, such as tachypnea (rapid breathing), hyperpnea (increased ventilation in proportion to metabolic demands), and hyperventilation (increased ventilation in excess of metabolic demands). These changes in the pattern of ventilation may occur concurrently with dyspnea but are not synonymous with it.[1]

PREVALENCE AND POPULATIONS AT RISK

Dyspnea is one of the most common human responses to real or potential health problems affecting both children and adults. Although the exact incidence has not been reported and is not known, it is a frequently reported symptom occurring in association with a wide variety of clinical states. The prevalence of this symptom can be estimated only from the prevalence of the diseases in which it occurs. Dyspnea occurs primarily with three major health problems: pulmonary disease, cardiac disease, and cancer of the lung.

At one time or another, most individuals with acute or chronic pulmonary disease will suffer from dyspnea. The most common chronic pulmonary diseases are obstructive, restrictive, or vascular in nature. The prevalence of chronic obstructive lung disease, including emphysema, bronchitis, and asthma, is increasing. Trends in COPD morbidity and mortality from 1979 to 1985 demonstrate that approximately 5.5 million Americans older than 55 years of age have chronic obstructive lung disease.[18] COPD is cited as the fifth leading cause of death and the second leading cause of disability. It is esti-

mated that 30,000 people with COPD die each year, another 2 million are handicapped, and 6 to 10 million suffer with clinical symptoms.[19] Chronic bronchitis is a common problem affecting 10 to 30 per cent of the adult population.[20] The prevalence of asthma in adults and children is rising worldwide and in the United States is estimated to affect 10 million people, of which 3 million are younger than age 18.[21] Dyspnea is a ubiquitous recurring symptom in these diseases.

Lung cancer is the leading cause of death from malignancy in men and in women 35 years of age or older. Dyspnea is estimated to occur in 29 to 74 per cent of patients with terminal lung cancer.[22] There has been greater attention given to the frequency of dyspnea in lung cancer, especially as a symptom occurring in association with pleural effusions and chemotherapy or radiation therapy.[23, 24]

The prevalence of COPD and lung cancer is steadily increasing. This rise has been accompanied by an increase in occupational lung diseases, such as the restrictive processes of silicosis, asbestosis, and other pneumoconioses. Interstitial lung diseases, a group of restrictive diseases involving the lung parenchyma and fibrosis of the alveolar interstitium, most probably play a large role in the prevalence of dyspnea. There are more than 130 defined interstitial lung diseases resulting from ingestion or inhalation of organic and inorganic dusts, drugs, gases and fumes, and poisons.[25] Dyspnea occurs in other restrictive diseases, such as pneumonia and *Pneumocystis carinii*; pneumonia affects 80 per cent of the persons infected with the human immunodeficiency virus (HIV), and the most common presenting symptoms are dyspnea, cough, and fever.[26] The prevalence of dyspnea also extends to less pathological states, such as obesity and anxiety, and to nonpathological states like pregnancy.

Shortness of breath also occurs in both right-sided and left-sided heart failure.[27, 28] Although dyspnea is reported in various forms of heart disease, it is most common in those associated with pulmonary congestion, such as congestive heart failure (CHF), valvular heart disease, and idiopathic cardiomyopathies. The dyspnea associated with idiopathic or primary pulmonary hypertension can be severe, constant, and disruptive of work and activities.[12] Chronic cor pulmonale, or right-sided heart failure due to chronic pulmonary disease, may be as prevalent as emphysema. Because heart disease remains the largest single cause of death in the United States, the prevalence of dyspnea suffered by those who have CHF should be assumed to be great.

SITUATIONAL AND DEVELOPMENTAL STRESSORS

Antecedent variables that may be situational or developmental stressors related to the experience of dyspnea have been categorized into personal, health status, and situational domains (some appear in Table 11–1).[16] Personal factors include correlates such as age, obesity, habits (including cigarette smoking and alcohol use), occupation, mood state (including anxiety and depression), and level of fatigue. The person's previous experience with the symptom and beliefs about the symptom affects one's tolerance for breathlessness. Aging leads to alterations in both respiratory and cardiovascular function that may result in the development of dyspnea. By far the greatest risk factor for the development of dyspnea is cigarette smoking. Large prospective epidemiological studies have shown a strong association between primary and secondary cigarette smoking and chronic bronchitis, emphysema, cancer of the lung, and coronary heart disease and therefore subsequent dyspnea.[29]

Health status stressors include pulmonary and cardiac diseases, concurrent illness, duration of illness, decreased exercise tolerance, and deconditioning. Dyspnea increases as people with pulmonary disease decrease their activity, thus increasing their deconditioned state. A cyclic pattern of inactivity increases dyspnea, which leads to more inactivity.[30] Changes in pulmonary physiological parameters, such as respiratory muscle fatigue, breathing pattern, hyperinflation, airflow obstruction, hypoxemia, and loss of lung compliance, also are physiological antecedents to dyspnea.[31–33] The development of infection concurrent with underlying disease may cause increasing dyspnea in the chronically ill patient.

Situational or contextual variables, such as air pollutants, allergies, altitude, life events, perception of illness severity, and changes in social support, may also exacerbate shortness of breath.[12] Environmental and occupational pollution, such as smoke, sulfur dioxide, or ozone, have been shown to trigger bronchoconstriction in asthmatic and atopic subjects.[34]

TABLE 11-1 SITUATIONAL AND DEVELOPMENTAL STRESSORS THAT PRECIPITATE DYSPNEA IN ADULTS AND CHILDREN

Personal factors
  Physical conditions
    Disease category
    Deconditioning of muscles
    Infections
    Abdominal distention
    Obesity
    Secretions
    Feeling too warm
    Fatigue
    Smoking
    Use of alcohol
  Mechanical behaviors
    Talking
    Eating
    Coughing
    Laughing
  Emotions or moods
    Upset
    Worry
    Anger
    Excitement
    Depression
Situational factors
  Specific situations
    Living arrangement
    Social circumstances
    High pressure or tension
    Life events
  Environmental conditions
    Altitude
    Seasonal variation
    Cigarette smoke-filled room
    Air pollution
    Weather: heat, cold, wind, fog
  Allergens
    Grasses
    Molds
    Dust
    Animal dander
  Precipitating activities
    Resting
    Lying flat
    Walking level or uphill
    Housework
    Exercise
    Sexual activity
    Stooping and bending
    Hurrying
    Dressing and bathing
    Carrying heavy objects

Adapted from Kohlman-Carrieri, V., Janson-Bjerklie, S. (1990). Coping and Self-Care Strategies. In D.A. Mahler (ed.), *Dyspnea* (p. 204). Mt. Kisco, NY: Futura Publishing; and Carrieri, V.K., Janson-Bjerklie, S., & Jacobs, S. (1984). The sensation of dyspnea: A review. Heart Lung *13*:436–447.

More than 50 risk factors specific to cardiac disease and, therefore, antecedents for dyspnea have been identified and studied. These vary from elevated serum lipid levels and obesity to sedentary living and psychosocial stress.[35] Obesity is associated with dyspnea in a subgroup, but not in all patients, with obesity-related hypoventilation syndrome. The reasons for this variation in the intensity of breathlessness in obese patients are not known.

Stressors Described by Persons with Dyspnea

Stressors listed in Table 11-1 (see p. 249) that adults and children describe as precipitants or risk factors for their dyspnea have been designated as personal factors, situational factors, and physical activities.[12, 13] Infection, abdominal distention, increased secretions, feeling too warm or too cold, fatigue, and the use of alcohol or cigarettes are reported personal physical conditions that precipitate dyspnea. For some people, dyspnea can be triggered by talking, eating, coughing, or laughing. Actual emotional arousal, of either positive or negative affect, such as being upset, worried, angry, anxious, or depressed, may trigger breathlessness. Certain emotions, such as panic, anger, or anxiety, appear to be direct correlates of acute dyspnea.[36] Whether emotions develop as a result of dyspnea or escalate the symptom, it is important to be aware of the significant contribution of emotions to the intensity and frequency of the distress of dyspnea.

Situational factors, such as allergens, cigarette smoke, weaning from a ventilator, and environmental conditions, all can trigger shortness of breath. Stressful or high-pressure situations are described by patients as frequent stressors that precipitate dyspnea. People with allergen-sensitive or extrinsic asthma may experience shortness of breath in different seasons from exposure to grasses and molds, pollen, animal dander, dust, or air pollutants. Characteristics of weather, such as extreme heat or cold, wind, and fog, can also initiate dyspnea.

Children have also identified stressors that precipitate their shortness of breath, and these are similar to those for adults. Personal factors for children included physical states, mechanical behaviors, and emotions or mood. Illness and fatigue, like "catching a cold," were reported as stressors that trigger dyspnea. Children spontaneously described emotional arousal and resultant behaviors, negative or positive, including excitement, anxiety, and crying as triggers for shortness of breath. Life stressors, such as "being punished" or "death of a parent," exacerbate breathlessness. The most frequent stressor described by asthmatic children in one study was physical activity: running, playing, and participating in sports.[13] Situations that bring on shortness of breath for children include animal and plant allergens and weather.

Clinical States

Dyspnea is caused primarily by pulmonary, cardiac, and neuromuscular diseases. These same diseases were found in a study of primary causes of unexplained dyspnea. One group of investigators found that in 72 consecutive patients referred by physicians, dyspnea was due to pulmonary disease in 26 patients (36 per cent), cardiac disease in 10 patients (14 per cent), hyperventilation in 14 patients (19 per cent), and extrathoracic causes in 3 patients, including thyroid dysfunction and metabolic acidosis.[37]

Pulmonary Diseases

Acute and chronic obstructive, restrictive, or vascular pulmonary diseases are the most frequent clinical states in which dyspnea is experienced. The proposed relationships between clinical states associated with dyspnea and mechanisms believed to trigger the symptom are presented in Table 11-2. The pulmonary clinical states in which dyspnea may be a prominent symptom are organized under two hypothesized causes of dyspnea: increased effort of breathing and increased respiratory drive.

People with chronic bronchitis and emphysema experience increased work of breathing as a result of loss of elasticity of the airways, increased secretions, and hyperinflation. Hyperinflation increases the work for inspiratory muscles by shortening the diaphragm, therefore causing the muscles to function at a disadvantageous position on the length-tension curve. Hyperinflation also decreases diaphragmatic curvature and increases thoracic cage elastic recoil. In cystic fibrosis,

TABLE 11-2   PROPOSED MECHANISMS AND CLINICAL STATES PRODUCING DYSPNEA

Stimulus	Receptors	Clinical Disease
Vascular Stimuli		
Right atrial pressure	Right atrial mechanoreceptors	Congestive heart failure
Right ventricular pressure	Right ventricular receptors	Congestive heart failure
Pulmonary artery pressure	Pulmonary artery baroreceptors	Primary pulmonary hypertension
Left atrial pressure	Left atrial mechanoreceptors	Mitral valve disease
Mechanical Stimuli		
Intercostal muscle length-tension inappropriateness	Muscle spindles	Pleural effusion Pneumothorax
Pulmonary hyperinflation	Stretch receptors (vagal)	Bullous emphysema
Deformation of lung interstitium	J receptors (vagal)	Pulmonary edema Pneumonia
Humoral Stimuli		
Hypoxemia	Carotid bodies	Lung diseases
Hypercapnia	Carotid bodies Central chemoreceptors	Chronic obstructive lung disease
Acidosis	Carotid bodies Central chemoreceptors	Cardiovascular disease
Movement of Extremities	Mechanoreceptors Ergoreceptors	None reported
Psychogenic	Cerebral cortex	Psychoneurosis

Adapted from Wasserman, K., & Casaburi, R. (1988). Dyspnea: Physiological and pathophysiological mechanism. *Annu Rev Med 39*:503–515.

excessive airway secretions and an increase in airway hyperreactivity cause dyspnea.

Asthma is an example of a clinical state in which the effort of breathing is increased owing to an expansion in the work of breathing caused by narrowing of the airways. Breathing against greater airway resistance results in an increase in the work of breathing, an increase in the effort perceived, and the sensation of dyspnea. In interstitial pulmonary fibrosis caused by occupational lung diseases or idiopathic processes, compliance of the lung is decreased, resulting in an increased work of breathing to produce the same alveolar ventilation and associated increased effort and shortness of breath.

HIV-associated diseases are sometimes associated with dyspnea, especially if the lungs are involved. The exact mechanisms causing dyspnea are unknown; however, the combination of decreased lung compliance secondary to the interstitial disease process and the hypoxemia that results from decreased alveolar ventilation in pneumonia is a probable cause.

When large amounts of the pulmonary capillary vascular bed are destroyed, as in pulmonary embolism and pulmonary hypertension, ventilation is wasted, resulting in an increased work of breathing. The clinical states of hypoxemia and acidosis also trigger increased minute ventilation. A greater minute ventilation is associated with an increase in work of breathing, perceived effort, and therefore increased dyspnea.[32]

Acute dyspnea is a symptom in airway obstruction resulting from acute bronchoconstriction or a foreign body in the airway. Dyspnea can also occur in trauma states, such as fractured ribs or flail chest, when there is increased effort of breathing resulting from an inefficient respiratory pump.[38] Acute dyspnea is typically caused by chest trauma, pulmonary edema, pulmonary embolism, spontaneous pneumothorax, and hyperventilation syndrome.

Clinical states that cause relative or absolute respiratory muscle weakness may also cause an increase in effort of breathing. Muscle myopathies and muscular dystrophy produce weakness of inspiratory muscles. Hyperinflation of the lung in emphysema or asthma and pleural effusions in cancer of the lung cause shortening of inspiratory muscles. This decrease in muscle length results in relative muscle weakness and a decrease in the amount of contraction of the respiratory muscles available for ventilation. Kyphoscoliosis causes an alteration in the configuration of the chest wall, producing a musculoskeletal dysfunction that may result in relative or absolute muscle weakness and an increase in the effort of breathing. Muscle fatigue with diminished mechanical work results in loss of lung volume for the same respiratory effort and increasing breathlessness.

Disease processes that increase respiratory drive can cause dyspnea either directly by stimulating central or peripheral neuroreceptors or indirectly by stimulating receptors in muscles and joints that send afferent signals to the brain. One example of a clinical state that stimulates chemoreceptors is hypoxemia in which afferent signals from carotid body receptors trigger an increased respiratory drive. Through neurostimulation, hypoxemia can elicit dyspnea even before there is an increase in ventilation.[14] In a similar way, hypercapnia and metabolic acidosis cause stimulation of chemoreceptors centrally and peripherally, resulting in an increased respiratory drive. In patients with pulmonary hypertension and interstitial lung disease, J receptors are suspected to send afferent signals via the vagus nerve to the central, higher brain centers and increasing respiratory drive and dyspnea.

Lung Cancer

Dyspnea is a major and prevalent symptom in cancer.[39] Lung cancer can cause either obstructive or restrictive changes. Localized airflow limitation occurs in lung cancer owing to specific airway obstruction caused by endobronchial tumor or by extrinsic compression of the airway due to tumor deposits or nodes. Pleural effusions are a common occurrence in malignancy and cause restriction of the lung. Pneumonia resulting from cancer or its treatment causes dyspnea by increasing metabolic demands, altering gas exchange, and decreasing lung compliance. Patients with cancer frequently have hypoxemia and radiographic infiltrates suggestive of the presence of pneumonitis secondary to treatment with radiation and chemotherapy. Patients with massive interpulmonary tumors lose efficiency of gas exchange and the ability to ventilate. The most dyspneic of patients with widespread cancer are those with lymphangitic carcinomatosis; these patients usually succumb within a short period of time and suffer unrelenting dyspnea.

Cardiac Disease

Dyspnea is reported frequently in various forms of heart disease but is most common in those diseases associated with pulmonary congestion, such as left ventricular dysfunction or mitral stenosis. Particular stimuli proposed to trigger dyspnea are increases in

right atrial pressure, right ventricular pressure, pulmonary artery pressure, and left atrial pressure.[40] These changes in pressure are thought to activate receptors in the right atrium and ventricle, the pulmonary artery baroreceptors, and the left atrial mechanical receptors.

Left ventricular dysfunction results in left ventricular hypertension and ultimately pulmonary capillary hypertension. Elevation of pulmonary capillary pressures increases congestion in the capillaries, interstitial spaces, and ultimately the alveoli, resulting in loss of compliance and distensibility of the lung. With chronic pulmonary hypertension there is fibrosis of the alveolar walls and anatomical changes in small arteries, including medial hypertrophy and proliferation of the intima. The cellular changes in vessel walls contribute to increased arterial pressures greater than might be expected with the elevation of pulmonary venous pressures. Loss of lung compliance then increases the work of breathing and results in dyspnea. Dyspnea secondary to cardiac disease usually begins with strenuous exercise and over the course of months or years progresses until the person is dyspneic at rest.

Anemia

Dyspnea during exercise occurs in patients with anemia, yet the exact mechanism for the symptom in this and other metabolic states, such as thyrotoxicosis, remains hypothetical.[40] The reduction in hemoglobin concentration is associated with a reduction in oxygen content, mixed venous blood oxygen saturation, and a fall in tissue oxygen pressure. If the heart cannot respond, as in severe anemia, heart failure may ensue. Tissue hypoxia may be responsible for the hyperventilation frequently seen in anemic states. This hyperventilation can be out of proportion to that which is required to meet tissue needs and therefore may produce dyspnea.

Pregnancy

It is estimated that 60 to 70 per cent of pregnant women complain of dyspnea at some time during their pregnancy.[41] Although it might be expected that mechanical restriction would be an important etiological factor, the complaint of dyspnea most frequently occurs for the first time in the first or second trimester before any increase in abdominal girth and may even improve as pregnancy progresses. The increased drive to breathe induced by progesterone has been suggested as one cause of dyspnea in pregnancy.[42]

Neuromuscular Diseases

Neurological diseases involving the spinal cord, peripheral nerves, and respiratory muscles often produce respiratory insufficiency and associated dyspnea. In general, the degree of dyspnea is related to the respiratory muscles affected and not to the amount of ventilation achievable; that is, patients with paralysis of the diaphragm who are dependent on high intercostal muscles are dyspneic whereas patients who can use the diaphragm for respiration are not dyspneic. In diseases such as muscular dystrophy, myasthenia gravis, and amyotrophic lateral sclerosis, dyspnea may be present at rest or only with activity.[43] The precise influence of higher cerebral centers on respiration and the sensation of dyspnea within the context of neurological disease is difficult to evaluate and remains unclear.

Psychological States

The perception of dyspnea can be increased in both acute and chronic anxiety states. Researchers have verified the association between anxiety and dyspnea in the patient with COPD.[44–47] The characteristic breathing pattern of the anxious patient can be normal and interspersed with deep sighing respirations or rapid in the form of the "hyperventilation syndrome."[48] Patients with the hyperventilation syndrome may have ventilation appropriate for metabolic needs during exercise but may hyperventilate at rest. Frequently, the dyspnea occurs while the patient is resting or sitting and tends to occur independent of exercise.[49] Often the patient complains of "smothering" or inability to take a deep breath, with associated symptoms of palpitations, dizziness, lightheadedness, and numbness of hands and feet.

Depression has also been associated with dyspnea.[50] It is not known whether the depression or dyspnea occurs first in chronically ill patients. Depression and associated negative feelings are thought to produce an altered central perception of incoming afferent sensations and may be related to the increasing perception of the intensity of dyspnea.[49] Depressed patients often experience episodic dyspnea that fluctuates within minutes, occurs at rest, bears little relationship to exercise, and is demonstrated by sighing and rapid shallow breathing.[44]

MECHANISMS

The mechanisms producing breathlessness are multifactorial, including personal, situational, psychological, and biological variables. In the past several years, a number of excellent reviews of the psychophysical mechanisms and related treatments of dyspnea have been published and should be consulted for a thorough understanding of dyspnea as a respiratory sensation.[3, 5, 14, 40, 51–54] Dyspnea is generated through a complex series of processes involving the activation of sensory receptors, the transmission of sensory signals to the central nervous system (CNS), and the processing of those signals by higher brain centers.[55] A schematic diagram of these components is shown in Figure 11–1.

It is hypothesized that dyspnea occurs when an individual perceives a discrepancy between the demand to breathe and the amount of ventilation actually achieved.[56, 57] At least three circumstances may produce such a discrepancy: (1) when more than normal respiratory effort is required to ventilate because of increased resistance to airflow and stretch or because of weak respiratory muscles; (2) when there is increased respiratory drive, such as in hypoxemia, changes in altitude, or anemia; and (3) when there is an increased central perception eliciting the symptom, for example, in anxiety states.[58]

Increased Respiratory Muscle Effort

The most important determinants of dyspnea intensity appear to be increasing respiratory muscle activity and the effort needed to breathe. The sensation of dyspnea is most closely related to a "sense of respiratory effort."[59] This sensation of effort is thought to be mediated by the stretching of muscle spindles and tendons in the inspiratory muscles, intercostal muscles, and diaphragm, which results in afferent signals to higher brain centers.[60, 61] When subjects have been asked

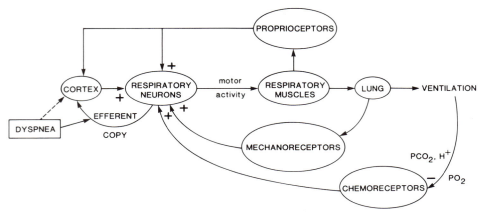

Figure 11–1. Factors postulated to produce dyspnea. (From Cherniack, N.S. [1988]. Dyspnea. In J.F. Murray & J.A. Nadel [eds.]. *Textbook of Respiratory Medicine* [p. 393]. Philadelphia: W.B. Saunders.)

to breathe against elastic and resistive ventilatory loads of increasing magnitude, there is a progressive increase in the intensity of the sensation, and this increasing intensity follows Stevens' psychophysical power law.[62, 63]

The intensity of the sensation, however, is not just a function of the magnitude of the added load. The sensation of load is based not only on the magnitude of the load but also on the level and duration of the force generated by the respiratory muscles.[64] The intensity of the sensation of respiratory force is primarily related to the tension developed by the contracting respiratory muscles; it is also related to the inspiratory time or breathing pattern.[32, 64]

With other stimuli such as bright light, when the stimulus is sustained for a prolonged period of time or presented repeatedly, adaptation takes place and the intensity of the stimulus perceived by the subject decreases.[65] Adaptation of respiratory sensations also occurs. After a person breathes against moderate loads for several minutes, the perceived intensity of the load decreases.[66] This process of adaptation may explain the decreased perception of ventilatory load in patients with COPD and the lack of breathlessness in some asthmatic persons with increased airway resistance.[67, 68]

Chronic lung disease can result in the increase of respiratory muscle effort from increased work of breathing or from weakness of the respiratory muscles. Hyperinflation of the lung and thorax in chronic lung disease causes shortening of the inspiratory muscles,

which decreases the efficiency of muscle contraction and increases the muscular effort needed to breathe the same volume of air. Research findings indicate that thoracic displacement and degree of lung inflation influence the intensity of dyspnea.[69] To overcome these changes, accessory muscles are needed to breathe. Accessory muscle use also increases the "sense" of respiratory effort and is correlated with increasing dyspnea.[70]

In emphysema, chronic bronchitis, cystic fibrosis, and asthma in both children and adults, increased airflow resistance and changes in airway caliber increase the work of breathing and produce dyspnea, presumably by altering the length-tension relationships of respiratory muscle and increasing the sense of respiratory muscle effort.[71]

Restrictive pulmonary diseases (pneumonia, pneumoconioses, cancer of the lung) and other restrictive processes (obesity, pregnancy, abdominal distention) cause a decrease in volume and compliance of the lung. In obese patients, the extra weight serves as a load to the respiratory muscles, especially the diaphragm, where muscle fibers are stretched beyond optimal length. The combination of shallow breathing, accumulation of sputum, and physical inactivity may result in atelectasis and further decreased pulmonary compliance. When lungs are "stiffer," more respiratory muscle effort is needed, more work is necessary, and dyspnea may occur even at rest. Undernutrition, hypoxemia, and pulmonary hypertension can all contribute to poor conditioning of peripheral skeletal and respiratory muscle. When increased muscle force is required to achieve increased ventilation in noncompliant lungs, the patient senses increased effort and dyspnea may result.

There is growing evidence, however, that the sense of respiratory effort is not sufficient to explain all the variance in the intensity of dyspnea. It has been suggested that if dyspnea were due solely to respiratory muscle effort, subjects would have the same degree of discomfort for a certain level of ventilation no matter what the stimulus was for the rapid or deep breathing.[51] However, subjects are more breathless with exercise[72] or with hypercapnia[73] than with voluntary hypercapnia. In addition, these authors suggest that the fact that patients with pulmonary vascular disease and interstitial disease frequently report more dyspnea than one would expect from their increased ventilation and the work of breathing is further evidence for mechanisms other than muscular effort.

Increased Respiratory Drive

The drive to breathe and presumably increased dyspnea can be stimulated by a variety of chemical and neural receptors.[74] Central processing and integration of afferent signals occur in higher brain centers; the theory of these processes are diagrammed in Figure 11–1. Central chemoreceptors in the brain and peripheral chemoreceptors in the carotid bodies respond to body and environmental changes in oxygen (PaO_2) and carbon dioxide ($PaCO_2$) tension. Hypoxia seems to be a specific dyspogen, with direct neural stimulation of the sensory cortex resulting from the peripheral chemoreceptors' response to a low PaO_2.[75] The relationship between hypercapnia and dyspnea is not as clear. Investigators have found that paralyzed patients or normal subjects could distinguish increasing $PaCO_2$ from normal levels, and this was associated with respiratory discomfort[76, 77]; other subjects reported no respiratory discomfort with elevation of $PaCO_2$.[78] In another study, investigators instructed subjects to maintain an elevated voluntary ventilation while surreptitiously increasing PCO_2; the subjects were able to detect elevated levels of PCO_2 and reported increasing dyspnea.[73] Therefore, these studies seem to indicate that hypercapnia by itself can increase dyspnea without being accompanied by increasing ventilation.

Numerous neural receptors in the upper and lower airways, parenchyma of the lung, and chest wall respond to changes in temperature, pressure, irritation, and stretch.[51, 79, 80] Irritant receptors in the epithelium of the airways are stimulated by dust and the irritating chemical gases of aerosols, contraction of bronchial smooth muscle, and stretch of the bronchial wall with large and sudden changes in lung volume. The impulses from irritant receptors are also increased in conditions with decreased lung compliance, such as pulmonary congestion and pulmonary embolism. The respiratory effects of stimulating intrapulmonary irritant receptors are hyperventilation, tachypnea, and bronchoconstriction mediated via vagal reflex pathways. Clinical situations in humans that result in stimulation of irritant receptors are also associated with difficult breathing, and therefore it has been proposed that these receptors may mediate the sensation of dyspnea.[79] Anesthesia of the upper airway increases dyspnea associated with rebreathing of carbon dioxide,[81] yet it may decrease the dyspnea of exercise.[82]

Receptors in the nasopharynx also affect breathlessness. Cold air has been shown to prolong breath-holding time,[83] and clinical studies have shown that improvements in dyspnea during oxygen administration via a nasal cannula[84] or transtracheal catheter[85] may be due to stimulation of receptors in the upper airways. In addition, stimulation of receptors in the distribution of the trigeminal nerve has been hypothesized to have a direct effect on dyspnea by authors who have shown that cold air to the face decreased breathlessness in normal subjects.[86]

These same authors suggest that studies showing that continuous positive airway pressure (CPAP) decreases breathlessness[87, 88] demonstrate that receptors may exist in the walls of airways. These receptors may be sensitive to the collapse of airways or to changes in the transmural pressure across the walls of bronchi modulating the level of dyspnea.[51] It has also been suggested that receptors in the oral mucosa may send information that modifies the intensity of breathlessness, since dyspnea was decreased in healthy subjects breathing through a mouthpiece and mask when topical 4 per cent lidocaine was applied to the oral mucosa.[89]

Information is conveyed from receptors in the lung parenchyma itself that transmit via the vagus nerve and may play a significant role in respiratory sensations associated with interstitial lung disease and congestive heart failure.[90] Irritant receptors in the lung may be responsible for the sense of "irritation" resulting from inhalation of noxious fumes. One group of investigators has found that inhaled lidocaine can reduce the dyspnea associated with bronchoconstriction but not the shortness of breath caused by external loading.[91] J receptors, presumed to be located near the capillary interstitium, are thought to be stimulated by respiratory loads caused by pulmonary congestion and microembolism and result in the stimulation of rapid, shallow breathing.[92] Other receptors in the joints, tendons, and muscles of the chest wall give information about the movement of the respiratory system and the respiratory muscles. The concept of "inappropriate" length of the muscle and the tension generated within the muscle as a mechanism of dyspnea was based on afferent information arising from muscles in the chest wall.[57] When the respiratory centers in the CNS are stimulated and the drive to breathe is increased, restriction of chest wall motion seems to make dyspnea worse.[51] Vibration of the chest wall during inspiration, used to increase the afferent information from the chest wall by stimulating skeletal muscle receptors, decreases this dyspnea in normal subjects.[93] Suggested receptors that may stimulate the respiratory drive are listed in Table 11–3.

Changes in Central Perception

In addition to the sensations of respiratory muscle effort and increased respiratory

TABLE 11–3 SUGGESTED RECEPTORS THAT STIMULATE THE SENSATION OF DYSPNEA

Chemoreceptors
  Central and peripheral
Mechanoreceptors
  Facial
  Nasopharyngeal
  Oral mucosal
  Upper and lower airway: irritant
  Lung: irritant, stretch, J receptors
  Chest wall: joints, tendons, muscles

Data from Killian, K.J., & Campbell, E.J.M. (1990). Mechanisms of dyspnea. In D.A. Mahler (ed.), *Dyspnea* (p. 61). Mt. Kisco, NY: Futura Publishing; Schwartzstein, R.M., Manning, H.L., Weiss, J.W., & Weinburger, S.E. (1990). Dyspnea: A sensory experience. Lung *168*:185–199.

drive, behavioral and contextual factors influence dyspnea. Anxiety, anger, and depression can cause variations in the pattern of breathing and are related to dyspnea.[44] Anxious persons experience greater dyspnea than nonanxious persons under experimentally induced conditions of respiratory loading. One investigator found significantly greater anxiety during periods of "high" dyspnea than in states of "low" dyspnea in hospitalized patients with asthma.[36]

A syndrome of disproportionately severe breathlessness occurred in subjects who are more socially isolated and younger and have more anxiety, stress, and more current psychiatric symptoms.[45] Some emotions are also accompanied by mechanical behaviors, such as yelling or crying, that stimulate afferent receptors that may trigger dyspnea by reflex mechanisms. Whether anxiety and depression precede, accompany, or are a result of dyspnea is unknown. However, patients with chronic dyspnea suffer from anxiety and depression, and these mood states may increase or decrease dyspnea.

PATHOLOGICAL CONSEQUENCES

Dyspnea occurs in a variety of pathological consequences, including physiological, psychological, social, and economical changes. Acute dyspnea associated with acute and severe hypoxemia may result in cerebral anoxia and brain injury. Dyspnea in association with hypoventilation can result in a dulling of sensory perception—the phenomenon of carbon dioxide narcosis. Patients with chronic lung disease, at risk for respiratory failure, are most likely to develop this clinical syndrome.

Chronic dyspnea may be severe and unrelenting, or it may be present at some tolerable level but punctuated with severe exacerbations of breathlessness. Both patterns result in profound physical, emotional, and social outcomes. Chronic dyspnea is frequently associated with overwhelming fatigue and physical inertia. The patient's ability and will to move out of the house and stay socially involved become seriously compromised. Many patients are unable to stay gainfully employed, as dyspnea limits their mobility. As these pervasive changes develop, people with chronic dyspnea become depressed and lose hope, reinforcing physical and social isolation.

RELATED PATHOPHYSIOLOGICAL CONCEPTS

The severity of breathlessness varies more than might be expected with a given degree of pulmonary dysfunction. Subjects may have marked changes in pulmonary function with no complaints of breathlessness, whereas others report uncomfortable breathing with little evidence of cardiopulmonary alterations.[94, 95] "Gold standard" pulmonary function variables, such as forced expiratory volume in 1 second (FEV_1) or static lung volumes, correlate only moderately with dyspnea in chronic obstructive pulmonary disease.[96]

The following physiological variables reflecting pulmonary mechanics, oxygenation, and ventilation correlate to some degree with shortness of breath and are listed in Table 11–7.

Hypoxemia and Hypercapnia

Hypoxemia is a specific dyspogen, with peripheral chemoreceptors responding to a low PaO_2 and subsequent direct neural stimulation of the sensory cortex.[75] Hypoxia during exercise produces higher ratings of respiratory difficulty and breathlessness than exercise alone.[75, 97, 98] Investigators have reported that hypercapnia itself may not be a specific stimulus for breathlessness, but rather the increased ventilation that accompanies the increasing $PaCO_2$ is most probably the trigger for dyspnea.[72, 73, 99]

Respiratory Mechanics and Breathing Pattern

The relationship between pulmonary dysfunction and the severity of dyspnea may be close only within individual disease entities. This specificity to a certain disease is seen by examining the pulmonary function tests that correlate with dyspnea in obstructive and restrictive pulmonary diseases. In emphysematous patients, maximal expiratory pressure (PEmax) ($r = .35$) and maximal inspiratory pressure (PImax) ($r = .34$) were the pulmonary function tests that had the highest correlation with dyspnea measured by the Baseline Dyspnea Index.[100] In another study with patients with COPD, forced vital capacity (FVC) and FEV_1 significantly correlated

in a range of .43 to .49 with three different measures of dyspnea.[101] Another investigator found a correlation as high as .71 between FEV_1 and dyspnea.[102] In this same study the maximal voluntary ventilation (MVV), the largest volume in liters that can be breathed per minute by voluntary effort, had the greatest correlation ($r = .78$) with dyspnea in obstructive diseases. A significant correlation between dyspnea and peak expiratory flow rates (PEFR) ($r = .85$) has been found with asthmatic patients.[103] All of these parameters measure airway obstruction and muscle force, important pathological changes that may affect dyspnea.

The pathology of a restrictive process decreases the FVC and impairs diffusion (DLCO). The resulting reduction in FVC ($r = -.41$) and DLCO ($r = -.50$) has been found to correlate moderately with severity of dyspnea in restrictive diseases.[100] Only PImax ($r = .51$) and FVC ($r = .44$) showed significant correlations with breathlessness in another study of patients with interstitial lung disease.[104]

LeBlanc and colleagues[32] found that 68 per cent of the variance or change in breathlessness in normal subjects and those with differing respiratory diseases was explained by the following regression equation:

$$\text{Breathlessness (Y)} = 3.0 \, (\text{Ppl/PImax}) \\ + 1.2 \, (\text{Vi}) + 4.5 \, (\text{VT/VC}) \\ + 0.13 \, (\text{Fb}) + 5.6 \, (\text{Ti/Ttot}) - 6.2$$

where Ppl is the pleural pressure, Vi is the inspiratory flow rate, VT/VC is the tidal volume expressed as a percentage of the vital capacity, Fb is the respiratory rate (RR), and Ti/Ttot is the duty cycle or the inspiratory time related to the total respiratory cycle.

Mahler and colleagues[33] tested the relationship of many of these variables to dyspnea in a group of patients with asthma who were exercising. The strongest predictors for dyspnea measured by the Borg scale were peak inspiratory flow ($P = .0005$) tidal volume ($P = .0009$), respiratory rate ($P = .0001$), and peak inspiratory mouth pressure ($P = .0001$). These four variables explained 63 per cent of the variance in the rating of dyspnea by these patients. Although minute ventilation (VE) was not a significant predictor, this measure did correlate significantly ($r = .67$, $P = .0001$). The fact that VE was not a predictor was attributed to its close relationship to the other variables.

The preceding studies suggest that the pattern of breathing is related to dyspnea. An increase in VE is related to dyspnea in normal subjects and in patients.[32, 105] An increase in respiratory rate alone has been associated with an increase in dyspnea in normal subjects and in hospitalized asthmatic subjects.[36] The length of inspiratory time was related to dyspnea in the previously discussed laboratory studies.[32, 33] Asynchronous breathing, ranging from some lag between rib cage and abdominal movement in paradoxical breathing, has been associated with dyspnea.[70] Therefore, the traditional assessment parameters of increased respiratory rate, I:E ratio, and paradoxical breathing all have been shown to be related to increasing shortness of breath in the laboratory or clinical setting.

Work of Breathing

The work of breathing is probably the closest physiological parameter related to dyspnea. In fact, dyspnea has been called the "clinical manifestation" of the work of breathing. Manifestations of increased work of breathing, such as the use of accessory neck and rib cage muscles of respiration, asynchronous breathing, facial frowning, and increased VE have all been related to dyspnea.[70, 106–108]

A more sensitive and reliable measurement of the work of breathing in the critically ill is being tested experimentally by a group of investigators with mechanically ventilated patients. These researchers have found a relationship between dyspnea and the pressure-time index (PTI). The PTI is a measure of the work of the respiratory muscles related to the oxygen consumption of the muscles.[109]

$$PTI = Pavg/Pmax \times Ti/Ttot$$

where Pavg is the average inspiratory pressure developed per breath, Pmax is the maximum pressure that can be developed by the patient, and Ti/Ttot is the duty cycle, or the fraction of the total breathing cycle spent in inspiration. The PTI is difficult to measure at the bedside. However, it has been suggested that the Ti/Ttot does not vary significantly in the spontaneously breathing patient; therefore, if this portion of the equation is disregarded, only the Pavg/Pmax

ratio has to be measured. The average inspiratory pressure developed per breath

$$(Pavg) = Vt \times E + Vi \times R$$

where Vt is tidal volume, E is the elastance of the respiratory system, Vi is the inspiratory flow rate, and R is the resistance to gas flow.[110] Each of these variables can be calculated at the bedside, but at present these parameters are not being measured in most intensive care units. This clinical measure of the work of breathing, however, is the most promising indirect clinical physiological correlate of dyspnea when the patient is unable to communicate.

Fatigue

One of the most frequent physical correlates of dyspnea that patients describe is fatigue. They complain of overwhelming weariness or say they are "all worn out." Indeed, some patients describe their dyspnea only in terms of fatigue. The degree of pervasive fatigue patients feel seems to correlate with increasing dyspnea. In a retrospective study of 68 patients with various obstructive, restrictive, and vascular pulmonary diseases, fatigue, as measured by the Profile of Mood States (POMS), was correlated positively ($r = .41$) with usual dyspnea.[12] Another investigator found that fatigue was a significant variable in a conceptual model relating dyspnea, severity, functional status, and quality of life in 45 adults with chronic bronchitis and emphysema.[111] When dyspnea severity increased, fatigue increased ($r = .47$), depression increased ($r = .67$), and quality of life decreased ($r = -.75$). In nine patients receiving ventilation for acute respiratory failure, fatigue, again measured by the POMS, was related to the preweaning dyspnea score. Those subjects who had the highest dyspnea scores had the highest fatigue and tension scores.[112] Fatigue, heart rate, somatization, and congestion were significantly elevated during high dyspnea when compared with times of lower dyspnea in another group of patients with asthma.[36]

ASSOCIATED PSYCHOSOCIAL CONCEPTS

Clinically, anxiety and depression frequently are associated with dyspnea. Patients in the hospital become more and more dyspneic as their anxiety increases, or anxiety may snowball as dyspnea increases. This clinically evident relationship has been shown in the laboratory and in patients hospitalized for COPD and asthma.[36, 44, 46, 47] Gift and colleagues measured emotional states during high, medium, and low dyspnea states in patients hospitalized for COPD.[46, 47] Anxiety was significantly raised during high or medium states of dyspnea than during low states. The severity of dyspnea was significantly related to the anxiety trait ($r = .34$) and depression trait ($r = .43$). The relationships among disease severity, dyspnea severity, depression and functional status, and quality of life were found to be significant and correlated in a group of patients with chronic bronchitis and emphysema.[113] Possible pathways between emotional factors and dyspnea are outlined and discussed in a review of emotional influences on breathing.[49]

MEASUREMENT AND MANIFESTATIONS

Dyspnea is a subjective phenomenon that can be rated only by the person who is experiencing it. Therefore, direct measurement of the symptom necessarily is subjective. Indirect or objective measures are important only if the patient cannot communicate.

Subjective Manifestations

Activity Scales

Historically, dyspnea has been measured indirectly by the minimum level of activity that is associated with shortness of breath. In chronic situations when people are active, the severity of breathlessness can be assessed by asking patients what level of activity brings on their shortness of breath (SOB).

Over the years, a variety of instruments have been developed to measure dyspnea by using the level of activity that brings on shortness of breath. The first of these was the Pneumoconiosis Research Unit Dyspnea Questionnaire, a five-point scale based on degrees of physical activities that trigger breathlessness.[114] This scale was adapted and used in the development of other instruments, such as the American Thoracic Society

Grade of Breathlessness Scale shown in Table 11–4.[115]

Another scale that integrates activity with dyspnea is the oxygen-cost diagram (OCD). The OCD is a 100-mm visual analogue scale with descriptive activities at various points along the line that correspond to oxygen requirements of different activities. The top of the vertical line represents "no breathlessness," and the bottom anchor is "the greatest breathlessness."[116] These various activity scales are illustrated and discussed in-depth elsewhere.[117]

Other measures of dyspnea based on activity are the Baseline Dyspnea Index (BDI) and Transition Dyspnea Index (TDI), which have been developed and tested extensively.[96, 117, 118] The BDI includes five grades that reflect increasing severity of dyspnea for each of three categories: functional impairment, magnitude of task, and magnitude of effort. Ratings for each category ranging from 0 to 4 are determined by an interviewer following specific criteria. The TDI is used to evaluate breathlessness ratings from the baseline condition (BDI) in each category. Ratings for each category of the BDI on the TDI range from +3 (major improvement) to −3 (major deterioration). This instrument has been tested for reliability and related to physiological lung function, oxygen consumption, and exercise capacity.[100, 101, 119] The

TABLE 11–4 AMERICAN THORACIC SOCIETY GRADE OF BREATHLESSNESS SCALE

Grade	Degree	
0	None	Not troubled with breathlessness except with strenuous exercise
1	Slight	Troubled by shortness of breath when hurrying on the level or walking up a slight hill
2	Moderate	Walks slower than people of the same age on the level because of breathlessness or has to stop for breath when walking at own pace on the level
3	Severe	Stops for breath after walking about 100 yards or after a few minutes on the level
4	Very severe	Too breathless to leave the house or breathless when dressing or undressing

From Brooks, S.M. (1982). Task group on surveillance for respiratory hazards in the occupational setting. ATS News *8*:12–16.

index also has been used to evaluate pharmacological and medical therapies such as theophylline and inspiratory muscle training.[120, 121] The BDI is illustrated in Table 11–5, while the TDI is illustrated elsewhere.[96]

Dyspnea Intensity

The simplest but least sensitive measure of dyspnea is to ask the patient whether he or she is short of breath. This yes-or-no categorical measurement probably is the most frequently used method of assessing dyspnea but gives no information about the severity of the sensation.

Investigators have increased the validity, reliability, and sensitivity of the measurement of dyspnea by using numerical scales or a visual analogue scale on which the person rates the actual dyspnea perceived. Borg developed a categorical scale in which words describing degrees of perceived exertion during work are anchored to numbers from 0 to 20.[122] An adaptation of the Borg scale was completed by Burdon and colleagues specifically to evaluate breathlessness in relationship to changes in pulmonary function parameters.[123] Since then, the Borg scale has been used extensively to measure dyspnea in the laboratory and in the clinical environment. It is presented in Table 11–6.

The visual analogue scale has also been used to measure dyspnea and is a vertical or horizontal line of 0 to 100 mm anchored at either end of the line by descriptive words such as "not at all breathless" to "worst imaginable breathlessness." It is illustrated in Figure 11–2. The subject marks the line at the point representing the degree of dyspnea felt.[124] The validity and reliability of the visual analogue scale for measuring breathlessness has been shown in both normal subjects and patients with chronic pulmonary disease.[97, 125, 126] The visual analogue scale has been presented horizontally or vertically with little difference in results[127] and has been used in correlational studies of dyspnea,[31] in studies of the mechanisms of dyspnea,[128] and in determining the effect of nursing care activities and therapeutic interventions on dyspnea.[129, 130] The visual analogue scale and Borg scale have been found to have similar properties and reproducibility.[131] A strong (r = .90) and significant correlation has been found between the two scales when used by critically ill patients.[132]

Magnitude estimation, a psychophysiological technique used to measure the subjective magnitude of a sensation, has been used in experimental studies of dyspneic thresholds. Subjects estimate the added loads to breathing from their own original reference point for the initial load. The technique is based on Stevens' power law, which states that a constant change in stimulus intensity produces a constant change in the magnitude of a sensation. Respiratory sensations have been found to follow Stevens' law and to be perceived in approximately the same quantitative manner as other sensory stimuli.[6] Magnitude estimation has been used predominantly in the laboratory study of the perception of added resistive and elastic loads to breathing and has been found to be a reliable measure of one dimension of dyspnea.[133] This technique requires patient learning and therefore is more appropriate for measuring chronic dyspnea.

Objective Manifestations

Measures of respiratory distress, which include behavioral manifestations that can be observed or physiological pulmonary function parameters, can be used as indirect measures of dyspnea if the patient is unable to communicate.

Behavioral Manifestations

Behavioral manifestations that are frequently observed when patients say they are short of breath include increased respiratory rate, restlessness, diaphoresis, use of accessory respiratory muscles, tremulousness, gasping breaths, pallor, interrupted or "staccato" speech, large staring eyes, professorial position or a frozen appearance, audible wheezing, and coughing. When asked, "How can other people tell when you are short of breath?", pulmonary patients named some of these same behaviors.[12] Labored breathing, wheezing, and a straight upright position with a frozen, immobile position were descriptions of behaviors they believed others could see. Other common manifestations listed in the literature, such as rapid and open mouth breathing, use of accessory muscles, and appearing withdrawn and uncommunicative, were corroborated by these patients. Use of learned strategies including pursed lips breathing may also be subjective manifestations of increasing breathlessness.

TABLE 11–5 BASELINE DYSPNEA INDEX

Functional Impairment

_____	Grade 4:	*No Impairment.* Able to carry out usual activities and occupation without shortness of breath.
_____	Grade 3:	*Slight impairment.* Distinct impairment in at least one activity but no activities completely abandoned. Reduction in activity at work or in usual activities that seems slight or not clearly caused by shortness of breath.
_____	Grade 2:	*Moderate impairment.* Patient has changed jobs or has abandoned at least one usual activity because of shortness of breath.
_____	Grade 0:	*Very severe impairment.* Unable to work and has given up most of all usual activities owing to shortness of breath.
_____	W:	*Amount uncertain.* Patient is impaired owing to shortness of breath, but amount cannot be specified. Details are not sufficient to allow impairment to be categorized.
_____	X:	*Unknown.* Information unavailable regarding impairment.
_____	Y:	*Impaired for reasons other than shortness of breath.* For example, musculoskeletal problem or chest pain.

Usual activities refer to requirements of daily living, maintenance or upkeep of residence, yard work, gardening, and shopping.

Magnitude of Task

_____	Grade 4:	*Extraordinary.* Becomes short of breath only with extraordinary activity such as carrying very heavy loads on the level, lighter loads uphill, or running. No shortness of breath with ordinary tasks.
_____	Grade 3:	*Major.* Becomes short of breath only with major activities such as walking up a steep hill, climbing more than three flights of stairs, or carrying a moderate load on the level.
_____	Grade 2:	*Moderate.* Becomes short of breath with moderate or tasks such as walking up a gradual hill, climbing less than three flights of stairs, or carrying a light load on the level.
_____	Grade 1:	*Light.* Becomes short of breath with light activities such as walking on the level, washing, or standing.
_____	Grade 0:	*No task.* Becomes short of breath at rest, while sitting, or lying down.
_____	W:	*Amount uncertain.* Patient's ability to perform tasks is impaired due to shortness of breath, but amount cannot be specified. Details are not sufficient to allow impairment to be categorized.
_____	X:	*Unknown.* Information unavailable regarding limitation of magnitude or task.
_____	Y:	*Impaired for reasons other than shortness of breath.* For example, musculoskeletal problem or chest pain.

Magnitude of Effort

_____	Grade 4:	*Extraordinary.* Becomes short of breath only with the greatest imaginable effort. No shortness of breath with ordinary effort.
_____	Grade 3:	*Major.* Becomes short of breath with effort distinctly submaximal but of major proportion. Tasks performed without pause unless the task requires extraordinary effort that may be performed with pauses.
_____	Grade 2:	*Moderate.* Becomes short of breath with moderate effort. Tasks performed with occasional pauses and take longer to complete than usual.
_____	Grade 1:	*Light.* Becomes short of breath with little effort. Tasks performed with little effort, or more difficult tasks performed with frequent pauses and taking 50 to 100% longer to complete than if done by the average person.
_____	Grade 0:	*No effort.* Becomes short of breath at rest, while sitting, or lying down.
_____	W:	*Amount uncertain.* Patient's exertional ability is impaired owing to shortness of breath, but amount cannot be specified. Details are not sufficient to allow impairment to be categorized.
_____	X:	*Unknown.* Information unavailable regarding limitation of effort.
_____	Y:	*Impaired for reasons other than shortness of breath.* For example, musculoskeletal problems or chest pain.

From Mahler, D.A. (1990). Clinical measurement of dyspnea. In D.A. Mahler (ed.), *Dyspnea* (pp. 75–76). Mt. Kisco, NY: Futura Publishing.

TABLE 11-6   MODIFIED BORG SCALE

0	Nothing at all
0.5	Very, very slight (just noticeable)
1	Very slight
2	Slight
3	Moderate
4	Somewhat severe
5	Severe
6	
7	Very severe
8	
9	Very, very severe (almost maximal)
10	Maximal

From Borg, G.A.V. (1982). Psychophysical bases of perceived exertion. Med Sci Sports Exerc *14:*377–381. © The American College of Sports Medicine.

Signs of respiratory distress in children can include nasal flaring, use of accessory muscles, sternal retractions, cyanosis, wheezing, cough, and rapid respiratory rate.

Indirect Physiological Measures of Dyspnea

As described in the discussion of the physiological correlates of dyspnea, many of the behaviors indicative of increased work of breathing or changes in breathing pattern have been shown in the laboratory and clinical setting to be related to shortness of breath. Accessory muscle use has been correlated with dyspnea in the laboratory and in the clinical setting. Healthy subjects and patients with COPD who used accessory, neck, and rib cage muscles for ventilation were more likely to report an increase in the sensation of dyspnea.[70, 108] Clinically, the pattern of ventilation is related to the sensation of dyspnea. An increase in minute ventilation is related to dyspnea in normal subjects and patients.[32, 33] An increase in respiratory rate alone has been associated with an increase in dyspnea in normal subjects and in hospitalized patients.[36] The length of inspiratory time is related to dyspnea in subjects in the laboratory.[105] Asynchronous breathing, ranging from some lag between rib cage and abdominal movement to paradoxical breathing, has been associated with dyspnea.[70]

Other correlates described in the previous portion of text that can be used in the indirect measure of dyspnea include changes in arterial blood gases, measures of work of breathing, and measures of decreases in muscle strength or endurance, such as peak inspiratory pressure or sustained inspiratory pressure. Pulmonary function parameters that can be used as indirect measures of dyspnea are listed in Table 11–7.

In summary, many of those parameters that have been observed clinically when patients are experiencing dyspnea now have been validated in the laboratory or clinical setting. If the patient is unable to rate shortness of breath, these indirect objective manifestations can be used to estimate the dyspnea felt by the patient.

SURVEILLANCE

In the chronically ill, dyspnea with changing activities and emotional situations can be monitored by the patient at home. A daily log to monitor shortness of breath has been used successfully.[135] For other illnesses, monitoring of the symptom has been shown to decrease the symptom.[136] If the patient is

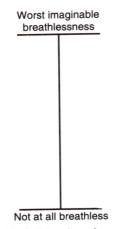

Worst imaginable
breathlessness

Not at all breathless

Figure 11–2. Visual analogue scale.

TABLE 11-7   PHYSIOLOGICAL VARIABLES RELATED TO DYSPNEA IN RESEARCH STUDIES

Position
Respiratory rate
Inspiratory time
Tidal volume
Minute ventilation
Accessory muscle use
Paradoxical and dysynchronous breathing
Hypoxia
Hypercapnia
Forced expiratory volume
Maximum inspiratory and expiratory pressures
Work of breathing
Fatigue

Adapted from Carrieri-Kohlman, V. (1991). Dyspnea in the weaning patient: Assessment and intervention. AACN Clin Issues Crit Care Nurs *2:*467.

seen by the nurse on an outpatient basis, these logs can be used to evaluate changes in the therapeutic regimen, to target breathing strategies, and to prescribe energy conservation, depending on the intensity of dyspnea and the triggers. At the initial visit, a baseline dyspnea measurement can be obtained with a visual analogue scale or Borg scale. The worst and usual dyspnea level with and without activity should be measured at each clinic visit to determine patterns over time, during different seasons, and with varying activities and environments.

Multiple measures of dyspnea, for instance, the baseline and transitional dyspnea index, dyspnea with activity log, and visual analogue scale, can be used at each visit to track changes in the symptom. Guyatt and colleagues developed a Chronic Respiratory Questionnaire that measures dyspnea with activities and includes measures of other concepts, such as mastery of the symptom, fatigue, and emotional factors. This instrument has been shown to be sensitive to changes in dyspnea after therapeutic regimens and can be used to measure the effect of dyspnea on quality of life.[137]

Baseline measurements recorded when patients are stable can be used to determine changes during acute exacerbations, especially if patients are unable to rate their own shortness of breath. In addition, during acute dyspnea, the patient can be asked to rate dyspnea on a visual analogue scale or Borg scale. Behavioral manifestations, measures of work of breathing, and pulmonary function are related to the rating of dyspnea, so that in the event that the patient's condition becomes severe and they are unable to rate the intensity of the sensation, these measures can be used to estimate indirectly the level of dyspnea.

Despite the individual variation and subjective nature of the symptom, the presence of breathlessness remains a clue or prodromal indicator that the patient is not tolerating a new procedure or that the treatment is not effective. More important than the type of instrument the nurse chooses to monitor dyspnea is that the symptom be monitored. If validated instruments are not used, the nurse can ask the patient to rate on a scale of 0 to 10 shortness of breath in response to a certain treatment, change in position, or strategy being implemented. Knowledge related to dyspnea has grown exponentially in the past several years. However, this knowledge of measurement is not reflected in practice, and dyspnea still is not being measured systematically in the majority of patients with chronic or acute shortness of breath. The measurement of dyspnea is an excellent method to determine whether nursing care is having an impact on the patient's actual work of breathing or perception of discomfort.

THERAPIES

The therapeutic goals for treating dyspnea are to decrease the distress of dyspnea and to increase exercise tolerance, physical and social well-being, and quality of life. Interventions for decreasing dyspnea are directed at altering one or more of the proposed causes of the symptom. Therefore, the discussion of therapies is organized by the proposed mechanisms: decreasing the sense of respiratory muscle effort, decreasing chemical or neurological respiratory drive, and altering the central perception of breathlessness. Strategies identified by adults and children who have experienced dyspnea will be included in the discussion.

Decreasing Respiratory Muscle Effort

Respiratory muscle effort can be decreased by limiting physical exertion, decreasing the effort of breathing, or using medications to decrease airway obstruction and inflammation.

Limiting Physical Exertion—Energy Conservation

The ultimate goal for patients with dyspnea is to find an optimal balance between activity and rest. Patients can be taught to use strategies to conserve energy, simplify work, and pace themselves. Activities and hobbies that are pleasurable but require less activity need to be substituted for strenuous work. Graduated exercise and activity to stay physically conditioned is stressed while at the same time emphasizing the need for a slower pace. Effort used for unnecessary tasks should be saved for energy that can be used for leisure activities and daily exercises, enhancing the efficiency of the muscles and increasing well-being. Advanced planning and careful scheduling of activities save energy and decrease dyspnea. Instructions on how to conserve energy and pace activities are published by the American Lung Association and in various pulmonary rehabilitation references.[138] Exemplary suggestions for energy conservation are discussed in-depth elsewhere.[139]

Decreasing the Effort of Breathing

Two breathing strategies—pursed lips breathing and diaphragmatic breathing—may decrease the effort of breathing and therefore dyspnea. Benefits of coordinating abdominal wall expansion with inspiration and slowing expiration have included an increased tidal volume, decreased respiratory rate, increased oxygen saturation, increased exercise tolerance, and less dyspnea for some patients.[143, 144] Pursed lips breathing decreases respiratory rate and increases tidal volume,[140, 141] with a resulting increase in ventilatory efficiency and oxygen saturation.[142] Other authors have found that airway compression and alteration in breathing pattern may contribute to the sensation of dyspnea and propose that pursed lips breathing decreases dynamic compression of the airways. Many patients report less dyspnea and describe a feeling of control of their dyspnea while using pursed lips breathing.[140] Patients with COPD often assume a position of leaning forward when they are short of breath. This position stabilizes the upper chest while allowing freedom of movement of the lower chest. The leaning forward position allows abdominal organs to drop away from the diaphragm and may decrease accessory muscle use, thus producing subjective relief of dyspnea by permitting better diaphragmatic excursion. Research has shown that in the leaning forward position dyspnea is decreased; an improvement in the diaphragm's length-tension ratio has been hypothesized as the reason for this.[145] It is important to remember that the patient with shortness of breath will assume the most comfortable position.[146]

The effort of breathing may also be decreased by increasing the efficiency of muscle work. Physical reconditioning or total body exercise training improves exercise tolerance, and evidence indicates that it also decreases dyspnea.[147–150] The proposed mechanisms for

exercise training producing these beneficial effects include improved aerobic capacity, increased motivation, desensitization to dyspnea, improved muscle coordination, and improved ventilatory muscle function.[151] Although pulmonary function parameters such as FEV_1 may not improve after physical reconditioning, patients may discover that they can walk farther. Movement becomes more efficient and requires lower oxygen consumption, thereby lowering required ventilation and dyspnea. One benefit of exercise may be that experiencing dyspnea in a secure situation decreases the anxiety associated with the symptom and actually "desensitizes" the patient to higher levels of dyspnea.[152] Patients are then able to tolerate greater dyspnea with less fear and thus accomplish more activities.

Because persons with chronic dyspnea often are more short of breath when they perform activities of daily living with unsupported arms, upper extremity training recently has been included in most pulmonary rehabilitation programs. One investigator reported decreased breathlessness after 6 weeks of upper extremity training with arm cycling and a series of low-resistance, high-repetition arm exercises.[153] Another therapy that appears to decrease the effort of breathing and "unload" the inspiratory muscles in patients with COPD is CPAP. Some authors have found that CPAP decreases dyspnea during exercise[87] and ventilator weaning[154]; others have found an improvement in only some patients.[155] The mechanism has been attributed to a reduction in inspiratory muscle effort and dynamic airway compression.

Investigators have studied both resting the respiratory muscles and training them with inspiratory muscle training. Early findings have suggested that if respiratory muscles are in a chronic fatigued state as indicated by tachypnea (greater than 30 breaths per minute), CO_2 retention (greater than 45 mm Hg), and a reduction in maximal inspiratory pressure (less negative than -50 cm H_2O in COPD), then these patients may benefit from rest.[58] Techniques to rest the muscles include a cuirass or body shell or a total body wrap, which provides negative pressure ventilation. Improvement in respiratory muscle function after a program of daily intermittent negative pressure ventilation has been found by some authors[156]; however, when dyspnea was measured by the OCD, it did not significantly improve compared with a control group.[157] Other investigators have found subjective improvement in dyspnea by patient report, but a valid instrument was not used to measure the dyspnea.[158, 159] In contrast, a program of inspiratory muscle training decreased dyspnea intensity in patients with chronic dyspnea.[160, 161] Patients with decreased respiratory muscle strength without severe hyperinflation are thought to be the group that would benefit the most from inspiratory muscle training.

In acutely ill patients, various modes of ventilation have been used to decrease the effort of breathing and dyspnea. Pressure support ventilation (PSV) has been found to increase patient "comfort."[162] It is unknown whether this comfort represents an actual decrease in dyspnea.[110]

Medications to Decrease Effort of Breathing

Medications to decrease the effort of breathing and dyspnea include bronchodilators, corticosteroids, and theophylline. Although there are few controlled studies, bronchodilators have been found to decrease dyspnea. Two investigators studied the effect of beta$_2$-adrenergic agonists on dyspnea in patients with COPD. Dullinger and associates found that two puffs of metaproterenol every 3 hours significantly decreased dyspnea measured by a visual analogue scale,[163] whereas Guyatt and colleagues found that two puffs of albuterol decreased dyspnea after a 6-minute walking test.[164] The use of salbutamol decreased dyspnea without changing ventilation in patients with asthma.[165]

Several investigators using well-designed studies reviewed by others[166] have found that theophylline decreases dyspnea with little improvement in standard pulmonary function tests.[164, 167, 168] This significant decrease in dyspnea may be due to improvement in the length-tension relationship of the diaphragm or improved respiratory muscle function.

Corticosteroids are used frequently for severe asthma and other diseases in which there is a significant degree of reversibility, such as chronic bronchitis, but they are of questionable value in the treatment of pure emphysema. Patients with severe dyspnea who have intermittent wheezing seem to benefit the most. Clinically, corticosteroids do seem to decrease shortness of breath by an unknown mechanism. Presumably, the reduction in perceived dyspnea is due to the decrease in inflammation and increase in bronchodilation. To date, the direct effect of corticosteroids on dyspnea has not been studied.

Decreasing Chemical or Neurological Respiratory Drive

Oxygen Therapy

Oxygen therapy decreases the respiratory drive and ventilation during rest and exercise. It may be for these reasons that investigators have found that subjects can walk farther and are less breathless when breathing oxygen.[169, 170] Oxygen may also decrease dyspnea in patients who do not have a P_{O_2} within guidelines for oxygen therapy.[171]

Medications

Medications that may reduce dyspnea by decreasing the respiratory drive or by altering the central perception of discomfort include opiates, benzodiazepines, and phenothiazines. During acute bronchoconstriction in asthmatics, the activity of endogenous opioids decreases ventilatory output and the sensation of dyspnea.[172] Opiates at low doses (dihydrocodeine and morphine) decrease dyspnea and increase walking distance without intolerable side effects.[173–175] However, higher doses of opiates caused greater side effects.[176] Routine administration of opiates is not advised by the authors at this time; however, the use of opiates in end-stage respiratory failure to provide comfort for the dying patient is recommended.[166] Benzodiazepines may modulate dyspnea by decreasing the patient's anxiety level or by depressing the ventilatory drive. Investigators using small samples with no control groups found that diazepam and alprazolam decreased dyspnea[177, 178]; however, three other investigators used controlled designs and found no change in dyspnea.[179–181] Promethazine, one type of phenothiazine, has been investigated with mixed results. Woodcock and associates reported a small decrease of breathlessness during exercise;[181] however, Rice and colleagues found no improvement in dyspnea.[182] These psychotropic medications should be used on an individual basis when anxiety is a primary mechanism of dyspnea.[166]

Bilateral removal of the carotid bodies reduces dyspnea and increases exercise tolerance in patients with severe COPD.[183, 184] The cost-benefit of this treatment for end-stage respiratory failure with extreme dyspnea remains controversial, and the treatment is not accepted practice.

Altering the Central Perception of Dyspnea

Management strategies that help to decrease the perception of dyspnea may be successful clinically. As with pain, strategies that help patients to feel in control of the symptom or that distract them from the symptom clinically seem to decrease the sensation.

Relaxation and Psychophysical Technique

If dyspnea is escalated and reinforced by anxiety, a strategy that decreases anxiety may also be expected to reduce the intensity and distress of dyspnea. In addition, it has been suggested that relaxation can increase the ability of persons to cope with a disease by helping them to exert greater control over associated symptoms. Most investigators who have systematically studied relaxation techniques have done so with asthmatic patients and have used progressive muscle relaxation to determine the effect of relaxation on anxiety, respiratory rate, flow rates, and lung volumes but not on dyspnea.[185–187] One investigator studied the effect of relaxation on dyspnea and found reduced dyspnea scores during treatment sessions but not at the end of the 4-week period.[188] In the laboratory setting, relaxation and biofeedback reduce respiratory rate and increase tidal volume in some patients.[189–191] However, these investigators did not measure dyspnea. Individualized tape recordings that describe specific solutions have been successfully used to coach some patients through relaxation techniques during times of panic when dyspnea occurs in the home.[192]

Other psychophysiological techniques that are used clinically to relax patients also slow breathing and presumably increase tidal volume. These interventions, such as visual imagery, meditation, and yoga, need to be tested for their effect on breathlessness.[193]

Increasing Knowledge and Education

Although the effect of knowledge on the intensity of dyspnea has not been studied, preparatory information about anticipated sensations similar to dyspnea has been shown to decrease anxiety and increase the patient's perception of control over impending distress.[194] Teaching by the nurse has reduced dyspnea in patients with COPD[195] and has been labeled the most important function by the nurse in dyspnea management.[196] Knowledge of risk factors or triggers of episodes of dyspnea enables the patient to manipulate environmental and personal situations by staying away from the precipitant, by taking preparatory medications, by relaxing, or by using strategies to minimize the distress of the event. Strategies that have been identified by patients as helpful in minimizing dyspnea can be combined with those that have been found by other patients to be successful. Tips for coping with acute and chronic dyspnea have been described elsewhere by the authors.[139]

Pulmonary Rehabilitation Programs

Patients who complete a pulmonary rehabilitation program experience a reduction in respiratory symptoms and increase their ability to carry out activities of daily living.[138, 197] Although various instruments and measurement time periods were used, selected studies have shown that pulmonary rehabilitation programs have a positive effect on the symptom of dyspnea.[147–150] However, it is difficult to determine the true effect of the multiple components of pulmonary rehabilitation programs on the intensity and frequency of dyspnea. Most rehabilitation programs include education, exercise, psychological support, breathing retraining, and social interaction. Controlled clinical trials are needed to determine the true effect of each of these components on the intensity and distress of dyspnea.

Strategies Reported by Patients with Dyspnea

The strategies actually used by patients to decrease shortness of breath have been described by nurse researchers. Barstow described general strategies such as postponing, prioritizing, and careful advanced planning.[198] A significant person in the household

(social support), financial well-being, posses-
sion of a car, and an efficacious medical
regimen were important factors that promoted adjustment for the patient with emphysema. Fagerhaugh identified money,
time, energy, "breathing stations," and "mobility assistants" as important determinants
of successful coping.[199]

Chalmers described three categories of
coping strategies used by patients with
COPD.[200] Behavioral strategies or actions to
deal with the effects of the disease included
taking medications, making environmental
alterations, and avoiding precipitants. Cognitive strategies included focusing on the
positive aspects of life, normalization or min-
imization, pacing activities, reminiscing and
reflection, and problem solving. Expressive
strategies consisted of verbalizing emotions
that helped the patient adjust to the disease.

Carrieri and Janson-Bjerklie described
strategies used by individuals who experience
dyspnea as a result of obstructive, restrictive,
or pulmonary vascular disease.[201] Successful
strategies focused more on problems than on
emotions. Asthmatic patients developed the
greatest number of coping strategies. The
strategies commonly taught to patients experiencing dyspnea were not always useful
for patients with restrictive and vascular disease. Adaptive strategies and changes in life
style used by persons with emphysema-bron-
chitis were very similar to those described
above. In general, these subjects made the
same types of changes in activities of daily
living, modifying and pacing their daily tasks.
They used advanced planning of activities,
resting places, complex medication regimens,
and avoidance of precipitating situations in
order to cope with shortness of breath. Very
specific strategies for reducing acute dyspnea
were described, such as turning on a fan or
sitting by an open window to allow cool air
to blow directly on the face. Cool air generated by fans to reduce dyspnea has been
tested with normal subjects.[202] (A summary
of these strategies is listed in Table 11–8.)
There were differences in the number and
type of immediate and long-term strategies
used by patients across disease categories.
The type and frequency of strategies were
determined by the frequency, periodicity,

TABLE 11–8 STRATEGIES USED BY CHILDREN AND ADULTS TO MANAGE DYSPNEA

	Problem-Focused	Emotion-Focused

Immediate Strategies	Position and motion
	  Move slower
	  Lie or sit down
	  Keep still
	  Positioning
	Breathing strategies
	  Pursed lip-breathing
	  Diaphragmatic breathing
	  Slow, deep breathing
	Physical distancing
	Medications and oxygen
	Fresh air/fans
	Fluids
	Health provider visit
		Self-isolation
		Relaxation
		Distraction/diversion
		Meditation
		Conscious "calming" of self
		Seeking of social support

Long-Term Strategies	Slow down
	Energy conservation
	Changes in activities of daily
	  living (ADL)
	Transfer of ADL to others
	Changes in living situation
	Activity modification, including
	  advanced planning, decrease
	  in activities, change in type
	  and time
	Health behaviors (e.g., lose
	  weight, exercise)
	Medications
	Oxygen
	Distancing from triggers
		Emphasis on positive (e.g.,
		  ignore it, don't think about it)
		Social support
		Relaxation
		Social isolation
		Avoiding being alone

Adapted from Carrieri, V.K. & Janson-Bjerklie, S. (1986). Strategies patients use to manage the sensation of dyspnea. West J Nurs Res 8:284. Reprinted by permission of Sage Publications, Inc.

and intensity of dyspnea experienced by the person.

REVIEW OF RESEARCH FINDINGS

Research related to dyspnea has focused on describing respiratory sensations in healthy subjects and in numerous pulmonary disease states, validating instruments to measure dyspnea, investigating the relationship of physiological and psychosocial correlates, and studying the effect of various therapies on the intensity of the symptom. There has been a renewed interest in dyspnea as a phenomenon of study, which has led to a proliferation of laboratory and clinical investigations that have been reviewed elsewhere.[14, 51–54] Only exemplary studies that are especially noteworthy or are conducted by nurse researchers will be discussed here.

A renewed focus on the "language of breathlessness" has prompted investigators to study the different respiratory sensations felt during a variety of stimuli used to mimic disease processes or perceived by patients who are experiencing the clinical state. To investigate whether breathlessness represents more than one sensation, Simon and colleagues studied 30 healthy subjects in whom breathlessness was induced by eight types of respiratory stress: breath-holding, carbon dioxide inhalation, carbon dioxide inhalation with ventilation voluntarily targeted below the level dictated by chemical drive, breathing with a resistive load, breathing with an elastic load, voluntary elevation of functional residual capacity, voluntary limitation of tidal volume, and exercise.[8] Subjects were asked to choose descriptions of their sensations from a questionnaire listing 19 descriptors. Distinct clusters of descriptors emerged, subjects could distinguish different sensations of breathlessness, and clusters were associated with certain stimuli. For example, the most frequent sensations during exercise were "rapid" and "heavy," while a resistive load was associated with "work" and "air hunger." Nine clusters of descriptors were identified, including rapid, exhalation, concentration, shallow, work, suffocating, hunger, heavy, and gasping. These same investigators modified this list of descriptors and studied 53 patients with different pulmonary conditions, such as COPD, pulmonary vascular disease, interstitial disease, and pregnancy.[9] Patients were asked to choose the phrases that best described their breathlessness. Certain clusters again grouped together, and there was an association between condition and descriptive cluster. These findings and those of others suggest different diseases may produce different sensations of breathlessness and may be mediated by different mechanisms. Patients could distinguish between different sensations of breathlessness, and there was an association between certain clusters of descriptors and the specific conditions. These researchers proposed that the term breathlessness encompasses multiple sensations. It was suggested that different types of dyspnea are mediated by different mechanisms.

Nurses have focused recent research efforts on the measurement of dyspnea and the relationship of selected variables with the symptom. A recent study explored the role of dyspnea in a test of a predictive model of asthma outcomes.[203] A sample of 95 adults with asthma was studied over 60 days with daily peak flow (PEFR) monitoring, symptom reporting, and three monthly interviews focused on coping with asthmatic episodes. In the theoretical model, three exogenous variable sets representing personal factors, disease severity, and coping factors were expected to exert indirect effects on psychosocial and morbidity outcomes through dyspnea intensity. Only dyspnea was expected to have a direct effect on the outcomes of depression, life satisfaction, and number of emergency room visits. The concept of dyspnea-related distress was also explored in the statistical test of the model. Results showed that 37 per cent of the variance in depression was explained by nocturnal asthma, dyspnea-related distress, and self-care strategies. Financial status and nocturnal asthma explained 24 per cent of the variance in life satisfaction. Twenty-seven per cent of the variance in morbidity as indexed by emergency room visits and hospitalizations was explained by dyspnea-related distress.

Another nurse scholar compared psychological and physiological variables during intense dyspnea with variables at no or low levels of dyspnea in 36 asthmatic patients.[36] In the emergency room when dyspnea was rated high, as determined by the patient respiratory rate, pulse, wheezing, and accessory muscle use were higher, whereas PEFR and oxygen saturation were lower. The psychological variables of anxiety, depression, psychological somatization, and hostility were higher during times of high dyspnea. More clinical signs were found to be different at high and low levels of dyspnea in this study than in previous studies by the same researchers.[46] These correlates are suggested as indicators that can be monitored to determine the effectiveness of interventions.

A group of nurse investigators used a path analysis model to examine interrelationships among significant variables related to dyspnea in 45 adults with chronic bronchitis and emphysema.[111] Dyspnea severity had strong but separate effects on functional status ($r = -.40$) and quality of life ($r = -.23$). Mastery, the individual's perceived ability to manage daily events, measured by the Quality of Life Questionnaire,[137] was highly related to dyspnea severity ($r = -.71$). Because the relationship between dyspnea and mastery was greater than that between dyspnea and disease severity, these authors suggested that dyspnea severity is associated with a psychological variable. Dyspnea may be affected by direct focus on psychological interventions to decrease depression and improve mastery. They proposed that reducing dyspnea severity may improve quality of life and functional status.

Steele and colleagues described two dimensions of dyspnea: a sensory component (perceptual sensitivity to breathing effort) and an affective component (perceptual sensitivity to breathing discomfort) in 27 subjects with COPD who were breathing added inspiratory muscle loads through an inspiratory muscle trainer.[204] Breathing effort and discomfort were measured with separate visual analogue scales. Effort had a significant effect on discomfort, the perceived effort was greater than perceived discomfort, and there was a greater rate of increase in discomfort than effort. It was determined that 12 out of 27 subjects were able to differentiate breathing discomfort from effort, and 8 of those 12 had greater "perceptual sensitivity" for discomfort than for effort. The authors suggest that dyspnea does have separate affective and sensory dimensions and that both dimensions should be measured.

Controlled studies related to the treatment of dyspnea are only beginning to be undertaken; therefore, findings are preliminary and scattered. The following studies relate examples of therapies that have been successful in decreasing dyspnea in small samples of COPD patients.

Strijbos and colleagues randomized 30 COPD subjects to a pulmonary rehabilitation program and 15 subjects to a control group that received no intervention.[149] The rehabilitation program consisted of relaxing exercises, breathing retraining, and exercise reconditioning twice a week for 2 hours for 12 weeks. During cycle ergometry and the 6-minute walk, the rehabilitation group significantly increased their exercise tolerance and significantly decreased their dyspnea, as rated on a Borg scale. The control group had no significant changes in any measured parameters. In this study the total rehabilitation program was tested; therefore, there is no way to evaluate its various components.

In contrast to the study of total body exercise, as reviewed earlier, other studies have evaluated the effect of an inspiratory muscle training program on the level of dyspnea. Harver and associates used a randomized, placebo-controlled design to study the effect of a targeted 8-week inspiratory muscle training program on 10 subjects with COPD.[161] The experimental group trained at six levels of inspiratory resistance while the controls trained at a constant small level of resistance. The experimental group showed significant improvement in all categories of the Transition Dyspnea Index (TDI), including function, task, and effort. The control group had minimal changes in dyspnea measured by the TDI after 2 months.

Oxygen therapy and opiates have been tested for their effect on dyspnea during exercise. In two reports the same authors studied the effect of oxygen and opiates on walking distance and dyspnea.[169, 173] Although other investigators have subsequently tested these modalities,[170, 171, 175] these early studies are exemplary of classic work in this area. Woodcock and colleagues compared the effects of air and oxygen in 10 patients with emphysema.[169] The use of supplemental oxygen increased walking distance and decreased dyspnea. These same authors demonstrated that a single dose of dihydrocodeine (1 mg/kg) after 45 minutes significantly decreased dyspnea and increased walking distance in 12 patients with COPD.[173]

ILLUSTRATIVE CASE STUDIES

The following descriptions of dyspnea are given by patients in four categories of pulmonary disease.

PULMONARY VASCULAR DISEASE

Nancy, a 26-year-old patient with severe pulmonary hypertension, described her dyspnea in this way: "I can't get enough oxygen. I feel dizzy, hot, and weak with discomfort in my chest. I feel heaviness in my chest. Coughing, walking, carrying things, bending over, talking, eating, and bathing all make my breathing worse. I try to suppress coughing because it just takes my breath away, but then I end up holding my breath and it's worse. Laughing, crying, and getting angry also make me short of breath. I can't do anything."

This patient believed that others could detect her shortness of breath easily because she looked blue, her neck muscles bulged, her chest moved noticeably, she sat very straight, and she often coughed when extremely breathless. Nancy's pronounced hyperventilation on exercise was quite typical of pulmonary hypertension. Her ratio of oxygen consumption to minute ventilation ($\dot{V}O_2/\dot{V}E$) was 1.22 compared with about 4.8 for healthy individuals. Pulmonary physiological dead space was greatly increased because of large numbers of ventilated alveoli that received little perfusion from her grossly hypertensive pulmonary circulation. The severity of this young woman's pulmonary hypertension was evident in measurements of pulmonary pressures: 60/32 mm Hg, with a mean pressure of 47 mm Hg in the pulmonary artery. A possible mechanism for dyspnea in this situation is the abnormally increased neural impulses from J receptors in the congested alveolar-capillary walls.

The overwhelming intensity of her dyspnea placed serious constraints on her daily functioning, but she had an extensive personal support system, as evidenced by close relationships with family and friends. She relied heavily on these people for both physical assistance and emotional support. When acutely short of breath, she found sips of water, oxygen therapy, sitting up straight, and slow, deep breathing to be useful strategies. Like many others with pulmonary hypertension, this young woman was not taught breathing or coping strategies by health professionals, nor was she referred to classes to learn more about breathing problems. Everything she knew was self-taught or learned from her sister, a registered nurse. This patient underwent cardiopulmonary transplantation for severe irreversible pulmonary hypertension. She died 2 weeks after her surgery.

EMPHYSEMA

George, who is 58 years old and has emphysema, lives on disability payments he has received for the past 17 years, when his illness caused him to retire from his job as an office manager. Notably, he has a 43 pack-year history of smoking. George is breathless dressing himself and relies on his wife for transportation, dressing, and any social activity. This severely ill man described his dyspnea episodes as "gasping for breath," "not getting enough air," and "all closed up." His shortness of breath, which is almost continuous, is aggravated by smoke and fumes, any physical exertion, such as walking from the bed to the bathroom in the morning, excessive humidity, or emotional arousal, such as anger and frustration. His FEV_1 is 1 L, with an FEV_1/FVC ratio of 46 per cent. His grade of breathlessness on the American Thoracic Society scale is 5, and he rates his usual daily dyspnea at 60 on a 100-mm visual analogue scale.

He describes behaviors that others see as leading to increased shortness of breath as changes in position, straining of neck muscles, especially on the left side, and sitting up straight or standing. If he is walking, he stops and doesn't move. George relies primarily on medications to decrease his symptoms. He has also learned pursed lips breathing and relaxation techniques to use when he is walking or during attacks of panic. A massage by his wife to any part of his body relieves the tension and helps him to relax and breathe easier. He has been taught in the past by a nurse in the hospital to wear loose clothes and conserve energy. When his regular medicine doesn't work, he describes trips to the hospital for a stay of 4 to 7 days, where he gets "more intensive treatment," like intravenous medications and a ventilator.

George's social space is confined to his home; in fact, he has no friends in particular. Although he "still feels as good about himself as ever," he doesn't believe that he contributes much to the world and this bothers him. He has given up most of his hobbies, like golf and trips, and has trouble finding alternative activities. He prefers not to talk about his shortness of breath because, as he emphasized, "I don't like to burden others, I feel it brings down other people's spirits, and I don't like to burden others, I feel it brings down other people's spirits, and I don't want sympathy or pity." George has begun to monitor his shortness of breath with a visual analogue scale during rest and activity and feels he has "greater control" of the symptom and, therefore, can tolerate the symptom more.

RESTRICTIVE DISEASE

Paul, 28 years old, was initially told that he had pneumonia, but after a year, a "specialist" confirmed the diagnosis of sarcoidosis. He is separated, lives alone, and continues to work as a record salesman. His dyspnea occurs "anytime, anywhere," and although he sometimes can disregard it, "it's always there." This young man describes his dyspnea as a "funny feeling, like you're going to pass out but know you're not. It's like putting salt on a sore—you know it's going to burn a little, pain down both sides of my back. I can feel fluid moving in my lungs, my heart beats fast, and I feel hot." Although physical exertion almost always brings on his shortness of breath, strong emotions, saunas, lying down, playing with his nephew, or energy required when he's concentrating may all increase his breathing difficulty. Sitting up straight, being quiet, or taking his prescribed diazepam (Valium) are strategies he uses to diminish the "overexcited feeling" he gets when he is short of breath. Others might notice his increasing shortness of breath because he is sweating and "I breathe after every 10 words compared to every 30 words for other people." Paul believes that his shortness of breath has "changed my life completely" and that he just has to deal with it; "it's a trip to change my life style and know I'll be under a doctor's care for the rest of my life."

Typical of his disease pattern, remissions have allowed Paul to maintain a job, perform activities of daily living, and take trips by car or plane that do not require walking too far. His pulmonary function parameters are typical of restrictive disease with all lung volumes decreased, with a 60 per cent of predicted vital capacity and 70 per cent predicted total lung capacity. Flow rates are normal. Paul has little or no social support. More than decreased energy from his dyspnea, his feelings about the symptom have limited communication and friendship with others. He describes it like this: "I'm jealous of other people: they can breathe, I can't. My friends have told me I've changed; they can't help me, so why talk about it. I wouldn't depend on anyone else for anything, it's just a crutch." Typically, this restrictive patient has never been taught strategies to help him cope with persistent shortness of breath. Although he receives daily steroid treatment, he believes that "nothing can make it better, I just have to live with it."

ASTHMA

Shortness of breath of long duration with periodic increases in intensity is evident in adult asthmatics with severe disease diagnosed in early childhood. Bill is 49 years old and has had asthma for 48 years. When he was a young child, his mother was advised by physicians not to allow him to play at all, since they believed that activity would make his asthma worse. As an adult attending school classes, he found that school pressures and commitments made his breathing worse. He described his dyspnea in association with wheezing as "tightness around my chest and shoulders, with a painful feeling in my chest." He stated that when an attack is developing, his breathing feels like great work and his chest is as "tight as a fiddlestring." As the attack progressed, he would have a severe headache and quickly become very tired.

This patient can identify precisely the stages of progression of his attacks. Stage 1 begins with tightness in the chest, followed by mild wheezing without shortness of breath. As stage 2 develops, he finds it harder to exhale and the tightening begins in his shoulders, chest, and back. Shortness of breath is noticeable now. If the attack progresses to stage 3, he finds that he can barely move air at all, his chest aches, and he feels as if he will pass out.

During acute episodes, his FEV_1 has been

as low as 0.8 L, with marked improvement after inhalation of albuterol. With many years of experience with dyspnea, Bill had developed a series of strategies to use at each stage of the attack. First, he tries to ward off attacks by avoiding allergens and staying in bed if he gets a cold. During stage 1 of an asthma attack, he uses guided relaxation exercises and diversional activities, like reading or watching television. If the attack progresses to stage 2, he assumes a leaning-forward position on the edge of a chair, with shoulders hunched, bracing himself with his arms on the seat of the chair. He uses extra medications at this point in amounts exceeding the usual daily dosage, such as extra theophylline and several extra puffs from his nebulizer. If the attack progresses to stage 3 and his breathing gets worse, he goes to the hospital emergency department immediately. More recently, Bill was provided with a peak flow meter and was taught to use it to monitor his response to inhaled bronchodilators during acute episodes. He has begun to keep daily records of peak flow measurements and is now able to detect impending asthmatic attacks earlier. Newer therapeutic approaches including inhaled corticosteroids to reduce airway inflammation decreased Bill's frequent exacerbations of asthma.

IMPLICATIONS FOR RESEARCH

Future research related to the sensation of dyspnea should include continued investigation of the precise physiological and psychological mechanisms, in-depth study of alternative methods for measuring both the sensory and affective components of this sensation, development and testing of therapies that modulate the symptom, and further exploration of the process of coping with this distressing symptom. Dyspnea or breathlessness is probably only one of several respiratory sensations with multifactorial causes that are just beginning to be identified. Receptors and neural pathways that are responsible for the transmission of relevant information need to be identified. Little is known about why the level of dyspnea varies among people with the same pathological changes in pulmonary function. The symptom of dyspnea needs to be studied in different populations,

such as in cardiac or neurological patients. Treatments have been tested primarily in pulmonary patients with chronic dyspnea, with little focus on acute dyspnea in other populations. Although many techniques have been used by the patient and the nurse to decrease dyspnea clinically, few have been systematically tested in controlled experiments; therefore, the efficacy of the techniques is unknown across populations. Health professionals have much to learn from "expert" patients who have lived with this distressing symptom on a daily basis. The knowledge about dyspnea is minimal. This is what is so unique about this symptom. Future research studies could target any aspect of dyspnea—whether that be the identification of the mechanisms at the basic science level, methods for measurement in a variety of settings, correlates that change the level of the symptom, or therapies to decrease the symptom in the acute or chronic phase.

REFERENCES

1. Comroe, J. H. (1965). Some theories of the mechanisms of dyspnea. In J. B. Howell & E. J. M. Campbell (eds.), *Breathlessness* (pp. 1–7). Boston: Blackwell Scientific.
2. Killian, K. J. (1988). Assessment of dyspnoea. Eur Respir J *1*:195–197.
3. Gold, W. M. (1983). Dyspnea. In R. S. Blacklow (ed.), *MacBryde's Signs and Symptoms* (6th ed. pp. 335–348). Philadelphia: J. B. Lippincott.
4. Killian, K. J., Gandevia, S. C., Summers, E., & Campbell, E. J. M. (1984). Effect of increased lung volume on perception of breathlessness, effort and tension. J Appl Physiol *57*:686–691.
5. Burki, N. K. (1980). Dyspnea. Clin Chest Med *1*:47–55.
6. Harver, A., & Mahler, D. A. (1990). The symptom of dyspnea. In D. A. Mahler (ed.), *Dyspnea* (pp. 1–53). Mt. Kisco, N. Y.: Futura Publishing.
7. Guz, A. (1977). Respiratory sensations in man. Br Med Bull *33*:175–177.
8. Simon, P. M., Schwartzstein, R. M., Weiss, J. W., Lahive, K., Fencl, V., & Teghtsoonian, J. M. (1989). Distinguishable sensations of breathlessness induced in normal volunteers. Am Rev Respir Dis *140*:1021–1027.
9. Simon, P. M., Schwartzstein, R. M., Weiss, J. W., Fencl, V. Teghtsoonian, M. & Weinberger, S. E. (1990). Distinguishable types of dyspnea in patients with shortness of breath. Am Rev Respir Dis *142*:1009–1014.
10. Elliott, M. W., Adams, L., Cockcroft, A., Macrae, K. D., Murphy, K., & Guz, A. (1991). The language of breathlessness: Use of verbal descriptors by patients with cardiopulmonary disease. Am Rev Respir Dis *144*:826–832.
11. Killian, K. J., Gandevia, S. C., Summers, E., & Campbell, E. J. M. (1984). Effect of increased lung volume on perception of dyspnea, effort and tension. J Appl Physiol *57*:686–691.

12. Janson-Bjerklie, S., Carrieri, V. K., & Hudes, M. (1986). The sensation of pulmonary dyspnea. Nurs Res *35*:154–159.
13. Carrieri, V. K., Kieckhefer, G., Janson-Bjerklie, S., & Sousa, J. (1991). The sensation of pulmonary dyspnea in school age children. Nurs Res *40*:81–85.
14. Adams, L., & Guz, A. (1991). Dyspnea on exertion. In C. Lenfant (ed.) *Pulmonary Physiology and Pathophysiology of Exercise* (pp. 449–494). New York: Marcel Dekker.
15. Altose, M. D. (1985). Assessment and management of breathlessness. Chest *88*:73S–77S.
16. Carrieri, V. K., Janson-Bjerklie, S., & Jacobs, S. (1984). The sensation of dyspnea: A review. Heart Lung *13*:436–447.
17. Wilson, R. C., & Jones, P. W. (1991). Differentiation between the intensity of breathlessness and the distress it evokes in normal subjects during exercise. Clin Sci *80*:65–70.
18. Woolcock, A. J. (1989). Epidemiology of chronic airway disease. Chest *96*(Suppl.):302S–306S.
19. Higgins, M. (1986). Epidemiology of COPD: State of the art. Chest *85*(Suppl.):3S–8S.
20. Higgins, I. T. T. (1988). Epidemiology of bronchitis and emphysema. In A. P. Fishman (ed.), *Pulmonary Diseases and Disorders* (2nd ed. pp. 1237–1246). New York: McGraw Hill.
21. National Health Survey, National Center for Health Statistics, December 1989.
22. Bruera, E., MacMillan, R., Pither, J., & MacDonald, R. N. (1990). Effects of morphine on the dyspnea of terminal cancer patients. J Pain Symptom Manage *5*:341–344.
23. Reuben, D. B., & Mor, V. (1986). Dyspnea in terminally ill cancer patients. Chest *89*:234–236.
24. Brown, M., Carrieri, V., Janson-Bjerklie, S., & Dodd, M. (1986). Lung cancer and dyspnea: The patient's perception. Oncol Nurs Forum *13*:19–24.
25. Interstitial Lung disease. In T. L. Petty & R. M. Cherniack, (series ed.) and M. Turner-Warwick (vol. ed.). *Seminars in Respiratory Medicine*. New York: Thieme-Stratton, 6:1984.
26. Hopewell, P. (1990). Pneumocystis carinii pneumonia. In M. A. Sande & P. A. Volberding (eds.) *The Medical Management of AIDS*. Philadelphia: W. B. Saunders.
27. Turino, G. M. (1988). The lungs and heart disease. In J. F. Murray & J. A. Nadel (eds.), *Textbook of Respiratory Medicine* (pp. 1883–1893). Philadelphia: W. B. Saunders.
28. Cabanes, L. R., Weber, S. N., Matran R., et al. (1989). Bronchial hyperresponsiveness to methacholine in patients with impaired left ventricular function. N Engl J Med *320*:1317–1322.
29. The Health Consequences of Smoking: Chronic Obstructive Lung Disease: A Report of the Surgeon General. (1984). Rockville, MD: Department of Health and Human Services, PHS Office on Smoking and Health.
30. Dudley, D. L., Glaser, E. M., Jorgenson, B. N., & Logan, D. L. (1980). Psychosocial concomitants to rehabilitation in chronic obstructive pulmonary disease. I. Psychosocial and psychological considerations. Chest *77*:413–420.
31. Janson-Bjerklie, S., Ruma, S. S., Stulbarg, M. S., & Carrieri, V. K. (1987). Predictors of dyspnea intensity in asthma. Nurs Res *36*:179–183.
32. LeBlanc, P., Bowie, D. M., Summer, E., Jones, N., & Killian, K. (1986). Breathlessness and exercise in patients with cardiorespiratory disease. Am Rev Respir Dis *133*:21–25.
33. Mahler, D. A., Faryniarz, K., Lentine, T., Ward, J., Olmstead, E. M., & O'Connor, G. T. (1991). Measurement of breathlessness during exercise in asthmatics. Am Rev Respir Dis *144*:39–44.
34. Bethel, R. A., Epstein, J., Sheppard, D., Nadel, J. A., & Boushey, H. A. (1983). Sulfur dioxide-induced, bronchoconstriction in freely breathing, exercising, asthmatic subjects. Am Rev Respir Dis *128*:987–990.
35. Davidson, D. M. (1991). *Preventive Cardiology*. Baltimore: Williams and Wilkins.
36. Gift, A. (1991). Psychologic and physiologic aspects of acute dyspnea in asthmatics. Nurs Res *40*:196–199.
37. De Paso, W. J., Winterbauer, R. H., Lusk, J. A., Dreis, D. F., & Springmeyer, S. C. (1991). Chronic dyspnea unexplained by history, physical examination, chest roentgenogram and spirometry: Analysis of a seven-year experience. Chest *100*:1293–1299.
38. Mahler, D. A. (1990). Acute dyspnea. In D. A. Mahler (ed.), *Dyspnea* (pp. 127–144). Mt. Kisco, NY: Futura Publishing.
39. Fishbein, D., Kearon, C., & Killian, K. J. (1989). An approach to dyspnea in cancer patients. J Pain Symptom Manage *4*:76–81.
40. Wasserman, K., & Cassaburi, R. (1988). Dyspnea: Physiological and pathophysiological mechanisms. Annu Rev Med *39*:503–515.
41. Milne, J. A., Howie, A. D., & Pack, A. I. (1978). Dyspnea during normal pregnancy. Br J Obstet Gynaecol *85*:260–263.
42. Cugell, D. W., Frank, N. R., Gaensler, E. A., & Badger, T. L. (1953). Pulmonary function in pregnancy. I. Serial observations in normal women. Am Rev Tuberculosis *67*:568–597.
43. Vicken, W., Elleker, M. G., & Cosio, M. G. (1987). Determinants of respiratory muscle weakness in stable chronic neuromuscular disorders. Am J Med *82*:53–58.
44. Dudley, D. L., Martin, C. J., & Holmes, T. H. (1968). Dyspnea: Psychologic and physiologic observations. J Psychosom Res *11*:325–339.
45. Burns, B. H., & Howell, J. B. L. (1969). Disproportionately severe breathlessness in chronic bronchitis. Q J Med *38*:277–294.
46. Gift, A. G., Plaut, M., & Jacox, A. (1986). Psychologic and physiologic factors related to dyspnea in subjects with chronic obstructive pulmonary disease. Heart Lung *15*:595–601.
47. Gift, A. G., & Cahil, C. A. (1990). Psychophysiologic aspects of dyspnea in chronic obstructive pulmonary disease: A pilot study. Heart Lung *19*:252–257.
48. Brashear, R. E. (1983). Hyperventilation syndrome. Lung *161*:257–273.
49. Bess, C., & Gardner, W. (1985). Emotional influences on breathing and breathlessness. J Psychosom Res *29*:599–609.
50. Sandhu, H. S. (1986). Psychosocial issues in chronic obstructive pulmonary disease. Clin Chest Med *7*:629–642.
51. Schwartzstein, R. M., Manning, H. L., Weiss, W. L., & Weinberger, S. E. (1990). Dyspnea: A sensory experience. Lung *168*:185–199.
52. Tobin, M. J. (1990). Dyspnea: Pathophysiologic

basis, clinical presentation, and management. Arch Intern Med *150*:1604–1613.

53. Sweer, L., & Zwillich, C. W. (1990). Dyspnea in the patient with chronic obstructive pulmonary disease. Clin Chest Med *11*:417–445.

54. Cherniack, N. S. (1988). Dyspnea. In J. F. Murray & J. A. Nadel (eds.), *Textbook of Respiratory Medicine* (pp. 389–396). Philadelphia: W. B. Saunders.

55. Altose, M. D., Cherniack, N. S., & Fishman, A. P. (1985). Respiratory sensations and dyspnea. J Appl Physiol *58*:1051–1054.

56. Campbell, E. J. M., & Howell, J. B. L. (1963). The sensation of breathlessness. Br Med Bull *19*:36–40.

57. Campbell, E. J. M. (1966). The relationship of the sensation of breathlessness to the act of breathing. In J. B. L. Howell & E. J. M. Campbell (eds.), *Breathlessness*. Oxford: Blackwell Scientific.

58. Stulbarg, M. S. (1986). The treatment of dyspnea: A physiologic approach. Clin Challenge Cardiopulmonary Med *7*:1–6.

59. Killian, K. J., & Campbell, E. J. M. (1990). Mechanisms of Dyspnea. In D. A. Mahler (ed.), *Dyspnea* (pp. 55–73). Mt. Kisco, NY: Futura Publishing.

60. Marsden, C. D., Merton, P. A., & Morton, H. B. (1976). Stretch reflex and servo action in a variety of human muscles. J Physiol *259*:531–560.

61. Wise, S. P., & Tanji, J. (1981). Neuronal responses in sensorimotor cortex to ramp displacements and maintained positions imposed on hindlimb of the unanesthetized monkey. Neurophysiol *45*:482–500.

62. Altose, M. D., & Cherniack, N. S. (1980). Respiratory sensation and respiratory muscle activity. Adv Physiol Sci *10*:111–120.

63. Killian, K. J., Mahutte, C. K., & Campbell, E. J. M. (1981). Magnitude scaling of externally added loads to breathing. Am Rev Resp Dis *123*:12–15.

64. Killian, K. J., Bucens, D. D., & Campbell, E. J. M. (1982). Effects of breathing patterns on the perceived magnitude of added loads to breathing. J Appl Physiol *52*:578–584.

65. Stevens, J. C., & Stevens, S. S. (1963). Brightness function: Effects of adaptation. J Opt Soc Am *53*:375–385.

66. Burdon, J. G. W., Killian, K. J., & Stubbing, D. G., et al. (1983). Effect of background loads on the perception of added loads to breathing. J Appl Physiol *54*:1222–1228.

67. Gottfried, S. B., Redline, S., & Altose, M. D. (1985). Respiratory sensation in chronic obstructive pulmonary disease. Am Rev Respir Dis *132*:954–959.

68. Sharp, J. T. (1985). The chest wall and respiratory muscles in obesity, pregnancy, and ascites. In C. Roussos & P. T. Macklem (eds.), *The Thorax* (part B, pp. 999–1021). New York: Marcel Dekker.

69. Chonan, T., Mulholland, M. B., Cherniak, N. S., & Altose, M. D. (1987). Effect of voluntary constraining of thoracic displacement during hypercapnia. J Appl Physiol *63*:1822–1828.

70. Breslin, E. H., Garoutte, B. C., Carrieri, V. K., & Celli, B. R. (1990). Correlations between dyspnea, diaphragm, and sternomastoid recruitment during respiratory resistive breathing in normal subjects. Chest *98*:298–302.

71. Killian, K. J., & Jones, N. L. (1988). Respiratory muscles and dyspnea. Clin Chest Med *9*:237–248.

72. Lane, R., Cockcroft, A., & Guz, A. (1987). Voluntary isocapnic hyperventilation and breathlessness during exercise in normal subjects. Clin Sci *73*:519–523.

73. Adams, L., Lane, R., Shea, S. A., Cockcroft, A., & Guz, A. (1985). Breathlessness during different forms of ventilatory stimulation: A study of mechanisms in normal subjects and respiratory patients. Clin Sci *69*:663–672.

74. Cherniack, N. S., & Altose, M. D. (1987). Mechanisms of dyspnea. Clin Chest Med *9*:237–248.

75. Chronos, N., Adams, L., & Guz, A. (1988). Effect of hyperoxia and hypoxia on exercise-induced breathlessness in normal subjects. Clin Sci *74*:531–537.

76. Banzett, R. B., Lansing, R., Reid, M. B., Adams, L., & Brown, R. (1989). Air hunger arising from increased PCO_2 in mechanically ventilated Cl-2 quadriplegics. Respir Physiol *76*:53–67.

77. Patterson, J. L., Mullinax, P. F., Bain, T., Kreuger, J. J., & Richardson, D. W. (1962). Carbon dioxide induced dyspnea in a patient with respiratory muscle paralysis. Am J Med *32*:811–816.

78. Campbell, E. J. M., Godfrey, S., Clark, T. J. H., Freedman, S., & Norman, J. (1969). The effect of muscular paralysis induced by tubocurarine on the duration and sensation of breath holding during hypercapnia. Clin Sci *36*:323–328.

79. Widdicombe, J. G. (1986). Reflexes from the upper respiratory tract. In A. P. Fishman, N. S. Cherniack & J. G. Widdicombe (eds.), *Handbook of Physiology* (pp. 363–394). Bethesda, MD: American Physiological Society.

80. Zechman, F. W., & Wiley, R. L. (1986). Afferent inputs to breathing: Respiratory sensation. In A. P. Fishman, N. S. Cherniack, J. G. Widdicomb, & S. R. Geiger (eds.), *Handbook of Physiology* (pp. 449–474), Bethesda, MD: American Physiological Society.

81. Hamilton, R. D., Winning, A. F., Perry, A., & Guz, A. (1987). Aerosol anesthesia increases hypercapnia ventilation and breathlessness in laryngectomized humans. J Appl Physiol *63*:2286–2292.

82. Winning, A. J., Hamilton, R. D., Shea, S. A., Knott, C., & Guz, A. (1985). The effects of airway anesthesia on the control of breathing and the sensation of breathlessness in man. Clin Sci *68*:215–225.

83. McBride, B., & Whitclaw, W. A. (1981). A physiologic stimulus to upper airway receptors in humans. J Appl Physiol *51*:1189–1197.

84. Liss, H. P., & Grant, J. B. (1988). The effect of nasal flow on breathlessness in patients with chronic obstructive pulmonary disease. Am Rev Respir Dis *137*:1285–1288.

85. Wesmiller, S. W., Hoffman, L. A., Sciurba, F. C., Ferson, P. F., Johnson, J. T., & Dauber, J. H. (1990). Exercise tolerance during nasal cannula and transtracheal oxygen delivery. Am Rev Respir Dis *141*:789–791.

86. Schwartzstein, R. M., Lahive, K., Pope, A., Weinberger, S. E., & Weiss, J. W. (1987). Cold facial stimulation reduces breathlessness induced in normal subjects. Am Rev Respir Dis *136*:58–61.

87. O'Donnell, D. E., Sanii, R., Giesbrecht, G., & Younes, M. (1988). Effect of continuous positive airway pressure on respiratory sensation in patients with chronic obstructive pulmonary disease during submaximal exercise. Am Rev Respir Dis *138*:1185–1191.

88. O'Donnell, D. E., Sanii, R., Anthonisen, N. R., & Younes, M. (1987). Effect of dynamic airway com-

pression on breathing pattern and respiratory sensation in severe chronic obstructive lung disease. Am Rev Respir Dis *135*:912–918.

89. Simon, P., Basner, R., Schwartzstein, R. M., Weinberger, S. E., Fencl, V., & Weiss, J. W. (1988). Oral mucosal stimulation modulates intensity of breathlessness induced in normal subjects. Am Rev Respir Dis *137*:A387.

90. Campbell, E. J. M., & Guz, A. (1981). Breathlessness. In T. F. Hornbein (ed.), *Regulation of Breathing* (pp. 1181–1195). New York: Marcel Dekker.

91. Taguchi, O., Kikuchi, Y., Hida, W., Iwase, N., Okabe, S., Satoh, M., Chonan, T., Inone, H., & Takashima, T. (1989). Effects of airway anesthesia on dyspnea during bronchoconstriction and loaded breathing in normal subjects. Am Rev Respir Dis *139*:A322.

92. Coleridge, H. M., & Coleridge, J. C. G. (1986). Reflexes evoked from tracheobronchial tree and lungs. In A. P. Fishman, N. S. Cherniack, & J. G. Widdicombe (eds.), *The Handbook of Physiology,* Section 3. Bethesda, MD: American Physiological Society.

93. Manning, H., Schwartzstein, R., Rand, C., Basner, R., Ringler, J., Fencl, V., Weinberger, S. E., & Weiss, J. W. (1989). Chest wall vibration reduces breathlessness in normals. Am Rev Respir Dis *139*:A320.

94. Rubinfeld, A. R., & Pain, M. (1976). Perception of asthma. Lancet *1*:882–884.

95. Rubinfeld, A. R., & Pain, M. (1977). Conscious perception of bronchospasm as a protective phenomenon in asthma. Chest *72*:154–258.

96. Mahler, D. A., Weinberg, D. H., Wells, C. K., & Feinstein, A. R. (1984). The measurement of dyspnea: Contents, interobserver agreement, and physiologic correlates of two new clinical indexes. Chest *85*:751–758.

97. Adams, L., Chronos, N., Lane, R., & Guz, A. (1985). The measurement of breathlessness induced in normal subjects: Validity of two scaling techniques. Clin Sci *69*:7–16.

98. Ward, S. A., & Whipp, B. J. (1989). Effects of peripheral and central chemoreflex activation on the isopneic rating of breathing in exercise in humans. J Physiol *411*:27–43.

99. Lane, R., Adams, L., & Guz, A. (1990). The effects of hypoxia and hypercapnia on perceived breathlessness during exercise in humans. J Physiol *429*:579–593.

100. Mahler, D. A., & Wells, C. K. (1988). Evaluation of clinical methods for rating dyspnea. Chest *93*:580–586.

101. Mahler, D. A., Rosiello, R. A., Harver, A., Lentine, T., McGovern, J. F., & Daubenspeck, J. A. (1987). Comparison of clinical dyspnea ratings and psychophysical measurements of respiratory sensation in obstructive airway disease. Am Rev Respir Dis *135*:1229–1233.

102. Epler, G. R., Sabec, F. A., & Goensler, E. A. (1980). Determination of severe impairment (disability) in interstitial lung disease. Am Rev Respir Dis *121*:647–659.

103. Gift, A. G. (1989). Validation of a vertical visual analogue scale as a measure of clinical dyspnea. Rehabil Nurs *14*:323–325.

104. Mahler, D. A., Harver, A., & Rosiello, R. A. (1989). Measurement of respiratory sensation in interstitial lung disease: Evaluation of clinical dyspnea ratings and magnitude scaling. Chest *96*:767–771.

105. Killian, K., Summers, E., Basalygo, M., & Campbell, E. (1985). Effect on frequency of perceived magnitude of added resistive loads to breathing. J Appl Physiol *58*:1616–1621.

106. Celli, B., Criner, G., & Rassulo, J. (1988). Ventilatory muscle recruitment during unsupported arm exercise in normal subjects. J Appl Physiol *64*:1936–1941.

107. Gilston, A. (1976). Facial signs of respiratory distress after cardiac surgery. Anaesthesia *31*:385–397.

108. Delgado, H. R., Braun, S., Skatrud, J. B., Reddan, W. G., & Pegelow, D. F. (1982). Chest wall and abdominal motion during exercise in patients with chronic obstructive pulmonary disease. Am Rev Respir Dis *126*:200–205.

109. Marini, J. J., Roussos, C. S., Tobin, M. J., MacIntyre, N. R., Belman, M. J., & Moxham, J. (1988). Weaning from mechanical ventilation. Am Rev Respir Dis *138*:1043–1046.

110. Knebel, A. R. (1990). Dyspnea intensity, psychological distress, anxiety, inspiratory effort: Effects on ventilator weaning. Ph.D. dissertation. San Francisco: University of California.

111. Moody, L., McCormick, K., & Williams, A. (1990). Disease and symptom severity, functional status, and quality of life in chronic bronchitis and emphysema (CBE). J Behav Med *13*:297–306.

112. Knebel, A. R. (1991). Dyspnea anxiety and inspiratory effort during weaning with intermittent mandatory ventilation (IMV) and pressure support ventilation (PSV) (abstract). Am Rev Respir Dis *143*(suppl.):A603.

113. Moody, L., McCormick, K., & Williams, A. R. (1991). Psychophysiologic correlates of quality of life in chronic bronchitis and emphysema. West J Nurs Res *13*:336–352.

114. Fletcher, C. M. (1952). Clinical diagnosis of pulmonary emphysema: An experimental study. Proc Royal Soc Med *45*:577–584.

115. Brooks, S. M. (1982). Task group on surveillance for respiratory setting. Surveillance for respiratory hazards. ATS News *8*:12–16.

116. McGavin, C. R., Artvinli, M., Naoe, H., & McHardy, G. J. R. (1978). Dyspnea, disability, and distance walked: Comparison of estimates of exercise performance in respiratory disease. Br Med J *2*:241–243.

117. Mahler, D. A., & Harver, A. (1990). Clinical measurement of dyspnea. In D. A. Mahler (ed.), *Dyspnea* (pp. 75–126). Mt. Kisco, NY: Futura Publishing.

118. Stoller, J., Ferranti, R., & Feinstein, A. (1986). Further specification and evaluation of a new clinical index for dyspnea. Am Rev Respir Dis *134*:1129–1134.

119. Mahler, D. A., & Harver, A. (1988). Prediction of peak oxygen consumption in obstructive airway disease. Med Sci Sports Exerc *20*:574–578.

120. Mahler, D. A., Matthay, R. A., Snyder, P. E., Wells, C. K., & Loke, J. (1985). Sustained-release theophylline reduces dyspnea in non-reversible obstructive airway disease. Am Rev Respir Dis *131*:22–25.

121. Harver, A., Mahler, D. A., & Daubenspeck, J. A. (1989). Targeted inspiratory muscle training improves respiratory muscle function and reduces dyspnea in patients with chronic obstructive pulmonary disease. Ann Intern Med *111*:117–124.

122. Borg, G. (1982). Psychophysical bases of perceived exertion. Med Sci Sports Exerc *14*:377–381.

123. Burdon, J., Juniper, E., Killian, K., Hargreave, F., & Campbell, E. (1982). The perception of breathlessness in asthma. Am Rev Respir Dis *126*:825–828.

124. Cockcroft, A., Adams, L., & Guz, A. (1989). Assessment of breathlessness. Q J Med *72*:669–676.

125. Stark, D. (1988). Dyspnea: Assessment and pharmacological manipulation. Eur Respir J *1*:280–287.

126. Wewers, M. E., & Lowe, N. K. (1990). A critical review of visual analogue scales in the measurement of clinical phenomena. Res Nurs Health *13*:227–236.

127. Gift, A. (1989). Visual analogue scales: Measurement of subjective phenomena. Nurs Res *38*:286–288.

128. Lane, R., Cockcroft, A., Adams, L., & Guz, A. (1987). Arterial oxygen saturation and breathlessness in patients with chronic obstructive airways disease. Clin Sci *72*:693–698.

129. Ruma, S. (1986). Dyspnea in the mechanically ventilated patient. M.S. thesis. San Francisco: University of California.

130. Woodcock, A. A., Gross, E. R., & Geddes, D. M. (1981). Oxygen relieves breathlessness in "pink puffers." Lancet *1*:907–909.

131. Wilson, R. C., & Jones, P. W. (1989). A comparison of the visual analogue scale and modified Borg scale for the measurement of dyspnoea during exercise. Clin Sci *76*:277–282.

132. Lush, M., Janson-Bjerklie, S., Carrieri, V., & Lovejoy, N. (1988). Dyspnea in the ventilator-assisted patient. Heart Lung *17*:528–535.

133. Nield, M., Kim, M. J., & Patel, M. (1989). Use of magnitude estimation for estimating the parameters of dyspnea. Nurs Res *38*:77–80.

134. Carrieri-Kohlman, V. (1991). Dyspnea in the weaning patient: Assessment and intervention. AACN Clin Issues Crit Care Nurs *2*:462–473.

135. Janson-Bjerklie, S., & Schnell, S. (1988). Effect of peak flow information on patterns of self-care in adult asthma. Heart Lung *17*:543–549.

136. Worth, R., Hoome, P. D., & Johnston, D. G. (1982). Intensive attention improves glycemic control in insulin-dependent diabetes without further advantage from home blood glucose monitoring: Results of a controlled trial. Br Med J *285*:1233–1240.

137. Guyatt, G. H., Berman, L. B., Townhead, M., Pugsley, S. O., & Chambers, L. W. (1987). A measure of quality of life for clinical trials in chronic lung disease. Thorax *42*:773–778.

138. Ries, A. L. (1990). Scientific basis of pulmonary rehabilitation: Position paper of the American Association of Cardiovascular and Pulmonary Rehabilitation. J Cardiopulmonary Rehabil *10*:418–441.

139. Kohlman-Carrieri, V., & Janson-Bjerklie, S. (1990). Coping and self-care strategies. In D. A. Mahler (ed.), *Dyspnea* (pp. 201–230). Mt. Kisco, NY: Futura Publishing.

140. Mueller, R. E., Petty, T. L., & Filley, G. F. (1970). Ventilation and arterial blood gas changes induced by pursed lips breathing. J Appl Physiol *28*:784–789.

141. Thoman, R. L., Stoker, G. L., & Ross, J. C. (1966). The efficacy of pursed-lips breathing in patients with chronic obstructive pulmonary disease. Am Rev Respir Dis *93*:100–106.

142. Tiep, B. L., Burns, M., Kao, D., Madison, R., & Herrera, J. (1986). Pursed lips breathing training using ear oximetry. Chest *90*:218–221.

143. Miller, W. F. (1954). A physiologic evaluation of the effects of diaphragmatic breathing training in patients with chronic pulmonary emphysema. Am J Med *17*:471–477.

144. Sinclair, J. (1955). The effect of breathing exercises in pulmonary emphysema. Thorax *10*:246–249.

145. Sharp, J. T., Drutz, W. S., Moisan, T., Foster, J., & Machnach, W. (1980). Postural relief of dyspnea in severe chronic obstructive pulmonary disease. Am Rev Respir Dis *122*:201–213.

146. Lareau, S., & Larson, J. L. (1987). Ineffective breathing pattern related to airflow limitation. Nurs Clin North Am *22*:179–191.

147. Cockcroft, A. E., Saunders, M. J., & Berry, G. (1981). Randomized controlled trial of rehabilitation in chronic respiratory disability. Thorax *36*:200–203.

148. Sinclair, D. J. M., & Ingram, C. G. (1980). Controlled trial of supervised exercise training in chronic bronchitis. Br Med J *280*:519–521.

149. Strijbos, J. H., Sluiter, H. J., Postma, D. S., Gimeno, F., & Koeter, G. H. (1989). Objective and subjective performance indicators in COPD. Eur Resp J *2*:666–669.

150. McGavin, C. R., Gupta, S. P., Lloyd, E. L., & McHardy, J. R. (1977). Physical rehabilitation of chronic bronchitis: Results of a controlled trial of exercises in the home. Thorax *32*:307–311.

151. Belman, M. J. (1986). Exercise in chronic obstructive pulmonary disease. Clin Chest Med *7*:585–597.

152. Belman, M. J., Brooks, L. R., Ross, D. J., & Mohsenifar, Z. (1991). Variability of breathlessness measurement in patients with chronic obstructive pulmonary disease. Chest *99*:566–571.

153. Ries, A. L., Ellis, B., & Hawkins, R. W. (1988). Upper extremity exercise training in chronic obstructive pulmonary disease. Chest *93*:688–692.

154. Petrof, B. J., Legare, M., Goldberg, P., Milic-Emili, J., & Gottfried, S. B. (1990). Continuous positive airway pressure reduces inspiratory work of breathing and dyspnea during weaning from mechanical ventilation in severe chronic obstructive pulmonary disease. Am Rev Respir Dis *141*:281–289.

155. Petrof, B. J., Calderini, E., & Gottfried, S. B. (1990). Effect of CPAP on respiratory effort and dyspnea during exercise in severe COPD. J Appl Physiol *69*:179–188.

156. Brown, N. M. T., & Marino, W. P. (1984). Effect of daily intermittent rest of respiratory muscles in patients with severe chronic airflow limitation (CAL). Chest *85*(suppl.):59S.

157. Martin, J. G. (1990). Clinical intervention in chronic respiratory failure. Chest *97*(suppl.):105S–109S.

158. Cropp, A., & Dimareo, A. F. (1987). Effects of intermittent negative pressure ventilation on respiratory muscle function in patients with severe chronic obstructive pulmonary disease. Am Rev Respir Dis *135*:1056–1061.

159. Celli, B., Lee, H., & Criner, G. (1989). Controlled trial of external negative pressure ventilation in patients with severe chronic airflow obstruction. Am Rev Respir Dis *140*:1251–1256.

160. Falk, P., Ericksen, A. M., Kolliker, K., & Andersen, J. B. (1985). Relieving dyspnea with an inexpensive

and simple method in patients with severe chronic airflow limitation. Eur J Respir Dis *66*:181–186.

161. Harver, A., Mahler, D. A., & Daubenspeck, J. A. (1989). Targeted inspiratory muscle training improves respiratory muscle function and reduces dyspnea in patients with chronic obstructive pulmonary disease. Ann Intern Med *111*:117–124.

162. MacIntyre, N. (1986). Respiratory function during pressure support ventilation. Chest *89*:677–683.

163. Dullinger, D., Kronenberg, R., & Niewoehner, D. E. (1986). Efficacy of inhaled metaproterenol and orally-administered theophylline in patients with chronic airflow obstruction. Chest *89*:171–173.

164. Guyatt, G. H., Townsend, M., Pugsley, S. O., Keller, J. L., Short, H. D., Taylor, D. W., & Newhouse, M. T. (1987). Bronchodilators in chronic air-flow limitation: Effects on airway function, exercise capacity, and quality of life. Am Rev Respir Dis *135*:1069–1074.

165. Stark, R. D., Gambles, S. A., & Chatterjee, S. S. (1982). An exercise test to assess clinical dyspnoea; estimation of reproducibility and sensitivity. Br J Dis Chest *76*:269–278.

166. Mahler, D. A. (1990). Therapeutic strategies. In D. A. Mahler (ed.), *Dyspnea* (pp. 231–263). Mt. Kisco, NY: Futura Publishing.

167. Chrystyn, H., Mulley, B. A., & Peake, M. D. (1988). Dose response relation to oral theophylline in severe chronic obstructive airways disease. Br Med J *297*:1506–1510.

168. Mahler, D. A., Matthay, R. A., Snyder, P. E., et al. (1985). Sustained-release theophylline reduces dyspnea in non-reversible obstructive airway disease. Am Rev Respir Dis *131*:22–25.

169. Woodcock, A. A., Gross, E. R., & Geddes, D. M. (1981). Oxygen relieves breathlessness in "pink puffers." Lancet *1*:907–909.

170. Davidson, A. C., Leach, R., George, R. J. D., & Geddes, D. M. (1988). Supplemental oxygen and oxygen ability in chronic obstructive airways disease. Thorax *43*:965–971.

171. Dean, N. C., Brown, J. K., Himelman, R. B., Doherty, J. J., Gold, W. M., & Stulbarg, M. S. (1992). Oxygen may improve dyspnea and endurance in patients with chronic obstructive pulmonary disease and only mild hypoxemia. Am Rev Respir Dis *146*:941–945.

172. Bellofiore, S., DiMaria, G. U., Privitera, S., Sapienza, S., Milic-Emili, J., & Mistretta, A. (1990). Endogenous opioids modulate the increase in ventilatory output and dyspnea during severe acute bronchoconstriction. Am Rev Respir Dis *142*:812–816.

173. Woodcock, A. A., Gross, E. R., Gellert, A., Shah, S., Johnson, M., & Geddes, D. M. (1981). Effects of dihydrocodeine, alcohol, and caffeine on breathlessness and exercise tolerance in patients with chronic obstructive lung disease and normal blood gases. N Engl J Med *305*:1611–1616.

174. Johnson, M. A., Woodcock, A. A., & Geddes, D. M. (1983). Dihydrocodeine for breathlessness in "pink puffers." Br Med J *286*:675–677.

175. Light, R. W., Muro, J. R., Sato, R. I., Stansbury, D. W., Fisher, C. E., & Brown, S. E. (1989). Effects of oral morphine on breathlessness and exercise tolerance in patients with chronic obstructive pulmonary disease. Am Rev Respir Dis *139*:126–133.

176. Woodcock, A. A., Johnson, M. A., & Geddes, D. M. (1982). Breathlessness, alcohol, and opiates (letter to the editor). N Engl J Med *306*:1363–1364.

177. Mitchell Heggs, P., Murphy, K., & Minty, K. (1980). Diazepam in the treatment of dyspnea in the "pink puffer" syndrome. Q J Med *49*:9–20.

178. Green, J. G., Pucino, F., & Carlson, J. D. (1989). Effects of alprazolam on respiratory drive, anxiety, and dyspnea in chronic airflow obstruction: A case study. Pharmacotherapy *9*:34–38.

179. Eimer, M., Cable, T., Gal, P., Rothenberger, L. A., & McCue, J. D. (1985). Effects of chorazepate on breathlessness and exercise tolerance in patients with chronic airflow obstruction. J Fam Pract *21*:359–362.

180. Man, G. C. W., Hsu, K., & Sproule, B. J. (1986). Effect of alprazolam on exercise and dyspnea in patients with chronic obstructive pulmonary disease. Chest *90*:832–836.

181. Woodcock, A. A., Gross, E. R., & Geddes, D. M. (1981). Drug treatment of breathlessness: Contrasting effects of diazepam and promethazine in pink puffers. Br Med J *283*:343–346.

182. Rice, K. L., Kronenberg, R. S., Hedemark, L. L., & Niewoehner, D. E. (1987). Effects of chronic administration of codeine and promethazine on breathlessness and exercise tolerance in patients with chronic airflow obstruction. Br J Dis Chest *81*:287–292.

183. Vermeire, P., DeBacker, W., Van Maele, R., Bal, J., & Van Kerckhoven, W. (1987). Carotid body resection in patients with severe chronic airflow limitation. Clin Respir Physiol *23*(Suppl. 11):S165–S166.

184. Stulbarg, M. S., & Winn, W. R. (1989). Bilateral carotid body resection for the relief of dyspnea in severe chronic obstructive pulmonary disease. Chest *95*:1123–1128.

185. Freedberg, P. D., Hoffman, L. A., Light, W. C., & Kreps, M. D. (1987). Effect of progressive muscle relaxation on the objective symptoms and subjective responses associated with asthma. Heart Lung *16*:24–30.

186. Acosta, F. (1988). Biofeedback and progressive relaxation in weaning the anxious patient from the ventilator: A brief report. Heart Lung *17*:299–301.

187. Erskine-Milliss, J., & Schonell, M. (1981). Relaxation therapy in asthma: A critical review. Psychosom Med *43*:365–372.

188. Renfroe, K. L. (1988). Effect of progressive relaxation on dyspnea and state anxiety in patients with chronic obstructive pulmonary disease. Heart Lung *17*:408–413.

189. Sitzman, J., Kamiya, J., & Johnson, J. (1987). Biofeedback training for reduced respiratory rate in chronic obstructive pulmonary disease. A preliminary study. Nurs Res *32*:218–223.

190. Holliday, J. E., & Hyers, T. M. (1990). The reduction of weaning time from mechanical ventilation using tidal volume and relaxation biofeedback. Am Rev Respir Dis *141*:1214–1220.

191. Acosta, F. (1988). Biofeedback and progressive relaxation in weaning the anxious patient from the ventilator: A brief report. Heart Lung *17*:299–301.

192. Horsman, J. (1978). Using tape recordings to overcome panic during dyspnea. Respir Care *23*:767–768.

193. Tandon, M. K. (1978). Adjunct treatment with

yoga in chronic severe airways obstruction. Thorax *33*:514–517.

194. Johnson, J. E. (1973). The effects of accurate expectations about sensations on the sensory and distress components of pain. J Pers Soc Psychol *27*:261–275.

195. Rosser, R., Denford, J., Heslop, A., Kinston, W., Macklin, D., Minty, K., Moynihan, C., Muir, B., Rein, L., & Guz, A. (1983). Breathlessness and psychiatric morbidity in chronic bronchitis and emphysema: A study of psychotherapeutic management. Psychol Med *13*:93–110.

196. Gift, A. G. (1990). Dyspnea. Nurs Clin North Am *25*:955–965.

197. Hodgkin, J. E. (1988). Pulmonary rehabilitation: Structure, components, and benefits. J Cardiopulmonary Rehabil *11*:423–434.

198. Barstow, R. (1974). Coping with emphysema. Nurs Clin North Am *9*:137–145.

199. Fagerhaugh, S. Y. (1973). Getting around with emphysema. Am J Nurs *73*:94–100.

200. Chalmers, K. L. (1984). A closer look at how people cope with chronic airflow obstruction. Can Nurse *80*:35–38.

201. Carrieri, V. K., & Janson-Bjerklie, S. (1986). Strategies patients use to manage the sensation of dyspnea. West J Nurs Res *8*:284–305.

202. Schwartzstein, R. M., Lahive, K., Pope, A., Weinburger, S. E., & Weiss, J. W. (1987). Cold facial stimulation reduces breathlessness induced in normal subjects. Am Rev Respir Dis *136*:58–61.

203. Janson-Bjerklie, S., Benner, P., & Becker, G. (In press). Predicting outcomes of living with asthma. Res Nurs Health. In press.

204. Steele, B., & Shaver, J. (1992). The dyspnea experience: Nociceptive properties and a model for research and practice. Adv Nurs Sci *15*:64–76.

12

Fatigue

Barbara F. Piper

DEFINITION

Because fatigue is a complex multicausal and multidimensional sensation,[1] it defies easy definition and explanation. No one definition has gained universal acceptance.[2] Fatigue has been defined by the investigator's interest or focus (e.g., neuromuscular versus subjective fatigue), by its proposed origin or cause (e.g., central versus peripheral, pathological versus psychological, or "attentional" fatigue), by the exclusion of all other diseases (e.g., chronic fatigue syndrome), by its response to electrical stimulation (e.g., high-frequency versus low-frequency fatigue), and by its duration (e.g., acute versus chronic fatigue).

It is generally accepted that subjective fatigue occurs on a continuum, ranging from tiredness to exhaustion.[3] Thus, the perception of fatigue's intensity and duration should be an essential component to any definition. The continuum of fatigue, however, should not be interpreted to imply that tiredness must always precede fatigue or exhaustion. Everyone experiences tiredness; it is a universal sensation that is expected to occur normally at certain times of the day (because of circadian rhythmicity) or after certain types of activity or exertion. It may be localized to a specific body part, such as the eyes, arms, or legs, or it may be generalized to the whole body. It usually has an identifiable cause, is short-lived, and is easily dissipated by a good night's sleep or rest.

In contrast to tiredness, subjective fatigue is perceived as unusual, abnormal, or excessive whole-body tiredness disproportionate to or unrelated to activity or exertion. It may be acute or chronic, it is not dispelled easily by sleep or rest, and it can have a profound, negative impact on the person's quality of life. Studies in the literature on fatigue suggest that differences exist between acute and chronic fatigue states.[4-13] Chronic fatigue is thought to last anywhere from 1 to 3 to 6 months or longer.[8, 10, 14-16]

Unfortunately, literature studies make no distinction between acute fatigue and tiredness states. As a consequence, what has been described in previous studies as acute fatigue may instead be the state of tiredness. Acute fatigue and tiredness may differ by severity and duration. As Carpenito states: "Fatigue is different from tiredness . . . a transient, temporary state. . . . Fatigue is a pervasive, subjective, drained feeling . . . not relieved by rest"[17] (pp. 362–363). Research studies need to clarify whether these distinctions exist and determine whether acute and chronic fatigue states can coexist simultaneously within the same individual as can acute and chronic pain states.[18] Table 12–1 summarizes characteristics that may enable the differential diagnosis to be made between tiredness and acute and chronic fatigue states.

Since muscle generates force, muscle physiologists define "neuromuscular fatigue" as the "failure to maintain force (or power output) during sustained or repeated contractions . . ."[19] (p. 120). Respiratory muscle fatigue is the failure "to continue generating the required force to sustain . . . movement of air into and out of the lungs"[20] (p. 6). While these definitions imply that the onset of fatigue is delayed and occurs only after some form of prolonged activity or exertion, physiological changes present at the onset rather than at the end of an activity may be more crucial to understanding what causes

TABLE 12–1 DIFFERENTIAL DIAGNOSIS: TIREDNESS AND SUBJECTIVE ACUTE AND CHRONIC FATIGUE STATES

Distinguishing Characteristics	Tiredness	Acute and Chronic Fatigue States
Purpose/function	Protective	Unknown, may no longer be protective
Populations at risk	Healthy individuals	Clinical populations
Etiology	Usually identifiable	May not be identifiable
	Single mechanism and cause	Usually multiple, additive causes
	Often experienced in relationship to some form of activity or exertion	Often experienced with no relationship to activity or exertion
Perception	Normal, usual	Abnormal, unusual
	Expected, anticipated	Excessive or disporportionate
	Pleasant or unpleasant	Unpleasant
	Localized or generalized	Generalized, whole-body sensation
Temporal		
Onset	Rapid or gradual	*Acute:* rapid; *Chronic:* a gradual cumulative, threshold model; insidious onset
Duration	Short, hours to days	*Acute:* short, less than 1 month
		Chronic: more than 1 month
Pattern	Circadian rhythmicity	Circadian rhythmicity may be absent
	Intermittent	Constant or recurrent
	Sporadic	Overwhelming
Relief	Usually relieved by a good night's sleep, adequate rest, attention to dietary, exercise, and stress management approaches	Acute fatigue may resolve quickly with proper treatment.
		Chronic fatigue may not be easily resolved
	Resolves quickly	A combination of approaches may be needed
Impact on activities of daily living/quality of life	Minor	Major negative impact

Adapted with permission from Piper, B. F. (1988). Fatigue in cancer patients: Current perspectives on measurement and management. In *Nursing Management of Common Problems: State of the Art. Proceedings of the Fifth National Conference on Cancer Nursing.* New York: American Cancer Society.

fatigue.[21, 22] From this "onset" perspective, neuromuscular fatigue is defined as "any reduction in the force generating capacity of the total neuromuscular system regardless of the force required in any given situation."[21] Exhaustion occurs when "the required force or exercise intensity can no longer be maintained"[22] (p. 691).

The Centers for Disease Control and Prevention, Division of Viral Diseases, has proposed a case definition for chronic fatigue syndrome (CFS) on the basis of specific sign and symptom criteria.[16] Two major and several minor criteria must be met before the diagnosis can be made (Table 12–2). The major criteria stipulate that fatigue must be new, persistent, or relapsing; cause a 50 per cent reduction or impairment in average daily activity for at least 6 months; and not be caused by any other diseases.

PREVALENCE

Figures on the exact incidence and prevalence of fatigue are unknown. Methodologi-

cal problems in defining and measuring fatigue are contributing factors.[23] Fatigue is the seventh most common complaint in primary care, accounting for an estimated 10 million office visits a year and more than $300 million in medical care costs.[24] Since fatigue often is chronic, its prevalence is much higher than its incidence.[25] In general medical clinics, 21 to 24 per cent of the adults indicate that fatigue is a major problem.[25]

Despite the current attention given to CFS, when the CDCP's stringent diagnostic criteria are used to determine its incidence, it is a relatively uncommon disorder.[26] CFS constitutes 10 per cent or less of those affected with persistent, chronic fatigue. It therefore represents only the tip of the iceberg for the more than 10 million Americans who seek treatment for chronic fatigue.[26] Even when extensive investigations are conducted, in at least one third of patients with chronic fatigue there is no identifiable cause.[25] For example, at one Connecticut fatigue clinic, only 6 per cent of 135 patients met the CDCP's definition for CFS, 67 per cent had active psychiatric disorders, 3 per cent were diagnosed with medically related disorders,

TABLE 12–2 DIAGNOSTIC CRITERIA FOR CHRONIC FATIGUE SYNDROME

Major Criteria*	Minor Criteria

1. Fatigue
  New
  Persisting or relapsing
  Reduction in activity by 50% or more
  Present for 6 or more months
 	
2. Absence of other illnesses
  Autoimmune disorders
  Cardiac, endocrine, gastrointestinal,
    hematological, hepatic, neuromuscular,
    pulmonary disorders
  Chronic inflammatory diseases
  Drug abuse, depending on side effects
  Infections: bacterial, fungal, parasitic, or
    viral, including HIV
  Malignancy
  Psychiatric disorders
  Toxic reactions
	3. Symptoms
	  Mild fever (37.5 to 38.6° C) *or* chills
	  Sore throat
	  Painful cervical or axillary lymph nodes
	  Muscle soreness or pain
	  Prolonged (24 hours or more) fatigue after
	    exercise
	  Headaches
	  Joint pain without swelling or redness
	  Neuropsychological symptoms
	    (photophobia, transient visual scotomata,
	    forgetfulness, excessive irritability,
	    confusion, difficulty thinking, inability to
	    concentrate, depression)
	  Sleep disturbance
	  Development of symptoms over a few
	    hours to a few days
	
	4. Signs†
	  Low-grade fever (37.6 to 38.6° C orally;
	    37.8 to 38.8° C rectally)
	  Nonexudative pharyngitis
	  Palpable or tender cervical or axillary
	    lymph nodes less than 2 cm in diameter

Adapted with permission from Holmes, G. P., Kaplan, J. E., Gartz, N. M., Komaroff, A. L., Schonbeyer, L. B., Straus, S. E., et al. (1988). Chronic fatigue syndrome: A working case definition. Ann Intern Med *108*:387–399.

*Both major criteria must be met and: (1) six or more symptoms and two or more signs or (2) eight or more symptoms without physical signs.

†Physical signs must be documented by a physician on at least two occasions at least 1 month apart.

and no cause of fatigue could be found in the remaining 24 per cent.[27]

Fatigue is more common in clinical populations. It frequently precedes or accompanies most major illnesses and treatments. In cancer patients, fatigue is a major clinical problem. In patients receiving chemotherapy, 80 to 96 per cent experience fatigue.[23] The incidence of and concern about fatigue increase over time for patients with cancer and their family members.[28] Cumulative fatigue, or fatigue that increases over time, occurs in the majority of patients receiving radiation therapy irrespective of treatment site.[23, 29, 30] Fatigue is a dose-limiting toxicity for many of the biological response modifiers, such as interferon.[31]

For family caregivers, fatigue is a major problem. In one study, moderate to severe fatigue occurred in 53 per cent of family caregivers of cancer patients.[32] In another study, family members identified their concern about fatigue second only to concerns about the future.[28]

Chronic fatigue is prevalent in patients undergoing hemodialysis, peritoneal dialysis, and renal transplantation,[33] with over 58 per cent of dialysis patients reporting moderate to severe fatigue.[34]

In postoperative patients, pronounced fatigue may persist for longer than 1 month following uncomplicated abdominal surgery.[35] Following major abdominal surgeries, approximately one third of patients will require 2 months to recover from their fatigue.[36]

Excessive fatigue and general malaise may precede 30 to 55 per cent of myocardial infarctions or sudden cardiac deaths.[37] Fatigue and dyspnea may be the most prominent symptoms of congestive heart failure.[38] In one study of congestive heart failure, 92 per cent of patients (n = 23) rated their fatigue as medium to high.[39]

Fatigue occurs in 76 to 87 per cent of patients with multiple sclerosis. Approximately one third initially have fatigue and identify it as their most troubling symptom.[40]

Fatigue is an almost universal complaint of patients with acquired immunodeficiency syndrome (AIDS), but few studies have documented its incidence. One study has suggested that fatigue may be more severe in AIDS than in bone marrow transplantation or malignant melanoma.[41]

Fatigue is also common in rheumatoid arthritis, but its prevalence has not been well documented. This is surprising, since the absence of fatigue is a criterion of disease remission.[42, 43] In one study, 19 of 20 patients experienced fatigue; more than half stated it was the most problematic symptom of their illness.[43]

POPULATIONS AT RISK

Developmental Stressors

Age, sex, and race have been postulated as risk factors for fatigue. Because data are limited and often conflicting, more prospective comparative studies are needed to identify the relationships between age, sex, race, and fatigue. Subjective fatigue is thought to be common in adolescents[44] and the elderly,[45] but few studies have documented the actual incidence. Premature infants and the elderly are at risk for respiratory muscle fatigue due to age-related muscle fiber differences.[20] Chronic fatigue syndrome primarily affects adults 20 to 44 years of age,[46] although studies document CFS in children as well.[47–50] No relationship between fatigue and age has been documented in renal dialysis[34] or cancer[51, 52] or in caregivers[32] of patients experiencing these treatments and diseases.

In family practice settings, women are twice as likely to report fatigue as men.[25, 53] Females are three times more likely to be diagnosed with CFS than males.[46] Some authors believe that the sex ratio is equal in childhood, doubles in adult women, and increases for both sexes in old age.[54] No sex differences have been documented in patients undergoing renal dialysis.[34]

Feeling tired is an almost universal complaint of women experiencing premenstrual syndrome (PMS), pregnancy, and postpartum states.[55] Fatigue increases significantly during labor[56] and may be more intense in pregnant black women who are anemic.[57] Of significance, fatigue is the most common postpartum symptom experienced by the male partners of these women.[55]

Nonwhite persons may report more fatigue in family practice settings,[53] whereas white patients are more likely to be affected by CFS than other groups.

Situational Stressors

Many situational factors increase the risk for fatigue. These include environmental factors, alterations in sleep and rest patterns, disruptions in work and activity or nutritional patterns, changes in psychological patterns, life events such as pregnancy, and socioeconomic and cultural factors.[1, 32, 40, 58, 59] For example, heat is known to worsen fatigue in multiple sclerosis.[40] In cancer, higher fatigue scores are associated with a poorer perception of health, poorer economic status, and lower perceived ability to manage side effects.[28] In family members caring for persons with cancer, the more the caregiver's schedule is perceived to be a burden, the greater the level of fatigue.[32]

Clinical States

Fatigue is so common in clinical populations that it is considered a universal precursor or sequela of disease progression.[1] In one study of patients with cancer, a positive correlation between subjective fatigue and disease activity, as measured by the tumor marker CA-125, was found. As tumor burden declined, so did subjective fatigue.[52] In arthritis, similar findings were documented. Fatigue was positively correlated to the number of joints that were inflamed.[60]

Higher fatigue levels are experienced by patients with multiple sclerosis and systemic lupus erythematosus in comparison to healthy controls.[61] Patients who have skeletal deformities of the spine or rib cage are at greater risk for respiratory muscle fatigue, as are nutritionally compromised persons; those who have neuromuscular, cardiac, or respiratory disease; and those who experience hypoxia and electrolyte disturbances.[20]

Fatigue is a common presenting symptom in depression. Sleep disturbances, such as insomnia, multiple awakenings during sleep, or early waking, are common in depression and may contribute to fatigue.[62] Diagnostic testing, anesthesia, and clinical therapies such as surgery, chemotherapy, radiation therapy, dialysis, and drug therapy used for symptom management are associated with fatigue.[1]

MECHANISMS

Despite the prevalence of fatigue in healthy and ill populations, little is known about the actual mechanisms of fatigue in healthy individuals; even less is known about how these normal fatigue mechanisms may be affected by disease or treatment. Demonstrating a direct cause and effect relationship is difficult because of fatigue's complexity and the problems inherent in the timing and measurement of fatigue.

For example, in neuromuscular fatigue a series of electrical, biochemical, and metabolic and mechanical events must occur between the central and peripheral nervous systems to produce a voluntary contraction. Given the many possible sites and mechanisms that are involved, it is not surprising that neuromuscular fatigue is incompletely understood and that controversy exists.[12, 63] Rather than a single cause, a spectrum of events probably occurs that varies by the type of muscle fiber activated; by the nature, duration, and intensity of the stimulus; and by the environmental conditions and the host's endurance capacity.[12, 21, 63] In addition, it is difficult to compare findings across studies because of the diversity of methods used to produce and measure skeletal muscle fatigue, the variations in the reliability and timing of measurements, and the different types and species of muscle preparations that have been studied. These measurement difficulties are compounded when studies attempt to correlate subjective and objective fatigue indicators in clinical populations.

Various models have attributed the development of fatigue to neurophysiological causes;[19] physiological, psychological, and situational factors;[10, 56] personality and environmental factors;[10] and response to stressor patterns.[64] A few of these models are reviewed next.

Central-Peripheral Model

Muscle physiologists have described a central-peripheral model for studying fatigue in which fatigue is produced by two types of neurophysiological mechanisms, central and peripheral (Fig. 12–1). These mechanisms may operate independently or together to produce fatigue, depending on the specific situation.[65] Most neuromuscular research addresses peripheral skeletal muscle fatigue in healthy subjects; less is known about central fatigue mechanisms.[66]

Central fatigue mechanisms are thought to include lack of motivation, impaired spinal

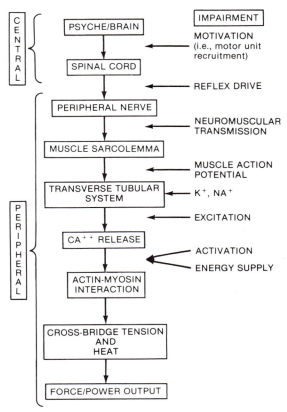

Figure 12–1. Central and peripheral mechanisms of fatigue. (Adapted with permission from Gibson, H., & Edwards, R. H. T. [1985]. Muscular exercise and fatigue. Sports Med 2:121.)

cord transmission or recruitment of motor neurons, inhibition of voluntary effort, or malfunction of nerve cells.[9, 19, 66] Many authors consider the action of sensory pathways on the reticular formation to be critical to understanding central fatigue.[3, 65] Chemoreceptors in fatigued muscles are thought to send feedback sensory impulses to the reticular formation in the central nervous system. These impulses result in "the inhibition of motor pathways anywhere from the voluntary centers in the brain to the spinal motor neurons"[65] (p. 320). This inhibition of voluntary effort may be overriden by feedback stimuli from nonfatigued muscles that stimulate the facilitatory portion of the reticular formation, resulting in decreased inhibition and decreased fatigue.[65]

Other central mechanisms posited include an increase in the plasma tryptophan-branched chain amino acid ratio that results in increased synthesis of 5-hydroxytryptamine, a central neurotransmitter.[67] Increased levels of brain ammonia (NH_3) that can occur during skeletal muscle exercise may cause fatigue.[66] These increased levels are thought to alter the concentration of neurotransmitters, reduce ATP, and cause postsynaptic inhibition and hyperpnea.[66]

Peripheral fatigue mechanisms include impaired peripheral nerve function, neuromuscular junction transmission, and fiber activation.[19] Impaired neuromuscular junction transmission causes fatigue in patients with myasthenia gravis.[22, 68] Disturbances in the neurotransmitter acetylcholine have been associated with fatigue in botulism.[58]

Metabolically, fatigue can be caused by the accumulation or depletion of certain metabolites.[69] In addition, structural or mechanical injury and inflammation can cause fatigue.[12] Because accumulation and depletion of energy substrates do not occur alone, a large degree of interaction between these mechanisms is thought to exist.[66] The accumulation of hydrogen ions (H^+), ammonia (NH_3), ammonium (NH_4), inorganic phosphate (Pi), monobasic phosphate (HPO_2), sodium (Na^+), and potassium (K^+)[12, 66, 70, 71] and the depletion of energy substrates such as adenosine triphosphate (ATP), phosphocreatine (PCr), muscle and liver glycogen, free fatty acids (FFA), intracellular K^+, and Pi have been implicated.[12, 22, 66]

Accumulation of H^+ and thus acidosis resulting from lactate production may impair muscle performance and cause fatigue by reducing enzyme activity (phosphofructokinase, hexokinase, phosphorylase, lactate dehydrogenase, and myosin-ATPase). This reduction in enzyme activity ultimately leads to the inhibition of glycolysis and a reduction in ATP resynthesis.[66] Accumulation of H^+ reduces calcium release by enhancing calcium binding by the sarcoplasmic reticulum. This results in decreased membrane excitability and conduction velocity.[66] In acidosis, depletion of PCr (a short-term energy substrate), decreased mobilization of FFA, and a reduction in the number of magnesium ion (Mg^{++}) complexes can occur.[66]

Because oxidation of FFA spares muscle glycogen reserves and delays the onset of fatigue due to glycogen depletion, any factor that interferes with oxidation or mobilization of FFA may cause fatigue. Inhibition of FFA mobilization occurs with beta blockers[72] and may be responsible for fatigue in patients receiving these drugs.[10] Declines in Mg^{++} complex concentrations are thought to inhibit ATP and ADP reactions.[66] Magnesium depletion may be a cause of fatigue in patients treated with cisplatin chemotherapy.

Since fatigue can occur in nonacidotic states such as McArdle's disease, not all fatigue can be explained by the accumulation of lactic acid and hydrogen ions.[63] The availibility and utilization of oxygen are important to the onset of fatigue. It is not clear whether it is the oxidative capacity of the muscle (mitochondrial respiratory capacity) or the oxygen-carrying capacity of the cardiovascular system that limits maximum oxygen consumption ($\dot{V}O_2max$) and thus endurance.[66] Probably an interplay of both mechanisms is important. Additional fatigue mechanisms posited include factors that negatively affect mitochondrial transport and enzymatic activity, trigger the production of free radicals,[66] or cause an increase in cellular water content that interferes with blood supply to contracting muscles.[22, 63]

Both central and peripheral mechanisms may be involved in the overwhelming subjective fatigue that patients experience with chronic fatigue syndrome, multiple sclerosis, or cancer therapies. It has been postulated that the central and peripheral release of cytokines and lymphokines by white blood cells may be responsible for fatigue in these patients.[31, 73] Cytokines are natural cell products or proteins, such as interferon, interleukin, and cachectin or tumor necrosis factor, that are released by leukocytes, lymphocytes, and macrophages in response to endogenous or exogenous stimuli such as viral infections. These cytokines carry messages that regulate other elements of the immune system and may even alter neuroendocrine secretion, brain electrical activity, and blood-brain barrier permeability.[31] In high amounts, these cytokines can be toxic and lead to persistent fatigue, aching muscles, swollen glands, and sometimes severe brain changes.[74] Viral infections have been implicated in the cause of CFS. Four out of five patients diagnosed with CFS show an overactive immune system and evidence of brain inflammation on magnetic resonance imaging. Seventy per cent show evidence of an active infection with human herpesvirus 6 compared with 20 per cent of controls.[75] A relationship between interleukins and multiple sclerosis has also been postulated.[73]

Childbirth Fatigue Model

Pugh has proposed a childbirth fatigue model that identifies physiological, psychological, and situational factors that may cause fatigue and influence performance factors during labor and delivery[56] (Fig. 12–2). Pugh studied 100 primiparous women from admission through labor and delivery. Fatigue was high in these women as a group and increased as labor progressed and as contraction patterns became stronger. Fatigue was most intense in women who had the longest labors, were more anxious, had less sleep, and received more pain medication.

During pregnancy, women may experience fatigue from the increased energy expenditure that results from the enormous physiological, metabolic, and psychological changes that occur (i.e., rapid fetal development, increased oxygen consumption, increased metabolic rate, and cardiovascular repiratory changes). Increased progesterone levels have also been implicated.[76]

Integrated Fatigue Model

An integrated fatigue model has been proposed[1, 18] that permits multiple disciplinary perspectives, definitions, and theories about fatigue to be analyzed (Fig. 12–3).

In the center of this framework are the subjective (perceptual) and objective (physiological, biochemical and metabolic, and behavioral) indicators of fatigue reported in the literature.[1, 18] Surrounding the center of the framework are the metabolic, neurophysiological, situational, and developmental stressor patterns that may cause or modulate the signs and symptoms of fatigue. The accumulation of various metabolites such as uremia in renal disease[33] and those previously discussed (see Central-Peripheral Model) may affect fatigue. Changes in energy production and availability of substrate that may occur in cachexia, anorexia, bulimia, infection, fever, hypoglycemia, and hyperthyroid or hypothyroid states may cause fatigue. In some cancer patients, abnormal levels of fructose biphosphate, a muscle enzyme, have been documented.[77] These abnormal levels may lead to accelerated energy expenditure in these patients.

Alterations in activity and rest patterns can play significant roles in the prevention, cause, and alleviation of fatigue. Unnecessary sedentariness, prolonged bedrest, and immobil-

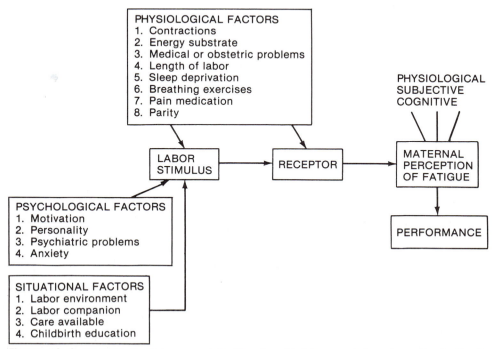

Figure 12–2. Childbirth fatigue model. (Reprinted with permission from Pugh, L. C. [1990]. *Psychophysiological Correlates of Fatigue During Childbirth* [p. 8]. Doctoral dissertation. Baltimore: University of Maryland.)

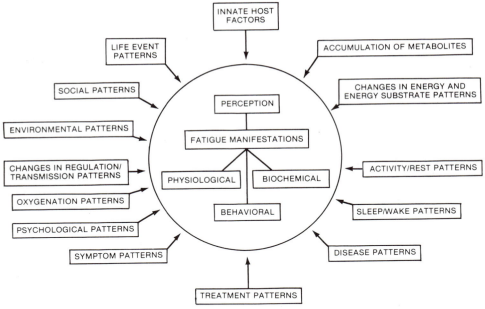

Figure 12–3. Integrated fatigue framework in healthy and clinical populations. (Redrawn with permission from Piper, B. F., Lindsey, A. M., & Dodd, M. J. [1987]. Fatigue mechanisms in cancer patients: Developing nursing theory. Oncol Nurs Forum *14*:18.)

ity contribute to weakness and fatigue. Skeletal muscle that is not exercised loses its oxidative capacity. More oxygen, therefore, is required for the performance of comparable work than that required by conditioned muscle. This factor alone can contribute significantly to the development of fatigue[20, 78, 79] and is one of the reasons why aerobic endurance exercise is often prescribed. With disuse, such as may occur during hospitalization and treatment, rapid and potentially irreversible losses in energy and functioning can occur as muscle enzymes are depleted and increased nitrogen excretion results.[80] For example, in multiple sclerosis, patients expend two to three times more energy in walking than healthy individuals. This high energy cost for walking, perhaps due to lack of endurance, may be an important cause of fatigue and dyspnea in multiple sclerosis.[81]

Sleep-wake patterns can influence fatigue. Lack of restful sleep at night can lead to increased sleepiness and fatigue during the day. This daytime fatigue increases the need for daytime napping and increased nighttime sleep.[82, 83] Various disease states, medical therapies, and symptoms are associated with fatigue. Frequently, symptom management may temporarily exacerbate fatigue. Ulti-

mately, however, effective symptom management should prevent or ameliorate it.

Any factor that alters or interferes with the ability to maintain adequate oxygen levels, such as anemia in renal disease,[33] can produce fatigue. Fluid and electrolyte imbalances and changes in neurohormone levels, such as melatonin and serotonin or cytokine release, can affect neurotransmission and cause fatigue. Decreased levels of corticotropin-releasing hormone and cortisol have been documented in CFS.[84]

Psychological factors, such as usual response to stressors, depression, anxiety, motivation, distraction, boredom, beliefs, and attitudes, may influence fatigue. Depression may be a principal cause of fatigue in patients who report being tired upon arising.[34] Other factors may include environmental patterns; life events, such as the common transitions associated with growth, development, and maturation (pregnancy, parenting, and divorce); and innate host factors, such as age, sex, race, and genetic make-up (i.e., type of muscle fibers and their predisposition to fatigue).

Social patterns, such as perceived quality and amount of social support, cultural beliefs, and economic factors, may influence fatigue. In one study, single parents with ovarian cancer who had no assistance at home had higher levels of fatigue than their married counterparts.[83] In another study, cultural beliefs were found to influence the type of fatigue symptoms experienced by women with breast cancer.[85] In this preliminary study comparing fatigue patterns in Korean and American women with breast cancer, Korean women were more likely than their American counterparts to attribute gastrointestinal symptoms, such as indigestion, constipation, and loss of appetite, to their fatigue.[85]

PATHOLOGICAL CONSEQUENCES

Fatigue is thought to have a protective function. In extreme forms of exercise, fatigue usually occurs before ATP is depleted and muscle contractures occur.[63] In some metabolic myopathies, this protection is lacking and painful muscle cramps, necrosis, myoglobinuria, and renal damage can result.[63, 68]

Although more prospective studies are needed to confirm the following findings, three studies suggest that the presence of fatigue at diagnosis may predict a negative treatment and disease outcome in patients with breast cancer,[86] lung cancer,[87] and malignant melanoma.[88] Feelings of fatigue also may be predictive of future myocardial infarctions (MIs) independent of the classic risk factors for an MI (i.e., blood pressure, smoking, cholesterol, age, and antihypertensive drugs).[37]

RELATED PHYSIOLOGICAL CONCEPTS

Several physiological concepts or states have been linked to fatigue. These include stress, immobility and activity intolerance, exertion, weakness and aesthenia, cachexia, and numerous signs and symptoms such as nausea and vomiting, pain, dyspnea, and insomnia.[89] Treatment of these states may prevent or ameliorate associated fatigue. Fatigue also may contribute to exacerbating these signs, symptoms, or states. Unfortunately, data that examine these relationships are limited.

A few studies have investigated fatigue and pain.[60, 90] In patients with chronic low back pain, fatigue (as measured by the Profile of Mood States, or POMS) not only was associated with pain intensity during a painful episode but also followed the painful episode 24 hours later.[90] In patients with rheumatoid arthritis, subjective fatigue was correlated positively with pain and negatively with perceived quality of sleep.[60]

Additional studies are needed to clarify the distinctions between subjective fatigue and aesthenia, which some authors define as a perceived state of fatigue (mentally and physically) and weakness.[91-93] For instance, in one study of multiple sclerosis, patients were able to distinguish subjectively between the two sensations of weakness and fatigue.[94] Also, weakness may not always accompany fatigue.

Subjective fatigue and perceived exertion also need to be differentiated. All too often the Borg scale, a measure of perceived exertion, is used to quantitate subjective fatigue when actually perceived exertion may differ from subjective fatigue.[95]

RELATED PSYCHOSOCIAL CONCEPTS

Various psychosocial concepts have been associated with fatigue. These include malaise, depression, quality of life, and social roles and responsibilities. Fatigue can influence negatively the quality of a person's life by interfering in the ability to perform the kinds of activities and roles that give meaning and value to life. Chronically fatigued individuals may not have the same energy reserves that they once had. Fewer activities are undertaken, and those that are performed may take longer to complete and require more effort.[18] In cancer patients, significant negative correlations are found between fatigue scores and quality of life.[96] Similar findings are documented in dialysis patients: the greater the level of fatigue, the lower the perceived quality of life.[33]

As chronic fatigue begins to alter what patients can do for themselves, family members or caregivers begin to assume many of the roles previously held by patients. These increased role demands can lead to fatigue in the caregiver.[97] Social isolation for both the patient and the caregiver can result.[18]

Studies are needed to distinguish malaise[98] and depression from fatigue, since management may vary.[1] Conflicting data exist about the relationship between depression and fatigue. Although direct comparisons cannot be made between studies that have used different instruments and populations, some studies have found positive correlations between depression and fatigue;[43, 60, 83, 91, 99] others have not.[33, 40, 52, 61]

MANIFESTATIONS

Subjective Manifestations

Subjective manifestations of fatigue may include physical, emotional, behavioral, and cognitive and mental symptoms. Physical symptoms may include expressions about physical exhaustion: experiencing tired arms, legs, eyes, and whole-body tiredness; having "no energy"; and feeling weary, "listless," or "worn out." Emotionally, fatigue may be described as being abnormal or unpleasant. The person may feel impatient, irritable, and disinterested and lack motivation. Behaviorally, the person may say that it takes longer to do things, that more effort is required, or that certain activities are no longer undertaken because of fatigue. The need to sleep and nap more is a common complaint. Mental or cognitive symptoms may include difficulties in concentration, memory, or ability to think clearly.

Subjective Measurement

Subjective fatigue has been measured as a component in instruments designed to measure other phenomena. These instruments include the Symptom Distress Scale,[100, 101] the Adapted Symptom Distress Scale,[102] and the long and short forms of the POMS.[103, 104] As more cross-cultural studies of fatigue are initiated, the difficulties in attempting to translate instruments directly from one culture to another must be considered.[105]

Several scales are available to measure subjective fatigue. Some are unidimensional in that they measure only one dimension of subjective fatigue such as intensity or degree of tiredness. Others are multidimensional in that they measure not only intensity but also severity and distress (severity dimension), sensory (cognitive and mental, physical, and emotional symptoms of fatigue), affective (emotional meaning of the fatigue), and temporal dimensions (timing, onset, and duration of fatigue).[99]

Unidimensional measures such as single visual analogue scales (VAS) and Likert-type scales have been used to measure the intensity of subjective fatigue. These single-item intensity measures correlate well with other multiple-item measures of intensity such as the POMS Fatigue-Inertia subscale[43] and the Pearson-Byars Fatigue Feeling Tone Checklist (PBF) described below.[33]

The PBF[106, 107] is a 10-item adjective rating scale originally developed to measure tiredness in airmen. Subjects are asked to indicate the degree to which they feel the "same as," "worse than," or "better than" each of the adjectives that have been placed on a continuum from "extremely peppy" to "ready to drop." The scale has been used and adapted in several clinical studies with comparable reliability and validity estimates.[33, 51, 58, 82, 83, 96, 108, 109]

The Fatigue Severity Scale is a nine-item self-report scale developed to measure the common features of fatigue in patients with multiple sclerosis or systemic lupus erythematosus.[61] Subjects select a number from one to seven that indicates the degree of agreement with each statement (1 = strongly disagree; 7 = strongly agree). The scale is internally consistent and correlates well with VAS measures. It is able to differentiate patients from controls and detects clinically predicted changes in fatigue over time.[61]

Another scale that measures fatigue severity is the Visual Analogue Scale to Measure Fatigue Severity, or VAS-F.[110] It is an 18-item scale consisting of visual analogue lines to rate severity of fatigue (13 items) and energy (5 items). It has good reliability and validity estimates in a variety of populations. A numerical version of the VAS-F is also available to facilitate scoring (K. Lee, personal communication, 1991).

Multidimensional measures include the Fatigue Symptom Checklist (FSCL) and the Piper Fatigue Scale (PFS). The FSCL is a 30-item checklist that measures three sensory dimensions of subjective fatigue symptoms: decline in motivation or concentration (mental fatigue) and general and specific feelings of fatigue incongruity. This checklist, originally developed to measure fatigue in Japanese industrial populations,[111–113] has been used in several clinical studies with comparable reliability and validity estimates.[33, 51, 82, 99, 108, 109, 114–116]

Symptoms reflecting general incongruity,

such as "wanting to lie down," "feeling tired in the legs," and "feeling tired in the body," are generally cited more frequently by subjects than the symptoms of mental fatigue or specific incongruity. Other common symptoms include "impatience" (mental fatigue) and having "stiff shoulders" (specific incongruity).[33, 51, 82, 99, 108] Feelings of thirst (specific incongruity) are more commonly mentioned by patients with cancer and multiple sclerosis,[33, 51, 99, 109] suggesting that symptoms may vary by disease or cause.[1, 33] In general, the more numerous the symptoms of fatigue, the greater the fatigue intensity.[33, 112]

The Piper Fatigue Scale is a 41-item VAS that measures four dimensions of subjective fatigue: temporal, severity, sensory, and affective. Three additional open-ended items measure perceived causes of fatigue, relief measures, and associated symptoms.[18, 99] The PFS has excellent reliability and validity estimates in patients receiving radiation therapy and chemotherapy and in pregnancy[57, 99, 115] and currently is undergoing testing in a variety of other clinical populations. The scale has been adapted for use as a clinical assessment and interview guide for subjective fatigue.[31]

Objective Manifestations

Objective manifestations of fatigue may include physiological indicators such as decreased hematocrit, blood glucose, thyroid, and oxygen saturation levels. Biochemical and metabolic indicators may include alterations in pH, electrolytes, lactate, and phosphate-containing compounds. Behaviorally, there may be changes in physical appearance, affect, and attitude and changes in communication and activity patterns.[117]

Objective Measurement

Studies of fatigue have investigated a variety of physiological, biochemical and metabolic, and behavioral indicators in an attempt to measure fatigue "objectively." Physiologically, neuromuscular fatigue has been measured in terms of loss of force or work-generating capacity, by shifts in the power spectrum of the electromyogram from higher to lower frequencies, by the slowing of muscle conduction velocity and contractile speed, and by hand-held bulb dynamometers and other indices of decreased strength.[96, 116]

Other physiological indicators have included changes in serum levels of melatonin,[118, 119] blood glucose, thyroid hormones, and cortisol[9] and changes in heart rate, oxygen consumption,[120] temperature,[109] and hematocrit levels.[18, 83, 115]

Biochemically and metabolically, fatigue has been measured by the accumulation or depletion of various metabolites[21] and by fluid and electrolyte shifts. As with subjective measures of fatigue, every objective method has its limitations. For example, serum levels may not always reflect intramuscular levels or pH changes.[12] Invasive muscle biopsy techniques have been used to measure metabolic changes and to identify specific types and distribution of muscle fibers that may place an individual at greater risk for muscle fatigue. Changes in phosphate-containing compounds, pH, and phosphocreatine levels can now be measured noninvasively in living, contracting tissue through the use of phosphorus 31 (^{31}P) nuclear magnetic resonance spectroscopy, or ^{31}P NMR.[19, 31, 71, 121]

Behaviorally, investigators have examined relationships between subjective fatigue and specific performance such as card sorting and bicycling.[59, 107, 109, 122, 123] A variety of neurobehavioral tests have also been used to measure the impact of fatigue on concentration, memory, visual-motor functioning, and motor performance.[124]

Rhoten developed an observational checklist to describe the behavioral manifestations of fatigue in five postoperative patients (Table 12–3).[117] Although this checklist has not been further tested, future research on refining it and testing other behavioral measures is warranted.[18] Videotaping fatigued subjects (M. Pitzer, personal communication, 1988) and conducting observational studies similar to those identifying pain behaviors may prove fruitful.[125]

Subjective and Objective Correlations

Many neuromuscular studies have focused solely on the measurement of peripheral mechanisms of fatigue; subjective perception is rarely measured. If perception is measured, perception of exertion and not of fatigue is more commonly the variable measured.

Few studies have documented correlations

TABLE 12–3 PEARSON-BYARS FATIGUE FEELING TONE CHECKLIST

INSTRUCTIONS: The statements to follow are to help you decide how you feel at this time—not yesterday, not an hour ago—but *right now*. For each statement you must determine whether you feel (1) "better than," (2) "same as," or (3) "worse than" the feeling described by that statement.

As an example, take a person who feels a little tired. He might respond to the following items as follows:

	Better Than	Same As	Worse Than	Statement
a	( )	( )	(X)	Extremely fresh
b	( )	(X)	( )	Slightly tired
c	(X)	( )	( )	Completely exhausted

In other words, this person feels worse than "extremely fresh," about the same as "slightly tired," but, on the other hand, better than "completely exhausted."

No.	Better Than	Same As	Worse Than	Statement
1.	( )	( )	( )	Very lively
2.	( )	( )	( )	Extremely tired
3.	( )	( )	( )	Quite fresh
4.	( )	( )	( )	Slightly pooped
5.	( )	( )	( )	Extremely peppy
6.	( )	( )	( )	Somewhat fresh
7.	( )	( )	( )	Petered out
8.	( )	( )	( )	Very refreshed
9.	( )	( )	( )	Fairly well pooped
10.	( )	( )	( )	Ready to drop

Reprinted from Pearson, R. G., & Byars, G. E., Jr. (1956). *The Development and Validation of a Checklist for Measuring Fatigue* (No. 56–115). Randolph AFB, TX: School of Aviation Medicine, USAF.

between subjective and objective measures of fatigue.[25] Differences in the timing and sensitivity of the measures may be contributing factors. Indicators of subjective and objective fatigue may have diurnal fluctuations that complicate the timing of measurement. Unfortunately, few studies describe the timing of fatigue measurement. When it is mentioned, it is usually in studies that use repeated measurements throughout the day to capture circadian patterns (i.e., on arising, at midday, late afternoon, and bedtime)[34, 58] or that control for the effects of treatment (i.e., always 2 hours after radiation therapy)[51] or control for circadian patterns (always at the same time of day).[99] Ideally, laboratory studies should be performed concurrently or within a few hours of subjective fatigue measurements.

With these limitations in mind, the following studies have demonstrated significant correlations between subjective and objective

indicators of fatigue. In women with breast[18] and ovarian cancers,[83] negative correlations between hematocrit levels and subjective fatigue have been documented when hematocrit values were calculated from the most recent blood specimens available.

In patients with congestive heart failure, negative correlations have been documented between subjective fatigue and pH, oxygen saturation, and cardiac ejection fractions.[39] In patients receiving radiation therapy, negative correlations between weight and subjective fatigue were documented.[51] No correlations have yet been found between subjective fatigue and hematocrit, blood urea nitrogen, and creatinine levels in patients undergoing dialysis.[34]

In uncomplicated abdominal surgical procedures, significant correlations have been found between postoperative fatigue and preoperative body weight,[126] postoperative increases in heart rate,[127, 128] and depression of muscle protein synthesis, as measured by serial muscle biopsies.[35] No significant correlations have been found between postoperative fatigue and age, gender, preoperative anxiety, anesthesia duration, weight loss, deterioration in nutritional status,[126, 128, 129] and changes in hematocrit and serum levels of lactate, noradrenaline, growth hormone, and alanine.[35, 129] Thus far, changes in oral and forehead temperature are the only physiological indicators to correlate with subjective fatigue in multiple sclerosis.[109]

Behaviorally, subjective fatigue in rheumatoid arthritis positively correlates with functional status and an interviewer's perceived rating of the patient's fatigue[43] and negatively correlates with physical activity and grip strength.[60]

SURVEILLANCE

Assessment

In order to identify individuals at risk for acute and chronic fatigue, the nurse needs to perform a thorough assessment of all subjective and objective factors that may influence fatigue while remaining sensitive to cross-cultural nuances.[18] In addition to assessing subjective dimensions of fatigue, the nurse should perform a baseline assessment of any changes that have occurred in usual life patterns that may affect fatigue, such as changes in activity or sleep patterns, nutritional status, or the onset of other symptoms such as pain or dyspnea (see Fig. 12–3). Family members should be asked about the patient's and their own patterns of fatigue. Documenting fatigue intensities for 1 day or longer (see Case Study No. 2) may help delineate patterns and diurnal variations.[18, 53] Since underreporting can be of concern when reliance is placed solely on self-report measures,[130] data collection should include a review of all laboratory, physical, and behavioral findings and the medical history to identify objective risk factors and indicators of fatigue.

Screening and Detection

Patients and family members considered at risk need to be monitored on an ongoing basis to prevent acute fatigue from becoming chronic (see Table 12–1). Those at risk for nutritional deficits should have accurate monitoring and recording of intake, calorie counts, changes in weight, and fluid and electrolyte balance for early recognition and detection of problems. Indirect calorimetry and dietary consultation may be helpful.[20]

The nurse must remain alert to early warning signs of fatigue in high-risk populations. For example, in patients being weaned from ventilators, the perception of respiratory distress may herald the onset of respiratory muscle fatigue.[20] Tachypnea (more than 30 breaths per minute) may be the first objective sign of inspiratory muscle fatigue in these patients.[20] This type of tachypnea typically occurs with or immediately following a shift in the power spectrum of the electromyogram. In these patients, the noninvasive monitoring of signs of abdominal paradox (inward displacement of the abdominal wall on inspiration) and respiratory alternans (alternate recruitment and nonrecruitment of diaphragm and inspiratory muscles) may allow for detection of hypercapnia and acidemia before they are determined by invasive arterial blood gas sampling.[20]

THERAPIES

Clinical therapies for fatigue include the ongoing surveillance of those at high risk, the prevention and early detection of acute and chronic fatigue states, the tailoring of therapies according to cause of fatigue, and

the continuing evaluation of treatment effectiveness. The following areas show the most promise for nursing interventions for fatigue: modulating activity and rest patterns, managing symptoms and alterations in nutrition and oxygenation patterns, reducing anxiety through patient teaching and counseling and referral, and modulating environmental factors to conserve energy and reduce disruption of sleep-wake cycles[64, 131, 132] (see Fig. 12–3).

Unfortunately, few studies have formally tested fatigue interventions. Based on data from these studies, however, the following interventions may be helpful under certain conditions.

Acid-Base Modulation

Since acidosis has been shown to enhance the development of fatigue and alkalotic states have been shown to reduce it, methods designed to reduce or prevent intracellular acidosis might hold promise for the management of fatigue.[71]

Aerobic Exercise

Aerobic exercise reduces fatigue via a number of different mechanisms. The primary effect is thought to be increased efficiency in using energy, which results from endurance training. For example, athletes who have undergone endurance training have enhanced malate-aspartate shuttle enzyme activity that may play a role in reducing the lactate accumulation during exercise.[12, 66] Endurance training also leads to an increase in intramuscular glycogen stores and an increase in carnitine palmitoyl transferase, an enzyme that transports free fatty acids into the mitochondria. This results in improved fat utilization as an energy source, sparing muscle glycogen stores and delaying the onset of fatigue.[12]

Table 12–4 summarizes the findings of three exercise studies.[123, 133, 134] In healthy adults, a brisk 10-minute walk produces higher levels of energy and for more sustained periods of time than the ingestion of a candy bar. Significantly less tension also occurs.[134] Decreased levels of fatigue and other benefits are experienced by patients with chronic obstructive pulmonary disease and cancer who exercise.[123, 133]

TABLE 12–4   EXERCISE STUDIES WITH FATIGUE FINDINGS

Author(s) and Purpose*	Subjects and Procedures	Major Findings
MacVicar & Winningham, 1986[123] Evaluate the effect of a progressive, 10 week, 3 times/week interval-training, cycle-ergometric exercise protocol on the physical and psychological responses of breast cancer patients (functional capacity and mood states)	Ten women with breast cancer receiving chemotherapy without cardiovascular disease and not taking doxorubicin (Adriamycin)-containing regimens Six exercising healthy age-matched controls	Exercising cancer patients demonstrated increases in oxygen uptake and vigor-activity and decreases in total mood disturbance scores. Decreased fatigue scores were reported for the exercising groups; an increased score was reported in the nonexercising patient group.
Pardue, 1984[133] Determine changes in fatigue and energy expenditure in chronic obstructive pulmonary disease patients who participate in a pulmonary rehabilitation program	82 chronic obstructive pulmonary disease patients 15-session, 5-week outpatient course with classes held for 2 hours, 3 days/week, consisting of didactic and practical applications (breathing, retraining, paced walking, individual exercise programs, energy conservation activities, relaxation training)	All subjects experienced significantly less fatigue following the rehabilitation program; the mean difference was greatest for the severe chronic obstructive pulmonary disease group and least for the moderate group. Mental and physical symptoms were reported less frequently than symptoms of general tiredness and decreased exercise tolerance; these symptoms improved as a result of the program.
Thayer, 1987[134] To compare self-rated energy, tiredness, and tension effects of a common sugar snack versus a rapid 10-minute walk	18 undergraduate students Random assignment of sugar snack (1.5 oz. candy) versus walk (10 minutes breathing deeply, swinging arms freely) over 12 experimental days in a 3-week period of time	Majority of subjects felt increased energy for at least 20 minutes; less energy was perceived at 1 and 2 hours after eating a snack. Authors concluded that a 10-minute rapid walk raises energy faster and to a greater degree than the sugar snack and avoids the unpleasant correlate of increased tension from the sugar snack.

Reprinted with permission from Piper, B. F. (1991). Alteration in energy: The sensation of fatigue. In S. B. Baird, R. McCorkle, & M. Grant (eds.), *Cancer Nursing: A Comprehensive Textbook* (p. 905). Philadelphia: W. B. Saunders.
*For complete citation, see the references at the end of the chapter.

In patients with systemic lupus erythematosus, fatigue is reduced significantly by an 8-week aerobic conditioning program.[135] In multiple sclerosis, however, vigorous exercise is thought to make fatigue worse whereas moderate exercise may be beneficial.[136] In one study of multiple sclerosis, a three-times-per-week aquatic exercise program over the course of 10 weeks reduced muscle fatigue in 10 patients.[137] More research is needed to document the effects of exercise on fatigue in clinical populations and to tailor exercise programs according to disease and treatment factors.[80, 138, 139]

Diversional-Distracting Activities

Activities such as reading, listening to music, doing crossword puzzles, and thinking about pleasant things have been identified consistently by patients as being effective in relieving fatigue.[39, 42, 99, 124, 140] These diversional or distracting activities are thought to produce an inflow of nerve impulses from the nonfatigued parts of the body to the facilitatory part of the reticular formation, thus shifting the balance between inhibition of voluntary effort and facilitation to one of facilitation.[65] Decreased "central" fatigue may result.

Experiments have shown that if subjects keep their eyes open during fatiguing activities, more "work" can be performed than if the work is performed with the eyes closed.[65] Alpha rhythms on electroencephalograms are characteristic of lowered arousal and occur when subjects close their eyes. Closing of the eyes is associated with central inhibition by the reticulum formation; opening of the eyes is associated with facilitation. Introducing diverting activities or "active rest" or performing "work" with the eyes open makes this characteristic alpha wave pattern associated with lowered arousal and central fatigue disappear.[65, 66, 141]

Although distraction is generally considered to be helpful in certain pain states, limited data exist on its role in fatigued states. Cimprich tested the effects of a "restorative" intervention program on "attentional capacity" or mental fatigue in women with breast cancer.[124] Subjects self-selected distracting or diversional activities that met certain criteria (i.e., catches a person's interest easily, is enjoyable or pleasureable, involves a change from daily routine, does not require someone else's assistance). Subjects selected activities that more often had to do with the environment or nature, such as gardening, walking in the park, or bird watching. They then contracted with the investigator to do one self-selected restorative activity for 30 minutes three times per week over the course of 3 months. Subjects assigned to the experimental restorative program showed greater gains in attentional capacity and perceived quality of life than did controls. While no measure of whole-body fatigue was used in this study, the results suggest that distracting enjoyable activities performed routinely three times per week for 30 minutes may alleviate mental fatigue and improve concentration and quality of life.[124]

Drug Therapies

A variety of drug therapies have been used to treat fatigue, but most published reports are anecdotal or are limited case study reports.[132] Few randomized clinical trials have been conducted to confirm efficacy of drugs in fatigued clinical populations such as chronic fatigue syndrome.[442] Additionally, drug therapies inevitably have associated side effects, thus limiting their efficacy in the treatment of fatigue. Table 12–5 summarizes data from five studies that have tested the effects of certain medications on subjective fatigue.[10, 143–147]

Amantidine consistently produces significant declines in fatigue in the majority of patients with multiple sclerosis.[146, 148, 149] Pemoline and amitriptyline hydrochloride may also be effective.[40] In healthy subjects and in patients with COPD, theophylline and ami-nophylline may enhance diaphragmatic contractility and reduce susceptibility to respiratory muscle fatigue, but these findings need to be confirmed prospectively in larger clinical samples.[20, 150] Fatigue in fibromyalgia syndrome may be reduced by the administration of serotonin (5-hydroxytryptophan).[151] Methylprednisolone and various amphetamines and their derivatives, such as methylphenidate (Ritalin), have been tested in cancer patients with varying responses.[92]

Energy-Conserving Activities

Qualitative studies consistently document the perceived efficacy of energy-conserving activities. Such activities may include pacing oneself, prescheduling activities, delegating responsibilities, using energy-saving equipment, and organizing the home or workplace to do activities more efficiently and with less effort.[33, 42, 43, 94, 99, 136, 152] Only one study actually tested the effects of a patient education energy conservation program on fatigue. In this study, no significant differences were found in fatigue levels between experimental and control groups.[153]

Energy-Enhancing Activities

Energy-enhancing activities generate increased levels of perceived energy and decreased levels of fatigue.[42] Examples include taking time-out from tiring activities or coworkers;[42] performing diversional activities, such as listening to music, reading, taking a nature walk, or performing a hobby,[124] chanting, socializing, and going for a car ride.[8] Other energy-enhancing activities include aerobic exercise and the interventions described in the following text.

Nutritional Interventions

In high-risk clinical populations, nutritional assessment, referral, and support are considered essential to fatigue management.[20] The reverse also may be true; treatment of fatigue may improve nutritional status in patients and families too tired to eat, shop, or prepare food.

Thirst is a common symptom of fatigue in several studies that have used the Fatigue

TABLE 12–5 DRUG STUDIES WITH FATIGUE FINDINGS

Author(s) and Purpose*	Subjects and Procedures	Major Findings
Ellis & Nasser, 1973[143] To determine if injections of vitamin B_{12} improve the well-being and perception of tiredness in patients who are experiencing fatigue but do not have a deficiency of the vitamin	14 patients and hospital staff with fatigue for which no organic cause could be found Crossover within subject design with random allocation of double-blind 5 mg hydroxycobalamin and placebo, both given intramuscularly	All criteria including the energy item showed a trend in favor of the vitamin B_{12} injections, but only improvement in well-being and happiness were statistically significant.
Hicks, 1964[144] To determine the effect of oral tablets of potassium and magnesium salts of aspartic acid on neuromuscular (chronic) fatigue, strength, and physical activity	145 office patients Double-blind study for 18 months, then code was broken	46% received Spartase (n = 66) 85% of these (n = 56) had a positive effect
McAdoo, Doering, Kraemer, Dessert,[145] Brodie, & Hamburg, 1978 To determine the effects of gonadotropin-releasing hormone (GNRH) given intravenously on human mood behavior and other psychological parameters	12 healthy male paid volunteers Double-blind random assignment design	There was a significant decrease in self-perceived fatigue and drowsiness as measured by the Profile of Mood States (POMS) and Aitkon scales apparent 6 hours after GnRH administration.
Murray, 1985[146] To characterize fatigue in multiple sclerosis patients and to evaluate the effects of various drug therapies on fatigue	40 patients were selected for the amantidine double-blind crossover study; 32 completed the study (6 weeks of drug or placebo, followed by a 1-week rest, followed by the drug or placebo)	Overall improvement was seen in 62.5% of patients taking amantidine and 21.8% taking placebo.
Potempa, 1986[147] To determine if perceptions of fatigue, rate of perceived exertion (RPE), and graded exercise performance differ among mildly hypertensive men	19 stage I and II white male hypertensives Double-blind randomized crossover design	There were no significant differences between mean RPE scores from placebo to drug groups or between drug treatment phases. Fatigue subscale of the POMS did not appear valid or reliable for study. Maximal exercise time did not vary significantly.

Reprinted with permission from Piper, B. F. (1991). Alteration in energy: The sensation of fatigue. In S. B. Baird, R. McCorkle, & M. Grant (eds.), *Cancer Nursing: A Comprehensive Textbook* (p. 904). Philadelphia: W. B. Saunders.

*For complete citation, see the references at the end of the chapter.

Symptom Checklist to measure subjective fatigue.[85] This suggests that there may be merit to "forcing fluids" in these patients to promote the excretion of cell destruction end-products thought to be associated with fatigue.[85]

In healthy subjects, a diet high in carbohydrates 3 days prior to or during prolonged exercise can delay fatigue by slowing the depletion of muscle glycogen stores and protecting against the effects of hypoglycemia.[154] A combination of carbohydrate loading and caffeine ingestion has been shown to improve endurance.[155] Caffeine ingestion may spare muscle glycogen depletion by stimulating free fatty acid mobilization, thus delaying the onset of fatigue,[66] although results from studies are conflicting.[156] Diets that eliminate additives and food allergens have been shown to reduce symptoms of tension and fatigue in children.[157] In an animal model, calcium-rich diets fed to rats delayed the onset of local muscle fatigue.[158] More research is needed in this area, particularly in fatigued clinical populations in whom oral intake or nutritional status may be compromised.

Oxygen Patterns

Enhancement of $\dot{V}O_2$ max occurs in healthy subjects following red blood cell reinfusion, suggesting that improvement in the oxygen-carrying capacity of the blood stream can improve fatigue.[159] Anecdotally, cancer patients report increased energy and decreased fatigue 24 to 36 hours after the administration of packed red blood cell (PRBC) transfusions. Studies are needed to evaluate the effects of PRBCs and erythropoietin[31] and respiratory muscle training programs on fatigue.

Patient and Family Teaching

Since patient and family teaching can enhance a sense of control and mastery over the unfamiliar and reduce anxiety, it follows that patient and family teaching should be able to reduce anxiety-induced fatigue. "Preparatory sensory information" about what patients can expect to feel, sense, or experience as they go through diagnostic testing or treatment has been shown to reduce anxiety in several studies.[160] Thus, "preparatory fatigue teaching" might be beneficial and needs to be tested as an intervention. Teaching should include the types of symptoms that may be experienced (mental and cognitive, physical, emotional, behavioral); when these symptoms might be expected to occur (onset, pattern, duration, and frequency); and what other individuals have found useful in the prevention and alleviation of fatigue.[18, 161] Emphasis should be placed on early recognition and reporting of unusual levels of fatigue so that interventions can be instituted immediately to prevent fatigue from becoming chronic.[161]

Teaching should also focus on enabling the patient or family member to think about personal energy stores as a bank.[1, 18] Deposits and withdrawals need to be made over the course of a day or week to ensure that a balance is achieved between energy expenditure and energy conservation and restoration.[1, 18] Conducting periodic "energy audits," the process by which a person takes stock of existing energy reserves and "parcels or rations" energy toward activities left to do, may be helpful.[42]

Psychological Patterns

Two prospective studies suggest that, at least in early stage malignant melanoma[41] and metastatic breast cancer,[162] weekly attendance at a professionally led psychological support group for 6 weeks or longer may decrease fatigue and increase survival time.[163]

Respiratory Muscle Training Programs

Ingersoll reviewed the efficacy of respiratory muscle training studies in the treatment of respiratory muscle fatigue and failure.[20] Several studies focused on resting the respiratory muscles while they recovered by using negative pressure body respirators or by administering positive pressure ventilation via tracheostomies; other studies focused on improving respiratory muscle strength and endurance by using maximal inspiratory breathing devices or repeated runs of normocapnic hyperventilation. Ingersoll concluded that additional studies were needed before respiratory training programs could be considered therapeutic for the treatment of respiratory muscle fatigue.[20]

Rest

Few research studies formally describe or measure different types of rest; no studies have determined the effects of rest on fatigue. Table 12–6 summarizes data from three rest studies.[164–166] Altieri found that the pressure-rate product (multiplying the heart rate times the systolic blood pressure and dividing the product by 100) was a useful way to pace activities and determine rest periods for cardiac patients.[164] More studies describing and quantifying rest such as these are needed. Although rest is frequently viewed as an energy-conserving or energy-enhancing activity, too much rest is considered detrimental, particularly if it leads to a cycle of decreased energy and increased inactivity.[80]

Sleep-Nap Patterns

Clinical studies continue to document anecdotally the perception that napping and resting are among the most frequently tried and useful self-initiated interventions for fatigue.[8, 39, 136] Unfortunately, studies in clinical populations linking fatigue with sleep are limited.[23]

TABLE 12–6   REST STUDIES

Author(s) and Purpose*	Subjects and Procedures	Major Findings
Altieri, 1984[164] Determine adequate rest periods after activities of daily living during the immediate post–myocardial infarction (MI) period	10 male MI patients 8–20 days after infarction ($\bar{x}$ = 13.5 days) Rest defined as the amount of time needed for 90% of the patient's pressure rate product (peak systolic blood pressure × heart rate) to return to baseline	Adequate rest periods: After showering, 30.5 minutes After stair climbing, 7 minutes After walking, 10 minutes Showering required greater use of arm work than either stair climbing or walking; therefore, greater blood pressure and heart rate changes were found with this activity, requiring a greater rest period for recovery.
Bruya, 1981[165] Determine the effects of planned rest periods versus no planned rest periods following specific nursing care activities on intracranial pressure in intensive care unit patients	20 patients; 17 were male Mean age: 33 years (males); 36 years (females) 10 minutes of uninterrupted rest between nursing activities of vital signs, hyperventilation, suction, oral care, and bed, bath, and hygiene routines for experimental group; 10 minutes of rest only after all three activities for control group	10-minute rest periods did not affect intracranial pressure as anticipated; increased intracranial pressure was reported during the rest periods. 10-minute rest periods may be an insufficient time period to provide "rest." What constitutes rest needs to be determined, because rest may be more than simply being left alone.
Daiss, Bertelson, & Benjamin, 1986[166] Investigate the effects of nap taking and resting on performance and mood	94 male and female university students in a sleep laboratory Habitual nappers and non-nappers (½ to 2 hours 3 times/week) were randomly assigned to each of three groups: napping, resting in bed without falling asleep, or watching a neutral videotape (control group)	Sleep itself may not be the critical variable; rather, the act of lying down and relaxing may help in decreasing negative affect. Nap taking may provide an outlet for daily stress, which may influence mood states.

Reprinted with permission from Piper, B. F. (1991). Alteration in energy: The sensation of fatigue. In S. B. Baird, R. McCorkle, & M. Grant (eds.), *Cancer Nursing: A Comprehensive Textbook* (p. 905). Philadelphia: W. B. Saunders.

*For complete citation, see the references at the end of the chapter.

CASE STUDIES

CASE STUDY NO. 1

A 34-year-old married Brazilian woman was interviewed in a San Francisco hospital through a translator after she had requested a consultation for her fatigue. She had been hospitalized for 3 weeks to receive chemotherapy for multiple myeloma. Her husband and two young children remained in Brazil. At the time she was interviewed, she was running high fevers with positive blood cultures and was receiving total parenteral nutrition (TPN) and multiple intravenous antibiotics.

She described her fatigue as having started 1 week prior to the interview, coincident with chemotherapy-induced bone marrow suppression. Her fatigue was very unusual for her, in that it was constant and did not seem to fluctuate during the

day. "There is no end to it; it is continuous" (temporal dimension). The intensity of fatigue was rated as "more than a 10" on a 0 to 10 scale. "My fatigue is different from tiredness; it is extreme." Her fatigue symptoms included an overwhelming sense of whole-body fatigue. "I have no strength or force. I can't open my eyes without a great deal of effort. I feel separated from things and feel that my mind and spirit can't fight this fatigue. I feel that I'm losing control over my own body" (sensory dimension).

"I think that the fever and infection are the primary causes of my fatigue at this point. The doctors keep wanting to tell me that it is all in my head; that it is psychological because I am depressed because I might die and because I am separated from my husband and children. But I know better. It is not in my head. It is a profound whole-body fatigue that is overwhelming me and is very frightening [affective dimension]. Trying to convince my doctors that there is a physical reason for my fatigue is making me very tired."

Nothing she had tried to do relieved her fatigue. She was afraid to use relaxation or visual imagery to treat her fatigue for fear that it might cause her to lose control over her body; that she already was fighting with everything that she could "mentally and spiritually." Medically, her fatigue began to subside as soon as her infection and fever responded to changes made in her antibiotic therapy.

This case illustrates the multicausal nature of fatigue, how medical therapies and effective symptom management can affect fatigue, and the importance of determining the patient's perspective about what is causing the fatigue. Perceived causes of fatigue frequently influence perceptions about the effectiveness of certain interventions. On the basis of her disease status and life style patterns, walking and swimming were recommended for this patient as the best forms of aerobic exercise to build endurance for subsequent cycles of chemotherapy.

CASE STUDY NO. 2

Margo, a 71-year-old woman living with her husband in a retirement community in Florida, complained of chronic fatigue since the diagnosis of non-A, non-B hepatitis 6 months prior to her consultation. Always a self-described "high-energy" person until her fatigue became chronic, Margo was severely bothered by her fatigue because it limited her activities. She had difficulty adjusting to this reduced energy level and pacing herself. On rare occasions, she was able to plan deliberately to take it "easier one day" so that she could do something that required extra energy the next day.

This difficulty in pacing herself is not uncommon in people who are tired; it is particularly common in people like Margo who describe themselves as high-energy people before their illnesses. This has obvious implications for nursing practice and future research. As another self-described "high energy" person with rheumatoid arthritis stated: "Most often my fatigue comes from overdoing. After all my years of living with rheumatoid arthritis, I still find it difficult to pace myself. I don't always heed the signals of pain and fatigue. I am generally driven to accomplish whatever I undertake; when I am feeling good, I push myself too hard"[42] (p. 68).

With minimal instruction, Margo was able to maintain a fatigue diary for 1 week to determine if there were any patterns to her fatigue or activity. In this diary, she recorded the intensity of fatigue upon awakening and continued to record intensities and activities at 2-hour intervals until she fell asleep. She also recorded any insights about her fatigue.

A visual graph of her intensity-activity patterns for the week revealed that she routinely became tired immediately before every meal, again at 4 p.m., and whenever she socialized with others. Her fatigue patterns did not vary by day of the week. She realized that her fatigue was accentuated during social activities by her wanting to make the extra effort to be her "usual self and not by accepting her current limitations." By gaining insight into these behaviors, she was able to sit down rather than stand up while socializing to conserve her energy. She increased her complex carbohydrate intake and began eating six smaller, more frequent meals per day to reduce her fatigue associated with hypoglycemia.

REVIEW OF RESEARCH FINDINGS

In addition to the research findings that have been integrated throughout this chapter, several review articles are particularly recommended for additional reading.[12, 20, 23, 66]

IMPLICATIONS FOR RESEARCH

Assessment and Measurement

There continues to be a need to develop and test valid and reliable measures for fatigue in order to compare patterns across clinically diverse populations, to identify cultural differences, and to differentiate between fatigue and related concepts such as weakness and aesthenia, malaise, exertion, and depression. Particularly, there is a need to develop instruments that can be used in clinical settings. Studies are needed to document circadian patterns of fatigue, to determine whether chronic fatigue has a circadian pattern or is continuous in nature, and confirm whether depressed subjects truly are more fatigued in the mornings upon awakening, as the literature suggests.

Priority should be given to collaborative, multidisciplinary studies that investigate correlations between subjective and objective indicators of fatigue. Cross-disciplinary publication of such findings is also needed to speed knowledge development.[18] Further research into the behavioral manifestations of fatigue is warranted.

Documentation of Patterns

While basic research must continue to investigate normal peripheral fatigue mechanisms, increased attention needs to be given to the study of central fatigue. Studies need to investigate how central and peripheral fatigue mechanisms interact and influence fatigue manifestations and to determine how normal fatigue mechanisms are affected by disease or treatment. More longitudinal, prospective studies are needed that compare clinical populations to matched, healthy controls over time and to distinguish between tiredness and acute and chronic fatigue states.

Intervention Studies

Lastly, intervention studies are needed to prevent or ameliorate fatigue. As discussed previously, studies that test interventions involving some form of activity modulation hold the most promise (rest, exercise, pacing, delegating, or prescheduling activities). Other promising avenues include modulating psychological patterns (testing diversional activities, preparatory sensory information, support groups), nutritional patterns (increasing complex carbohydrate intake, forcing fluids), and symptom cluster patterns (exploring relationships between fatigue and pain and dyspnea and cachexia and determining how effective treatment of these states may affect fatigue patterns). In conclusion, although much has occurred since this chapter appeared in the first edition of this book in 1986,[167] much more work needs to be done to effectively recognize and treat fatigue in clinical populations.

REFERENCES

1. Piper, B. F., Lindsey, A. M., & Dodd, M. J. (1987). Fatigue mechanisms in cancer patients: Developing nursing theory. Oncol Nurs Forum *14*:17–23.
2. Eidelman, D. (1980). Fatigue: Towards an analysis and unified definition. Med Hypotheses *6*:517–526.
3. Grandjean, E. P. (1970). Yant memorial lecture. Am Industrial Hygiene Assoc J *31*:401–411.
4. Bartley, S. H., & Chute, E. (1947). *Fatigue and Impairment in Man*. New York: McGraw-Hill.
5. Cameron, C. (1973). A theory of fatigue. Ergonomics *16*:633–648.
6. McFarland, R. A. (1971). Understanding fatigue in modern life. Ergonomics *14*:1–10.
7. Muncie, W. (1941). Chronic fatigue. Psychosom Med, *3*:277–285.
8. Piper, B. F. (1988). Fatigue in cancer patients: Current perspectives on measurement and management. In *Nursing Management of Common Problems: State of the Art. Proceedings of the Fifth National Conference on Cancer Nursing*. New York: American Cancer Society.
9. Poteliakhoff, A. (1981). Adrenocortical activity and some clinical findings in acute and chronic fatigue. J Psychosom Res *25*:91–95.
10. Potempa, K., Lopez, M., Reid, C., & Lawson, L. (1986). Chronic fatigue. Image, *18*:165–169.
11. Riddle, P. K. (1982). Chronic fatigue and women: A description and suggested treatment. Women Health *7*:37–47.
12. Roberts, D., & Smith, D. J. (1989). Biochemical aspects of peripheral muscle fatigue. Sports Med *7*:125–138.
13. Rockwell, D. A., & Burr, W. D. (1977). The tired patient. J Fam Pract *5*:853–857.
14. Kirk, J., Douglass, R., Nelson, E., Jaffe, J., Lopez, A., Ohler, J., Blanchard, C., Chapman, R., McHugo, G., & Stone, K. (1990). Chief complaint of fatigue: A prospective study. J Fam Prac *30*:33–41.
15. Komaroff, A. L., & Goldenberg, D. (1989). The chronic fatigue syndrome: Definition, current studies and lessons for fibromyalgia research. J Rheumatol *19*(Suppl.):23–27.
16. Holmes, G. P., Kaplan, J. E., Gantz, N. M., Komaroff, A. L., Schonberger, L. B., Straus, S. E., Jones, J. F., Dubois, R. E., Cunningham-Rundles, C., Pahwa, S., Tosato, G., Zegans, L. S., Purtilo, D. T., Brown, N., Schooley, R. T., & Brus, I. (1988). Chronic fatigue syndrome: A working case definition. Ann Intern Med *108*:387–389.
17. Carpenito, L. J. (1992). *Nursing Diagnosis: Application to Practice* (4th ed.). Philadelphia: J. B. Lippincott.
18. Piper, B. F. (1991). Alterations in energy: The sensation of fatigue. In S. B. Baird, R. McCorkle, & M. Grant (eds.), *Cancer Nursing: A Comprehensive Textbook* (pp. 894–908). Philadelphia: W. B. Saunders.
19. Gibson, H., & Edwards, R. H. T. (1985). Muscular exercise and fatigue. Sports Med *2*:120–132.
20. Ingersoll, G. L. (1989). Respiratory muscle fatigue

research: Implications for clinical practice. Appl Nurs Res 2:6–15.

21. Bigland-Ritchie, B., & Woods, J. J. (1984). Changes in muscle contractile properties and neural control during human muscular fatigue. Muscle Nerve 7:691–699.

22. Vollestad, N. K., & Sejersted, O. M. (1988). Biochemical correlates of fatigue. Eur J Appl Physiol 57:336–347.

23. Irvine, D. M., Vincent, L., Bubela, N., Thompson, L., & Graydon, J. (1991). A critical appraisal of the research literature investigating fatigue in the individual with cancer. Cancer Nurs 14:188–199.

24. Cypress, B. K. (1977). Office visits to internists: National ambulatory medical survey, United States 1975. *Advance Data, from Vital and Health Statisics.* (No. 16. DHEW publication No. [PHS] 78-1250.) Hyattsville, MD: National Center for Health Statistics.

25. Kroenke, K., Wood, D. R., Mangelsdorff, A. D., Meier, N. J., & Powell, J. B. (1988). Chronic fatigue in primary care: Prevalence, patient characteristics, and outcome. *JAMA* 260:929–934.

26. Manu, P., Lane, T. J., & Matthews, D. A. (1988). The frequency of the chronic fatigue syndrome in patients with symptoms of persistent fatigue. Ann Intern Med 109:554–556.

27. Lane, T. J., Manu, P., & Matthews, D. (1988). Prospective diagnostic evaluation of adults with chronic fatigue (abstract). Clin Res 316:714.

28. Piper, B. F., Dibble, S., & Dodd, M. J. (1991). Fatigue patterns and theoretical model testing in cancer patients receiving chemotherapy (Abstract 190A). Oncol Nurs Forum 18:348.

29. Lee, E. H. (1991). A study on the change in degree of fatigue with the elapse of radiation therapy in cancer patients. M.A. thesis. Yonsei University, Seoul, Korea.

30. King, K. B., Nail, L. M., Kreamer, K., Strohl, R. A., & Johnson, J. E. (1985). Patients' descriptions of the experience of receiving radiation therapy. Oncol Nurs Forum 12:55–61.

31. Piper, B. F., Rieger, P. T., Brophy, L., Haeuber, D., Hood, L. E., Lyver, A., & Sharp, E. (1989). Recent advances in the management of biotherapy-related side effects: Fatigue. Oncol Nurs Forum 16:27–34.

32. Jensen, S., & Given, B. A. (1991). Fatigue affecting family caregivers of cancer patients. Cancer Nurs 14:181–187.

33. Srivastava, R. H. (1989). Fatigue in end-stage renal disease patients. In S. G. Funk, E. M. Tournquist, M. T. Champagne, L. A. Copp, & R. A. Weise (eds.) *Key Aspects of Comfort: Management of Pain, Fatigue, and Nausea* (pp. 217–224). New York: Springer.

34. Cardenas, D. D., & Kutner, N. G. (1982). The problem of fatigue in dialysis patients. Nephron 30:336–340.

35. Petersson, B., Wernerman, J., Waller, S. O., von der Decken, A., & Vinnars, E. (1990). Elective abdominal surgery depresses muscle protein synthesis and increases subjective fatigue: Effects lasting more than 30 days. Br J Surg 77:796–800.

36. Kehlet, H. (1988). Anesthetic technique and surgical convalescence. Acta Chir Scand Suppl 550: 182–191.

37. Appels, A., & Mulder, P. (1988). Excess fatigue as a precursor of myocardial infarction. Eur Heart J 9:758–764.

38. Feinstein, A. R., Fisher, M. B., & Pigeon, J. G. (1989). Changes in dyspnea-fatigue ratings as indicators of quality of life in the treatment of congestive heart failure. Am J Cardiol 64:50–55.

39. Schaefer, K. M. (1990). A description of fatigue associated with congestive heart failure: Use of Levine's conservation model. In M. Parker (ed.), *Nursing Theories in Practice* (pp. 217–237). New York: N.L.N. Pub. No. 15-2350.

40. Krupp, L. B., Alvarez, L. A., LaRocca, N. G., & Scheinberg, L. C. (1988). Fatigue in multiple sclerosis. Arch Neurol 45:435–437.

41. Fawzy, F. I., Cousins, N., Fawzy, N. W., & Kemeny, M. E. (1990). A structured psychiatric intervention for cancer patients. Arch Gen Psychiatry 47:720–725.

42. Tack, B. B. (1990). Fatigue in rheumatoid arthritis: Conditions, strategies, and consequences. Arthritis Care Res 3:65–70.

43. Tack, B. B. (1990). Self-reported fatigue in rheumatoid arthritis. Arthritis Care Res 3:154–157.

44. Cavanaugh, R. M. (1987). Evaluating adolescents with fatigue. Am Fam Physician 35:163–168.

45. Klumpp, T. (1976). Some thoughts on fatigue in older patients. Med Times 104:87–93.

46. Cassel, W., & Archer-Duste, H. (1989). The new epidemic: Chronic fatigue syndrome. Calif Nurse 89:6–7.

47. Bell, K. M., Cookfair, D., Bell, D. S., Reeses, P., & Cooper, L. (1991). Risk factors associated with chronic fatigue syndrome in a cluster of pediatric cases. Rev Infect Dis 13(Suppl. 1):S32–8.

48. DeFreitas, E., Hilliard, B., Cheney, P. R., Bell, D. S., Kiggundu, E., Sankey, D., Wroblewska, Z., Palladino, M., Woodward, J. P., & Koprowski, H. (1991). Retroviral sequences related to human T-lymphotropic virus type II in patients with chronic fatigue immune dysfunction syndrome. Proc Natl Acad Sci USA 88:2922–2926.

49. Marshall, G. S., Gesser, R. M., Yamanishi, K., & Starr, S. E. (1991). Chronic fatigue in children: Clinical features, Epstein-Barr virus and human herpesvirus 6 serology and long-term follow-up. Pediatr Infect Dis J 10:287–290.

50. Smith, M. S., Mitchell, J., Corey, L., Gold, D., McCauley, E. A., Glover, D., & Tenover, F. C. (1991). Chronic fatigue in adolescents. Pediatrics 88:195–202.

51. Haylock, P. J., & Hart, L. K. (1979). Fatigue in patients receiving localized radiation. Cancer Nurs 2:461–467.

52. Pickard-Holley, S. (1991). Fatigue in cancer patients: A descriptive study. Cancer Nurs 14:13–19.

53. Valdini, A. F., Steinhardt, S., Valicenti, J., & Jaffe, A. (1988). A one-year follow-up of fatigued patients. J Fam Pract 26:33–38.

54. Ridsdale, L. (1989). Chronic fatigue in family practice. J Fam Pract 29:486–488.

55. Fawcett, J., & York, R. (1986). Spouses' physical and psychological symptoms during pregnancy and the postpartum. Nurs Res 35:144–148.

56. Pugh, L. C. (1989). *Psychophysiological Correlates of Fatigue During Childbirth.* Doctoral dissertation. Baltimore: University of Maryland.

57. Pitzer, M. (1991). Patterns of fatigue and physiological factors during pregnancy: Their relationship to preterm labor/birth. *Proceedings of the 1991*

International Research Conference: Nursing Research: Global Health Perspectives (p. 429). Kansas City: ANA Council of Nurse Researchers.

58. Cohen, F. L., & Hardin, S. B. (1989). Fatigue in patients with catastrophic illness. In S. G. Funk, E. M. Tournquist, M. T. Champagne, L. A. Copp, & R. A. Weise (eds.), *Key Aspects of Comfort: Management of Pain, Fatigue, and Nausea* (pp. 208–216). New York: Springer.

59. Putt, A. M. (1977). Effects of noise on fatigue in healthy middle-aged adults. Commun Nurs Res 8:24–34.

60. Tack, B. B. (1991). Fatigue in rheumatoid arthritis: Dimensions and correlates. In *Proceedings of the 1991 International Nursing Research Conference: Nursing Research: Global Health Perspectives* (p. 407). Kansas City: ANA Council of Nurse Researchers.

61. Krupp, L. B., LaRocca, N. G., Muir-Nash, J., & Steinberg, A. (1989). The fatigue severity scale: Application to patients with multiple sclerosis and systemic lupus erythematosus. Arch Neurol 46:1121–1123.

62. Blumenthal, M. D. (1980). Depressive illness in old age: Getting behind the mask. Geriatrics 35:34–43.

63. Fatigue. (1988). Lancet (editorial). 2:546–548.

64. Aistars, J. (1987). Fatigue in the cancer patient: A conceptual approach to a clinical problem. Oncol Nurs Forum 14:25–30.

65. Asmussen, E. (1979). Muscle fatigue. Med Sci Sports Exerc 11:313–321.

66. Maclaren, D. P. M., Gibson, H., Parry-Billings, M., & Edwards, R. H. T. (1989). A review of metabolic and physiological factors in fatigue. Exerc Sport Sci Rev 17:29–66.

67. Newsholme, E. A., Acworth, I. N., & Blomstrand, E. (1987). Amino acids, brain neurotransmitters and a functional link between muscle and brain that is important in sustained exercise. In G. Benzi (ed.), *Advances in Myochemistry* (pp. 127–133), London: John Libbey.

68. Edwards, R. H. T., & Jones, D. A. (1983). Diseases of skeletal muscle. In D. Peachey, R. H. Adrian, & S. R. Geiger (eds.), *Handbook of Physiology: Skeletal Muscle* (pp. 633–672), Baltimore: Williams & Wilkins.

69. Simonson, E. (1971). *Physiology of Work Capacity and Fatigue*. Springfield, IL: Charles C Thomas.

70. Friedland, J., & Paterson, D. (1988). Potassium and fatigue. Letter to the editor. Lancet 2:961–962.

71. Miller, R. G., Boska, M. D., Moussavi, R. S., Carson, P. J., & Weiner, M. W. (1988). 31P nuclear magnetic resonance studies of high energy phosphates and pH in human muscle fatigue. J Clin Invest 81:1190–1196.

72. Simpson, W. T. (1977). Nature and effects of unwanted effects with atenolol. Post Med J 53 (Suppl. 3):162–167.

73. Rosse, R. B. (1989). Fatigue in multiple sclerosis. (Letter to the editor.) Arch Neurol 46:841–842.

74. Fatigue disorder linked to immune response: Overactive T-cells may cause syndrome (1991). *San Francisco Chronicle*, Sept. 20, p. A2.

75. Unraveling chronic fatigue. (1992) *Marin Independent Journal*, Jan. 15, p. A 6.

76. Poole, C. J. (1986). Fatigue during the first trimester of pregnancy. J Obst Gynecol Neonatal Nurs 15:375–379.

77. Church, J. M., Choong, B. Y., & Hill, G. L. (1986). Abnormal muscle fructose biphosphatase activity in malnourished cancer patients. Cancer 58:2448–2452.

78. Astrand, P., & Rodahl, K. (1986). *Textbook of Work Physiology* (3rd ed.). New York: McGraw-Hill.

79. Wegner, N. K. L., & Hellerstein, H. K. (1984). *Rehabilitation of the Coronary Patient*. New York: John Wiley.

80. Winningham, M. L. (1991). Walking program for people with cancer: Getting started. Cancer Nurs 14:270–276.

81. Oligati, R., Jacquet, J., & Di Prampero, P. E. (1986). Energy cost of walking and exertional dyspnea in multiple sclerosis. Am Rev Respir Dis 134:1005–1010.

82. Hart, L. K. (1978). Fatigue in the patient with multiple sclerosis. Res Nurs Health 1:147–157.

83. Jamar, S. C. (1989). Fatigue in women receiving chemotherapy for ovarian cancer. In S. G. Funk, E. M. Tournquist, M. T. Champagne, L. A. Copp, & R. A. Weise (eds.), *Key Aspects of Comfort: Management of Pain, Fatigue, and Nausea* (pp. 224–233). New York: Springer.

84. Demetriack, M. A., Dale, J. K., Straus, S. E., Laue, L., Listwak, S. J., Kruesi, M. J. P., Chrousos, G. P., & Gold, P. W. (1991). Evidence for impaired activation of the hypothalamic-pituitary-adrenal axis in patients with chronic fatigue syndrome. J Clin Endocrinol Metabol 73:1224–1234.

85. Piper, B. F., Lee, H. O., Kim, O., Pak, Y., & Kim, O. (1991). Fatigue—Transcultural implications for nursing interventions. In A. P. Pritchard (ed.), *Cancer Nursing: The Balance. Proceedings of the Sixth International Conference on Cancer Nursing, Amsterdam* (pp. 140–144). Middlesex, England: Scutari Press.

86. Levy, S. M., Herberman, R. B., Maluish, A. M., Schlien, B., & Lippman, M. (1985). Prognostic risk assessment in primary breast cancer by behavioral and immunological parameters. Health Psychol 4:99–113.

87. Kukell, W. A., McCorkle, R., & Driever, M. (1986). Symptom distress, psychosocial variables, and survival from lung cancer. J Psychosocial Oncol 4:91–104.

88. Temoshok, L. (1987). In consultation: Discussion of psychosocial factors related to outcome in cutaneous malignant melanoma: A matched samples design. Oncol News/Update 2:6–7.

89. Norris, C. M. (1982). Synthesis of concepts: Evolving an umbrella concept-protection. In C. M. Norris (ed.), *Concept Clarification in Nursing* (pp. 385–403). Rockville, MD: Aspen Systems.

90. Fuerstein, A. I. A., Carter, R. L., & Papciak, A. S. (1987). A prospective analysis of stress and fatigue in recurrent low back pain. Pain 31:333–344.

91. Bruera, E., Brennis, C., Michaud, M., Rafter, J., Magnan, A., Tennant, A., Hanson, J., & MacDonald, R. N. (1989). Association between nutritional status, lean body mass, anemia, psychological status, and tumor mass in patients with advanced breast cancer. J Pain Symptom Manage 4:59–63.

92. Bruera, E., & MacDonald, R. N. (1988). Overwhelming fatigue in advanced cancer. Am J Nurs 88:99–100.

93. Theologides, A. (1982). Asthenia in cancer. Am J Med 73:1–3.

94. Monks, J. (1989). Experiencing symptoms in

chronic illness: Fatigue in multiple sclerosis. Int Disabil Stud *11*:78–82.

95. Borg, G. A. V. (1962). *Physical Performance and Perceived Exertion*. Copenhagen: Ejnor Munksgaard.

96. Rieger, P. T. (1986). Interferon-induced fatigue. M.A. thesis. Houston: University of Texas Health Science Center.

97. Goldstein, V., Regnery, G., & Wellin, E. (1981). Caretaker role fatigue. Nurs Outlook *29*:24–30.

98. Kobashi-Schoot, J. A. M., Hanewald, G. J. F. P., Van Dam, F. S. A. M., & Bruning, P. F. (1985). Assessment of malaise in cancer patients treated with radiation therapy. Cancer Nurs *8*:306–313.

99. Piper, B. F., Lindsey, A. M., Dodd, M. J., Ferketich, S., Paul, S. M., & Weller, S. (1989). The development of an instrument to measure the subjective dimension of fatigue. In S. G. Funk, E. M. Tournquist, M. T. Champagne, L. A. Copp, & R. A. Weise (eds.), *Key Aspects of Comfort: Management of Pain, Fatigue, and Nausea* (pp. 199–208). New York: Springer.

100. McCorkle, R., Benoliel, J. Q., & Donaldson, G. (1979–1981). *A Manual of Data Collection Instruments*. Seattle: University of Washington, Community Health Care Systems.

101. McCorkle, R., & Young, K. (1978). Development of a symptom distress scale. Cancer Nurs *5*:373–378.

102. Rhodes, V. A., Watson, P. M., & Johnson, M. H. (1984). Development of reliable and valid measures of nausea and vomiting. Cancer Nurs *6*:33–41.

103. McNair, D. M., Lorr, M., & Droppleman, L. F. (1971). *Profile of Mood States*. San Diego: Education and Testing Service.

104. Shachem, S. (1983). A shortened version of the Profile of Mood States. J Pers Assess *47*:305–306.

105. Lee, H. O. (1991). Fatigue—Transcultural issues in assessment and measurement. In A. P. Pritchard (ed.), *Cancer Nursing: The Balance. Proceedings of the Sixth International Conference on Cancer Nursing, Amsterdam* (pp. 138–140). Middlesex, England: Scutari Press.

106. Pearson, R. G. (1957). Scale analysis of a fatigue checklist. J Appl Psychol *41*:186–191.

107. Pearson, R. G., & Byars, G. E. (1956). *The Development and Validation of a Checklist for Measuring Subjective Fatigue* (pp. 56–115). Randolph AFB, TX: Texas School of Aviation Medicine, USAF.

108. Davis, C. A. (1984). Interferon-induced fatigue. Oncol Nurs Forum *11*(Suppl.):872. Abstract No. 72.

109. Freel, M. I., & Hart, L. K. (1977). *Study of Fatigue Phenomena of Multiple Sclerosis Patients* (USDHEW Grant No. 5R02-NU-00524-02). Iowa City: University of Iowa, Division of Nursing.

110. Lee, K. A., Hicks, G., & Nino-Murcia, G. (1991). Validity and reliability of a scale to assess fatigue. Psychiatry Res *36*:291–298.

111. Yoshitake, H. (1969). Rating the feelings of fatigue. J Sci Labour *45*:422–432.

112. Yoshitake, H. (1971). Relations between the symptoms and the feeling of fatigue. Ergonomics *14*:175–186.

113. Yoshitake, H. (1978). Three characteristic patterns of subjective fatigue symptoms. Ergonomics *21*:231–233.

114. Milligan, R. (1989). Maternal fatigue during the first three months of the postpartum period. Ph.D. dissertation. Baltimore: University of Maryland.

115. Piper, B. F., Friedman, L., Hartigan, K, Post, B., Smith, J., Coleman, C. A., Gilman, N., Dodd, M. J., Lindsey, A. M., & Paul, S. (in review). Fatigue patterns over time in women receiving CMF chemotherapy for breast cancer.

116. Pugh, L. C. (1991). The measurement of a multidimensional concept: Fatigue. *Proceedings of the 1991 International Nursing Research Conference: Nursing Research: Global Health Perspectives* (p. 428). Kansas City: ANA Council of Nurse Researchers.

117. Rhoten, D. (1982). Fatigue and the postsurgical patient. In C. M. Norris (ed.), *Concept Clarification in Nursing* (pp. 277–300). Rockville, MD: Aspen Systems.

118. Akerstedt, T., Gillberg, M., & Witterberg, L. (1982). The circadian covariation of fatigue and urinary melatonin. Biol Psychiatry *17*:547–554.

119. Arendt, D., Borbely, A. A., Franey, C., & Wright, J. (1984). The effects of chronic, small doses of melatonin given in the late afternoon on fatigue in man: A preliminary study. Neurosci Lett *45*:317–321.

120. Burton, R. R. (1980). Human responses to repeated high G simulated aerial combat maneuvers. Aviat Space Environ Med *51*:1185–1192.

121. Miller, R. G., Giannini, D., Milner-Brown, H. S., Layzer, R. B., Koretsky, A. P., Hooper, D., & Weiner, M. W. (1987). Effects of fatiguing exercise on high-energy phosphates, force and EMG: Evidence for three phases of recovery. Muscle Nerve *10*:810–821.

122. Heuting, J. E., & Sarphati, H. R. (1966). Measuring fatigue. J Appl Physiol *50*:535–538.

123. MacVicar, M. G., & Winningham, M. L. (1986). Promoting functional capacity of cancer patients. Cancer Bull *38*:235–239.

124. Cimprich, B. E. (1990). Attentional fatigue and restoration in individuals with cancer. Ph.D. dissertation. Ann Arbor: University of Michigan.

125. Wilkie, D. J., Lovejoy, N., Dodd, M. J., & Tesler, M. D. (1989). Pain control behaviors of patients with cancer. In S. G. Funk, E. M. Tournquist, M. T. Champagne, L. A. Copp, & R. A. Weise (eds.), *Key Aspects of Comfort: Management of Pain, Fatigue, and Nausea* (pp. 119–126). New York: Springer.

126. Christensen, T., Hougard, F., & Kehlet, H. (1985). Influence or pre- and intra-operative factors on the occurence of postoperative fatigue. Br J Surg *72*:63–65.

127. Christensen, T., Bendix, T, & Kehlet, H. (1982). Fatigue and cardiorespiratory function following abdominal surgery. Br J Surg *69*:417–419.

128. Christensen, T., Stage, J. G., Galbo H., Christensen, N. J., & Kehlet, H. (1989). Fatigue and cardiac and endocrine metabolic response to exercise after abdominal surgery. Surgery *105*:46–50.

129. Christensen, T., Nygaard, E., & Kehlet, H. (1988). Skeletal muscle fiber composition, nutritional status and subjective fatigue during surgical convalescence. Acta Chir Scand *154*:335–338.

130. Leikin, L., Firestone, P., & McGrath, P. (1988). Physical symptom reporting in type A and type B children. J Consult Clin Psychol *56*:721–726.

131. Hart, 1. K., Freel, M. I., & Milde, F. K. (1990). Fatigue. Nurs Clin North Am *25*:967–976.

132. Piper, B. F. (1989). Fatigue: Current bases for practice. In S. G. Funk, E. M. Tournquist, M. T.

Champagne, L. A. Copp, & R. A. Weise (eds.), *Key Aspects of Comfort: Management of Pain, Fatigue, and Nausea* (pp. 187–198). New York: Springer.

133. Pardue, N. H. (1984). Energy expenditure and subjective fatigue of chronic obstructive pulmonary disease patients before and after a pulmonary rehabilitation. Doctoral dissertation. Washington, D.C.: Catholic University.

134. Thayer, R. E. (1987). Energy, tiredness, and tension effects of a sugar snack versus moderate exercise. J Pers Soc Psychol 52:119–125.

135. Robb-Nicholson, L. C., Daltroy, L., Eaton, H., Gall, V., Wright, E., Hartley, L. H., Schur, P. H., & Liang, M. H. (1989). Effects of aerobic conditioning in lupus fatigue: A pilot study. Br J Rheumatol 28:500–505.

136. Freal, J. F., Kraft, G. H., & Coryell, J. K. (1984). Symptomatic fatigue in multiple sclerosis. *Arch Phys Med Rehabil* 65:135–138.

137. Gehlsen, G. M., Grigsby, S. A., & Winant, D. M. (1984). Effects of an aquatic fitness program on the muscular strength and endurance of patients with multiple sclerosis. Phys Therapy 64:653–657.

138. MacVicar, M. G., Winningham, M. L., & Nickel, J. L. (1989). Effects of aerobic interval training on cancer patients' functional capacity. Nurs Res 38:348–351.

139. Piper, B. F. (1991). The effect of exercise on fatigue, depression and mood states in women with breast cancer receiving radiation therapy. In *Proceedings of the 1991 International Nursing Research Conference: Nursing Research: Global Health Perspectives* (p. 408). Kansas City: ANA Council of Nurse Researchers.

140. Namir, S., Wolcott, D. L., Fawzy, F. I., & Alumbagh, M. J. (1987). Coping with AIDS: Psychological and health implications. J Appl Psychol 17:309–328.

141. Rojtbak, A. J., & Dedabrishvili, C. M. (1959). On the mechanism of active rest. Dik Akad Nauk USSR 124:957–960.

142. Gantz, N. M., & Holmes, G. P. (1989). Treatment of patients with chronic fatigue syndrome. Drugs 38:855–862.

143. Ellis, F. R., & Nasser, S. (1973). A pilot study of vitamin B-12 in the treatment of tiredness. Br J Nutr 30:277–283.

144. Hicks, J. T. (1964). Treatment of fatigue in general practice: A double-blind study. Clin Med 71:85–90.

145. McAdoo, B. C., Doering, C. H., Kraemer, H. C., Dessert, N., Brodie, H. K. H., & Hamburg, D. A. (1978). A study of the effects of gonadotropin-releasing hormone on human mood and behavior. Psychosom Med 40:199–209.

146. Murray, T. J. (1985). Amantidine therapy for fatigue in multiple sclerosis. Can J Neurol Sci 12:251–254.

147. Potempa, K. M. (1986). A comparison of exercise performance and fatigue in hypertensive men over 50 years of age taking propanolol and pindolol. Ph.D. dissertation. Chicago: Rush University.

148. Cohen, R. A., & Fisher, M. (1989). Amantidine treatment of fatigue associated with multiple sclerosis. Arch Neurol 46:676–680.

149. Rosenberg, G. A., & Appenseller, O. (1988). Amantidine, fatigue and multiple sclerosis. Arch Neurol 45:1104–1106.

150. Landsberg, K. F., Vaughan, L. M., & Heffner, J. E. (1990). The effect of theophylline on respiratory muscle contractility and fatigue. Pharmacotherapy 10:271–279.

151. Caruso, I., Puttini, P. S., Cazzola, M., & Azzolini, V. (1990). Double-blind study of 5-Hydroxytryptophan versus placebo in the treatment of primary fibromyalgia syndrome. J Int Med Res 18:201–209.

152. Rhodes, V. A., Watson, P. M., & Hanson, B. M. (1988). Patients' descriptions of the influence of tiredness and weakness on self-care abilities. Cancer Nurs 11:186–194.

153. Gerber, L., Furst, G. Shulman, B., Smith, C., Thornton, B., Liang, M., Cullen, K., Stevens, M. B., & Gilbert, N. (1987). Patient education program to teach energy conservation behaviors to patients with rheumatoid arthritis: A pilot study. Arch Phys Med Rehabil 68:442–445.

154. Bergstrom, J., Hermansen, L. Hultman, E., & Saltin, B. (1967). Diet, muscle glycogen and physical performance. Acta Physiol Scand 71:140–150.

155. Maclaren, D. P. M., & Ricketts, S. (1983). Effect of glycogen loading and caffeine on endurance performance. J Sports Sci 1:141–142.

156. Williams, J. H., Signorile, J. F., Barnes, W. S., & Henrich, T. W. (1988). Caffeine, maximal power output and fatigue. Br J Sports Med 22:132–134.

157. Valverde, E., Vich, J. M., Garcia-Calderon, J. V., & Garcia-Calderon, P. A. (1980). In vitro response of lymphocytes in patients with tension-fatigue syndrome. Ann Allergy 45:185–188.

158. Richardson, J., Palmerton, T., & Chenan, M. (1980). The effect of calcium on muscle fatigue. J Sports Med 20:149–151.

159. Williams, M. H., Wesseldine, S., Somma, T., & Schuster, R. (1981). The effects of induced erythrocythemia upon 5-mile treadmill run time. Med Sci Sports Exerc 13:169–175.

160. McHugh, N. G., Christman, N. J., & Johnson, J. E. (1982). Preparatory information: What helps and why. Am J Nurs 82:780–782.

161. Piper, B. F. (1991). Alteration in comfort: Fatigue. In McNally, J. C., Somerville, E. T., Miaskowski, C., & Rostad, M. (eds.), *Guidelines for Oncology Nursing Practice* (2nd. ed, pp. 155–162). Philadelphia: W. B. Saunders.

162. Spiegel, D., Bloom, J. R., & Yalom, I. D. (1981). Group support for metastatic cancer patients: A randomized prospective outcome study. Arch Gen Psychiatry 38:527–533.

163. Spiegel, D., Bloom, J. R., Kraemer, H. C., & Gottheil, E. (1989). Effect of psychosocial treatment on survival of patients with metastatic breast cancer. Lancet 2:888–891.

164. Altieri, C. A. (1984). The patient with myocardial infarction: Rest prescriptions for activities of daily living. Heart Lung 13:355–360.

165. Bruya, M. A. (1981). Planned periods of rest in the intensive care unit: Nursing care activities and intracranial pressure. J Neurosurg Nurs 13:184–194.

166. Daiss, S. R., Bertelson, A. D., & Benjamin, L. T., Jr. (1986). Napping versus resting: Effects on performance and mood. Psychophysiology 23:82–88.

167. Piper, B. F. (1986). Fatigue. In V. K. Carrieri, A. M. Lindsey, & C. M. West (eds.), *Pathophysiological Phenomena in Nursing: Human Responses to Illness* (pp. 219–243). Philadelphia: W. B. Saunders.

13

Pain

Kathleen Puntillo
Mary D. Tesler

DEFINITION

Since the beginning of time, pain has been a part of life, a subject of myths, and a part of religions.[1, 2] Yet pain's complexity and its attribute as a private subjective experience challenge our understanding and even its definition.

Pain has been described as a multidimensional phenomenon with sensory, affective, and cognitive dimensions.[3] Its expression is influenced by numerous individual, experiential, and situational variables; it cannot be measured directly but can be assessed only indirectly by others' evaluation of an individual's report of pain or through manifested behaviors. Two definitions serve both clinicians and researchers. The first, that "pain is whatever the experiencing person says it is, existing whenever he says it does"[4] is often identified as the clinical definition because it emphasizes the importance of individual input. The second definition, formulated by the International Association for Study of Pain (IASP), states that "pain is an unpleasant sensory and emotional experience associated with actual or potential tissue damage, or described in terms of such damage."[5, 6] This definition considers the two essential elements of pain: sensory perception of the actual or potential tissue damage and the accompanying unpleasant emotions.

PREVALENCE AND POPULATIONS AT RISK

Prevalence

Pain is estimated to cost Americans more than $100 billion a year; in 1984 it cost $55 billion and accounted for 4 billion workdays, making it a major health and economic problem.[7] In 1985 Bristol Meyers commissioned a study of pain prevalence and severity and their impact on the individual's work using a cross section of 1254 individuals older than 18 years of age. Findings, published as the Nuprin Report, showed that in the preceding 12 months the respondents had experienced the following: headaches, 73 per cent; backaches, 56 per cent; muscle aches, 53 per cent; and stomach aches, 46 per cent; 40 per cent of the women reported menstrual and premenstrual pain. Excluding joint pain, those older than 65 years of age reported less pain.[7] Bailit found that 20 to 30 per cent of 5- to 61-year-olds reported dental pain in the preceding 3 months, with the highest incidence in nonwhite, low-income individuals.[8] Findings from the National Ambulatory Care Survey indicated that about 70 million of 1.2 billion patient visits to physicians' offices were for "new pain."[9] In another study 16 per cent of patients in a family practice group had experienced pain in the previous 2 weeks, and 66 per cent had not sought medical care.[10] These large surveys and workman's compensation statistics demonstrate the prevalence of pain in the general population.

These reports of pain prevalence omit the entire population of children, whose pain until recently has been largely ignored, disbelieved, untreated, and unstudied. However, exciting advances have been made in the field, and study results of infants undergoing surgery without analgesics have raised both professional and public concern and outcry.[11, 12]

Populations at Risk

Employment-Related Pain

The workplace is a frequent setting for painful encounters. Back injuries constitute a major industrial medicine problem and account for 15 to 18 per cent of all industrial injuries.[13] Long hours in front of a video display terminal now constitute a major cause of carpal tunnel disease and neck pain. Health professionals are not immune to work-related injuries. Mior and Diakow found that 74 per cent of chiropractors suffered work-related back pain.[14] In addition, employment-related pain can be underestimated; 78 per cent of nurses with work-related low back pain did not report it.[15]

Postoperative Pain

More than 21 million surgical procedures are performed in the United States each year, and many are associated with pain.[16] Pain associated with thoracic, abdominal, spinal, and joint surgery is reported to be particularly severe.[17] Yet despite advances in analgesics and newer methods of their administration, the incidence of postoperative pain in children and adults is astounding. In fact, adult postsurgical patients who remained in hospitals longer than 4 days experienced increased pain.[18] A study of medical-surgical patients showed that 79 per cent had experienced pain during hospitalization, and the average amount of medication given was less than one fourth of what was ordered.[19] The postoperative pain management of children has been consistently poor. Children, when compared to adults, are still prescribed and administered inadequate doses of analgesics and are at high risk for suffering pain.[20–23]

Chronic Nonmalignant Pain

The distinguishing features of this complex pain are resistance to treatment and duration. It is arbitrarily defined as lasting 30 or more days in the Nuprin Pain Report.[7] However, chronic pain can start in the acute period by unexplained delays in healing.[17] The most commonly reported types of chronic pain are headaches, low back pain, joint pains, arthritis, and rheumatism.[13] In addition to duration and treatment resistance, chronic pain is frequently associated with anxiety and depression in children and adults. It can incapacitate individuals, causing loss of work and untold personal and family suffering. Paradoxically, advances in health care can often lead to pain. Patients surviving organ transplantation, major surgeries, and chemotherapy are often left with serious conditions and pain. They may experience painful therapies and additional surgeries and treatments.

Chronic pain in children has not been well documented, but 7.5 million children younger than age 18 are estimated to have a chronic illness; 10 per cent are severely affected. Another 9 million are afflicted with less severe forms of illness, many of them associated with pain: asthma, sickle cell disease, and juvenile rheumatoid arthritis. It is sad that the resources for the management of children's chronic pain are limited and shrinking.[24]

Cancer Pain

It is estimated that more than 3 million people throughout the world suffer from cancer pain each day.[25] In 65 to 78 per cent of cancer patients, the pain is due to the disease itself; the severity of the pain ranges from moderate to excruciating in 80 per cent of this population.[26] In a group of 92 children and young adults 6 months to 24 years of age, 78 per cent had pain as a presenting symptom of their cancer.[27] Yet, over one quarter who reported their pain to be moderate to severe had received no analgesics in their cancer treatment to date. Cancer treatments themselves, such as surgery, chemotherapy, and radiation therapy, generate pain in 20 to 50 per cent of patients.[28]

Cancer pain intensity can affect an individual's life style and interfere with sleep, mood, and activity. Of special concern are the views of society and health professionals toward cancer.[29] When cancer is viewed as implying impending death and its accompanying pain is seen as inevitable and unmanageable, a complete pain alleviation goal may not be set.

Iatrogenically Induced Pain

Paradoxically, pain often results from therapeutic efforts to support life, monitor patient progress, and relieve pain itself. Critical care patients reported pain from chest tubes and pulmonary artery catheters[30] as well as from other treatments and unexplained procedures.[31] Nurses have identified central and peripheral lines and Foley catheter insertions as painful procedures for their patients.[32] These same types of treatments cause pain in neonates and children. Yet, infants may often undergo surgical procedures such as circumcisions and tube insertion or removal with no analgesics.[33, 34] Children's assessment of pain intensity associated with routine procedures ranged from 2.0 to 4.7 on a 0 to 5 scale.[35]

Many doctors and nurses who use neuromuscular blocking agents in critically ill patients are unaware that these blocking agents are neither analgesics nor sedatives.[36] Therefore, the paralyzed patient not treated with analgesics is at great risk for suffering needless iatrogenic pain.

Social Behavior and Pain

Changes in societal behavior have created new sources of pain. The increased interest in health and exercise has resulted in a rise in injuries from both single-impact macrotrauma and microtrauma overuse injuries that cause pain.[37] The increase in sexual experimentation and activity and recreational drug use has resulted in a dramatic rise in the incidence of sexually transmitted diseases and acquired immunodeficiency syndrome (AIDS). Pelvic inflammatory disease causes many women to suffer pain from both the disease and the therapy. Pain associated with abortion and methods to reduce it are now receiving research attention.[38] Regrettably, little research has been reported on the incidence of pain in AIDS, yet pain was the second most common presenting symptom in 54 per cent of patients hospitalized for AIDS; 41 per cent suffered chest pain and 28 per cent mouth pain.[39] Strafford and associates found pain and agitation at death in all 12 children who died of AIDS and that the source of the disease-related pain was neurological, pulmonary, gastrointestinal, and dermatological complications.[40]

DEVELOPMENTAL DIMENSIONS

Although not widely disseminated, knowledge of the physiological basis of infant pain has grown in the last few years, challenging the skeptical attitudes regarding infant pain. Anand and his colleagues described the developmental neuroanatomy, physiology, and neurochemistry that explains nociception and stimulus transmission in the earliest stages of life.[41, 42] The concurrent development of the cutaneous sensory system and the synaptic connections at the spinal cord between incoming sensory fibers and receptive neurons starts at 6 to 7 weeks' gestation. By 20 weeks' gestation the mechanics for sensory perception of stimuli from mucous and cutaneous tissues is complete. By 30 weeks' gestation dorsal horn cell differentiation, synaptic interconnections, and formation of neurotransmitter vesicles lead to the formation of mature spinal cord dorsal horns.[43] This concurrent development allows for the transmission of nociception. However, because their descending pain control mechanism is incomplete, infants are unable to modulate nociceptive transmission as do adults.[41] Nociception is not translated as pain in infants, but the infant has the capacity to respond to noxious stimulation with the same endocrine, hormonal, and stress responses as adults. The detrimental hormonal-metabolic consequences of unrelieved pain on the cardiovascular and neural systems of premature neonates jeopardize their recovery.[41]

Term infants are clearly able to respond to nociceptive input on the first day of life; the intensity of their responses is influenced by the stage of the sleep-wake state.[44, 45] However, memory for painful events, as manifested by anticipatory crying, is not evident until 6 months.[46] Pain responses after this early period are correlated with cognitive development. The ability to discriminate levels of pain intensity increases over the years from ages 3 to 6. Belter and associates found that younger children tended to discriminate only low and high levels of pain while older children could identify a broader range of levels that included no pain, little pain, and a lot of pain.[47] Pain thresholds of 5- to 18-year-olds increase with age.[48] This knowledge provides further support to treat the pain of very young infants.

During the preschool years, the child often associates pain with misbehavior and may feel guilt in addition to pain. School-aged children can relate pain to bodily injury, although they see no value to pain as a protective mechanism and only appreciate its relief from duties.[49] It is not until 10 to 12 years of age that psychological causes of pain begin to be verbalized and adult concepts of pain as a protective function are identified.[50, 51] Older adolescents, because they can anticipate the future, are often fearful of the implications of their pain. However, like their younger counterparts, they often believe that a nurse automatically knows they are in pain.

A group of age-specific syndromes of recurrent pain is associated with the growing years and plagues many children and their families.[52] Colic, seen in early infancy, usually resolves by the third month and is followed by teething pains. Otitis media is a problem of late infancy and toddlerhood. Recurrent abdominal and leg pains are seen in middle childhood, and the adolescent years are marked by migraines and chest pain in both boys and girls. Premenstrual and menstrual pains are problems for many adolescent girls, and juvenile rheumatoid arthritis is seen throughout childhood. Pain associated with these conditions is difficult to manage as emotional components begin to overlay the physical aspects of pain.[53, 54]

Young and middle-aged adults suffer varying degrees of acute pain from trauma or surgery, and women experience pain associated with childbearing. Adults can also become afflicted with one or another of the chronic pain conditions, most commonly musculoskeletal and chest pain and cancer pain.

Like members of other age groups, elderly individuals are at risk for developmentally related painful conditions such as arthritic disorders, cardiovascular problems, cancer, and osteoporosis.[17] However, there is inconclusive evidence of the effect of aging on the perception of pain. Some research has shown that threshold for radiant heat pain increases with age in both sexes.[55, 56] This may be due to age-related changes in nociceptors or to a decrease in skin thickness resulting in a dispersion of thermal energy via the vascular network.[55]

Research on the influence of age on analgesic effectiveness[57] shows that the increased effectiveness resulted from increased analgesic duration due to prolonged plasma clearance of morphine. Physiologically, changes in drug metabolism may be influenced by changes in body composition such as increased or decreased levels of fat in subcutaneous tissues or of serum proteins that affect drug binding. Elderly postoperative patients have required smaller dosages of opiates to achieve the same level of analgesia as younger patients achieve.[58] Considerably more work is needed before

the pain relief needs of the elderly are understood. Issues such as the effect of aging on pain sensitivity, the manifestations of pain in patients with communication difficulties associated with hearing and vision loss, mental confusion and pain, and the role of depression in elderly individuals with pain all need to be examined.

MECHANISMS

While the experience of and interest in pain has existed for centuries, much of the knowledge about pain physiology has been derived from the results of adult and animal studies conducted during the past 25 years. One way of organizing the current knowledge of pain physiology is to discuss the transduction, transmission, perception, and modulation of pain. Such a process allows for synthesis of what is known, identification of gaps in the understanding of pain, and formulation of a framework for therapeutic interventions. Box 13–1 provides a glossary of terms useful to the understanding of pain.

Transduction

Transduction is the process by which a noxious stimulus is changed into an electrical stimulus on a cell membrane.[59] A noxious stimulus, one that actually or potentially causes tissue damage, may originate from chemical, thermal, or mechanical sources. Biochemical substances are released from damaged cells that in turn sensitize nerve endings, which leads to nerve cell membrane depolarization. Biochemical substances believed to be released from or activated by cell damage include bradykinins, histamine, hydrogen ions, and potassium ions.[60] In addition, prostaglandins, biochemical substances synthesized from arachidonic acid, also mediate pain. Substance P, an amino acid released from peripheral nerve terminals, and serotonin (5-HT), released from platelets, also sensitize nociceptors[59] (Fig. 13–1).

The nerve cells that are depolarized by these events are peripheral afferent neurons and are called nociceptive fibers because they are receptive to noxious stimuli. If depolarization is strong enough to generate an action potential, the nerve impulse will travel along these afferent nociceptive fibers from the periphery (that is, from skin, somatic struc-

BOX 13–1

Acute pain—complex constellation of unpleasant sensory, perceptual, and emotional experience associated with autonomic, psychological, and emotional response that follows tissue injury.[17]

Addiction—a psychological dependence, a pattern of compulsive drug use characterized by continued craving for an opioid and need to use the opioid for other than pain relief.[184]

Chronic pain—pain not due to malignant disease and persisting beyond the expected healing time or pain associated with a chronic pathophysiological process.[17]

Deafferentation pain—pain due to loss of sensory input into the central nervous system.[89]

Neuropathic pain—pain resulting from dysfunction or injury to the peripheral or central nervous system.[88]

Nociceptor—a receptor preferentially sensitive to a noxious stimulus or to a stimulus that could become noxious if prolonged.[6]

Noxious stimulus—one that is damaging to normal tissues.[6]

Pain threshold—the least amount of pain that a subject can recognize.[6]

Pain tolerance—the greatest level of pain that a subject is prepared to tolerate.[6]

Physical dependence—state when discontinuance of an opioid or administration of opioid antagonist produces an abstinence syndrome characterized by withdrawal symptoms.[184]

Suffering—a state of anguish experienced by the individual who bears pain, injury, or loss.[296]

Tolerance—larger dose of opioid analgesia required to maintain original analgesia effect.[184]

Transmission

Impulses originating in peripheral receptors can actually travel in two directions: (1) in an antidromic fashion, that is, in an unexpected direction back toward the periphery near where the original impulse was generated and (2) in an orthodromic direction, toward the central nervous system (CNS), where integration, transmission, modulation, and perception of pain occur (Fig. 13–1).

Antidromic Transmission

Antidromic impulses may cause the release of additional pain-producing substances in the periphery. Hyperalgesia may develop, which is an increased sensitivity to pain that occurs when the threshold to a noxious stimulus is lowered.[5] In addition to antidromic impulses in nociceptive nerve fibers, efferent sympathetic impulses to the periphery can also help to maintain pain sensation long after the initial pain stimulus.[63] Proposed mechanisms of sympathetically mediated pain will be discussed later.

Orthodromic Transmission

Cutaneous noxious impulses are transmitted to the gray matter of the spinal cord by small-diameter myelinated A delta fibers as well as by smaller-diameter unmyelinated C fibers.[64] Cutaneous A delta-fiber activity results in a sharp pain that elicits a rapid response.[65] Impulses from deep somatic structures such as ligaments, muscles, tendons, joints, and fascia as well as from viscera

tures, or viscera) to the spinal cord.[61] Impulses along afferent fibers from the face are transmitted to the medulla.[62]

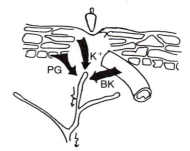

NOCICEPTOR ACTIVATION

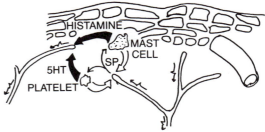

Figure 13–1. Biochemical mediators of nociception. PG, prostaglandins; K+, potassium ions; BK, bradykinins; 5HT, serotonin; SP, substance P. Lower figure depicts both antidromic and orthodromic transmission of nerve impulse. (Modified from Fields, H. L. [1987]. *Pain: Mechanisms and Management* [p. 36]. New York: McGraw-Hill.)

seem to be predominantly through C fibers.[66, 67] C-fiber impulses transmit pain that is described as diffuse, dull, and delayed,[65] making the pain difficult to localize.

The phenomenon of pain referral also accounts for the difficulty in localizing pain at times. Because deep somatic, visceral, and cutaneous fibers often converge on the same spinal neuron, pain may be referred to an anatomical site other than its real site of origin[68] (Fig. 13–2).

Peripheral afferent C fibers and A delta fibers carrying noxious sensations terminate in different layers, called laminae, of the spinal cord gray matter (Fig. 13–3). Most C fibers terminate in lamina II, the substantia gelatinosa, which also contains numerous small interneurons[69] that participate in communicating, integrating, modulating, or inhibiting noxious peripheral input. Afferent A delta fibers and their branches terminate in laminae I and V, respectively. Nociceptive impulses from the face or oral cavity are primarily transmitted via A delta and C fibers through the three branches of the trigeminal nerve to the nucleus caudalis of the medulla.[62] As depicted in Figure 13–3, there are A alpha fibers that transmit sensations other than pain to the spinal cord dorsal horn. The influence of these "nonpain" A alpha or A beta fibers on inhibition of pain transmission will be presented in a later discussion of the gate control theory of pain.

Ascending Transmission from Spinal Cord to Brain

Noxious stimuli from primary afferent neuron fibers that originate in the periphery

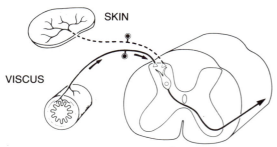

Figure 13–2. A model of referred pain. Afferent fibers from the viscus converge on the same pain projection neurons in the spinal cord as afferent fibers from somatic structures (such as skin) do. Thus, visceral pain may be perceived as somatic pain. (Modified from Fields, H. L. [1987]. *Pain: Mechanisms and Management* [p. 91]. New York: McGraw-Hill.)

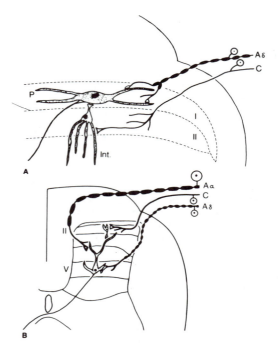

Figure 13–3. *A*, Noxious input per A delta and C fibers to spinal cord laminae 1 and 2, respectively. *B*, Non-noxious fibers, such as A alpha, and noxious A delta and C fibers synapse with spinal cord interneurons. (From Fields, H. L. [1987]. *Pain: Mechanisms and Management* [p. 55]. New York: McGraw-Hill.)

are transmitted to secondary neurons originating in the spinal cord. Some of these secondary neuron fibers are nociceptive specific while others receive multiple sensations, both noxious and non-noxious. These latter multisensory neurons are termed wide-dynamic range (WDR) neurons.[68] The secondary spinal cord nociceptive neurons are contained in fiber tracts that ascend to multiple brain sites where perceptive, evaluative, emotional, and cognitive responses to pain originate (Fig. 13–4).

The neospinothalamic tract is a major ascending projection system that receives fibers both directly from primary afferent peripheral fibers or by way of lamina II interneurons.[70] This tract, terminating in contralateral thalamic nuclei,[71] purportedly transmits sensory-discriminative aspects of pain.[72]

The paleospinothalamic tract is a second major ascending system that projects to both the ipsilateral and contralateral brain stem reticular formation as well as to other areas of the limbic system.[59] Other fibers then project from these multiple sites to the thalamus.

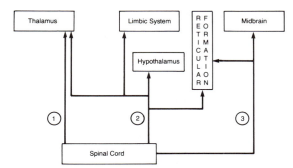

Figure 13–4. Diagram showing projection tracts from spinal cord to brain centers. Final pathways will be to cortex, where pain perception occurs. 1, Neospinothalamic tract system. 2, Paleospinothalamic tract system. 3, Spinomesencephalic tract system. (Reprinted from *Pain in the Critically Ill: Assessment and Management* by K. A. Puntillo, p. 16, with permission of Aspen Publishers, Inc., © 1991.)

This tract is involved in motivational-affective pain dimensions and has also been referred to as the spinoreticulothalamic pathway.

A third important ascending projection system from the spinal cord is the spinomesencephalic tract. Its cells of origin, in spinal cord laminae I and V, project to midbrain reticular formation and midbrain periaqueductal gray [matter] (PAG).[71] The PAG, medulla, and spinal cord dorsal horn are immensely important areas where pain transmission can be affected and pain can be modulated, that is, influenced or inhibited. These sites contain endorphins, whose role in pain inhibition is discussed later.

Perception

A noxious sensation becomes pain when that sensation reaches conscious levels.[59] Perception of pain and the evaluation of its meaning, therefore, are believed to be cortical processes. Yet, it has been difficult to localize pain to any one particular cortical site. It appears that many cortical areas become activated as a result of a painful stimulus.[73] The somatosensory cortex within and posterior to the central fissure is particularly responsive to noxious stimuli.[74]

Modulation

The Gate Control Theory

Pain modulation can occur in many areas along the CNS. According to the gate control theory, the spinal cord dorsal horn is an extremely important site for pain modulation.[3, 75] The hypothesis of the gate control theory is that there is a balance of activity between large diameter, nonpain fibers, and smaller-diameter pain fibers that synapse on the same central transmission cells in the spinal cord (Fig. 13–5). Transmission cells are excitatory fibers believed to be responsible for central transmission of noxious information from spinal cord to brain. They represent the spinal cord-to-brain tracts described earlier that are involved with motivational-emotional and sensory-discriminative dimensions of pain.

Lamina II substantia gelatinosa inhibitory interneurons are thought to influence the central transmission cells by interrupting the balance between large (nonpain) and smaller-diameter (pain) fiber activity. The smaller pain fibers are believed to inhibit substantia gelatinosa interneurons, allowing transmission cells to remain active. Thus, the gate to pain is opened, and there is central transmission of pain. Conversely, large nonpain fibers activate substantia gelatinosa cells that in turn inhibit transmission cell activity, thus closing the "pain gate." Higher CNS control processes can also influence the gate control system by delivering descending inhibitory messages to the spinal cord. Some goals of therapy then are to stimulate descending CNS central control inhibitory processes and to stimulate large peripheral nonpain fibers, both of which are thought to close the pain gates. The gate control theory is not considered to be entirely accurate or complete[76]; however, it helps explain the effects of some current pain therapies, which are discussed later.

Descending Endogenous Analgesia Modulating Systems

Pain modulation also occurs through endogenous analgesia opioid and nonopioid systems. Endogenous opioid analgesia is mediated primarily through actions of endorphins, while monoamines mediate nonopioid analgesia.

The Opioid System of Endogenous Analgesia. Endogenous opioids, generically referred to as endorphins, are synthesized and released from numerous CNS sites. There are at least three classes of endorphins: beta-endorphin, enkephalin, and dynorphin. Beta-endorphins have been located in hypo-

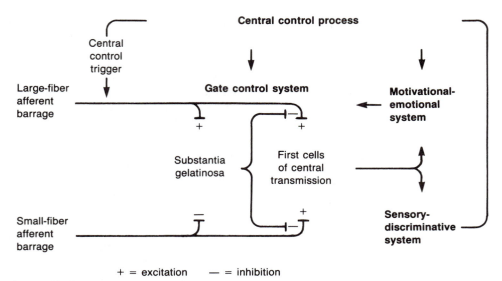

Figure 13–5. Gate control model. See text for explanation. (From Chapman, C. R., & Bonica, J. J. [1983]. *Current Concepts: Acute Pain* [p. 11]. Kalamazoo, MI: The Upjohn Company.)

thalamic and midbrain PAG neurons.[59, 77] In fact, when the PAG was electrically stimulated during classic rat experimentations,[78] the rats became profoundly analgesic. It is now believed that beta-endorphins serve as at least one of the substrates for this endogenous analgesia and that they may be released during acupuncture and transcutaneous electrical nerve stimulation (TENS) as well as by stress and pain.[79] The other two endorphins, enkephalins and dynorphin, have been located in midbrain, brain stem, and spinal cord nuclei. Activation of neural pathways that descend from the PAG to nuclei in the rostroventral medulla and thence to the spinal cord dorsal horn leads to enkephalin release and subsequent nociceptive inhibition.[80]

The action of endogenous opioids is contingent upon their binding to specific receptors.[81] These receptors differ as to the type of opioid that attaches to each and in the physiological response to the attachment. Most opiate drugs, such as morphine, fentanyl, alfentanil, and sufentanil, are mu receptor ligands.[82] Opiates, their receptors, and their clinical effects will be discussed in a subsequent section.

The Nonopioid System of Endogenous Analgesia. The nonopioid system of endogenous analgesia uses the monoamines serotonin and norepinephrine as substrates. Serotonin is believed to be a major pain-

inhibiting neurotransmitter of medulla-to-spinal cord neurons. In fact, tricyclic antidepressants such as amitriptyline that prolong the actions of serotonin by blocking its neuronal re-uptake are used to treat chronic pain.[83] Norepinephrine, contained in neurons located in the pons that project to the spinal cord dorsal horn, attaches to spinal cord alpha$_2$-adrenergic receptors. When clonidine, an alpha$_2$-agonist, is administered spinally, nociception is inhibited.[59] Research has shown that administration of clonidine intrathecally and of morphine sulfate subcutaneously provided a synergistic analgesia in rats.[84]

Numerous factors such as pain, stress,[85] fear, restraint, and hypoglycemia[80] appear to activate endogenous analgesia systems. Conversely, differences in the perceived intensity of pain may be due to alterations in function of these pain-inhibitory systems.[86] Pharmacological, nonpharmacological, and surgical enhancement of endogenous analgesia system activity is currently a major focus of research and clinical interventions. They are discussed later.

Mechanisms of Chronic Pain

The previous discussion is an explanatory model for the mechanisms of pain of an acute nature. Acute pain is due to activation of nociceptive systems and pathways and thus is also referred to as nociceptive pain. Although chronic pain at times can be due to persistent nociceptive activation, this is not the model for many types of chronic pain. In these other cases, pain is not a response to real or potential tissue damages but is, rather, its own separate disease process.[87] Neuropathic pain is the term used for this type of pain, and it occurs as a result of dysfunction or injury to the peripheral or central nervous system.[88]

Various categories of neuropathic pain have been devised according to the predominant pathophysiological features of each. The first of these is deafferentation pain, resulting from damage to peripheral or central somatosensory pathways. This may occur, for example, after traumatic injury to a nerve root.[89] As a result of the injury, the flow of nerve impulses is partially or completely interrupted.[90] However, instead of becoming less sensitive, neurons become abnormally sensitive and excitable. The increased sensitivity can involve the second-order WDR CNS neurons described earlier that respond to both noxious and non-noxious stimuli.[63] Non-noxious stimuli such as touch may now spontaneously excite the WDR neurons and generate pain.

A second category of neuropathic pain is mediated by the sympathetic nervous system (SNS). Other terms used to describe sympathetic-maintained pain are reflex sympathetic dystrophy and causalgia.[87] It is hypothesized that in some cases non-noxious peripheral fibers that activate WDR neurons are stimulated by norepinephrine released from efferent SNS neurons.[63] The exact mechanism by which sympathetic nerve impulses to the periphery generate firing of nociceptive neurons to cause pain is unclear.[87]

Another proposed mechanism for chronic pain is loss of pain inhibition by nonpain fibers whose hypothesized actions were explained by the gate control theory[59] or loss of inhibition normally produced by descending endogenous analgesic systems.[91] These proposed explanations for the persistence of pain—loss of inhibition—serve as a basis for the selected treatments that will be discussed later.

Clinical management of chronic neuropathic types of pain is quite challenging. Some types of neuropathic pain may be resistant to opioids. Since nociceptors are not always activated with neuropathic pain, endogenous opioid systems may not be in-

volved.[88] However, the responsiveness of neuropathic pain to opioids may be dose-dependent, suggesting that opioid therapy may still be attempted.[92] Other treatments have been used with variable degrees of success for neuropathic pain. See Table 13–1 for a differentiation of effects of acute versus chronic pain.

Mechanisms of Cancer Pain

The causes of cancer pain are many, although the mechanisms for this pain are not entirely understood.[25] The disease itself and the bony metastases that frequently occur account for a great deal of cancer pain. Most often, bones are invaded by a primary or metastatic tumor.[93] These tumors serve as mechanical stimuli or, alternatively, stimulate the production of chemicals such as prostaglandins; both of these activate nociceptors[25] and initiate afferent noxious impulses. In addition, tumors frequently have an area of inflammation surrounding them that may add to the mechanical compression of nerves or spinal cord.[94] Tumors may also invade peripheral nerves, nerve plexuses, or nerve roots. They may spread along the nerve root, infiltrate various structures of the spinal cord and compress it.[93] Therefore, the pain experienced may be due to nerve compression or destruction and development of deafferentation pain.[94] In addition to pain due to bony or nerve involvement by tumors, cancer

TABLE 13–1 CHARACTERISTICS OF ACUTE AND CHRONIC PAIN

Acute	Chronic
Sympathetic-adrenergic response	Habituation of sympathetic response
+ Heart and respiratory rate	+ Vegetative signs
+ Blood pressure	+ Sleep disturbances
− Gastrointestinal motility	+ Irritability
+ Oxygen consumption rates	+ Fatigue and exhaustion
+ Muscular tension and motility	− Pain tolerance
+ Pupillary dilation	Changes in eating patterns
+ Palmar and plantar sweating	+ Alterations in mood, self-concept, thinking
+ Increased anxiety	+ Social isolation
	+ Depression

Data from Sternbach, R. A. (1990). Acute versus chronic pain. In Melzack, R., & Wall, P. (eds.), *Textbook of Pain* (pp. 242–246.) New York: Churchill Livingstone.
Key: + = increased; − = decreased.

pain can be from invasion of somatic, visceral, or soft tissue structures.[25, 93] Muscle spasms[94] or pathological fractures[93] are sometimes secondary responses to the cancer's effects.

RELATED PATHOPHYSIOLOGICAL CONCEPTS

Motor, Respiratory, and Sympathetic Nervous System Consequences of Pain

Regardless of the origin of noxious stimuli (i.e., cutaneous, deep somatic, or visceral structures), segmental synapsing in the spinal cord and subsequent efferent output through reflex motor neurons lead to adverse physiological responses.[66, 95] Reflex motor activity is due to direct or indirect (through interneurons) synapsing of noxious fibers onto lower motor neurons originating in the anterior spinal cord dorsal horn.[96] This reflex activity may result in contraction of skeletal muscles in the area where the noxious stimulus originated. For example, after abdominal surgery or trauma, abdominal pain may lead to reflex abdominal skeletal muscle spasms, affect diaphragmatic excursion, and alter respiratory mechanics. The individual may voluntarily avoid coughing, deep breathing, or moving, maneuvers that help prevent respiratory impairment.[97]

Increased SNS activity is another physiological consequence of acute pain. Visceral afferent nociceptive fibers synapse with interneurons to preganglionic cell bodies of the SNS or the parasympathetic nervous system (PNS) located in spinal cord lamina VII.[98] Suprasegmental input to these preganglionic cell bodies is through a series of descending pathways from the hypothalamus, medulla, and other higher cortical centers.[61] SNS responses to pain can significantly alter cardiovascular parameters. Myocardial oxygen consumption is increased because of increased heart rate and contractility from the inotropic effects of SNS activation. Afterload, increased as a result of peripheral vasoconstriction, also increases the workload of the heart. Adequate blood flow to myocardial tissues may be impaired owing to coronary artery vasoconstriction. Thus, the person with acute pain may experience increased blood pressure, pulse rate, and diaphoresis. In the presence of chronic pain, however, these responses may not be present,[99] owing to a "dampening" of SNS physiological responses over time. It is important, therefore, for caregivers to avoid equating pain with increased SNS activity and diminishing the importance of the self-reports of persons with chronic pain when SNS responses are absent or diminished.

The Physiological Stress of Pain

Although it has been demonstrated that stress can induce an analgesic response to nociception,[85] this response has primarily been observed under short-term experimental conditions. As a painful condition persists, pain acts as a physiological stressor. It appears to do so through a spinal cord-to-pons-to-cortex feedback loop. This action may be mediated by norepinephrine-containing neurons that project from the pons to cortex. At the cortex, signals of potential danger are received and vigilance and behavioral arousal increase.[61, 100]

Physiologically, the stress of pain activates neuroendocrine mechanisms that are primarily integrated through homeostatic hypothalamic feedback loops. Severe pain can lead to profound reflex physiological stress responses.[101] Endocrine and metabolic stress responses, such as increased cortisol, catecholamines, antidiuretic hormone synthesis, glycolysis and hyperglycemia, increased protein catabolism, decreased plasma insulin, and increased lipolysis, may all be related to the extent of tissue injury. Eventually, the stress of pain can tax the body's homeostatic mechanisms.

Sleep, Fatigue, and Pain

Sleep disturbances and fatigue frequently accompany pain. However, the physiological bases for these relationships have not been clearly established. Sleep alterations have been identified as modulating variables associated with some chronic pain disorders such as osteoarthritis and fibromyalgia.[102] One endogenous peptide known to induce sleep, delta-sleep–inducing peptide (DSIP), has been demonstrated to have an antinociceptive effect in animals,[103] which suggests a relationship between sleeplessness and pain. It appears that the actions of this peptide, when injected into certain limbic and forebrain areas, are mediated at opioid receptors. Furthermore, the antinociceptive effect of DSIP is reversed by naloxone, an opioid antagonist, and diminished in morphine-tolerant animals.

Clinical studies have supported a relationship between pain, fatigue, and sleeplessness. For example, there were significantly more complaints of sleep disturbances in hospitalized patients with painful rheumatic diseases than in patients with other nonpainful medical disorders.[104] Fatigue accompanied and followed episodes of pain in chronic back pain and was related to pain intensity.[105] Researchers studying these relationships have suggested that the secondary fatigue experienced after an episode of pain may contribute to pain maintenance and disability. Treatments for pain, fatigue, and sleep disturbances may include use of analgesics, tricyclic antidepressants, and aerobic fitness programs.[102]

ASSOCIATED PSYCHOLOGICAL CONCEPTS

Fear, anxiety, anger, and depression have been described both as responses to and as mediators of pain. Attempts to determine the direction of causality have been inconclusive; what emerges is the reciprocal relationship between emotional distress and pain.[106, 107] Price states that "pain sensation, arousal, meanings and emotional responses exist simultaneously and moment by moment as an integrated experience"[108] (p. 5). These manifestations of the affective-motivational dimension of pain are in synchrony with the sensory-discriminative and the cognitive-evaluative components, each influencing and being influenced by the other.

Fear and Anxiety

Given the function of acute pain as the body's warning system of impending danger, the natural responses to it are fear and anxiety. Findings in studies of postoperative, childbirth, dental, and pediatric pain indicate that anxiety was the most reliable psychological variable associated with high intensity levels of acute pain. The most consistent predictor of fear about dental procedures was fear of pain.[109, 110]

The fear of needles is pervasive throughout childhood, causing children to deny pain to avoid an injection, and is the source of anxiety for many adults who experience needle phobia associated with dental care. In fact, Pawlicki found that the most frequent emotions expressed in dentist offices were fear and anxiety, which amplified and complicated pain perception.[111] Individuals who do not acquire dental fear either never had a painful dental experience or experienced delay between the first dental care and the painful encounter.[112] It is estimated that 6 to 7 per cent of adults and 16 per cent of children experience fear of pain severe enough to inhibit their seeking health care.[113]

Fear and anxiety are concomitant with hospitalization. Patients exhibit high levels of anxiety at all points; before admission, during the hospitalization, and afterward.[107, 114] Most patients fear anesthesia, altered body integrity and functions, and the ability to cope with pain.[107] Complex technology and environmental stressors associated with care in acute and critical care units increase the fear and pain of patients and families.[115, 116] Although life-saving machines may reassure the patient by providing better monitoring, they also emphasize the ever present risk to life.

Anger

Anger becomes associated with pain early in life. Responses of infants 2 to 19 months of age to immunizations assessed with the Maximally Discriminative Facial Movement Coding System (MAX)[117] included both pain and anger.[118] Expressions of pain decreased and those of anger increased with age and infants who were slow to soothe displayed greater duration of anger. The relationship between pain and anger is not reported extensively, probably because anger is not considered a socially appropriate response. Yet reports of nonmalignant chronic pain, AIDS, and cancer pain all identify anger as a response. In one study, 53 per cent of patients with intractable pain reported "bottling up anger" and 33 per cent reported "getting angry easily." Those who reported bottling up their anger also saw their illness as deserved retribution for their proneness to pain, which they saw as psychological rather than physiological.[119] Family members may also feel angry about pain they cannot help.

Portenoy found that adequately treating the terminally ill patient's pain lifted from the family the burden of anger associated with unrelieved pain.[120]

Depression

Depression and illness are commonly associated; reports show that between 10 and 15 per cent of hospitalized patients will manifest major depression and another 20 to 30 per cent will endure serious depressive symptoms.[121] Depression is variously described as a series of vegetative symptoms that include loss of appetite and libido, sleep disturbances, lack of interest, decreased pleasure, despair, hopelessness, prolonged malfunction, weakening of relationships, and increased somatic preoccupation.[122, 123]

Depression is most commonly associated with chronic intractable and indeterminate pain, although the relationship between depression and pain is unclear. Some believe that chronic pain without identifiable organ pathology is part of a larger depressive disorder; others feel that depression is the natural consequence of having to live with chronic pain.[124] The potential for becoming depressed, withdrawn, irritable, and preoccupied with pain may be related to the duration of pain.[106]

The reported incidence of depression in patients with chronic pain ranges from 10 to 87 per cent while pain in depressed patients ranges from 27 to 100 per cent.[125] Several research reviews examining the relationship between chronic pain and depression and the wide discrepancies in prevalence reports have identified problems with study designs.[123, 125, 126] Some sampling techniques did not include general population control groups to compare with the pain or depression groups, thus compromising the ability to identify the prevalence of chronic pain or depression in the general population. As a result, the characteristics of patients with chronic pain without depression or depressed patients without pain cannot be determined from the studies. Other design problems include varied study-specific definitions of depression and the use of a wide range of instruments measuring different components of depression, thus limiting the potential for repeatedly measuring the presence or degree of depression. These studies have also not adequately delineated chronic pain. Study findings are influenced by these design flaws and limit our knowledge of this important issue.

Fortunately, current investigators use more stringent criteria for determining depression. More definitive tools, such as the Research Diagnostic Criteria (RDC)[127] or the *Diagnostic and Statistical Manual of Mental Disorders*, 3rd edition (DSM-III-R),[128] are enabling investigators to identify and study similar depressed populations. France and associates identified subtypes of depression in 80 patients with chronic pain and reported significant differences in the depressive symptoms among major depressive, intermittent depressive, and not depressed patients.[129] Rudy and associates reported that while there was no significant link between pain and depression, the perceived interference with life and self-control were significant variables that intervened between pain and depression.[130] Pain was also identified as the critical factor in the relationship between physical illness and depression by Williams and Schulz.[131] These new investigative efforts may clarify the relationship between pain and depression as unique qualities of both conditions are made more specific and clear.

MANIFESTATIONS

Pain is generally manifested by three categories of responses: verbal, behavioral, and physiological. Manifestations vary from individual to individual and from time to time in the same individual, depending on the physiological and emotional state, cultural demands, and acuity or chronicity of pain.

Self-Reports of Pain

Self-reports of pain can describe the location, pattern, and sensory, affective, and evaluative qualitative aspects of a particular pain, such as constant, burning, pounding, nauseating, or excruciating.[132] Preverbal children and infants vocally communicate their pain through a characteristic cry that has been described as long, high pitched, shrill, and tense followed by breath holding, then a lower-pitched, more rhythmic cry comes in bursts. These cries have been studied by both sound acoustics and with voice spectrographs.[133–135] Other vocalizations such as whimpering, moaning, and groaning can be observed both in weakened or stressed adults and children in prolonged pain. Unless the caretaker is alert to this behavior, it can be easily missed.

Assessment of pain may be achieved by an evaluation of any or all of its manifestations. Because it is a subjective experience, eliciting an individual's self-report of the pain and its characteristics is a priority. Descriptions and quantification are important to its management.

Numerous instruments are available to clinicians and researchers for collection of self-reported data. However, in busy patient care units, pain intensity is the dimension most frequently assessed. Unidimensional pain intensity scales of either vertical or horizontal lines may be anchored only at either end, with words such as "no pain" or "worst possible pain," or they may have qualifying words, numbers, or marks along the line to assist in quantification. Many of these scales have reasonable or good validity and reliability in both adults and children.[136, 137] The individual places a mark along the line at the point that designates the intensity of the pain, and the value is determined by measuring the distance from the beginning of the scale to the mark. See Figure 13–6 for examples of pain intensity scales. Instruments for children for intensity or unpleasantness have also employed pictures or cartoons with smiling to distressed faces and colors.[138–140]

More knowledge about the multiple components of a person's pain can be obtained with the use of multidimensional tools. See Table 13–2 for useful unidimensional and multidimensional instruments. One example is the Memorial Pain Assessment Card (MPAC).[141] This instrument has a measure for intensity as well as mood associated with the pain. It also measures degree of pain relief to evaluate interventions. Finally, the person can select a word from a sample of words provided to more graphically describe the pain. An example of a multidimensional questionnaire for children is the Adolescent Pediatric Pain Tool (APPT) that measures location, intensity, and quality of the pain.[137, 142, 143] Investigators are developing a temporal component to add to the instrument. Another pediatric multidimensional tool is the Pediatric Pain Questionnaire (PPQ).[144]

Self-reports of pain are influenced by an individual's cognitive and language development and abilities, culturally influenced prescriptions for reporting pain, physical ability, and the willingness and opportunity to report pain. Most often self-reports are verbalized. Yet even if an individual is unable to verbalize (such as during mechanical ventilation) a nonverbal report is possible through the use of appropriate instruments.

Behavioral Manifestations of Pain

Behaviors associated with pain are both conscious and unconscious, including char-

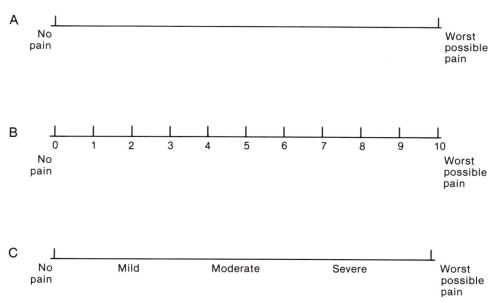

Figure 13–6. Examples of three pain scales. *A*, Visual analogue scale. *B*, Numerical rating scale. *C*, Word graphic / rating scale.

TABLE 13–2 PAIN ASSESSMENT TOOLS

Instrument	Appropriate Developmental Age	Completion Time	Description	Dimension Measured	Validity	Reliability	Principal Investigator*
Self-Report/ Unidimensional Rating Tools							
Visual Analogue Scale (VAS)	> 5 years	<3 seconds	10-cm line anchored at either end with "no pain" and "worst possible pain"	I	Concurrent Construct	Varied reports	Scott & Huskisson, 1976[136]
"Oucher"	3–12 years		Six photographs of child showing increasing distress placed at regular intervals; 0–100 scale for older children	I	Content Construct Descriminant Convergent	Yes	Aradine, Beyer, & Tompkins, 1988[145] Beyer, 1984, 1989[138]
Poker Chip	4–12 years	NR	Four red poker chips, each representing a piece of hurt	I	Concurrent Construct	Yes	Hester, 1979[146] Hester, Foster, & Kristensen, 1990[147]
Self-Report Tools/ Questionnaires							
McGill/Melzack Pain Questionnaire (MPQ)	> 12 years	15 minutes	78 descriptors (S,A,E,M), 9 pattern descriptors, front and back body outlines, verbal intensity scale	S,A,L,I, P,E,M	Content Concurrent Predictive	Test-retest	Melzack, 1975,[132] 1983[148]
McGill (MPQ) Short Form	> 12 years	2–5 minutes	11 sensory, four affective descriptors, VAS, verbal scale	S,A,I	Concurrent	NR	Melzack, 1987[149]
Pain Perception Profile (PPP)	Adults	NR	Three-column adjective list, 15 intensity, 13 sensory, 11 reactive words	I,S,A	Content Concurrent	NR	Tursky et al., 1982[150]
Memorial Pain Assessment Card (MPAC)	Adults	< 20 seconds (experienced person)	Folded 8.5 × 11 inch card VAS on three sides to score intensity, relief, and mood; fourth side pain adjectives	S,A,I	Construct; correlation among subscales and with McGill Pain Questionnaire	NR	Fishman et al., 1987[141]
Adolescent Pediatric Pain Tool (APPT)	8–17 years	3–10 minutes	67 descriptors (S,A,E,T,M), body outline, word-graphic rating scale	S,A,L,I E,M	Scale: content construct Words: content body outline concurrent	Test-retest Test-retest Alternate forms	Tesler et al., 1991[137] Savedra et al., 1989[142] Wilkie et al., 1990[143]
Pediatric Pain Questionnaire (PPQ)	4–19 years	NR	Three parts completed by child, parent, and physician, pain descriptors, body outline, VAS	I,S,A,E,L	NR	NR	Varni, Thompson, & Hanson, 1987[144]

TABLE 13–2 PAIN ASSESSMENT TOOLS *Continued*

Instrument	Appropriate Developmental Age	Completion Time	Description	Dimension Measured	Validity	Reliability	Principal Investigator*
Behavioral Rating Scales							
Children's Hospital of Eastern Ontario Pain Scale (CHEOPS)	1–7 years	NR	Rate on 0–4 intensity scale, six behaviors: cry, facial expression, verbal expression, torso, touch, and legs	I	NR	NR	McGrath et al., 1985[151]
Neonatal Infant Pain Scale (NIPS)	Premie-newborn	NR	Rate on 0–2 intensity scales, facial expression, cry, breathing, arm and leg movements, arousal state	I	NR	NR	Lawrence et al., 1991[152]

Modified from Puntillo, K. A., & Wilkie, D. J. (1991). Assessment of pain in the critically ill. In K. A. Puntillo (ed.), *Pain in the Critically Ill: Assessment and Management* (pp. 45–64). With permission of Aspen Publishers, Gaithersburg, MD.

*For complete citation, see references at the end of the chapter.

A, affective; E, evaluative; I, intensity; L, location; M, miscellaneous; NR, not reported; P, pattern; S, sensory; T, temporal.

acteristic facial expressions and varying degrees of movement or immobilization of torso and limbs. The facial configuration associated with acute pain in infants and adults is that of brows drawn together and down, eyes shut, deepening of the nasolabial folds and open mouth.[44, 117, 153, 154]

Body responses to acute pain in children include torso and limb movement or guarding. Very young children manifest a total body response that becomes more refined, guarded, and protective as the child grows older.[155, 156] More conscious types of behavior by patients with chronic and cancer pain have been described as body position changes (sitting, reclining, and standing), body movement (walking and shifting), and pain communication actions (guarding, bracing, rubbing, grimacing, and sighing).[157] Additional behaviors include analgesic use, distraction, pressure manipulation, use of heat, attitude alteration, sleeping, eating, and drinking.[158] Scales that assess behaviors associated with pain have been developed for infants and preverbal children. These instruments usually focus on characteristic facial expressions, body and limb movements, dimensions of cry, and physiological measures of heart and respiratory rates, blood pressure, and sweating. Facial expression was the most consistent indicator of infant pain.[134]

Physiological Responses

Acute pain often activates a sudden SNS response that includes elevation of heart and respiratory rates and blood pressure, pallor, perspiration, flushing, pupil dilation, and drops in levels of transcutaneous oxygen saturation lasting a few minutes to an hour. Very intense and brief pain can be followed by a rebound parasympathetic response. While the sympathetic response may be the only indicator of pain in a pharmacologically paralyzed patient, it is nonspecific and needs to be assessed in the context of potentially painful encounters. Physiological responses are also influenced by attention, habituation, distraction, or predictability.[159, 160]

Mediators of Pain

Manifestations of pain are mediated by personal and situational factors that may account for the differences seen among the responses of individuals experiencing a similar noxious insult. The subjective nature of pain, its intimate association with emotions, and the meaning the individual assigns to it influence how it is exhibited.

Personal Mediators

Pain threshold is relatively stable among individuals[59]; however, *pain tolerance* varies greatly from individual to individual and sometimes in the same individual, depending on the situation. The significance ascribed to a painful experience influences an individual's affective or emotional response. For example, Price found that unlike patients with back and labor pain, cancer patients rated the affective dimension of their pain significantly higher than the sensory dimension.[161] Personal mediators include the individual's own personality characteristics: position on the neuroticism-extroversion continuum, learning and coping style, dependence-independence, and emotional history and state.[162] Although not conclusive, high scores on the neuroticism-extroversion scales have been associated with patients who readily report pain and with higher pain scores.[163]

Individuals are socialized to express emotions and pain by their specific culture's and family's "display rules," which determine how and when to display emotions and pain.[164] This learning occurs through role modeling of acceptable behaviors and behavior modification by significant others.[113] Role modeling has been used successfully to prepare children for painful encounters by having a child initially portray fear and then model adaptive coping behaviors to deal with the painful encounter.[165]

Situational Mediators

Pain responses are also influenced by the situation in which the individual experiences the pain. A classic example is Beecher's comparison of expressions of pain in wounded soldiers and civilian surgical patients.[166] Soldiers with more severe wounds, seeing their injuries as a reprieve from danger, required less analgesia than surgical patients with less severe wounds. Athletes, dancers, and others often ignore their pain to complete their task. Hospital units, like the home culture, impose a set of "display rules" that reflect the beliefs of the physicians and nurses about pain, its manifestations, and relief. Beliefs about opiate usage and how much pain should be tolerated are readily communicated to patients.[167] Regrettably, this is still the situation in many hospitals. However, in 1989 representatives from the Children's Hospital at Johns Hopkins University announced on the national television program "20/20" that their goal for the year was to have a pain-free hospital. This message is very different than one described by Cohen in which only 3 per cent of the nurses had a goal of total pain relief.[168]

SURVEILLANCE

Surveillance for effective pain management requires a conscious vigilance attuned to the dynamic interaction between the patient's pain, its physiological and emotional consequences, therapeutic efficacy, and the patient's idiosyncratic responses. All need to be examined within the context of patient and staff biases that influence pain assessment and relief.

Pain management should be the joint responsibility of patient and staff. The patient needs to report pain and pain relief as accurately as possible, and the staff needs to make frequent and careful assessments and appropriate interventions. The staff also should create a milieu in which patients feel comfortable reporting pain in their own manner.[167] This has been termed "pain work" that the staff must balance with the work of carrying out procedures and treatments and other care-taking tasks. Nurses must assume responsibility and accountability for the assessment and management of patient pain. They must carefully evaluate the problems of unrelieved pain and establish pain work as a priority.

CLINICAL THERAPIES

Therapeutic Goals

The goal of pain management is to relieve pain completely; or, if that is not possible, to relieve it to a degree that the individual can function comfortably. Actions to achieve this goal include the following: (1) when feasible, developing contracts with patients for pain relief based on individual goals; (2) using knowledge of the pathophysiology and trajectory of pain as the basis for various interventions; (3) assessing pain routinely using appropriate instruments, both before and after interventions; (4) using a wide range of pharmacological and nonpharmacological pain relief measures; and (5) documenting pain characteristics and intervention effectiveness.

Two groups, the Oncology Nursing Society and the Agency for Health Care Policy and Research of the U.S. Department of Health and Human Services, Public Health Service,[169, 170] have published a position paper on cancer pain and a definitive guide for the management of acute pain that can help nurses, physicians, and patients design and implement effective strategies for the management of these two common and pervasive sources of pain. The guides clearly explicate nursing responsibilities for assessing and managing pain in both adults and children and emphasize the benefits of pain prevention and control.[169, 170, 170a] In addition, an IASP manual on acute pain management has been published.[170b]

Regrettably, in many situations there are major barriers to adequate pain management. The following are three such barriers:

1. Serious knowledge deficits exist among many physicians and nurses regarding the pathophysiology of pain and the physiological and psychological consequences of unrelieved pain. Many do not understand the difference in mechanisms of acute and chronic pain and why they should be treated differently. There is also limited understanding of the basis for and methods of providing both pharmacological and nonpharmacological relief.[171]

2. Inadequate and incorrect information and current societal attitudes regarding the use of opioids influence the treatment of pain. This results in inappropriate concerns about drug addiction and respiratory depression that adversely influence the treatment of terminally ill patients and those with intractable pain,[172, 173] postoperative pain,[168] and medical pain[174, 175] and of children's pain.[20, 21, 23] Foster and Hester found that administered analgesic doses to children ranged from 10 per cent below to 200 per cent above weight-determined pediatric doses.[22]

3. There is limited practice of routine pain assessments. When assessments are done, there is a limited use of any of the currently available psychometrically adequate pain assessment tools, thus compromising the ability to communicate in common terms about the pain. Assessments may be quite variable and offer little direction for intervention.[176] Foster and Hester found that there was only a moderate association between high pain ratings and analgesic administration and that nurses' pain assessments gave little direction for interventions.[22] Hospital quality assurance committees and administrative and clinical specialists in many institutions are now developing strategies and protocols to assist nurses in assuming accountability for appropriate pain management. Therapeutic interventions can be based on the knowledge of relevant pain anatomy, physiology, and psychology. Figure 13–7 depicts sites of actions for various pharmacological and nonpharmacological therapies.

Pharmacological Therapies

Nonopioid Analgesia: Nonsteroidal Anti-inflammatory Drugs

Nonsteroidal anti-inflammatory drugs (NSAIDs) consist of a heterogeneous group of about 60 chemically diverse compounds generally considered weaker analgesics. These drugs are most commonly used to treat mild-to-moderate, low-grade acute, chronic, inflammatory, and cancer-related pain. Because of their widespread use, both their effectiveness and their side effects are underestimated. All have varying degrees of analgesic, antipyretic, and (except for acetaminophen) anti-inflammatory actions.

These peripherally acting drugs produce analgesia by blocking the synthesis of prostaglandins from their arachidonic acid precursor at the site of tissue injury. Arachidonic acid is released from injured cell membranes and is metabolized through two enzyme-mediated pathways, the cyclo-oxygenase and lipo-oxygenase routes. Cyclo-oxygenase metabolism results in the production of prostaglandins, most importantly PGE_1, PGE_2, and prostacyclin (PGI_2). These sensitize nociceptors and work synergistically with other inflammatory products such as bradykinin and histamine to produce hyperalgesia at the tissue damage site. Aspirin and most NSAIDs inhibit cyclo-oxygenase and interrupt prostaglandin synthesis.[177, 178] The actions of NSAIDs, however, are complex and do not work only through their cyclo-oxygenase inhibition mechanism; there may be NSAID membrane-stabilizing activity as well. Their effects on blood cells and the immune system are now a major focus of study.

Acetaminophen (Tylenol) is the most

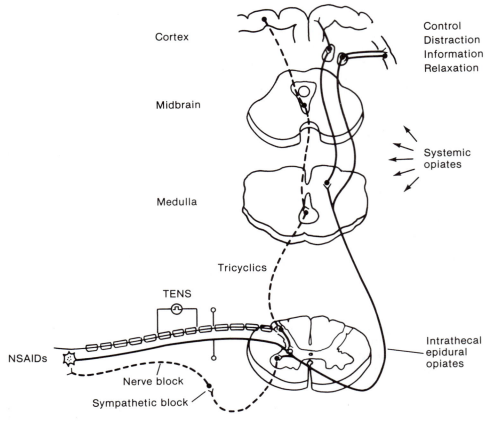

Figure 13–7. Pain therapies and their proposed action sites. (Modified with permission from Fields, H. L., & Levine, J. D. [1984]. *Pain: Mechanisms and Management.* West J Med *141*:347–357.)

widely used pediatric drug in the United States as well as a popular adult analgesic.[179] It is an effective drug for all ages, including premature infants.[180] Although it is thought to selectively inhibit prostaglandin synthesis in the brain,[181] its mode of action is still poorly understood. Since it doesn't inhibit peripheral cyclo-oxygenase, it has no effect on platelet aggregation or gastric and renal prostaglandin, thus avoiding the bleeding or gastric irritation and renal problems associated with other NSAIDs.

The most commonly used and generally least valued of these drugs is aspirin, which actually proved to provide better analgesia than eight other marketed drugs for a group of cancer patients.[182] When combined with weak opioids, aspirin provides significantly greater analgesia than when used alone. The introduction of the newer nonsteroidal drugs, among them ibuprofen (Motrin, Advil), fenoprofen (Nalfon), naproxen (Naprosyn), indomethacin (Indocin), sulindac (Clinoril), tolmetin (Tolectin), and lastly ketorolac tromethamine (Toradol) (which can be administered intramuscularly as well as orally) has enhanced the range of nonopioid choices available for therapy. These drugs have different half-lives and peak actions, which enable the individualization of timing and dosage. However, the selection process is often difficult, since each may act differently in different individuals.[183] Of the NSAIDs, only aspirin, tolmetin, naproxen, and acetaminophen are approved for pediatric use. An exception is indomethacin, which is approved for pediatric use only to close the patent ductus in neonates.[178]

For individuals with asthma, peptic ulcers, or bleeding disorders and for surgical patients, the use of most NSAIDs is not innocuous.[184] Aspirin-induced asthma is thought to result because the lipo-oxygenase–mediated metabolism of arachidonic acid is only variably inhibited by most NSAIDS in current use. When arachidonic acid is shunted from the cyclo-oxygenase to the lipo-oxygenase pathway during therapy with NSAIDS, there is an increased production of some broncho-constricting leukotrienes, the end-products of lipo-oxygenase metabolism.[185] However, ketoprofen (Orudis) appears to influence both pathways.[186] Gastric and renal irritation and bleeding may result from inhibition of prostaglandin synthetase, which also decreases the synthesis of desirable prostaglandins that are protective to stomach and kidneys.

NSAIDs differ from opioid analgesics in the following ways:

1. They exhibit a ceiling analgesic effect; that is, increasing the dosage above a certain level usually results in no increased analgesic action and only in a slight prolongation of analgesia with the added risk of toxic actions.

2. They do not result in tolerance and only rarely produce side effects. Dependence on these drugs is being questioned; however, most researchers discount it and attribute dependence to behavioral changes that result from pain relief.[175, 183]

3. They have antipyretic properties.

4. They are most commonly administered orally.

5. They may be combined with weak opioids such as codeine.[184]

Opioid Analgesia

Opium derivatives of the poppy plant have been used throughout history for their analgesic, sedative, and euphoric effects.[187] They continue to be the standard of pharmacological therapy for moderate-to-severe acute, chronic, and cancer pain. The actual mechanisms of opioid action have become more clear since the discovery and localization of endogenous opioid receptors.[188] Exogenous opioid ligands such as morphine interact with these opioid receptors and exert a biological response similar to the effects of endogenous opioids; that is, they have agonist action. Conversely, when opioid antagonists such as naloxone attach to an an opioid receptor, they prevent the binding of an agonist.[189] Some opioids such as butorphanol (Stadol) are classified as mixed agonist-antagonists, since they have agonist effects at one receptor type and antagonist effects when binding to a second type.[190]

Opioid receptors have been located in areas of the limbic system, the PAG and thalamus, the spinal cord gray matter, and the gut. This localization accounts for the alterations in mood, involvement of descending pain inhibitory systems, blockage of spinal pain transmission, and interruption of gastrointestinal motility, respectively, that occur with opioid analgesic therapy. Spinal cord opiate receptors are found predominantly in the substantia gelatinosa, the hypothesized site of gate control. Here opiates act presynaptically, binding to receptors on the cell body and terminals of primary afferents and inhibiting release of noxious transmitter substances such as substance P. Opiates may also act postsynaptically,[191] thus interfering with ascending transmission through secondary neurons.

Opioid actions can depend on the type of receptor to which they attach. Many different types of receptors have been discovered, some of which have subtypes.[192] Table 13–3 presents a list of the opioid receptor types believed to be involved in opiate analgesia. Most opiates have an affinity for mu receptors. Mu receptors are of two subtypes, mu-1 and mu-2. Mu-1 receptors are located in many supraspinal sites and mediate the analgesia effects of opiates. Mu-2 receptors may, in turn, mediate the respiratory depressant and gastrointestinal effects (e.g., consti-

TABLE 13–3 OPIOID RECEPTORS AND THEIR AGONISTS

Opiod Receptor Type	Clinical Effects	Agonist
Mu	Analgesia (supra-spinal) (mu-1)	Morphine and enkephalin (mu-1) Morphine (mu-2)
	Respiratory depression (mu-2)	Fentanyl Alfentanil
	Bradycardia	Sufentanil
	Euphoria	Lofentanil
Kappa	Sedation Analgesia (spinal) Low/no respiratory depression Low addiction	(Ethyl) ketocyclazocine Bremazocine Nalbuphine Butorphanol Nalorphine U-50488II
Delta	Respiratory depression Analgesia (spinal cord)	D-Ala-D-leu-enkephalin (DADL) Enkephalin

Modified from Veselis, R. A. (1988). Sedation and pain management for the critically ill. Crit Care Clin 4:168.

pation) of opiates.[192, 193] Knowledge of the differential opioid responses to mu-1 or mu-2 receptor attachment has clinical relevance. For example, development of analgesics with preferential affinity for mu-1 receptors may reduce unwanted side effects mediated at mu-2 receptors, such as respiratory depression and constipation.

A second type of opioid compound—D-Ala-D-leu-enkephalin (DADL)—has delta-receptor affinity properties. It has been used investigationally to treat pain in morphine-tolerant cancer patients with some degree of success,[194] since the two drugs act at different opiate receptors. Finally, kappa-selective compounds may mediate spinal cord level analgesia[59] and therefore have little or no respiratory depressant properties.

Opioid Tolerance, Physical Dependence, and Addiction. Development of tolerance, dependence, and addiction to opioids is a matter of great concern to patients and health care professionals alike. An understanding of the differences between these states is essential to the appropriate assessment and management of patients in pain. Tolerance is a physiological state in which greater amounts of opiates are required to achieve a similar analgesic effect.[184] Development of tolerance seems to vary across species,[195] individuals,[190] and types of opioid. In fact, fentanyl tolerance was reported to develop within hours after intravenous administration in a critically ill patient.[196] Catalano suggests that cross-tolerance between different opioids may be incomplete.[197] This provides a theoretical basis for substituting other opiates when a particular one has lost its effectiveness.

Physical dependence is also a physiological phenomenon in which a withdrawal syndrome is precipitated upon termination of analgesic use.[190] Opioid withdrawal behaviors are believed to result from rebound CNS noradrenergic activity that is depressed by chronic opioid use.[198] An exciting area for future research is the relationship of physical opioid dependence to receptor typology and the development of receptor-selective drugs[192] to avoid or counteract dependence.

Addiction, or psychological dependence, occurs when an individual shows evidence of compulsive, drug-seeking behavior.[184] Physical dependence and addiction are not the same; however, the addicted individual usually also has physical opioid dependence. It

is imperative that health care professionals recognize the differences between tolerance, physical dependence, and addiction in order to provide appropriate interventions. Development of addiction is extremely rare when opioids are used to treat patients in pain.[199, 200] Thus, limiting use of analgesics simply out of concern about addiction development is generally unwarranted and may, in fact, be negligent.

Modes and Sites of Opioid Analgesia Therapy. Tremendous advances have been made in opioid administration and methods. A direct result of the experimental knowledge developed about spinal cord receptor sites has been the administration of opioids spinally, either intrathecally (i.e, into the subarachnoid space) or epidurally. Since the drug is administered close to receptor sites, less drug is needed and duration of effect is longer than when given intravenously.

Although it is beyond the scope of this chapter to present a detailed discussion of spinal analgesia, it is important to note the diverse patient populations in which spinal analgesia has been used with success. Spinal opioids have been used to relieve postoperative pain in adults[201] and children.[202] However, respiratory depression in children may be prolonged, requiring close monitoring.[202, 203] Labor pain[204] and cancer pain[205] have also been managed with spinal opioids. Certain properties of specific opiates influence the onset, spread, and duration of analgesia obtained. A very important property is the drug's lipid solubility. Fentanyl, sufentanil, and alfentanil are very lipid soluble. Therefore, they will have a more rapid onset of action than morphine, which is one of the least lipid-soluble opioids.[206] In addition to their lipid solubility, the duration of action seen with opioids is influenced by the dose and spread of the drug, the pain stimulus, and the individuality of the patient.[206]

Side effects associated with spinal opioids may include respiratory depression, nausea, vomiting, constipation, pruritus, urinary retention, and ineffective analgesia.[191, 206] People who are receiving long-term opioid infusions, such as for cancer pain, often develop tolerance to the respiratory effects of the opioids.[197]

Delivery modes for spinal analgesics include bolus or continuous administration through catheters placed in the subarachnoid or epidural space. Analgesics may also be administered through implantable systems that deliver continuous specified volumes and concentrations of analgesics.[207] The latter modes are generally used for management of cancer pain when the goal of management includes the ability to be managed at home and cost efficiency[208] in addition to effective analgesia and safety. A second major method of opioid analgesia delivery is patient-controlled analgesia systems, which are discussed later.

Use of Local Anesthetics for Pain Control

Local anesthetics such as bupivacaine (Marcaine) block nerve conduction in primary afferent fibers, thus inhibiting the transmission of pain from a particular region. Specifically, they act by decreasing cell membrane permeability to sodium, thus preventing cellular depolarization.[209] The block can involve pain as well as other sensory (e.g., touch, pressure, and vibration), sympathetic, and motor fibers, depending on the amount, concentration, and type of local anesthetic used. Small, unmyelinated noxious and sympathetic fibers are usually affected by the block before involvement of larger, myelinated motor fibers.[210] The sympatholytic vasodilatation effect of local anesthetics may be an undesirable side effect if hypotension results.[209] Yet, this vasodilatation may be a desirable response if pain is due to diminished peripheral blood flow.[211] In fact, both pain reduction and increased regional blood flow are desired beneficial effects of use of regional anesthesia for reimplantation of severed extremities.[212] Axillary brachial plexus, supraclavicular, interscalene, stellate ganglion, or epidural blocks may be employed, depending on the reimplantation site. Intercostal[213, 214] and intrapleural[215] nerve blocks have been employed to relieve both pediatric[214] and adult[215] postoperative pain. Local anesthetics have also been administered spinally for pain in myocardial infarction.[216] Short-term use of local anesthetics may reverse opioid tolerance that develops with chronic opioid use by allowing opioid receptors to redevelop sensitivity.[207]

Surgical Ablative Procedures for Pain Relief

Many procedures have been performed to destroy nerve tissues, nerve fibers, or nerve tracts believed to be involved in, or the source of, pain. For example, lesions have been made in dorsal nerve roots, primary afferent fibers have been severed or destroyed with neurotoxic substances such as alcohol, ascending spinothalamic and trigeminal tracts have been severed, and and lesions have been made in nuclei in various brain sites.[217, 218] All of these procedures have had variable degrees of success in relieving pain. Anterolateral cordotomies, performed for relief of cancer and less often chronic pain usually have high degrees of initial success. In these procedures, spinoreticulothalmic tracts, which ascend in the anterolateral column of the spinal cord, are severed.[219] Because pain may recur over time after cordotomies, they are usually reserved for cancer pain. In fact, pain may recur in individuals who undergo any of these ablative procedures, demonstrating the complexity of a pain experience as well as our lack of complete knowledge of the anatomy and mechanisms of pain. These procedures can be accompanied by serious side effects, such as paresthesia or other serious neurological deficits.[218]

Neurostimulation Procedures

Peripheral Nerve Stimulation

Peripheral nerve stimulation has been used to relieve chronic causalgic, neuralgic, or phantom limb pains, with a success rate approximated at 46 per cent.[91] Stimulation, transmitted through electrodes placed near the peripheral pain site, may increase the pain threshold or inhibit spontaneous central discharges. The mechanism of pain relief from peripheral nerve stimulation is not entirely clear.

Spinal Cord Neurostimulation

The dorsal column of the spinal cord has been a site of intervention in cases of chronic pain, especially when the pain is neurogenic or vascular in origin.[91] Electrical stimulation of the dorsal column through an electrode placed in the vertebral canal rostral to the pain site[218] sometimes has been successful in long-term relief of pain.[91] There have been a number of proposed physiological mechanisms to explain chronic pain suppression resulting from dorsal column stimulation. These include stimulation of peripheral nonpain fibers at the spinal cord level, inhibition of sympathetic efferents, stimulation of descending pain inhibition pathways, and neurohormonal involvement.[91]

Deep Brain Neurostimulation

Knowledge gained about endogenous analgesic systems through experimental animal model research has led to the development and refinement of techniques designed to activate these systems electrically in cases of intractable pain. Electrodes are placed in specific brain sites, and a neuropacemaker apparatus is used to activate these electrodes.[218] A number of structures along the endogenous analgesic pathways have been stimulation sites. For example, periaqueductal gray (PAG) and periventricular gray (PVG) stimulation have been successful for pains of peripheral origin such as chronic low back pain, while stimulation of somatosensory areas such as the thalamus and internal capsule has controlled deafferentation pain in some cases.[220] The overall degree of success from these deep brain stimulation techniques has been estimated to be 55 per cent.[91] The mechanism for analgesia produced by electrical stimulation of these CNS sites is not clear. PAG and PVG stimulation-induced analgesia has led to increased endorphin release and probable activation of monoamine systems. The mechanism of thalamic stimulation success, on the other hand, is not understood. However, it does not appear to be opioid-mediated, since the analgesic effect from stimulation is not blocked by the opioid antagonist naloxone.[91]

Nonpharmacological Interventions for Pain

The gate control theory[3] serves as a theoretical basis for some nonpharmacological interventions. These interventions either inhibit or modulate the ascending transmission of a noxious stimulus from the periphery or stimulate descending inhibitory control from the brain. Their advantages are noninvasiveness, usual uncomplicated administration, and often economy. Patients may be taught to use them independently, which provides them a measure of control. Patients need to be encouraged to continue the treatment long enough for it to work. These measures may not cure painful conditions but may make them tolerable.[221]

Peripheral interventions that influence ascending impulse transmission include cutaneous stimulation such as massage, exercise, vibration, transcutaneous electrical nerve stimulation (TENS), acupuncture, acupressure, and heat or cold. Strategies inhibiting transmission by descending control include relaxation, distraction, information, patient control, guided imagery, and hypnosis. Some of these strategies will be described briefly.

Peripheral Interventions

Cutaneous Stimulation. Stimulation of large, non-nociceptive fibers is postulated to inhibit noxious impulse transmission at the spinal cord.[3] Firm stimulation may also cause release of endorphins and other pain-inhibiting neurotransmitters as well. The most common strategies are rubbing or massage. Rubbing or massaging may be accomplished with differing amounts of pressure and can use acupuncture or trigger points that are distributed throughout the body. Cutaneous stimulation is often facilitated by use of lubricant to reduce friction, and if performed by a caring person, it adds the additional dimension of emotional support.

Transcutaneous Electrical Nerve Stimulation. TENS is physician-prescribed and taught to patients. The TENS unit consists of a small battery power source with frequency, waveform, amplitude controls, and electrodes that, when activated, lead to selective and repetitive stimulation of the large non-nociceptive A alpha and beta fibers that inhibit nociceptive impulse transmission. Stimulation pulsations may vary, but electrode placement must take into consideration anatomical and physiological factors, pain source, and dermatomal distribution.[221, 222] Like acupuncture, TENS may also stimulate endorphin and serotonin release.[222]

Eland reported relief of therapy-related pain in eight children with cancer and phantom limb pain using TENS by applying electrodes at either acupuncture point or points determined by pain location.[223] In a study that examined patient, stimulator, and outcome variables in chronic pain, TENS reduced pain by more than half in 47 per cent of patients. Analgesia was attained within a half-hour in 75 per cent of the patients. Post-TENS analgesia lasted less than 30 minutes in 51 per cent and more than 1 hour in 30 per cent.[224] On the other hand, patients with low back pain treated with sham stimulation or TENS did not get significant relief from TENS.[225] Use of TENS is contraindicated in patients with demand cardiac pacemakers and in those who are susceptible to contact dermatitis, pregnant, emotionally unstable, or opioid dependent (opiates reduce effectiveness of TENS).[222]

Heat and Cold. Cold is hypothesized to relieve pain by causing vasoconstriction and decreasing conduction velocity of small unmyelinated fibers and by altering cellular permeability, thus reducing cellular metabolism, oxygen need, and edema.[226] It is useful in treating post-traumatic injuries, swelling, rheumatoid arthritis, muscle spasms, and low back pain. The effectiveness of commonly used cold packs is limited because the body can compensate for the slow temperature drop. Ice massage with an ice popsicle is reported to be more effective.[221] An ice popsicle, made by freezing a stick in a cup of water, is wrapped in a towel and rubbed over the area. Ice massage at trigger points or over the pain area was equal to TENS in reducing low back pain.[227] In contrast to heat, cold penetrates deeper into tissues without causing tissue damage. Precautions should be taken to avoid frostbite with all ice therapy, and it should not be used in individuals with compromised circulation. Early ambulation should be encouraged to avoid muscle stiffness.[221]

Heat produces vasodilation resulting in increased local blood flow, which improves tissue nutrition and removes algesic metabolic products. It is used to reduce muscle spasms, induce relaxation, and facilitate therapy and is especially useful for those who cannot tolerate cold. Heat is delivered by either conduction (heat pads, lamps, and paraffin dip), convection (whirlpool and steam cabinets), or conversion (shock wave diathermy and ultrasound). Tissue injury should be prevented by monitoring the temperature of the unit. Tissues should be protected by limiting treatments to 30 minutes three to four times daily.[221, 226] McCaffery and Beebe describe an electrically operated device that has various sized blankets and can be switched from heat to cold.[160] Caution is required when using heat for injuries in limited body spaces, since swelling can occur.

Centrally Acting Interventions

Relaxation. This strategy is designed to interrupt the pain-stress-pain cycle in which pain and stress reinforce each other, producing ever-increasing episodes of painful muscle spasms.[97] Relaxation may use progressive or individual muscle relaxation, deep breathing exercises, and attention focusing.[160]

Horowitz and associates compared pain in three groups of postoperative cardiac patients.[228] One group practiced local jaw relaxation training, the second practiced general relaxation training, and the third was a control group. Resting pain intensity did not differ among groups; however, both relaxation groups had lower pain distress scores, and the general relaxation group reported significantly lower distress scores and less pain when ambulating. Relaxation also reduced incisional pain, analgesic consumption, and body distress in another group of postoperative patients.[229] In two adaptations of relaxation procedures for children, one asked children to pretend to be a tire and breathe in slowly to inflate it and then slowly breathe out to deflate.[230] The second is the "He-Who" breathing exercise described by McCaffery.[231] The following directions can be used to teach relaxation: (1) get into a comfortable position and close the eyes; (2) starting at the feet, relax the muscles up to and including the face; and (3) breathe through the nose and say one while breathing in and breathe out while counting two.[232] A 20-minute session is advised, although individuals should not be concerned if they cannot last that long. The lack of success reported in some relaxation studies in clinical settings has been attributed to how well the patient learned the procedure. Mast and associates developed a three-unit self-learning module to teach and use relaxation techniques.[233]

When relaxation is successful, in addition to pain relief, patient responses may include decreases in heart and respiratory rates and blood pressure and reduced oxygen consumption, muscle tension, anxiety, and stress. Although relaxation is desirable for most patients, a few may find it difficult. Depressed persons and those who need to maintain control or have cardiac or respiratory irregularities may not benefit from relaxation and should have physician evaluation prior to the intervention.[233]

Distraction. Distraction interventions reduce pain by focusing the individual's attention away from pain onto another stimulus. This is based on the belief that when two separate stimuli are presented, focusing on one will negate the other.[160] When pain moves to the edge of consciousness, its intensity is reduced, and it becomes more tolerable. However, the complexity of the distraction needs to be increased as the intensity of the pain increases. A major misconception about distraction held by patients and professionals alike is that if the person is able to be distracted the pain is not real. Children often are victims of this belief. Young children with their shorter attention spans can easily distract themselves or be distracted; professionals observing children at play are unlikely to believe the presence of pain. Most individuals can distract their pain by visiting with friends, reading, watching television, or listening to radio. Such actions can minimize the perception of pain intensity while the activity is going on, but the pain may seem more severe when the distraction stops.

Listening to favorite music reduced analgesic requirements 30 per cent in patients experiencing pain[234] and reduced musculoskeletal and nerve pain reactions in gynecological patients who listened to 15 minutes of music every 2 hours.[235] Infants' use of nonnutritive sucking for heel stick pain has been successful.[236, 237]

Information. Information about impending events, including anticipated pain, is designed to reduce their unknown and frightening aspects and enable the individual to develop strategies to deal with them.[238] Many prehospitalization and preprocedural preparation programs have been developed with this goal in mind.[239–242] Many studies use behavioral distress as a measure that encompasses both pain and anxiety.[155] Three types of information are generally provided: procedural (what will happen and when), sensory (what it feels like), and instructional (what to do to help yourself during the event). Providing both procedural and sensory information increased pain tolerance[243] and reduced the amount of pain medication needed.[244] Visintainer and Wolfer added an instructional component to procedural and sensory information at specific stress points.[245] Children receiving information had lower distress scores at blood drawing and required less analgesics postoperatively.

Filmed modeling of a child, initially frightened, but using suggested techniques to cope with anxiety and potential painful encounters proved more effective than a "mastery"

model in which the patient shows no fear.[240] The timing for providing information appears to be critical. Melamed and associates[239] found that information helped reduce physiological arousal in older children and those whose surgery was the next day. Younger children and those whose information and surgery were on the same day had higher levels of arousal.

Individual coping styles, anxiety levels, and fear influence the success of information in reducing stress or pain. Patients, identified as "copers" or "sensitizers," use information to develop approaches to manage the event. On the other hand, providing information to "avoiders," who use denial as a coping strategy, may increase stress, postsurgical analgesia needs, and complaints.[246, 247]

Kim described the relationship between anxiety levels and the use of information on postoperative pain scores.[248] She found that providing information to individuals with high physical danger trait anxiety resulted in higher postoperative pain scores. Conversely, patients with low physical danger trait anxiety reported lower pain scores than a "no information" group.

Control. Control over life activities is achieved slowly throughout childhood and is the benchmark of adulthood. Extent of control over an adverse event can directly determine an individual's reaction to it; individuals who feel lack of control experience it as more anxious or painful. Control or perceived control thus becomes a significant factor in determining the reactive response to pain,[249, 250] and providing an individual with the opportunity to exercise control over pain may decrease its intensity.

Patient-controlled analgesia (PCA) is an analgesic delivery system that has become a popular method for relieving pain. With PCA, patients administer themselves a predetermined analgesic dose when they need it (within physician-specified parameters) via a special pump. The recommended dose of analgesic is divided into microdoses that are administered more frequently than the usual timed protocol, thus maintaining drug plasma levels within the narrow therapeutic window. Dubois reported that PCA adjusts for individual variation in analgesic needs and provides titration that maintains therapeutic levels.[251] The PCA system gives patients control and breaks the cycle of pain associated with analgesia peaks and valleys of the usual protocols. Postoperative patients generally use more analgesia during the first several days, but as pain intensity decreases, so does the analgesic use.

Many patients do not titrate for total relief but balance the intensity of their pain against undesired effects of the opioids. Ferrante and associates found that more PCA patients titrated to moderate pain than patients receiving intramuscular analgesics.[252] Albert and Talbot reported better analgesia with less sedation, and less drug use and that the shortened stays compensated for the higher cost of PCA.[253] In another study eight terminally ill cancer patients used PCA over a 48-hour period to titrate their analgesics. They managed their pain successfully with minimum sedation and no respiratory depression. They were then switched to oral analgesics using the PCA dosing guide with the same satisfactory results.[254] Although sedation and respiratory depression are concerns for patients and health care professionals, both issues have been manageable and patient safety has not been compromised.

PCA use with children, whose needle fears are a major concern, has also been successful. Samples in most studies, however, have been small, and most have included mainly older children.[255, 256] Gaukroger and associates found in a sample of 40 postsurgical patients, including eight who were 6 to 7 years old, that the scoliosis surgery patients required significantly more morphine than the general surgery patients.[257] Patients with sickle cell disease needed high doses early in the sickling crisis; however, drug use tapered off when the crisis was resolved, dispelling concerns of drug abuse.[258] PCA and PCA-plus patients reported lower pain scores in a study that compared intramuscular morphine, PCA morphine, and PCA plus continuous low-dose morphine. There was less sedation in the PCA-plus patients than in the intramuscular group.[259]

Further study is needed about the characteristics of patients who refuse or are unsuccessful in using PCA. It is not clear whether there are fears related to drug addiction or overdose or whether patients who have greater dependency needs do not want control.

ILLUSTRATIVE CASE STUDIES

PEDIATRIC CASE STUDY

A.D., a 20-kg, 10-year-old boy, was admitted after emergency surgery for correction of midgut volvulus malrotation, a tumor resection, and an appendectomy. He was pale, and his breath sounds were decreased in the lower bases. His heart rate ranged from 110 to 130, and respirations were between 20 and 24 throughout the night. He received 1.0 mg of morphine intravenously (IV) twice, then 1.5 mg every 3 to 5 hours throughout the night and the next day for complaints of pain, after which he reported relief. However, his breath sounds continued to be diminished. On the morning of postoperative day 2, he was found lying stiffly in bed, pale, perspiring, moaning quietly, face contorted, and refusing to deep breathe or get out of bed. Respirations were 28, heart rate was 124, and blood pressure was 118/80 mm Hg. He was placed on PCA with a basal rate of morphine of 0.015 mg/kg/hour and a patient control dose of 0.3 mg with a lockout period of 10 minutes. During the next 4 hours, he administered himself three doses on six attempts, then two doses on three attempts during the next 4 hours, followed by a 7-hour period with no attempts while he slept soundly. Total time on PCA was 72 hours with infrequent and clustered dosing. His respirations and heart rate returned to normal, and he willingly coughed, walked, and did deep breathing.

This case illustrates several problems in pediatric pain management. Although medicated on a routine basis when he complained of pain, the intensity of his pain or relief was never measured, a common problem on units that have not adopted a protocol for measuring pain. Second, the p.r.n. analgesic dose was inadequate for his weight. Considering the extent of his surgery, by the time he received the analgesics, the pain was out of control and it was difficult to catch up. Although he reported "relief" after medication, his heart and respiratory rates continued to be rapid, his respiratory function was inadequate, and he was still in pain as manifested by his behaviors. This child received more analgesics than many postoperative children, but it was not until he received a continuous infusion of morphine supplemented by additional morphine as needed that his pain was controlled.

ADULT CASE STUDY

Mr. H. was a 71-year-old patient in the intensive care unit after undergoing a four-vessel coronary artery bypass graft (CABG). His first few postoperative recovery days were relatively stable except for a heart rhythm of atrial fibrillation-flutter that was difficult to manage. His nurses noted Mr. H. to be quite hypervigilant, that is, overly attentive to bedside activity such as conversations with and between hospital personnel. His heart rate increased when staff moved about as they performed procedures. On the third postoperative day Mr. H. was supposed to have his chest tube removed, and he was told of this plan. Thirty minutes prior to the chest tube removal, Mr. H. expressed significant concern about this procedure. He told his nurse, "I'm not ready for this. Why don't we wait till tomorrow?" The nurse held Mr. H.'s hand and noted that it was diaphoretic. She gave him information about the procedure—what he should expect to feel, how long it would take—while stroking his hand. The nurse then asked him to close his eyes and take slow, deep breaths. She used distraction by talking about the patient's family and his leisure activities. Mr. H.'s heart rate decreased. At that time the medical team arrived and removed Mr. H.'s chest tube. Afterward he said that the procedure was much easier than he expected, yet Mr. H. rated the pain intensity of the chest tube removal procedure as 7 on a 0 to 10 numerical rating scale. He said that pain medications really helped him cope with the procedure; however, he had not received any medication since 3 mg of morphine had been administered over 11 hours earlier! Mr. H. appeared to respond positively to the distraction, relaxation, and imagery techniques instituted by the nurse; that is, his heart rate decreased and he believed the procedure was easier than he had anticipated. However, if nonpharmacological pain management techniques had been reinforced with appropriate types and amount of analgesics, pain management may have been improved and pain intensity decreased.

REVIEW OF NURSING RESEARCH FINDINGS

Pediatric Pain

Research in children's pain has grown dramatically since 1985, reflecting the interest and work of nurses, psychologists, and physicians. A dedicated cadre of investigators and clinicians has emerged and organized themselves as the Pediatric Pain Interest Group of the IASP. Four books devoted exclusively to children's pain have been published.[260–263] The breadth and depth of these works have added immeasurably to the understanding of children's pain and have raised both consciousness and excitement.

Nursing research launched this knowledge revolution with Eland's and Anderson's report of the marked discrepancy between the amount of analgesics prescribed and the amount administered to children and adults matched for diagnosis.[21] Six years later, Beyer and associates replicated this study with cardiac surgery patients and reported that compared with adults, children were still being woefully undermedicated.[20] The undermedication of children was reported again by Foster and Hester.[22]

The lack of developmentally appropriate valid and reliable tools to assess pain in children was identified in these early studies. Nurses, physicians, and psychologists responded to this need. In addition to tool development across the pediatric age range, nursing research has focused on variables and attitudes that influence nursing decisions to medicate children for pain as well as beginning intervention studies.

A variety of tools with acceptable to excellent psychometric values that use both verbal reports and behaviors have been reported. Hester and associates developed and tested the Poker Chip tool, which enabled children 4 to 13 years to report their pain intensity by the number of chips selected.[146, 147] Two years later, Eland described a color scale in which children selected their own colors to quantify their pain and developed individual color scales.[264] These scales were used in conjunction with body outline to report the location and intensity of pain. Beyer published the "Oucher," a two-scale tool that features a 0 to 100 scale for older children able to count to 100 and a faces scale showing increasing distress for the younger child.[138] It has been tested for its validity and reliability in a number of studies.[145] This tool is currently being adapted and tested for black and Hispanic children.[265] The cultural influence on pain assessment was also examined by Adams, who found that reliability coefficients between reported pain scores and observed behaviors were lower in Hispanic than Anglo children who underwent invasive oncological procedures.[266] Abu-Saad reported on the development and testing of a tool in Dutch children.[267]

Savedra and associates developed and tested a multidimensional pain assessment tool, the Adolescent Pediatric Pain Assessment Tool (APPT) described previously.[268] Among other less tested tools are a pain ladder,[269] a pain thermometer,[280] and a smiling-to-sad cartoon faces scale.[140] All these approaches attempt to capture a child's interest and developmental ability to report pain.

Others tackled assessing pain in infants, and their work has provided useful guidelines, although with limited psychometric reports for assessing pain in this vulnerable population. Franck used a photogrammetric method in which the videotapes of the heel sticks were replayed against a grid to measure the motor response of infants to the sticks.[271] She later reported on infant behaviors observed by nurses as indicators of infant pain and interventions the nurses used to relieve pain.[272] Lawrence and associates developed the Neonatal Infant Pain Scale (NIPS) that enables assessment of facial expression, cry, respirations, movement, and infant state.[152] Johnston and Strada used a multidimensional approach and reported physiological responses and changes in cry and facial expression by infants undergoing heel sticks.[134] Infant cries have been the focus of special study, and Fuller and associates identified specific changes in infant cry acoustics that indicate pain.[133]

Intervention studies for pediatric pain are only just beginning. Field and Goldson[237] and Campos[236] examined the influence of non-nutritive sucking on infants' response to painful stimuli. Fowler-Kerry and Ramsey-Lander found that distraction (music) and suggestion resulted in significantly lower pain scores in 54- to 74-month-old children to injection pain.[273] Brennen reported on the identification of 68 strategies used by nurses

to assist children during invasive procedures.[274]

A series of studies have attempted to identify and describe the variables that influence nurses' decisions to medicate children for pain.[275–278] This issue is a major focus of concern, since current research indicates that despite the advances made in the recognition of children's pain and the development of appropriate assessment tools, physicians still underprescribe and nurses still administer less analgesic than ordered. Decisions not to medicate are not based on pain assessment. In fact, Foster and Hester found that the nurses' assessment of a child's pain did not relate to the decision to administer analgesia.[22] Tesler and associates found similar results.[279] Variables identified as influencing decisions to medicate and how much analgesic to administer include the nurse's age (younger nurses administer medications more frequently) and education (the greater the nurse's education the more likely that analgesia will be provided). Also, nurses reported having children of their own and experiencing severe pain in the past as positively influencing their decision to medicate for pain.

Adult Pain

Although there is little doubt that nurses have long been concerned about patient pain, nursing research on the pain of adults began in earnest just over 2 decades ago. At that time, a number of nurse researchers were interested in investigating inferences that people make about pain and suffering in others.[280–283] These inferences, it was found, are influenced by the cultures of both patients and nurses, the length of time in nursing, and the occupation of the individual doing the pain assessment. For example, social workers who evaluated patient pain scenarios felt patients had more physical pain than did the nurses and physicians who evaluated the same scenarios.[280] Researchers later reinforced an earlier finding that length of time in nursing negatively correlated with nurses' impression about the amount of physical pain being experienced by patients.[284] Others found that nurses attributed significantly less pain in patients whose physical pathological findings were negative and when the pain was chronic.[285] Ratings were least positive for patients with chronic low back pain versus those with headaches or joint pain. On the other hand, nurses who personally experienced intense pain themselves have inferred significantly more patient physical suffering due to pain.[286] From these studies awareness of factors that can influence a nurse's assessment of patient pain may help to keep biases and prejudices in check to the benefit of patients.

Early nurse researchers were also interested in exploring the effect of nurses' interactions with patients on patients' pain relief.[287–290] Generally, deliberative nursing actions, such as positive comments, distracting statements, or involvement of patients in decision making, worked positively to help relieve pain. However, nurses have often not intervened adequately in the pharmacological relief of pain, partly because of their inaccurate and incomplete knowledge of analgesic actions.[168]

Recognizing that pain is a multidimensional experience, nurse researchers have been able to differentiate successfully between a patient's pain sensation and the distress associated with it through development and use of specific instruments.[229–293] However, few instruments have been developed and used in nursing research to assess patients' verbal, behavioral, and physiological responses to pain.[235, 287] Unfortunately, the validity and reliability of multidimensional instruments such as these have not been well established. Yet, currently there is work on the refinement of an instrument that quantifies both sensory and affective dimensions of pain as well as pain intensity.[294, 295]

Some nurse researchers have valued the importance of exploring the breadth of patients' pain experience. These explorations have included the percentage of patients in various populations who suffer pain, what the pain and suffering are like for them, and how it is assessed and treated.[19, 296–299] Medical-surgical,[19] cancer,[298] and critical care[299] patients have reported experiencing intense pain unrelieved by pharmacological and nonpharmacological pain-relief measures. A major reason for this may be that most of the time nurses never ask patients anything about their pain.[298, 300] Certainly, identification of pain is an important prerequisite to its treatment. Patients in research studies who have been willing to describe their suffering and methods by which they cope with their suffering[296, 297] give health professionals di-

rection for the use of specific relief interventions.

In fact, the most dominant category of nursing research of adult patients in pain has been in the area of nursing therapeutics. For example, nurses have taught patients about the type of pain sensations to expect from procedures or surgery[291, 301] in an attempt to decrease pain and suffering and increase coping. They have also tested various nonpharmacological methods of pain control that would help to decrease pain. For example, various pain coping strategies have been evaluated in nulliparous women for their potential effectiveness for childbirth pain.[302] Relaxation techniques and information have been used with variable degrees of success in decreasing postoperative pain and distress.[229, 293, 301] Relaxation techniques have also decreased pain, while not affecting functional ability, in women with rheumatoid arthritis.[303] Music has also decreased pain intensity, sensations, and affective responses during wound dressing changes[304] and has had a positive influence on pain and anxiety reduction in intensive care unit patients.[305] Research on nonpharmacological interventions for pain relief, such as information, relaxation techniques, and music, may stimulate further research and clinical use of these nursing therapeutics.

IMPLICATIONS FOR FURTHER RESEARCH

Pain in Children

The research thus far has set the stage for intervention studies in children's pain. Several investigators have stressed the need for developing strategies for using the tools that have been developed. Of crucial importance is the need to identify methods to reduce the unreasonable fears about opioids and to help health professionals, families, and children to understand the difference between the therapeutic and the recreational use of opioids. This involves a delicate balance between antidrug education and the need for pain relief. Myths need to be dispelled and a pharmacological knowledge base needs to be developed to make professionals and families feel comfortable with these analgesics.

Both pharmacological and nonpharmacological pain management interventions need to be tested in a variety of settings and with different populations. Testing the feasibility and effectiveness of different routes of medication administration for different age children is crucial. A major area of concern is the management of iatrogenic pain in the various settings in which children receive care, especially in trauma units. Although professionals are recognizing the pervasiveness of children's painful encounters, expediency often negates appropriate pain preventive measures. Chronically ill children need to have their pain recognized and assessed and managed appropriately. The need for the assessment and management of the pain of developmentally delayed and handicapped children who may not be able to communicate their pain adequately is imperative. The consequences of unrelieved and frequent pain on infants' and children's emotional development and their ability to handle future painful encounters also need to be studied.

Pain in Adults

Considerable nursing research on pain has been published in the past 20 years. An analysis of these studies shows that nurses have been particularly interested in researching the efficacy of nursing therapeutics. As a result, researchers have favored correlational and experimental research designs and have for the most part neglected studies of a qualitative nature. Qualitative studies could add a contextual component to the individual's pain experience and could increase understanding of the meaning of pain and suffering to patients.

Many different instruments have been used by nurses to measure pain, sometimes at the expense of accuracy and validity. Studies on instrumentation could improve validity and reliability of results and thereby increase confidence in research findings.

There is a particular value to the development of cluster studies, particularly those that extend, replicate, and refine prior work. For example, one cluster of studies used an analogue of labor pain to evaluate preparatory interventions for labor pain.[302, 306-308] This type of research enhances the development and extension of theory and can support the advancement of nursing science.[309]

Finally, conceptual frameworks, particularly those using pain physiology, have often not been well developed by nurses. Present knowledge of the physiological mechanisms of pain offers considerable support for the development and testing of both descriptive and interventional studies. Furthermore, nursing theories have been omitted in the conceptualization of most nursing pain research. Using nursing theory within the framework of pain studies could highlight nursing's unique ability to help the person in pain.

REFERENCES

1. Fülöp-Miller, R. (1938). *Triumph Over Pain*. New York: The Literary Guild of America.
2. Procacci, P., & Maresca, M. (1984). Pain concepts in western civilization: A historical review. In C. Benedetti, C. R. Chapman, & G. Moricca (eds.), *Advances in Pain Research and Therapy: Vol. 7* (pp. 1–11). New York: Raven Press.
3. Melzack, R., & Wall, P. D. (1965). Pain mechanisms: A new theory. Science *150*:971–977.
4. McCaffery, M. (1979). *Nursing Management of the Patient with Pain* (p. 11). Philadelphia: J. B. Lippincott.
5. International Association for Study of Pain. (1979). Pain terms: A list with definitions and notes on usage. Pain *6*:249–252.
6. International Association for Study of Pain Subcommittee on Taxonomy. (1986). Classification of chronic pain: Descriptions of chronic pain syndromes and definitions of pain terms. Pain (Suppl. 3), S216–S221.
7. Sternbach, R. A. (1986). A survey of pain in the United States: The Nuprin Pain Report. Clin J Pain *2*:49–53.
8. Bailit, H. L. (1987). The prevalence of dental pain and anxiety: Their relationship to "Quality of Life." NY State Dent J Aug-Sept:27–30.
9. Knapp, D. A., & Koch, H. (1984). The management of new pain in office-based ambulatory care. In National Ambulatory Medical Care Survey 1980 and 1981. Advance data from vital and health statistics (No. 97, DHHS. Pub No. 84-1250, p. 1). Hyattsville, MD: Public Health Service.
10. Crook, J., Rideout, E., & Browne, G. (1984). The prevalence of pain complaints in a general population. Pain *18*:299–314.
11. Anand, K. J. S., Sippell, W. G., & Aynsley-Green, A. (1987). Randomised trial of fentanyl anaesthesia in preterm babies undergoing surgery: Effects on the stress response. Lancet Jan 31, 243–248.
12. Fischer, A. (1987). Special medical report: Babies in pain. Redbook, Oct, 124–125, 183–187.
13. Kelsey, J. L., White A. A., Pastides, H., & Bisbee, G. E. (1979). The impact of musculoskeletal disorders on the population of the United States. J Bone Joint Surg *61-A*:959–964.
14. Mior, S. A., & Diakow, P. R. (1987). Prevalence of back pain in chiropractors. J Manipulative Physiol Ther *10*:305–309.
15. Cato, C., Olson, D. K., & Studer, M. (1989). Incidence, prevalence and variables associated with low back pain in staff nurses. AAOHN J *37*:321–327.
16. Oden, R. V. (1989). Acute postoperative pain:

Incidence, severity, and the etiology of inadequate treatment. Anesthesiol Clin North Am 7:1–15.

17. Bonica, J. J. (1990). Postoperative pain. In J. J. Bonica (ed.), *The Management of Pain* (2nd ed., pp. 461–480). Philadelphia: Lea & Febiger.

18. Melzack, R., Abbott, F. V., Zackon, W., Mulder, D. S., & Davis, M. W. L. (1987). Pain on a surgical ward: A survey of the duration and intensity of pain and the effectiveness of medication. Pain 29:67–72.

19. Donovan, M., Dillon, P., & McGuire, L. (1987). Incidence and characteristics of pain in a sample of medical-surgical inpatients. Pain 30:69–78.

20. Beyer, J. E., DeGood, D. E., Ashley, L. C., & Russell, G. A. (1983). Patterns of postoperative analgesic use with adults and children following cardiac surgery. Pain 17:71–81.

21. Eland, J. M., & Anderson, J. E. (1977). The experience of pain in children. In A. K. Jacox (ed.), *Pain: A Source Book for Nurses and Other Health Professionals* (pp. 453–473). Boston: Little, Brown & Co.

22. Foster, R. L., & Hester, N. O. (1989). The relationship between assessment and pharmacologic intervention for pain in children. In S. G. Funk, E. M. Tornquist, M. T., Champagne, L. A. Copp, & R. A. Wiese (eds.), *Key Aspects of Comfort: Management of Pain, Fatigue, and Nausea* (pp. 72–79). New York: Springer.

23. Schechter, N. L., Allen, D., & Hanson, K. (1986). Status of pediatric pain control: A comparison of hospital analgesic usage in children and adults. Pediatrics 77:11–15.

24. Gale, C. A. (1989). Inadequacy of health care for the nation's chronically ill children. J Pediatr Health Care 3: 20–27.

25. *Cancer Pain Relief.* (1986). Geneva: World Health Organization.

26. Bonica, J. J. (1985). Treatment of cancer pain: Current status and future needs. In H. L. Fields, R. Dubner, & F. Cervero (eds.), *Advances in Pain Research and Therapy: Vol. 9* (pp. 589–616). New York: Raven Press.

27. Miser, A. W., Dothage, J. A., Wesley, R. A., & Miser, J. S. (1987). The prevalence of pain in a pediatric and young adult cancer population. Pain 29:73–83.

28. Adler, R. H., & Hürny, C. (1988). Differential diagnosis of pain in cancer patients. In H. J. Senn, A. Glaus, & L. Schmid (eds.), *Supportive Care in Cancer Patients* (pp. 1–7). Berlin: Springer-Verlag.

29. Dicks, B. (1988). Treatment of pain in the cancer patient: The role of the nurse. In H. J. Senn, A. Glaus, & L. Schmid (eds.), *Supportive Care in Cancer Patients* (pp. 33–38). Berlin: Springer-Verlag.

30. Paiement, B., Boulanger, M., Jones, C. W., & Roy, M. (1979). Intubation and other experiences in cardiac surgery: The consumer's views. Can Anesthetists' Soc J 26:173–180.

31. Patacky, M. G., Garvin, B. J., & Schwirian, P. M. (1985). Intra-aortic balloon pumping and stress in the coronary care unit. Heart Lung 14:142–148.

32. Harrison, M., & Cotanch, P. H. (1987). Pain: Advances and issues in critical care. Nurs Clin North Am 22:691–697.

33. Barr, R. G. (1989). Pain in children. In P. D. Wall & R. Melzack (eds.), *Textbook of Pain* (pp. 568–588). Edinburgh: Churchill Livingstone.

34. Marshall, R. E. (1989). Neonatal pain associated with caregiving procedures. Pediatr Clin North Am 36:885–903.

35. Wong, D. L., & Baker, C. M. (1988). Pain in children: Comparison of assessment scales. Pediatr Nurs 14:9–17.

36. Loper, K. A., Butler, S., Nessly, M., & Wild, L. (1989). Paralyzed with pain: The need for education. Pain 37:315–316.

37. Micheli, L. J. (1989). Common painful sports injuries: Assessment and treatment. Clin J Pain 5(Suppl. 2): S51–S60.

38. Wells, N. (1989). Management of pain during abortion. J Adv Nurs 14:56–62.

39. Lebovits, A. H., Lefkowitz, M., McCarthy, D., Simon, R., Wilpon, H., Jung, R., & Fried, E. (1989). The prevalence and management of pain in patients with AIDS: A review of 134 cases. Clin J Pain 5:245–248.

40. Strafford, M., Cahill, C., Schwartz, T., Yee, J., Sethna, N., & Berde, C. (1991). Recognition and treatment of pain in pediatric patients with AIDS. J Pain Symptom Manage 6(abstr. 15):146.

41. Anand, K. J. S., & Hickey, P. R. (1987). Pain and its effects in the human neonate and fetus. N Engl J Med 317:1321–1329.

42. Anand, K. J. S., & Carr, D. B. (1989). The neuroanatomy, neurophysiology and neurochemistry of pain, stress and analgesia in newborns and children. Pediatr Clin North Am 36:795–822.

43. Rizvi, T., Wadhwa, S., & Bijlani, V. (1987). Development of spinal substrate for nociception (abstract). Pain (Suppl. 4): S195.

44. Grunau, R. V. E., & Craig, K. D. (1987). Pain expression in neonates: Facial action and cry. Pain 28: 395–410.

45. Owens, M. E., & Todt, E. H. (1984). Pain in infancy: Neonatal reaction to a heel lance. Pain 20:77–86.

46. Levy, D. M. (1960). The infant's earliest memory of inoculation: A contribution to public health procedures. J Genet Psychol 96:3–46.

47. Belter, R. W., McIntosh, J. A., Finch, A. J., Jr., & Saylor, C. F. (1988). Preschoolers' ability to differentiate levels of pain: Relative efficacy of three self report measures. J Clin Child Psychol 17:329–335.

48. Haslam, D. R. (1969). Age and the perception of pain. Psychonomic Sci 15:86–87.

49. Tesler, M. D., Wilkie, D. J., Savedra, M. C., Wegner, C., & Gibbons, P. *What's Good About Pain?* Unpublished data.

50. Savedra, M., Gibbons, P. T., Tesler, M., Ward, J. A., & Wegner, C. (1982). How do children describe pain? A tentative assessment. Pain 14:95–104.

51. Gaffney, A., & Dunne, E. A. (1986). Developmental aspects of children's definitions of pain. Pain 26:105–117.

52. Schechter, N. L. (1984). Recurrent pains in children: An overview and approach. Pediatr Clin North Am 31:949–968.

53. Lavigne, J. V., Schulein, M. J., Hannan, J. A., & Hahn, Y. S. (1987). Pain and the pediatric patient: Psychological aspects. In J. Echternach (ed.), *Pain Clinics in Physical Therapy* (pp. 267–296). New York: Churchill Livingstone.

54. McGrath P. J., & Craig, K. D. (1989). Developmental and psychological factors in children's pain. Pediatr Clin North Am 36:823–836.

55. Procacci, P., Bozza, G., Buzzelli, G., & Della Corte, M. (1975). The cutaneous pricking pain threshold

in old age. In M. Weisenberg (ed.), *Pain: Clinical and Experimental Perspectives* (pp. 117–120). St. Louis: Mosby.

56. Sherman, E. D., & Robillard, E. (1960). Sensitivity to pain in the aged. Can Med Assoc J *83*:944–947.

57. Kaiko, R. F., Wallenstein, S. L., Rogers, A. G., Grabinski, P. Y., & Houde, R. W. (1982). Narcotics in the elderly. Med Clin North Am *66*:1079–1089.

58. Ready, L. B., Chadwick, H. S., & Ross, B. (1987). Age predicts effective epidural morphine dose after abdominal hysterectomy. Anesth Analg *66*:1215–1218.

59. Fields, H. L. (1987). *Pain: Mechanisms and Management*. New York: McGraw-Hill.

60. Levine, J. (1984). Pain and analgesia: The outlook for more rational treatment. Ann Intern Med *100*:269–276.

61. Noback, C. R., & Demarest, R. J. (1981). *The Human Nervous System: Basic Principles of Neurobiology* (3rd ed.). New York: McGraw-Hill.

62. Chapman, C. R., & Bonica, J. J. (1985). *Current Concepts: Chronic Pain*. Kalamazoo, MI: The Upjohn Company.

63. Roberts, W. J. (1986). A hypothesis on the physiological basis for causalgia and related pains. Pain *24*:297–311.

64. Meyer, R. A., Campbell, J. N., & Raja, S. N. (1985). Peripheral neural mechanisms of cutaneous hyperalgesia. In H. L. Fields, R. Dubner, & F. Cervero (eds.), *Advances in Pain Research and Therapy: Vol. 9* (pp. 53–71). New York: Raven Press.

65. Torebjörk, E. (1985). Nociceptor activation and pain. In A. Iggo, L. L. Iverson, & F. Cervero (eds.), *Nociception and Pain* (pp. 227–234). London: The Royal Society.

66. Cervero, F. (1985). Visceral nociception: Peripheral and central aspects of visceral nociceptive systems. In A. Iggo, L. L. Iverson, & F. Cervero (eds.), *Nociception and Pain* (pp. 107–120). London: The Royal Society.

67. Mense, S., & Schmidt, R. F. (1974). Activation of group IV afferent units from muscle by algesic agents. Brain Res *72*: 305–310.

68. Jänig, W. (1987). Neuronal mechanisms of pain with special emphasis on visceral and deep somatic pain. Acta Neurochir *38*(Suppl.):16–32.

69. Iggo, A., Steedman, W. M., & Fleetwood-Walker, S. (1985). Spinal processing: Anatomy and physiology of spinal nociceptive mechanisms. In A. Iggo, L. L. Iverson, & F. Cervero (eds.), *Nociception and Pain* (pp. 235–252). London: The Royal Society.

70. Price, D. D., Hayashi, H., Dubner, R., & Ruda, M. A. (1979). Functional relationships between neurons of marginal and substantia gelatinosa layers of primate dorsal horn. J Neurophysiol *42*:1590–1608.

71. Willis, W. D. (1985). Nociceptive pathways: Anatomy and physiology of nociceptive ascending pathways. In A. Iggo, L. L. Iverson, & F. Cervero (eds.), *Nociception and Pain* (pp. 253–268). London: The Royal Society.

72. Melzack, R., & Casey, K. L. (1968). Sensory, motivational, and central control determinants of pain. In D. R. Kenshalo (ed.), *The Skin Senses* (pp. 423–443). Springfield, IL: Thomas.

73. Andersson, S. A., & Rydenhag, B. (1985). Cortical nociceptive systems. In A. Iggo, L. L. Iverson, &

F. Cervero (eds.), *Nociception and Pain* (pp. 347–355). London: The Royal Society.

74. Kenshalo, D. R., Jr., & Isensee, O. (1983). Responses of primate SI cortical neurons to noxious stimuli. J Neurophysiol *50*:1479–1496.

75. Melzack, R., & Wall, P. (1983). *The Challenge of Pain*. New York: Basic Books.

76. Hoffert, M. (1986). The gate control theory revisited. J Pain Symptom Manage *1*: 39–41.

77. Terenius, L. (1984). The endogenous opioids and other central peptides. In P. D. Wall & R. Melzack (eds.), *Textbook of Pain* (pp. 133–141). Edinburgh: Churchill Livingstone.

78. Reynolds, D. V. (1969). Surgery in the rat during electrical analgesia induced by focal brain stimulation. Science *164*:444–445.

79. Chapman C. R., & Bonica, J. J. (1983). *Current Concepts: Acute Pain*. Kalamazoo, MI: The Upjohn Company.

80. Basbaum, A. I., & Fields, H. L. (1984). Endogenous pain control systems: Brainstem spinal pathways and endorphin circuitry. Annu Rev Neurosci *7*:309–338.

81. Goldstein, A. (1976). Opioid peptides (endorphins) in pituitary and brain. Science *193*:1081–1086.

82. Veselis, R. A. (1988). Sedation and pain management for the critically ill. Crit Care Clin *4*:167–181.

83. Butler, S. (1984). Present status of tricyclic antidepressants in chronic pain therapy. In C. Benedetti, C. R. Chapman, & G. Moricca (eds.), *Advances in Pain Research and Therapy* (vol. 7, pp. 173–197). New York: Raven Press.

84. Drasner, K., & Fields, H. L. (1988). Synergy between the antinociceptive effects of intrathecal clonidine and systemic morphine in the rat. Pain *32*:309–312.

85. Watkins, L. R., & Mayer, D. J. (1982). Organization of endogenous opiate and nonopiate pain control systems. Science *216*:1185–1192.

86. Fields, H. L. (1988). Sources of variability in the sensation of pain. Pain *33*:195–200.

87. Portenoy, R. K. (1989). Mechanisms of clinical pain: Observations and speculations. Neurol Clin *7*:205–230.

88. Meyerson, B. A. (1990). Neuropathic pain: An overview. In S. Lipton, E. Tunks, & M. Zoppi (eds.), *Advances in Pain Research and Therapy* (vol. 13, pp, 193–199). New York: Raven Press.

89. Davar, G., & Maciewicz, R. J. (1989). Deafferentation pain syndromes. Neurol Clin *7*:289–304.

90. Tasker, R. R. (1984). Deafferentation. In P. D. Wall & R. Melzack (eds.), *Textbook of Pain* (pp. 119–132). Edinburgh: Churchill Livingstone.

91. Gybels, J., & Kupers, R. (1987). Central and peripheral electrical stimulation of the nervous system in the treatment of chronic pain. Acta Neurochir *38*(Suppl.): 64–75.

92. Portenoy, R. K., Foley, K. M., & Inturrisi, C. E. (1990). The nature of opioid responsiveness and its implications for neuropathic pain: New hypotheses derived from studies of opioid infusions. Pain *43*:273–286.

93. Foley, K. M. (1984). A review of pain syndromes in patients with cancer. In *Symposium on the Management of Cancer Pain* (pp. 7–16). New York: H. P. Publishing.

94. Twycross, R. G. (1988). The management of pain

in cancer: A guide to drugs and dosages. Oncology 2:35–44, 47.

95. Cervero, F. (1983). Supraspinal connections of neurones in the thoracic spinal cord of the cat: Ascending projections and effects of descending impulses. Brain Res 275:251–261.

96. Kandel, E. R., & Schwartz, J. H. (1984). *Principles of Neural Science*. New York: Elsevier/North-Holland.

97. Bonica, J. J., & Benedetti, C. (1980). Postoperative pain. In R. E. Condon & J. J. De Cossee (eds.), *Surgical Care: A Physiologic Approach to Clinical Management* (pp. 394–414). Philadelphia: Lea & Febiger.

98. Ganong, W. F. (1985). *Review of Medical Physiology* (12th ed.). Los Altos, CA: Lange Medical Publications.

99. Bonica, J. J. (1979). Important clinical aspects of acute and chronic pain. In R. F. Beers, Jr., & E. G. Bassett (eds.), *Mechanisms of Pain and Analgesic Compounds* (pp. 15–29). New York: Raven Press.

100. Reiser, M. F. (1984). *Mind, Brain, Body* (p. 101). New York: Basic Books.

101. Kehlet, H. (1986). Pain relief and modification of the stress response. In M. J. Cousins, & G. D. Phillips (eds.), *Acute Pain Management* (pp. 49–75). New York: Churchill Livingstone.

102. Moldofsky, H. (1989). Sleep influences on regional and diffuse pain syndromes associated with osteoarthritis. Semin Arthritis Rheum 18 (Suppl. 2): 18–21.

103. Nakamura, A., Nakashima, M., Sugao, T., Kanemoto, H., Fukumura, Y., & Shiomi, H. (1988). Potent antinociceptive effect of centrally administered delta-sleep-inducing peptide (DSIP). Eur J Pharmacol 155: 247–253.

104. Leigh, T. J., Bird, H. A., Hindmarch, I., & Wright, V. (1987). A comparison of sleep in rheumatic and non-rheumatic patients. Clin Exp Rheumatol 5:363–365.

105. Feuerstein, M., Carter, R. L., & Papciak, A. S. (1987). A prospective analysis of stress and fatigue in recurrent low back pain. Pain 31: 333–344.

106. Craig, K. K. (1989). Emotional aspects of pain. In P. D. Wall, & R. Melzack (eds.), *Textbook of Pain* (pp. 220–230). Edinburgh: Churchill Livingstone.

107. Egan, K. J. (1989). Psychological issues in postoperative pain. Anesthesiol Clin North Am 7:183–192.

108. Price, D. D. (1988). *Psychological and Neural Mechanisms of Pain* (p. 5). New York: Raven Press.

109. McNeil, D. W., & Berryman, M. L. (1989). Components of dental fear in adults. Behav Res Ther 27:233–236.

110. Peck, C. L. (1986). Psychological factors in acute pain management. In M. J. Cousins & G. D. Phillips (eds.), *Acute Pain Management* (pp. 251–274). New York: Churchill Livingstone.

111. Pawlicki, R. (1987). Psychologic interventions for the anxious dental patient. Anesthesiol Progress 34:220–227.

112. Davy, G. C. L. (1989). Dental phobias and anxieties: Evidence for conditioning processes in the acquisition and modulation of a learned fear. Behav Res Ther 27:51–58.

113. Craig, K. D. (1986). Social modeling influences: Pain in context. In R. A. Sternbach (ed.), *The Psychology of Pain* (2nd ed., pp. 67–95). New York: Raven Press.

114. Johnston, M. (1980). Anxiety in surgical patients. Psychol Med 10:145–152.

115. Cousins, N. (1979). *Anatomy of an Illness As Perceived by the Patient*. New York: Norton.

116. Puntillo, K. A. (1988). The phenomenon of pain and critical care nursing. Heart Lung 17:262–271.

117. Izard, C. E. (1979). The Maximally Discriminative Facial Movement Coding System (MAX). Newark, DE: University of Delaware, Instructional Resources Center.

118. Izard, C. E., Hembree, E. A., & Huebner, R. R. (1987). Infants' emotional expressions to acute pain: Developmental change and stability of individual differences. Dev Psychol 23:105–113.

119. Pilowsky, I., & Spence, N. D. (1976). Pain, anger and illness behavior. J Psycho Res 20:411–416.

120. Portenoy, R. K. (1988). Practical aspects of pain control in the patient with cancer. CA 38:327–352.

121. Buckwalter, K. D., & Babich, K. S. (1990). Psychologic and physiologic aspects of depression. Nurs Clin North Am 25:945–954.

122. Osterweis, M., Kleinman, A., & Mechanic, D. (1987). *Pain and Disability: Clinical, Behavioral and Public Policy Perspectives*. Institute of Medicine Committee on Pain, Disability, and Chronic Illness Behavior. Washington, DC: National Academy Press.

123. Roy, R., Thomas, M., & Matas, M. (1984). Chronic pain and depression: A review. Comp Psychiatry 25:96–105.

124. Roy, R. (1989). *Chronic Pain and the Family: A Problem Centered Perspective*. New York: Human Sciences Press.

125. Romano, J. M., & Turner J. A. (1985). Chronic pain and depression: Does the evidence support a relationship? Psychol Bull 97:18–34.

126. Magni, G. (1987). On the relationship between chronic pain and depression when there is no organic lesion. Pain 31:1–21.

127. Spitzer, R. I., Endicott, J., & Robins, E. (1975). *Research Diagnostic Criteria*. New York: Biometrics Research.

128. *Diagnostic and Statistical Manual of Mental Disorders* (3rd ed., revised). (1987). Washington, DC: American Psychiatric Association.

129. France, R. D., Skott, A., Krishnan, R. R., Urban, B., & Houpt, J. L. (1988). Subtypes of depression in patients with chronic pain. South Med J 81:485–488.

130. Rudy, T. A., Kerns, R. D., & Turk, D. C. (1988). Chronic pain and depression: Toward a cognitive-behavioral mediation model. Pain 35:129–140.

131. Williams, A. K., & Schulz, R. (1988). Association of pain and physical dependency with depression in physically ill middle-aged and elderly persons. Phys Ther 68:1226–1230.

132. Melzack, R. (1975). The McGill Pain Questionnaire: Major properties and scoring methods. Pain 1:277–299.

133. Fuller, B. F., Conner, D., & Horii, Y. (1990). Potential acoustic measures of infant pain and arousal. In D. C. Tyler & E. J. Krane (eds.), *Advances in Pain Research and Therapy: Vol. 15, Pediatric Pain* (pp. 137–145). New York: Raven Press.

134. Johnston, C. C., & Strada, M. E. (1986). Acute pain response in infants: A multidimensional description. Pain 24:373–382.

135. Porter, F. L., Miller, R. H., & Marshall, R. E.

(1986). Neonatal pain cries: Effects of circumcision on acoustic features and perceived urgency. Child Dev *57*:790–802.

136. Scott, J., & Huskisson, E. C. (1976). Graphic representation of pain. Pain *2*:175–184.

137. Tesler, M. D., Savedra, M. C., Holzemer, W. L., Wilkie, D. J., Ward, J. A., & Paul, S. M. (1991). The word-graphic rating scale as a measure of children's and adolescents' pain intensity. Res Nurs Health *14*:361–371.

138. Beyer, J. E. (1984, 1989). *The Oucher: A User's Manual and Technical Report.* Denver, CO: University of Colorado Health Sciences Center, School of Nursing.

139. McGrath, P. A., de Veber, L. L., & Hearn, M. T. (1985). Multidimensional pain assessments in children. In H. L. Fields, R. Dubner, & F. Cervero (eds.), *Advances in Pain Research and Therapy: Proceedings from the 4th World Congress on Pain* (vol. 9, pp. 387–393). New York: Raven Press.

140. Whaley, L., & Wong, D. L. (1987). Wong-Baker faces pain rating scale. In L. Whaley & D. Wong (eds.), *Nursing Care of Infants and Children* (p. 1070). St. Louis: C. V. Mosby.

141. Fishman, B., Pasternak, S., Wallenstein, S. L., Houde, R. W., Holland, J. C., & Foley, K. M. (1987). The Memorial Pain Assessment Card. Cancer *60*:1151–1158.

142. Savedra, M. C., Tesler, M. D., Holzemer, W. L., Wilkie, D. J., & Ward, J. A. (1989). Pain location: Validity and reliability of body outline markings by hospitalized children and adolescents. Res Nurs Health *12*:307–314.

143. Wilkie, D. J., Holzemer, W. L., Tesler, M. D., Ward, J. A., Paul, S. M., & Savedra, M. C. (1990). Measuring pain quality: Validity and reliability of children's and adolescents' pain language. Pain *41*:151–159.

144. Varni, J. W., Thompson, K. L., & Hanson, V. (1987). The Varni/Thompson Pediatric Pain Questionnaire. I. Chronic musculoskeletal pain in juvenile rheumatoid arthritis. Pain *28*: 27–38.

145. Aradine, C. R., Beyer, J. E., & Tompkins, J. M. (1988). Children's pain perception before and after analgesia: A study of instrument construct validity and related issues. J Pediatr Nurs *3*:11–23.

146. Hester, N. O. (1979). The preoperational child's reaction to immunization. Nurs Res *28*:250–255.

147. Hester, N., Foster, R., & Kristensen, K. (1990). Measurement of pain in children: Generalizability and validity of the Pain Ladder and the Poker Chip Tool. In D. C. Tyler & E. J. Krane (eds.), *Advances in Pain Research and Therapy: Vol. 15, Pediatric Pain* (pp. 79–84). New York: Raven Press.

148. Melzack, R. (1983). The McGill Pain Questionnaire. In R. Melzack (ed.), *Pain Measurement and Assessment* (pp. 41–47). New York: Raven Press.

149. Melzack, R. (1987). The short form McGill Pain Questionnaire. Pain *30*:191–197.

150. Tursky, B., Jamner, J. D., & Friedman, R. (1982). The pain perception profile: A psychophysical approach to the assessment of pain report. Behav Ther *13*:376–394.

151. McGrath, P. J., Johnson, G., Goodman, J. T., Schillinger, J., Dunn, J., & Chapman, J. A. (1985). CHEOPS: A behavioral scale for rating postoperative pain in children. In H. L. Fields, R. Dubner, & F. Cervero (eds.), *Advances in Pain Research and Therapy: Proceedings from the 4th World Congress on Pain: Vol. 9, Pediatric Pain* (pp. 395–402). New York: Raven Press.

152. Lawrence, J., Alcock, D., Kay, J., & McGrath, P. J. (1991). The development of a tool to assess neonatal pain. J Pain Symptom Manage *6*:Abstract 159.

153. Ekman, P., & Friesen, W. V. (1978). *Facial Action Coding System.* Palo Alto, CA: Consulting Psychologist Press.

154. LeResche, L., & Dworkin, S. F. (1988). Facial expressions of pain and emotions in chronic TMD patients. Pain *35*:71–78.

155. Katz, E. R., Kellerman, J., & Siegel, S. E. (1980). Behavioral distress in children with cancer undergoing medical procedures: Developmental considerations. J Consult Clin Psychol *48*:356–365.

156. Mills, N. (1989). Pain behaviors in infants and toddlers. J Pain Symptom Manage *4*:184–190.

157. Keefe, F. J. (1982). Behavioral assessment and treatment of chronic pain: Current status and future directions. J Consult Clin Psychol *50*:896–911.

158. Wilkie, D., Lovejoy, N., Dodd, M. J., & Tesler, M. D. (1989). Pain control behaviors of patients with cancer. In S. G. Funk, E. M. Tornquist, M. T. Champagne, L. A. Copp, & R. A. Wiese (eds.), *Key Aspects of Comfort: Management of Pain, Fatigue, and Nausea* (pp. 119–126). New York: Springer Publishing.

159. Barr, R. G. (1983). Variations on the theme of pain: Pain tolerance and developmental changes in pain perception. In M. D. Levine, W. B. Carey, A. C. Crocker, & R. T. Gross (eds.), *Developmental, Behavioral Pediatrics* (pp. 505–512). Philadelphia: W. B. Saunders.

160. McCaffery, M., & Beebe, A. (1989). *Pain: Clinical Manual for Nursing Practice.* St. Louis: C. V. Mosby.

161. Price, D. D. (1988). *Psychological and Neural Mechanisms of Pain.* New York: Raven Press.

162. Eysenck, H. J. (1970). The questionnaire measurement of neuroticism and extraversion In H. J. Eysenck (ed.), *Theoretical and Methodological Issues* (pp. 100–127). New York: Wiley-Interscience.

163. Parbrook, G. D., Dalrymple D. G., & Steel, D. F. (1973). Personality assessment and postoperative pain and complications. J Psychosom Res *17*:277–285.

164. Ekman, P., & Friesen, W. V. (1969). The repertoire of nonverbal behavior: Categories, origins, usage, and coding. Semiotica *1*:49–98.

165. Melamed, B. G., & Siegel, L. J. (1975). Reduction of anxiety in children facing hospitalization and surgery by use of filmed modeling. J Consult Clin Psychol *43*:511–521.

166. Beecher, H. K. (1956). Relationship of significance of wound to pain experienced. JAMA *161*:1609–1613.

167. Fagerhaugh, S. Y., & Strauss, A. (1977). *Politics of Pain Management: Staff-Patient Interaction.* Menlo Park, CA: Addison-Wesley.

168. Cohen, F. L. (1980). Postsurgical pain relief: Patients' status and nurses' medication choices. Pain *9*:265–274.

169. Spross, J. A., McGuire, D. B., & Schmitt, R. M. (1990). Oncology Nursing Society Position Paper on Cancer Pain. Oncol Nurs Forum *17*:4–6, 595–614, 751–760, 943–955.

170a. Acute Pain Management Guideline Panel. (1992). Acute pain management: Operative or medical procedures and trauma. Clinical Practice Guidelines (AHCPR Pub. No. 92-0032). Rockville, MD: Agency for Health Care Policy and Research, Public Health Service, U.S. Department of Health and Human Services.

170b. Task Force on Acute Pain (1992). Ready, L. B., & Edwards, W. T. (eds.), *Management of Acute Pain: A Practical Guide*. International Association for Study of Pain. Seattle

171. Edwards, W. T. (1990). Optimizing opioid treatment of postoperative pain. J Pain Symptom Manage 5(Suppl. 1):S24–S36.

172. Freidman, D. P. (1990). Perspectives on the medical use of drugs of abuse. J Pain Symptom Manage 5(Suppl. 1):S2–S5.

173. Joranson, D. (1989, October). Purposes, patterns and consequences of state regulation of opioids. In DuPont Pharmaceuticals Pain Update, *Relieving Patient Pain in a Regulated Environment: A Medical Dilemma for the 90's*. Phoenix, AZ: American Pain Society Pain Update Session.

174. Marks, R. M., & Sachar, E. J. (1973). Undertreatment of medical inpatients with narcotic analgesics. Ann Intern Med 78:173–181.

175. Donovan, M. I. (1988). Relieving pain: The current basis for practice. In S. Funk, E. M. Tornquist, M. T. Champagne, L. A. Copp, & R. A. Wiese (eds.), *Key Aspects of Comfort: Management of Pain, Fatigue, and Nausea* (pp. 25–31). New York: Springer Publishing.

176. Rankin, M. A., & Snider, B. (1984). Nurses' perceptions of cancer patients' pain. Cancer Nurs 7:149–155.

177. Lee, V. C. (1989). Non-narcotic modalities for the management of acute pain. Anesthesiol Clin North Am 7:101–131.

178. Mortensen, M. E., & Rennebohm, R. M. (1989). Clinical pharmacology and use of nonsteroidal anti-inflammatory drugs. Pediatr Clin North Am 36:1113–1139.

179. Shannon, M., & Berde, C. B. (1989). Pharmacologic management of pain in children and adolescents. Pediatr Clin North Am 36:855–871.

180. Berde. C. B. (1989). Pediatric postoperative pain management. Pediatr Clin North Am 36:921–939.

181. Flower, R. J., & Vane, J. R. (1972). Inhibition of prostaglandin synthetase in brain explains the antipyretic activity of paracetamol (4-acetamidophenol). Nature 240:410–411.

182. Moertel, C. G., Ahmann, D. L., Taylor, W. F., & Schwartau, N. (1972). A comparative evaluation of marketed analgesic drugs. N Engl J Med 286:813–815.

183. Catalano, R. B. (1987). Pharmacologic management in the treatment of cancer pain. In D. McGuire & C. H. Yarbro (eds.), *Cancer Pain* (pp. 151–201). Orlando, FL: Grune & Stratton.

184. *Principles of Analgesic Use in the Treatment of Acute Pain and Chronic Cancer Pain: A Concise Guide to Medical Practice* (2nd ed.). (1989) Skokie, IL: American Pain Society.

185. Boynton, C. S., Dick, C. F., & Mayor, G. H. (1988). NSAIDs: An overview. J Clin Pharmacol 28:512–517.

186. Williams, R. L., & Upton, R. A. (1988). The clinical pharmacology of ketoprofen. J Clin Pharmacol 28:S13–S22.

187. Benedetti, C. (1987). Intraspinal analgesia: An historical overview. Acta Anaesthesiol Scand 31(Suppl. 85):17–24.

188. Pert, C. B., & Snyder, S. H. (1973). Opiate receptor: Demonstration in nervous tissue. Science 179:1011–1014.

189. Carmody, J. J. (1987). Opiate receptors: An introduction. Anaesth Inten Care 15:27–37.

190. Inturrisi, C. E. (1989). Clinical pharmacology of opioid analgesics. Anesthesiol Clin North Am 7:33–49.

191. Sabbe, M. B., & Yaksh, T. L. (1990). Pharmacology of spinal opioids. J Pain Symptom Manage 5:191–203.

192. Pasternak, G. W. (1988). Multiple morphine and enkephalin receptors and the relief of pain. JAMA 259:1362–1367.

193. Pasternak, G. W. (1986). Multiple morphine and enkephalin receptors: Biochemical and pharmacological aspects. In D. D. Kelly (ed.), *Stress-Induced Analgesia* (pp. 130–139). New York: The New York Academy of Sciences.

194. Moulin, D. E., Max, M. B., Kaiko, R. F., Inturrisi, C. E., Maggard, J., Yaksh, T. L., & Foley, K. M. (1985). The analgesic efficacy of intrathecal D-Ala²-D-Leu⁵-Enkephalin in cancer patients with chronic pain. Pain 23:213–221.

195. Yaksh, T. L. (1987). Spinal opiates: A review of their effect on spinal function with emphasis on pain processing. Acta Anaesthesiol Scand 31(Suppl. 85):25–37.

196. Shafer, A., White, P. F., Schuttler, J., & Rosenthal, M. H. (1983). Use of a fentanyl infusion in the intensive care unit: Tolerance to its anesthetic effects? Anesthesiology 59:245–248.

197. Catalano, R. B. (1985). Pharmacology of analgesic agents used to treat cancer pain. Semin Oncol Nurs 1:126–140.

198. Gossop, M. (1988). Clonidine and the treatment of the opiate withdrawal syndrome. Drug Alcohol Depend 21:253–259.

199. Perry, S., & Heidrich, G. (1982). Management of pain during debridement: A survey of U.S. burn units. Pain 13:267–280.

200. Porter, J., & Jick, H. (1980). Addiction rare in patients treated with narcotics. N Engl J Med, 302:123.

201. Logas, W. G., El-Baz, N., El-Ganzouri, A., Cullen, M., Staren E., Faber, L. P., & Ivankovich, A. D. (1987). Continuous thoracic epidural analgesia for postoperative pain relief following thoracotomy: A randomized prospective study. Anesthesiology 67:787–791.

202. Attia, J., Ecoffey, C., Sandouk, P., Gross, J. B., & Samii, K. (1986). Epidural morphine in children: Pharmacokinetics and CO_2 sensitivity. Anesthesiology 65:590–594.

203. Krane, E. J. (1988). Delayed respiratory depression in a child after caudal epidural morphine. Anesth Analg 67:79–82.

204. Wuitchik, M., Bakal, D., & Lipshitz, J. (1990). Relationship between pain, cognitive activity and epidural analgesia during labor. Pain 41:125–132.

205. Nitescu, P., Appelgren, L., Linder, L., Sjöberg, M., Hultman, E., & Curelaru, I. (1990). Epidural versus intrathecal morphine-bupivacaine: Assessment of consecutive treatments in advanced cancer pain. J Pain Symptom Manage 5:18–26.

206. Gregg, R. (1989). Spinal analgesia. Anesthesiol Clin North Am 7:79–100.

207. Paice, J. A. (1987). New delivery systems in pain management. Nurs Clin North Am *22*:715–726.

208. Cherry, D. A. (1987). Drug delivery systems for epidural administration of opioids. Acta Anaesthesiol Scand *31*(Suppl. 85):54–59.

209. Ritchie, J. M., & Greene, N. M. (1985). Local anesthetics. In A. G. Gilman, L. S. Goodman, T. W. Rall, & F. Murad (eds.), *Goodman & Gilman's The Pharmacological Basis of Therapeutics* (7th ed. pp. 302–321). New York: Macmillan.

210. Covino, B. G., & Scott, D. B. (1985). *Handbook of Epidural Anaesthesia and Analgesia.* Orlando, FL: Grune & Stratton.

211. Zenz, M. (1988). Epidural opiates and nerve blocks. In H. J. Senn, A. Glaus, & L. Schmid (eds.), *Supportive Care in Cancer Patients* (pp. 18–27). Berlin: Springer-Verlag.

212. Shanahan, P. T. (1989). Replantation of extremities. Anesthesiol Clin North Am *7*:675–692.

213. Engberg, G. (1978). Relief of postoperative pain with intercostal blockade compared with the use of narcotic drugs. Acta Anaesthesiol Scand Suppl *70*:36–38.

214. Fleming, W. H., & Sarafian, L. B. (1977). Kindness pays dividends: The medical benefits of intercostal nerve block following thoracotomy. J Thorac Cardiovasc Surg *74*:273–274.

215. Symreng, T., Gomez, M. N., & Rossi, N. (1989). Intrapleural bupivacaine v. saline after thoracotomy—Effects on pain and lung function—A double-blind study. J Cardiothorac Anesth *3*:144–149.

216. Toft, P., & Jorgensen, A. (1987). Continuous thoracic epidural analgesia for the control of pain in myocardial infarction. Intens Care Med *13*:388–389.

217. Sano, K. (1987). Neurosurgical treatments of pain: A general survey. Acta Neurochir Suppl *38*:86–96.

218. Siegfried, J. (1988). Electrostimulation and neurosurgical measures in cancer pain. In H. J. Senn, A. Glaus, & L. Schmid (eds.), *Supportive Care in Cancer Patients* (pp. 28–32). Berlin: Springer-Verlag.

219. Sindou, M., & Daher, A. (1988). Spinal cord ablation procedures for pain. In R. Dubner, G. F. Gebhart, & M. R. Bond (eds.), *Proceedings of the Fifth World Congress on Pain* (pp. 477–495). Amsterdam: Elsevier.

220. Hosobuchi, Y. (1980). The current status of analgesic brain stimulation. Acta Neurochir Suppl *30*:219–227.

221. Mehta, M. (1986). Current views on non-invasive methods of pain relief. In M. Swerdlow (ed.), *The Therapy of Pain* (2nd ed., pp. 115–131). Boston: MTP Press.

222. Choi, J. J., & Tsay, C. L. (1987). Technology of transcutaneous electrical nerve stimulation. In W. Wu & L G. Smith (eds.), *Pain Management: Assessment and Treatment of Chronic and Acute Pain Syndromes* (pp. 137–165). New York: Human Sciences Press.

223. Eland, J. M. (1989). The effectiveness of transcutaneous electrical nerve stimulation (TENS) with children experiencing cancer pain. In Funk, S. G., Tornquist, E. M., Champagne, M. T., Copp, L. A., & Wiese, L. A. (eds.), *Key Aspects of Comfort: Management of Pain, Fatigue, and Nausea* (pp. 87–100). New York: Springer Publishing.

224. Johnson, M. I., Ashton, C. H., & Thompson, J. W. (1991). An in-depth study of long-term users of transcutaneous electrical nerve stimulation (TENS). Implications for clinical use of TENS. Pain *44*:221–229.

225. Deyo, R. A., Walsh, N. E., Martin, D. C., Schoenfeld, L. S., & Ramamurthy, S. (1990). A controlled trial of transcutaneous electrical nerve stimulation (TENS) and exercise for chronic low back pain. N Engl J Med *322*:1627–1634.

226. Tepperman, P. S., & Devlin, M. (1983). Therapeutic heat and cold. A practitioner's guide. Postgrad Med, *73*:69–76.

227. Melzack, R., Jeans, M. E., Stratford, J. C., & Monks, R. C. (1980). Ice massage and transcutaneous electrical stimulation: Comparison of treatment for low back pain. Pain *9*:209–217.

228. Horowitz, B. F., Fitzpatrick, J. J., & Flaherty, G. G. (1984). Relaxation techniques for pain relief after open heart surgery. Dimen Crit Care Nurs *3*:364–371.

229. Flaherty, G. G., & Fitzpatrick, J. J. (1978). Relaxation technique to increase comfort level of postoperative patients: A preliminary study. Nurs Res *27*:352–355.

230. Jay, S. M., Elliott, C. H., Ozolins, M., Olson, R. A., & Pruitt, S. D. (1985). Behavioral management of children's distress during painful medical procedures. Behav Res Ther *23*:513–520.

231. McCaffery, M. (1977). Pain relief for the child. Problem areas and selected nonpharmacological methods. Pediatr Nurs *3*:11–16.

232. Benson, H., Kotch, J. B., & Crassweller, K. D. (1977). The relaxation response: A bridge between psychiatry and medicine. Med Clin North Am *61*:929–938.

233. Mast, D., Meyers, J., & Urbanski, A. (1987). Relaxation techniques: A self-learning module for nurses: Units I, II, III. Cancer Nurs *10*:141–147, 217–225, 279–285.

234. Herth, K. (1978). The therapeutic use of music. Supervisor Nurse *9*:22–23.

235. Locsin, R. (1981). The effect of music on the pain of selected postoperative patients. J Adv Nurs *6*:19–25.

236. Campos, R. G. (1989). Soothing pain-elicited distress in infants with swaddling and pacifiers. Child Dev *60*:781–792.

237. Field, T., & Goldson, E. (1984). Pacifying effects of nonnutritive sucking on term and preterm neonates during heelstick procedures. Pediatrics *74*:1012–1015.

238. Siegel, L. J. (1976). Preparation of children for hospitalization: A selected review of the research literature. J Pediatr Psychol *1*:26–30.

239. Melamed, B. G., Meyer, R., Gee, C., & Soule, L. (1976). The influence of time and type of preparation on children's adjustment to hospitalization. J Pediatr Psychol *1*:31–37.

240. Peterson, L., & Shigetomi, C. (1981). The use of coping techniques to minimize anxiety in hospitalized children. Behav Ther *12*:1–14.

241. Reading, A. E. (1979). The short term effects of psychological preparation for surgery. Soc Sci Med *13A*:641–654.

242. Johnson, J. E., Rice, V. H., Fuller, S. S., & Endress, M. P. (1978). Sensory information, instruction in a coping strategy and recovery from surgery. Res Nurs Health *1*:4–17.

243. Staub, E., & Kellet, D. S. (1972). Increasing pain

tolerance by information about aversive stimuli. J Pers Soc Psychol *21*:198–203.

244. Johnson, J. E., & Leventhal, H. (1974). Effects of accurate expectations and behavioral instruction on reactions during noxious medical examinations. J Pers Soc Psychol *29*:710–718.

245. Visintainer, M. A., & Wolfer, J. A. (1975). Psychological preparation for surgical pediatric patients: The effect of children's and parents' stress responses and adjustment. Pediatrics *56*:187–202.

246. Andrew, J. (1970). Recovery from surgery with and without preparatory instruction for three coping styles. J Pers Soc Psychol *15*:233.

247. Cohen, F., & Lazarus, R. S. (1973). Active coping processes, coping dispositions, and recovery from surgery. Psychosom Med *35*:375–389.

248. Kim, S. (1990). *A Contingency Model of Preparatory Information, Anxiety and Pain.* Presented at Research Meeting, UCSF School of Nursing, San Francisco, February.

249. Egan, K. J. (1990). What does it mean to a patient to be "in control." In F. M. Ferrante, G. W. Ostheimer, & B. G. Covino (eds.), *Patient-Controlled Analgesia* (pp. 17–26). Boston: Blackwell Scientific.

250. Bowers, K. S. (1968). Pain, anxiety, and perceived control. J Consult Clin Psychol *32*:596–602.

251. Dubois, M. (1989). Patient-controlled analgesia for acute pain. Clin J Pain *5*(Suppl. 1):S8–S15.

252. Ferrante, F. M., Orav, E. J., Rocco, A. G., & Gallo, J. A. (1988). A statistical model for pain in patient-controlled analgesia and conventional intramuscular opioid regimens. Anesth Analg *67*:457–461.

253. Albert, J. M., & Talbot, T. M. (1988). Patient-controlled analgesia vs. conventional intramuscular analgesia following colon surgery. Dis Colon Rectum *31*:83–86.

254. Baumann, T. J., Batenhorst, R. L., Graves, D. A., Foster, T. S., & Bennett, R. L. (1986). Patient controlled analgesia in the terminally ill cancer patient. Drug Intelligence Clin Pharmacol *20*:297–301.

255. Brown, R. E., Jr., & Broadman, L. M. (1987). Patient-controlled analgesia (PCA) for postoperative pain control in adolescents. Anesthes Analg *66*(Suppl.):S1–S191, S22.

256. Rodgers, B. M., Webb, C. J., Stergios, D., & Newman, B. M. (1988). Patient-controlled analgesia in pediatric surgery. J Pediatr Surg *23*:259–262.

257. Gaukroger, P. B., Tompkins, D. P., & Van der Walt, J. H. (1989). Patient-controlled analgesia in children. Anesth Intens Care *17*:264–268.

258. Schechter, N. L., Berrien, F. B., & Katz, S. M. (1988). The use of patient-controlled analgesia in adolescents with sickle cell pain crisis: A preliminary report. J Pain Symptom Manage *3*:109–113.

259. Berde, C. B., Lehn, B. M., Yee, J. D., Sethna, N. F., & Russo, D. (1991). Patient-controlled analgesia in children and adolescents: A randomized, prospective comparison with intramuscular administration of morphine for postoperative analgesia. J Pediatr *18*:460–466.

260. McGrath, P. A. (1990). *Pain in Children: Nature, Assessment and Treatment.* New York: Guilford Press.

261. McGrath, P. J., & Unruh, A. M. (1987). *Pain in Children and Adolescents.* Amsterdam: Elsevier.

262. Ross, D. M., & Ross, S. A. (1988). *Childhood Pain: Current Issues, Research, and Management.* Baltimore: Urban & Schwarzenberg.

263. Tyler, D. C., & Krane, E. J. (1990). *Advances in Pain Research and Therapy: Vol. 15, Pediatric Pain.* New York: Raven Press.

264. Eland, J. M. (1981). Minimizing pain associated with pre-kindergarten intramuscular injections. Issues Pediat Nurs *5*:361–372.

265. Denyes, M. J., Beyer, J. E., Villarruel, A. M., & Neuman, B. M. (1991). Issues in validation of culturally sensitive pain measure for young children. Paper presented at 2nd International Symposium on Pediatric Pain, Montreal.

266. Adams, J. (1990). A methodological study of pain assessment in Anglo and Hispanic children with cancer. In D. C. Tyler & E. J. Krane (eds.), *Advances in Pain Research and Therapy: Vol. 15, Pediatric Pain* (pp. 43–51). New York: Raven Press.

267. Abu-Saad, H. (1990). Toward the development of an instrument to assess pain in children: Dutch study. In D. C. Tyler & E. J. Krane (eds.), *Advances in Pain Research and Therapy: Vol. 15, Pediatric Pain* (pp. 101–106). New York: Raven Press.

268. Savedra, M. C., Tesler, M. D., Ward, J. A., Holzemer, W. L., Wilkie, D. J., & Ward, J. A. (1990). Testing a tool to assess postoperative pediatric and adolescent pain. In D. C. Tyler & E. J. Krane (eds.), *Advances in Pain Research and Therapy: Vol. 15, Pediatric Pain* (pp. 85–93). New York: Raven Press.

269. Hay, H. (1984). The measurement of pain intensity in children and adults—a methodological approach. Unpublished Masters research. Montreal: McGill University.

270. Molsberry, D. (1979). Young children's objective quantification of pain following surgery. Unpublished Masters thesis. Iowa City, IA: University of Iowa.

271. Franck, L. S. (1985). A new method to quantitatively describe pain behavior in infants. Nurs Res *35*:28–31.

272. Franck, L. S. (1987). A national survey of the assessment and treatment of pain and agitation in the neonatal intensive care unit. JOGGN *16*:387–393.

273. Fowler-Kerry, S., & Ramsay-Lander, J. (1990). Utilizing cognitive strategies to relieve pain in young children. In D. C. Tyler & E. J. Krane (eds.), *Advances in Pain Research and Therapy: Vol. 15, Pediatric Pain* (pp. 247–253). New York: Raven Press.

274. Brennen, A. (1991). The nursing care of children during intrusive procedures (abstr 85). J Pain Symptom Manage *6*:170.

275. Burokas, L. (1985). Factors affecting nurses' decisions to medicate pediatric patients after surgery. Heart Lung *14*:373–379.

276. Davis, K. L. (1990). Postoperative pain in toddlers: Nurses' assessment and intervention. In D. C. Tyler & E. J. Krane (eds.), *Advances in Pain Research and Therapy: Vol. 15, Pediatric Pain* (pp. 53–61). New York: Raven Press.

277. Gonzales, J., & Gadish, H. (1990). Nurses' decisions in medicating children postoperatively. In D. C. Tyler & E. J. Krane (eds.), *Advances in Pain Research and Therapy: Vol. 15, Pediatric Pain* (pp. 37–41). New York: Raven Press.

278. Page, G. G., & Halverson, M. (1991). Pediatric nurses: The assessment and control of pain in preverbal infants. J Pediatr Nurs, *6*:99–106.

279. Tesler, M. D., Wilkie, D. J., Savedra, M. C., Holzemer, W. L., & Ward, J. A. Postoperative anal-

gesics for children and adolescents: Prescription and administration. (In press).

280. Baer, E., Davitz, L. J., & Lieb, R. (1970). Inferences of physical pain and psychological distress. In relation to verbal and nonverbal patient communication. Nurs Res 19:388–392.

281. Davitz, L. J., & Pendleton, S. H. (1969). Nurses' inference of suffering. Nurs Res 18:100–106.

282. Lenburg, C. B., Burnside, H., & Davitz, L. J. (1970). Inference of physical pain and psychological distress. III. In relation to length of time in the nursing education program. Nurs Res 19:399–401.

283. Lenburg, C. B., Glass, H. P., & Davitz, L. J. (1970). Inference of physical pain and psychological distress. II. In relation to the stage of the patient's illness and occupation of the perceiver. Nurs Res 19:392–399.

284. Mason, D. J. (1981). An investigation of the influences of selected factors on nurses' inferences of patient suffering. Int J Nurs Stud 18:251–259.

285. Taylor, A. G., Skelton, J. A., & Butcher, J. (1984). Duration of pain condition and physical pathology as determinants of nurses' assessments of patients in pain. Nurs Res 33:4–8.

286. Holm, K., Cohen, F., Dudas, S., Medema, P. G., & Allen, B. L. (1989). Effect of personal pain experience on pain assessment. Image 21:72–75.

287. Chambers, W. G., & Price, G. G. (1967). Influence of nurse upon effects of analgesics administered. Nurs Res 16:228–233.

288. Diers, D., Schmidt, R. L., McBride, A. B., & Davis, B. L. (1972). The effect of nursing interaction on patients in pain. Nurs Res 21:419–428.

289. McBride, M. A. (1967). Nursing approach, pain, and relief: An exploratory experiment. Nurs Res 16:337–341.

290. Moss, F. T., & Meyer, B. (1966). The effects of nursing interaction upon pain relief in patients. Nurs Res 15:303–306.

291. Johnson, J. E. (1972). Effects of structuring patients' expectations on their reactions to threatening events. Nurs Res 21:499–504.

292. Johnson, J. E., & Rice, V. H. (1974). Sensory and distress components of pain: Implications for the study of clinical pain. Nurs Res 23:203–209.

293. Wells, N. (1982). The effect of relaxation on postoperative muscle tension and pain. Nurs Res 31:236–238.

294. Gaston-Johansson, F., & Asklund-Gustafsson, M. (1985). A baseline study for the development of an instrument for the assessment of pain. J Adv Nurs 10:539–546.

295. Gaston-Johansson, F., Fridh, G., & Turner-Nor-vell, K. (1988). Progression of labor pain in primiparas and multiparas. Nurs Res 37:86–90.

296. Copp, L. A. (1974). The spectrum of suffering. Am J Nurs 74:491–495.

297. Copp, L. A. (1985). Pain coping model and typology. Image J Nurs Sch 17:69–71.

298. Donovan, M. I., & Dillon, P. (1987). Incidence and characteristics of pain in a sample of hospitalized cancer patients. Cancer Nurs 10:85–92.

299. Puntillo, K. A. (1990). Pain experiences of intensive care unit patients. Heart Lung 19:526–533.

300. McGuire, D. B. (1987). The multidimensional phenomenon of cancer pain. In D. B. McGuire & C. H. Yarbro (eds.), Cancer Pain Management (pp. 1–20). Orlando: Grune & Stratton.

301. Ziemer, M. M. (1983). Effects of information on postsurgical coping. Nurs Res 32:282–287.

302. Geden, E., Beck, N., Hauge, G., & Pohlman, S. (1984). Self-report and psychophysiological effects of five pain-coping strategies. Nurs Res 33:260–265.

303. Dulski, T. P., & Newman, A. M. (1989). The effectiveness of relaxation in relieving pain of women with rheumatoid arthritis. In S. G. Funk, E. M. Tornquist, M. T. Champagne, L. A. Copp, & R. A. Wiese (eds.), Key Aspects of Comfort: Management of Pain, Fatigue, and Nausea (pp. 150–154). New York: Springer Publishing.

304. Angus, J. E., & Faux, S. (1989). The effect of music on adult postoperative patients' pain during a nursing procedure. In S. G. Funk, E. M. Tornquist, M. T. Champagne, L. A. Copp, & R. A. Wiese (eds.), Key Aspects of Comfort: Management of Pain, Fatigue, and Nausea (pp. 166–172). New York: Springer Publishing.

305. Stone, S. K., Rusk, F., Chambers, A., & Chafin, S. (1989). The effects of music therapy on critically ill patients in the intensive care setting. In Proceedings of the 16th Annual National Teaching Institute of the American Association of Critical-Care Nurses (p. 624). Atlanta.

306. Geden, E., Beck, N. C., Brouder, G., Glaister, J., & Pohlman, S. (1985). Self-report and psychophysiological effects of Lamaze preparation: An analogue of labor pain. Res Nurs Health 8:155–165.

307. Geden, E., Beck, N., Brouder, G., & O'Connell, E. (1983). Identifying procedural components for analogue research of labor pain. Nurs Res 32:80–83.

308. Manderino, M. A., & Bzdek, V. M. (1984). Effects of modeling and information on reactions to pain: A childbirth-preparation analogue. Nurs Res 33:9–14.

309. Brown, J. S., Tanner, C. A., & Padrick, K. P. (1984). Nursing's search for scientific knowledge. Nurs Res 33:26–32.

14

Hunger

Karen R. Williams

"I'm hungry!" How often have we heard this or said it ourselves? But what does it really mean? What are we really feeling?

"I'm starved!" cried Jim as he burst through the door after school and charged over to the refrigerator. He loaded his arms nonselectively with a variety of the foods closest to his reach and sat down with his afternoon snack. Kathleen entered the house soon after Jim, set her books down and announced, "I've been craving a nice crisp apple all day, sure hope we have one."

Janet came home a little later, exclaiming, "I'm so hungry I could eat a horse. But we're having my favorite tonight so I'm going to wait for dinner."

Jim, Kathleen, and Janet were all expressing their desire for food but what did they really mean? Was Jim really starving? Why did Kathleen crave a specific item? What was Janet feeling? Were they all experiencing the same sensations but expressing them differently? What internal events prompted their statements? How could Janet be really hungry yet delay eating?

Jim, Kathleen, and Janet were not concerned with these questions. They simply responded to their feelings and did not worry about any deeper meaning. Their feelings of hunger signaled a required action, and they carried it out.

Nurses caring for patients who are unable to express or respond to their feelings must consider these questions in order to intervene appropriately. To do so requires an increased awareness, which begins with definition of the problem.

DEFINITION

Hunger is defined as a compelling desire, need, or yearning[1] and has several uses. Psy-chologically, one may hunger for affection, recognition, or attention. Physiologically, a person with dyspnea may be said to have air hunger. The term "hunger disease" has been used to mean the effects of starvation as a result of the unavailability of an adequate food supply.[2]

While these other uses of the word have been recognized, the definition of hunger used in this chapter is the stimulus to obtain and ingest nutrients to meet metabolic demands; a subjective and involuntary instinct that impels an individual to seek out and ingest food. The feeling and expression of hunger is the sum of several internal processes. The sensation of hunger signals the physiological need for food; "appetite" reflects a psychological or cerebral desire for food. Appetite is a function of a person's mind, a learned mechanism expressed according to personal preferences of taste, social conditioning, mores, and taboos. Hunger and appetite are often used interchangeably, but they really reflect different conditions and are satisfied in different ways (See Related Physiological, Pathophysiological, and Psychosocial Concepts).

Hunger, thus defined, is a normal biological process and a protective mechanism that maintains homeostatic functioning, providing that one is able to respond to these feelings. Hunger may result in psychological or physiological complications when persons are unable to respond to their feelings, when the desire to eat is thwarted or denied by others, or when food is withheld from the individual. It is this unrequited hunger that presents a challenge to nurses and thus is addressed in this chapter.

PREVALENCE

The prevalence of unrelieved hunger in hospitalized patients is unknown. The only study to examine hunger in hospitalized patients was reported by Jordan and colleagues, who observed 18 patients on total parenteral nutrition (TPN).[3] Most of the patients reported hunger in spite of daily intakes as high as 4800 kcal. The meaning of the reported hunger was not investigated.

Although not specifically studying hunger, Padilla and associates found that the three most commonly reported distressing psychosensory experiences during enteral tube feeding were related to oral deprivation.[4] Patients complained of an unsatisfied appetite for food; deprivation of tasting, chewing, or swallowing food or drinking fluids; and deprivation of regular food.

The inability to eat was also a major stress in nonhospitalized patients on long-term TPN. Several studies have reported that frustration with the loss of eating and drinking caused the major stress in the patient's life.[5-9] No studies have specifically examined the meaning of hunger in hospitalized patients, and none of these studies has investigated the possibility of hunger as a physiological phenomenon. They do, however, reflect the recognition of hunger as a legitimate health concern. The inability to respond to feelings of hunger would seem to be stressful to the hospitalized patient as well as the patient receiving enteral tube feedings or home TPN, but no studies have been done to confirm this.

POPULATIONS AT RISK

Patients who are dependent on others to provide for their nutritional needs are at the greatest risk of suffering unrequited hunger. This category includes patients who need to be fed because of physical limitations and patients who require either enteral or parenteral tube feeding. Nutritional requirements are calculated based on preset criteria, and the subjective sensations of these patients are not considered. Yet, if hunger is "that set of internal signals that stimulate the acquisition and consumption of food,"[10] exploring the meaning of a patient's expression of hunger is of paramount importance to nursing. The presence of hunger sensations may indicate inadequate nutritional intake, which, if unchecked, will lead to malnutrition.

Another risk group consists of patients who are allowed nothing by mouth (nil per os [NPO]). Most patients can tolerate NPO status for brief periods without risk for diagnostic tests or surgical procedures. However, patients who are maintained on NPO status for an extended period of time (longer than 5 to 7 days), whether for diagnostic or treatment purposes, are at increased risk.

Patients who are advised to limit their intake of some component, whether it is sodium, fat, or calories, and those who require food with an altered consistency, such as puréed, soft, or liquid, are another group at risk. Diets may become unpalatable with these restrictions and may lead to reduced intake, frequently below the necessary caloric requirements. Patients with caloric restrictions often find their diet insufficient and may be distressed by continued and unrelieved feelings of hunger.

Those whose energy output is greater than their caloric intake are another group of patients at risk. Energy requirements are increased with stress, infection, fever, wound healing, and higher activity levels. Hunger may develop if the caloric intake of these patients does not reflect these increased needs.

Patients who are exposed to external inducements, such as the sight and smell of food, television or magazine advertisements, or even the discussion of food,[11] may experience an increased desire for food. When these patients are unable to respond to this desire, feelings of anxiety and oral deprivation may result. The patient may complain of hunger, but most likely the feeling is probably triggered by appetite.

Patients with altered psychological states such as depression and anxiety often have alterations in their desire for food.[12] These may be reflected by an increase or decrease in food intake (see Behavioralist Theories).

Because the prevalence of hunger is unknown, the nurse must maintain a high index of suspicion for these populations at risk of unrequited hunger.

MECHANISMS

The precise mechanisms involved in signaling hunger, that is, the event that impels an organism to seek out and ingest food, are unknown. Several theories have been proposed, and some have been tested scientifically; however, there does not seem to be any single event that heralds the sensations and expression of hunger. The hunger system contains several control mechanisms and built-in redundancies; if any one of the control sites is bypassed or altered, other mechanisms take over and apparently normal regulation ensues.

The primary purpose of hunger is to impel an organism to eat in order to ensure a continued supply of nutrients for cellular functioning. However, this basic physiological drive can be overridden by conscious mental control or psychological and emotional factors. The fact that numerous and varied factors impinge on the act of eating confound and complicate investigations into the control of hunger.

The field of research in the control of food intake has attempted to answer questions from two different but related approaches: (1) What signals the ingestion of food, and what controls the expression of hunger? (2) What causes one to stop eating, and what causes the feelings of satiety?

For purposes of organization, the theories of the control of hunger and satiety are divided into four major sections. In the first two sections, the physiological centralist and peripheralist theories regarding the sites of control are reviewed with the inclusion, where appropriate, of possible control mechanisms. The behavioralist theories, which deal with psychological, emotional, and conditioned learning aspects of hunger and satiety, are presented in the third section. A synthesis and integration of these various theories are presented in the fourth section.

Hunger and appetite are frequently used interchangeably in the following review of the literature. Measurements of hunger ratings in humans have often been equated with appetite, and appetite in turn has been equated with quantity consumed. However, these two terms are probably different mechanisms (see Related Physiological, Pathophysiological, and Psychosocial Concepts). Rowland and Carlton suggest caution when reviewing research studies that used appetite and hunger interchangeably.[13] They concluded that until the normal mechanisms of hunger and appetite are understood, research into the causes and controls of ingestive behavior will remain elusive.

Eating behavior of animals is often used as a dependent variable to measure hunger and appetite, with the amount of food consumed reflecting the intensity of the feelings.[14]

Centralist Theories

The centralist theories focus upon the role of the central nervous system as the center for regulation of hunger and satiety. The traditional view emphasizing the role of the hypothalamus as the control site is still viable, with the realization that the input to the hypothalamus may come from other centers in the brain.

Ventromedial Hypothalamus

It had long been noted that brain tumors led to obesity,[15] but the area of the brain responsible for this development, whether the pituitary or the hypothalamus, was unknown. Hetherington and Ranson reported the results of studies that first presented the role of the ventromedial hypothalamus (VMH) as the satiety center.[16, 17]

Although it had been shown that VMH damage would produce obesity, the reason for this—how these lesions produced obesity—was undetermined. Evidence that these lesions produced obesity by overeating was presented in 1943, with the results of two experiments.[18] Brobeck and coworkers induced electrolytic lesions in the VMH of rats and compared their intake with that of a control group of rats offered the same diet.[18] They then studied 12 groups of pair-fed rats, with one rat of each pair given electrolytic lesions of the VMH. The free-feeding rats with VMH lesions ate more than the control group and became obese; the pair-fed lesioned rats gained only as much weight as their mates. Anesthetization of the VMH with procaine hydrochloride (HCl) led to hyperphagia and provided additional evidence for the VMH as the satiety center.[19] This role of the VMH was further supported when electrical stimulation of the VMH suppressed intake.[20, 21]

Lateral Hypothalamus

The role of the lateral hypothalamus (LH) as the feeding center was proposed by Anand and Brobeck with the finding that electrolytic lesions of the LH in rats produced aphagia and adipsia.[22] Stricker and associates used injections of kainic acid to destroy selectively the cell bodies of the LH in rats while preserving the axons (fibers of passage through the LH).[23] They found that these rats ate less food than did a control group. Epstein found that anesthetization of the LH with procaine HCl suppressed eating whereas hypertonic saline injections elicited eating.[19]

The schema in Table 14–1 summarizes the results of these studies. Arrows indicate the change in feeding behavior with each treatment.

The Dual Center Hypothesis

The dual center hypothesis posits that the LH, which initiates feeding, is inhibited by the VMH as a result of unspecified body changes after feeding. When these signals are depleted, the LH becomes active again. The "feeding center" in the LH is responsible for the urge to eat, while the VMH, or some "structure in its neighborhood" exerts an inhibitory control.[22] Morley and Levine postulated that there is a tonic signal impelling animals to eat and that appetite regulation is mainly involved in inhibiting this signal.[24]

Refutation of the LH and VMH as Discrete Control Centers

Most arguments against hypothalamic control of hunger and satiety center around the fact that alterations in other sensory-motor behaviors are also produced by lesion or stimulation, and these "side effects" play a more important role in the ingestive behavior observed. Brobeck suggested the possibility that lesions of the hypothalamus resulted in the interruption of fibers passing to other areas of the brain.[15] Behavioral changes seen in LH damage are not confined to ingestive behavior but extend to most aspects of motivation,[25] and lesions of the amygdala produce behavioral changes and alterations in feeding patterns similar to hypothalamic damage.[26] It has been suggested that the

TABLE 14–1 SUMMARY OF THE RESULTS OF HYPOTHALAMIC STUDIES

	Ventromedial Hypothalamus	Lateral Hypothalamus
Stimulation	↓	↑
Depression	↑	↓

Arrows indicate the change in feeding behavior with each treatment.

Increased intake (↑) is observed with stimulation of the lateral hypothalamus (LH) or depression of the ventromedial hypothalamus (VMH). Decreased intake (↓) is seen with stimulation of the VMH or depression of the LH.

TABLE 14–2 EFFECTS OF MONAMINES ON FEEDING BEHAVIOR

	Lateral Hypothalamus* (Feeding)	Ventromedial Hypothalamus (Satiety)
Norepinephrine	−	−
Epinephrine	−	
Dopamine	−	
Serotonin		+

*The lateral hypothalamus (LH) initiates feeding while the ventromedial hypothalamus (VMH) induces satiety. In the LH, catecholamines act to inhibit feeding. In the VMH, norepinephrine inhibits satiety, while serotonin facilitates it. Destruction of the catecholamine pathways to the VMH causes decreased food intake, whereas destruction of the catecholamine pathways to the LH results in overeating. Depletion of serotonin in the VMH inhibits the satiety center and results in overeating.

Key: − = inhibition; + = stimulation.

decreased intake seen with LH lesions may be due in part to damage or interruption of trigeminal or olfactory cortex nerve fibers and, possibly, other sensory input.[27] However, the LH neurons have been selectively damaged, producing aphagia without other behavioral changes.[28–30]

Controversy remains about the site of CNS regulation, with evidence mounting for more diffuse excitatory and inhibitory systems regulating it rather than discrete anatomical areas. This appreciation has led to studies attempting to identify the substances and pathways involved in communication between these excitatory and inhibitory systems and the method of communication with the periphery.

Central Neurochemical Mediators

Monamines. The catecholamines (norepinephrine, epinephrine, and dopamine) are synthesized from tyrosine (TYR), while serotonin (5-hydroxytryptamine) is derived from tryptophan (TRP). Studies of the effects of these monamines on feeding behavior have used various techniques to alter the concentration of monamines, including intracerebral injections, selective depletion of the putative transmitter, destruction of the monamine pathway with lesions or neurotoxins, increasing the availability of the amino acid precursor, or inhibiting the monamine oxidase system that catabolizes the monamine.[25] The results of these studies are summarized in Table 14–2.

Just how the brain receives input resulting in an increase or decrease of these mediators to affect feeding is undetermined. Normal dietary intake probably does not have a great influence on brain concentrations of serotonin, norepinephrine, epinephrine, or dopamine, but it has been shown that acute alterations in diet can influence these levels.[31, 32] The amino acid precursors to these neurotransmitters compete with other neutral amino acids (NAA) for active transport across the blood-brain barrier.[33] Because tryptophan is present in only small amounts in foods, an increase in protein intake does little to increase serotonin synthesis. However, insulin stimulated by a meal rich in carbohydrate lowers the concentration of the other amino acids, causing a relative increase in the blood level of tryptophan, thus facilitating its transport into the brain, and increasing serotonin levels.[34] Patients with diabetes mellitus, possibly because of a lack of this insulin response, have been reported to have decreased TRP/NAA ratios.[35] The decreased availability of tryptophan results in decreased serotonin synthesis, thus preventing normal satiety signals, resulting in overeating and obesity. Lean diabetic patients have been shown to have normal TRP/NAA ratios.[36]

Certain disease states may alter the blood-brain barrier and the competitive uptake of precursors. Jeppson and associates compared two groups of rats by inducing sepsis in one group by puncturing the cecum, with sham-operated rats serving as the control group.[37] They found that the brain uptake of labeled neutral amino acids was increased in the septic rats when compared with the control group. Krause and coworkers found elevated concentrations of brain tryptophan and increased levels of serotonin in tumor-bearing rats.[38]

Studies in which the role of the brain concentration of precursors on monamine synthesis has been examined have used monamine oxidase inhibitors or large doses of the amino acid.[30] Whether the availability of these substrates is subject to variations with the ingestion of normal meals in normal individuals has been questioned. Wolever and associates found a positive correlation between the expression of hunger and fasting ratios of tryptophan to tyrosine in nonobese diabetic subjects.[36] They concluded that the serum amino acid ratios are normal in diabetics and that their findings were consistent with the hypothesis that "the TRP/NAA ratio is involved in the regulation of the long-term perception of hunger in different individu-

als" (p. 137). Peters and Harper used animals as subjects to study the relationship between protein and calorie intake, plasma ratios of tryptophan and tyrosine to other neutral amino acids, and brain concentrations of serotonin, dopamine, and norepinephrine; they failed to find any correlation.[39] Fernstrom also found no effect on brain concentrations of neurotransmitters with the ingestion of a mixed diet.[40] Curzon concluded that the synthesis of critical substances in the brain is too important to be easily influenced by changes in diet and probably is altered only by extreme changes.[41]

Amphetamines exert their anorexic effect probably by releasing catecholamines that inhibit the LH. Tricyclic antidepressants increase the concentration of norepinephrine and serotonin by blocking their reuptake; norepinephrine inhibits the VMH while serotonin induces satiety. Because these two effects should cancel each other, resulting in a zero net change, the increased feeding seen with antidepressants[42, 43] may be due to a greater effect of norepinephrine or may be a result of improved mental outlook. Yeragani and associates concluded that the antidepressants produce increased appetite by their pharmacological action rather than by an improvement of depression.[44] However, their study of 180 patients receiving antidepressant therapy for conditions other than depression was a retrospective chart analysis and relied on the reporting of carbohydrate craving and increased appetite. The weight gain seen in their subjects may have been due to other effects. Fernstrom and coworkers reported a decreased metabolic rate in patients treated with antidepressants, and this response may account for the increased weight seen in the other studies.[45]

The efferent pathways from the brain affecting feeding behavior are unknown.

Peptides

Until it was demonstrated that many peptides are synthesized by and widely distributed in the brain,[46] the interest in peptides as modulators of brain activity was largely pharmacological, since peptides normally do not cross the blood-brain barrier. Numerous regulatory peptides have been demonstrated in the mammalian central nervous system.[47]

Cholecystokinin (CCK) is the peptide that has been studied the most, using central as well as peripheral administration. Studies have concluded that CCK and its active fragment, CCK-8, suppress intake when given as a continuous infusion either intraventricularly, intravenously, or intraperitoneally. Central administration required only 5 per cent of the peripheral dose to suppress intake.[48–50]

Della-Fera and Baile hypothesized that the mechanism of the effect of centrally administered CCK is separate from that of peripheral administration.[50] Moran and McHugh proposed that CCK reduces food intake by contributing to gastric distention by decreasing gastric emptying.[51] They found that peripheral administration of CCK in monkeys was more effective when the subjects had been given a gastric preload. Muurahainen and associates monitored gastric emptying while intravenous CCK-8 was administered to 12 healthy volunteers.[52] They also found decreased gastric emptying with CCK-8 and concluded that "CCK may amplify satiety signals in proportion to the fullness of the stomach" (p. 645).

Additionally, endogenous opiates have been studied as influencing control mechanisms for hunger and satiety. Opiate agonist injections increased intake, while opiate antagonists decreased intake.[53–56] Morley and Levine offered a teleological explanation for the role of endogenous opiates in inducing feeding, stating that "it would be of use to an animal when hungry and forced to encounter danger to find food to have some protection against pain"[55] (p. 760).

However, high doses of opiates decrease intake in laboratory animals as a result of depressive effects. Nurses anecdotally report that the administration of exogenous opiates to patients results in a decreased desire for food. In other words, patients who are in pain and receive narcotic relief often forgo or reduce their next meal. Whether this behavior is due to pain or the sedative effect of the drug is undetermined but illustrates the importance of the differential effects between pharmacological and physiological dosages of putative regulators of hunger and satiety.

Additional study is necessary to answer questions about how (or whether) the hormones from the peripheral system interact with the central system or whether these hormones affect naturally motivated feeding behavior under physiological conditions.

Peripheralist Theories

The peripheralist theories of the control of food intake focus upon the origin of signals of hunger and satiety arising outside the central nervous system. Some theories maintain that purely peripheral events are responsible, while other theories suggest a peripheral sensor with input into the central nervous system.

Gastrointestinal Tract

Novin and VanderWeele described how the earliest theory of the mechanisms of hunger and satiety, that the gastrointestinal (GI) tract controlled food intake, began in ancient Greece.[57] It was posited that hunger pangs arising from contractions of an empty stomach initiated feeding and the sensation of fullness terminated it. The first experiment testing this hypothesis in humans was performed by Cannon and Washburn.[58] Washburn swallowed a tube with pressure balloons to record gastric motility while he indicated when he experienced the sensation of hunger. An invariable correlation between gastric contractions and the expression of hunger was noted. It was concluded that the periodic activity of the gastrointestinal tract is the sole source of hunger pangs. However, Wangensteen and Carlson provided evidence in 1931, with a case study of a patient with a total gastrectomy, that the stomach is not essential in the expression of hunger.[59]

In more recent times, studies of the GI tract have focused more on its role in producing satiety than on its role in signaling hunger and initiating food intake; investigators are looking at those factors that terminate feeding rather than affect its onset. This approach is consistent with the idea that the urge to eat is dominant and would exist at all times unless inhibited by some satiety factor.

Pregastric Phase: Visual, Olfactory, and Orosensory

Studies in which the role of the pregastric segment in feeding in animals has been examined have concluded that normal feeding is enhanced by sensations arising from this segment but that they are neither sufficient nor essential. Epstein and Teitelbaum eliminated orosensory input by means of direct gastric infusions in rats and found that they were able to regulate food intake.[60] However, in humans direct intragastric infusions of varying amounts and caloric dilutions of oral preloads led to overeating during a test meal. The overeating, according to the authors, was due to insufficient oral stimulation.[61] This view is supported by Rodin, who stated: "Internal signals do not guide eating behavior unless cognitive or external cues are present"[62] (p. 231).

The subjects in the study conducted by Walike and others received no cues, visual or tactile, because the intragastric preloads were out of the subjects' view and the caloric value of the oral preloads was disguised.[61] Over a longer period of time, both humans and animals are able to adjust their oral intake when given direct gastric infusions of varying percentages of their baseline intake.[63, 64] However, the observation that overeating occurs initially when oral feedings are combined with intragastric feedings demonstrates the importance of oropharyngeal sensations for proper metering of intake.[65] The fact that monkeys,[66] dogs,[67] and rats[68, 69] are better able to regulate their oral intake than humans[70, 71] perhaps underscores the importance of learning, which is greater in humans than in lower animals, in the regulation of food intake. In the above studies, animal subjects were able to compensate for intragastric nutrient loads and reduce their spontaneous intake to a much greater degree than were humans. Rolls and associates gave test meals with disguised caloric content to normal subjects who were then asked to rate their degree of hunger and fullness and were offered additional foods.[72] They found no effect of the caloric density on the perception of hunger or fullness or in the amount of additional food consumed. They concluded that there is a sensory-specific satiety independent of the energy density of foods.

Gastric Phase

Several studies have concluded, and it is generally accepted, that gastric distention induces satiety and meal termination in both humans and laboratory animals.[66, 68, 71, 73–81] The mechanism responsible, the signal from the distended stomach, has not been identified; it is unclear whether or not it is the vagus. Kraly and Gibbs concluded that the signal for gastric distention was not mediated by the vagus when a bilateral subdiaphrag-

matic vagotomy failed to block the satiating effect of food in the stomach of rats.[78] In contrast, however, Gonzales and Deutsch reported that subdiaphragmatic vagotomy did abolish the satiating effect of gastric distention in rats.[79] With the finding that vagotomized rats were able to compensate as well as controls for the removal of nutrients from the stomach, Deutsch and Ahn concluded that "The signals concerning distention travel to the central nervous system via the vagus. The route taken by nutrient signals remains unknown except that it cannot be the vagus"[80] (p. 47).

In a study in which rats were fed via a denervated stomach that had been transplanted from another rat and yet demonstrated satiety, Koopmans and Maggio also concluded that neural signals were not responsible for gastric satiety.[68] They theorized that "some humoral signal must be involved" (p. 52). They further proposed that release of this signal requires a combination of chemical stimulation of the gastric surface and gastric distention, the mechanisms of which are also unknown.

Although the role of gastric distention, especially with nutritive substances, in eliciting satiety is well accepted, it is also well accepted that gastrectomized humans and animals are able to regulate their intake. This finding points out the probable redundancy in the system controlling food intake; there is no one mechanism with total control, and in the absence of one signal, others are capable of taking over.

Intestinal Phase

The role of the intestines in eliciting satiety seems to be centered in the upper duodenum, but whether this occurs in response to the osmotic or nutrient load or both is inconclusive. Yin and Tsai concluded that it was the osmotic effect of the intestinal load.[81] When isotonic infusions reduced intake, Campbell and Davis concluded that the nutritional load elicited satiety.[82] Leibling and others instilled a liquid diet in varying amounts and osmolalities into the duodenum of rats and found that it was the intestinal load (concentration times volume) rather than either concentration or volume alone that was the stimulus for intestinal satiety.[69] Welch and associates found that while both ileal and jejunal infusions of a corn oil emulsion reduced food intake in healthy volunteers, only jejunal infusions alleviated feelings of hunger.[83] The presence of fat in the jejunum retards gastric emptying by stimulating the release of CCK. The authors proposed that the jejunal control of hunger was not related to gastric distention, because the stomach was empty, and that hunger and satiety are mediated by CCK.

Combined Pregastric, Gastric, and Intestinal Phases

Pregastric and intestinal mechanisms for satiety are probably synergistic, over and above the function of pregastric stimuli acting alone as a cue to prepare the intestines.[84] Moran and McHugh suggest that the rate of gastric emptying into the duodenum provides the link between these two phases.[85]

Adipose Tissue

The role of adipose tissue in the regulation of food intake was first proposed by Kennedy[86] and expanded by Brobeck.[87] This theory states that the clearance rate of circulating metabolites by fat depots influences hunger and satiety. If fat is being synthesized, the satiety signal produced by feeding will be increased; if fat is not being synthesized, the signal will be diminished and feeding will continue longer.

VanderWeele and associates tested this theory in relation to insulin as the satiety signal in rats and found a decrease in food intake with infused insulin, which affected nutrient clearance from the blood into the adipose tissue.[88] Woods and others also tested Kennedy's theory with baboons.[89] They supported the role of insulin by citing the fact that insulin is secreted in direct relationship to adiposity. They hypothesized that insulin in the cerebral spinal fluid signals the state of adiposity and influences food intake via a central mechanism. They infused insulin intraventricularly, at varying intervals, for several weeks, with a significant reduction of food intake and body weight without an effect on plasma insulin or glucose levels.

Role of fat stores is also implicated in the long-term control of body weight. This is discussed below in the text on integration of theories.

Liver

The hepatostatic theory, which places the liver as the site of regulation of food intake, was first proposed by Russek and associates.[90] This theory states that there are hepatic receptors monitoring glucose availability, relating both to glucose delivered to the liver and liver glycogen stores. Thus, when absorption from the intestine is reduced and liver glycogen is depleted, hunger is signaled. Absorption will restore liver glycogen and liver pyruvate and induce satiety.[91]

Campbell and Davis infused glucose into the portal vein of rats and found decreased intake of an oral glucose solution.[82] They concluded that this effect was specific to glucose when isovolumetric infusions of urea or saline produced no effect. Friedman and Stricker supported this hypothesis: "Hunger usually is associated with a decreased supply of fuels from the intestines (and adipose tissue) . . . when the availability of fat is relatively low, the need for exogenous fuels increases. The liver is the organ that is most responsive to differences of this kind in the supply of metabolic fuels from both endogenous and exogenous sources"[92] (p. 428). However, support is not unanimous, and thus this theory remains controversial.[93–96]

Postabsorptive Signals and Mechanisms

The preabsorptive mechanisms have been mentioned above. Postabsorptive mechanisms could be mediated by one of the several hormones secreted by the stomach, intestines, or pancreas. The most studied of these are CCK, bombesin (BBS), and insulin.

Cholecystokinin, as discussed previously, decreases intake when injected intraperitoneally or intravenously. This action is enhanced by other satiety factors, such as force of habit or central mechanisms.[97] CCK seems to act locally rather than centrally, since abdominal or gastric vagotomy blocks its effects while lesions of the VMH do not.[98]

Bombesin injected intraperitoneally in rats decreased intake,[99] but controversy exists as to whether this decreased intake was due to malaise rather than actual satiety.[100] Other hormones studied (gastrin, secretin, and gastric inhibitory peptide) have demonstrated no effect on satiety.[101]

The effects of insulin are equivocal. Insulin injections produced hunger sensations in normal human subjects, but only in those who developed abnormal hypoglycemia (42 mg/dl); when blood glucose levels were returning to normal, hunger subsided at 61 mg/dl, still below normal levels.[102] Increased insulin responses to sights and sounds of food have been implicated in the development of obesity in humans, leading them to eat more to balance the increased level of insulin.

Inoue and Bray found that hyperinsulinemia from VMH lesions in rats led to excessive fat deposition, resulting in obesity.[103] However, it is not thought that insulin causes obesity by leading to overeating because pair feeding in rats failed to block the obesity seen with VMH lesions.[104] The rats developed hyperinsulinemia but were not allowed to overeat and yet they still gained weight.

Opposite results, in which insulin is a satiety hormone, have been obtained in rats and baboons, as discussed above, and in pigs.[77] Anika and associates infused insulin intravenously in pigs in doses that approximated physiological responses, according to the authors, and found that it depressed food intake.[77] Woo and others infused insulin intravenously in human volunteers while maintaining normal blood glucose levels and concluded that a rise in plasma insulin levels without a fall in glucose levels does not influence food intake or satiety.[105] The prevailing hypothesis, in spite of these conflicting results, is that insulin is a satiety signal because its inhibitory effects on satiety appear only after severe hypoglycemia and that this effect is nonphysiological.[106] This is in keeping with the observations that insulin increases serotonin levels in the brain and that serotonin induces satiety.

Behavioralist Theories

Clearly, hunger and satiety are signaled by physiological mechanisms, but it is also evident that the findings of the studies regarding these mechanisms are inconsistent. Although physiological events have been identified, their precise causation (input) and mode of action (output) have yet to be determined. The control of food intake in humans is more complex than that of other animals because of the greater influence of non-nutritional factors, such as psychological and emotional states, sociocultural and religious backgrounds, economic status, the amount of work required to obtain food, the aesthetic appeal of the food and the environment in which it is served, and the overriding cognitive aspects.

Behavioral aspects play a significant role even in laboratory animals. Friedman and Stricker have observed that "animals with

nutritional needs may not choose to eat, and that animals with no such needs may eat anyway"[92] (p. 424). Perhaps this observation could account for the inconsistent findings in a group of four retriever dogs who received the same type of vagotomy; all dogs were tested for completeness of vagotomy yet "these four dogs, having undergone apparently identical denervation, showed a range of response to food ranging from completely normal to completely abnormal; moreover, these responses were specific to each dog and consistent throughout the study period"[107] (p. 361).

Fonberg also cautioned that social factors play a significant role not only in humans but also in animals.[26] She studied the effects of hypothalamic damage versus amygdalar lesions on feeding and emotional states of various species and found that the more social the animal (e.g., dogs and cats as compared to rats), the more effective amygdalar lesions were in producing behavioral and food intake changes. The role of the amygdala was suggested in contributing to the conditioning, which varies from species to species as well as from person to person.[108] DeCastro[109] and DeCastro and DeCastro[110] studied free-living adults who kept a detailed diary of their intake and subjective sensations. They concluded that the presence of other people may override or prevent normal regulation and suggested that "species differences may be due to the social context of observation"[110] (p. 651).

In humans, it is well known that a party or social gathering improves appetite and one may eat even though not hungry because the social stimuli add to the reward of eating. In the dog, an animal that is accustomed to having humans provide its food, these social relations probably also have an alimentary component. "This may influence the results of many experiments performed on ingestive behavior in which social factors are not taken into account; these factors should not be omitted but incorporated into the study"[26] (p. 26). None of the experimental studies reviewed in this chapter had done so.

Much of the work on the nonphysiological aspects of human feeding behavior has been reported in the obesity literature.* The

*The definitions of obesity used in these studies were based on reference to published height-weight tables; the term "statistical overweight" refers to these actuarial tables. These tables are open to criticism on a number of points and must be viewed with these limitations in mind.

prominent theories of obesity are interrelated. The "externality" theory embraces features of the "restrained-eating" theory, and both are related to the "set-point" theory. The hypotheses underlying these theories are reviewed below, with the admonition to bear in mind that numerous nonphysiological factors are involved in the regulation of food intake, including psychological, sociocultural, emotional, environmental, cognitive, and ethnological,[111] and that there is probably not one theory that explains all aspects of feeding behavior.

Externality Theory

Although almost everyone responds to external cues, such as the appearance, aroma, and taste of food, numerous investigators have observed that obese individuals are more affected by these non-nutritional factors than leaner individuals.[62] This "externality" theory was first proposed by Schachter and associates on the basis of results of studies in which obese subjects ate more than lean subjects in response to visual and sensory cues. The criteria for determining obesity were not presented.[112]

Pliner also found that obese people appeared to be more responsive to external factors and ate more when presented with palatable food served in an appealing manner whereas lean people tended to respond more to their internal, physiological states.[113]

Stunkard corroborated this theory when he found that obese subjects seemed to be unaware of their internal signals.[114] He placed tubes with pressure balloons in the stomachs of obese subjects and even though frequent and large gastric contractions were recorded, reflecting "hunger pangs," the subjects did not express hunger and denied it when questioned. The results of the study by Mayer and associates[115] found that while gastric contractions were a frequent symptom in hunger, they were not universal; Stunkard's subjects may not have *been* hungry, rather than denying hunger.

The responsiveness of the obese to external events was also studied by Rodin.[62, 116] However, she cautioned that the Schachterian hypothesis is too simplistic in many respects. The factors leading to weight gain may be quite different than those that determine the level of body weight one finally reaches and maintains (see Set-Point, below).[62] Not all overweight people are overly responsive to external cues, and lean people as well are often tempted by aromas, sights, and thoughts of food.[117]

Restrained-Eating Theory

Schachter's hypothesis that the obese tend to eat on the basis of external cues and ignore their internal, physiological signals was tested by Herman and Polivy.[118] Under the pretense of a test of tactile stimulation on taste, subjects were seated near an electrical apparatus, presented with three flavors of ice cream, told to taste as much as they wanted, and were left alone for 10 minutes. Anxiety was created in half of the 42 subjects with the suggestion that the tactile stimulation would be an electric shock. A restraint scale, developed by the authors to assess the individual's concern for dieting and keeping weight down, was correlated with the amount eaten. Restrained eaters ate more than unrestrained eaters, whether obese or lean. Unrestrained normal-weight individuals ate significantly less when anxious than restrained eaters.

Set-Point Theory

Nisbett posed the theory that the difference in eating behavior between the obese and the lean had more to do with the degree of underweight than the degree of overweight.[119] He hypothesized that obese people might be statistically and socially overweight but biologically underweight; their increased number of adipocytes generate hunger signals, while social and cultural pressures tend to inhibit weight gain. Thus, these obese individuals exhibit the behaviors of people who are food-deprived.[120] Normal-weight individuals who are constantly dieting to maintain their weight resemble the obese who limit their intake. They would gain weight if they would "let themselves go." Once this self-control is breached, the restraint is removed and eating continues.

Bromberg and Bernstein studied cephalic phase insulin release as a measure of desire to eat by the sight, smell, or thought of food in women with anorexia nervosa.[121] A control group of lean, age-matched, nondieting women showed no insulin response to the presentation of a palatable food, while the anorexic group demonstrated a 31 per cent increase. However, the anorexic women reported lower hunger levels than the control group, and when offered food, ate less than the control group. The authors theorize that patients with anorexia either misinterpret or deny their feelings of hunger or have a high degree of restraint. Because other groups of dieters studied with the same design did not show this insulin response, the authors suggested that the combination of high restraint and low body weight somehow enhanced this response.[122]

Anxiety

The alterations seen with anxiety are highly individual. Some people react with increased intake; others find it "impossible to eat anything." Anxiety has been hypothesized to affect the eating habits of obese and lean individuals differently.[112] The physiological basis for this theory is that anxiety produces symptoms that are similar to those following food intake (e.g., increased blood glucose levels) and that leaner individuals, responsive to their internal states, reduce their intake, while the obese, who are not responsive to these internal states, are not as affected. The observation that obese individuals increase their intake in response to anxiety has been reported in several studies.[116–119] The physiological basis for this observation is unknown. According to these theories, anxiety would decrease eating in normal-weight individuals by inhibiting gastric contractions and releasing glucose into the circulation; obese individuals who are relatively insensitive to their internal signals would be unaffected. Restrained-eaters, when presented with tempting food, respond to anxiety with increased intake. These theories have been questioned, however, and more research in this area is needed.[122]

Depression

Depression also affects ingestive behaviors. The effect of depression is usually in the direction of decreased desire for and enjoyment of food.[122] Many of the self-report inventories for assessing depression include items about weight loss.[123, 124] Weight loss has been recognized as a feature of depression since 1904,[125] but more recent studies have demonstrated that depression induces eating in restrained eaters.

Frost and associates[126] and Lowe and Maycock[122] experimentally induced various mood states in student volunteers and counted the number of M & M candies eaten during the sessions. Prior to the procedures, subjects were given the restrained-eating questionnaire; their responses to the three different moods (depressed, neutral, or elated) were classified according to their level of restraint.

High-restraint subjects who were induced into a depressed mood ate more than high-restraint subjects induced into neutral or elated moods or low-restraint subjects induced into a depressed mood. The authors stated that these results provided strong support for the restrained-eating theory. Depression interfered with self-control of the high-restraint person and once the dietary restraint was removed, the subject's eating behavior was uninhibited. The major drawback of this study was that the moods were artificially induced; the investigators read a series of statements that were either "depressing, neutral, or cheerful." This presupposes that all people would respond in a like manner to the same statement. Also, using only one food item as the dependent variable might have skewed the results if subjects did not find the item palatable.

Polivy and Herman suggested that certain people may gain rather than lose weight when depressed.[127] They administered a questionnaire regarding symptoms of depression, especially weight changes, and their restraint questionnaire to 12 moderately depressed outpatients. As discussed previously, it is thought that high-restraint persons are characterized by an overconcern with dieting and food-related issues and by substantial weight fluctuations.[128] Herman and Polivy found that depressed, low-restraint subjects experienced typical weight loss during the course of their depression, while high-restraint subjects recalled weight gain during depression.[118]

Paykel examined the relationship of appetite and depression in 208 psychiatric patients.[129] Appetite was rated on a scale of 0 to 12; each gradation was labeled, with 12 being "severe, little food eaten" and 0 being "severe increase in intake and preoccupation with food." Level of depression was assessed with an interview by the author and rated on a scale from 1 to 7. Sixty-six per cent of the 208 subjects reported a decrease in appetite, 20 per cent reported no change, and only 14 per cent reported an increase.

Thus, although the presence of physiological determinants and signals of hunger have been acknowledged, there are numerous ways in which behavioral events contribute to or influence the regulation of food intake.

Conditioned Response

Some linkages between the results of physiological and behavioral studies have been made. Stunkard[130] and Booth[131, 132] argue that satiety is a conditioned response. This explanation attempts to reconcile the inadequate mechanisms proposed in purely physiological studies. Clearly, the role of food intake is to assure adequate energy for metabolic functioning, but it is also obvious that a distended stomach cannot sense calories and that satiation occurs before adequate digestion and absorption into the blood could signal metabolic events. Therefore, there must be some conditioning that has taken place in response to eating similar foods on other occasions. Canon and Washburn stated that "Habit no doubt plays an important role"[58] (p. 452).

Results of a study by Rolls and associates[72] lend support to this hypothesis. Subjects responded to familiar foods in a similar way regardless of the disguised energy density. "The beliefs about the foods appeared to be so strong that foods with little energy content reduced hunger for the hour after consumption" (p. 732). The conditioned response hypothesis does not address the issue of initiation of eating, that is, those factors that signal hunger or appetite.

Integration—Energostatic Theory

The main problem with both the pure peripheralist and centralist theories is that none of the control sites discussed seems essential to maintenance of regulation. There are many redundancies in the system, and back-up mechanisms exist to replace those that are lost. The elimination of information from peripheral sites (with the exception of adipose tissue, which has not been scientifically tested), has had little long-term effect on feeding. Normal regulation of food intake apparently ensues. Animals with LH or VMH damage do eventually recover and maintain their body weight, although at a different level.

The discrepancies among the findings of various studies may be reconciled if the control of hunger and satiety is viewed as a system whose main goal is to regulate the body's energy supply (energostatic theory). This involves adjustments in ingestion as well as adjustments in the expenditure of energy. This regulation probably has two components, one for short-term (meal-to-meal) intake and one for long-term (daily, weekly) adjustments. It is well established that animals and humans regulate and defend their body weight quite effectively.[58, 133] How, where, or when the defended body weight is established is undetermined. Various investigators hypothesize a "ponderostat" or "set-point."[66, 119, 134] Keesey and coworkers reported experimentally induced shifts in the regulated body weight of rats with LH lesions.[135] When allowed control of its own intake, each animal successfully maintained a stable body weight, although at a different level than before the operation. After dietary-induced shifts in weight, an animal increased or decreased intake and returned to prediet baseline weight.[135]

Body weight is maintained at a stable level when energy input equals energy expenditure, and the two must not be considered separately.[136] Keys and others found decreased metabolic rates with chronic underfeeding in humans.[120] Landsberg and Young found changes in metabolic rate with changes in both acute and chronic intake.[137] Keesey cited a classic study, conducted by Neuman in 1902, in which he overate for 3 years, accounting for almost an additional 400,000 calories during this time. Theoretically, he should have gained about 100 pounds (45.4 kg), yet he reported a gain of only several pounds. Clearly, in view of the fact that the expected weight gain did not occur, marked increases in his rate of energy expenditure must have taken place.

The energostatic theory does not account for all aspects of food intake, however. "While it appears that the behavioral event of feeding is essentially controlled by ischymetric (power production of substrates monitored at intracellular level) mechanisms, these are modulated by both specific appetite and 'oral need' factors"[137] (p. 668).

Conscious Control

Despite the overwhelming evidence offered in support of specific mechanisms or an interplay of mechanisms, the overriding role of conscious control of food ingestion is unquestioned. Herman and Mack found that the cognitive element was more potent than the physiological one—hunger.[128] This is demonstrated when hunger strikers consciously refuse to eat regardless of internal physiological and emotional states as well as external pressures. This ultimate control is also readily apparent in *Ordeal by Hunger*[138] and *Alive*[139] which document the cannibalistic behavior of some of the stranded and starving individuals. However, the fact that some people were unable to resort to this type of food in order to prolong their life points out the underlying conscious control, because of personal, cultural, or religious beliefs, over the physiological need for food.

Many patients with anorexia nervosa *do* admit to feelings of hunger and admit to an intense desire for food when questioned but suppress their expression of hunger and refuse to eat.[140] Thus, it is possible to elicit feelings of hunger and appetite even though the person refuses to eat when presented with food.

Conversely, people who are not operationally hungry (those who have just finished a meal or are not energy-depleted) can still have a desire for and ingest food. This is commonly seen when a tempting dessert is offered after a satisfying meal. These observations may underscore the importance of the social context of eating or may reflect a stimulus-induced response to previous experiences and pleasures,[141] or they are illustrative of the difference between hunger and appetite (see Related Physiological, Pathophysiological, and Psychosocial Concepts). Nevertheless, one is still able to retain conscious control over the choice to accept or refuse the dessert, albeit with difficulty at times.

PATHOLOGICAL CONSEQUENCES

The hunger that occurs with extreme food deprivation happens in the United States today only under exceptional circumstances, but the physical and emotional effects of such starvation and unrelieved hunger have been well documented.

Winick compiled the results of studies by a group of Jewish physicians in the Warsaw ghetto during World War II.[2] These physicians documented the effects of undernutrition and malnutrition as they developed in the prisoners who sought their services. Keys and associates reported the results of a monumental series of experiments performed on

healthy volunteers (conscientious objectors during World War II) who were subjected to varying degrees and duration of caloric restriction and various refeeding schedules.[120] These populations differed in that the first group, in addition to suffering from hunger and malnutrition, suffered also from the extremes of war and other deprivations, such as lack of housing and clothing, and lived with constant fear and disease; the other group knew that the experiment would eventually end and were otherwise well cared for and comfortable. Yet, both groups exhibited the depression, apathy, disorientation, and physiological deterioration seen with chronic undernutrition and hunger. These psychological and physiological changes, including gradual physical wasting and death, are consequences of prolonged hunger and form yet another phenomenon.

A patient's inability to respond to hunger sensations may lead to malnutrition unless caretakers provide proper surveillance and timely interventions. Normally nourished persons can withstand a brief period of fasting (3 to 5 days) without apparent ill effects, but those with pre-existing nutritional deficiencies and those whose fasting will be prolonged should be identified early and provided with adequate nutritional intake enterally or parenterally.

A patient's inability to respond to hunger sensations may also lead to psychological stress. Those on weight-reducing diets who are taking in fewer calories than their setpoint may indeed be physically hungry and not just expressing an appetite. They are in a state of starvation and may undergo the same psychological deterioration documented by Winick[2] and Keys[120]: depression, lethargy, apathy, poor thinking, disorientation, and incoherence.

When one is able to respond to individual signals for food ingestion, the distinction between hunger and appetite may be just a confusion of terms. When one is not able to respond to these sensations, the expression of these feelings must be sought out and interpreted by others, especially if the sensations of hunger and appetite are regulatory systems.

It is not known to what extent the sensations of hunger and appetite are merely an awareness that the regulatory processes are operating or to what extent they participate in and control the regulation of food intake.

In lower forms of animals, the urge to eat is probably a primitive instinct that exists at all times unless inhibited, and regulation is mainly involved in inhibiting this signal.[55] The higher the organism on the phylogenetic scale, the more important the sensations of hunger and appetite become.[26, 108] Even though these sensations seem to be dispensable in regulating intake, the unrequited feelings of hunger and appetite may be distressful to those who are not allowed oral intake because of disease or anatomical structural abnormalities.

No study has yet adequately addressed the complex problem of interpreting patients' complaints of hunger. However, the surprising frequency of malnutrition in hospitalized patients, which may have developed from disordered or ignored hunger mechanisms, has been well documented.[142–144]

Patients may be in danger of developing malnutrition if their reports of hunger are not explored and properly interpreted or if their cries of "I'm hungry!" are dismissed out of hand. Inadequate nutritional repletion can result when nurses, believing patients to be ingesting adequate amounts of food, dismiss their expressions of hunger as "natural" without further investigation. Psychological distress may also develop if patients are unable to respond to their internal signals of hunger.

A lack of normal hunger mechanisms or expression also places patients at risk for malnutrition (see discussion in Chapter 5, Anorexia).

RELATED PHYSIOLOGICAL, PATHOPHYSIOLOGICAL, AND PSYCHOSOCIAL CONCEPTS

Hunger, appetite, satiety, and anorexia are often considered to be gradations in the urge or drive for food, with appetite being the first, more gentle stimulus to nutrient ingestion and anorexia being the antithesis, an unwillingness or inability to eat (total lack of desire for food).

Although these concepts are all associated with food—thinking about it, seeking it out, initiating the ingestion of it, terminating the ingestion of it, or absolute refusal of it—they are fundamentally different. To say that these concepts are on a continuum is an oversimplification, implying that the only difference between each is in the *quantity* of feelings. Quality, not quantity, is really the differentiating factor, with the quality and meaning of the sensations giving rise to the expression of the various conditions. These represent different but related concepts.

Appetite

The concept of appetite is most closely related to hunger. The sensation of "hunger" signals the physiological need for food; "appetite" reflects a psychological or cerebral desire for food. These two sensations can occur together or singly. The difference between these two concepts is in the etiology of the sensations and the intervention strategies for each. Appetite is a function of a person's mind, a learned mechanism expressed according to personal preferences of taste, social conditioning, mores, and taboos. As individuals experiencing these sensations, we instinctively know which intervention to choose for ourselves, whether to grab any available food to assuage our hunger or to seek out a specific food to satisfy our appetite. As nurses designing interventions for patients, we must elicit these distinctions of sensation from the individual patient.

Appetite has been presented as the first gentle urge to eat, and as deprivation continues, the feelings intensify and appetite becomes hunger.[145] In this view, appetite, as the earlier impetus for food ingestion, is related to the selection of specific foods guided by personal preferences. If food is not eaten in response to the feeling of appetite at this point, and as the length of time of deprivation continues, the sensation intensifies and becomes hunger. If hunger and appetite were on a continuum, the presence of hunger would preclude a sensation of appetite as shown in Figure 14–1.

Depending on the point along the continuum at which appetite becomes hunger, with the sensations of appetite and hunger overlapping, the diagrammatic representation may look like the illustration in Figure 14–2. A major consideration in the conceptualization of hunger and appetite in Figure 14–2 is the point, or area, at which appetite and hunger overlap. It is tempting to view the area of overlap at the midpoint of appetite (point a) such that appetite continues to exist along with hunger for a period of time, influencing the selection of food, even when

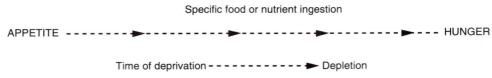

Figure 14–1. Appetite and hunger viewed on a continuum. In this interpretation, appetite is presented as a cluster of pleasant sensations that provide the first gentle urge to eat; specific selected food may be ingested at this stage. As deprivation continues over time, the sensations intensify and become less pleasant, evolving into hunger, which is viewed as a cluster of unpleasant feelings and sensations. In the beginning stages, a person is more particular about the food selected; as deprivation continues, the person becomes less particular and will seek out any food.

eaten in response to hunger signals. The presence of *both* appetite and hunger would have to be within the area of overlap (i.e., between point a and point b in the diagram). Figure 14–3 represents the view of the relationship between hunger and appetite as two discrete but related sensations.

Although the terms appetite and hunger are often used interchangeably, once they are defined, people are usually able to distinguish between hunger and appetite and indicate the intensity of each of the sensations.[120, 146]

The etiology of hunger and the etiology of appetite are separate and distinct entities, not two poles of one continuum. The nature of these subjective signals for food ingestion has been of interest to scientists and philosophers for centuries, and debate over semantics of these terms has raged equally long.[146]

In their classic study of the nature of hunger signals, Cannon and Washburn refuted the then commonly held view that appetite was the first stage of hunger.[58] They concluded that the two were fundamentally different in etiology, localization of sensations, and psychic elements. "Hunger may be satisfied while the appetite still calls" (p. 454).

Grossman differentiated between hunger and appetite, relating hunger to a physiolog-

ical need and appetite to an affective desire.[147] Janowitz and Grossman wrote that although many authors had advocated the banishment of the terms hunger and appetite as separate sensations, "Their [the terms'] stubborn longevity appears to this observer to mean that there is some basis of reality for the distinction drawn between hunger and appetite in every day speech"[148] (p. 327). Mayer distinguished between hunger and appetite yet adopted the earlier view of a continuum.[145, 149] He defined appetite as the first pleasant complex of sensations by which one is aware of a need for food and hunger as the complex of unpleasant sensations, felt after a period of prolonged deprivation, which impels the organism to seek food. "The passage from appetite to hunger is dependent on duration of deprivation, rate of energy expenditure, etc"[145] (p. 474).

Clearly, there is not a consensus in the literature regarding hunger and appetite. Authorities who distinguish between hunger and appetite have defined hunger as a subjective reflection of a physiological need for nutrient intake that is evoked by various individualized sensations, moods, and feelings. Appetite is defined as a subjective reflection of a *psychological* desire, urge, or craving for a specific food or nutrient. It is based

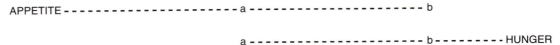

Figure 14–2. Appetite and hunger viewed as overlapping sensations. This view presents appetite and hunger as two distinct sensations having a period of overlap, where the two can exist at the same time. In this interpretation, appetite and hunger guide ingestive behavior as a discrete impetus, or together they guide ingestive behavior so that appetite continues to exist along with hunger for a period of time, influencing the selection of food even when food is eaten in response to hunger signals. The degree of influence each sensation has on eating is individual. Appetite and hunger can be experienced together only in the area of overlap (between point a and point b).

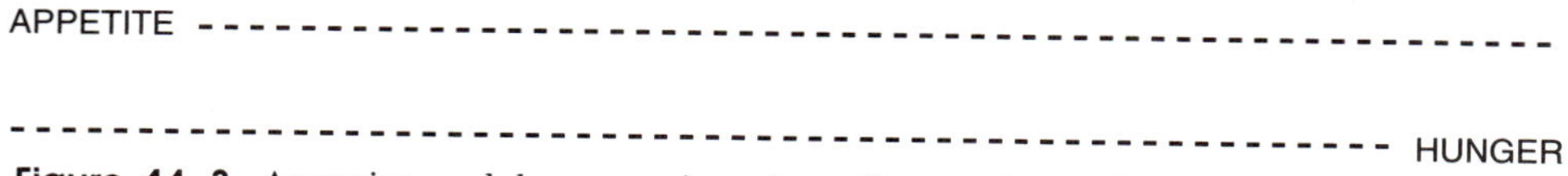

APPETITE -

- HUNGER

Figure 14–3. Appetite and hunger viewed as discrete but related sensations. In this perspective, appetite and hunger are related but are not on the same continuum. This depiction best represents the view of hunger and appetite developed in this chapter, in which appetite and hunger can exist separately or simultaneously, with any magnitude of expression. Hunger and appetite can influence ingestive behavior either singly or together.

on prior learning and preferences of taste and smell or remembered feelings and moods that accompanied previous ingestion, often rooted in cultural and religious customs. These are the definitions used in this chapter and depicted in the model in Figure 14–4.

An unsatisfied appetite can be just as severe or urgent as hunger but does not have the same physiological consequences. Those who are denied a desired food item because of lack of availability or because of restricted intake (such as those on reducing diets who crave forbidden foods) find an unrequited appetite just as psychologically distressing as unfulfilled hunger.

Bruch provided a nice example of this distinction:

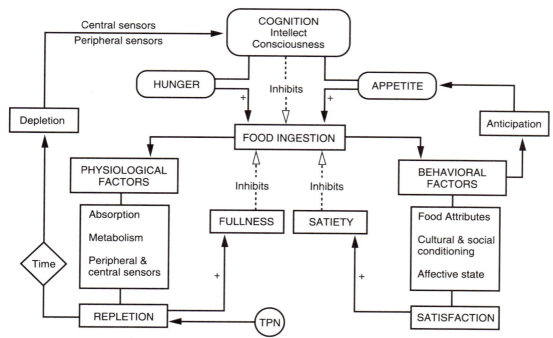

Figure 14–4. Conceptual model of hunger and appetite. Hunger and appetite have the same function of initiating food ingestion but are different in physiological basis and psychological elements. Hunger and appetite may operate singly or in combination. Note that total parenteral nutrition (TPN), since it bypasses the other factors, operates only via metabolites and repletion of energy stores to inhibit food ingestion. Although TPN bypasses the gastrointestinal (GI) tract structurally, some GI factors may still be operational owing to hormonal responses. Feelings of hunger and increased appetite may be distressing to patients on TPN, since the ability to satisfy these feelings is not usually available to them. Even though these feelings may be intense, the conscious control of food choice, guided by likes and dislikes and social restraints, prevents the patient from eating "just anything" to avoid starvation.

The Thanksgiving holiday may serve as an illustration of the many ways in which food and emotions are interrelated. There is every reason to doubt that the sudden desire for turkey which overcomes the people of the United States on that day is related to a physiologic need, or to a deficiency not noticeable during the rest of the year. Yet those who must go without turkey and all the traditional trimmings will feel unjustly treated, dissatisfied, and left out[150] (p. 68).

Hunger can be assuaged by eating a hamburger on Thanksgiving day, but the appetite (craving) for turkey with all the trimmings and meaning would not be satisfied. The difference between hunger and appetite is further elucidated by Mayer.

Terribly hungry people want food, not a specific kind of food, even though cultural standards may compel them at least for a time to starve in the presence of food which human beings otherwise conditioned would find acceptable, even attractive. But, usually, the hungrier one becomes, the less particularized the demands become. Only a few brief days of deprivation in the foodless individual separate a yearning for steak from a prayerful eagerness to devour any substance, however aesthetically and morally repulsive it had seemed before. Appetite, even in the grossest feeder, is certainly a more civilized matter than hunger. Appetite has conspicuous nuances of taste, sight, and smell"[149] (p. 10).

Satiety

Satiety is related to hunger as an opposing affective state signifying a lack of desire to eat or, more precisely, a desire not to eat.[151] It is not just a decrease in food intake but a cluster of sensations reflecting satisfaction and fulfillment. Satiety cannot be implied simply because one stops eating; humans can consciously avoid ingestion when hungry or experiencing appetite or may be incapable of eating even though hungry.[120] Also, it is possible to have feelings of hunger without an appetite for food[152] when, for instance, one knows that hunger exists but "nothing sounds good."

Anorexia

Anorexia is an abnormal state in which intake is vastly reduced. It may be accompa-nied by a lack of appetite or desire to eat ("nothing tastes good") or diminution of hunger ("I don't feel like I need to eat"). Anorexia may also, however, be accompanied by feelings of hunger and appetite that are denied. Bruch reported case studies of patients with anorexia nervosa who, with probing, admitted to feeling hungry but attempted to ignore their feelings[153] (see Chapter 5, Anorexia).

Cachexia

Cachexia is malnutrition associated with chronic illnesses and is characterized by bodily wasting and emaciation. It may be the ultimate result of disordered hunger sensations in that the person does not feel hunger even though energy demands are not being met. Cachexia may also result with an intact hunger mechanism; however, even with seemingly adequate intake, malnutrition ensues. Cachexia also develops with prolonged semistarvation regimens or fasting (see Chapter 6, Cancer Cachexia).

Other Related Concepts

Alterations in eating habits are commonly associated with alterations in moods such as depression and anxiety.[123, 154, 155] These variations usually center around the desire for food or changes in the expression of hunger and appetite and were discussed previously.

MANIFESTATIONS

Objective Manifestations

It is well known that salivary flow increases with the thought, sight, or smell of palatable food. In an attempt to find an objective, valid, and sensitive physiological measure of hunger, quantification of the salivation response to food has been proposed and tested.[156] Dry cotton dental rolls were first weighed then placed in the subject's mouth. The dependent variable (food) was then presented to the subject, and the dental rolls removed and reweighed. The amount of saliva present was then quantified as a reflection of the degree of the subject's hunger. However, for salivation to be a valid measure, the subjects must be sufficiently hungry; be able to view, recognize, and want the food; and think that they will be able to eat it. This method works well in the laboratory setting but would not be feasible to use with patients who are on NPO status and unable to eat. In addition, salivation is not a measure of hunger or specific to the desire for food and is influenced by thirst or emotional states having no consistent relationship to ingestive behaviors[157] or is a side effect of various medications.

Other objective data, such as body weight, laboratory test results, and anthropometric measurements, are reflective of the consequences of unmet hunger—malnutrition—rather than hunger per se.

Subjective Manifestations

The realization that one is hungry is a private process based on the recognition and integration of various sensations. In only one study has the array of sensations of hunger been examined. Mayer and associates surveyed approximately 800 people with a self-administered, structured questionnaire consisting of eight single and 70 multiple-choice questions "designed to help the subjects recollect their sensations or moods."[115] Subjects were asked to describe their physical sensations and moods during extreme hunger (as they were remembered) and to respond to the questions during eating as well as 2 hours and one-half hour before and after a current meal.

Manifestations of hunger reported in this study were grouped into (1) gastric sensations (emptiness, rumbling, ache, pain, tenseness, nausea), (2) mouth and throat sensations (emptiness, dryness, salivation, pleasant or unpleasant taste or sensation), (3) cerebral sensations (headache, dizziness), and (4) general overall sensations (weakness, fatigue, restlessness, coldness, warmth). Moods were categorized as (1) negative active mood (irritable, nervous, tense), (2) negative passive mood (depressed, apathetic), (3) positive passive mood (calm, relaxed, contented), and (4) positive active mood (cheerful, excited). Preoccupations with thoughts of food were graded as (1) not at all preoccupied (no thoughts of food), (2) mildly preoccupied (only occasional thoughts of food), (3) moderately preoccupied (many thoughts of food but can easily concentrate on other things),

and (4) quite preoccupied (most of thoughts are on food and it is difficult to concentrate on other subjects).

The authors concluded that gastric sensations appeared to be the most sensitive indicators of hunger.[115] This view of contraction of an empty stomach initiating feedings has been held for a long time, probably since the time of ancient Greece.[63] Other investigators have looked at single sensations as the operational definition of hunger, namely gastric "hunger pangs," emptiness, or dull aches. Cannon and Washburn recognized other affective states as appearing in hunger but noted that these are individualized and negligible and that "the dull, pressing (epigastric) sensation is the constant characteristic, the central fact . . ."[58] (p. 442).

Even though the stomach appears to be the central site of hunger sensations, it is well known that humans can still recognize hunger after gastrectomy or gastric denervation.[59, 158] Therefore, a complex of sensations and behavioral responses must motivate hunger. The private aspects of this complex may include gastric or other specific sensations, but these are highly variable and individual.

In summary, determination of the presence of hunger or appetite relies on the individual experiencing some sensations or processes, integrating these, and defining them as hunger or appetite according to the individual's own experience. Thus, measurement and quantification of the degree of hunger must rely on self-reports. Several tools to quantify these feelings have been tested.

Questionnaires

Various questionnaires have been used to evaluate the degree of hunger, but the lack of consistency in their structure or use makes them unreliable for clinical use. Some investigators have attempted to quantify responses such as "some," "none," and "severe" by assigning each response a numerical rating. Scales on questionnaires have ranged from a 0 to 4 rating system to a 0- to 100-point spread.[3, 61, 70, 159] Even within a consistent scale, each subject may have an individual interpretation and definition of the spacing between categories; in addition, subjects are restricted to the investigator's boundaries.

Tape Measure

To overcome the bias in questionnaires and scoring systems using the investigator's definition and numbering system, the use of an adjustable tape measure was suggested.[160] Subjects were given a tape measure and asked to pull out the length of tape corresponding to the intensity of their feelings. Critics pointed out the fact that the other end of the tape was not visible and that this "floating" reference point could produce highly variable results.[161] No reliability or validity of this instrument has been reported.

Visual Analogue

The visual analogue scale (VAS) (Fig. 14–5) has been proven to be a reasonably reliable, valid, and sensitive tool to assess the degree of hunger and appetite.[161–166]

The VAS is a self-reporting device utilizing a straight line usually 100 mm long for ease of measurement (but unmarked when given to subjects), with statements of the extremes of the concept being measured at each end of the line. The subject is asked to place a mark at the point along the line that best corresponds to the feelings being elicited.

Reliability. The use of the VAS to assess hunger has been shown to have both test-retest and between-subject reliability by Silverstone and Fincham[166] and Robinson and associates.[167]

Validity. To assess validity of a measurement, there must be some objective standard to which to compare the results. Because there is no objective measurement of hunger, the next best correlation is a comparison of the subject's responses on the VAS to the amount of food ingested by a subject after completing the VAS. Robinson and associates[167] and Silverstone and Stunkard[168] found a valid relationship between the intensity of VAS ratings and the amount of food subsequently ingested.

The VAS is simple for the patient to mark and requires little time. The degree of the patient's hunger or any other sensation can be quantified by measuring the distance between the left hand end of the line to the patient's mark along the line.

Because this tool has only been used in research studies, the critical values for patients are unknown, but the individual results, compared from time to time, provide an objective assessment of the presence of hunger. Research studies using patients as subjects are needed to provide guidelines for interpreting this important concept.

SURVEILLANCE

Is the patient indicating hunger, a physiological need, or appetite, a craving or desire for a specific food? Until definitive questionnaires can be developed to determine the degree of hunger as differentiated from appetite, the implications of and interventions for patients' expressing hunger are uncertain. It can be said, however, that patients' expressions of hunger warrant further investigation and that this is a fertile field for nursing research. Until studies provide specific guidelines, using the VAS as a rough estimate of the presence of hunger and appetite can be recommended. Any marks to the right of midline on the VAS warrant

HUNGER

Not at all   Hungriest
physically hungry   ever felt

APPETITE

No appetite   Severe appetite
(no cravings)   (severe cravings)

Figure 14–5. Visual analogue scales.

TABLE 14–3 THE HARRIS-BENEDICT BASAL ENERGY EXPENDITURE EQUATION (BEE)

Females: 655.10 + 9.56W + 1.85H − 4.68A
Males: 66.47 + 13.75W + 5.00H − 6.76A   where

W = weight (kg); use actual body weight for maintenance and the ideal body weight for those who are depleted or overweight; H = height (cm); and A = age (years).

1. Convert weight to kilograms: pounds ÷ 2.2 = kg.
2. Convert height to centimeters: height (in inches) × 2.14 = cm.
3. Take patient's age using closest year.

Complete equation as follows:

	Females			Males	
1.	Given number	= 655.10		Given number	= 66.47
2.	Wt. in kg × 9.56	=		Wt. in kg × 13.75	=
3.	Ht. in cm × 1.85	=		Ht in cm × 5.00	=
4.	Add lines 1, 2, 3	=		Add lines 1, 2, 3	=
5.	Age × 4.68	=		Age × 6.76	=
6.	Subtract line 5 from line 4 to get BEE	=		Subtract line 5 from line 4 to get BEE	=

Data from Harris, J. A., & Benedict, F. G. (1919). *A Biometric Study of Basal Metabolism in Man* (Pub. No. 279). Washington, D.C., Carnegie Institute of Washington.

further investigation. Even the simple questioning of a patient about the presence of hunger or appetite provides some information and is better than ignoring this aspect of patient care.

When the presence of hunger has been established, further assessment is needed to ensure adequacy of the patient's nutritional intake. Patients should be referred to a dietitian for a calorie count to compare their actual intake to their requirements. Energy requirements may be estimated by indirect calorimetry or calculated with the Harris-Benedict basal energy expenditure (BEE) equation (Table 14–3).

If the patient is receiving formula feedings, it should be relatively easy to determine the energy intake by multiplying the amount of formula received during the past 24 hours by the number of calories per milliliter. This information is printed on the container of most enteral formulas and appears on the label of parenteral nutritional solutions, or it can be obtained from the pharmacist or dietitian. In addition to the calorie count, the adequacy of nutritional intake may be determined by nitrogen balance studies.

Nitrogen Balance Studies. Nitrogen must be provided in sufficient amounts to meet the protein-building needs of the body (for tissue, muscles, enzymes, and hormones). A well-nourished adult with an adequate nutritional intake will have a normal nitrogen balance; that is, the amount of ingested protein will be equal to the amount of protein metabolized. The amount of protein metabolized can be calculated from the amount of nitrogen (protein metabolite) excreted in the urine (Box 14–1).

When nitrogen intake equals nitrogen out-

BOX 14–1

Formula for Calculating Nitrogen Balance

Nitrogen balance = [protein intake (grams) / 6.25] − (UUN + 3)

Urinary urea nitrogen (UUN) is measured on an aliquot of a 24-hour urine collection and is used to provide an estimate of nitrogen losses. Protein intake is estimated based on a 24-hour intake analysis that includes any oral or intravenous protein given during the 24-hour period in which urine is collected. Dividing the protein value by 6.25 converts it to the value for nitrogen concentration. Non-urea nitrogen loss through the feces and skin is considered to be approximately 3 g/day. Because only average values are used for skin and fecal losses, they will be increased substantially by diarrhea or fistula loss. When protein anabolism exceeds protein catabolism, nitrogen balance is positive; when excretion exceeds intake, nitrogen balance is negative.

put, there is no net tissue gain and no body protein is being used for energy. Healthy adults with an adequate diet excrete the same amount of nitrogen as they ingest: Cells are being replaced, but no net synthesis occurs.

When nitrogen intake exceeds output, nitrogen is retained for protein synthesis and the individual is in a positive nitrogen balance. Growing children have a positive nitrogen balance: They retain some of the nitrogen to synthesize new cells and tissues. Protein is required for tissue anabolism. Nutritionally depleted patients exhibit a nitrogen balance curve similar to growing children and require a greater nitrogen intake to meet their needs.[169] Patients with increased metabolic activity owing to illness or stress exhibit a reduced protein economy and also require an increased amount of nitrogen.[169] It is generally accepted that a malnourished or stressed patient requires almost double the amount of nitrogen as a healthy individual to remain in nitrogen balance.[170] The absence of positive nitrogen balance in a malnourished person indicates inadequate nutritional intake and not malnutrition itself. A positive nitrogen balance of 4 to 6 g per day represents a gain of 25 to 37.5 g of protein and a synthesis of 120 to 180 g of lean tissue.[171]

When nitrogen intake is less than nitrogen output (when nitrogen losses exceed intake), endogenous protein is being metabolized. Negative nitrogen balance indicates catabolism of body protein sources, and additional protein intake should be assured.

Glucose is the major body fuel, but if glucose is not available in sufficient amounts, amino acids will be used for energy. The amino acids are derived from metabolism of ingested protein or mobilization of body protein and can be used directly for energy or converted to glucose in the liver (gluconeogenesis). Provision of sufficient energy to sustain vital functions with restoration or maintenance of adequate protein and body cell mass is vital for optimum functioning.

Patients should be monitored at intervals, with the results compared over time in order to note individual trends.

THERAPIES

Expressions of hunger and appetite in patients may indicate inadequate caloric intake. Whether physiological or psychological interventions or both are offered to the patient depends on the cause of these subjective states. Psychological interventions (such as reassurance) may be appropriate for those who state that they have an appetite, but those who express feelings of hunger may be indicating that they are receiving inadequate levels of calories.

Patients expressing hunger and who have been identified as receiving inadequate nutritional repletion (by a clinical dietitian, nutritional support nurse, or nutritional support team) should have their intake adjusted. Those patients who express hunger but are unable to eat must be fed by tube, either enterally or parenterally, as their condition warrants. Those who are receiving enteral or parenteral nutrition should have their formula changed or the amount of formula increased. A clinical dietitian or nutritional support team should be involved in these decisions.

Patients who are hungry and able to eat but have no appetite may be given oral supplements. Liquid, high-caloric formula may be used, or puddings or milkshakes can be reinforced with calories or protein sources. Food from an outside vendor may provide enough variety to appeal to the patient. Familiar food brought from home may stimulate an appetite.

Other interventions are appropriate for those patients receiving adequate nutritional repletion (in positive or zero nitrogen balance and maintaining or gaining weight) but expressing an appetite. If the patient is placed on NPO status but is allowed *some* intake, hard candies or gum can help to satisfy the oral cravings. Patients who have an appetite for a forbidden item, such as salty or fatty foods, may benefit from varied seasonings and textures of allowable foods. Advertisements would lead one to believe that consuming large amounts of liquids or increasing the bulk in the diet helps to decrease these feelings. This strategy has not been supported by experimental studies, however.

Those patients who express an unsatisfied appetite and are unable to eat anything orally to satisfy it should be protected from situations that may aggravate their appetite. Nurses can discuss the meaning of the sensations: Are the feelings distressing? Are they of some concern? Explore solutions with each patient, involving the members of the nutrition support team if at all possible. A private room, away from the area of food preparation, may afford some respite from the sights, odors, and sounds of food. Perhaps watching television advertisements and reading magazines about food may increase feelings of appetite; however, some persons on dietary restrictions may receive a little satisfaction by collecting recipes, planning meals, and otherwise being involved with food.[120]

Until definitive questionnaires can be developed to assist nurses in determining the degree of hunger as differentiated from appetite, the implications of and interventions for patients expressing hunger are variable. However, patients' expressions of hunger warrant further investigation and this is a fertile field for nursing research.

REVIEW OF RESEARCH FINDINGS

The terms hunger and appetite are used synonymously by most authors in the review of the literature that follows and are used interchangeably to denote eating behavior itself, the size of the meal reflecting the intensity of the feelings.[14] Measurements of hunger ratings in humans have often been equated with appetite, and appetite in turn has been equated with quantity consumed (i.e., meal size). These inferences should, however, be treated with caution.[172] Rowland and Carlton concluded that until the normal mechanisms of hunger and appetite are understood, research into the causes and controls of ingestive behavior will remain elusive.[13]

The effects of the caloric density of infused liquid diets on voluntary food intake have been examined in a number of studies. Investigators using animals as research subjects have noted that the animals will eat more to compensate for a reduction in calories infused either parenterally or enterally.[64, 66–69, 82, 173]

DeSomery and Hansen investigated the effects of parenteral nutrition on the number of calories orally ingested by two monkeys.[174] After recovery from surgery to implant intravenous catheters and gastric strain gauges, baseline determinations of each monkey's usual caloric intake were made, using a complete liquid diet delivered through a feeding machine to which the monkeys had become accustomed. TPN was given at varying levels of the subject's baseline intake while the subjects were allowed access to the liquid oral diet. In the two monkeys, voluntary intake

was reduced in response to the increasing levels of the TPN infusion. The total caloric intake of one monkey was generally above baseline for all levels of infusion, while the other monkey overate only at the lower infusion levels and ceased oral feedings completely when 100 per cent of his baseline intake was being given as TPN. Motility data (reported only on the second monkey) showed that the motility pattern usually associated with hunger was absent at the high levels of TPN infusion. Suppression of oral intake continued after cessation of TPN for nine and 21 days. In another report using the results of this study, the authors hypothesized that hunger might be a danger signal indicating inadequate repletion.[175]

Nicolaides and Rowland studied the effect of various intravenous (IV) nutrients on the oral (PO) intake of regular chow in rats and found a direct correlation between less nutritionally complete infusions and the largest oral intake.[176] They concluded that the residual oral food intake resulted from a specific appetite for a missing element in the diet. They cited the results of Adair and associates, who offered rats the same diet orally that was infused intravenously and found marked hypophagia.[177] Had Nicolaides and Rowland offered the rats a varied oral diet, the rats' intake might have increased. Nicolaides and Even[178] extended the work of Nicolaides and Rowland and devised a system in which rats learned to press a lever for intravenous self-injection of liquid diet when oral food was not available. Intakes were low but regulated and were sufficient to balance energy expenditures, although at a lower body weight. They concluded their report by stating: "Systemic receptors alone are thus adequate to motivate feeding behavior and meter the caloric yield of the intravenous injections" (p. 589).

Some evidence supports the hypothesis that humans also respond to varying levels of caloric intake. Walike and associates studied the effects of disguised oral preloads from a hidden reservoir on subsequent meal intake and subjective ratings of hunger in 17 normal volunteers.[61] All caloric preloads reduced intake of the test meal, and the greater the preload, the greater the depression of intake. The accuracy of the compensation was inconsistent, however, and some subjects overate their baseline at the test meal. Hunger, rated from 0 (not hungry) to 9 (hungriest ever), varied with the caloric value of the preload; the lowest caloric preload produced the greatest hunger rating, which diminished as the caloric value increased, but hunger was never completely eliminated. Again, hunger and appetite were not differentiated, and the subjects may have been indicating an appetite for solid food during the liquid meals, rather than a physiological hunger.

Geliebter administered varying caloric preloads to 12 healthy men after a 13 hour fast.[70] Subjects were asked to indicate their feelings of hunger on a scale from 0 (not at all hungry) to 100 (extreme hunger) and satiety on a similar scale. The amount of a liquid diet taken through a straw from a hidden container was measured 1 hour later. The higher caloric preloads tended to suppress intake more than the noncaloric ones, but there were no differences in hunger ratings before or after the preload or between the caloric and noncaloric preloads. The investigator did not differentiate between hunger and appetite and defined appetite as "the subjective evaluation of hunger and satiety" (p. 271). Subjects gargled with a lidocaine solution for 7 minutes before the preload and wore a noseclip during ingestion to disguise taste and consistency of the preload. It is conceivable that these would adversely affect a subject's feeling of appetite, in that nothing would seem tasty. However, feelings of hunger may not have been as affected as appetite by the dulled sensations of taste and smell. Had the investigator differentiated between hunger and appetite, different conclusions may have been drawn.

In the single study in which the subject's expressions of hunger *and* appetite rather than food intake were the dependent variable, Durrant and Royston reported increased claims of hunger in obese patients when given a disguised low calorie preload compared with a high calorie preload.[179] They gave preloads of either 100 or 300 calories 1 hour before a meal to 18 obese subjects on a metabolic unit. The subjects were asked to indicate the degree of hunger (physiological signals) and appetite (mental signals) they felt immediately after the preload and again 1 hour later. The subjects were unable to estimate the energy content of the preload but were significantly more hungry with the low-calorie preloads than with the high-calorie preloads ($P < .02$). Appetite ratings did not correlate with the energy content of the

preloads. It would have been interesting, if intake of subsequent meals had been measured, to observe whether subjects compensated for the caloric content of the preload and whether the magnitude of intake correlated with hunger ratings. The results of this study are significant because the subjects were able to distinguish between hunger and appetite and because hunger, a physiological signal, *did* vary with the energy load, while appetite, a mental urge, did not.

In the only reported study of hunger in patients receiving TPN, Jordan and colleagues administered a questionnaire to assess hunger and appetite.[3] They observed 18 patients receiving TPN from 10 to 85 days (mean = 31) to assess the degree of hunger felt during therapy and its relationship to the amount of food ingested during the transition to oral feedings. The investigators found that most patients reported hunger during TPN in spite of daily intakes as high as 4800 kcal and that even the hungriest patients had difficulty eating when oral diets were introduced. The authors concluded that the patients' reports of hunger "reflected a need for some oral stimulation, or satisfaction, rather than a need to actually ingest the food" (p. 153).

There are several methodological difficulties in interpreting Jordan and colleagues' data. The questionnaire used to assess hunger and satiety can be criticized on the basis of some items containing more than one condition or feeling but requiring a "yes" or "no" response, making it unclear to which item the answer referred. Also, assessments of hunger were not obtained concurrently with measurements of metabolic state (e.g., blood glucose levels) or correlated with the adequacy of caloric intake. The subjects in this study had diagnoses that included pelvic abscesses with septic enterocutaneous fistulas and inflammatory bowel disease and perhaps had caloric requirements greater than 4800 kcal per day. In their conclusion, the authors in essence doubted the validity of the patients' expression of hunger when they were able to consume only a small amount of food. However, TPN leads to hypoplasia of the stomach and small intestine, with decreased absorptive abilities.[180–183] These anatomical and physiological changes may account for early satiety in spite of feelings of appetite or hunger.

The study is of interest, however, because

TABLE 14–4   SUMMARY OF RESULTS OF PILOT STUDY

Patient Number	Age	Height (cm)	Weight (kg)	BEE (1)	Activity Factor*	Injury Factor†	Calories Required‡	Calories Received§	Score on Hunger VAS‖
1	46	180	77 (75)	1714 (1686)¶	1.3	0	2228 (2192)	2975	22
2	32	193	68 (83	1750 (1956)	1.3	1.2	2730 (3152)	2550	80
3	36	183	70 (76)	1701 (1783)	1.3	0	2210	3060	90
4	53	167	55 (64)	1299 (1423)	1.2	0	1599 (1708)	3150	17
5	28	172	61	1576	1.3	1.2	2458 (2630)	2125	75

*Basal energy expenditure (BEE) calculated from the Harris-Benedict formula (see Table 14–3).
†Adjustments to the BEE for injury and activity as given in Table 14–5.
‡Caloric requirements determined from the BEE with adjustments for activity and injury as given in Table 14–5.
§Number of calories received by the patient in the 24 hours before hunger assessment.
‖Hunger score was measured from the left-hand side of the visual analogue scale (VAS) to the patient's mark in millimeters (see Fig. 14–5).
¶The values given in parentheses are the patient's ideal body weight and calculated BEE and caloric requirements using the *ideal* body weight.

it is the only study of hunger in humans receiving TPN. It points out the magnitude of the problem: 16 of 18 patients reported hunger during therapy. Based only on patients' inability to eat normal amounts when presented with food, the authors considered the patients' complaints psychologically induced and advocated the practice of reassuring patients that there is no need to worry about nutrition. Further research is required before such feelings are dismissed as a natural occurrence with TPN, especially when the adequacy of intake is unknown or undetermined.

Oral deprivation with artificial feeding has been considered a psychological phenomenon. Padilla and associates reported findings from a study of 30 patients receiving nasogastric tube feedings.[4] The three most commonly reported distressing psychosensory experiences were related to oral deprivation: (1) an unsatisfied appetite for food; (2) deprivation of tasting, chewing, or swallowing food or drinking fluids; and (3) deprivation of regular food. Physiological aspects of hunger and appetite were not pursued. According to several other authors, the inability to respond to feelings of hunger or appetite was the major stress in patients receiving home TPN.[5-9] It seems that this limitation would be distressing to the hospitalized patient as well, but no studies have explored this situation.

The following case study helps to illustrate some of the points covered in this chapter. Table 14–4 is a summary of data from a pilot study of the expression of hunger in patients receiving TPN.[184]

CASE STUDY

All of the patients in this sample were adult males who were receiving TPN and who were also on NPO status. The TPN solution consisted of 25 per cent glucose and 4 per cent amino acids with electrolytes, vitamins, and minerals. In addition, two of the patients received a 10 per cent intravenous fat emulsion: Patient No. 1 received 500 ml twice a week, and Patient No. 4 received 500 ml every day. Both patients had received an infusion of fat in the 24-hour period before hunger was assessed. All patients had at least one roommate who was eating a regular diet and all had access to television and magazines. All of these patients were receiving TPN for nonmalignant disease and were afebrile, alert, and cooperative. They were asked to indicate their degree of hunger by placing a mark on the hunger visual analogue scale in the early afternoon between 1 p.m. and 3 p.m.

Patients who had a rating on the hunger VAS of 51 mm or greater were categorized as hungry; the higher their score, the greater their degree of hunger. Those with scores of 50 or lower were categorized as not hungry; the lower the score the lower their degree of hunger. The data in this sample can be examined in several different ways.

Body weight and fat stores. Patients 2, 3, and 5 were all below their ideal body weight and all expressed hunger; Patient 2, who was the most depleted, expressed the most hunger. Patient 4, at 9 kg below his ideal weight, was also depleted but expressed no hunger. Patient 1 was the only subject who weighed more than his ideal body weight, and he also expressed no hunger.

Adequacy of caloric intake. Caloric intake was calculated as a percentage of the estimated calculated requirement. Energy requirements were calculated using the Harris-Benedict equation for basal energy expenditure[185] (see Table 14–3), with adjustments for the patient's disease, injury, and activity according to Long and others[186] (Table 14–5).

This method has had widespread acceptance and use.[187, 188] The results showed that Patients 1 and 4, who were receiving 134 and 184 per cent, respectively, of their calculated requirements reported no hunger, while Patients 2 and 5, who were receiving 84 and 81 per cent, respectively, were hungry. Patient 3 was receiving greater than 100 per cent of his calculated requirements yet reported hunger.

Intravenous fat. Jordan and associates reported that the infusion of fat intravenously seemed to decrease hunger sensations.[3] The two patients in this study, numbers 1 and 4, who received fat infusions prior to hunger assessment also reported no hunger. Because these patients were also receiving greater than 100 per cent of their calculated caloric

requirements, no conclusions can be drawn about the effect of intravenous fat infusions on hunger.

Even though this pilot study produced more questions than answers, it is tempting to form some tentative conclusions: The more depleted the patient's fat stores, the more hunger is expressed. The feeling of hunger can be depressed by the infusion of intravenous fat, regardless of the patient's fat stores. Patients who receive fewer calories than they require will express hunger, while those receiving more calories will not express hunger. Patient 3, however, received more calories than his calculated requirements and yet expressed hunger. He was receiving TPN for inflammatory bowel disease and was in the recovery phase. He was beginning to gain weight, and perhaps his caloric requirements were actually higher than calculated. The results of nitrogen balance determinations would have helped in this evaluation.

IMPLICATIONS FOR FURTHER RESEARCH

The results of the pilot study listed in Table 14–1 suggest additional questions and implications for research. Why did some of the patients report hunger? Why did some of the patients who were receiving no nutrients via the gastrointestinal tract not feel hungry? How does TPN, which bypasses the intestinal lumen, prevent hunger? Does this rule out the importance of mechanical events in the gastrointestinal tract in the control of hunger? It is well known that intravenous infusion of glucose stimulates pancreatic insulin release, but the effect of infused nutrients on gut hormones is inconclusive.[189, 190] Perhaps the stimulation of some gut hormone is responsible for suppressing hunger, yet the most studied gut hormone in relation to hunger and satiety, cholecystokinin, is not stimulated with TPN.[191]

The most depleted patients as determined by comparing actual body weight with the ideal body weight (patients 2, 3, and 5 in Table 14–4) expressed the most hunger. Does the amount of adipose tissue influence hunger? Can the provision of calories in excess of requirements suppress hunger regardless of fat stores? Can hunger be sup-

TABLE 14–5 ACTIVITY AND INJURY FACTOR ADJUSTMENTS TO THE BASAL ENERGY EXPENDITURE (BEE)

Factor	Factor × BEE
Activity	
1. Confined to bed	1.2
2. Out of bed	1.3
Injury	
3. Minor operation	1.2
4. Skeletal trauma	1.35
5. Major sepsis	1.6
6. Severe thermal burns	2.1

From Long, C. L., Schaffel, N., Geiger, J. W., Scheller, W. R., & Blakemore, W. S. (1979). Metabolic response to injury and illness: Estimation of energy and protein needs from indirect calorimetry and nitrogen balance. J Parenter Enter Nutr 3:452–456.

pressed by the infusion of intravenous fat, regardless of the patient's nutritional status?

Hunger as a phenomenon of interest to nurses is just beginning to be addressed. Perhaps the most important questions are what nursing interventions are appropriate for use with patients complaining of hunger? What is the meaning of hunger in patients receiving nutrition by artificial methods? Is the expression of hunger an indication of inadequate caloric repletion? When one is able to respond to individual signals for food ingestion, the distinction between hunger and appetite may be "just a confusion of terms." But when patients are *not* able to respond to their sensations, how others interpret these feelings may be vital. Research studies using patients as subjects are needed to discover simpler and more accurate methods of measuring hunger and distinguishing hunger from appetite. Further studies are also needed to define the meaning of these sensations and to provide guidelines for responding to patients' expressions or complaints of hunger and appetite.

REFERENCES

1. Stein, J., & Su, P. Y. (eds.). (1988). *The Random House Dictionary*. New York: Random House.
2. Winick, M. (ed.). (1979). *Hunger Disease. Studies by the Jewish Physicians in the Warsaw Ghetto*. New York: John Wiley.
3. Jordan, H. A., Hamilton, M., MacFayden, B. V., Jr., & Dudrick, S. J. (1969). Hunger and satiety in humans during parenteral hyperalimentation. Psychosom Med 36:144–155.
4. Padilla, G. V., Grant, M., Wong, H., Hansen, B. W., Hanson, R. L. Bergstrom, N., & Kubo, W. R. (1979). Subjective distresses of nasogastric tube feeding. J Parenter Enter Nutr 3:53–57.
5. MacRitchie, K. H. (1978). Life without eating or drinking. Total parenteral nutrition outside hospital. Can Psychiatr Assoc J 23:373–379.
6. Perl, M., Hall, R. C., Dudrick, S. J., Englert, D. M., Stickney, S. K., & Gardner, E. R. (1980). Psychological aspects of long-term home hyperalimentation. J Parenter Enter Nutr 4:554–560.
7. Perl, M., Peterson, L. G., Dudrick, S. J., & Benson, D. M. (1981). Psychiatric effects of long-term home hyperalimentation. Psychosomatics 22:1047–1063.
8. Price, B. S., & Levine, E. L. (1979). Permanent TPN: Psychological and social responses of the early stages. J Parenter Enter Nutr 3:48–52.
9. Robinovitch, A. E. (1981). Home TPN: A psychosocial viewpoint. J Parenter Enter Nutr 5:522–525.
10. Castonguay, R. W., Applegate, E. A., Upton, D. E., & Stern, J. S. (1984). Hunger and appetite: Old concepts/new distinctions. In *Nutrition Reviews: Present Knowledge in Nutrition* (5th ed.). Washington, D.C.: The Nutrition Foundation.
11. Feldman M., & Richardson C. T. (1986). Role of thought, sight, smell, and taste of food in the cephalic phase of gastric acid secretion in humans. Gastroenterology 90:428–433.
12. Reed, K. (1982). Descriptive aspects of depression. Texas Med 78:55–57.
13. Rowland, N. E., & Carlton, J. (1986). Neurobiology of an anorectic drug: Fenfluramine. Prog Neurobiol 27:13–62.
14. Bolles, R. C. (1980). Historical note on the term "appetite." Appetite 1:3–6.
15. Brobeck, J. R. (1946). Mechanism of the development of obesity in animals with hypothalamic lesions. Physiol Rev 26:541–559.
16. Hetherington, A. W., & Ranson, S. W. (1939). Experimental hypothalamico-hypophyseal obesity in the rat. Proc Soc Exp Biol Med 41:465–466.
17. Hetherington, A. W., & Ranson, S. W. (1940). Hypothalamic lesions and adiposity in the rat. Anat Rec 78:149–152.
18. Brobeck, J. R., Tepperman, J., & Long, C. N. H. (1943). Experimental hypothalamic hyperphagia in the albino rat. Yale J Biol Med 15:831–853.
19. Epstein, A. N. (1960). Reciprocal changes in feeding behavior produced by intrahypothalamic chemical injections. Am J Physiol 199:969–974.
20. Krasne, F. B. (1962). General disruption resulting from electrical stimulus of the ventromedial hypothalamus. Science 138:822–823.
21. Grossman, S. P. (1960). Eating or drinking elicited by direct adrenergic or cholinergic stimulation of the hypothalamus. Science 132:301–302.
22. Anand, B. K., & Brobeck, J. R. (1951). Hypothalamic control of food intake in rats and cats. Yale J Biol Med 24:123–140.
23. Stricker, E. M., Swerdloff, A. F., & Zigmond, M. J. (1978). Kainic acid injections selectively destroy LH neurons. Brain Res 158:470–473.
24. Morley, J. E., & Levine, A. S. (1980). Stress-induced eating is mediated through endogenous opiates. Science 209:1259–1260.
25. Krasne, F. B. (1962). General disruption resulting from electrical stimulus of the ventromedial hypothalamus. Science 138:822–823.
26. Fonberg, E. (1981). Amygdala and emotions. In L. A. Cioffi, W. P. T. James, & T. B. Van Itallie (eds.), *The Body Weight Regulatory System: Normal and Disturbed Mechanisms*. New York: Raven Press.
27. Ziegler, H. P., & Karten, H. J. (1974). Central trigeminal structures and the lateral hypothalamic syndrome in the rat. Science 186:636–638.
28. Grossman, S. P., Dacey, D., Halaris, A. E., Collier, T., & Routtenberg, A. (1978). Aphagia and adipsia after preferential destruction of nerve cell bodies in the hypothalamus. Science 202:537–539.
29. Stricker, E. M., Swerdloff, A. F., & Zigmond, M. J. (1978). Intrahypothalamic injections of kainic acid produce feeding and drinking defects in rats. Brain Res 158:470–473.
30. Park, I. R. A., Himms-Hagen, J., & Coscina, D. V. (1986). Long-term effects of lateral hypothalamic lesions on brown adipose tissue in rats. Brain Res Bull 17:643–651.
31. Wurtman, R. J. (1982). Nutrients that modify brain function. Sci Am 246:50–59.
32. Wurtman, R. J., Larin, S., Mostafapour, S., & Fernstrom, J. D. (1974). Brain catecholamine synthesis: Control by brain tyrosine concentration. Science 185:183–184.
33. Bender, D. A. (1978). Regulation of 5-hydroxytryptamine synthesis. Proc Nutr Soc 37:167–171.

34. Fernstrom, J. D., & Wurtman, R. J. (1974). Nutrition and the brain. Sci Am 230:84–91.

35. Ashley D. V. M., Fleury, M. O., Golay, A., Maeder E., & Leathwood P. D. (1985). Evidence for diminished brain 5-hydroxytryptamine biosynthesis in obese diabetic and non-diabetic humans. Am J Clin Nutr 42:1240–1245.

36. Wolever, T. M., Jenkins, D. J. A., Josse, R. G., Wong, G. S., Lee, R., & Anderson, G. H. (1988). Relationship between fasting serum tryptophan/large neutral amino acid ratio and reported hunger in subjects with diabetes. Diabetes Res 9:131–137.

37. Jeppsson, B., Freund, H. R., Gimmon, Z., James, J. H., von Meyenfeldt, M. F., & Fischer, J. E. (1981). Blood-brain barrier derangement in sepsis: Cause of septic encephalopathy? Am J Surg 141:136–142.

38. Krause, R., James, J. H., Humphrey, C., & Fischer, J. E. (1979). Plasma and brain amino acids in Walker 256 carcinosarcoma-bearing rats. Cancer Res 39:3065–3069.

39. Peters, J. C., & Harper, A. E. (1981). Protein and energy consumption, plasma amino acid ratios, and brain neurotransmitter concentrations. Physiol Behav 27:287–298.

40. Fernstrom, J. D. (1982). Acute effects of tryptophan and single meals on serotonin synthesis in the rat brain. In B. T. Ho (ed.), Serotonin in Biological Psychiatry. New York: Raven Press.

41. Curzon, G. (1978). Influence of nutritional state on transmitter synthesis. Proc Nutr Soc 37:155–157.

42. Stein, E. M., Stein, S., & Linn, M. W. (1985). Geriatric sweet tooth. A problem with tricyclics. J Am Geriatr Soc 33:687–692.

43. Berken, G. H., Weinstein, D. O., & Stern, W. C. (1984). Weight gain. A side effect of tricyclic antidepressants. J Affective Disord 7:133–138.

44. Yeragani, V. K., Pohl, R., Aleem, A., Balon, R., Sherwood, P., & Lycaki, H. (1988). Carbohydrate craving and increased appetite associated with antidepressant therapy. Can J Psychiatry 33:606–610.

45. Fernstrom, M. H., Epstein, L. H., & Spiker, D. G. (1985). Resting metabolic rate is reduced in patients treated with antidepressants. Biol Psychiatry 20:688–692.

46. Leibowitz, S. F. (1980). Neurochemical systems of the hypothalamus in control of feeding and drinking behavior and water-electrolyte excretion. In P. J. Morgane & J. Panskepp (eds.), Handbook of the Hypothalamus. New York: Marcel Dekker.

47. Roberts, G. W., Crow, T. J., & Polak, J. M. (1981). Neuropeptides in the brain. In S. R. Bloom & J. Polak (eds.), Gut Hormones (2nd ed.). New York: Churchill Livingstone.

48. Gibbs, J., Falasco, J. P., & McHugh, P. R. (1976). Cholecystokinin-decreased food intake in Rhesus monkeys. Am J Physiol 230:15–18.

49. Pi-Sunyer, F. X., Kissileff, H. R., Thornton, J., & Smith, G. P. (1981). Cholecystokinin-octapeptide decreases food intake in man. In L. A. Cioffi, W. P. T. James, & T. B. Van Itallie (eds.), The Body Weight Regulatory System: Normal and Disturbed Mechanisms. New York: Raven Press.

50. Della-Fera, M. A., & Baile, C. A. (1980). Cerebral ventricular injections of CCK octapeptide and food intake: The importance of continuous injection. Physiol Behav 24:1133–1138.

51. Moran, T. H., & McHugh, P. R. (1982). Cholecystokinin suppresses food intake by inhibiting gastric emptying. Am J Physiol 242:R491–R497.

52. Muurahainen, N., Kissileff, H. R., Derogatis, A. J., & Pi-Sunyer, F. X. (1988). Effects of cholecystokinin-octapeptide (CCK-8) on food intake and gastric emptying in man. Physiol Behav 44:645–649.

53. Baile, C. A., Keim, D. A., Della-Fera, M. A., & McLaughlin, C. L. (1981). Opiate antagonists and agonists and feeding in sheep. Physiol Behav 25:1019–1023.

54. Trenchard, E., & Silverstone, T. (1983). Naloxone reduces the food intake of normal human volunteers. Appetite 4:43–50.

55. Morley, J. E., & Levine, A. S. (1982). The role of the endogenous opiates as regulators of appetite. Am J Clin Nutr 35:757–761.

56. Melchior, J.-C., Fantino, M., Rozen, R., Igoin, L., Rigaud, D., & Apfelbaum, M. (1989). Effect of a low dose of naltrexone on glucose-induced alliesthesia and hunger in humans. Pharmacol Biochem Behav 32:117–121.

57. Novin, D., & VanderWeele, D. A. (1977). Visceral involvement in feeding: There is more to regulation than the hypothalamus. In J. M. Sprague & A. N. Epstein (eds.), Progress in Psychobiology and Physiological Psychology (Vol. 7). New York: Academic Press.

58. Cannon, W. B., & Washburn, A. L. (1912). An explanation of hunger. Am J Physiol 31:441–454.

59. Wangensteen, O. H., & Carlson, H. A. (1931). Hunger sensations in a patient after total gastrectomy. Proc Soc Exp Biol Med 28:545–547.

60. Epstein, A., & Teitelbaum, P. (1962). Regulation of food intake in the absence of taste, smell and the oropharyngeal sensations. J Comp Physiol Psychol 55:753–759.

61. Walike, B. C., Jordan, H. A., & Stellar, E. (1968). Preloading and the regulation of food intake in man. J Comp Physiol Psychol 68:327–333.

62. Rodin, J. (1980). The externality theory today. In A. J. Stunkard (ed.), Obesity. Philadelphia: W. B. Saunders.

63. Jordan, H. A. (1969). Voluntary intragastric feeding: Oral and gastric contributions to food intake and hunger in man. J Comp Physiol Psychol 68:498–506.

64. McHugh, P. R., & Moran, T. (1979). Calories and gastric emptying: A regulatory capacity with implications for feeding. Am J Physiol 236:R254–R260.

65. Kraly, F. S., & Smith, G. P. (1978). Combined pregastric and gastric stimulation by food is sufficient for normal meal size. Physiol Behav 21:405–408.

66. Hansen, B. C., Jen, K.-L. C., & Brown, N. (1981). Regulation of food intake and body weight in Rhesus monkeys. In L. A. Cioffi, W. P. T. James, & T. B. Van Itallie (eds.), The Body Weight Regulatory System: Normal and Disturbed Mechanisms. New York: Raven Press.

67. Share, I., Martyniuk, E., & Grossman, M. I. (1952). Effect of prolonged intragastric feeding on oral food intake in dogs. Am J Physiol 169:229–235.

68. Koopmans, H. S., & Maggio, C. A. (1978). The effects of specified chemical meals on food intake. Am J Clin Nutr 31:S267–S272.

69. Leibling, D. S., Eisner, J. D., Gibbs, J., & Smith, G.

P. (1975). Intestinal satiety in rats. J Comp Physiol Psychol 89:955–965.

70. Geliebter, A. A. (1979). Effects of equicaloric loads of protein, fat, and carbohydrate on food intake in the rat and man. Physiol Behav 22:267–273.

71. Burks, T. F., & Villar, H. V. (1980). Gastric distention and satiety. In Christensen, J. (ed.), *Gastrointestinal Motility*. New York: Raven Press.

72. Rolls, B. J., Hetherington, M., & Burley, V. J. (1988). The specificity of satiety: The influence of foods of different micronutrient content on the development of satiety. Physiol Behav 43:145–153.

73. Davis, J. D., & Campbell, C. S. (1973). Peripheral control of meal size in the rat: Effect of sham feeding on meal size and drinking rate. J Comp Physiol Psychol 83:379–387.

74. Deutsch, J. A., Young, W. G., & Kalogers, T. J. (1978). The stomach signals satiety. Science 201:165–166.

75. Deutsch, J. A. (1985). The role of the stomach in eating. Am J Clin Nutr 42:1040–1043.

76. Geliebter, A. (1988). Gastric distension and gastric capacity in relation to food intake in humans. Physiol Behav 44:665–668.

77. Anika, S. M., Houpt, T. R., & Houpt, K. A. (1980). Insulin as a satiety hormone. Physiol Behav 25:21–23.

78. Kraly, F. S., & Gibbs, J. (1980). Vagotomy fails to block the satiating effect of food in the stomach. Physiol Behav 44:665–668.

79. Gonzalez, M. F., & Deutsch, J. A. (1981). Vagotomy abolishes cues of satiety produced by gastric distension. Science 212:1283–1284.

80. Deutsch, J. A., & Ahn, S. J. (1986). The splanchnic nerve and food intake regulation. Behav Neural Biol 45:43–47.

81. Yin, T. H., & Tsai, C. T. (1973). Effects of glucose on feeding in relation to routes of entry in rats. J Comp Physiol Psychol 85:258–264.

82. Campbell, C. S., & Davis, J. D. (1974). Licking rate of rats is reduced by intraduodenal and intraportal glucose infusion. Physiol Behav 12:357–365.

83. Welch, I., Sepple, K., & Read, N. W. (1985). Effect of ileal and intravenous infusions of fat emulsions on feeding and satiety in human volunteers. Gastroenterology 89:1293–1297.

84. Epstein, A., & Teitelbaum, P. (1962). Regulation of food intake in the absence of taste, smell and the oropharyngeal sensations. J Comp Physiol Psychol 55:753–759.

85. Moran, T. H., & McHugh, P. R. (1981). Distinctions among three sugars in their effects on gastric emptying and satiety. Am J Physiol 241:R25–R30.

86. Kennedy, C. C. (1953). The role of depot fat in the hypothalamic control of food intake in the rat. Proc R Soc London [Biol] 140:578–592.

87. Brobeck, J. R. (1975). Nature of satiety signals. Am J Clin Nutr 28:806.

88. VanderWeele, D. A., Haraczkiewics, E., & Van Itallie, T. B. (1982). Elevated insulin and satiety in obese and normal-weight rats. Appetite 3:99–109.

89. Woods, S. C., Porte, D., Jr., Bobbioni, E., Ionescu, E., Sauter, J.-F., Rohner-Jeanrenaud, F., & Jeanrenaud, B. J. (1985). Insulin: Its relationship to the central nervous system and to the control of food intake and body weight. Am J Clin Nutr 42:1063–1071.

90. Russek, M., Rodriguez-Zendejas, A. M., & Pina, S. (1968). Hypothetical liver receptors and the anorexia caused by adrenaline and glucose. Physiol Behav 3:249–257.

91. Russek, M. (1981). Current status of the hepatostatic theory of food intake control. Appetite 2:137–143.

92. Friedman, M. I., & Stricker, E. M. (1976). The physiological psychology of hunger: A physiological perspective. Psychol Rev 83:409–431.

93. Bellinger, L. L. (1981). Commentary on "The current status of the hepatostatic theory of food intake control." Appetite 2:144–145.

94. Louis-Sylvestre, J. (1981). Hepatic glucoreceptors do exist but do not control food intake. Appetite 2:146–148.

95. Niijima, A. (1981). Neurophysiological evidence for hepatic glucose-sensitive afferents. Commentary on "The current status of hepatic theory of food intake control." Appetite 2:151–152.

96. Novin, D., Robinson, K., Culbreth, L. A., & Tordoff, M. G. (1985). Is there a role for the liver in the control of food intake? Am J Clin Nutr 42:1059–1062.

97. Schallert, T., Pendergrass, M., & Farrar, S. B. (1982). Cholecystokinin-octapeptide effects on eating elicited by "external" versus "internal" cues in rats. Appetite 3:81–90.

98. Smith, G. P., Jerome, C., Cushin, G. J., Eterno, R., & Simansky, K. J. (1981). Abdominal vagotomy blocks the satiety effects of cholecystokinin in the rat. Science 213:1036–1037.

99. Gibbs, J., Fauser, D. J., Rowe, E. A., Rolls, B. J., Rolls, E. T., & Maddison, S. P. (1979). Bombesin suppresses feeding in rats. Nature 282:209–210.

100. Deutsch, J. A. (1980). Bombesin—satiety or malaise? Nature 285:592.

101. Schanzer, M. D., Jacobson, E. D., & Dafny, N. (1978). Endocrine control of appetite: Gastrointestinal hormonal effects on CNS appetitive structures. Neuroendocrinology 25:329–342.

102. Janowitz, H., & Ivy, A. C. (1949). Role of blood sugar levels in spontaneous and insulin induced hunger in man. J Appl Physiol 1:643–645.

103. Inoue, S., & Bray, G. A. (1981). Ventromedial hypothalamic obesity and autonomic nervous system: An autonomic hypothesis. In L. A. Cioffi, W. P. T. James, & T. B. Van Itallie (eds.), *The Body Weight Regulatory System: Normal and Disturbed Mechanisms*. New York: Raven Press.

104. Cox, J. E., & Powley, R. L. (1981). Intragastric pair feeding fails to prevent VMH obesity or hyperinsulinemia. Am J Physiol 240:E566–E572.

105. Woo, R., Kissileff, H. R., & Pi-Sunyer, F. X. (1979). Is insulin a satiety hormone? Fed Proc 38:547.

106. Hernandez, L., & Hoebel, B. G. (1980). Basic mechanisms of feeding and weight regulation. In A. J. Stunkard (ed.), *Obesity*. Philadelphia: W. B. Saunders.

107. Reverdin, N., Hutton, M. R., Ling, A., Thompson, H. H., Wingate, D. L., Cristofides, N., Adrian, T. E., & Bloom, S. R. (1980). Vagotomy and the motor response to feeding. In J. Christensen (ed.), *Gastrointestinal Motility*. New York: Raven Press.

108. Rodin, J. (1981). Social and environmental determinants of eating behavior. In L. A. Cioffi, W. P. T. James, & T. B. Van Itallie (eds.), *The Body Weight Regulatory System: Normal and Disturbed Mechanisms*. New York: Raven Press.

109. DeCastro, J. M. (1988). A microregulatory analysis of spontaneous fluid intake by humans: Evidence

that the amount of liquid ingested and its timing is mainly governed by feeding. Physiol Behav 43:705–714.

110. DeCastro, J. M., & DeCastro, E. S. (1989). Spontaneous meal patterns of humans: Influence of the presence of other people. Am J Clin Nutr 50:237–247.

111. Psychological Aspects of Feeding Group Report. (1976). In T. Silverstone (ed.), *Dahlem Workshop on Appetite and Food Intake*. Berlin: Abakon Verlagsgesellschaft.

112. Schachter, S., Goldman, R., & Gordon, A. (1968). Effects of fear, food deprivation and obesity on eating. J Pers Soc Psychol 10:91–97.

113. Pliner, P. (1978). Influence of psychological (exogenous) and endogenous factors in the regulation of nutritional uptake. In H. M. Katzen, & R. J. Mahler (eds.), *Advances in Modern Nutrition. Diabetes, Obesity, and Vascular Disease. Metabolic and Molecular Interrelationships* (Vol. 2). Washington, D.C.: Hemisphere Publishing.

114. Stunkard, A. J. (1959). Obesity and the denial of hunger. Psychosom Med 21:281–289.

115. Mayer, J., Monello, L. F., & Seltzer, C. C. (1965). Hunger and satiety sensations in man. Postgrad Med 37:A97–A102.

116. Rodin, J. (1976). The relationship between external responsiveness and the development and maintenance of obesity. In D. Novin, W. Wyrwicka, & G. Bray (eds.), *Hunger: Basic Mechanisms and Clinical Implications*. New York: Raven Press.

117. Rolls, B. J. (1981). Palatability and food preference. In L. A. Cioffi, W. P. T. James, & T. B. Van Itallie (eds.), *The Body Weight Regulatory System: Normal and Disturbed Mechanisms*. New York: Raven Press.

118. Herman, C. P., & Polivy, J. (1975). Anxiety, restraint, and eating behavior. J Abnorm Psychol 84:666–672.

119. Nisbett, R. E. (1972). Hunger, obesity, and the ventromedial hypothalamus. Psychol Rev 79:433–453.

120. Keys, A., Brozek, J., Henschel, A., Mickelsen, O., & Taylor, H. L. (1950). *Biology of Human Starvation*. Minneapolis, MN: University of Minnesota Press.

121. Bromberg, D. J., & Bernstein, I. L. (1989). Cephalic insulin release in anorexic women. Physiol Behav 45:871–874.

122. Lowe, M. R., & Maycock, B. (1988). Restraint, disinhibition, hunger and negative affect eating. Addict Behav 13:369–377.

123. Zung, W. W. K. (1965). A self-rating depression scale. Arch Gen Psychiatry 12:63–70.

124. Beck, A. T., Ward, C. H., Mendelson, M., Mock, J., & Erbaugh, J. (1961). An inventory for measuring depression. Arch Gen Psychiatry 4:561–571.

125. Weissenburger, J., Rush, A. J., Giles, D. E., & Stunkard, A. J. (1986). Weight change in depression. Psychiatry Res 17:275–283.

126. Frost, R. O., Goolkasian, G. A., Ely, R. J., & Blanchard, F. A. (1982). Depression, restraint, and eating behavior. Behav Res Ther 20:113–117.

127. Polivy, J., & Herman, C. P. (1976). Clinical depression and weight change: A complex relation. J Abnorm Psychol 85:338–341.

128. Herman, C. P., & Mack, D. (1975). Restrained and unrestrained eating. J Pers 43:647–660.

129. Paykel, E. S. (1977). Depression and appetite. J Psychosom Res 21:401–405.

130. Stunkard, A. J. (1975). Satiety is a conditioned reflex. Psychosom Med 37:383–387.

131. Booth, D. A. (1977). Satiety and appetite are conditioned reactions. Psychosom Med 39:76–81.

132. Booth, D. A. (1976). Approaches to feeding control. In T. Silverstone (ed.), *Dahlem Workshop on Appetite and Food Intake*. Berlin: Abakon Verlagsgesellschaft.

133. McHugh, P. R., & Moran, T. (1978). Accuracy of the regulation of caloric ingestion in the Rhesus monkey. Am J Physiol 235:R29–R34.

134. Keesey, R. E. (1980). A set-point analysis of the regulation of body weight. In A. J. Stunkard (ed.), *Obesity*. Philadelphia: W. B. Saunders.

135. Keesey, R. E., Boyle, P. C., Kemmitz, J. W., & Mitchel, J. S. (1976). The role of the lateral hypothalamus in determining the body weight set point. In D. J. Novin, W. Wyrwicka, & G. Bray (eds.), *Hunger: Basic Mechanisms and Clinical Implications*. New York: Raven Press.

136. James, W. P. T., Trayhune, P., Davies, H., Crisp, T., & Ravenscroft, C. (1981). Interactions of food intake and energy expenditure: An overview. In L. A. Cioffi, W. P. T. James, & T. B. Van Itallie (eds.), *The Body Weight Regulatory System: Normal and Disturbed Mechanisms*. New York: Raven Press.

137. Landsberg, L., & Young, J. B. (1981). Diet-induced changes in sympathoadrenal activity: Implications for thermogenesis and obesity. Obesity Metabol 1:5–33.

138. Stewart, G. R. (1936). *Ordeal by Hunger*. Boston: Houghton Mifflin.

139. Read, P. P. (1974). *Alive*. London: Churchill Livingstone.

140. Crisp, A. H. (1978). Disturbances of neurotransmitter metabolism in anorexia nervosa. Proc Nutr Soc 37:201–209.

141. Cornell, C. E., Rodin, J., & Weingarten, H. (1989). Stimulus-induced eating when satiated. Physiol Behav 45:695–704.

142. Butterworth, C. E. (1974). The skeleton in the hospital closet. Nutr Today March/April:4–8.

143. Weinsier, R. L., Hunker, E. M., Krumdieck, C. L., & Butterworth, C. E., Jr. (1979). Hospital malnutrition. A prospective evaluation of general medical patients during the course of hospitalization. Am J Clin Nutr 32:418–426.

144. Young, R. C., & Blass, J. P. (1982). Iatrogenic nutritional deficiencies. Annu Rev Nutr 2:201–227.

145. Mayer, J. (1972). The dimensions of human hunger. Sci Am 235:40–49.

146. Bolles, R. C. (1980). Historical note on the term "appetite." Appetite 1:3–6.

147. Grossman, M. I. (1955). Integration of current views on the regulation of hunger and appetite. Ann NY Acad Sci 63:76–91.

148. Janowitz, H., & Grossman, M. I. (1948). Effect of parenteral administration of glucose and protein hydrolysate on food intake in the rat. Am J Physiol 155:28–32.

149. Mayer, J. (1968). *Overweight: Causes, Cost and Control*. Englewood Cliffs, NJ: Prentice Hall.

150. Bruch, H. (1955). Role of the emotions in hunger and satiety. Ann NY Acad Sci 63:68–75.

151. Booth, D. A., Fuller, J., & Lewis, V. (1981). Human control of body weight: Cognitive or physiological? Some energy-related perceptions and misperceptions. In L. A. Cioffi, W. P. T. James, & T. B. Van

Itallie (eds.), *The Body Weight Regulatory System: Normal and Disturbed Mechanisms.* New York: Raven Press.

152. Sclafani, A. (1976). Appetite and hunger in experimental obesity syndromes. In D. J. Novin, W. Wyrwicka, & G. Bray (eds.), *Hunger: Basic Mechanisms and Clinical Implications.* New York: Raven Press.

153. Bruch, H. (1978). *The Golden Cage.* Cambridge, MA: Harvard University Press.

154. Abramson, E., & Wunderlich, R. (1972). Anxiety, fear and eating: A test of the psychosomatic concept of obesity. J Abnorm Psychol 79:317–321.

155. McKenna, R. J. (1972). Some effects of anxiety level and food cues on the eating behavior of obese and normal subjects: A comparison of the Schachterian and psychosomatic conceptions. J Per Soc Psychol 22:311–319.

156. Wooley, O. W., & Wooley, S. C. (1981). Relationship of salivation in humans to deprivation, inhibition and the encephalization of hunger. Appetite 2:370–372.

157. Booth, D. A., Fuller, J., & Lewis, V. (1981). Human control of body weight: Cognitive or physiological? Some energy-related perceptions and misperceptions. In L. A. Cioffi, W. P. T. James, & T. B. Van Itallie (eds.), *The Body Weight Regulatory System: Normal and Disturbed Mechanisms.* New York: Raven Press.

158. Grossman, M. I., & Stein, I. F., Jr. (1948). Vagotomy and the hunger-producing action of insulin in man. J Appl Physiol 1:263–269.

159. Grinker, J., Cohn, C. K., & Hirsch, J. (1971). The effects of intravenous administration of glucose, saline, and mannitol on meal regulation in normal-weight human subjects. Commun Behav Biol 6:203–208.

160. Teghtsoonian, M., Becker, E., & Edelman, B. (1981). A psychophysical analysis of perceived satiety: Its relation to consumatory behavior and degree of overweight. Appetite 2:217–229.

161. Kissileff, H. R. (1981). Getting satiety taped: Comments on Teghtsoonian, Becker & Edelman. Appetite 2:235–236.

162. Rosen, J. C., Hunt, D. A., Sims, E. A. H., & Bogardus, C. (1982). Comparison of carbohydrate-containing and carbohydrate-restricted hypocaloric diets in the treatment of obesity: Effects on appetite and mood. Am J Clin Nutr 36:463–469.

163. Silverstone, T. (1975). Anorectic drugs. In T. Silverstone (ed.), *Obesity: Its Pathogenesis and Management.* Acton, MA: Publishing Sciences Group.

164. Silverstone, T. (1980). Techniques for evaluating antiobesity drugs in man. In P. Bjorntorp, M. Cairella, & A. N. Howard (eds.), *Recent Advances in Obesity Research: III.* London: John Libbey.

165. Stacher, G., Bauer, H., & Steinringer, H. (1979). Cholecystokinin decreases appetite and activation evoked by stimuli arising from the preparation of a meal in man. Physiol Behav 23:325–331.

166. Silverstone, T., & Fincham, J. (1978). Experimental techniques for the measurement of hunger and food intake in man for use in the evaluation of anorectic drugs. In S. Garrattini & R. Samanin (eds.), *Central Mechanisms of Anorectic Drugs.* New York: Raven Press.

167. Robinson, R. G., McHugh, P. R., & Folstein, M. F. (1975). Measurement of appetite disturbances in psychiatric disorders. J Psychiatry 12:59–68.

168. Silverstone, T., & Stunkard, A. J. (1968). The anorectic effect of dexamphetamine sulfate. Br J Pharmacol Chemother 33:513–522.

169. Wilmore, D. W. (1977). Energy requirements for maximum nitrogen retention. In H. L. Greene, M. A. Holliday, & H. N. Munro (eds.), *Symposium on Clinical Nutrition Update, Amino Acids.* Chicago: American Medical Association.

170. Peters, C., & Fischer, J. E. (1980). Studies on calorie to nitrogen ratio for TPN. Surg Gynecol Obstet 151:1–8.

171. Bistrian, B. R. (1981). Assessment of protein energy malnutrition in surgical patients. In G. L. Hill (ed.), *Nutrition and the Surgical Patient.* London: Churchill Livingstone.

172. Smith, G. P., & Gibbs, J. (1979). Postprandial satiety. In J. M. Sprague & A. N. Epstein (eds.), *Progress in Psychobiology and Physiological Psychology* (Vol. 8). New York: Academic Press.

173. Martyn, P. A., Hansen, B. C., & Jen, K.-L. C. (1984). The effects of parenteral nutrition on food intake and gastric motility. Nurs Res 33:336–342.

174. DeSomery, C. H., & Hansen, B. W. (1978). Regulation of appetite during total parenteral nutrition. Nurs Res 27:19–21.

175. Hansen, B. W., DeSomery, C. H., Hagedorn, P. K., & Kalnasy, L. W. (1977). Effects of enteral and parenteral nutrition on appetite in monkeys. J Parenter Enter Nutr 1:83–88.

176. Nicolaides, S., & Rowland, N. (1976). Metering of intravenous vs oral nutrients and regulation of energy balance. Am J Physiol 231:661–668.

177. Adair, E. R., Miller, N. E., & Booth, D. A. (1968). Effects of continuous intravenous infusion of nutritive substances on consumatory behavior in rats. Commun Behav Biol 2(Part A):25–37.

178. Nicolaides, S., & Even, P. (1985). Physiological determinant of hunger, satiation, and satiety. Am J Clin Nutr 42:1083–1092.

179. Durrant, M. L., & Royston, P. (1979). Short-term effects of energy density on salivation, hunger and appetite in obese subjects. Int J Obes 3:335–347.

180. Feldman, E. J., Dowling, R. H., McNaughton, J., & Peters, T. J. (1976). Effects of oral versus intravenous nutrition in intestinal adaptation after small bowel resection in the dog. Gastroenterology 70:712–719.

181. Gliner, M., Kawashima, Y., & Meguid, M. (1987). Effect of TPN on food intake in rats offered a choice of foods. American Society of Parenteral and Enteral Nutrition, 11th Clinical Congress Abstracts, 5S.

182. Greenberg, G. R., Wolman, S. L., Christofides, N. D., Bloom, S. R., & Jeejeebhoy, K. N. (1981). Effect of total parenteral nutrition on gut hormone release in humans. Gastroenterology 80:988–993.

183. Levine, G. M., Mullin, J. L., & O'Neill, F. (1980). Effect of TPN on gastric acid secretion. Dig Dis Sci 25:284–288.

184. Williams, K. R. (1988). Unpublished data.

185. Harris, J. A., & Benedict, F. G. (1991). *A Biometric Study of Basal Metabolism in Man* (Pub. No. 279). Washington, D.C.: Carnegie Institute of Washington.

186. Long, C. L., Schaffel, N., Geiger, J. W., Scheller, W. R., & Blakemore, W. S. (1979). Metabolic response to injury and illness: Estimation of energy and protein needs from indirect calorimetry and

nitrogen balance. J Parenter Enter Nutr 3:452–456.

187. Leff, M. L., Hill, J. O., Yates, A. A., Cotsonis, G. A., & Heymsfield, S. B. (1987). Resting metabolic rate: Measurement reliability. J Parenter Enter Nutr 11:354–359.

188. Rainey-MacDonald, C. G., Holliday, R. L., & Wells, F. A. (1982). Nomograms for predicting resting energy expenditure of hospitalized patients. J Parenter Enter Nutr 6:59–60.

189. Cornell, C. E., Rodin, J., & Weingarten, H. (1979). Effects of various diets on colonic growth in rats. Gastroenterology 77:658–663.

190. Read, N. W., McFarlane, A., Kinsman, R. I., & Bloom, S. R. (1984). Effect of infusion of nutrient solutions into the ileum on gastrointestinal transit and plasma levels of neurotensin and enteroglucagon. Gastroenterology 86:274–280.

191. Hughes, C. A., Bates, T., & Dowling, H. (1978). Cholecystokinin and secretin prevent the intestinal mucosal hypoplasia of total parenteral nutrition in the dog. Gastroenterology 75:34–41.

15

Nausea, Vomiting, and Retching

Patricia Larson
Pat Halliburton
Janet Di Julio

DEFINITION

The nausea, vomiting, and retching experience consists of the subjective sensations of throat tightness and abdominal queasiness or heaviness that gradually or suddenly end in emesis.[1] Clinically, these sensations are often approached as one phenomenon. However, as Rhodes notes, this leads to confusion and inadequate understanding, measurement, and management in practice and research.[2] In this chapter, both the specific aspects and the interrelationship of the three phenomena are presented to aid in the understanding and management of these challenging patient experiences.

The literature presents varied definitions of nausea. Rhodes indicates that it is a subjective, nonobservable phenomenon of an unpleasant sensation experienced in the back of the throat and epigastrium that may or may not culminate in vomiting.[2] Borison states that nausea is the subjective recognition of the desire to vomit, manifested as an unpleasant wave-like sensation in the epigastric area, at the back of the throat, or throughout the abdomen.[3] Nausea is defined as a subjective individual experience, not observable by another, wherein the individual perceives visceral discomfort and an unpleasant sensation in the back of the throat.

A commonly accepted definition of vomiting is that it is the forceful expulsion, through the mouth, of the contents of the stomach, duodenum, or jejunum. The force is created by the squeezing of abdominal contents between the muscles of the diaphragm and abdomen.[4] With vomiting, the person often assumes the posture of head down and shoulders hunched forward. There is a momentary cessation of respiration, which is quickly followed by the forceful ejection of emesis.[5] Vomiting is defined as the expulsion of the contents (emesis) of the stomach, duodenum, or jejunum through the mouth. It may or may not be preceded by or followed by nausea or retching. In illness, it is important to note the amount, content (e.g., undigested food or blood), and pattern of the vomiting episodes.

Retching has been defined as a rhythmic activity that precedes vomiting.[4, 6] However, it is also perceived as occurring after vomiting, when the stomach contents have been emptied, and not ceasing until the source of the stimulation has been removed.[7] Rhodes defines it as the attempt to vomit and uses the common lay terms of "dry heaves" or "not being able to bring anything up" to convey the sensation it creates.[2] In this chapter, retching is defined as the rhythmic activity of the muscles of vomiting without production of emesis. From clinical experience, it is known that retching can occur prior to or after vomiting. In this chapter, retching is incorporated in the discussion of vomiting, since there is a lack of agreement on the time sequence of retching and because in the research literature discussion of retching is frequently subsumed under the vomiting act.

Terms that are commonly associated with nausea, vomiting, and retching include regurgitation, gagging, and "spitting up." Regurgitation is the return of solids or food to the mouth from the stomach. There is no nausea or abdominal, diaphragmatic muscular contraction and no ejection of emesis through the mouth.[5, 6] However, Norris perceives regurgitation as a vomiting episode and reports it as such.[6] Others equate retching with the sensation of gagging. However, gagging is usually limited to a sensation in the back of the throat, predominantly associated with inability to handle saliva. On occasion this may lead to nausea and vomiting. Spitting up is usually associated with infants, and as Norris[6] points out, may represent overfeeding or overstimulation and may not truly be representative of vomiting.

PREVALENCE AND POPULATIONS AT RISK

Nausea, vomiting, and retching are associated with a variety of medical conditions and typical life events. Overindulgence of food and drink, excitement, fear, pain, dizziness, or motion sickness can suddenly induce nausea, retching, and vomiting. The actual incidence of these events is not known. If the events are not problematic enough for the individual to bring them to the attention of others, they may be viewed as only passing unpleasantness. It is when they become so bothersome that the individual must miss work or seek medical attention that they are truly viewed as problematic. Other than the common cold, nausea and vomiting cause more employee absenteeism than any other single factor.[8] Nausea, along with pain and fatigue, has been identified as causing the most human suffering, affecting persons with both acute and chronic conditions as well as the terminally ill.[9]

In studies focusing on "morning sickness" of the first trimester of pregnancy, nausea was estimated to affect 80 per cent of women, with over 50 per cent also experiencing vomiting.[10–15] Hyperemesis gravidarum, a more severe, persistent vomiting of early pregnancy, affects approximately 1 in 1000 women.[16]

Patients experiencing myocardial infarction or gastrointestinal system disease are at high risk for nausea and vomiting. It has been found that 47 to 50 per cent of patients with a diagnosis of myocardial infarction ex-

perienced nausea or vomiting at the onset of their cardiac episode.[17, 18] The incidence of nausea and vomiting associated with intra-abdominal disorders is so high that it defies meaningful tabulation and categorization.[19] Gastrointestinal disorders that cause local distention may initiate episodes of vomiting because of the afferent impulses sent to the vomiting center.

A third population at risk are surgical patients. The postoperative incidence of nausea and vomiting has been reported as 27 to 80 per cent in patients receiving anesthesia.[20] Factors associated with postoperative nausea and vomiting include anesthetic techniques and agents, narcotics, type of surgical procedures, and pain.[21] The characteristics that predispose patients to postoperative nausea and vomiting include age (younger patients have increased risk), gender (females have increased incidence), obesity, and general predisposition to nausea and vomiting.[21]

The prevalence and severity of nausea and vomiting associated with cancer chemotherapy have resulted in the most extensive work on nausea and vomiting. The magnitude of this problem is linked to the incidence of cancer and the number of cancer patients who receive chemotherapy. Annually, there are approximately 1 million new cancer cases, and of these, 400,000 will receive some form of chemotherapy.[22] The incidence of nausea and vomiting associated with chemotherapy is affected by the type of chemotherapy and the type of antiemetic and consistency with which it is administered.

The actual incidence of nausea and vomiting from chemotherapy is difficult to ascertain because there is no required or common reporting mechanism. Experientially, patient and care provider often tell of the challenges of nausea and vomiting control. In a study of 1733 chemotherapy patients, Morrow reported a 50 per cent incidence of nausea with consistent antiemetic therapy and a 70 per cent incidence when antiemetics were inconsistently prescribed.[23] Other studies have reported a similar incidence in patients undergoing chemotherapy.[24–26] In a study that examined both nausea and vomiting episodes, 29 per cent of 309 outpatients experienced nausea and vomiting after chemotherapy. Of these, 34 per cent experienced nausea, 19 per cent experienced nausea distress, 17 per cent experienced bouts of vomiting, and 5 per cent had latent vomiting distress, a low amount of vomiting distress for 36 hours after chemotherapy and increasing abruptly at 48 hours.[27] Anticipatory nausea and vomiting, in which the person receiving chemotherapy experiences nausea or vomiting prior to actually receiving the chemotherapy, has been reported to range from 33 per cent (n = 121) to 65 per cent (n = 34) to 42 per cent (n = 149).[28-30] These studies indicate that the variation in incidence of nausea and vomiting may have been affected by differences in cancer type, disease status, chemotherapy agents, and antiemetic protocols. How nausea and vomiting were defined and assessed may also have influenced how the study results were interpreted.

Nausea and vomiting have been cited as one set of symptoms that established symptom management as a priority for the National Institutes of Health National Center for Nursing Research.[31] The importance of these phenomena for nursing care is further verified by the number of chapters in nursing texts and journals that focus on nausea and vomiting.[5, 27, 32-40]

SITUATIONAL STRESSORS

Clinical States

Nausea and vomiting can be induced by a variety of clinical states. Organic, systemic, and gastrointestinal disorders can produce an acute isolated nausea and vomiting episode or chronic nausea and vomiting.[3, 41-45] Clinical states that initiate nausea or vomiting range from pregnancy to infections.

Emesis gravidarum, commonly referred to as morning sickness, is an uncomfortable experience of nausea and vomiting for many women during their first trimester of pregnancy. It generally occurs upon rising or when the stomach is empty. For most women, morning sickness is self-limiting and ends when the woman enters her second trimester. Interestingly, morning sickness of the first trimester is associated with decreased risk of spontaneous abortion during the first 20 weeks of gestation and with increased birth weight.[46, 47] In a study of women in their first trimester of pregnancy (n = 825), those at lowest risk for experiencing morning sickness included women older than 35 years with a history of infertility and women without a history of morning sickness in other pregnancies.[46]

In contrast, the disorder hyperemesis gravidarum, in which there is almost continuous episodes of vomiting throughout much of the pregnancy, often has a negative impact on the outcome of pregnancy. This is especially true when this type of nausea and vomiting is accompanied by maternal weight loss and electrolyte disturbance. Further, fetal growth retardation and anomalies have been reported.[47]

Nausea and vomiting are common side effects of the postoperative period. This was documented early in the anesthesia literature and persists even today for many surgical patients.[48-51] The most frequently identified causes are anesthesia and anesthesia techniques.[52, 53] Other factors associated with postoperative nausea and vomiting are a previous history of postoperative emesis and the type of surgical procedure. Especially problematic are surgical procedures that involve middle ear manipulation, gastrointestinal trauma, peritoneal irritation, or increased gastric pressure from swallowed blood or secretions.[54]

Infectious processes associated with nausea and vomiting episodes include fever, which is particularly common among infants and small children.[55] Inflammatory conditions of the gastrointestinal tract, such as cirrhosis and acute and chronic pancreatitis, are frequently accompanied by nausea and vomiting.

Iatrogenic causes of nausea and vomiting are often associated with pharmacological agents.[56] For example, nausea is one of the first signs of cardiac glycoside toxicity. As noted, anesthetic agents often initiate nausea and vomiting in the postoperative period. Among the most notable iatrogenic causes of nausea and vomiting is the emetic-potentiating chemotherapy used in the treatment of cancer. How chemotherapy agents cause nausea and vomiting is not well understood. It appears that each class of antineoplastics may initiate nausea and vomiting by stimulating different body systems, for example, the vomiting center, which is known to be instrumental in inducing vomiting (see Mechanisms).[57] *Acute* nausea and vomiting occur within a few minutes to several hours after chemotherapy, whereas *delayed* nausea and vomiting can occur as late as 24 to 48 hours after completion of treatment. *Anticipatory* nausea and vomiting is the presence of nausea and vomiting prior to chemotherapy.[58, 59] The anticipatory symptoms do not usually occur until the third or fourth chemotherapy treatment and are quite resistant to standard antiemetic therapy.[60, 61]

Medical States

A number of disease states often present with varying degrees of nausea and vomiting. Of note are the nausea and vomiting associated with myocardial infarction. The autonomic vagal ganglions act as receptors to changes in myocardial ischemia or infarction. These changes are then relayed to the reticular formation, where the vomiting center is located, and produce the sympathetic manifestations of diaphoresis, increased salivation, the urge to defecate, and nausea and vomiting.[62] Myocardial infarction of the inferior wall is hypothesized to initiate vomiting because of the local irritation of the diaphragm.[63] Disorders of the labyrinth apparatus, such as Ménière's disease, frequently produce symptoms of nausea and vomiting. Cerebral conditions that commonly have nausea and vomiting as a part of their symptomatology include medulloblastomas, migraine headaches, and increased intracranial pressure.[64] Vomiting associated with central nervous system disorders is often projectile without any nausea sensations.[65] Central neurological lesions of the vestibular nuclei, especially those that impinge on the floor of the fourth ventricle, for example, medulloblastomas or ependymomas, also produce episodes of nausea and vomiting.[66]

In addition to patients receiving chemotherapy, other cancer populations at risk for nausea and vomiting include patients with malignant involvement of the gastrointestinal tract or with metastatic disease to the cerebrum. Metabolic abnormalities due to either the malignancy or the therapy will also increase the likelihood of nausea and vomiting, as will irradiation of the gastrointestinal tract.

DEVELOPMENTAL DIMENSIONS

There are no studies of the natural history of nausea and vomiting through the developmental stages. Norris proposed a developmental typology of the emotional origin of nausea and vomiting.[6] Her typology starts with the "spitting up" of infancy, which she believes may not be a true developmental aspect of nausea and vomiting but rather a matter of an overfed infant who may have been additionally overstimulated. On the other hand, she notes that the "spitting up" of infancy may be the precursor of vomiting, indicating that there may be a neural developmental aspect associated with the formation of the vomiting center (see Mechanisms). Emotionally, the child may learn to use vomiting to control feelings of helplessness, perhaps vomiting to gain attention, or refusing to vomit to demonstrate ability to control one's actions. Often the child receives approval for not vomiting. By the time adolescence occurs, very few children choose to vomit in the presence of others. Nausea with vomiting becomes for most adults a very private experience; therefore, when it occurs in front of others, it usually causes embarrassment. In contrast, some adults may use vomiting as a means to control, manipulate, and get attention.[6]

In illness, younger patients are more likely to experience nausea and vomiting than are older patients.[66, 67] This is particularly true in chemotherapy-related nausea and vomiting, in which younger patients report a higher incidence of nausea and vomiting than older patients.[68–72] Other research indicates that age is also a factor. Studies showed that subjects 55 years and younger experienced more nausea and vomiting than older individuals,[70, 71] while another study revealed less vomiting for those younger than 65 years.[72] It is not known whether the influence of age is related to physiological mechanisms, whether the younger patient experiences more emotional distress from the symptoms, or, conversely, whether the normal process of aging produces more tolerance to the adverse phenomenon.

MECHANISMS

Physiological Mechanisms

The mechanism of nausea, vomiting, and retching is complex and highly dependent on the evoking stimulus. Some physiologists describe the triad of symptoms in evolutionary terms, implying that they are protective mechanisms to guard against the danger of ingested toxins.[73, 74] This is particularly true of vomiting and less so of nausea and retching. Norris describes the phenomenon of nausea and vomiting as an adjustment and adaptive response dependent on the nature of the cause.[6]

Vomiting and retching occur when the vomiting center, located in the dorsolateral reticular formation of the medulla, has been sufficiently stimulated.[75] Afferent pathways carry the impulse from the gastrointestinal tract via the vagal and sympathetic nerves; the cerebral cortex; vestibulocerebellar afferents; the limbic system; or the chemoreceptor trigger zone.[76] The vomiting center was originally thought to be a discrete center that controlled the vomiting act.[77, 78] However, it now appears more likely that it is an area of effector cell nuclei that serves separate output functions of the vomiting act.[76]

The chemoreceptor trigger zone is a specialized chemosensitive organ that, as a result of its location on the surface of the brain, is exposed to both blood and cerebral spinal fluid. It is hypothesized that the chemoreceptor trigger zone performs a sensory role in identifying agents that are harmful to the organism.[75, 76] How the actual communication occurs between the chemoreceptor trigger zone and the vomiting center is not fully understood; however, several endogenous neurotransmitters have been implicated in the communications between neurons. The neurotransmitters or neuromodulators that have been identified in the nucleus tractus solitarius of the area postrema are the biogenic amines (dopamine, norepinephrine, serotonin, histamine) and neuropeptides (endorphins, enkephalins, substance P, vasopressin, neurotensin, somatostatin, gastrin, vasoactive intestinal peptides, cholecystokinin).[3, 79]

Stimulation of the vomit center and initiation of retching and vomiting are relayed by impulses from the afferent pathways through phrenic nerves to the diaphragm and to the abdominal muscles and viscera via the spinal neurons. In contrast to vomiting and retching, the mechanism of nausea is not known.[80] It is associated with decreased functional activity of the duodenum and small intestine and, when present, precedes retching and vomiting. Just as retching and vomiting can occur in isolation, so too can nausea.[6] Although nausea is a subjective experience, it may be accompanied by the vasomotor phenomena pallor, increased salivation, increased perspiration, and feelings of hot and cold.[3, 71, 79, 81, 82] Figure 15–1 represents the mechanisms of nausea, vomiting, and retching.

Initiation of the vomiting act results first in several protective events to decrease the risk of aspiration. These include taking a deep breath, raising the hyoid bone, closing the glottis, and lifting the soft palate to close the nares. These protective events are followed by a strong downward contraction of the diaphragm and a simultaneous contraction of the abdominal muscles. Intragastric pressure is raised owing to the squeezing of the stomach between two sets of muscles. The gastric esophageal sphincter relaxes, allowing expulsion of gastric content upward through the esophagus.[81] Once the vomiting act has begun, it is an all-or-nothing event. Repeated episodes will continue with the same force and pattern despite the fact that stomach contents have diminished until the evoking stimulus has been removed.[7, 83]

Drug studies have provided the most information about the causative mechanisms of nausea, vomiting, and retching. Of the categories of drugs studied, the antineoplastics have received the most attention. Therefore, these drugs will be used to further elucidate the hypothesized mechanisms of nausea, vomiting, and retching.

The antineoplastic drugs that have the highest emetic potential primarily inhibit ribonucleic acid (RNA) and protein synthesis. These drugs are also associated with the most rapid onset of vomiting; however, this can range from 1 to 12 hours after administration. If the sensing of the drug by the chemoreceptor trigger zone is the only mechanism to induce vomiting, the occurrence should be almost immediate, since peak serum levels are reached within minutes of intravenous administration. This delay suggests that there may be secondary mechanisms for drug-induced vomiting. Currently, there is only speculation on what these mechanisms might be. One possible explanation is that the cytotoxic drug interferes with the synthesis of a key enzyme in the emetic pathway. Inhibition of the enzyme would allow accumulation of a neurotransmitter that at sufficient levels would stimulate the emetic response. Enkephalins are the transmitters most often mentioned as the likely cause of chemotherapy-induced nausea and vomiting.[81, 84]

The role of serotonin (5-hydroxytrypta-

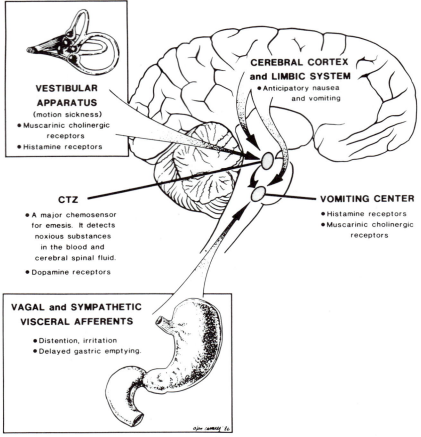

Figure 15–1. Mechanisms of nausea, vomiting, and retching. (Adapted from Goodman, M. [1987]. Management of nausea and vomiting induced by outpatient cisplatin (Platend) therapy. Semin Oncol *3*([Suppl. 1]:25.)

mine) in chemotherapy-induced nausea and vomiting has been investigated. Serotonin receptors (5-hydroxytryptamine M-receptors) are present in both the area postrema and the gastrointestinal tract. More than 90 per cent of the total body serotonin can be found within the enterochromaffin cells of the gastrointestinal mucosa.[81] Chemotherapy and radiation therapy are both thought to cause cell damage, degeneration, and necrosis in the gastrointestinal tract. Serotonin is released from the enterochromaffin cells and activates the S3 receptors on the visceral afferent fibers. This afferent input via the vagal and greater splanchnic nerve fibers is thought to converge on the area postrema and the vomiting center.[85] Clinical trials with serotonin antagonists have shown increased efficacy in controlling the severe nausea and vomiting usually associated with cisplatin.[85–87]

When the associated events related to nausea and vomiting are perceived as particularly aversive, the vomiting center may be activated via the afferent pathways from the cerebral cortex. This stimulation by previously neutral stimuli in the environment, such as sights, sounds, or smells, results in anticipatory nausea and vomiting, a form of classical conditioning.

The nausea, vomiting, and retching of chemotherapy can have two distinct patterns. These patterns are anticipatory[88–91] and post-chemotherapy.[67, 92, 93] Within the postchemotherapy pattern, the response may be acute, occurring 1 to 2 hours after chemotherapy and controlled within 24 hours. Delayed or persistent symptoms occur later in the course of therapy and may be caused by a variety of factors. For example, nausea and vomiting related to cyclophosphamide administration occur 6 to 12 hours after administration and are thought to be due to hepatic metabolism of the drug, with the resulting metabolites responsible for the nausea and vomiting.[94, 95] A second explanation is that once activated by serotonin, the afferent neurons remain activated for a long period of time. A third possibility is that a high rate of serotonin synthesis is maintained, which would stimulate vomiting over several hours.[86]

Inventory of Causes

Inquiry into the causes of nausea, vomiting, and retching reveals a multitude of complex and diverse mechanisms. Many of the causes can be subsumed under the heading of disease state, gastric irritants, internal toxins, pressure states, and psychological states. Figure 15–2 is a survey of the causes.

The actual mechanisms that initiate vomiting are still largely speculative. For example, it is hypothesized that myocardial infarction of the inferior wall initiates vomiting because of local irritation.[6] In contrast, drugs, particularly chemotherapeutic agents, may exert their effect directly on the chemoreceptor trigger zone, or they may cause the release of chemical mediators such as serotonin, which initiate the vomiting act.[96] Gastrointestinal disorders that cause local distention may initiate episodes of vomiting because of the afferent impulses that are sent to the vomiting center. It has been found that distention of the pyloric pouch with pressures of 30 to 35 m/mg always results in vomiting, regardless of the substance causing the distention.[81] In cholecystitis when there is distention of the gallbladder ducts, the nausea and vomiting experience is worse than when only the gallbladder is involved.[66]

RELATED PATHOPHYSIOLOGICAL CONCEPTS

Nausea and vomiting are not isolated phenomena. For example, patients receiving chemotherapy often experience alopecia, fatigue, mucositis, anorexia, weight change, and toxicities that adversely affect the liver, lungs, and kidneys. In the process of destroy-

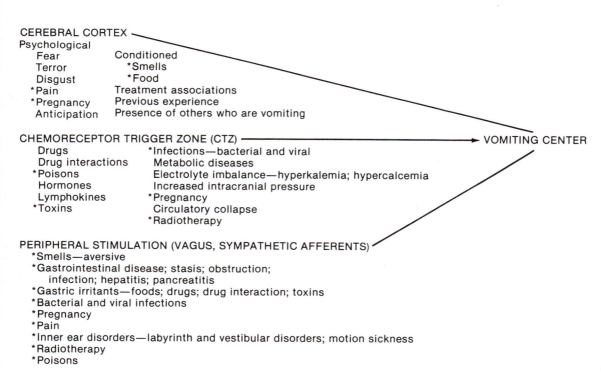

Figure 15–2. Inventory of causes of nausea and vomiting and pathways for stimulation of the vomiting center.

ing the cancer cells, chemotherapy also affects normal-functioning cells. The cells that are primarily adversely affected are the rapidly proliferating cells, such as mucous membranes, hemopoietic cells, and hair follicles.[97] Although patients may experience one or more of these manifestations while undergoing chemotherapy, there does not seem to be a definitive physiological interrelationship among them; that is, nausea and vomiting have not been proved to be directly related to the onset of any of these other phenomena, nor does the treatment of one directly alter any other.

Although the nausea and vomiting associated with the administration of chemotherapy is problematic, patients often find the management of anticipatory and delayed symptoms of nausea and vomiting additionally taxing. It has been estimated that two thirds of patients receiving cisplatin, a highly emetogenic agent, experience after three to four courses what is called anticipatory nausea and vomiting.[98] This is believed to be a conditioned response in which a particular smell, sight, or image associated with chemotherapy may suddenly cause nausea or spontaneous vomiting. Premedication with antiemetics 24 hours prior to treatment is often tried in an attempt to prevent the problem. However, the majority of patients who experience anticipatory emesis have also experienced poor control with antiemetics during the treatment period as well.[99]

Delayed-onset nausea and vomiting usually occur after three to four treatment-associated nausea and vomiting experiences that were ineffectively or marginally controlled by antiemetics. Delayed nausea and vomiting usually start about 24 hours after chemotherapy, when essentially there should be no residual systemic effect of the chemotherapeutic agents.[100] Management centers on aggressive standard antiemetic regimens during administration of chemotherapy followed by a single antiemetic for another 6 to 7 days. The nurse who has an ongoing interaction with the patient receiving chemotherapy must assist the physician in determining the most effective antiemetic regimen for each patient. Studies have found that antiemetics are both underprescribed by physicians and underused by patients.[101]

Research on the experience of chemotherapy treatment does indicate that there are other physiological parameters with a relationship to nausea and vomiting. These include age, extent of disease, susceptibility to motion sickness, fatigue, and patterns of sleep and food intake[71, 101-105] (see Indications for Further Research).

Other consequences also occur as a result of nausea and vomiting. For example, persons who experience nausea and vomiting frequently reduce the intake of food and fluids, putting them at risk for dehydration and possible starvation. If there is inadequate fluid intake by the cancer patient receiving renal toxic agents (e.g., cisplatin), irreversible kidney damage may occur.[106] The cancer patient receiving cyclophosphamide and ifosfamide is also at risk from inadequate fluid intake. Hemorrhagic cystitis will occur if fluid intake is not sufficient to maintain high urine flow.[107]

Consequences of prolonged nausea and vomiting can result in several pathophysiological states, including hypovolemia, hypokalemia, alteration in acid-base balance, and starvation.[83] As hydrogen is excreted into gastric juice and lost during vomiting, there is a shift of bicarbonate ions into the plasma. To maintain the electric neutrality of the blood, chloride is excreted into the gastric juice. Concentration of bicarbonate in the plasma is maintained by the loss of both chloride and sodium in the emesis. Furthermore, an inverse relation exists between the concentration of hydrogen ion and sodium in the emesis. As plasma bicarbonate rises, the body compensates by increasing the rate of renal excretion of bicarbonate and reducing the rate and depth of respirations to maintain the acid-base ratio. The blood pH may remain normal while the urine becomes alkaline because of bicarbonate excretion. With continued vomiting, the plasma and extracellular potassium is decreased as a result of the increased quantities of potassium excreted in the urine in exchange for sodium because the hydrogen ions have been depleted by the vomiting. Adrenal cortical stimulation intensifies the potassium loss and potentiates absorption of bicarbonate in the renal tubules. Extracellular and intracellular potassium concentration is reduced, and sodium cations shift into the cell. In order to conserve sodium, an acid urine is formed despite generalized alkalosis in the system. This sets up a vicious circle that intensifies the alkalosis. The fluid loss results in a reduction of circulating blood volume, and if vomiting is prolonged, cellular breakdown will occur as a consequence of starvation.[83]

When vomiting is sustained over a long period of time, there is risk of weight loss and severe malnutrition. As noted with women who experience hyperemesis gravidarum, there is an additional risk to the fetus. A rare but serious complication of retching is Mallory-Weiss tear syndrome, a tear of the esophagus.[108] Abnormalities of fluid and electrolyte balance may result, and hospitalization may be necessary for correction.

When nausea and vomiting are severe, patients may be forced to reduce or to discontinue drugs essential to treating their underlying disease state. For example, patients receiving chemotherapy who experience uncontrolled nausea and vomiting must often have their chemotherapy dose reduced by half or they may skip a dose that originally was viewed as being vital to their treatment protocol. To what extent this affects the opportunity for cure or prolonged remission of the disease has not been determined, but any reduction in chemotherapy is not advantageous. Antiemetics, while effective in controlling nausea and vomiting, also produce sedative side effects that may interfere with the patients' ability to function normally.

ASSOCIATED PSYCHOSOCIAL CONCEPTS

Nausea and vomiting are often associated with psychosocial-related issues. First, most people do not like to share their experiences of nausea and vomiting. Because of personal style, cultural influences, or the etiquette of aesthetics, people have a tendency to "hide" when they are experiencing nausea and vomiting. Thus, preferentially and socially, most people view the experience of nausea and vomiting as a very private experience. Second, society often views nausea and vomiting as the result of "emotions." For example, the nausea and vomiting of the first trimester of pregnancy and the nausea and vomiting that occur at the time of a sudden emotional or physical crisis are often ascribed to the emotional state of the person. This may be because not everyone experiencing these events also experiences nausea and vomiting. This is also true with the nausea and vomiting associated with chemotherapy. Not all cancer patients experience nausea and vomiting

from their chemotherapy, and for those who do, it is often not with the same intensity and/or severity. Why such diverse responses exist is not known.

Other psychological dimensions that decrease in intensity when the patient's nausea is held in check include anger and depression.[109] Expectation of treatment side effects and psychosocial adjustment have also been investigated in studies of nausea and vomiting. Patients who anticipated that chemotherapy would make them nauseated were more likely to have post-treatment nausea at greater intensity and for longer periods of time.[103, 104]

The interaction between many of these related concepts is of great interest to both clinicians and theorists. Norris[6] and Jacox[110] have noted that there is a tendency for one phenomenon to influence the other, and when one is reduced, it is hypothesized that the other will likewise be tempered. Because of these occurrences, it is often necessary to assess and manage several events in order to control one particular dimension. More research is needed on the interrelatedness of both physical and psychosocial concepts associated with nausea, vomiting, and retching.

MANIFESTATIONS

The manifestations of these phenomena are both subjective and objective. Manifestations of vomiting and retching are objective; either the person experiencing these phenomena or someone observing the person can report the occurrence. With vomiting, the type and amount of emesis produced is observable and measurable. Nausea, in contrast, is a subjective experience. The impact of the nausea may, however, produce objective manifestations. For example, dehydration and alterations in nutrition may be manifestations of severe or prolonged nausea if the person cannot eat or drink. Observable acute manifestations include pallor, cold sweats, increased salivation, swallowing, tachycardia, gastric relaxation, diarrhea, posturing, and abdominal muscle contraction.[43] Although nausea and vomiting are usually associated with each other, they can occur independently. Independent vomiting, for example, is associated with increased intracranial pressure. Vomiting is sudden and projectile with no preceding nausea.[74, 111, 112] Anticipatory vomiting related to chemotherapy is a second example.[101] The person experiences no nausea but suddenly vomits when confronted with a sensation or experience associated with chemotherapy.

SURVEILLANCE AND MEASUREMENT

Guidelines for management of nausea and vomiting include an assessment of nutritional parameters, nausea and vomiting status (including history), current and recent treatment, and antiemetic efficacy.[113] Specifically, the assessment of nausea and the review of the vomiting history need to include the risk for anticipatory nausea, relationship between nausea and vomiting, etiology, frequency, duration, and pattern. Measures used to successfully or unsuccessfully relieve the discomfort of nausea and vomiting also need to be assessed. Morrow indicates that it is especially important to determine whether a patient faces increased risk for anticipatory nausea and vomiting related to chemotherapy.[114] Risk factors include age younger than 50 years, susceptibility to motion sickness, and greater than "moderate" nausea and vomiting, warm or hot sensations, sweating, or weakness after the first chemotherapy treatment. This information can help identify patients who are likely to experience difficult emetic control.

Because of the differential aspects of nausea and vomiting, the clinician has to evaluate their frequency, duration, and intensity separately.[22] Other schemata for assessment of nausea and vomiting include decision trees,[115] nursing diagnoses,[116] and a chemotherapy diary.[117] Such assessment techniques help

both patient and clinician to monitor nausea and vomiting patterns, effectiveness of control measures, degree of distress, and sequelae (e.g., malnutrition, fluid and electrolyte loss).

Surveillance of nausea and vomiting during chemotherapy is particularly important. Treatment protocols usually require patients to receive chemotherapy for 6 to 12 monthly cycles, making it critically important that the emetic potential of drugs is assessed. Such assessment includes the emetogenicity of the agent (both onset and duration) plus the efficacy and duration of antiemetics. Differences occur in both emetic potential and onset among various drugs, even among those structurally related or with similar cytotoxicity.[67] Antineoplastic agents are grouped according to relative emetic potential. Table 15-1 lists commonly used chemotherapeutic agents ranked by their emetogenic potential. Patterns of nausea and vomiting range from acute to delayed and will depend on the drug, dosage, and time and route of administration. For example, cyclophosphamide and doxorubicin may not cause nausea and vomiting until 12 to 24 hours later, long after the patient has left the treatment setting[118] (see Mechanisms). With combination chemotherapy, the emetic pattern of each individual agent requires evaluation. However, there are often wide variations in nausea and vomiting among persons receiving the same chemotherapy protocol.

The nursing skills of assessment, psychosocial interaction, and exploration of individual patient needs are essential in ensuring that the patient is receiving the greatest assistance in preventing or realistically managing

TABLE 15–1   EMETIC POTENTIAL OF ANTINEOPLASTIC DRUGS

High (90%)	Moderately High (60–90%)	Moderate (30–60%)	Moderately Low (10–30%)	Low (10%)
Amsacrine	Actinomycin	Asparaginase	Cytarabine	Androgen
Cisplatin	Carmustine	Azacitidine	Etoposide	Bleomycin
Cytarabine*	Cyclophosphamide*	Daunorubicin	5-Fluorouracil	Busulfan
Dacarbazine	Methotrexate*	Doxorubicin	Melphalan	Corticosteroids
Mechlorethamine	Plicamycin	Hexamethylmelamine	Mitomycin C	Estramustine
Mitoxantrone	Procarbazine	Hydroxyurea		Estrogen
Streptozocin		Ifosfamide		Mercaptopurine
				Methotrexate†
				Progesterone
				Thioguanine
				Vinblastine
				Vincristine

*High-dose therapy.
†Low-dose therapy.

nausea and vomiting. It is vitally important that the nurse involved with the care of patients receiving chemotherapy have a foundation in the basis of antiemetic therapy. This includes knowledge about the major drugs that are used in antiemetic therapy, the rationale of the behavioral interventions, and an understanding of other measures, such as diet, that patients commonly use along with their prescribed regimens.

Clinicians and researchers need valid and reliable measures to determine the effectiveness of pharmacological and nonpharmacological interventions for nausea and vomiting. Some researchers use a visual analogue scale (VAS) to rate severity of pretreatment and post-treatment nausea and vomiting.[59, 101] A VAS is a self-report device used to measure phenomena such as pain, fatigue, dyspnea, quality of life, nausea, and vomiting.[59, 101, 119, 120] The VAS uses a 10-cm (100-mm) vertical or horizontal line with anchoring words like "not at all" and "extremely." The patient reports the magnitude of the phenomenon by placing a mark on this line. Kris and associates found the VAS reliable and associated with convergent validity in their antiemetic clinical trials.[121]

Another self-report tool, the Duke Descriptive Scale (DDS), additionally incorporates an activity level as a criterion for severity of nausea and vomiting. However, the broad grading scale one (1) through four (4) reduces this tool's sensitivity for studies in which it is critical to measure more minute parameters of nausea and vomiting.[122, 123] The Morrow Assessment of Nausea and Emesis (MANE), an index using a self-report Likert scale, separately measures the frequency, severity, and duration of nausea and vomiting.[124] Studies of the prevalence, correlates, and treatment of anticipatory nausea and vomiting support the efficacy of the MANE.[28, 30, 114, 125]

The eight-item Rhodes Index of Nausea and Vomiting (INV-Form 2) measures separately the duration, frequency, and distress of nausea; the frequency, distress, and amount of vomiting; and the frequency and distress from dry heaves or retching.[1, 27, 92] Items on this five-point Likert scale contain a 12-hour time frame reference. Researchers report that the INV-Form 2 is a reliable and valid measure of chemotherapy-induced nausea and vomiting.[126–128] Rhodes and associates used the INV-Form 2 to identify four post-

chemotherapy symptom occurrence patterns (minimal, declining, sustained, and peak).[27] Seventy-five per cent of the sample (n = 309) experienced minimal symptom occurrence 48 hours after therapy. Symptom occurrence pattern was defined as the occurrence (frequency and amount and duration) of nausea and vomiting as measured by the INV-Form 2. Symptom experience (occurrence and distress) at 12 hours after therapy did increase over six cycles, a finding that emphasized the importance of time since chemotherapy administration in planning nursing interventions.[27]

CLINICAL THERAPIES

The management of nausea and vomiting has primarily centered on three approaches: pharmacological, behavioral, and dietary. The management of nausea and vomiting of pregnancy with pharmacological approaches poses difficult problems because of the risk to the fetus. Therefore, dietary and behavioral approaches are the primary clinical therapies for these women. Increasing rest and changing eating patterns to high-carbohydrate, low-fat meals may provide symptom relief.[129, 130] Clinical therapies for gastrointestinal disorders, myocardial infarction, and postoperative nausea and vomiting are almost always single-agent antiemetics. Since the cause of these symptoms is usually self-limiting, there has been less research on clinical therapies for these conditions.

The nausea and vomiting of chemotherapy, because of the frequency of occurrence and the length of time the patient must deal with these experiences, have generated the most pharmacological and behavioral management research.

Pharmacological Management

The management of nausea and vomiting for patients undergoing chemotherapy with known emetogenic potential primarily focuses on regimens using multi-antiemetic drug therapy. The antiemetics work by blocking the dopamine receptors in the chemoreceptor trigger zone and the histamine and muscarinic cholinergic receptors in the vomiting center.[118] The antiemetics are individualized for each patient based on the (1) emetic potential and anticipated onset and duration of nausea and vomiting of the various chemotherapy agents the patient is receiving, (2) the known effectiveness and length of action of these antiemetic agents, (3) the anticipated side effects of the antiemetic agents, and (4) patient characteristics, such as age, prior experience with chemotherapy, and history of motion sickness. Table 15–2 provides a list of commonly prescribed agents in use.

The diverse factors involved in initiating nausea and vomiting and the fact that the different antiemetics have varied mechanisms, sites of action, and side effects make it obvious that a combination antiemetic regimen is most effective in controlling nausea and vomiting for the patient receiving multiple-dose chemotherapy protocols. Until recently, most patients received a combination of at least three antiemetic agents prior to and during the day of their chemotherapy. In addition, depending on the potential for ongoing or postchemotherapy bouts of nausea and vomiting, patients may be instructed to take antiemetics for longer periods of time.

TABLE 15–2 COMMONLY PRESCRIBED AGENTS IN ANTIEMETIC REGIMENS FOR ACUTE NAUSEA AND VOMITING

Drug	Dosage
Dexamethasone (Decadron)	Oral: 10–40 mg every 3 hr IV: 8–20 mg every 3 hr
Diphenhydramine (Benadryl)	Oral: 25–50 mg IV: 25–50 mg
Droperidol (Inapsine)	IM: 2.5 mg every 4–6 hr IV: 2.5 mg every 3 hr
Haloperidol (Haldol)	Oral: 1–2 mg every 12 hr IM: 1–2 mg every 12 hr
Lorazepam (Ativan)	Oral: 1–2 mg IV: 1–2 mg
Metoclopramide (Reglan)	Oral: 0.5–1 mg/kg every 2 hr IV: 1–2 mg/kg every 2–3 hr for two to six doses
Ondansetron (Zofrin)	Oral: not available IV: 0.15 mg/kg 30 minutes prior to chemotherapy and every 8 hr for two doses
Prochlorperazine (Compazine)	Oral: 10–20 mg every 4 hr 30 mg spansules every 12 hr p.r.: 25 mg every 4–6 hr IM: 5–10 mg every 4–6 hr IV: 10–30 mg every 4–6 hr
Thiethylperazine (Torecan)	Oral: 10–20 mg every 4 hr p.r.: 10 mg every 4–6 hr IM: 10 mg every 4 hr

Adapted from Fischer, D., & Knobf, M. (1989). *The Cancer Chemotherapy Handbook* (3rd ed., pp. 506–507). Chicago: Year Book Medical.

IM, intramuscular; IV, intravenous; p.r., per rectum.

With the advent of the serotonin antagonist ondansetron, the pharmacological management of the acute nausea and vomiting of chemotherapy has been changed. Ondansetron administered 30 minutes prior to chemotherapy and every 2 to 4 hours after chemotherapy for two additional doses is sufficient to control the acute nausea and vomiting associated with highly emetic agents such as cisplatin.[85] However, for patients who experience nausea and vomiting after the acute period, it is unclear whether the causative mechanism is serotonin or a different mechanism.

Additionally, clinicians need to assess the patient's acceptance and experience of the antiemetics with the side effects. Initially, most patients are willing to deal with the side effects of the antiemetics as long as the drugs control the nausea and vomiting, but after two or three cycles of chemotherapy (and many cycles continue for 6 to 12 months, some for as long as 18 months), patients find the side effects of antiemetics problematic. For example, if one of the phenothiazines is being prescribed, patients may find that the resulting sedation causes them too much "down time," and often complain that the antiemetic drugs essentially control their life. Also, akathisia, a disconcerting form of extreme restlessness, has been so troublesome with intravenous administration of metoclopramide that clinicians have been forced to quickly explore ways to alleviate the problem. Clinicians now administer metoclopramide slowly over time and have added benzodiazepines to prevent akathisia and diamenhydrinate to decrease systemic reactions.[66] This has greatly reduced the problem of akathisia.

Clinicians must work closely with the patient to continually evaluate the effectiveness of the prescribed regimen and, when necessary, to explore new approaches. Patients who have experienced profound problems with nausea and vomiting are very tempted to discontinue their chemotherapy even when they know that without such therapies their cancer will progress.

Behavioral Management

Patients have demonstrated an interest in becoming more active participants in their plan of care and thus exert more control over their treatment-related problems.[131] Nurses have long recognized the problems of relying solely on pharmacological interventions for control of nausea and vomiting.[132, 133] Many nurses believe a more holistic approach in which a variety of measures are used, such as antiemetic therapy and behavioral interventions, would be more beneficial to the patient.

Behavioral management of nausea and vomiting is of great interest to clinicians and patients alike. The problems associated with anticipatory and delayed nausea and vomiting have been a prime motivator in increasing the exploration of behavioral approaches. A study of women undergoing outpatient chemotherapy for breast cancer is representative of the issues associated with nausea and vomiting: 70 per cent of the patients experienced nausea and vomiting after treatment; of these, 57 per cent experienced anticipatory symptoms by the sixth treatment.[103]

The occurrence of nausea and vomiting in anticipation of chemotherapy is an example of a conditioned response.[134] Previously neutral stimuli, such as sights, sounds, and persons, as well as stimuli associated with the chemotherapy may prompt a sudden bout of nausea and vomiting.[134-136] Behavioral interventions are based on the premise that the conditioning response can be attenuated by interrupting the negative association by replacing it with a more positive connection.

Behavioral interventions used with patients undergoing chemotherapy include distraction, relaxation, guided imagery, hypnosis, and biofeedback. The latter two (hypnosis and biofeedback) require professional training and certification. The other behavioral interventions, although requiring an understanding of their rationale as well as preparation and experience, are within the scope of nursing practice. They are inexpensive, easy to learn, self-induced by the patient, readily available, and essentially free from side effects.

Relaxation, in which the person concentrates on relaxing muscle groups in a systematic manner, has been suggested as a means of preventing nausea and vomiting either through the inhibition of muscular activity necessary to produce the vomiting or through reduction of physiological arousal and anxiety. Distraction, or guided imagery, focuses the patient's attention away from the nausea to a more pleasant memory and may work in a similar fashion as relaxation.[60] Systematic desensitization is a technique in which the patient achieves a deep state of relaxation,[137] then recalls a negative event, such as nausea, and then imagines a positive mental image to resolve the negative experience. Patients who have used these behavioral approaches also report experiencing a feeling of greater control and well-being.[60, 138]

Studies have explored the effectiveness of behavioral interventions, including relaxation with guided imagery,[60, 109, 139] progressive muscle relaxation with imagery,[140] electromyographic feedback with relaxation and imagery,[109] systematic desensitization,[141] and attentional and cognitive distraction in children.[103] However, the rather small sample sizes, lack of randomization, and at times lack of equally comparative control groups precluded generalizations to all chemotherapy populations. The studies did, however, demonstrate rather clinically impressive reductions in anticipatory nausea and vomiting.

Dietary Strategies

Another self-care approach used by patients in managing nausea and vomiting associated with chemotherapy is dietary. They try eating bland food, such as soda crackers and carbonated beverages, taken in small amounts over the course of the day.[126, 142, 143] The effectiveness of these dietary manipulations has not been well documented, however, because they are basically benign and believed to be somewhat effective and within the control of the patient and family. These are supported and promoted by most nurses.

ILLUSTRATIVE CASE STUDY

The case of a young woman undergoing extensive chemotherapy for Hodgkin's disease who participated in a research study on the experience of therapy illustrates the effect of nausea and vomiting.[144] Laurie, a 24-year-old college student sharing an apartment with a friend, underwent an 8-month course of chemotherapy consisting of nitrogen mustard, vincristine, procarbazine, doxorubicin, vinblastine (Velban), bleomycin, and prednisone. In anticipation of nausea and vomiting, her physician prescribed prochlorperazine (Compazine), diphenhydramine (Benadryl), acetaminophen (Tylenol), and lorazepam

(Ativan) on the premise that she would have several medications available if one or more of them did not control her nausea and the vomiting that was expected to occur for 3 to 4 days after therapy.

Laurie reported that following her first two cycles of therapy she had taken the prescribed antiemetics and had experienced very little nausea and no vomiting. She did, however, experience lethargy and fatigue. After her second cycle of therapy, she found it difficult to concentrate and felt very restless and somewhat depressed. She stated that with all the medication (chemotherapy and antiemetics) she felt "like there's a chemical warfare going on inside me." She had tried imagery and relaxation suggested by a friend but found that because of her inability to concentrate she was unable to establish a positive mind-set to follow through on the processes required for relaxation and imagery. She wondered whether she could go through the additional cycles of chemotherapy. She was so discouraged she finally called the nurse at the clinic.

It was determined that Laurie had been taking lorazepam, prochlorperazine, and diphenhydramine on a daily basis for 7 days. Laurie, wanting to prevent any experience with nausea, used her prescribed antiemetics beyond the 3 to 4 days her physician anticipated she should use them. Her physician and clinic nurse clarified the time frame for her nausea control in subsequent cycles of therapy. For cycle three of chemotherapy, the physician had her take prochlorperazine and lorazepam just prior to therapy. She took only the specified antiemetic for the 4 days after chemotherapy, and she experienced minimal nausea and no vomiting. She did, however, continue to experience varying bouts of depression and sleeplessness.

Prior to her fourth cycle of chemotherapy, she moved to her mother's house because of fatigue. Following this cycle of therapy, she began to experience increasing bouts of nausea (but minimal vomiting) on a continuous basis. Her mother, an advocate of a naturalistic approach to health, encouraged Laurie to maintain a vegetarian diet and use herbal teas, relaxation, and imagery to counter these bouts of nausea. Her mother believed the antinausea medications were not helping prevent Laurie's nausea, only increasing her fatigue and depression.

For her fifth cycle of therapy Laurie decided not to take her pre-chemotherapy antinausea medications. She felt that she was being overmedicated. However, on the day following this fifth cycle of chemotherapy, her mother had to take her to the local emergency department because of severe nausea, vomiting, and shortness of breath that occurred during the periods of retching accompanying the vomiting. Laurie was treated with diphenhydramine and trimethobenzamide. This bout of nausea, retching, and vomiting also brought about a new reality for Laurie: now her nausea "could be triggered just by someone saying something, by a smell, by a certain sight, it's become an unconscious reflex." Although she did relaxation and took antiemetic drugs, she could not control her severe nausea. She began to dread the thought of going for chemotherapy.

She still had three cycles of chemotherapy to complete. She was very miserable, living alone at times, with her mother for other times, and not seeing friends or going to college. She found her life centered on chemotherapy and nausea. She stated at this point, "I fear I'm losing control over the nausea . . . it permeates all of my thoughts and often enters into my conversations with friends. I often just ramble on about it. They [the friends] imply I'm making something big out of nothing. But, just anticipating the nausea gets me depressed." She made a list of words, sights, and sounds that seemed to trigger her nausea in the hope that by "confronting them" she could gain control and prevent the nausea. Then, in spite of her anticipation and dread, she decided that beginning with her sixth cycle of chemotherapy she would only take her antiemetics immediately after chemotherapy. She said she did not like her life being totally controlled by drugs.

The nausea and vomiting associated with her last cycles of chemotherapy (six, seven, and eight) consisted of several hours (usually four) of nausea and several episodes of retching followed by vomiting during the immediate period after chemotherapy. At cycle seven, she began to experience difficulty with her saliva. If she swallowed the saliva, it increased the nausea and caused her to gag and then vomit. She found it disgusting, but effective, to just keep her mouth open and drool the saliva onto a towel. Once the four hours passed, the nausea and resulting drooling ended. There was no ongoing nausea. Further, her fatigue was lessening in both degree and duration.

For her final cycle of chemotherapy, she refused any antiemetics and declined to discuss the issue of nausea, stating, "This is my last time, I'll get by."

Once her therapy was complete, Laurie began to re-establish a normal life for herself. She returned to college, found a new job, and began to enjoy the evidence that her Hodgkin's disease was controlled. She recalled her "battle" with her side effects, including the nausea and vomiting, but conceded that for the most part all of these were fading from her memory.

This case study of Laurie, representing the subjective and objective experience of nausea and vomiting associated with chemotherapy, presents several salient aspects of the phenomena of nausea and vomiting. Laurie's experience highlights the impact nausea often has on a person.

REVIEW OF RESEARCH FINDINGS

The basis of this chapter is to present, whenever possible, the issues of nausea and vomiting from the scientific perspective. In keeping with this goal, there are several critical issues that warrant additional emphasis based on the findings of empirical research. In particular, there is a need to highlight the behavioral and pharmacological interventions that have potential for controlling the nausea and vomiting of early pregnancy, postoperatively, and during chemotherapy. Nurses need to be aware of what is available or has potential to control this high-incidence, challenging experience.

Interventions to Control Nausea and Vomiting of Pregnancy

Nonpharmacological interventions are the primary approach to control the nausea and vomiting of pregnancy because antiemetic drugs pose a risk to the fetus. DiIorio and van Lier studied the various interventions used by first-trimester women (n = 19) to control nausea and vomiting.[35] The women indicated intermittent rest periods, especially when they experienced nausea, were the most effective in relieving nausea and preventing vomiting. The authors did not find increased emphasis on performing interventions early in the day helpful, since the majority of women either had great time variation in their bouts of nausea or experienced an evening peak of nausea. In a similar study, DiIorio found that 46 per cent of a sample of women (n = 44) with first-trimester nausea used lying down to control bouts of nausea and 26 per cent of the women ate dry crackers as a means to control nausea.[15] This is in keeping with the findings of other research that a low-fat, high-carbohydrate diet was effective in controlling the nausea associated with the first trimester.[12] In contrast, three other studies found that dietary manipulation was not particularly effective in controlling the nausea of pregnancy.[15, 16, 145]

Jenkins and Shelton evaluated the effectiveness of self-care actions in reducing morning sickness.[8] More than 70 per cent of the women (n = 37) managed by adjusting their resting, eating, and cooking and increasing their emotional support. Increasing rest periods was perceived as being the most effective in controlling nausea.

Thus, it seems that the traditional methods of rest and small amounts of carbohydrate-rich food are helpful to women who experience nausea in the first trimester. Research findings indicate that it is important to explore ways in which women can increase their rest periods during this period. This is particularly important in light of the many women who remain in the work force throughout their pregnancy. Further research is needed to determine effective, non-tetrogenic approaches to the control of the nausea of pregnancy.

Interventions to Control Nausea and Vomiting Postoperatively

Postoperative nausea and vomiting are common after general anesthesia. Reported frequencies range from 38 to 92 per cent.[146, 147] Leeser and Lip observed the use of ondansetron in a randomized double-blind, placebo-controlled study in 84 patients undergoing a gynecological operation who received the same general anesthetic.[148] The group (n = 421) receiving ondansetron had significantly less nausea and vomiting (P < .005). These differences were maintained over a 24-hour period. Jorgensen and Coyle evaluated the use of low-dose and moderate-dose droperidol in controlling postoperative nausea and vomiting in postoperative patients who had received an alfentanil-based anesthetic.[49] Sixty adults undergoing short surgical procedures were randomly assigned to one of three groups. The control group received normal saline (n = 20), the second group received droperidol at 10 mcg/kg (n = 20), and a third group (n = 20) received droperidol at 20 mcg/kg. The frequency of nausea and vomiting was significantly less (P < .05) for the group receiving droperidol at 20 mcg/kg than for the other two groups.

Interventions to Control the Nausea and Vomiting of Chemotherapy

Nonpharmacological interventions have been most widely studied in patients with anticipatory nausea and vomiting associated with chemotherapy. This classic conditioned response, in which previously neutral stimuli become the conditioned stimuli for evoking the nausea and vomiting response, is very challenging to clinicians and researchers to control.

Burish and Lyles, in a study of patients with anticipatory nausea and vomiting, used a two-group design to test the effectiveness of guided relaxation imagery.[109] A control group (n = 8) received the usual antiemetic therapy, and the experimental group (n = 8) received an antiemetic and participated in progressive muscle relaxation plus guided relaxation imagery. Measurement was based on patient and nurse perceptions of the patient's nausea. There was a significant reduction of nausea in the experimental group compared with the control group.

Cotanch used progressive muscle relaxation in a single group of patients (n = 12) experiencing anticipatory nausea and vomiting. At the first measurement period (48 hours after chemotherapy), nausea had decreased for nine of the patients and all 12

were able to eat. However, by the end of the study, 6 months after patients began chemotherapy, six of the 12 patients had dropped out. The data on this small sample indicate that a behavioral approach has initial potential to reduce this form of chemotherapy-associated nausea.[123] The attrition of study subjects makes it unclear whether this behavioral approach is sustained and accepted by patients over time.

Exercise has been postulated as a mechanism to control postchemotherapy nausea and vomiting. Winningham and MacVicar reported on the effects of aerobic exercise on nausea in 42 women receiving cyclophosphamide, methotrexate, and 5-fluorouracil protocols for breast cancer.[149] None of the patients was receiving antiemetics. Results suggest that moderate exercise may be beneficial as an adjunctive self-care measure to antiemetics. Relaxation was also effective in Morrow's study of 92 patients with anticipatory nausea.[137] In addition, Scott and associates' study of behavioral and pharmacological modalities in 17 women with ovarian cancer showed that the drug regimen was effective in reducing peak emesis but the total emetic period was 4 hours shorter with relaxation.[139] These research studies strongly indicate that behavioral approaches are an option for emetic control. However, researchers need to carefully monitor and enforce their interventions and to increase their sample sizes to prove definitively that behavioral approaches work.

The most common studies of nausea and vomiting are the trials of antiemetics with either placebos or standard antiemetic therapy in chemotherapy-induced nausea and vomiting. There has been an exponential growth in these studies related primarily to the more aggressive approach to the treatment of malignancies with highly emetic chemotherapy.

In a double-blind, randomized trial, Kris and associates compared placebo, dexamethasone alone, and metoclopramide plus dexamethasone in 91 patients receiving high-dose cisplatin.[121] Patients who had not previously received chemotherapy and who had a Karnovsky performance status greater than 50 per cent were eligible. They used a self-report patient log, VAS, and investigator observation or questioning to assess delayed nausea and vomiting for 4 consecutive days. Forty-eight per cent of the subjects who received the two-drug combination experienced delayed vomiting as opposed to 65 per cent for dexamethasone alone and 89 per cent for placebo ($P = .006$).

In a similar study, 67 patients received metoclopramide, droperidol, and dexamethasone as prophylaxis for cisplatin chemotherapy.[150] No patients were excluded on the basis of prior chemotherapy experience or performance status. The severity of nausea was determined by the level of activities of daily living. In this sample, 76.1 per cent experienced no nausea or vomiting during their first course of treatment and 62.7 per cent in all their treatment courses (26 had three or more courses). The addition of diphenhydramine to prevent an extrapyramidal reaction secondary to metoclopramide and droperidol was deemed effective.

Of further interest is the investigation of a new class of antiemetic agents that block serotonin receptors, specifically serotonin (5-hydroxytryptamine). Addleman and associates completed a phase I and II trial of granisetron, a novel serotonin antagonist, in 24 first-time chemotherapy patients receiving any combination of doxorubicin and cisplatin.[151] Nausea was assessed by VAS, patient log, and independent observation. Nausea prophylaxis was achieved for 32 per cent of the sample during the first 24 hours after chemotherapy. Fifty-two per cent had no vomiting. The investigators concluded that granisetron shows promise as a well-tolerated and effective antiemetic.

Other researchers compared the efficacy and safety of ondansetron, a selective antagonist of serotonin receptors, with those of a placebo in 28 patients receiving cisplatin.[85] Study criteria excluded patients with previous chemotherapy and a Karnofsky score of less than 60 per cent. Nausea and vomiting were markedly diminished in the group given ondansetron. No adverse effects were noted. A trained observer recorded treatment response, that is, frequency and intensity of emesis. Patients used a VAS to assess the severity of their nausea. A patient log and interview supplemented these methods.

The control of nausea and vomiting associated with chemotherapy and pharmacological agents is important because it presently offers the most efficacious approach to this major health care dilemma. The advent of the serotonin antagonists is especially important because the data clearly indicate their effectiveness in controlling the nausea and vomiting of most patients receiving emetic potentiating chemotherapy. Clinically, patients and health care providers alike are very impressed with their effect. There are countless stories of patients, previously experiencing nausea and vomiting, who upon receiving ondansetron for the first time call their nurses and physicians to express their unbelievable relief that they are no longer experiencing nausea and vomiting after chemotherapy. Ondansetron is not a panacea for all, however. Many patients still experience anticipatory nausea and vomiting in spite of receiving ondansetron, and for all patients the cost of these serotonin antagonists remains at three figures for each dose.

IMPLICATIONS FOR FURTHER RESEARCH

There are numerous opportunities for nurses to advance the knowledge of the incidence and management of nausea and vomiting. To assist the practitioner in addressing the areas that need further study, a conceptual model is presented (Fig. 15–3). The model was developed through a review of relevant research studies, theoretical literature, and personal experience.[71] Because the prevalent literature of nausea and vomiting concerns cancer and cancer treatment, the model draws heavily from this literature.

Evoking Stimulus

The model first considers the nature of the evoking stimulus. Using chemotherapy drugs as an example, one would need to consider the emetic potential of the drugs, the dosage, and the route of administration. Studies could then be done to document the difference in response between oral and intravenous administration of certain agents as well as the time of onset of the nausea and vomiting. This approach could also be used in the study of postoperative nausea and vomiting with regard to anesthetics and other drugs given in the perioperative period.

Patient Characteristics

The second area for study identified in the model is patient characteristics. Numerous

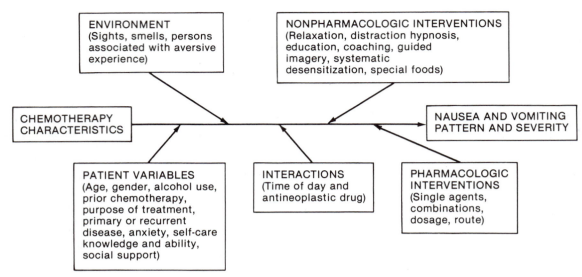

Figure 15–3. Model for assessment of nausea and vomiting. (From DiJulio, J., 1991, unpublished.)

patient variables have been identified as potential modifiers of nausea and vomiting. Of these variables, age has been well studied, and it has been documented that patients younger than age 50 experience more nausea and vomiting than older patients. However, other variables such as gender, performance status, anxiety, predisposition to motion sickness, and a history of heavy alcohol usage need further delineation in the role they might play in nausea and vomiting. With chemotherapy, it is important to know whether patients being treated for cure respond differently than those patients being treated for control of disease. Do patients receiving chemotherapy for the first time exhibit less nausea and vomiting than those patients receiving repeated treatments? Many of these variables have some support in the literature in the role they play in nausea and vomiting, but the studies are far from definitive.

Self-Care Behavior

Many practitioners believe that if the patient participates in the management of side effects, the outcome will result in better management and less distress. The variable of self-care behavior by patients to modify their experience of side effects has been investigated by Dodd in a series of studies.[143, 152–155]

Patients in these studies on the whole reported few self-care behaviors; however, those who did evaluated the behaviors as moderately effective. In a replication and extension of Dodd's work, Musci found that patients receiving chemotherapy over three cycles reported low self-care behavior scores and rated side effects as severe.[156] Severity of side effects, however, appears to limit the patient's self-care ability. In a study by Musci and Dodd, 42 patients and 40 family members were followed for three cycles of chemotherapy.[157] Side effects reported most frequently by the patients were nausea (90 per cent), fatigue (65 per cent), vomiting (62 per cent), mouth sores (31 per cent), and weakness (31 per cent). The two most distressing side effects were vomiting and fatigue. According to the study, patients did not delay in initiating self-care behaviors for more than 24 hours after treatment; however, as the severity of the side effects increased, delays in initiating self-care behaviors increased from one to several days.

Social Support

Social support has been identified as a variable that can impact health outcomes.[158–160] Lazarus' and Folkman's theories of stress, coping, and adaptation[161] have been used to develop the framework of social support as a coping strategy in stressful situations. An individual, when faced with stressors, engages in behaviors that result in the receipt of emotional, appraisal, informational or instrumental support.[162] Although social support has not been studied specifically with regard to the nausea and vomiting associated with chemotherapy, there is strong theoretical support for doing so.

Environment

Clinical experience with patients receiving chemotherapy has contributed to the knowledge about nausea and vomiting through anecdotal reports of environmental factors that have triggered the nausea and vomiting response. These factors are more frequently related to the conditioned response of anticipatory nausea and vomiting and serve as the replacement stimulus for the chemotherapeutic agent.[91, 101, 141] Most research with environmental factors has dealt with behavioral interventions to modify the anticipatory response.[60, 109, 141, 163] Documentation of the magnitude of the problem and the environmental triggers needs further study.

Interactions

The model next considers interactions, of which there are undoubtedly numerous cases that need to be studied. For example, the interaction of age and antiemetics is a major concern for nurses. Younger patients (under 30 years of age) tend to experience more acute dystonic reactions from dopamine receptor blockers such as metoclopramide.[66, 163, 164] Allen and associates summarized the experience of 500 patients receiving metoclopramide and found that trismus or torticolis occurred only 2 per cent of the time in those patients older than age 30.[66] In contrast, patients younger than 30 years had a 27 per cent incidence of dystonic reactions. Furthermore, for patients receiving dopamine-blocking antiemetics on a daily schedule for chemotherapy, the incidence was even higher.

Age is also a factor in antiemetic trials using cannabinoids (delta-9-tetrahydrocannabinol [THC], marijuana). Researchers studying the effect of THC have shown greater efficacy in controlling nausea and vomiting in younger patients.[165, 166] Support of age-related central nervous system toxicity in older patients appears more often in anecdotal reports than in controlled clinical trials.[69, 80] Carey and colleagues have suggested that the depersonalization reaction that occurs during a THC "high" may be desirable to the younger patient but that older patients may find this experience emotionally devastating.[80]

The relationship between the time of day that chemotherapeutic drugs are administered and the nausea and vomiting experienced is a possible second interaction. Hrushesky reported that when administering doxorubicin in the evening and cisplatin in the morning, patients experienced much more toxicity than those patients receiving the opposite schedule.[167] In a study of circadian timing of cisplatin and vomiting effects, patients who received cisplatin at 0600 hours had significantly more vomiting episodes than those who received cisplatin at 1800 hours.[168] Moore[169] and Headley[127] each studied administration time of protocols containing cisplatin. No significant correlation between the time of administration and the nausea and vomiting response was found. Nurses are in an ideal position to study these interactions as well as others not yet identified.

Pharmacological Interventions

Pharmacological interventions are the next area of the model that have many implications for nursing research. The addition of the serotonin antagonists has changed the acute management of nausea and vomiting in the chemotherapy patient and is currently being studied in the postoperative population.[148] Nurses need to be able to manage both the acute and chronic side effects that may occur. Unfortunately, little is known at this time about the delayed incidence of nausea and vomiting in patients receiving the serotonin antagonists. It is also unclear as to which, if any, antiemetics should be used for either prevention or control of delayed side effects.

Nonpharmacological Interventions

Nursing practice is rich with nonpharmacological interventions for the relief of nausea and vomiting. The effectiveness of the behavioral interventions has been studied by nurses and psychologists alike. Unfortunately, many of the studies involved a small sample size, lacked randomization, and did not always control for antiemetic administration. Because many of these studies are carried out by nurses, it is important to continue this line of study.

Dietary modifications are another non-pharmacological intervention that has received little study. Nurses are well equipped to pursue this area of research and can do so in a variety of populations.

Patterns and Severity

The final area of the assessment model concerns the patterns and severity of the nausea and vomiting. Perhaps the most fruitful area of research for nurses is the documentation of these patterns. This is particularly important because much of patient care is carried out in an outpatient setting and these phenomena are not readily observed by a nurse. The pattern of anticipatory nausea and vomiting appears to have several patient characteristics[134] that could lead to a predictive model for nursing that would allow for early intervention and treatment.

REFERENCES

1. Rhodes, V., Watson, P., & Johnson, M. (1984). Development of reliable and valid measures of nausea and vomiting. Cancer Nurs 7:33–41.
2. Rhodes, V. (1990). Nausea, vomiting, and retching. Nurs Clin North Am 24:885–901.
3. Borison, H., & McCarthy, L. (1983). Neuropharmacologic mechanisms of emesis. In J. Laszlo (ed.), Antiemetics and Cancer Chemotherapy (pp. 6–20). Baltimore: Williams & Wilkins.
4. Tortorice, P., & O'Connell, M. (1990). Management of chemotherapy-induced nausea and vomiting. Pharmacotherapy 10:129–145.
5. Gold, M. I. (1969). Postanesthetic vomiting in the recovery room. Br J Anaesth 41:143–149.
6. Norris, C. M. (1982). Nausea and vomiting in concept clarification. In C. M. Norris (ed.), Nursing (pp. 81–110). Rockville, MD: Aspen.
7. Borison, H. L. (1986). Anatomy and physiology of the chemoreceptor trigger zone and area postrema. In C. J. Davis, G. V. Lake-Bakaar, & D. G. Grahame-Smith (eds.), Nausea and Vomiting: Mechanisms and Treatment (pp. 10–17). Berlin: Springer-Verlag.
8. Jenkins, M., & Shelton, B. J. (1989). The effectiveness of self-care actions in reducing morning sickness. In S. G. Funk, E. M. Tornquist, M. T. Champagne, L. A. Copp, & R. A. Weise (eds.), Key Aspects of Comfort. Management of Pain, Fatigue, and Nausea (p. 267). New York: Springer.
9. Funk, S. G., Tornquist, E. M., Champagne, M. T., Copp, L. A., & Weise, R. A. (eds.), (1989). Key Aspects of Comfort. New York: Springer.
10. Brandes, J. (1967). First-trimester nausea and vomiting as related to outcome of pregnancy. Obstet Gynecol 30:429.
11. Vellacott I., Cooke E., & James C. (1988). Nausea and vomiting in early pregnancy. Int J Gynecol Obstet 27:57–62.
12. Fairweather, D. V. I. (1986). Mechanisms and treatment of nausea and vomiting in pregnancy. In C. J. Davis, G. V. Lake-Bakaar, & D. G. Grahame-Smith (eds.), Nausea and Vomiting: Mechanisms and Treatment. Berlin: Springer-Verlag.
13. Jaenfelt-Samsloe, A., Samslow G., & Velinder, G. (1983). Nausea and vomiting in pregnancy—a contribution to this epidemiology. Gynecol Obstet Invest 16:221–229.
14. Klebanoff, M., Koslowe, P., Kaslow, R., & Rhoads, G. (1985). Epidemiology of vomiting in early pregnancy. Obstet Gynecol 66:612–616.
15. DiIorio, C. (1988). The management of nausea and vomiting in pregnancy. Nurs Pract 13:23–28.
16. Walters, W. A. (1987). The management of nausea and vomiting during pregnancy. Med J Aust 147:290–291.
17. Ahmad, S. (1978). Significance of nausea and vomiting during acute myocardial infarction. Am Heart J 95:671.
18. Ingram, D. A., Fulton, R., Portal, R., & Aber, C. P. (1980). Vomiting as a diagnostic aid in acute ischemic cardiac pain. Br Med J [Clin Res] 281:636.
19. McGuigan, J. & Wolfe, M. (1983). Anorexia, nausea, and vomiting. In R. Blacklow (ed.), MacBryde's Signs and Symptoms (6th. ed., pp. 361–373). Philadelphia: J. B. Lippincott.
20. Wilkinson A., Frampton, C., Glover, P., & Davis, F. M. (1989). Preoperative transdermal hyoscine for the prevention of postoperative nausea and vomiting. Anaesth Inten Care 17:285.
21. Muir, J. J., Warner, M. A., Offord, K. P., Buck, C. F., Harper, J. V., & Kunkel, S. E. (1987). Role of nitrous oxide and other factors in postoperative nausea and vomiting: A randomized and blinded prospective study. Anesthesiology 66:513–518.
22. California Cancer Facts & Figures. (1992) Oakland, CA: American Cancer Society.
23. Morrow, G. (1989). Chemotherapy-related nausea and vomiting: Etiology and management. CA Cancer J Clin 39:89–104.
24. Morrow, G. (1991). Predicting development of anticipatory nausea in cancer patients: Prospective examination of eight clinical characteristics. J Pain Symptom Manage 6:215–223.
25. Jacobson, P., & Redd, M. (1988). The development and management of chemotherapy-related anticipatory nausea and vomiting. Cancer Invest 6:329–336.
26. Krasnow, S. (1991). New directions in managing chemotherapy-related emesis. Oncology 5(Suppl.): 19–24.
27. Rhodes, V., Watson, P., Johnson, M., Madsen, R., & Beck, N. (1987). Patterns of nausea, vomiting, and distress in patients receiving antineoplastic drug protocols. Oncol Nurs Forum 14:35–44.
28. Stefanek, M., Sheidler, V., & Fetting, J. (1988). Anticipatory nausea and vomiting: Does it remain a significant clinical problem? Cancer 62:2654–2657.

29. Coons, H., Leventhal, H., Nerenz, D., Love, R., & Larson, S. (1987). Anticipatory nausea and emotional distress in patients receiving cisplatin-based chemotherapy. Oncol Nurs Forum *14*:31–35.

30. Cohen, R., Blanchard, E., Ruckdeschel, J., & Smolen, R. (1986). Prevalence and correlates of post treatment and anticipatory nausea and vomiting in cancer chemotherapy. J Psychosom Res *30*:643–654.

31. Hinshaw, A., Heinrick, J., & Block, D. (1988). Evolving clinical nursing research priorities: A rational endeavor. J Prof Nurs *4*:458–459.

32. Grant, M. (1987). Nausea and vomiting. In *Nursing Management of Common Problems*. American Cancer Society: Atlanta.

33. Nolan, E. (1985). Nausea, vomiting, and dehydration. In M. Jacobs & W. Geels (eds.), *Signs and Symptoms in Nursing. Interpretation and Management* (pp. 373–401). Philadelphia: J. B. Lippincott.

34. Cotanch, P. (1989). Management of nausea: Current bases for practice. In S. Funk, E. Tornquist, & M. Champagne, L. A. Copp, & R. A. Weise (eds.), *Key Aspects of Comfort, Management of Pain, Fatigue, and Nausea* (pp. 243–248). New York: Springer.

35. DiIorio, C., & van Lier, D. (1989). Nausea and vomiting in pregnancy. In S. G. Funk, E. M. Tornquist, M. T. Champagne, L. A. Copp, & R. A. Weise (eds.), *Key Aspects of Comfort. Management of Pain, Fatigue, and Nausea* (pp. 259). New York: Springer.

36. Ehlke, G. (1988). Symptom distress in breast cancer patients receiving chemotherapy in the outpatient setting. Oncol Nurs Forum *15*:343–346.

37. Pole, L. (1989). Relieving nausea: A discussion. In S. Funk, E. Tornquist, M. Champagne, L. A. Copp, & R. A. Weise (eds.), *Key Aspects of Comfort. Management of Pain, Fatigue, and Nausea* (pp. 276–280). New York: Springer.

38. Pervan, V. (1990). Practical aspects of dealing with cancer therapy-induced nausea and vomiting. Semin Oncol Nurs *6*:3–5.

39. Ouwerkerk, J., & Keizer, H. (1990). Psychologic aspects of the treatment of emesis in cancer nursing. Semin Oncol Nurs *6*(Suppl. 1):6–9.

40. Maher, M. (1990). The conduct of clinical trials in the area of emesis control. *Semin Oncol Nurs 6*(Suppl. 1):10–13.

41. Cookson, R. F. (1986). Mechanisms and treatment of post-operative nausea and vomiting. In C. J. Davis, G. V. Lake-Bakaar, & D. G. Grahame-Smith (eds.), *Nausea and Vomiting: Mechanisms and Treatment*. Berlin: Springer-Verlag.

42. Alexander, G. D., Skupski, J. N., & Brown, E. M. (1984). The role of nitrous oxide in postoperative nausea and vomiting. Anesth Analg *63*:175.

43. Peroutka, S., & Snyder, S. (1982). Antiemetics: Neurotransmitter receptor binding predicts therapeutic actions. Lancet *1*:658–659.

44. Yasko, J. (1985). Holistic management of nausea and vomiting caused by chemotherapy. Top Clin Nurs *7*:26–38.

45. Burish, T., Carey, M., Krozely, M., & Greco, F. A. (1987). Conditional side effects induced by cancer chemotherapy: Prevention through behavioral treatment. J Consult Clin Psychol *55*:42–48.

46. Weigel, M., & Weigel, R. (1989). Nausea and vomiting in early pregnancy outcome. A meta-analytical review. Br J Obstet Gynecol *96*:1312–1318.

47. Gross, S., Librach, C., & Cecutti, A. (1989). Maternal weight loss associated with hyperemesis gravidarum: A predictor of fetal outcome. Am J Obstet Gynecol *160*:906–909.

48. Buckler, H. (1914). Prophylaxis of post anesthetic vomiting. Am J Surg, Quart Suppl Anesth Analg *28*:13–15.

49. Jorgensen, N. H., & Coyle, J. P. (1990). Intravenous droperidol decreases nausea and vomiting after alfentanil anesthesia without increasing recovery time. J Clin Anesth *2*:312–316.

50. Mecca, R. S. (1989). Postanesthesia recovery in clinical anesthesia. In P. G. Barish, B. F. Cullan, & R. K. Stoelting (eds.), Clin Anesth (pp. 1419–1420). Philadelphia: J. B. Lippincott.

51. Dent, S. J., Ramachandra, V., & Stephen, C. R. (1958). Post-operative vomiting: Incidence, analysis and therapeutic measures in 3,000 patients. Anesthesiology *16*:564–572.

52. Kottila, K., Kausti, A., & Aavinen, M. (1979). Comparison of droperitol, and metoclopprenude in the prevention and treatment of nausea and vomiting after balance general anesthesia. Anesthesia *41*:16–20.

53. Dundee, J. W., Kilwan, M. J., & Clark, R. S. J. (1965). Anesthesia and premedication as factors in postoperative vomiting. Acta Anesthesiol Scand *9*:223–231.

54. Bellville, J. W., Bross, I. P. J., & Howlands, W. S. (1959). Postoperative nausea and vomiting. IV. Factors related to postoperative nausea and vomiting. Anesthesiology *21*:186–193.

55. Palazzo, M. G. A., & Strunin, L. (1984). Anesthesia and emesis. Can Anaesth Soc J *31*:178–187.

56. Lasley, K., & Ignaffo, R. (1981). *Manual of Oncology Therapeutics*. St. Louis: C. V. Mosby.

57. Button, D. (1990). Recent developments in the management of emesis with the 5-HT_3 antagonist granisetron. Semin Oncol Nurs *6*(Suppl. 1):14–19.

58. Andrykowski, M. (1988). Defining anticipatory nausea and vomiting: Differences among cancer chemotherapy patients who report pretreatment nausea. J Behav Med *11*:59–69.

59. Jacobson, P., Andrykowski, M., Redd, W., Die-Trill, M., Hakes, T., Kaufman, R., Currie, V., & Holland, J. (1988). Nonpharmacologic factors in the development of post-treatment nausea with adjuvant chemotherapy for breast cancer. Cancer *61*:379–385.

60. Redd, W. H., & Andrykowski, M. A. (1982). Behavioral intervention in cancer treatment: Controlling aversion reactions to chemotherapy. J Consult Clin Psychol *50*:14–19.

61. Olafsdottir, M., Sjoden, P. I., & Westling, B. (1986). Prevalence and prediction of chemotherapy related anxiety, nausea and vomiting in cancer patients. Behav Res Ther *24*:59–66.

62. Minow, S. (1982). Nausea and the patient with myocardial infarction. In C. Norris (ed.), *Concept Clarification in Nursing* (pp. 111–132). Rockville, MD: Aspen.

63. Hanson, J., & McCallum, R. (1985). The diagnosis and management of nausea and vomiting: A review. Am J Gastroenterol *80*:210–218.

64. Billings, V. (1985). *Outpatient Management of Advanced Cancer: Symptom Control, Support, and Hospice-in-the-Home*. Philadelphia: J. B. Lippincott.

65. Plum R., & Posner, J. (1980). *The Diagnosis of Stupor and Coma* (3rd ed.). Philadelphia: F. A. Davis.

66. Allen, J., Gralla, R. & Reilly, C. (1985). Metoclopramide: Dose-related toxicity and preliminary an-

tiemetic studies in children receiving cancer chemotherapy. J Clin Oncol *3*:1136–1141.

67. Gralla, R., Kris, M. G., Tyson, L. B. & Clark, R.
A. (1988). Controlling emesis in patients receiving
cancer chemotherapy. Recent Results Cancer Res
108:89–101.

68. Krasnow, S. (1989). Problems in antiemetic trial
design and interpretation. Oncology *3*(Suppl.):5–
9.

69. Olver, N., Simon, R. M., & Aisner, J. (1986).
Antiemetic studies: A methodological discussion.
Cancer Treat Rep *70*:555–563.

70. Redd, W. J., Jacobsen, P. B., Die-Trill, M., Der-
matis, H., McEvoy, M., & Holland, J. C. (1987).
Cognitive/attentional distraction in the control of
conditioned nausea. J Consult Clin Psychol
55:391–395.

71. DiJulio, J., Dodd, M., Larson, P., & Dibble, S.
(1991). Identification of variables related to chemotherapy induced nausea and vomiting. Oncol
Nurs Forum *18*(2), 335 (Abstract No. 64A).

72. Reuben, D., & Mor, V. (1986). Nausea and vomiting in terminal cancer patients. Arch Intern Med
146:2021–2023.

73. Davis, C. J., Harding, R. K., Leslie, R. A., &
Andrews, P. L. R. (1986). The organization of
vomiting as a protective reflex: A commentary. In
C. J. Davis, G. V. Lake-Bakaar, & D. G. Grahame-
Smith (eds.), *Nausea and Vomiting: Mechanisms and
Treatment*. Berlin: Springer-Verlag.

74. Laszlo, J. (1983). Emesis as limiting toxicity in
cancer chemotherapy. In Laszlo, J. (ed.), *Antiemetics
and Cancer Chemotherapy*. Baltimore: Williams &
Wilkins.

75. Borison, H., & Wang, S. (1953). Physiology and
pharmacology of vomiting. Pharmacol Rev *5*:192–
230.

76. Miller, A. D., & Wilson, V. J. (1983). Vomiting
center reanalyzed: An electrical stimulation. Brain
Res *270*:154–158.

77. Borison, H. L., & Wang, S. C. (1949). Functional
localization of the central coordinating mechanism
for emesis in the cat. J Neurophysiol *12*:305–313.

78. Borison, H. L., & Wang, S. C. (1950). The vomiting
center. Arch Neurol Psychiatry *63*:928–941.

79. Grahame-Smith, D. G. (1986). The multiple causes
of vomiting: Is there a common mechanism? In C.
J. Davis, G. V. Lake-Bakaar, & D. G. Grahame-
Smith (eds.), *Nausea and Vomiting: Mechanisms and
Treatment*. Berlin: Springer-Verlag.

80. Carey, M., Burish, T., & Brenner, D. (1983). Delta
9-tetra-hydrocannabinal in cancer chemotherapy:
Research problems and issues. Ann Intern Med
99:106–114.

81. Guyton, A. (1981). *Textbook of Medical Physiology*
(6th. ed.). Philadelphia: W. B. Saunders.

82. Cohen, S. E., Woods, W. A., & Wyner, J. (1984).
Antiemetic efficacy of droperidol and metoclopramide. Anesthesiology *60*:67–70.

83. Schwartz, S. I. (1989). Manifestations of G.I. disease. In S. I. Schwartz, G. T. Shina, & F. C. Spencer
(eds.), *Principles of Surgery* (pp. 1067–1070). New
York: McGraw-Hill.

84. Harris, A., & Cantwell, B. (1986). Mechanisms and
treatment of cytotoxic-induced nausea and vomiting. In C. J. Davis, G. V. Lake-Bakaar, & D. G.
Grahame-Smith (eds.), *Nausea and Vomiting: Mechanisms and Treatment* (pp. 78–93). Berlin: Springer-
Verlag.

85. Cubeddu, L. S., Hoffman, I. S., Fuenmayor, N.
T., & Finn, A. L. (1990). Efficacy of Ondansetron
(Gr 38032F) and the role of serotonin in cisplatin-
induced nausea and vomiting. N Engl J Med
322:810–816.

86. Andrews, P. L., Rapeport, W. G., & Sanger, G. J.
(1988). Neuropharmacology of emesis induced by
anti-cancer therapy. Trends in Pharmacological
Sciences *9*:331–341.

87. Marty, M., Pouillart, P., Scholl, S., Droz, J. P.,
Azab, M., Brion, N., Pujade-Lauraine, E., Paule,
B., Paes, D., & Bons, J. (1990). Comparison of the
5-hydroxytryptamine 3 (serotonin) antagonist ondansetron (GR 38032F) with high-dose metoclopramide in the control of cisplatin-induced emesis.
N Engl J Med *322*:816–820.

88. Andrykowski, M. (1989). Prescription and use of
antiemetics among cancer chemotherapy outpatients. J Psychosoc Oncol *7*:141–157.

89. Love, R. R., Nerenz, R. R., & Leventhal, H. (1982).
The development of anticipatory nausea during
cancer chemotherapy. Proc Am Soc Clin Oncol
1:47.

90. Morrow, G. R. (1982). Prevalence and correlates
of anticipatory nausea and vomiting in chemotherapy patients. J Nat Cancer Inst *68*:585–588.

91. Nesse, R. M., Carli, T., Curtis, G. C., & Kleinman,
P. D. (1980). Pretreatment nausea in cancer che-
motherapy: A conditioned response? Psychosom
Med *42*:33–36.

92. Rhodes, V., & Watson, P. (1987). Final Report of
US PHS grant #5 R01 NU01154-02. Nausea, vom-
iting and anxiety in cancer patients. Columbia,
MO: University of Missouri School of Nursing.

93. Wickham, R. (1989). Managing chemotherapy-related nausea and vomiting: The state of the art.
Oncol Nurs Forum *16*:563–574.

94. Fetting, J. H., Grochow, L. B., Folstein, M. F.,
Ettinger, D. S., & Colvin, M. (1982). The course of
nausea and vomiting after high dose cyclophosphamide. Cancer Treat Rep *66*:1487–1493.

95. Friedman, O. M., Myles, A., & Colvin, M. (1979).
Cyclophosphamide and related phosphoramide
mustards: Current status and future prospects. In
A. Rosowsky (ed.), *Advances in Cancer Chemotherapy*
(pp. 143–204). New York: Marcel Dekker.

96. Gralla, R. (1989). Nausea and vomiting. In V.
DeVita, S. Hellman, & S. Rosenberg (eds.), *Cancer*
(3rd ed.). Philadelphia: J. B. Lippincott.

97. Dorr, R. T., & Fritz, W. L. (1980). *Cancer Chemotherapy Handbook*. New York: Elsevier.

98. Zaglama, N. E., Rosenblum, S. L., & Sartiano, G.
P. (1986). Single, high-dose intravenous dexameth-
asone as an antiemetic in cancer chemotherapy.
Oncology *43*:27–32.

99. Wilcox, P., Fetting, J., Nettesheim, K., et al. (1982).
Anticipatory vomiting in women receiving cyclophosphamide methotrexate and 5-FU (CMF) adjuvant chemotherapy for breast carcinoma. Cancer
Treat Rep *66*:1601–1604.

100. Strum, S., McDermed, J. E., Abrahano-Umali, R.,
& Sanders, P. (1985). Management of cisplatin-
induced delayed-onset nausea and vomiting: Preliminary results with two drug regimens. Proc Am
Soc Clin Onocol *4*:263.

101. Andrykowski, M., & Redd, W. (1981). Longitudinal
analysis of the development of anticipatory nausea.
J Consult Clin Psychol *55*:36–41.

102. Morrow, G. (1985). The effect of a susceptibility
to motion sickness on the side effects of cancer
chemotherapy. Cancer *55*:2766–2770.

103. Redd, W., Jacobsen, P, & Andrykowski, M. (1989). Behavioral side effects of adjuvant chemotherapy. Recent Results Cancer Res *115*:272–278.

104. Scogma, D. M., & Smalley, R. V. (1979). Chemotherapy induced nausea and vomiting. Am J Nurs *79*:1562–1564.

105. Zook, D., & Yasko, J. (1983). Psychologic factors: Their effect on nausea and vomiting experienced by clients receiving chemotherapy. Oncol Nurs Forum *10*:76–81.

106. Javadapour, N. (1985). Pharmacologic and clinical application of cis-platinium. Urology *25*:155–160.

107. Fischer, D., & Knobf, M. (1989). *The Cancer Chemotherapy Handbook*, (3rd ed., pp. 506–507). Chicago: Year Book Medical.

108. Fishman, M., Thirlwell, M., & Daly, D. (1983). Mallory-Weiss tear: A complication of cancer chemotherapy. Cancer *52*:2031–2032.

109. Burish, T. G., & Lyles, J. N. (1981). Effectiveness of relaxation training in reducing adverse reactions to cancer chemotherapy. J Behav Med *4*:65–78.

110. Jacox, A. K. (1979) Pain assessment. Am J Nurs *79*:895–900.

111. Barton, M. D., Libonati, M., & Cohen, P. J. (1975). The use of haloperidol for treatment of postoperative nausea and vomiting: A double-blind placebo-controlled trial. Anesthesiology *42*:508–512.

112. Parkes, J. D. (1986). A neurologist's view of nausea and vomiting. In C. J. Davis, G. V. Lake-Bakaar, & D. G. Grahame-Smith (eds.), *Nausea and Vomiting: Mechanisms and Treatment*. Berlin: Springer-Verlag.

113. Hall, B., Hardesty, I., & Hogan, R. (1991). Nutrition alteration: In less than body requirements related to nausea and vomiting. In J. McNally, E. Somerville, C. Miaskowski, & M. Rostad (eds.), *Guidelines for Oncology Nursing Practice* (2nd ed., pp. 173–178). Philadelphia: W. B. Saunders.

114. Morrow, G. (1988). Anticipatory nausea. Cancer Invest *6*:327–327.

115. Baird, S. (1988). *Decision Making in Oncology Nursing*. Toronto: B. C. Decker.

116. Carnevali, D., & Reiner, A. (1990). *The Cancer Experience: Nursing Diagnosis and Management*. Philadelphia: J. B. Lippincott.

117. Goodman, M. (1987). Management of nausea and vomiting induced by outpatient cisplatin therapy. Semin Oncol Nurs *3*:23–35.

118. Merrifield, K., & Chaffee, B. (1989). Recent advances in the management of nausea and vomiting caused by antineoplastic agents. Clin Pharmacol *8*:187–199.

119. Gift, L. (1989). Visual analog scales: Measurement of subjective phenomena. Nurs Res *28*:286–288.

120. Lee, K., & Kieckhefer, G. (1989). Measuring human responses using visual analogue scales. West J Nurs Res *11*:128–132.

121. Kris, M., Gralla, R., Tyson, L., Clark, R., Cirrincione, C., & Groshen, S. (1989). Controlling delayed vomiting: Double-blind, randomized trial comparing placebo, dexamethasone alone, and metoclopramide plus dexamethasone in patients receiving cisplatin. J Clin Oncol *3*:1379–1384.

122. Cotanch, P. (1988). Measuring nausea and vomiting. In M. Frank-Stromborg (ed.), *Instruments for Clinical Nursing Research* (pp. 313–322). East Norwalk, CT: Appleton & Lange.

123. Cotanch, P., & Strum, S. (1987). Progressive muscle relaxation as antiemetic therapy for cancer patients. Oncol Nurs Forum *14*:33–37.

124. Morrow, G. (1984). The assessment of nausea and vomiting: Past problems, current issues, and suggestions for future research. Cancer *53*:51–62.

125. Gard, D., Harris, J., Edwards, P., & McCormack, G. (1988). Sensitizing effects of pretreatment measures on cancer chemotherapy nausea and vomiting. J Consult Clin Psychol *56*:80–84.

126. Rhodes, V., Watson, P., & Hansen, B. (1988). Patients' descriptions of the influence of tiredness and weakness on self-care abilities. Cancer Nurs *11*:186–194.

127. Headley, J. A. (1987). The influence of administration time on chemotherapy-induced nausea and vomiting. Oncol Nurs Forum *14*:43–47.

128. McMillan, S., Johnston, L., Tedford, K., & Harley, C. (1989). Measurement of chemotherapy-induced nausea and vomiting. Appl Nurs Res *2*:93–95.

129. DiIorio, C. (1985). First trimester nausea in pregnant teenagers: Incidence, characteristics, intervention. Nurs Res *34*:372–374.

130. Iatrakis, G., Sakellaropoulos, G., Kourkoubas, A., & Kabounia, S. (1988). Vomiting and nausea in the first 12 weeks of pregnancy. Psychother Psychosom *49*:22–24.

131. Larson, P., & Dodd, M. (1991). The cancer treatment experience: Family models of caring. In D. Gaut & M. Leininger (eds.), *Caring: The Compassionate Healer*. New York: National League for Nursing.

132. Oberst, M. T. (1984). Methodology in behavioral and psychosocial cancer research. Patients' perception of care. Measurement of quality and satisfaction. Cancer *54*(Suppl. 10):2366–2375.

133. Frank, J. G. (1985). The effects of music therapy and guided visual imagery on chemotherapy-induced nausea and vomiting. Oncol Nurs Forum *12*:47–52.

134. Morrow, G., Lindke, J., & Black, R. M. (1991). Anticipatory nausea development in cancer patients: Replication and extension of a learning model. Br J Psychol *82*:61–72.

135. Morrow, G. (1986). Behavioral management of chemotherapy-induced nausea and vomiting in the cancer patient. Clin Oncol *1*:11–14.

136. Weddington, W., Miller, N., & Sweet, D. (1982). Anticipatory nausea and vomiting associated with cancer chemotherapy. N Engl J Med *307*:825–826.

137. Morrow, G. (1986). Effect of the cognitive hierarchy in the systematic desensitization treatment of anticipatory nausea in cancer patients: A component comparison with relaxation only, counseling and no treatment. Cog Ther Res *10*:421–446.

138. Cotanch, P. H. (1983). Relaxation for control of nausea and vomiting in patients receiving chemotherapy. Cancer Nurs *6*:277–283.

139. Scott, D., Donahue, D., Mastrovito, R., & Hakes, T. (1986). Comparative trial of clinical relaxation and an antiemetic drug regimen in reducing chemotherapy-related nausea and vomiting. Cancer Nurs *9*:178–187.

140. Lyles, J., Burish, T., Krozely, M., & Oldham, R. K. (1982). Efficacy of relaxation training and guided imagery in reducing the aversiveness of cancer chemotherapy. J Consult Clinical Psychol *50*:509–524.

141. Morrow, G. R., & Morrell, B. S. (1982). Behavioral treatment for the anticipatory nausea and vomiting induced by cancer chemotherapy. N Engl J Med *307*:1476–1480.

142. Dodd, M. J. (1986). Self-care in patients with cancer. In R. McCorkle & G. Hongladorum (eds.), *Issues and Topics Cancer Nursing*, (pp. 143–169). East Norwalk, CT: Appleton-Century-Crofts.

143. Dodd, M. J. (1988). Patterns of self-care in cancer patients with breast cancer receiving chemotherapy. West J Nurs Res *10*:7–24.

144. Larson, P., Koetters, T., & Benner, P. (1992). Final Report of Oncology Nursing Foundation grant. *Clinical Ethnography of Two Cancer Trajectories*. Unpublished manuscript, University of California, San Francisco, Dept. of Physiological Nursing.

145. Voda, A., & Randall, M. (1982). Nausea and vomiting of pregnancy: "Morning sickness." In C. Norris (ed.), *Concept Clarification in Nursing*. Rockville, MD: Aspen.

146. Bodner, M., & White, P. F. (1991). Antiemetic efficacy of ondansetron after outpatient laparoscopy. Anesth Analg *73*:250–254.

147. Larjani, G. E., Gratz, I., Afshar, M., & Minassian, S. (1991). Treatment of postoperative nausea and vomiting with ondansetron: A randomized, double-blind comparison with placebo. Anesth Analg *73*:246–249.

148. Leeser, J., & Lip, H. (1991). Prevention of postoperative nausea and vomiting using ondansetron, a new selective, 5-HT3 receptor antagonist. Anesth Analg *72*:751–755.

149. Winningham, M., & MacVicar, M. (1988). The effect of aerobic exercise on patient reports of nausea. Oncol Nurs Forum *15*:447–450.

150. Sridhar, K., & Donnelly, E. (1988). Combination antiemetics for cisplatin chemotherapy. Cancer *61*:1508–1517.

151. Addelman, M., Erlichman, C., Fine, S., Warr, D., & Murray, C. (1990). Phase I/II Trial of Granisetron: A novel 5-hydroxytryptamine antagonist for the prevention of chemotherapy-induced nausea and vomiting. J Clin Oncol *8*:337–341.

152. Dodd, M. J. (1982). Assessing patient self-care for side effects. Cancer Nurs *5*:447–451.

153. Dodd, M. J. (1983). Self-care for side effects of cancer chemotherapy: An assessment of nursing interventions. Cancer Nurs *6*:63–67.

154. Dodd, M. J. (1984). Measuring informational intervention for chemotherapy and self-care behaviors. Res Nurs Health *7*:43–50.

155. Dodd, M. J. (1984). Patterns of self-care in cancer patients receiving radiation therapy. Oncol Nurs Forum *10*:23–27.

156. Musci, E. C. (1983). Relationship between family coping strategies and self-care during cancer chemotherapy treatment. Doctoral dissertation. University of California, San Francisco.

157. Musci, E. C., & Dodd, M. J. (1990). Predicting self-care with patients and family members' effective states and family function. Oncol Nurs Forum *17*:394–400.

158. Bruhn, J. G., & Phillips, B. O. (1984). Measuring social support: A synthesis of current approaches. J Behav Med *7*:151–169.

159. Cobb, S. (1976). Social support as a moderator of life stress. Psychosom Med *38*:300–314.

160. Norbeck, J. S., Lindsey, A. M., & Carrieri, V. L. (1981). The development of an instrument to measure social support. Nurs Res *30*:4–9.

161. Lazarus, R. S., & Folkman, S. (1984). *Stress Appraisal and Coping*. New York: Springer.

162. Tilden, V. P. (1985). Issues of conceptualization and measurement of social support in the construction of nursing theory. Res Nurs Health *8*:199–206.

163. Cotanch, R., Hockenberry, M., & Herman, S. (1985). Self-hypnosis as antiemetic therapy in children receiving chemotherapy. Oncol Nurs Forum *12*:41–46.

164. Kris, M. G., Tyson, L. B., Gralla, R. J., Clark, R. A., Allen, J. C., & Reilly, L. K. (1983). Extrapyramidal reactions with high-dose metoclopramide. N Engl J Med *309*:433.

165. Sallan, S., Zinberg, N., & Frei, E. (1975). Antiemetic effect of delta-9-tetrahydrocannabinol in patients receiving cancer chemotherapy. N Engl J Med *293*:795.

166. Sallan, S., Cronin, C., Zelen, M., & Zinberg, N. (1980). Antiemetics in patients receiving chemotherapy for cancer: A randomized comparison of delta-9-tetrahydrocannabinol and prochlorperazine. N Engl J Med *302*:135.

167. Hrushesky, W. (1985). Circadian timing of cancer chemotherapy. Science *288*:73–75.

168. Hrushesky, W., Vukelich, M., Halberg, F., Levi, F., Langevin, T., Kennedy, D. J., Gergen, J., Goetz, F. & Theologidis, A. (1981). Optimum circadian treatment time reduces cis-diamminedichloroplatinum-induced vomiting. Int J Chemobiol *7*:64.

169. Moore, J. (1982). The influence of time of administration on cisplatinum-induced nausea and vomiting. Oncol Nurs Forum *9*:26–32.

III

ALTERATIONS IN PROTECTION

Protection, viewed as a life process, involves numerous complex mechanisms, host-environment interactions, and reactions. Protection as a process results in shielding the individual from stressors or in altering the impact of the stressors. Like the life process regulation, the process of protection encompasses interactions that promote and maintain homeostasis, that is, ensuring an environment conducive to the normal functioning of the total organism. Protective mechanisms are physiological, psychological, and sociological. However, the major foci of the chapters in this section are alterations in the physiological mechanisms of protection.

Physiological protective mechanisms are pervasive throughout the body and are the structural and functional defenses that serve to protect the individual against such stressors as physical and chemical injury, mutagens, carcinogens, foreign bodies, and microorganisms. Examples of the wide range of protective mechanisms operating in the individual include detoxification of drugs and other potentially harmful chemicals by the liver, the cough reflex that protects the respiratory tract from foreign bodies, the thick mucus barrier that protects the stomach against the corrosive effects of hydrochloric acid, the increased production of red blood cells to protect body tissues from hypoxia, the finely tuned neuromotor reflexes that remove the body from harmful stimuli to avoid injury, and the first line of defense, the skin, which shields the internal structures from the external environment. Alterations in the body's protective mechanisms can have local or systemic effects, and the consequences can range from minor to fatal.

The five chapters in this section discuss alterations in protection that manifest the wide diversity, effects, and consequences discussed above. They are the stress response, immunosuppression, impaired wound healing, altered clotting, and impaired sleep.

The stress response is viewed as an adaptive, protective mechanism that occurs when endogenous or exogenous stimuli are sensed as threatening to the individual. Stimuli include psychological and physiological stressors; a myriad of responses result to allow the individual to respond to danger or to protect adaptive processes.

Immunosuppression can result from many therapies and clinical conditions. Immunocompetence is essential to protect against infectious organisms, foreign bodies or tissue, and antigens. Alterations in immunocompetence can result in serious consequences for the individual.

Infection results when protective mechanisms have been compromised. The alterations in protection, that is, etiologic explanations for the infection, may range from a very simple wound to multiple traumatic injuries occurring in a leukemic child with bone marrow suppression.

Alterations in clotting reflect a state of imbalance in one or more of the multiple factors and processes involved in the mechanisms of hemostasis. Alterations in any of these mechanisms result in potential impairment of tissue oxygenation and metabolism.

Sleep disturbances are reflected in alterations in the sleep stages; these range from a minor occasional problem to a severe condition in which the individual becomes dysfunctional or disoriented.

In each chapter, populations at risk for alterations in protection are identified as well as commonly encountered diagnoses and clinical states that compromise one or more of the protective mechanisms. The professional nurse must be aware of individuals whose protective mechanisms may be impaired and who require therapeutic interventions. The mechanisms for each alteration and the pathological consequences to the individual are presented. Manifestations of the alterations are delineated, and various parameters for monitoring the patient's state of protection and response to therapies over time are identified.

Understanding the mechanisms by which alterations in protection occur provides the means for developing instruments to measure and assess these human responses and for implementing appropriate management strategies. In this way, nursing practice is influenced by the state of knowledge about the phenomena.

16

Stress Response

Ada M. Lindsey
Virginia Carrieri-Kohlman
Gayle Giboney Page

DEFINITION

Much has been written about stress; the primary approaches used have included stress as a response to a severe injury, explication of stress and coping paradigms, delineation of stressful life events, and suggestions for stress reduction therapies. In more recently published literature on stress, there has been considerably less confusion about the differences between stressors and the resulting stress response. In earlier reports, these two notions frequently were described interchangeably. In the nursing literature, there still is a paucity of work describing stress from a physiological response perspective. The focus of this chapter is the stress response as a physiological response to biopsychosocial stressors.

A variety of definitions have been given to the phenomenon, and the emphasis depends on the approach or framework being posited. Sociologists, psychologists, physiologists, and nurses have studied the effects of multiple stressors and have used a variety of parameters to determine the resulting stress response. The nature of each of these disciplines and the individual work done have, to some extent, influenced the approaches used, leading to rather disparate bodies of information about stress. Although the intent is to describe the stress response from a physiological perspective, the following definition has been created to encompass the salient, distinguishing characteristics of the phenomenon.

Stress is a sociopsychophysiological phenomenon. It is a composite of intellectual, behavioral, metabolic, immune, and other physiological responses to a stressor (or stressors) of endogenous or exogenous origins. The stressors may involve thoughts and feelings or may be a perceived threat (actual or potential) or some afferent input signaling injury, illness, or other conditions such as cold. The response generally serves a protective, adaptive function. It is graded; that is, the extent of the response depends on the magnitude (intensity and duration) of the afferent signals (stimuli). It is an integrated hypothalamic response that in addition to being subject to the strength and temporal characteristics of the stimulus is further modified by individual characteristics such as genetic endowment, age, gender, previous experiences, and concurrent illness. The multiple components included in this definition are addressed within this chapter.

PREVALENCE AND POPULATIONS AT RISK

There are no specific reports on the prevalence or incidence of the stress response. Inasmuch as stressors, whether from sociological, psychological, or physiological sources, are ubiquitous (when considering life in general), it becomes obvious that the prevalence of the stress response is great. According to the definition, it is important to acknowledge that although the response generally serves a protective, adaptive function, it is a graded response, such that there is a point at which it may even result in death. What remains somewhat difficult to quantify precisely is the varying magnitude of these responses and the specific circumstances in which they occur.

Studies in which attempts have been made to measure the stress response have used a variety of parameters to indicate the magnitude of this response. Anxiety scales, heart rate, blood pressure, levels of plasma and urinary catecholamines and cortisol, antibody production, and natural killer cell activity are examples of the variety of these parameters. Studies have also used different samples and different stimuli (stressors) as independent variables as well as the different measurement parameters (as indicators of the dependent-outcome variable, the stress response). It is not possible to be more definitive about the prevalence of the stress response; however, it is a common phenomenon and it is of varying magnitude with varying consequences.

Individuals experiencing the situational or developmental stressors described below represent populations at risk. People who are at risk for the greater stress response are those who are already compromised in some way. For example, if someone were in a serious auto accident, had multiple traumatic injuries, had undergone surgery, and then developed a wound infection, this subsequent infection might escalate the stress response. In contrast, individuals in whom the hypothalamic-pituitary-adrenal axis is not intact or is compromised may have a diminished capacity for responding to stressors. Clinical examples include patients who have adrenal or pituitary gland dysfunction or who have undergone adrenalectomy.

Concurrent sociological, psychological, or pathophysiological problems place the individual at risk for a greater stress response when some other stimulus or insult is encountered. Those with diminished or compromised physiological reserves, such as premature infants, older adults, or people with multiple traumatic injuries or concurrent illness, are at greater risk for having a less than adequate response to encountered significant stressors. If the magnitude of the stressors remains great and the existing reserves requisite for the stress response are compromised or diminished or remain untreated in cases in which the hypothalamic-pituitary-adrenal axis is dysfunctional, death may occur.

SITUATIONAL AND DEVELOPMENTAL STRESSORS

Multiple situational stressors are encountered in the day-to-day environment. These can be the daily hassles of finding a parking place, receiving unexpected news, or experiencing a cold environment, or they can be of a more severe nature, such as being involved in an accident, being informed that surgery is necessary, receiving a diagnosis of cancer, or sustaining a burn. Infection, shock, starvation, pain, surgery, emotional arousal, such as fear and anxiety, and even exercise are situational stressors. Plasma levels of cortisol, adrenocorticotropic hormone (ACTH), epinephrine, and norepinephrine are increased with strenuous exercise, and when there is a sense of competition to win an event, the stress may be heightened.

Events that occur along the developmental or age continuum may be perceived as stressors; for example, the multiple developmental tasks associated with the adolescent period or the period of adulthood when children leave home or a job change in adulthood may be stressors. Major life events, such as moving, divorce, and death of a loved one, have been studied as stressors. The individual's perception and interpretation (appraisal) of the stressors influence the magnitude of the response. The response is further modified by a number of other circumstances, such as the individual's age, gender, previous experiences, social support available, and concurrent illness.

A great deal of stress-related research uses animals, with the intention of modeling the phenomenon of stress in humans. The responses of animals subjected to a stressful experience can be compared to animals in the same environment without the stressor; in this way, outcomes may be directly attributed to the stressful situation. Stressors used in animal research may be painful or nonpainful. Nonpainful stressors include forced swim stress, restraint stress, and predator exposure stress; painful stressors include surgical stress (e.g., laparotomy and hind limb amputation) and footshock or tailshock stress.

The prevailing thought is that the human response to stressors is an individual phenomenon. The same stressor does not have the same effect on all individuals experiencing that particular stressor, although some outcomes of some stressors, such as surgery, are similar among individuals.

Clinical States or Diagnoses

In addition to the examples given above, a myriad of reports are associated with other clinical states and stress.[1-10] Some may be viewed as evidence of stress or as pathological consequences of the stress response. These include migraine headaches, peptic and duodenal ulcers, obesity, drug and alcohol abuse, compromised immunocompetence, assorted cardiovascular problems such as angina and hypertension, and even the occurrence of cancer. The extent to which stressors and the stress response contribute to or result in these clinical states remains a circumstance of association, as there is, as yet, no absolute or definitive proof. There are, however, data that strongly suggest these relationships.

Other clinical states are viewed as being the stressor that results in a stress response. For example, clinical states that are potent afferent stimuli and that result in increased sympathetic nervous system discharge are acute hypovolemia, acute hypoglycemia, and hypoxia.[5] In each of these states there is a deficiency in a required central nervous system (CNS) substrate. A stress response to emotional arousal, such as fear or anxiety, which may occur with the thought of impending surgery or other circumstances, may augment or exceed the concurrent physiological response to the illness or injury. Some cases of fibrillation following myocardial infarction have been postulated to be the result of a stress response.

Cohen and Williamson have proposed two models suggesting the role of stress in influencing infectious disease pathology and illness behaviors.[11] While acknowledging that there are stressor-induced health-promoting behaviors, they primarily propose a model to explain stress-induced illness behaviors. They focus on the negative stressful events and affective states and view stress as a state of psychological distress. They suggest that the relationship between stress and susceptibility to infection is mediated through immune system function as modulated via the neuroendocrine hormones that are released in response to stress. This response may result in immunosuppression; what remains unknown is whether or not the magnitude or duration of the suppression and the types of cells involved are changed sufficiently to alter host resistance significantly. Another unanswered question is related to the time course; what is the length of time required, that is, exposure to a stressor, before negative biological changes result?

A review of studies in which stress and infection or stress and illness behaviors are examined shows that the evidence is insufficient to support a relationship between onset of upper respiratory infections and stress; however, there is evidence of an association between stress and illness behaviors.

Another clinical state is risk taking or thrill seeking. This raises other questions. Are there pleasurable and enjoyable stressors, and, if so, do the responses to these stressors contribute to the same changes that result from unpleasant or harmful stressors? Tache and Selye have commented that "it is not what happens to you but how you take it."[12] The following excerpt written by Vaillant clearly exemplifies this idea.

> Last spring, I was watching a loop-the-loop roller coaster. I knew that for me such rides are stressful, and I contemplated the physiologic wear and tear that would ensue were I to make the ride. Undoubtedly, the experience would sequester calcium in my bursae, erode the lining of my stomach, deposit cholesterol in the intima of my arteries, compromise my immune system with an outpouring of corticosteroids and, metaphorically at least, take years off my life. But as I watched the excited passengers gather speed, sweep up the loop and hang suspended upside-down with their arms waving, I saw that for them the experience was one of joy, release and even relaxation. By what alchemy had their central nervous system mitigated an experience that should have been noxious to their health? The difference between them and myself, had I ventured to join them, would not have been the external stress and the imposed helplessness. The difference would have been in the ways by which our minds distorted the experience.
>
> If many environmental stimuli endanger health only because of the symbolic meaning the recipient attaches to them, others, like the roller coaster, are made safe because of unconscious mechanisms of adaptation. As the power of the placebo illustrates, man's capacity for ingenious self-deception seems infinite, and the wisdom of the body may be no match for the benign alchemy of the mind[13] (p. 732).

Teleologically, the stress response has evolved for the benefit it has for survival. Modern society has imposed new values that are perceived by some as important for "survival" and as more or less stressful, for example, achieving greater social or educational status. These new stressors are predominantly psychological in nature, yet they elicit "old world" physiological survival responses. This idea is conveyed by the following quote from Tache and Selye: "Taking an exam does not have the same survival significance as . . . facing a pack of wolves, yet we have not learned to respond in a different way to those stressors"[12] (p. 21). Events or hassles encountered every day may not be life-threatening, but they still may be perceived as stressors. Pleasurable social occasions also may be stressors.

Stress as a response of people to their social environment is given as an explanation for the occurrence of an illness or has been shown to be associated with the onset of illness.[14–17] Stress is important to acknowledge not only because of the expressed general feelings of discomfort but also because of its potential influence on the onset of illness as well as its augmenting influence on concurrent illness. Perceptions regarding the controllability and predictability of the stressor have been shown to be of some importance in studies examining the effects of stress on the immune systems in animals. These relationships are too variable to draw conclusions at this point, but there are sufficient data to support the notion that the psychological attributes of a stressor can differentially affect immune function.[18]

MECHANISMS

The response to a stressor involves multiple mechanisms.[5, 6, 19–26] As noted in the definition, the response is integrated through the hypothalamus and is a graded response, depending on the individual and the magnitude of the afferent signals. The systems participating in the stress response are depicted in Figure 16–1. The process requires many feedback loops (not shown in Fig. 16–1), and the response results in an altered physiological equilibrium.

As shown in Figure 16–1, the afferent input that is generated from sensory or psychological stimuli (stressors) is processed locally and then ultimately within the central nervous system. Neural information is forwarded to the hypothalamus. Through hypothalamic integration, an orderly response is achieved; that is, the hypothalamus coordinates the homeostatic adjustments. Hypothalamic output influences three major responses: (1) the sympathetic nervous system discharge via the autonomic nervous system, (2) the release of selected anterior pituitary hormones via stimulation from hypothalamic-releasing or release-inhibiting factors, and (3) release of vasopressin in the posterior pituitary from hypothalamic neurons.

As one continues to the next level depicted in Figure 16–1, it is important to recognize that sympathetic nervous system discharge influences responses in other systems and organs. Increased palmar sweat is an example of an exocrine gland response. There are responses to the sympathetic discharge in several major organs (e.g., liver, pancreas, spleen, bone marrow, and kidney) and in other peripheral tissues innervated with sympathetic nerve endings. The adrenal medulla also responds to sympathetic discharge. Because the processes involved in these responses are multiple and complex, complete explication is beyond the scope of this chapter; they are described simply and briefly.

Release of norepinephrine by the sympathetic nerve endings results in glycogenolysis in the liver (i.e., conversion of stored glycogen to glucose), decrease in insulin and increase in glucagon secretion in the pancreas, inhibition of glucose uptake by peripheral tissues, release of renin by the kidney, increase in vascular smooth muscle contraction, and a number of other cardiopulmonary responses, including increased heart rate and contractility. Two central notions are that both substrate and energy metabolism and cardiovascular functions are affected. The net effects of the release of norepinephrine are the increase in blood glucose levels, the peripheral catabolism of protein and fat, and the increase in cardiac output (and consequently increased myocardial oxygen demand), heart rate, respiratory rate, and blood pressure. These changes occur, presuming that these systems are not compromised, and are capable of responding to the sympathetic discharge.

In response to the sympathetic discharge, epinephrine is released primarily from the adrenal medulla. Circulating epinephrine inhibits the uptake of glucose by peripheral

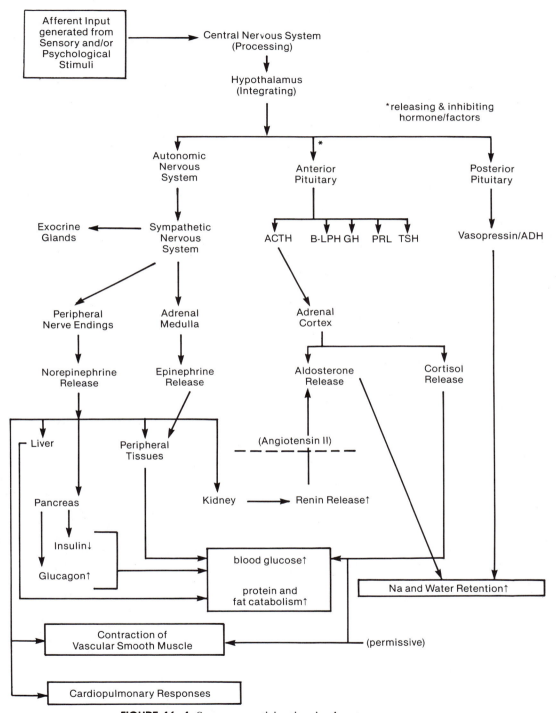

FIGURE 16–1. Systems participating in the stress response.

tissues, thus contributing to the increased levels of blood glucose. Epinephrine also promotes the peripheral catabolism of protein and fat for conversion to energy substrate. Epinephrine also contributes to the observed cardiopulmonary responses.

Increased secretion of ACTH from the anterior pituitary is the most dramatic pituitary response. Corticotropin-releasing factor (CRF) is secreted from hypothalamic neurons in response to stressors; in response to CRF, ACTH and other peptides such as beta-lipotropin and its subunit, beta-endorphin, are released from the anterior pituitary. As noted in Figure 16–1, release of other anterior pituitary hormones (growth hormone, prolactin, and thyroid-stimulating hormone) also occurs in the stress response. ACTH primarily stimulates release of cortisol and to a much lesser extent (when ACTH secretion is great) aldosterone from the adrenal cortex. Aldosterone is secreted in response to sodium and potassium levels and to angiotensin II (a product resulting from the action of renin on precursor molecules).

Increased cortisol secretion from the adrenal cortex is the most notable response to increased ACTH. Cortisol influences a great many processes; it has a potentiating effect on the actions of epinephrine and glucagon, with the net effect resulting in an increased blood glucose level. Cortisol exerts a permissive effect, resulting in the sustained vascular smooth muscle response (contraction) to catecholamines (epinephrine and norepinephrine). Without cortisol, this response would not be sustained.

Increased cortisol alters the immune and inflammatory responses. In animals, thymicolymphatic involution, eosinopenia, and immune deficiency have been observed as a response to prolonged, increased cortisol levels. In humans, decreased lymphocytes have been reported in response to minor surgery and psychologically based stress; a decrease in both T-cell and B-cell lymphocytes has been observed in response to major surgery. In response to tissue damage or infection, peptide-labeled lymphokines are secreted; a number of lymphokines are under the regulatory influence of glucocorticoids.

Heavy exercise induces leukocytosis, granulocytosis, and lymphocytosis and increases the number of natural killer cells; these alterations are variable by type and duration of exercise and condition of individual and

are relatively transient.[24] Some of the findings suggest that exercise results in a transient suppression of immune function. It is not known whether the exercise itself results in the observed immune system changes or whether the alterations are caused by the neuroendocrine (hormonal) response to the stressor.

The precise mechanisms of the effects of stress on immunity are largely unknown; however, research focusing on this issue is at the forefront of psychoneuroimmunology, the study of relationships between the nervous and immune systems. Most evidence to date suggests that the nervous system can modulate the immune system. Potential sources for this "direction" of communication include catecholamines, steroids, and other hormones such as endorphins. Signals from the brain and neuroendocrine system are transported to the immune system via the autonomic nervous system and hormonal secretion, and the immune system communicates with the brain via cytokines. There is considerable evidence that the thymus, spleen, and bone marrow are innervated by the autonomic nervous system, the sympathetic branch in particular. The existence of adrenergic receptors on T cells, B cells, and macrophages supports the likely presence of sympathetic innervation of immune organs, although the functional role of such innervation is not clear. Corticosteroids such as cortisol are well known to exert immunosuppressive effects, but stimulatory effects have been reported as well.[25, 26]

Target tissue for aldosterone action is the renal tubule cells, with the net result being retention of sodium and excretion of potassium. Vasopressin (antidiuretic hormone [ADH]) is released from hypothalamic neurons terminating in the posterior pituitary. Target tissue for vasopressin action is also renal tubule cells, but the net result is resorption of water from the renal tubules. Thus, in the kidney, secretion of renin in response to the sympathetic discharge, retention of sodium in response to adrenal cortex secretion of aldosterone, and retention of water in response to ADH participate in the net defense of fluid volume.

A summary of the actions of the glucoregulatory hormones involved in altering substrate metabolism in the stress response is given in Table 16–1. The net effect of insulin is to lower blood glucose levels; however, in

TABLE 16–1 GLUCOREGULATORY HORMONES

Hormone	Action
Insulin*	Inhibits hepatic glucose production Enhances glucose and AA uptake by peripheral tissues Enhances glycogen synthesis
Glucagon	↑ Hepatic glucose production (gluconeogenesis) Glycogenolytic
Catecholamines	↑ Hepatic glucose production Glycogenolytic Inhibits insulin secretion → ↑ AA from muscle Stimulates lipolysis → ↑ FFA ↑ Peripheral uptake of glucose
Cortisol	Potentiates effects of glucagon and catecholamines on hepatic glucose production
Growth hormone (somatotropin)	In periphery, antagonizes effects of insulin Resets response to glucose Stimulates release of FFA

*The net effect of insulin is to lower the blood glucose level. The net effect of other regulatory hormones is to increase the blood glucose level (hyperglycemia). Each of the counter regulatory hormones antagonizes one or more of the effects of insulin.

Abbreviations: AA, amino acids; FFA, free fatty acids.
Key: ↑ , increase; →, leads to or results in.

response to the sympathetic discharge, less insulin is secreted. In addition, there is an increased secretion of the other glucoregulatory hormones that antagonize the effects of insulin. If the stress is of sufficient magnitude, hyperglycemia results.[2, 5, 27]

The stress response is a neuroendocrine response that is generally protective and homeostatic. It is a response to threatening external stimuli or to changes originating from the individual's internal environment. There is some evidence that repeated exposure to stressors results in adaptive changes. For example, in rats subjected to repeated stimuli, an increase in adrenal tissue levels of tyrosine hydroxylase occurred.[28] Tyrosine hydroxylase is an enzyme that catalyzes the process of synthesis of norepinephrine and epinephrine; thus, elevated levels of tyrosine hydroxylase increase the capacity for synthesis of the catecholamines involved in the stress response. It is apparent, even from this very cursory overview, that a number of systems and a number of complex, interrelated mechanisms are involved in the stress response. The net effects are the increased availability of energy substrate and maintenance of adequate blood volume and pressure. A summary of the neuroendocrine responses, the metabolic processes, and the net results is provided in Table 16–2. Stressors elicit integrated neuroendocrine responses involving complex interactions; this stress response is protective and adaptive. Characteristics of the stress response are summarized in Table 16–3.

A reparative phase follows the stress response. Without a change in nitrogen intake, a decrease in the excretion of urinary nitrogen signals the occurrence of the reparative phase. The time for reparation of nitrogen loss is dependent on the extent of the loss;

TABLE 16–2 SUMMARY OF NEUROENDOCRINE STRESS RESPONSES AND RESULTING EFFECTS

Neuroendocrine	Effects on Metabolic Processes	Net Results
↑ Catecholamines ↑ Glucocorticoids ↑ Glucagon ↑ Growth hormone ↓ Insulin	Glycogenolysis Gluconeogenesis Lipolysis Proteolysis	Provision of substrate for energy
↑ Catecholamines ↑ Glucocorticoids ↑ Vasopressin (ADH) ↑ Aldosterone	Sodium and water retention	Defense of fluid volume
Reparative Phrase ↑ Insulin ↓ Glucagon ↑ Growth hormone and other growth factors ↑ Thyroid hormones		*Net Results* Protein synthesis Cell proliferation Restoration of fat deposits

Key: ↑ , increase; ↓ , decrease.

TABLE 16–3 CHARACTERISTICS OF THE STRESS RESPONSE

Stress response is natural and generally protective and adaptive.

There are normal responses to stressors (stressors encountered in everyday circumstances increase catecholamine excretion).

Physical and emotional stressors trigger similar responses (specificity versus nonspecificity: magnitude and patterns may differ).

Magnitude and duration of stressors may be so great that homeostatic mechanisms for adjustment fail, leading to death; there are limits in ability to compensate.

Repeated exposure to stimuli results in adaptive changes, that is, tissue levels of tyrosine hydroxylase increase capacity for synthesis of norepinephrine and epinephrine.

There are individual differences in response to the same stressors, although some stressors, such as major surgery, result in a very similar pattern of hormonal and immune consequences.

the rate of restoration is approximately 3 to 5 g of nitrogen per 70 kg/day. After nitrogen balance is achieved, restoration of fat deposits occurs.[5] The entire reparative phase may continue for several weeks to several months. During the reparative phase, there is an anabolic pattern resulting in protein synthesis, cell proliferation, and eventually fat deposition. Table 16–2 summarizes the reparative phase.

One cannot consider the stress response without acknowledgment of the very early work of Hans Selye in describing the "nonspecific" effects of the stress response. From animal experiments, he labeled the responses observed as the "general adaptation syndrome" (GAS); this GAS is characterized by three phases: an alarm reaction, resistance and adaptation, and exhaustion. After continued exposure to stressors, a triad of pathological consequences occurs: adrenal gland enlargement, thymus gland involution, and gastrointestinal ulcerations.[21] Review of current empirical work provides evidence that refutes many of Selye's theories. Work by Mason and others suggests that the stress response is specific, given the particular properties of the stressful stimulus; that is, the characteristics of the stress response vary with the type of stressor.[29–34] This is in contrast to Selye's early work and presents the continuing refinement of the phenomenon. Selye reported his later views on this controversy in the field of stress research.[35] For further examples and explanation of these

ideas, refer to the review articles by Mason and others.[29–34]

Moore provides a historical summary of the contributions of early scientists to the current understanding of the homeostatic responses to stressors such as trauma and surgery.[5] These scientists include Charles Darwin, Claude Bernard, Walter Cannon, Harvey Cushing, David Cuthbertson, and Hans Selye. Moore also reviews the physiological responses that occur with acute injury.

In a review of the physiological functions of glucocorticoids in stress, Munck and colleagues hypothesize and make a case that the net result of glucocorticoid action is to suppress rather than enhance normal defense mechanisms.[34] They suggest that this inhibition occurs after an initial increase in these defense mechanisms and that this inhibition is protective; that is, the defense mechanisms are "damped or switched off" after the initial increase. If the defense mechanisms are activated for a prolonged period, they may cause damage or otherwise compromise survival. This proposed damping effect of glucocorticoids prevents a prolonged response that would threaten homeostatic balance.[34]

Pathological Consequences

Clinical states such as migraine headaches, asthmatic attacks, obesity, and hypertension may, in some circumstances, be considered pathological consequences of stress. Direct evidence of pathological causation remains problematic; the evidence to date is rather one of association. There are situations, however, in which pathological consequences do result from the stress response. The response to a severe traumatic injury is an example.[2, 5] With moderate to severe trauma, lipolysis, proteolysis, gluconeogenesis, and ureagenesis occur. Amino acids are mobilized primarily from skeletal muscle. The liver converts the carbon fragments to new glucose and forms urea from the nitrogen residues that are excreted as urinary nitrogen. The nitrogen loss is related to the size of the injury and other influencing factors such as poor nutritional intake and lack of muscle activity. Because glycogen stores in the liver are limited, the gluconeogenesis increases or maintains serum glucose levels. This protective response is requisite to preserve the function of glucose-dependent tissues. With lipolysis of triglycerides, the free fatty acids cannot be converted to glucose but the glycerol moieties can be used through the Krebs cycle to provide an energy source and the fatty acids can be used as an energy source by some tissues.

If there is negligible or insufficient nutrient intake beyond a few days following a situation that produces a profound stress response, mobilization of fat stores will provide the energy source for those tissues in which glucose is not obligatory. Glucose as the energy source is provided via gluconeogenesis, primarily at the expense of body protein. This catabolic response (proteolysis) to injury or other stressors is characterized by hyperglycemia and increased urinary nitrogen; thus, the pathological consequence occurring in critically stressed individuals is the loss of muscle mass and nitrogen. Weight loss, although not an obligatory factor, reflects the difference between the energy required and the substrate provided exogenously.

Surgery is a physiological stressor. The surgical stress response prominently includes neuroendocrine, metabolic, and inflammatory responses to the acute injury. ACTH levels increase markedly by 1 hour following the start of surgery. Further, the plasma concentrations of ACTH and cortisol seem to have no predictable relationship during a typical perioperative period. Peak concentrations of cortisol are reached within a few hours of surgery, and the duration of elevated plasma cortisol levels varies. The magnitude of hypercortisolism generally correlates with the invasiveness of the surgery. As can be seen in Figure 16–1, hypothalamic activation of the autonomic nervous system results in a cascade of effects on metabolism and the cardiovascular system.[36, 37] The surgically stressed system is thrust into a hypermetabolic state in which there is increased demand for nutrients to promote healing, and there is accelerated metabolism resulting from the physiological stress of surgery. It is important to know that the very young, including neonates, are capable of mounting a stress response to surgery.[38]

Some evidence suggests that the endogenous opioid system plays a role in the stress response to surgery. It is known that the mu-opioid and kappa-opioid receptors affect the hypothalamic-pituitary-adrenal (HPA) axis in surgical stress, and beta-endorphin (core-leased with ACTH at the anterior pituitary) levels may negatively impact homeostasis.[39, 40]

An example from animal research illustrates the interaction between hormones and immunity. Rats undergoing painful footshock stress exhibit an analgesic state referred to as stress-induced analgesia (SIA). One measure of the magnitude of SIA is the duration the animal will stand on a hot plate (53° C) compared with their own pre-SIA state without exhibiting a characteristic hind paw lick, at which time they are removed from the plate. Footshock was found to result in both SIA and suppression of NK cell activity. However, when animals were injected with naltrexone (an opioid antagonist that blocks both morphine analgesia and some forms of SIA) before footshock, they exhibited no SIA and NK cell activity that was equivalent to that of control animals that did not undergo footshock. Additionally, it was found that injection of very large, and very probably stressful, doses of morphine (30 and 50 mg/kg) resulted in NK activity suppression as well. These results support the hypothesis that the immunosuppressive effects of some forms of stress are mediated by opioid peptides.[41]

Some pain relief interventions have been shown to attenuate, and in some cases, block the surgical stress response. High-dose narcotic anesthesia suppresses the stress response during surgery in adults and neonates as long as blood opiate concentrations remain high; the endocrine and metabolic responses to surgery emerge as opiate concentrations decrease.[42, 43] Regional anesthesia, such as epidural administration of local anesthetics (e.g., bupivacaine), largely prevents the stress effects of lower abdominal and lower extremity surgery. The endocrine and metabolic responses that are inhibited include the following: levels of ACTH, ADH, thyrotropin-releasing hormone, circulating beta-endorphins, cortisol, aldosterone, renin, and catecholamines. Increased levels of blood glucose and free fatty acid may be attenuated as well, with improvement in plasma nitrogen balance. Regional anesthetic techniques are less successful in inhibiting the stress response resulting from upper abdominal and thoracic surgery.[43–45] Postoperative epidural analgesia administration has been shown to be an effective pain relief strategy; however, no significant modulation of hyperglycemia or hypercortisolism has been demonstrated.[46, 47] These findings suggest that some mechanism not dependent on pain is involved in promoting the stress response to surgery.

The immune consequences of stress have been demonstrated in humans and in animals, and there is a growing body of literature reporting this research. Major surgery in humans results in a decrease in the absolute numbers of circulating lymphocyte subpopulations (T, T_h, T_s, T_c, NK, and B) for several days, with normal levels returning by the seventh postoperative day. Although minor surgery results in a similar reduction of lymphocyte subpopulations, these changes are of a lesser magnitude and of shorter duration.[48] Major surgery also depresses significantly the ability of lymphocytes to proliferate in response to an antigen and to suppress the function of NK cells.[49, 50] (Refer to Chapter 17, Immunosuppression, for the functions associated with the above-mentioned cell populations.)

Similar immunosuppression has been demonstrated in animals undergoing surgery.[51, 52] A biologically significant outcome unique to animal research is the impact of surgery on tumor metastasis. NK cell activity plays a critical role in the immune defense against metastatic growth.[53–55] Several animal studies have documented the tumor-enhancing effects of surgery.[52, 56–61] Although both tumor development and immunity are affected by surgical stress, it is not clear that changes in immune function mediate the surgical effect on tumor development. Although there is evidence of correlational relationships between immunosuppression and tumor development, many other mechanisms may be involved; for example, several stress hormones are known to increase tumor development directly.[62]

In summary, there are limits to the individual's ability to respond to stressors; if the stressors are sufficiently great, the adaptive mechanisms may fail and death will occur. The response requires energy and metabolic reserves. If these reserves are insufficient or if the response is at the maximum rate of energy production (related to maximum oxygen consumption) and additional stressors such as infection occur, no greater adaptive response may be possible.[5, 7] Although the stress response is protective, pathological consequences occur when the magnitude of the stressor taxes the homeostatic mechanisms.

RELATED PATHOPHYSIOLOGICAL CONCEPTS

The physiological concepts related to the stress response consist of antecedent conditions, the associated clinical states, or the symptoms reported in association with perceived stress. Examples of conditions antecedent to the stress response and clinical states are multiple traumatic insult, ischemia, hypoxia, burns, surgery, sepsis, loss of a loved one, or some other catastrophic sociopsychological loss. But none of these conditions or states constitutes a concept exactly parallel or similar to the stress response. Starvation is a condition that results in some of the same adaptive mechanisms seen as part of the stress response, but deficient nutrient intake is the antecedent to the response, not the response.

ASSOCIATED PSYCHOSOCIAL CONCEPTS

In studies in which the variable of stress is of interest, the most frequently used measures tap the concept of anxiety.[33, 63–68] In the psychosocial and nursing literature, anxiety is frequently used in referring to stress and as an indirect measure of stress. In some cases, it is used interchangeably. From the perspective of the multiple and complex interrelated mechanisms involved in the stress response, anxiety as a concept does not encompass or convey the same scope of mechanisms. However, emotional arousal does trigger the stress response and may indeed be a severe response.[1, 4, 69–71]

Another similarly related notion is work stress. The term "burnout" is used as a concept to convey a response to work stress. Attention to promotion of activities to prevent burnout is increasing.[72, 73]

Coping is another psychosocial concept associated with stress.[3, 10, 64–67, 74] Coping patterns, strategies, styles, and behaviors are described variously by the multitude of investigators who are defining the concept and developing instruments to measure it.[3, 10, 64–68, 75–79] An individual's coping abilities and resources are perceived to moderate or ameliorate the severity of the perceived stressors and to influence the magnitude of the stress response.

Further description of these related psychosocial concepts is beyond the scope of this chapter. There is a large and growing body of articles and books in which these concepts are reviewed in detail.[33, 65, 79]

MANIFESTATIONS

The stress response is characterized by increased adrenergic activity and a shift in flow of substrates from an anabolic to a catabolic pattern. Because the stress response involves multiple mechanisms, is graded, and is modified by the individual's characteristics, there is no single manifestation or parameter that can be used alone to indicate the response. Use of multiple parameters is necessary.

Objective Physiological Manifestations

It is important to recognize that there are differences in the manifestations of the stress response given the many possible characteristics of the stressor itself and the many temporal possibilities for relating the stressor to outcome measures. Different stressors result in different configurations of the stress response, and the success in detecting these objective measures depends on the ability to "capture" the effect by optimally timing measurement of the outcome variable. In other words, different hormonal effects peak at different points in time given the same stressor. For example, ACTH peaks at about 1 hour and cortisol peaks several hours following major surgery.

Hyperglycemia (increased blood glucose levels) occurs early in the postoperative recovery period after major surgery, and if the response has a prolonged duration, the loss of muscle and adipose tissue becomes obvious and weight loss may occur. Loss of energy may be characterized by slow or weak movements and by difficulty in turning, in getting up, or even in breathing if the response is sufficiently severe and prolonged to involve deterioration of the muscles of respiration, for example, the diaphragm and intercostals. With loss of muscle from proteolysis and mobilization of amino acids, an increase in urinary nitrogen excretion is observed.

The most dramatic increases in the hormones participating in the stress response are observed in the plasma levels of ACTH and cortisol (and their metabolites) and catecholamines. In response to increased circulating catecholamines, cardiopulmonary changes, such as increases in blood pressure, heart rate, and respiratory rate, are seen. Many other factors can contribute to changes in these cardiopulmonary parameters, such as position, change in position, caffeine and alcohol consumption, blood volume, and a variety of pharmacological agents. With regard to these other factors, the cardiopulmonary parameters alone are not reliable indicators of the stress response, but certainly, given probable cause, the increases in the stress-related hormone levels and their accompanying cardiopulmonary changes are likely manifestations of the stress response. Measurement of multiple parameters is necessary; there is no one direct measure, and the context is also of importance in considering the objective measures.[2, 23, 24, 29, 32, 33, 71]

Measurement of galvanic skin resistance and of palmar sweat have been used as indicators of stress. With increased palmar sweat, a decrease in skin resistance is observed. These changes also are indicative of sympathetic discharge; in fact, general diaphoresis or cold hands and feet may be observed. Increased gastric secretions, bronchial and pupil dilation, and tremors are other physiological manifestations of the response.

The catecholamines norepinephrine and epinephrine or their metabolites, primarily vanillylmandelic acid (VMA), can be determined in plasma and urine; increases in catecholamines are observed with the stress response. However, the half-life of the catecholamines is very short, on the order of a very few minutes, and the plasma catecholamine levels change within seconds in response to sympathetic stimulation. Thus, a single determination of catecholamine levels is inadequate as an indicator of the stress response.

Timing for collection of the sample also is important. If the sample is from urine, the catecholamine levels obtained will represent a composite or average over the time the urine has been accumulating in the bladder. A plasma sample would more accurately characterize the response to some specific transient stressful event. Timing of the sample collection is not as critical if one is attempting to assess the response to a prolonged or chronic stressor.

Cortisol and one of its metabolites, 17-hydroxycorticosteroid (17-OHCS), can be measured in plasma and in urine. These are increased in response to stressors. The magnitude and duration of the response are graded in relation to the magnitude of the stressors and in relation to the individual's characteristics and the physiological state.

A ratio of urinary sodium to potassium excretion levels has been used in determining the stress response.[80, 81] A decreased ratio suggests sodium retention and potassium excretion in response to aldosterone. This is not a rapid response, as a number of processes are involved and synthesis of aldosterone requires time. Also, the level of sodium excretion can be influenced by other factors, such as blood volume and the renal glomerular filtration rate. Urinary creatinine excretion should be measured concomitantly to account for the contribution of these latter variables, and the urinary sodium:potassium ratio should be considered in relation to urinary creatinine excretion.

Other measures of objective manifestations that indirectly indicate a stress response include muscle tension. Primarily, muscle tension has been measured in the study of biofeedback for stress management.[82, 83] Increased levels of prolactin (anterior pituitary hormone) have been observed in the stress response.[32] The response of prolactin secretion to psychological influences is rapid and marked. Increased serum levels of beta-endorphins have been observed in response to stressors.[34, 84] Additional studies are needed to confirm these observations, but measurement of muscle tension, prolactin, or beta-endorphins may become useful indicators of the stress response.

The emergence of psychoneuroimmunology has contributed several objective physiological manifestations to the battery of hormonal and metabolic assessments already used. Immune outcomes are believed to be a consequence of the cascade of hormonal changes brought about by stress. Outcomes include lymphocyte subpopulation distribution, lymphocyte proliferation response to antigenic challenge, NK cell cytotoxicity measurements in vitro, and resistance to disease and metastatic growth in the whole organism (animal studies).[85] Caren reviews a number of studies demonstrating the effects of exercise as a stressor on human immune system responses.[24] The results suggest that the effects of exercise vary, depending on whether or not an individual is trained and conditioned.

These parameters are only indicators of the response and not a precise direct measure. They are influenced by a variety of other factors, the responses of individuals to the same stimuli (stressors) may be different, and the levels of the various parameters will vary in relation to the progression of the response. For all these reasons, it is important to use a battery or combination of parameters to assess the existence, magnitude, and duration of the stress response. All of the above cited objective manifestations of the stress response are nonspecific responses to stressors, that is, the increased sympathetic activity and adrenomedullary activity resulting in increased catecholamine secretion, the adrenocortical hyperactivity resulting in increased glucocorticoids and aldosterone, and the protein catabolism resulting in increased urinary nitrogen.

Objective Behavioral Manifestations

Some individuals seem to be able to exert more control and others less control over the behavioral responses that are frequently associated with stress. Observable manifestations may be a reflection of the coping behaviors assumed by individuals. Examples of observable behaviors that may suggest the presence of stress are vomiting, fainting, trembling, tapping of fingers, kicking or swinging movement of lower extremities while sitting, sitting on the edge of a chair, clenched fists, other evidence of muscle tension, pitch of voice, speed of talk, crying, pacing, and being immobilized or nonfunctional; perhaps excessive eating, smoking, and drinking may also be indicators. In observing such behaviors, one should not make assumptions about the basis for the behavior. From either a clinical or a research point of view, additional verification of the observed behaviors, the attending circumstances, and other data are necessary.

Subjective Manifestations

In today's world, a number of people freely acknowledge feeling stressed. The feeling is frequently attributed to job demands or the sociopsychological environment or even to the state of physical health. Burnout is a word that has been derived to convey this general feeling of stress. Some report more specific manifestations, such as headaches, nausea, anorexia or hunger, fatigue, problems with sleep and concentration, sensations of uneasiness, and gnawing or burning sensations in the gut; some report palpitations, angina, and difficulty breathing. These reported subjective manifestations may, in fact, suggest stress, or they may be related to some other condition. These are examples of the subjective sensations more commonly associated with stress.

Several psychometric instruments have been used as indirect measures to reflect the level of stress or stressors.[33, 76, 79, 86–100] Examples of these instruments include anxiety scales and life events scales. Individuals are requested to complete these scales; their responses are taken as the subjective measure of the variable. Spielberger's State-Trait Anxiety Inventory is designed to determine the individual's anxiety as an inherent trait and anxiety in relation to the current period of time.[91] The Profile of Mood States (POMS) includes anxiety as one of six subscales.[92] A number of other scales have been designed to measure anxiety.[79]

Measurement of psychosocial stressors has included both daily hassles and major life events.[94, 95, 97, 98] The Social Readjustment Rating Scale, developed originally by Holmes and Rahe, has been used as an indicator to quantify the individual's stressful life events.[86, 87] This instrument has been revised and has been adapted by a number of other investigators. Sarason and colleagues developed the Life Experiences Survey to capture both positive and negative life events.[88, 93]

Recognizing that frequent minor aggravations may contribute to stress, a daily hassles scale has been used.[97, 98] Stokes and Gordon developed a 104-item instrument to measure stress in the older adult.[99] They identified stressors from the gerontology literature, from interviews with healthy individuals who were 65 years or older, and from a review of the items by experts in gerontological nursing. The items generated make this instrument most useful in determining psychosocial stressors perceived by elderly individuals.

Benoliel and colleagues developed a 74-item instrument, the nurse stress checklist, to measure the stress of clinically employed nurses.[100] The instrument measures five components of stress: personal reactions, personal concerns, work concerns, role competence, and work completion concerns. This too represents a measure of the individual's perception of stressors and does not measure a physiological response. However, personal reaction items include some behaviors suggestive of physiological alterations.

Standardized instruments, for example, the Jenkins Activity Scale, are used to classify people's behaviors into what is called type A or type B behaviors.[96] A positive relationship between type A behaviors and proneness to myocardial infarction has been shown.[101–103] This relationship is strengthened when other cardiac risk factors are also present. "Impatient," "time-conscious," "ambitious," "competitive," and "aggressive" are some of the descriptors given to characterizing type A behavior. Matthews reviews in depth the work done on characterizing the type A behavior pattern and the measures used in quantifying this coronary-prone behavior.[104] Whether or not these type A behaviors reflect stress and the extent to which stress results in infarction remain unclear. However, this is one example of the important theoretically posed links between stress and illness for which there is no direct empirical evidence as yet. The current evidence does show an association.

There are, of course, other measures. These are all indirect measures used to tap the subjective dimensions, that is, the person's perception of the variable being measured. None of these are designed specifically to measure the stress response but to tap characteristics reflective of or associated with the phenomenon.

SURVEILLANCE AND MEASUREMENT

From a broad perspective, surveillance includes identification of and, if possible, assessment of the intensity of the stressors over time. From a narrower perspective, surveillance of the stress response includes consideration of the multiple parameters specified above. The professional nurse can have a primary role in monitoring parameters associated with both the stressors and the stress response. Insulin and blood glucose levels, urinary excretion of nitrogen, nitrogen balance, indicators of loss of muscle, ACTH and cortisol levels, heart rate, respiratory rate, and blood pressure are the more commonly monitored parameters reflecting changes in the stress response. Immune function may become an important parameter to consider. Subjectively reported sensations also need to be noted (refer to Manifestations).

Given that the nature of the stress response is generally protective, adaptive, and homeostatic, if the stressor is transient and the individual's resources are adequate, with time the response diminishes and normal values for the parameters are observed. The professional nurse should be alert to changes in urinary excretion of nitrogen as well as other indicators of loss of muscle protein, such as specific behaviors reflecting muscle weakness. Noting either an increase or a decrease in these parameters is an important nursing observation. If the response has been prolonged owing to the magnitude of the stressors, a decrease in excretion of urinary nitrogen is the signal indicating the reparative phase. If the response results from more chronic or psychological stressors, surveillance of the behavioral manifestations and the subjectively reported sensations may be the more important parameters for the professional nurse to use in surveillance of the stress response. Evidence of compromise in immune status may be another critical indicator of the presence of a stress response. (Refer to more detailed descriptions of these parameters in the discussion in Manifestations.) Several reviews provide additional information on psychological and neuroendocrinological measures to monitor the stress response.[33, 71, 88, 95]

CLINICAL THERAPIES

An immediate therapeutic goal is to eliminate, ameliorate, or—at the very least—diminish the stressors. This presumes that the stressors are known or identifiable and that they are more than a transitory event. In some instances, however, the precipitating stressors may be an event, such as a traumatic accident or loss of a loved one. Therapies used to decrease the stressor are as variable as the stressors. They can be directed very specifically to eliminate the stressor, such as use of an antibiotic selected for its effectiveness in the treatment of an infection from a specific causative organism, or the therapies can be more general, such as patient education to enhance coping abilities, use of resources, or stress management techniques.

If the magnitude of the stressors and the stress response is great (e.g., multiple traumatic injuries), subsequent therapeutic goals include provision of substrate and maintenance of fluid volume to complement the adequacy of the response. Following the more immediate phases of the response, therapies are directed toward restoration of tissue and of the individual. The professional nurse has an important role in all of these therapies.

Current therapies include (1) administration of glucose, potassium, and insulin intravenously; (2) administration of blood, blood components, or other fluids; (3) administration of glucocorticoids; (4) administration of total parenteral nutrition; (5) use of protective environments; and (6) use of technologically developed life-supporting systems. The specific role of the nurse is dependent on the nature of the stressors, the extent of the stress response, and the therapies instituted. Therapies for a variety of circumstances precipitating the stress response are reviewed by others.[5, 105–109]

For those with a more psychologically derived stress response, therapies are designed to assist the individual in dealing with the stress-producing situations, to enhance stress management techniques such as guided imagery and relaxation strategies, and to develop coping behaviors to ameliorate the stress-producing effects of various situations.[3, 10, 64, 66, 68, 73, 75, 79] Biofeedback has been used with some success as a therapy in diminishing the stress response.[82, 83] There is no best or definitive therapy that is effective for preventing the response to sociopsychological stressors or for treating the response. The characteristics of persons for which specific therapies would be most effective are also unknown. Therapies are explored primarily on an individual trial basis. To date, there are insufficient data available about the effectiveness of these therapies and the treatments have not been standardized across studies. Thus, comparison of findings with the potential for deriving practice implications remains problematic. Professional nurses can continue to make contributions to this field as they investigate the effectiveness of the therapies in diminishing the stress response.

ILLUSTRATIVE CASE STUDY

The course of Mr. F.'s illness provides an illustration of the changes that occur during an acute physiological stress response. Mr. F., a 55-year-old executive, was driving home on a rainy, stormy evening, having left his office after an argument with one of his associates. Tired, worried, and under much psychological stress in the last month because of a business failure, Mr. F. was driving faster than the freeway speed limit in a hurry to get home. Suddenly, a car swerved in front of him; he was unable to react quickly enough, and his car crashed into the other car. Not wearing a seat belt, he was thrown from the car onto the freeway. Mr. F. suffered multiple fractures, lacerations, and a lacerated spleen. After being transported to the emergency department by paramedics, he was taken to surgery, where he underwent an exploratory laparotomy and repair of the ruptured spleen and fractures. Postoperatively, Mr. F. was admitted to the surgical intensive care unit. During the first 24 hours of recovery, vital signs and laboratory values exemplified those changes expected to occur during a physiological stress response.

For the first 24 hours, Mr. F.'s heart and respiratory rates and temperature were elevated, accompanied by a slight hypotension. These responses (except hypotension) demonstrated the increased secretion of both epinephrine and norepinephrine. Serum sodium levels were moderately elevated with decreasing sodium excretion in the urine; there also was evidence of conservation of the extracellular fluid volume. The blood loss had augmented aldosterone secretion normally seen with stress as well as the release of vasopressin, the antidiuretic hormone. Serum potassium, phosphate, and sulfate levels were decreased, reflecting the loss of electrolytes and other cellular contents resulting from cell lysis. Increased levels of urine creatine, creatinine, and urea nitrogen occurred, and with a decreased intake, a negative nitrogen balance resulted. A dramatic initial finding was the hyperglycemia resulting from the net effects of norepinephrine, epinephrine, and cortisol secretion. There was a decrease in insulin secretion and an increase in glucagon secretion. Under normal circumstances, insulin secretion would be increased in

response to hyperglycemia, but under conditions of stress, insulin secretion is suppressed, resulting in a net hyperglycemia with a decreased ability for glucose utilization. Mr. F.'s increased blood cortisol and 17-hydroxycorticosteroid levels were evidence that ACTH had stimulated the adrenal cortex to produce glucocorticoids, typical of the stress response following traumatic injury. Although Mr. F. was a candidate for hypoxemia resulting from ventilation-perfusion abnormalities with abdominal incisional pain and multiple fractures, he was in the expected mixed state of metabolic and respiratory alkalosis with hyperventilation.

Over the next 7 days, Mr. F. was treated with vigorous respiratory therapy and intravenous fluids. Despite the use of parenteral substrates, he continued to remain in an acute catabolic state. He lost 5 pounds and continued to lose phosphorus and nitrogen and showed consistent elevated levels of urine creatine and creatinine. Serum sodium levels also remained elevated. With treatment, the potassium and phosphorus levels were only slightly decreased. A wound infection developed that contributed to a persistent slightly elevated temperature. Levels of plasma and urinary corticosteroids remained increased. In several days, Mr. F. was given a high-protein, high-caloric oral diet and his intake progressively approached his caloric expenditure.

During the next 2 weeks, metabolic and electrolyte values returned to normal. Following augmented antibiotic therapy, the abdominal wound healed; the patient began walking with crutches and was discharged home on a high-protein and high-caloric diet. With the complex compensatory physiological stress response to a multiple traumatic injury, homeostatic balance was restored. Table 16–4 is a summary of the metabolic changes following Mr. F.'s accident.

The professional nurse has many responsibilities in caring for an individual such as Mr. F. This case example is only a summarization of the more characteristic changes that occur as a result of an acute stress response. The important parameters to be monitored were included as well as examples of the direction of change to be

TABLE 16–4   SUMMARY OF METABOLIC CHANGES OBSERVED IN A PATIENT (MR. F.)

	Postoperative Period		
	24 Hours	7 Days	21 Days
Temperature	↑	↑	↔
Glucose (blood)	↑	↑	↔
Potassium (serum)	↓	↓ ↔	↔
Sodium (serum)	↑	↑	↔
Phosphorus (serum)	↓	↓	↔
Urine creatine, creatinine, and nitrogen	↑	↑	↔
Cortisol	↑	↑	↔
17-Hydroxycortico-steroid	↑	↑	↔
Weight	↔	↓	↓

Key: ↑, increased; ↓, decreased; ↔, normal.

expected in similar clinical circumstances. In addition, there were nursing responsibilities inherent in the therapies administered in wound care and in assisting Mr. F. in interpersonal and physical activities associated with his clinical state and recovery process.

REVIEW OF RESEARCH FINDINGS

Numerous studies about stressors and stress responses have been reported.[30, 31, 69, 78, 80, 81, 110] The approaches used are varied. The following briefly described examples characterize the range of studies.

Mild tail pinching was applied several times a day to rats as the stressor and the resulting behavior was an immediate eating response.[111]

A longitudinal study was conducted with parents of leukemic children; measurement of urinary 17-OHCS levels was used to quantify the stress response.[112] Those parents with low 17-OHCS levels were identified as using denial. In a war-time situation, no significant increase in urinary 17-OHCS was found in severely wounded soldiers; this finding, similar to the one described above for the parents, indicated that some mental mechanisms may be operating to alter the stress response.[113]

With chronic repeated periods of immobilization stress in rats, increased adrenal medulla tissue levels of the enzyme tyrosine hydroxylase were found.[28] This enzyme catalyzes the rate-limiting step in the synthesis of catecholamines. This adaptive response of increasing tyrosine hydroxylase levels enhances the capacity for synthesis of the catecholamines.

Using monkeys as subjects, Mason demonstrated some specificity in the stress response; that is, the response varied according to the stimulus used as the stressor.[4, 29] This is in contrast to the work of Selye, which demonstrated a general response to stressors.[21, 22, 35] Mason exposed monkeys to a variety of noxious agents, such as fasting, heat or cold exposure, muscular exercise, and hemorrhage. When psychological influences were minimized during the experiment, no increase in urinary 17-OHCS occurred in response to fasting or in response to exposure to heat. Different patterns of release of other hormones also were observed in response to the various stressor situations. This work suggests that there may be specificity in the stress response. However, it is also possible that these stressors are a test of different levels, intensity or magnitude, and that the difference in responses may be attributed to those differences rather than to the specificity of the stressor. Mild stressors may not activate all the reactions characterizing the full stress response seen with severe stressors.

Dimsdale and Moss studied ten young physicians to examine the catecholamine response to the psychological stress of public speaking.[69] Recognizing the rapid transient changes in catecholamine levels, they used a portable nonobtrusive pump to withdraw blood samples periodically through a catheter inserted in the antecubital vein of each subject. A baseline sample was obtained and two samples were withdrawn as the physicians spoke publicly, one sample within the first 3 minutes and the second sample 15 minutes into the speaking time. They reported no significant difference in the norepinephrine values for the two times during speaking but found a significant difference in the epinephrine levels for the two times. The greatest elevation occurred during the first 3 minutes of speaking. The design of this study shows the effect of timing on the response observed and thus the importance of timing in the collection of blood samples for measurement of the response to a transient stressful event. They concluded that epinephrine release is the more sensitive indicator of emotional stress.

Studies using stressful events as the emotional arousal stressor and determination of plasma lipid levels as the dependent variable indicating the stress response were reviewed by Dimsdale and Herd.[70] The findings showed that plasma lipid levels are influenced by situations of transient emotional arousal, such as taking an exam or viewing a disturbing film. Elevated free fatty acid levels as well as an increase in cholesterol levels were found. They acknowledged that some of these studies were conducted before the current sophisticated technology was available and suggested that additional studies investigating responses to psychological stressors need to be conducted.

One study frequently cited in the stress literature was conducted by Hale and colleagues to characterize and quantify the stress experienced by air traffic controllers while working at Chicago's O'Hare International Airport.[80] To quantify stress, the investigators used multiple parameters, including urinary levels of epinephrine, norepinephrine, 17-OHCS, urea, sodium, and potassium. They studied 20 air traffic controllers daily for two 5-day periods of work. Control values for these same parameters were determined using seven of the investigator team. Three samples were collected daily: one at the end of sleep, one in the middle of the work session, and one near the end of the work session. They reported increased urinary catecholamine levels during the work periods as well as a direct relationship of this parameter to work load. Differences were observed in the values of the parameters according to the work period, that is, morning shift versus evening shift. They concluded that the stress experienced by these air traffic controllers exceeded that induced by other stress-related events.

Giuffre and colleagues explored the impact of several hormones, including beta-endorphin, on ACTH and corticosterone levels and survival following surgical stress in rats. Animals undergoing laparotomy with ether anesthesia followed by withdrawal of 7 ml blood (approximately 50 per cent of blood volume in the animals used) were premedicated with rabbit antisera to human beta-endorphin or normal rabbit serum.[40] Animals who received anti-beta-endorphin sera had improved survival rates and significantly lower ACTH levels at the end of surgery than did the controls receiving normal rabbit serum. These findings suggest that increases in beta-endorphin levels resulting from surgical stress may have

a negative impact on homeostasis. The large blood withdrawal in addition to the surgical stress is a concern in citing this study, as there was no volume replacement at any time. The paradigm used by Giuffre and colleagues may be more applicable to stress associated with trauma. The real importance here is the finding that beta-endorphin release in response to some stressors may negatively affect the outcome.

The effects of patient-controlled analgesia (PCA) on plasma catecholamines, cortisol, and glucose levels following cholecystectomy have been examined.[114] Sixteen otherwise healthy patients scheduled for elective cholecystectomy made up the population for this study. All received the same anesthesia protocol using oral diazepam preoperatively and fentanyl intraoperatively. All patients received 0.7 mg/kg of morphine in the recovery room. The group using PCA received a continuous fentanyl infusion of 40.5 μg/50 kg per hour with patient controlled boluses of fentanyl 9 μg/50 kg; they also received 0.5 ml saline subcutaneously as a placebo. The control group received isotonic saline via PCA infusion pump with morphine injections (0.7 mg/kg) subcutaneously on request. Both groups received additional morphine injections (5 mg/70 kg) subcutaneously on request for insufficient pain relief. Patients were observed for the first 12 hours following surgery.

The pain intensity scores 2 to 12 hours after surgery (on a 10 cm visual analogue scale) for the group using PCA were significantly lower than those of the control group. Cortisol levels were significantly lower in the PCA group compared with those of the control group 4 to 12 hours following surgery, with no differences between groups before 4 hours. Plasma glucose and epinephrine levels were similar and constant in both groups; however, the PCA group exhibited consistently lower plasma norepinephrine levels than the control group (a statistically significant difference only at 6 hours following surgery).[114]

There are three broad points to be made regarding this study. First, the route of delivery of the preponderance of pain relief medication for each group was different, that is, intravenous versus subcutaneous by group (PCA group versus control group, respectively). By virtue of the property of subcutaneous absorption, the blood level of narcotic will vary over time, whereas the intravenous route is constant. Thus, one might expect differences in pain intensity scores related to the route of narcotic administration alone. Second, the impact of the drug regimen itself (the dynamics of absorption) on cortisol may be different. The oscillation between peak and trough plasma levels of narcotic may be a stressor that is eliminated by PCA. Finally, the two groups received different drugs; thus, the differences in cortisol and norepinephrine may be related to their mode of action rather than the adequacy of pain relief per se.

While the above points are issues with this particular study, it is doubtful that optimal pain relief per se would be sufficient to have a clinically relevant modulatory effect on the surgical stress response. Kehlet believes that very large doses would be necessary to affect significantly the neuroendocrine response to surgery.[45]

Tonnesen examined the effects of coronary bypass grafting and the resulting stress response on NK cell activity, lymphocyte subpopulation distribution, and phytohemagglutinin (PHA)-induced lymphocyte transformation in 20 patients.[49] Two different anesthesia regimens were used, one with high-dose fentanyl administered just prior to cardiac bypass. Serum catecholamine levels increased severely during the bypass procedure, with a gradual return to control values in the early postoperative period; cortisol levels rose more gently and remained significantly increased through postoperative day 6. PHA-induced lymphocyte transformation was significantly depressed from coronary bypass through postoperative day 1 or 3 (high-dose and low-dose fentanyl, respectively); there were no significant differences between groups. There was generalized leukopenia with significant decreases in all T-cell subpopulations and in NK cells, while the number of B cells remained unchanged. NK activity was significantly suppressed after bypass and remained so through postoperative day 1 or 3 (low-dose and high-dose fentanyl, respectively); there were no significant differences between groups. Tonnesen and colleagues proposed that NK cell activity changes result from a complex interaction involving epinephrine and cortisol.[49]

Recent findings validate that surgery enhances metastatic growth in rats and suggest a role for pain in mediating these effects.[115]

Page and colleagues used a mammary adenocarcinoma tumor (MADB106) syngeneic to the inbred Fischer 344 rat. This tumor metastasizes to the lungs when injected intravenously and is sensitive to NK cell activity for the first day following injection. These characteristics match what is known about the process of metastatic growth and therefore make this model useful for studying the impact of stress on metastatic spread. The findings of this research demonstrate that rats undergoing standard abdominal surgery under halothane anesthesia exhibit a twofold increase in the number of pulmonary metastases compared with untreated controls or animals given halothane anesthesia only. Further analgesic doses of morphine attenuated the surgery-induced enhanced metastatic growth. This finding suggests that pain does play a role in mediating surgery-induced enhanced metastasis. If similar relationships among pain, stress, and metastasis occur in humans, then pain control must be considered a vital component of postoperative care.[115]

Another interesting study conducted by a nurse determined the relationship between exposure to resuscitation procedures on other patients in a coronary care unit (CCU) and stress.[63] The stress response was measured by continuous heart rate recording. The sample was 37 myocardial infarction patients in a CCU; 12 were considered a control group, that is, having no exposure to resuscitation procedures on other patients, and 25 were experimental subjects. The heart rates for control subjects were obtained at 4-hour intervals over 3 uneventful days. The heart rates for the experimental subjects were taken before resuscitation, during a resuscitation procedure on another patient, and 4 hours after exposure to the resuscitation procedure. The investigator reported little change in heart rate for the control subjects whereas exposure to resuscitation procedures on other patients resulted in significant increases in the heart rate of the experimental subjects. This increase remained greater than baseline for 4 hours after exposure for 11 of the subjects. After witnessing resuscitation procedures on another patient, two subjects experienced cardiac arrest (without recovery). Premature ventricular contractions and chest pains were reported by some of the subjects during exposure to resuscitation. Sczekalla concluded from her findings that exposure to resuscitation on other patients was a stress-inducing event.[63] Again, one needs to examine aspects of this study in more detail, for example, the influence on heart rate of other events or factors that might have occurred, medication regimens involved, severity of the infarct, length of time after the infarct, and other concomitant conditions.

Lanuza and Marotta studied the endocrine and psychological responses of patients to cardiac pacemaker implantation.[116] Twenty-eight patients were assigned either to a treatment group or a control group. The treatment group received a structured teaching program. The physiological stress-related measures included determination of levels of urinary cortisol, epinephrine, norepinephrine, and 3-methoxy-4-hydroxy-phenylethylene glycol (MHPG). The structured teaching program did not lower the neuroendocrine responses over the 5-day preoperative-postoperative period.

Randolph exposed 60 female college students to a stressful film and treated the experimental group with therapeutic touch and the control group with physical touch to assess the effects on the stress response.[117] The response was measured using skin conductance, peripheral skin temperature, and muscle tension as indicators. No difference was found between therapeutic touch and physical touch on these dependent variables. One major problem is to verify that in fact the touch designed to be therapeutic is perceived by the recipients to be therapeutic. Alternative explanations for the findings are provided in the research report.

Doswell reviewed a decade of nursing research relevant to physiological responses to stress.[110] The 19 studies reviewed were categorized into four groups: life events, vocal stress, hospital-environmental stressors, and miscellaneous. Many of the dependent physiological response measures in these studies were cardiovascular (e.g., blood pressure, heart rate, cardiac output). Other physiological variables measured as dependent variables were levels of plasma catecholamines, urinary cortisol, blood glucose, insulin, and free fatty acids and skin conductance. From her review, Doswell concluded there is confusion in conceptual definitions of stress used by nurse researchers and that the studies are too varied and the number too small to provide any definitive conclusions. She also suggested the need to use multiple measures to capture the phenomenon and the proposed relationships.

These few examples of studies were selected to illustrate the diverse nature of research on stress, to include some studies conducted by nurse investigators, to cross clinical areas of interest, to acknowledge work completed, and to recognize the scope of work yet to be accomplished in the field of stress. Critical analysis of these studies is beyond the scope of this chapter.

IMPLICATIONS FOR FURTHER RESEARCH

One notable observation is that findings in these sample studies cannot be compared; the purposes are different, samples are different, measures used to quantify the variables of interest are different, the interventions are different, and even the conceptualization of the stress response is described differently. This observation provides the basis for considering the implications for further research.

Lowrey presents some theoretical and methodological issues confronting researchers studying stress.[118] Primarily, she makes a case for the need for nurse researchers to examine carefully the articulation and relevance of the framework, physiological variables, and measures selected. To develop the knowledge base for the field, similar studies need to be conducted using similar samples with sufficient number of subjects, similar interventions, and similar measures. Future studies need to extend the work of previous studies. Currently, there are too few examples in the stress field in which this systematic building is occurring. There are more specific and sensitive biochemical assays available for measurement of levels of catecholamines and other hormones and metabolites in blood and urine samples; thus, the study of the stress response now can be more precise and reliable. It is also possible to consider using several of the immune function measures as indicators or to examine stress response relationships. It is obvious, even from the few studies included as examples, that considerably more research is required to achieve the understanding of stress necessary to establish clinically appropriate and effective interventions. Considering the very broad range of stressors, their ubiquitous nature, and the influence of the individual's characteristics on the response, it is not a simple problem; there are and will continue to be multiple and diverse findings.

REFERENCES

1. Frankenhaeuser, M. (1975). Sympathetic-adreno-medullary activity, behavior and the psychosocial environment. In P. Venables & M. Christie (eds.), *Research in Psychophysiology*. New York: John Wiley.
2. Ganong, W. F. (1981). Neuroendocrine responses to injury and shock. Adv Physiol Sci 26:35–44.
3. Lazarus, R. (1974). Psychological stress and coping in adaptation and illness. Int J Psychiatry Med 5:321–333.
4. Mason, J. (1975). Psychologic stress and endocrine function. In E. J. Sachar (ed.), *Topics in Psychoneuroendocrinology*. New York: Grune & Stratton.
5. Moore, F. D. (1977). Homeostasis: Bodily changes in trauma and surgery. In D. C. Sabiston (ed.), *Textbook of Surgery* (11th ed.). Philadelphia: W. B. Saunders.
6. Wilmore, D. W., Long, J. M., Mason, A. D., & Pruitt, B. A., Jr. (1976). Stress in surgical patients as a neurophysiologic reflex response. Surg Gynecol Obstet 142:257–269.
7. Schumer, W. (1976). Metabolism during sepsis and shock. Heart Lung 5:416–421.
8. Sparacino, J. (1982). Blood pressure, stress and mental health. Nurs Res 31:89–94.
9. Hyman, R., & Woog, P. (1982). Stressful life events and illness onset: A review of crucial variables. Res Nurs Health 5:155–163.
10. Holroyd, K. A., & Lazarus, R. S. (1982). Stress, coping and somatic adaptation. In L. Goldberger & S. Breznitz (eds.), *Handbook of Stress: Theoretical and Clinical Aspects* (pp. 21–35). New York: Free Press.
11. Cohen, S., & Williamson, G. M. (1991). Stress and infectious disease in humans. Psychol Bull 109:5–24.
12. Tache, J., & Selye, H. (1978). On stress and coping mechanisms. Stress Anxiety 5:3–24.
13. Vaillant, G. (1979). Health consequences of adaptation to life. Am J Med 67:732–734.
14. Cassel, J. (1976). The contribution of the social environment to host resistance. Am J Epidemiol 104:107–123.
15. Hurst, M., Jenkins, D., & Rose, R. (1976). The relation of psychological stress to onset of medical illness. Annu Rev Med 27:301–312.
16. Syme, S. L., & Berkman, L. F. (1976). Social class, susceptibility, and sickness. Am J Epidemiol 104:1–8.
17. Rahe, R. H., & Arthur, R. H. (1978). Life change and illness studies. J Human Stress 4:3–15.
18. Bohus, B., & Koolhaas, J. M. (1991). Psychoimmunology of social factors in rodents and other subprimate vertebrates. In R. Ader, D. L. Felten, & N. Cohen (eds.), *Psychoneuroimmunology* (2nd ed., pp. 807–830). San Diego: Academic Press.
19. Ganong, W. F. (1980). Participation of brain monoamines in the regulation of neuroendocrine activity under stress. In E. Usdin, R. Kvetnansky, & I. J.

Kopin (eds.), *Catecholamines and Stress: Recent Advances* (pp. 115–124). New York: Elsevier North-Holland.
20. Kopin, E. J. (1976). Catecholamines, adrenal hormones, and stress. Hosp Pract 11:49–55.
21. Selye, H. (1956). *The Stress of Life*. New York: McGraw-Hill.
22. Selye, H. (1956). A syndrome produced by diverse noxious agents. Nature 72:138.
23. Ciaranello, R., & Lipton, M. (1982). Panel Report on Biological Substrates of Stress. In G. R. Elliott & C. Eisdorfer (eds.), *Stress and Human Health: A Study by the Institute of Medicine/National Academy of Sciences* (pp. 189–254). New York: Springer.
24. Caren, L. D. (1991). Effects of exercise on the human immune system. BioSci 41:410–415.
25. Dantzer, R., & Kelley, K. W. (1989). Stress and immunity: An integrated view of relationships between the brain and the immune system. Life Sci 44:1995–2008.
26. Dunn, A. J. (1989). Psychoneuroimmunology for the psychoneuroendocrinologist: A review of animal studies of nervous system-immune system interactions. Psychoneuroendocrinology 14:251–274.
27. DeFronzo, R. A., Sherwin, R. S., & Felig, P. (1980). Synergistic interactions of counter-regulatory hormones: A mechanism for stress hyperglycemia. Acta Chir Scand Suppl 498:33–42.
28. Kvetnansky, R., Weise, V. K., & Kopin, I. J. (1970). Elevation of adrenal tyrosine hydroxylase and phenylethanolamine-N-methyl transferase by repeated immobilization of rats. Endocrinology 87:744–749.
29. Mason, J. (1974). Specificity in the organization of neuroendocrine response profiles. In P. Seeman, & G. M. Brown (eds.), *Frontiers in Neurology and Neuroscience Research* (pp. 68–80). First International Symposium of The Neuroscience Institute, University of Toronto, Canada.
30. Mason, J. W. (1975). A historical view of the stress field (Part I). J Hum Stress 1:6–12.
31. Mason, J. W. (1975). A historical view of the stress field (Part II). J Hum Stress 1:22–36.
32. Lenox, R., Kant, G., Sessions, G., Pennington, L., Mougey, E., & Meyerhoff, J. (1980). Specific hormonal and neurochemical responses to different stressors. Neuroendocrinology 30:300–308.
33. Baum, A., Grunberg, N., & Singer, J. (1982). The use of psychological and neuroendocrinological measurements in the study of stress. Health Psychol 1:217–236.
34. Munck, A., Guyre, P. M., & Holbrook, N. J. (1984). Physiological functions of glucocorticoids in stress and their relations to pharmacological actions. Endocr Rev 5:25–44.
35. Selye, H. (1975). Confusion and controversy in the stress field. J Hum Stress 1:37–44.
36. Anand, K. J. S. (1986). The stress response to surgical trauma: From physiological basis to therapeutic implications. Prog Food Nutr Sci 10:67–132.
37. O'Neal, K., & Waxman, K. (1987). Mediators of altered perioperative physiology. Crit Care Clin 3:359–371.
38. Anand, K. J. S., Brown, M. J., Causon, R. C., Christofides, N. D., Bloom, S. R., & Aynsley-Green, A. (1985). Can the human neonate mount an

endocrine and metabolic response to surgery? J Pediatr Surg *20*:41–48.

39. Cover, P. O., & Buckingham, J. C. (1989). Effects of selective opioid-receptor blockade on the hypothalamo-pituitary-adrenocortical responses to surgical trauma in the rat. J Endocrinol *121*:213–220.

40. Giuffre, K. A., Udelsman, R., Listwak, S., & Chrousos, G. P. (1988). Effects of immune neutralization of corticotropin-releasing hormone, adrenocorticotropin, and β-endorphin in the surgically stressed rat. Endocrinology *122*:306–310.

41. Shavit, Y., Lewis, J. W., Terman, G. W., Gale, R. P., & Liebeskind, J. C. (1984). Opioid peptides mediate the suppressive effect of stress on natural killer cell cytotoxicity. Science *223*:188–190.

42. Anand, K. J. S., & Hickey, P. R. (1992). Halothane-morphine compared with high-dose sufentanil for anesthesia and postoperative analgesia in neonatal cardiac surgery. N Engl J Med *326*:1–9.

43. Kehlet, H. (1984). The stress response to anaesthesia and surgery: Release mechanisms and modifying factors. Clin Anaesthesiol *2*:315–339.

44. Kehlet, H. (1988). The stress response to surgery: Release mechanisms and the modifying effect of pain relief. Acta Chirurg Scand *550*:22–28.

45. Kehlet, H. (1989). Surgical stress: The role of pain and analgesia. Br J Anaesth *63*:189–195.

46. Schulze, S., Roikjaer, O., Hasselstrom, L., Jensen, N. H., & Kehlet, H. (1988). Epidural bupivacaine and morphine plus systemic indomethacin eliminates pain but not systemic response and convalescence after cholecystectomy. Surgery *103*:321–327.

47. Scott, N. B., Mogensen, T., Bigler, D., Lund, C., & Kehlet, H. (1989). Continuous thoracic extradural 0.5% bupivacaine with or without morphine: Effect on quality of blockade, lung function and the surgical stress response. Br J Anaesth *62*:253–257.

48. Lennard, T. W. J., Shenton, B. K., Borzotta, A., Donnelly, P. K., White, M., Gerrie, L. M., Proud, G., & Taylor, R. M. R. (1985). The influence of surgical operations on components of the human immune system. Br J Surg *72*:771–776.

49. Tonnesen, E., Brinklov, M. M., Christensen, N. J., Olesen, A. S., & Madsen, T. (1987). Natural killer cell activity and lymphocyte function during and after coronary artery bypass grafting in relation to the endocrine stress response. Anesthesiology *67*:523–533.

50. Tonnesen, E. (1989). Immunological aspects of anaesthesia and surgery—with special reference to NK cells. Danish Med Bull *36*:263–281.

51. Pollock, R. E., & Lotzova, E. (1987). Surgical-stress-related suppression of natural killer cell activity: A possible role in tumor metastasis. Nat Immun Cell Growth Regulat *6*:269–278.

52. Saba, T. M., & Antikatzides, T. G. (1976). Decreased resistance to intravenous tumour-cell challenge during reticuloendothelial depression following surgery. Br J Cancer *34*:381–389.

53. Gorelik, E., Wiltrout, R. H., Okumura, K., Habu, S., & Herberman, R. B. (1982). Role of NK cells in the control of metastatic spread and growth of tumor cells in mice. Int J Cancer *30*:107–112.

54. Hanna, N. (1985). The role of natural killer cells in the control of tumor growth and metastasis. Biochim Biophys Acta *780*:213–226.

55. Wiltrout, R. H., Herberman, R. B., Zhang, S., Chirigos, M. A., Ortaldo, J. R., Green, K. M., &

Talmadge, J. E. (1985). Role of organ-associated NK cells in decreased formation of experimental metastases in lung and liver. J Immunol *134*:4267–4275.

56. Buinauskas, P., McDonald, G., & Cole, W. H. (1958). Role of operative stress on the resistance of the experimental animal to inoculated cancer cells. Ann Surg *148*:642–645.

57. Hattori, T., Hamai, Y., Harada, T., Ikeda, H., & Ikeda, T. (1977). Enhancing effect of thoracotomy and/or laparotomy on the growth of ascitic tumor in rats. Jpn J Surg *7*:258–262.

58. Hattori, T., Hamai, Y., Harada, T., Ikeda, H., & Ikeda, T. (1977). Enhancing effect of thoracotomy and/or laparotomy on the development of the lung metastases in rats after intravenous inoculation of tumor cells. Jpn J Surg *7*:263–268.

59. Lewis, M. R., & Cole, W. H. (1958). Experimental increase of lung metastases after operative trauma (Amputation of limb with tumor). Arch Surg *77*:621–626.

60. Lundy, J., Lovett, E. J., Hamilton, S., & Conran, P. (1978). Halothane, surgery, immunosuppression and artificial pulmonary metastases. Cancer *41*:827–830.

61. Page, G. G., Ben-Eliyahu, S., Yirmiya, R., & Liebeskind, J. C. (1991). Surgical stress promotes metastatic growth and suppresses natural killer cell function in rats. J Pain Symptom Manage *6*:180.

62. Welsch, C. W., & Nagasawa, H. (1977). Prolactin and murine mammary tumorigenesis: A review. Cancer Res *37*:951–963.

63. Sczekalla, R. M. (1973). Stress reactions of CCU patients to resuscitation procedures on other patients. Nurs Res *22*:65–69.

64. Lazarus, R. S. (1981). The stress and coping paradigm. In C. Eisdorfer, D. Cohen, A. Kleinman, & P. Maxim (eds.), *Models for Psychopathology* (pp. 173–209). New York: Spectrum.

65. Folkman, S., & Lazarus, R. S. (1980). An analysis of coping in a middle-aged community sample. J Health Soc Behav *21*:219–239.

66. Folkman S., Schaefer, C., & Lazarus, R. S. Cognitive processes as mediators of stress and coping. In V. Hamilton, & D. M. Warburton, (eds.), *Human Stress and Cognition: An Information Processing Approach* (pp. 265–298). London: John Wiley and Sons.

67. Pearlin, L. I., & Schooler, C. (1978). The structure of coping. J Health Soc Behav *19*:2–21.

68. Weinberger, D., Schwartz, G., & Davidson, R. (1979). Low-anxious, high-anxious, and repressive coping styles: Psychometric patterns and behavioral and physiological responses to stress. J Abnorm Psychol *88*:369–380.

69. Dimsdale, J., & Moss, J. (1980). Short-term catecholamine response to psychological stress. Psychosom Med *42*:493–497.

70. Dimsdale, J., & Herd, J. (1982). Variability of plasma lipids in response to emotional arousal. Psychosom Med *44*:413–430.

71. Frankenhaeuser, M. (1975). Experimental approaches to the study of catecholamines and emotion. In L. Levi (ed.), *Emotions: Their Parameters and Measurement*. New York: Raven Press.

72. Grout, J. (1980). Stress and the nurse: A selected bibliography. J Nurs Ed *19*:58–59.

73. Donovan, M. (1981). Study of the impact of relax-

ation with guided imagery on stress among cancer nurses. Cancer Nurs *4*:121–126.

74. Robinson, L. (1990). Stress and anxiety. Nurs Clin North Am *25*:935–943.

75. Gal, E., & Lazarus, R. S. (1975). The role of activity in anticipating and confronting stressful situations. J Human Stress *1*:4–19.

76. Jalowiec, A., & Powers, M. J. (1981). Stress and coping in hypertensive and emergency room patients. Nurs Res *30*:10–15.

77. Lazarus, R., & Launier, R. (1978). Stress-related transactions between person and environment. In A. Pervin & M. Lewis (eds.), *Perspectives in Interactional Psychology*. New York: Plenum.

78. Cohen, S. (1980). After effects of stress on human performance and social behavior: A review of research and theory. Psychol Bull *87*:578–604.

79. Stone, C. G., Cohen, F., & Adler, N. (eds.) (1979). *Health Psychology: A Handbook*. San Francisco: Jossey Bass.

80. Hale, H. B., Williams, E. W., Smith, B. N., & Melton, C. E., Jr. (1971). Excretion patterns of air traffic controllers. Aerospace Med *42*:127–138.

81. Foster, S. B. (1974). An adrenal measure for evaluating nursing effectiveness. Nurs Res *23*:118–124.

82. Meichenbaum, D., & Jaremko, M. E. (eds.) (1983). *Stress Reduction and Prevention*. New York: Plenum Press.

83. Anchor, K. N., Beck, S. E. Sievking, N., & Adkins, J. (1982). A history of clinical biofeedback. Am J Clin Biofeedback *5*:3–16.

84. Santiago, T. V., Remolina, C., Scoles, V., & Edelman, N. H. (1981). Endorphins and control of breathing: Ability of naloxone to restore the impaired flow-resistive load compensation in COPD. N Engl J Med *34*:1190–1195.

85. Baltrusch, H. J. F., Stangel, W., & Titze, I. (1991). Stress, cancer, and immunity. Acta Neurol, *13*:315–327.

86. Holmes, T., & Rahe, R. (1967). The social readjustment rating scale. J Psychosom Res *11*:213–218.

87. Holmes, T., & Masuda, M. (1974). Life change and illness susceptibility. In B. S. Dohrenwend & B. P. Dohrenwend (eds.), *Stressful Life Events: Their Nature and Effect*. New York: John Wiley.

88. Sarason, I., deMonchaux, C., & Hunt, T. (1975). Methodological issues in the assessment of life stress. In L. Levi (ed.), *Emotions: Their Parameters and Measurement*. New York: Raven Press.

89. Volicer, B. J., & Bohannon, M. W. (1975). A hospital stress rating scale. Nurs Res *24*:352–359.

90. Volicer, B. J. (1975). Stress factors in the experience of hospitalization. Commun Nurs Res *8*:53–67.

91. Spielberger, C. D., Gorsuch, R. L., & Lushene, R. E. (1970). *STAI Manual for the State-Trait Anxiety Inventory*. Palo Alto: Consulting Psychologists Press.

92. McNair, D. M., Lorr, M., & Droppleman, L. F. (1971). *POMS Manual for Profile of Mood States*. San Diego: Educational and Industrial Testing Service.

93. Sarason, I. G., Johnson, J. H., & Siegel, J. M. (1978). Assessing the impact of life changes: Development of the life experiences survey. J Consult Clin Psychol *46*:932–943.

94. Dohrenwend, B. S., & Dohrenwend, B. P. (eds.) (1974). *Stressful Life Events: Their Nature and Effects*. New York: Wiley Press.

95. Tausig, M. (1982). Measuring life events. J Health Soc Behav *23*:52–64.

96. Jenkins, C. D., Rosenman, R. H., & Friedman, M. (1967). Development of an objective psychological test for the determination of the coronary prone behavior pattern in employed men. J Chron Dis *20*:371–379.

97. DeLongis, A., Coyne, J. C., Dakof, G., Folkman, S., & Lazarus, R. S. (1982). Relationship of daily hassles, uplifts, and major life events to health status. Health Psychol *1*:119–136.

98. Kanner, A. D., Coyne, J. C., Schaefer, C., & Lazarus, R. S. (1981). Comparison of two modes of stress measurement: Daily hassles and uplifts versus major life events. J Behav Med *4*:1–39.

99. Stokes, S. A., & Gordon, S. E. (1988). Development of an instrument to measure stress in the older adult. Nurs Res *37*:16–19.

100. Benoliel, J. Q., McCorkle, R., Denton, T., & Spitzer, A. (1990). Measurement of stress in clinical nursing. Cancer Nurs *13*:221–228.

101. Rosenman, R. H., Braud, R. V., Sholtz, R. I., & Friedman, M. (1976). Multivariate prediction of coronary heart disease during 8.5 year follow-up in the Western Collaborative Group Study. Am J Cardiol *37*:903–910.

102. Jenkins, C. D. (1976). Recent evidence supporting psychologic and social risk factors for coronary disease, Part 1. N Engl J Med *294*:987–994.

103. Jenkins, C. D. (1976). Recent evidence supporting psychologic and social risk factors for coronary disease, Part 2. N Engl J Med *294*:1033–1038.

104. Matthews, K. A. (1982). Psychological perspectives on the type A behavior pattern. Psychol Bull *91*:293–323.

105. Long, C., & Blakemore, W. (1979). Energy and protein requirements in the hospitalized patient. J Parenter Enter Nutr *3*:69–71.

106. Brennan, M. (1981). Total parenteral nutrition in the cancer patient. N Engl J Med *305*:375–382.

107. Wilmore, D. (1976). Alimentation in injured and septic patients. Heart Lung *5*:791–792.

108. Blackburn, G. (1979). Hyperalimentation in the critically ill patient. Heart Lung *8*:67–70.

109. Lumb, P., Dalton, B., Bryan-Brown, C., & Donnelly, C. (1979). Aggressive approach to intravenous feeding to the critically ill. Heart Lung *8*:71–80.

110. Doswell, W. M. (1989). Physiological responses to stress. Annu Rev Nurs Res *7*:51–69.

111. Morley, J. E., & Livine, A. S. (1980). Stress-induced eating is mediated through endogenous opiates. Science *209*:1259–1269.

112. Wolff, C. T., Friedman, S. B., & Hofer, M. A. (1964). Relationship between psychological defense and mean urinary 17-OHCS excretion rates. I. A predictive study of parents of fatally ill children. Psychosom Med *26*:576–591.

113. Wolf, C., Friedman, S., Hofer, M., & Mason, J. (1964). Relationship between psychological defenses and mean urinary 17-hydroxycorticosteroid excretion rates. Psychosom Med *26*:596–608.

114. Moller, I. W., Dinesen, K., Sondergard, S., Knigge, U., & Kehlet, H. (1988). Effect of patient-controlled analgesia on plasma catecholamine, cortisol and glucose concentrations after cholecystectomy. Br J Anaesth *61*:160–164.

115. Page, G. G., Ben-Eliyahu, S., & Liebeskind J. (1991). Morphine attenuates the enhanced meta-

static effects of surgery in rats. Society for Neuroscience Abstracts 21st Annual Meeting *17*:829.

116. Lanuza, D. M., & Marotta, S. F. (1987). Endocrine and psychologic responses of patients to cardiac pacemaker implantation. Heart Lung *16*:496–505.

117. Randolph, G. (1984). Therapeutic and physical touch: Physiological response to stressful stimuli. Nurs Res *33*:33–41.

118. Lowrey, B. J. (1987). Stress research: Some theoretical and methodological issues. Image *19*:42–46.

17

Immunosuppression

Pat Halliburton

DEFINITION

Immunosuppression is the reduction of the immune response. In addition to the application of therapeutic maneuvers to depress or eliminate the immune response (immunosuppressive therapy), specific immune disorders also reduce the host reaction to molecules it identifies as foreign. Immune disorders are generally classified according to their immune cellular defect, for example antibody (B-cell) immunodeficiency disorders. A variety of immunological abnormalities, however, occur in a large number of clinical states or diseases, such as diabetes mellitus, alcoholic cirrhosis, anesthesia, and burns, and limits classification by a singular defect. In addition, the severity of a disease and its treatment and factors such as aging and malnutrition may also compromise an individual's immune response. The term immunocompromised host, irrespective of the cause, refers to a person predisposed to infection or with an impaired resistance to infection.[1]

According to the American Nurses Association, nursing practice addresses phenomena that are often multiple, episodic or continuous, fluid and varying, and less discrete or circumscribed than medical diagnostic categories.[2] Immunosuppression may be subtle or severe and possibly transient, with treatment of the cause or dose reduction of therapy restoring normal immune response. Its frequent insidious onset and complicated pathogenesis further increase the complexity of immunosuppression. The pervasive nature of immunosuppression makes the study of this phenomenon particularly relevant for clinical practice, whatever the specialty. In keeping with standard usage, the term immunodeficiency in this chapter refers to a specific diagnostic category and immunocompromised to host immune status.

PREVALENCE

The overall prevalence of immunosuppression is not known, and estimates must frequently substitute for actual figures. For example, although the prevalence of X-linked infantile hypogammaglobulinemia in the United States is unknown, estimates in the United Kingdom suggest that it is one case per 100,000 population.[3] Other congenital immunodeficiencies, such as ataxia-telangiectasia and Wiskott-Aldrich syndrome, are also considered rare. The immunosuppression caused by many current treatments, however, has resulted in a large and growing number of individuals with decreased resistance to infection.[1] In fact, modern medical techniques are credited for the current era of opportunistic infections,[4, 5] which are usually considered the consequence of a reduced immune response.

Nurses care for more immunocompromised patients than in the past because of the increase in broad-spectrum antimicrobials, cytotoxic therapies, prolonged duration of indwelling catheters, parenteral nutrition, organ transplantation, and acquired immunodeficiency syndrome (AIDS). Specifically regarding transplantation, in 1987 more than 1100 liver and 1500 heart transplants were performed in the United States.[6] After renal transplantation, the average incidence of infection as determined by antibody titer or virus isolation was 71 per cent in 15 studies.[7] In fact, infection is the most common postoperative complication.[8] Recognition of the immunocompromised patient is assuming greater importance. The American Cancer Society estimates that about 83 million Americans now living, one in three of the U. S. population, will eventually have cancer.[9] These estimates are based on incidence rates from the National Cancer Institute Surveillance, Epidemiology and End Results (SEER) program for 1986 to 1988 applied to 1992 Census population projections. The SEER program collects data from nine cancer registries, covering about 10 per cent of the U.S. population. To potentiate cure for this new cancer population, the use of newer classes of drugs, preoperative chemotherapy (neoadjuvant treatment), and bone marrow transplantation will increase as important treatment options.

The most common cause of immunodeficiency worldwide is malnutrition, and one of the most alarming and rapidly growing causes is human immunodeficiency virus (HIV) infection.[10] According to the Centers for Disease Control (CDC),[11] 206,171 adult and adolescent AIDS cases were reported in the United States through January 1992. From February 1991 through January 1992,

the major exposure category for male cases was homosexual contact (62 per cent), followed by injecting drug use (21 per cent) then the combination category, homosexual contact and injecting drug use (6 per cent); and for female cases, injecting drug use (48 per cent) and heterosexual contact (37 per cent). Throughout this same period, 133,554 deaths attributed to AIDS occurred, a 64.8 per cent case-fatality rate.

SITUATIONAL STRESSORS

Clinical States and Medical Diagnoses

Numerous clinical states and diagnoses are associated with a reduction in the number or function of immune components and therefore in the reduction of the immune response (Table 17–1). For example, decreased in vitro cell-mediated (T-cell) responsiveness and phagocytic migration (chemotaxis) occur with such chronic diseases as diabetes mellitus and alcoholic cirrhosis.[12] Anesthesia causes T-cell suppression and reduces the engulfment of

TABLE 17–1   EXAMPLES OF CLINICAL STATES AND MEDICAL DIAGNOSES

Diagnoses	T Cell	B Cell	Phagocytosis
Burns	Decreased delayed hypersensitivity, lymphopenia	Decrease in all immunoglobulins, normal antibody response	Decreased phagocytic function, decreased chemotaxis
Cancer (nonlymphoid)	Suppression of PHA, MLC, T cells; immunosuppressive factors	Variable immunoglobulin levels	Normal
Hepatitis	Decreased delayed hypersensitivity, decreased lymphocyte cytotoxicity, decreased T cells	Immunoglobulins increased	Unknown
Infection			
Chronic	Usually normal	Increased immunoglobulins	Decreased chemotaxis
Viral	Lymphopenia, decreased T cells, depressed helper-to-suppressor cell ratio	Normal	Normal
Leukemia (acute)	Decreased delayed hypersensitivity, PHA	Variable immunoglobulin levels	Normal
Rheumatoid arthritis	Decreased delayed hypersensitivity, decreased PHA, MLC	Immunoglobulin levels usually increased, normal antibody response to antigens	Normal
Systemic lupus erythematosus (SLE)	Decreased delayed hypersensitivity, decreased T cells, PHA, MLC, and suppressor cells in animal models and in humans	Immunoglobulins usually elevated, increased antibody titers to multiple antigens	Normal

Adapted with permission from Ammann, A. (1984). Immunodeficiency diseases. In D. Stites, J. Stobo, J. Wells (eds.), *Basic and Clinical Immunology* (6th ed., pp. 348–350). Los Altos, CA: Lange Medical.
PHA, phytohemagglutinin stimulation of lymphocytes; MLC, allogeneic cell stimulation of lymphocytes.

microorganisms by leukocytes (phagocytosis); this type of immunosuppression may last several weeks. Another acute event, a major thermal burn, results in a decrease in all immunoglobulins, the number of T cells, and in both chemotaxis and phagocytosis. As a consequence, systemic sepsis resulting from invasive infection remains the leading cause of mortality in burn patients.[13-16] In contrast, although splenectomy for splenic trauma reduces phagocytosis and clearance of microorganisms, postsplenectomy sepsis is rare.[16]

Immunosuppression is also severe in cancer of the lymphoid system, which includes the acute and chronic leukemias and the lymphomas. As previously noted, treatment may also produce immune abnormalities. Corticosteroids, cytotoxic drugs, and specific immunosuppressive agents (e.g., cyclosporine) can reduce cell-mediated and antibody-mediated responses to antigens and phagocytosis. Such a reduction is drug- and dose-dependent, variable with the use of cytotoxic agents, and occurs only temporarily during corticosteroid therapy because of sequestration of T cells. Data do not exist supporting a general immunosuppressive effect for other therapy, including the ultraviolet radiation used to treat dermatological problems. The special relationship between antimicrobials and infection is discussed in Manifestations (p. 429).

Diverse clinical states and diagnoses cause similar immune disorders. For example, the number of T cells, particularly CD4 cells, decreases in viral infections (e.g., HIV infection), nonlymphoid cancer, and chronic active hepatitis. Acute leukemia and the autoimmune diseases rheumatoid arthritis and chronic persisting (active) hepatitis are associated with relative anergy, a reduction in delayed hypersensitivity. Chronic infection will suppress the nonspecific immune response, chemotaxis. The development of such immunopathology, and that of other disorders, including AIDS, is discussed in Mechanisms (next page).

DEVELOPMENTAL DIMENSIONS

Infants are relatively immunologically immature. Morphological studies show that the weight and volume of the neonatal thymus increase for the first 6 months before stabilizing.[17] Neonatal T cells possess the functional capability of adult T cells but are hampered by lower levels of effector T-cell precursors and deficiencies of accessory or antigen-presenting cells. Monocytosis also occurs until about 1 month of age, whereas complement in newborn sera ranges from 60 to 90 per cent of adult values before rising steadily for 2 years. Maternally acquired antibody lessens but does not prevent the rate of infection for the first 6 months.[17, 18] The pattern of certain infections after 6 months of age illustrates the effectiveness of this protection. For example, the period of greatest susceptibility to primary herpes infection occurs between 6 months and 2 years. In addition, a period of hypogammaglobulinemia occurs at approximately 5 to 6 months of age, and recurrent respiratory infections then develop.[3] As expected, the immune antibody response is highly variable in infants, depending on antigen exposure. The oral unresponsiveness of the adult mucosal immune system to antigens is also reduced in young children and results in hypersensitivity to milk proteins.[19]

Pregnancy itself is characterized by a depression in cellular immune response.[18] Total lymphocyte counts fall, the maximum decrease occurring at mid pregnancy, and a reversed CD4-CD8 ratio occurs (see Mechanisms). In vitro tests of T-cell function show a decrease during gestation. The pregnant woman resembles a patient with selective immunosuppression; she has a diminished ability to defend against certain infectious agents (e.g., hepatitis A, *Neisseria gonorrhoeae*) controlled primarily by the cell-mediated immune response. Steroid hormones produced in pregnancy may have some responsibility for these infections.

Many cell- and antibody-mediated responses decline or change with advanced age; this is known as immune senescence. Cellular activation and differentiation, especially of the CD4 T-cell subset, and its product interleukin-2 (IL-2) are markedly decreased.[20] The principal clinical evidence for immune senescence is the high cancer incidence in the aged.[21] The immune senescence is a mild to moderate decrease in cellular immune functions that appears early at the onset of sexual maturation and progresses throughout the life span as the thymus continues to involute.

The magnitude of immune responses, however, does vary between individuals. For example, in one study, lymphocytes from 30 per cent of the elderly subjects mounted vigorous proliferative responses in vitro.[22] The elderly may be a less homogeneous group than other populations. Variance in the data of an aged sample may also suggest that immune senescence is determined by multiple factors and is not simply a result of aging. Regarding specific age-related infection, the elderly host does show a susceptibility to varicella-zoster virus (shingles)[22] and an impaired ability to lyse the fungus Candida.[20]

MECHANISMS

The development of immunosuppression results in a decline in the protective functions of the immune system. This discussion provides an overview of the immunological components involved in a protective reaction, their regulation and responsiveness, and the sequence of events that results in an immune response. See Therapies for a review of non-immunological defenses, that is, host defenses at body surfaces, inflammation, and fever.

The immune system consists of a large network of organs and varied cell types, some with highly specialized subpopulations that carry out interrelated functions. Immunological reactions require lymphoid organs and tissues such as the thymus, bone marrow, spleen, lymph nodes, and lymphoid cells. The predominant cellular components of the immune system are the T lymphocytes, which differentiate mainly in the thymus, and the B lymphocytes, which differentiate in the bone marrow. Other immunological cells, such as the phagocytic mononuclear cells, macrophages (derived from bone marrow monocytes), polymorphonuclear neutrophils (PMNs), and the natural killer (NK) cells, also play a role in the immune response. The NK cells exhibit cytotoxicity without prior sensitization. The heterogeneous T lymphocytes are classified according to their distinct functions, such as cytotoxic, helper (i.e., amplification), suppressor (i.e., inhibition), and delayed-type hypersensitivity cells. Delayed hypersensitivity reactions require time for the synthesis and release of cell products (cytokines) and for their actions to become manifested.

The immune response also involves the B-cell product, immunoglobulin (Ig). Immunoglobulins are the protein molecules that carry antibody activity and account for ap-proximately 20 per cent of the total plasma proteins. IgG constitutes approximately 75 per cent of the total serum Ig and is capable of fixing the serum protein complement, a primary mediator of antigen-antibody reactions. The sequential activation of complement, a system of 25 proteins, causes lysis of cells during the immune response. Macrophages can function in a cytotoxic fashion when they bind with subclasses of IgG. Since IgA is the principal Ig in membrane secretions, it provides the primary defense against some local infections. IgM participates in most early immune responses to antigens and is necessary in certain antibody responses, such as blood group antibodies. The main function of IgD is not known. Upon combination with certain specific antigens called allergens, IgE antibodies trigger immediate hypersensitivity reactions.

The immune response is primarily a cellular event with secondary formation of cytokines that defer to immune cell function. The normal immune system distinguishes "self" from "not self" and reacts to foreign substances through immunologically specific components (T and B lymphocytes). The nonspecific (innate) elements such as monocytes and macrophages, PMNs, and complement amplify and modify specific (acquired) immune responses. The immune system has specificity, memory, mobility, replicability, and cooperativity.[23] Antigen-specific receptors on the surfaces of T lymphocytes, and Ig on B cells, provide specificity for immune responses. The system obtains memory after first contact, and a rechallenge with the antigen results in a heightened response. Because both specific and nonspecific elements circulate, immune reactions become systemic. Specific and nonspecific cellular components can also replicate and thereby amplify responses. Finally, lymphocytes and cell products (Ig and cytokines) interact with each other and nonlymphoid elements to maintain optimal functioning of the system.

A stepwise review of the immune response, from initial encounter with an antigen to its elimination, clarifies a host reaction consisting of a complex sequence of events (Fig. 17–1). Activation of the cell-mediated response requires the T-cell receptor to interact with an antigenic determinant (i.e., epitope) presented by another cell, usually a macrophage. The receptor recognizes the epitope together with a part of the major histocompatibility complex (MHC), a gene cluster in a chromosomal region. In other words, the T cell "sees" the epitope together with self-MHC on the antigen-presenting cell (APC).[24, 25]

The immune response also involves non-specific soluble mediators (cytokines). Those that act between leukocytes are called inter-leukins; for example, the APC produces interleukin-1 (IL-1) when it presents antigen to the T cell. An activated T cell then secretes IL-2. IL-2 increases T-cell and B-cell clonal expansion, the synthesis of cells through the cloning of a single lymphoid cell. In addition, IL-2 induces cytotoxic T-lymphocyte activity, increases NK cell activity, and monocyte cytotoxicity.[26] Virally infected cells will produce another cytokine, alpha- or beta-interferon (IFN), that interferes with superinfection by another virus. These same antiviral proteins also have potent immunomodulatory activities, for example, activation of macrophages.[27]

Mobilization of the cell-mediated response and its regulation involves various T-cell subpopulations (Fig. 17–1). Cytotoxic T lymphocytes recognize only antigens together with class 1 MHC antigens on the surfaces of other cells. The cytotoxic lymphocytes express the cell surface marker CD8 (i.e., cluster of differentiation), as do suppressor T cells. Suppressor T cells inhibit the immune response. Delayed-type hypersensitivity cells "see" antigen in the context of the class II MHC and are designated CD4. Helper T cells, also CD4 cells, control the development of T and B lymphocytes. In addition, T cell–B cell interactions result in efficient antibody production to T cell–dependent antigens. The T cell recognizes antigen-MHC on the B cell and triggers B-cell development and clonal expansion, and therefore antibody production results.[25, 28] The mature B cell uses its surface IgM as a receptor for the antigen. The primary response (first contact) involves "Ig class switching"; that is, the first B cells make IgM, but later in the response, the predominant Ig isotype classes are IgG, IgA, and sometimes IgE.[17, 29] This allows for the generation of Ig with identical specificity but diverse function.

As noted, helper T cell–B cell interaction initiates the antibody-mediated response. B cells expand clonally and differentiate into antibody-secreting cells. Antibody binds specifically to the antigen (antigen-antibody com-

plex), enhancing macrophage action and therefore phagocytosis. The complex may induce activation of the complement system. The coating by complement and antibody (opsonization) also promotes phagocytosis. Binding by IgM or IgG initiates the classical complement pathway, a cascading, sequential activation of complement (C1-C9) that amplifies as it proceeds.[7] In the absence of specific antibody, C3 is activated directly (alternative pathway). Antibody may opsonize tumor cells or virally infected cells, facilitating cytolysis by NK cells, macrophages, or PMNs (antibody-dependent, cell-mediated cytotoxicity, or ADCC).[29] The cytokines secreted during specific responses also stimulate the nonspecific responses, that is, NK cytolysis and PMN phagocytosis.

Some aspects of the biology of the immune system are relatively established, others require more investigation. For example, why the T-cell receptor recognizes a foreign peptide only in the context of the self-MHC molecule is not known. Still tentative is the division of CD4 and CD8 cells into functional subsets on the basis of various cell surface markers.[24] The mode of action of suppressor cells is controversial.[24, 25] A "T suppressor circuit" may exist and involve more than a single cell. In vitro research shows that MHC class I–restricted CD8 T cells may participate in protection against intracellular organisms by lysing infected target cells and producing gamma IFN.[31] Interestingly, some immunologists propose that a layered immune system, in which several types of hematopoietic stem cells evolve sequentially at specified times, may explain functional differences among immune cells.[32]

The mechanisms of immunosuppression with various clinical states and diagnoses reflect these continual refinements in the field of immunology. In addition, an overview of the reduced immune response with AIDS, trauma, autoimmune disease, cancer, and immunosuppressive therapy provides insight into the scope of immunopathogenesis and the significance of immunosuppression for clinical practice.

Acquired Immunodeficiency Syndrome

Infection with HIV causes a gradual suppression of immune function, eventually resulting in widespread immunosuppression and diverse opportunistic diseases.[33] HIV is

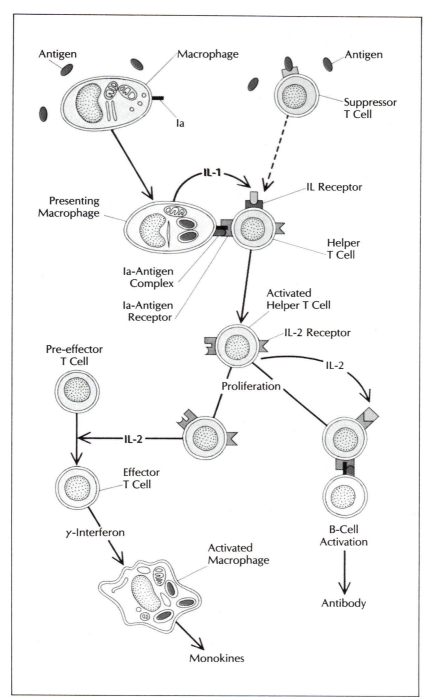

Figure 17–1. Components of the cell-mediated response. (Ia, leukocyte antigen; IL-2, interleukin-2; IFN-γ, gamma-interferon.) (Reprinted with permission from Young, L. [1989]. Infections in patients with cellular immunodeficiency. Hosp Pract [Aug. 15], *24*:191.)

a retrovirus, an enveloped virus possessing the enzyme reverse transcriptase. HIV is sub-classified as a lentivirus, a retrovirus whose viral expression is restricted in vivo. A long latency period from infection to the onset of clinical features occurs. The interaction between HIV and the host involves various mechanisms that result in the destruction of CD4 T cells.[33, 34] This selective depletion of the CD4 helper subset reverses the usual T cell ratio of approximately 2:1 of CD4 to CD8 T cells.[34, 35] The CD4 functions as the receptor for HIV, and HIV fuses to the cell membrane, enters the cell, and replicates. This disrupts other CD4 MHC class II interactions, such as those with antigens and macrophages. The binding of both MHC class II and HIV to CD4 may also result in autoantibodies and an autoimmune reaction.[33, 36] The attachment of HIV to the surface of uninfected CD4 T cells may target these cells for antibody-dependent cellular cytotoxicity. As a result, CD4 T-cell responses decrease, including T-cell cytotoxicity, cytokine release (IL-2), and T cell–B cell interaction for Ig synthesis.[37]

HIV seems to have the ability to use normal immune processes to reproduce.[33] Activation of HIV-infected CD4 cells or monocytes and macrophages during normal immune responses may result in activation of HIV from a latent or low replication state. Certain subsets of monocytes and macrophages, although low in numbers do express the CD4 surface molecule and bind to HIV. Restriction of viral expression, the adaption of a form an immunologically responsive host cannot recognize, is a feature of lentiviruses and may occur after the enzyme reverse transcriptase converts the HIV viral RNA to DNA.[17] In addition to undergoing latency, the HIV mutates rapidly, thus resisting the immune responses that usually control viral infections. Of primary importance, the depletion and dysfunction of CD4 T cells cause a reduction in clonal expansion, the replication method used by antigen-specific cells. Profound immunosuppression of the cell-mediated response results.

Trauma

Patients sustaining major injuries develop reductions in the function of lymphocytes, macrophages, neutrophils, Ig levels, and the concentration and activity of complement as well as in the reticuloendothelial system (RES), plasma fibronectin, and opsonic activity.[12, 38] The RES consists of the fixed macrophages of the liver, spleen, and lymph nodes and clears the blood of circulating bacteria. Macrophages secrete fibronectin and utilize this protein as opsonin and for cell adhesion. Research shows that the magnitude of such immunosuppression is directly related to the extent of the injury, including thermal injuries. Reduction of chemotaxis, consumption of complement factors, and deficient production of colony-stimulating factor (CSF) by monocytes, and, therefore, granulocyte production occur after thermal injuries.

For these reasons, the inflammatory response, a nonspecific response to infection, has often been considered the most important immune alteration in seriously burned patients. A large surgical study (n = 606), however, found no significant relationship between PMN adherence or chemotaxis and septic mortality.[39] Another surgical study (n = 14) demonstrated PMN-enhanced activity and no correlation with increased susceptibility to infection. The delineation of the nonspecific immune modifications during various trauma requires further study.

Any dysfunction of the specific immune response, however, is important, since one of its major roles is to amplify and focus the nonspecific response. In burns, suppressor lymphocytes or inadequate IL-2 may cause the decrease in B cells, primarily in IgG levels.[14] The release of suppressive substances during burns, such as circulating toxins, histamines, prostaglandins, and endotoxins, may activate the suppressor lymphocytes. Researchers have also identified immunoreactive prostaglandin E_2 as the link in the dysfunctional monocyte–T cell network after trauma.[40] Another study using the mouse model found that fluid from 10-day old healing murine wounds inhibited lymphocyte mitogenesis.[41] The different mechanisms exhibited during trauma may reflect the limitations of in vitro data or even local reactions to tissue injury. Whatever the mechanism, numerous research studies support the finding that anergy does predict an infectious outcome after injury.[39, 42, 43]

Autoimmune Disease

Autoimmune disease is characterized by an increased immune response but decreased suppression that results in the functional loss of tolerance to self-antigens. In systemic lupus erythematosus (SLE), an organ-non-specific autoimmune disease, the defective suppressor T-cell activity may be due to anti–T-cell antibody activity, that is, defective immune regulation, and not to a primary cell deficiency.[17, 44] In fact, suppressive factors themselves cannot regulate self–non-self discrimination; it is a characteristic of T-cell help. In addition to a genetic susceptibility defect, factors in the immunological pathogenesis of SLE include double-stranded DNA and T-lymphocytotoxic antibodies. Also, in a study of 33 patients with SLE, data demonstrated deficient IL-2 activated killer (LAK) cell cytotoxicity, an activity dependent on activated T cells.[45] Patients with SLE, therefore, lack an essential first step in the immune response, autorecognition, and thus SLE effectively illustrates a disease of disordered immune regulation.

Cancer

All components of the immune system have the potential to eradicate tumor cells. Natural killer (NK) cells, macrophages, and PMNs destroy by spontaneous, nonspecific cytotoxicity, a reaction enhanced by antibody (i.e., ADCC). NK cells may provide the first line of defense against the intravascular spread of tumor cells and, therefore, metastasis.[46] In the presence of complement, both IgM and certain types of IgG directly lyse tumor cells; however, ADCC may be the more important mechanism. T cells also lyse cells or function through cytokines. For example, IL-2 increases the number and lytic activity of NK cells and IFN stimulates macrophage and NK cell activity. Most tumor cells express class I but not class II MHC antigens; therefore, T-helper cells, which recognize class II MHC, depend on APCs such as macrophages.[28, 47]

Tumor cells may escape from an immune response by several mechanisms. For example, as these cells generate, they may become weakly immunogenic or nonimmunogenic (antigen-negative).[46, 47] The surface membrane glycoproteins may change during cell division, affecting antigenic detection of tumors,[28] as does the possible shedding or internalizing of tumor surface antigen. Specific immune responses may also contribute to ineffective tumor cell lysis. In human B-cell tumors and leukemias, the initial immune response modulates antigenic expression. Antibodies change the concentration and distribution of the tumor antigens.[48] Noncytolytic, non–antigen-specific antibody may also bind to the antigen and interfere with recognition by cytolytic, antigen-specific antibodies or T cells.[47]

Suppressor T cells may further inhibit immune reactivity with cancer, as demonstrated in animals with progressive tumors when a secondary, highly immunogenic tumor challenge is not rejected.[47] In patients with melanoma, the nodes nearest the tumor contained suppressor cells and were suggested as a factor in the generation of metastatic disease. The immune response does not effectively[47] eliminate a large tumor burden, whatever the specific mechanisms.

Immunosuppressive Therapy

Glucocorticoids interfere at many steps in the immune response, for example, transitory reduction of circulating lymphocytes and monocytes and suppression of IL-1 and IL-2 production.[49, 50] Leukopenia results from both an altered release from the bone marrow and exodus from the circulation, while those neutrophils circulating have reduced adherence.[28, 51] The glucocorticoid inhibition of cytokines also suppresses granulopoiesis. Particularly important, clones of helper T cells show more sensitivity to these drugs than cytotoxic T cells.[52]

Another drug, cyclosporin A, a fungal metabolite given to prevent organ transplant rejection, blocks helper T cells while sparing memory cells, resting cells, and dividing cells in the bone marrow.[28] In some cases, cyclosporin has even contributed to the development of specific suppressor T cells and therefore maintained host tolerance to the immune response.

Cytotoxic agents such as azathioprine, cyclophosphamide (an alkylating agent), and methotrexate (an antimetabolite) block cell replication and preferentially kill dividing tumor cells.[28] Cyclophosphamide, a nitrogen mustard derivative, kills cells during the mitotic phase; azathioprine and methotrexate, a folic acid antagonist, kill cells during the DNA synthesis phase of the cell cycle. Lymphocytes are also destroyed by these agents, such as low-dose cyclophosphamide, during the proliferative stage after antigen stimulation. Interestingly, low-dose cyclophospha-mide, may restore immune response by re-ducing tumor-related immunosuppression.[52] Researchers attribute this immunopotentiat-ing effect to selective elimination of suppres-sor cell activity and possibly to enhancement of IL-2 production.[53]

An important consequence of these thera-pies is that tumors develop in immunosup-pressed hosts (i.e., transplant recipients), al-though tumors of lymphoreticular origin predominate. The drugs employed that di-rectly target the lymphoreticular system may explain the incidence of these cancers in this population.[28] Allotransplant recipients who receive immunosuppressive therapy have at least a 100-fold increase in cancer risk com-pared with that of an age-corrected general population.[54] A high percentage of these, as noted, are lymphoreticular cancers, particu-larly central nervous system lymphoma; Ka-posi's sarcoma and epithelial cancers also develop. Kaposi's sarcoma and B-cell lym-phoma occur with AIDS. According to epi-demiological studies, acute nonlymphocytic leukemia is the most frequently reported second cancer following aggressive cancer chemotherapy.[55]

RELATED PHYSIOLOGICAL CONCEPTS

The physiological concepts related to im-munosuppression are infection and malnu-trition. A close interrelationship exists be-tween infection and immune function. Infection is considered an expression or con-sequence of a reduction in the immune re-sponse (see Manifestations). In fact, con-trolled studies are difficult to perform in this area, since malnutrition, infection, and im-munosuppression commonly coexist, making it virtually impossible to establish which is the primary causative agent. Consideration of the interrelation of these concepts to immuno-suppression is further discussed in Thera-pies.

Malnutrition is viewed as predisposing the individual to a compromised immune status. Both deficiency and imbalance of the many nutrients that regulate lymphoid cellular ac-tivity can produce adverse immunological consequences. For example, protein-calorie malnutrition has been associated with a re-duction in thymic hormone activity, resulting

in inadequate differentiation of the T lym-phocyte and thus an increase in immature T cells and a decreased CD4 cell subset.[56] A deficiency of nutrients also adversely affects complement reactions and phagocytosis. Studies of nutritional modulation (the appli-cation of single nutrients) or of specific mal-nourished populations (e.g., the elderly) pro-vide evidence of a relationship between nutrition and immune function.

In one postoperative study, supplementa-tion with arginine, a semi-essential amino acid, resulted in an enhanced T lymphocyte response and augmented the numbers of CD4 cells.[57] Other studies also showed that arginine prevented or lessened immuno-suppression after injury.[57, 58] Research fur-ther suggested that an increased intake of vegetable oil, omega-6 fatty acids, alters membrane fluidity, and thus the struc-ture and function of receptor binding sites, and the initiation of the immune re-sponse.[59–61]

In contrast, the inclusion of omega-3 fatty acids (i.e., fish oil) may alter prostaglandin synthesis and therefore enhance macrophage function. According to preliminary data, combination nutritional modulation using ar-ginine and omega-3 fatty acids did reduce infection morbidity in 50 seriously burned patients,[62] and improved in vitro lymphocyte proliferation in 20 patients in an intensive care unit.[63] Modification of current diet ther-apy, however, must await replication of these very early data.

In the elderly, nutritional supplements providing an extra 500 kcal per day and the recommended allowances of essential micro-nutrients for 8 weeks resulted in improved skin test response, in vitro lymphocyte prolif-eration, and T-lymphocyte numbers.[64] About one third of another sample of elderly pa-tients who were anergic (i.e., lacking skin reactivity to antigens) showed positive skin reactions after receiving 50 mg of zinc daily for 8 weeks.[56] Three months of zinc supple-mentation, however, did not significantly al-ter immune response in a study of 103 ap-parently healthy elderly subjects.[65] Of note, it is known that the crucial role of zinc is clinically manifested during protein or pro-tein-calorie malnutrition.[66] Goodwing and Garry concluded from their research that subtle nutritional deficiencies do not contrib-ute to the immunosuppression of aging.[67] Again, future clinical trials will determine whether nutritional modulation will restore the immune response of this high-risk population.

ASSOCIATED PSYCHOSOCIAL CONCEPTS

The possible impact of stress on the immune response, although nebulous, requires some attention by clinicians. Stress may directly influence the immune system through hypothalamic pituitary peptides and the sympathetic nervous system.[68, 69] Feedback regulatory loops may also exist and provide bi-directional communications between the immune system and the central nervous system and between the immune system and the endocrine system.[70] Hormones primarily may facilitate this two-way flow of information through closely interlocked systems. For example, even though glucocorticoids and catecholamines are immunosuppressive, corrective feedback signals exist that can interfere with their sustained release and reduce the magnitude of their immune modulation.[71]

Immune alterations associated with stress (i.e., decreased lymphocytes and in vitro response) may not be specific biological correlates of stress but only occur in subgroups such as the elderly.[72] Factors such as attitudes, spiritual resources, hopes, and ideals can neutralize the effects of stress,[73] whereas alcohol and drug abuse and poor nutrition and health status may potentiate immune alterations.[74] Research has shown that extremely small amounts of the cytokine IL-1 acting in the brain suppress cellular immune responses very rapidly and for a prolonged period of time.[75, 76] The relationship of brain IL-1 to the immunosuppression produced by stressful conditions, however, still needs to be determined.

MANIFESTATIONS

The manifestations of immunosuppression relate to infection. The epidemiology of infections in compromised hosts encompasses a large and variable group, for example, nosocomial (hospital-acquired) and opportunistic infections (e.g., latent microbes). A clear picture of trends in infectious disease in immunocompromised patients, however, is hindered by changing supportive care practices as well as new therapies for the underlying disease, difficulties in isolating the causative organism, and simultaneous infection by several pathogens.

Table 17–2 lists the general characteristics of infection seen in the immunocompromised host. As noted earlier, a compromised host is a person susceptible to infections or in whom a particular infection follows an unexpectedly severe clinical course. This susceptibility results in the frequent and recurrent infections commonly seen with immunosuppression.[17] Resistance to antimicrobials, incomplete response to therapy, and a failure to heal between infectious episodes all contribute to the chronicity of these infections. A reactivation of latent and controlled organisms and an absence of signs of inflammation, except fever, are also characteristic of infection in the immunocompromised host.[77, 78]

Whatever the specific cause, immunosuppression will result in an enhanced susceptibility to infection, a manifestation related to both the degree of reduction in the immune response and the immunological components affected. Patients with cell-mediated immunodeficiency are more susceptible to intracellular pathogens, but differences in the host (e.g., presence of latent organisms) and the therapies used can predispose the host to variable organisms.[79] For example, trimethoprim-sulfamethoxazole used as a prophylactic against *Pneumocystis carinii* pneumonia can induce neutropenia in patients with AIDS and overwhelming infection with encapsulated bacteria or *Pseudomonas aeruginosa* may result. Organisms that infect individuals with cell-mediated defects may be exogenous or endogenous or both. Endogenous infections include the common latent infections with organisms that may be reac-

TABLE 17–2   CHARACTERISTICS OF INFECTION

1. Unusual pathogens
   a. Opportunistic
   b. Endogenous
   c. Low virulence
2. Reactivation of latent and controlled organisms
3. Frequent
4. Chronic and recurrent
5. Failure to clear between episodes
6. Incomplete response to therapy
7. Resistant to antimicrobials
8. Dissemination to distant sites
9. Absence of signs of inflammation except fever

tivated, such as herpes simplex, varicella-zoster, cytomegalovirus, *Candida, P. carinii,* and *Toxoplasma gondii.*[79] Antibody-mediated defects, in contrast, characteristically result in recurrent sinopulmonary tract infections, usually with encapsulated bacteria, such as otitis media, bronchitis, pneumonia, and gastrointestinal infections.[29]

As noted, cell-mediated mechanisms limit infection with intracellular organisms, including control of latent organisms. Reactivation of herpesvirus occurs in immunocompromised patients. In one institution, 85 per cent of patients undergoing bone marrow transplantation experienced reactivation of herpes simplex virus type 1 (e.g., aphthous stomatitis, or fever blisters), and 15 per cent experienced reactivation of herpes simplex virus type 2 (e.g., genital herpes).[80] Immunosuppression increases the mean healing time from days to approximately 3 weeks; the natural history of the infection is more severe. Herpes simplex virus also frequently reactivates in patients receiving intensive chemotherapy for leukemia, with a median onset of 17 days after treatment. In addition, in other patients with cancer who receive chemotherapy, herpes simplex virus reactivates after each chemotherapy cycle.[80]

Varicella-zoster virus (shingles), the reactivated form of the chickenpox virus, also causes substantial morbidity in the immunocompromised host. Skin or visceral dissemination of varicella-zoster virus may accompany acute lymphoblastic leukemia, SLE, organ transplantation, cytotoxic drugs, and steroids.[81, 82] In one study of 712 patients with localized varicella-zoster virus,[83] significant risk factors for dissemination included the diagnosis of Hodgkin's disease, advanced age, chemotherapy within 6 months of varicella-zoster virus infection, and extensive tumor at initial diagnosis.

Hospitalized patients in general are especially susceptible to exogenous transmission. The bacterium remains the most common pathogen responsible for hospital-acquired infections.[4] A 6-month study at a general hospital found a significant association between nosocomial enterococcal infections and antimicrobial therapy.[84] More specifically, the use of cephalosporins may selectively predispose patients to the increased risk of enterococcal superinfections, that is, infections occurring up to 1 week after administration of antimicrobials. In fact, enterococcal infec-

tions of wounds and the lower respiratory tract occurred almost one half as commonly as those due to *Staphylococcus aureus.* However, there has been a significant increase in nosocomial fungal infections, especially those due to *Candida* species, which progress rapidly and are refractory to therapy.[4]

Candida species, part of the indigenous microbial flora of the gastrointestinal tract, upper respiratory tract, buccal cavity, and vaginal tract, are normally suppressed by other microorganisms.[85] Alterations in host defense, for example, alterations in skin and mucous membranes, result in colonization and infection by this opportunistic fungus. Studies of intravenous catheters have shown a 2 to 8 per cent colonization rate by *Candida* species and an 18 per cent risk of fungemia after catheter colonization.[4] Disseminated candidiasis can result once colonization occurs, particularly in patients undergoing chemotherapy with persistent neutropenia. *Candida* organisms will multiply rapidly in many organs, especially if the host lacks systemic immune defenses.[85] In addition, *Candida* species in infected tissues are predominantly in the mycelial phase (M-phase) and more resistant to phagocytosis than in the Y phase (yeast phase). Burned patients who are immunosuppressed and receiving antibiotics to treat bacterial infections are also ideal hosts for early development of septicemia due to *Candida* species.[13] Of primary importance, several studies attribute an excessive mortality (38 per cent) to nosocomial candidemia.[86]

In opportunistic infections, the infecting organism may be common or rare but generally it is a pathogen (virus, bacteria, fungus, or protozoa) that lacks virulent properties and therefore causes disease only when the host's resistance is impaired.[17] Patients with cancer and prolonged neutropenia, many with indwelling catheters, and patients with AIDS and both T-cell and B-cell deficits exemplify the spectrum of compromised hosts. Neutropenia in the patient with cancer results from the chemotherapy, radiation therapy, or tumor invasion of the bone marrow.[87] This single most important defect makes the patient highly susceptible to bacterial and fungal infections.[77, 88] In this population, other interrelated defects increase the infection risk, such as defective neutrophil, T-cell and B-cell, and macrophage and monocyte function. Nutritional deficiencies, impaired physical barriers (skin, mucosal surfaces), and colonization by exogenous organisms further complicate the cancer infection risk profile.

Clinicians generally use an absolute granulocyte count of 500/mm[3] or less as an arbitrary criterion of neutropenia.[77, 78, 87] In neutropenic patients with cancer, particularly those with indwelling intravenous catheters, centers report gram-positive organisms (*S. aureus* and *S. epidermidis*) as the predominant bacterial isolates.[77, 78] In a cancer population with central venous catheters (n = 452), the gram-positive coagulase-negative staphylococcus accounted for the majority of the 88 episodes of catheter-related sepsis.[89] In contrast, Kiehn identified gram-negative rods Enterobacteriaceae as the cause of bacteremia in one series of 209 patients.[88] In addition, fungal overgrowth, mainly with *Candida* species, frequently accompanies the empiric antibiotic therapy required by these immunocompromised patients.[77, 90]

The incidence of opportunistic pathogens causing infection in AIDS differs from that reported for patients with neoplastic disease. Epidemiological data associate intracellular parasites that often cause latent infections with AIDS. For example, in 780 patients with AIDS, recurring or relapsing *P. carinii* infection developed in approximately half.[91] In fact, *P. carinii* pneumonia remains the most common infectious complication in AIDS.[34, 88, 92] Most humans by the age of 4 years develop antibody to *P. carinii*, a cyst-forming organism previously thought to be a protozoon and recently reclassified as a fungus.[93, 94] In the presence of immunosuppression, this pathogen multiplies, causing clinical disease. *P. carinii*, although generally confined to the lungs, can disseminate to the skin, eyes, spleen, and bone marrow.

In 336 patients with AIDS at one large center, *Mycobacterium avium*, also with an affinity for lung tissue, was the most frequent cause of bacteremia.[91] However, primarily *S. aureus*, *Streptococcus pneumoniae*, and *Escherichia coli* caused community-acquired bacteremia in a retrospective study of 38 AIDS patients.[95] In addition to the high incidence of *M. avium*, the opportunistic cytomegalovirus (CMV) persists as a common infection in AIDS. Close to 100 per cent of AIDS patients are seropositive for CMV, and longitudinal studies show a pattern of recurrent or chronic infection.[38] In an extensive study on AIDS (n = 780),[91] 224 patients developed CMV infection, but in some series this infection occurred in nearly all patients with AIDS.[88] As noted with other opportunistic organisms in AIDS, this organism usually causes chronic disseminated infection.

SURVEILLANCE AND MEASUREMENT

Clinicians need to identify patients who cannot respond adequately to an antigenic challenge. There are many more patients with a decreased resistance to infection than in the past, although data predicting which patients are more susceptible remain fragmented and controversial. The elucidation of risk factors prior to the onset of an infection, however, will decrease morbidity. For instance, people with nutritional deficits and those who experience stress, such as the hospitalized and the chronically ill, exemplify diverse populations susceptible to infections. Malnutrition and stress are clinically more varying and numerous and less discrete than medical diagnoses. Thus, early recognition of immunocompromised patients depends on assessing each patient for the presence of malnutrition and stress in addition to clinical states and diagnoses. The very young and elderly also require particular attention.

The manifestations of immunosuppression relate to infection; therefore, signs of infection further identify the immunocompromised host. Surveillance of fever, which is initiated by monocytes,[96] over time is important, although the frequency of monitoring is not established. Elevated body temperature, as a host defense, directs and accelerates the inflammatory response to the infection site and thereby limits its spread. Temperatures of 38° and 39° C dramatically augment the action of IL-1 and thus T-cell proliferation, cytolytic T-cell generation, and B-cell activity, including Ig synthesis. These febrile temperatures also adversely affect the replication of certain viruses and bacteria. NK activity, however, is substantially reduced.

The specific characteristics of infection (Table 17–2) and common infectious syndromes of skin, mucous membranes, gastrointestinal tract, or lungs assist in the identification of a compromised host. Mild pharyngeal inflammation and perianal tenderness in the absence of swelling or erythema require particular attention,[77] as do such signs occurring in the axilla. These areas are prone to infection in neutropenic patients who may not exhibit all the typical signs of inflammation when tissue infection occurs. Immunological tests will further identify immunosuppressed patients.

Immunological testing is particularly useful in monitoring immunosuppression, since there is lack of agreement on both the frequency and specific pathogens that indicate abnormal host resistance. Analysis of immunocompetent cells, however, remains hampered by difficulties in test standardization, biological variability, the imprecise nature of many assays, and the complexity and expense of the procedures.[97] Table 17–3 lists tests used to screen for general immune competence. Clinicians must use their own laboratory's normal values for comparison and avoid interpreting the level of the immunological component with functional competence.

Immunodiffusion techniques determine the levels of each of the major immunoglobulins (IgG, IgM, IgA). Quantification of serum Ig evaluates antibody-mediated immunity; however, test interpretation must reflect the large degree of variability in Ig levels that exists in the normal population. The total hemolytic complement (CH_{50}) test requires that all the nine major complement components (C1-C9) be intact.[98] Each component must activate sequentially in order for a complement reaction to progress. The antibody-mediated hemolysis of erythrocytes in the presence of an intact complement system is a crude screening test (CD_{50}) for complement activity, since a drastic reduction in complement components (> 50 per cent) is necessary to produce a reduction in this assay. The simpler immunochemical determination of the third complement component (C3), the component necessary for all types of complement activity, is more useful.[97] Values for normal CH_{50} and C3 can

vary greatly, depending on test conditions, and require cautious interpretation.

The differential white blood cell count measures total lymphocytes and neutrophils. An absolute neutrophil count below $500/mm^3$ is classified as neutropenia, and infection is likely to occur.[77] The nitroblue tetrazolium (NBT) dye reduction test assesses the overall metabolic integrity of phagocytosing neutrophils. Substituting the more sensitive chemoluminescence process to measure metabolic events of neutrophils during phagocytosis is occurring more frequently. Assessment of neutrophil function, however, must always take into account its essential dependence on both the antibody- and cell-mediated immune response.

The delayed hypersensitivity (DHS) skin test, a relatively simple intradermal test, is very valuable in the overall assessment of immunosuppression.[97–100] The in vivo DHS reaction is actually the result of a series of complex phenomena, including antigen recognition, lymphocyte-macrophage interaction, release of soluble lymphocyte mediators, and changes in vascular permeability. Inability to react to a battery of recall antigens to which patients are commonly sensitized (e.g., streptokinase/streptodornase, *Candida albicans*, trycophyton, mumps) is termed anergy. Anergy is associated with numerous clinical states and diseases, including malnutrition, surgery, and cancer.[42, 43, 101] Sequential skin testing monitors more accurately an immune-compromised host, although the appropriate or optimal timing remains undocumented.

In vitro assessment of lymphocyte response to nonspecific mitogens, or to specific antigens, is not indicated for routine use. Only when the in vivo skin test results suggest possible cell-mediated immune response alterations should cell function be explored in vitro. In vitro tests clarify and elaborate on cell types. This is also true for assays of T and B lymphocytes, which help characterize cellular markers and the proportional relationship of one group of cells to another. They do not identify, however, the cause of the abnormality or provide sufficient information on immune status.

After immunocompromised hosts are identified, an ongoing assessment of their immune status is necessary. The characteristics of infection that identified these patients as immune compromised also guide in their surveillance. For example, chronic therapy-

TABLE 17–3 TESTS OF GENERAL IMMUNE COMPETENCE

Antibody-mediated immunity
   Quantitative immunoglobulin levels
Cell-mediated immunity
   Differential white blood cell count
   Delayed hypersensitivity skin test
Phagocytosis
   Differential white blood cell count
   Nitroblue tetrazolium dye reduction test (NBT) or
     chemoluminescence
Complement
   Hemolytic complement quantitation (CH_{50})
   Third complement component (C3) level

resistant infections occur in this population and monitoring the response of the patient to infection and its treatment can detect persistent immunosuppression.

Tests of general immune competence (Table 17–3) can help evaluate changes in the quality or quantity of an immune response. Multiparameter and sequential testing yield the most useful information, especially since, as noted previously, neither the results of a specific test nor a battery of tests is documented as indicative of immunosuppression. Continual use of the in vivo DHS test also needs emphasizing. In vitro tests remove the immune component under study from the host and address only a single immune component or part of the host response. Such isolation does not consider the complex interdependency of the various components of the immune system.

THERAPIES

Prevention of infection is a high priority in immunocompromised patients. Nurses may make an invaluable contribution to their care through the initiation of infection prevention measures.[87, 102] One approach to the development of such measures considers four separate but interrelated strategies: (1) reducing damage to mechanical barriers, (2) preventing acquisition of organisms, (3) suppressing organisms currently colonizing the patient, and (4) augmenting host defenses.[77] An effective protocol includes all four strategies.

An infectious agent challenges multiple host defenses, including the potent, although relatively nonspecific, body surface defenses. The mucociliary action of the respiratory tract, local production of chemical antimicrobial factors, presence of normal body flora, and mucosal activity preventing epithelial attachment and penetration all provide surface defense. These external host defenses act at the site of microbial attack and protect tissues from invasion.[77] Specifically, the skin, nasopharynx, oropharynx, eyes, and respiratory, gastrointestinal, and genitourinary tracts act as the mechanical barriers to infection. Interruption of these barriers through, for example, vascular access devices or chemotherapy-induced mucositis allows various microbes to become pathogenic and produce infection.

The respiratory tract is in constant contact with the environment, and its defenses (mucociliary apparatus, pulmonary macrophages, nasal hairs, and cough reflex) play a critical role in defending the body against a hostile environment.[103, 104] Lung defenses are particularly important against opportunistic infections, such as the predominantly extracellular pathogen *P. carinii*. This infection virtually never occurs unless the host is immunocompromised, and even then it is usually confined within the lung, suggesting an organism of low-invasive potential.[103] Nurses protect the healthy respiratory tract from infection by monitoring respiratory function, initiating pulmonary hygiene, and educating the patient about predisposing factors and reportable signs and symptoms.[102, 105–107]

The National Institutes of Health Consensus Development Conference on Oral Complications of Cancer Therapy explicitly advocated early oral care to prevent mucositis.[108] Most oral care protocols that reduce alterations in oral integrity include systematic mouth inspections, cleansing by various agents (e.g., saline, sodium bicarbonate), maintenance of good dental hygiene and adequate nutrition, and early treatment of infectious complications.[109–111] There is no general agreement about the frequency of oral care or what tools (e.g., brushes, sponges) or agents to use.[112] Perineal care, preventing pressure sores, and avoiding invasive procedures (enemas, venipunctures, and bladder catheterizations) also prevent damage to mechanical barriers.

Another strategy of infection prevention, reducing the acquisition of and colonization by new organisms from the environment, involves measures that vary in their complexity. Often simple but effective ones, such as careful hand washing are often overlooked.[77, 79, 102, 113] Meticulous hand washing prevents transmission of both endogenous and exogenous nosocomial infections, since organisms are transmitted on the hands of personnel. Researchers observing 986 hand washes found that the hand-washing practices of individual oncology nurses varied significantly and were not necessarily associated with the extent of patient contact.[114] Evidence also exists that the main causative agents of hospital-acquired infection (i.e., *S. aureus*, gram-negative bacilli) reach susceptible patients via direct contact, predominantly on the hands of hospital staff, rather than via the airborne route.[115] The Centers for Disease Control recommends universal precautions, body substance isolation, for all patients. This infection control measure focuses on isolating body substances from the hands of personnel, primarily by increased use of gloves and hand washing, and provides a consistent approach to preventing the transmission of potentially infectious agents.[116]

Cost factors limit the utility of protective isolation, a measure that protects patients from nosocomial microbial flora and includes a ventilation system to remove microorganisms from the air (laminar airflow), room decontamination, low-microbial diets, and the exclusion of raw fruits and vegetables to decrease gut colonization.[106, 107] In addition to measures previously discussed, traditional neutropenic precautions may also include a private room, reduced room clutter, no flowers or plants, and visitor restriction, especially of infected individuals.[102, 105–107] Systematic patient teaching regarding these measures must start before their initiation and is reinforced as needed. As noted, hospitalization results in increased colonization and minimalizing hospitalizations and lengths of stay should result in decreased nosocomial infection rates. Current supportive data, however, do not exist. Also, some measures to reduce respiratory colonization, such as sterile tracheostomy suctioning techniques, and specific methods to reduce resuscitation equipment contamination require further research.[113] The standard protective measures, such as hand washing and a private room, therefore still remain important modalities in effectively preventing the acquisition of new organisms.

Suppression of aerobic microorganisms with preservation of the anaerobic flora, and thus host resistance to colonization, might prove beneficial in infection prophylaxis. Anaerobic bacteria reside throughout the body and are particularly in high concentrations in the gastrointestinal tract as part of the normal flora. Current regimens contain either nonabsorbable multiple drugs that act locally on the digestive tract (e.g., vancomycin, gentamicin, polymyxin, nystatin, colistin) or absorbable agents such as trimethoprim-sulfamethoxazole, erythromycin, or nalidixic acid that act both locally and systemically.[106, 107, 117] The oral nonabsorbable agents, however, are unpalatable and together with the side effects of nausea, vomiting, and diarrhea

contribute to patient compliance problems. Prophylactic efficacy and costs are other unsolved difficulties associated with this measure.

Some clinicians advocate selective decontamination of the digestive tract to control colonization of the oral cavity and the gastrointestinal tract in patients undergoing mechanical ventilation.[118] This technique uses nonabsorbable topical antibiotics (polymyxin B, tobramycin, amphotericin B) applied to the oropharynx and instilled into the stomach and a short course of intravenous cephalosporin. Dose-related nephrotoxicity and rigors, however, accompany empiric amphotericin B therapy used for undocumented fungal infections.[119, 120]

Similarly, Niederman recommends re-evaluating aerosolized or topically applied antibiotics (e.g., polymixin B, tobramycin) to prevent colonization of the airways and thus nosocomial respiratory infections in high-risk patients.[121] He suggests that confining this technique to only very-high-risk patients should reduce the problem of emerging bacterial resistance. Long-term prophylaxis with local antibiotics could result in increased antibiotic resistance.[122, 123] The superinfection of antimicrobial prophylaxis occurs when prolonged use of antimicrobials alters the normal flora, suppressing the susceptible organisms and favoring the growth of drug-resistant ones.[17] Specifically, in intensive care units the most prevalent isolates, *S. epidermidis*, *P. aeruginosa*, enterococcus, and *Candida* species, all exhibit multiple drug resistance.[124] Antibiotic resistance genes carried in extrachromosomal DNA not only facilitate transmission of the resistant gene from organism to organism within the environment but also confer resistance to multiple antibiotics.

Reducing damage to the host augments host defenses and can bolster resistance to infection. For example, maintaining adequate blood perfusion is critical to host defenses because ischemic tissue is poorly resistant to infection. Decreased perfusion reduces the circulation of immune components and impairs the oxygen-dependent microbicidal mechanisms of neutrophils. The prophylaxis and treatment of stress ulcers, mainly in critically ill patients, by antacids such as sucralfate that maintain the gastric pH between 1 and 2 demonstrate another measure that enhances host resistance. Antacids (magnesium or aluminum hydroxide) or H_2 blockers (e.g., cimetidine) that reduce gastric acidity neutralize natural chemical barriers and allow overgrowth of gastric flora.[124, 125] This results in microbe migration up the esophagus to the pharynx, their continual aspiration, and pneumonia.

Infection itself can alter host resistance not only to the primary infection but also to a secondary infection. Plasma Ig concentration increases during infection, but antibody response to an unrelated antigen is depressed.[12] Similarly, the number of circulating PMNs increases but chemotaxis, phagocytosis, and bactericidal activity are impaired. Acute infections may result in a transient immunosuppression, possibly mediated by suppressor T cells. This reduction in host resistance to a secondary infection makes early detection of infection and prompt intervention a major nursing responsibility.

In addition, improving the nutritional status can optimize the host's metabolic response to infection. Once activated, immune cells are metabolically very active. Nutritional deficits, however, alter cellular synthesis and the immune response.[60] These effects may be long-term but reversible or irreversible, depending on the severity and duration of the malnutrition; therefore, inadequate nutritional support must be avoided. Nurses, in consultation with the dietitian, need to consistently evaluate nutritional assessment data and individual energy and protein requirements in determining the most appropriate nutritional regimen for the malnourished patient.[87, 102]

Clinical trials are currently evaluating the efficacy of immunomodulators, drugs that directly change specific immune reactions to augment host defense (e.g., interferons, interleukins, and colony-stimulating factors).[77] These agents are also referred to as biological response modifiers (BRMs). Specific tumors (chronic myelogenous leukemia) and viral infections (HIV, hepatitis B virus, and herpesvirus) respond to alpha-interferon, although most patients develop an influenza-like syndrome.[126–128] This syndrome includes fever, chills, nausea and vomiting, and headache, requiring dose adjustment for severe reactions.

A more significant toxicity, however, accompanies the use of IL-2 alone or in combination with lymphokine-activated killer (LAK) cells for cancer therapy.[129] LAK cells, generated from lymphoid cells incubated in IL-2, can lyse a broader range of tumor cells (adoptive immunotherapy) than NK cells. Tumor-infiltrating lymphocytes (TILs), another type of activated lymphocytes, are isolated from tumors then expanded by culture in IL-2 to give them more specificity than LAK cells. Patients with melanoma show a therapeutic response when treated with TILs.[130] Researchers are also testing the response of LAK cells and IL-2 in combination with monoclonal antibody, identical copies of antibody, as a colorectal cancer therapy.[130] The acute cardiovascular, renal, and pulmonary toxicities of IL-2 therapy are affected by dose, route, and schedule. Nurses from the National Biotherapy Study Group developed specific symptom management strategies for intravenous, intracavitary, and intraarterial activated lymphocyte administration.[131]

In contrast to the tumor cytolytic properties of IL-2, granulocyte and granulocyte-macrophage colony-stimulating factors (G-CSF, GM-CSF) promote the proliferation of earlier hematopoietic precursors, lessening the neutropenia associated with cancer chemotherapy.[132, 133] Treatment with both G-CSF and GM-CSF at effective doses generally is well tolerated. The Oncology Nursing Society, projecting future nursing involvement with patients receiving BRMs, developed recommendations for nursing education and practice.[134] These guidelines stress the importance of the patient-family-nurse triad reporting and documenting the occurrence of biotherapy-induced reactions.

REVIEW OF RESEARCH FINDINGS

A review of several research studies (excluding drug trials), some previously cited, illustrates the current state of clinical research in the area of immunosuppression. The complexity of the immune system and the multifaceted etiology of immunosuppression, and thus its diverse mechanisms and manifestations, limit not only the number of clinical studies but also the research questions asked and the conclusions made by investigators. Clinical studies focus on identifying predictors of infection in various immunocompromised populations or on its prevention. The lack of methodological standards in the documentation of infection, however, frequently hinders an analysis of findings across studies.

Talcott and associates examined the medical records of 184 cancer patients admitted for fever and neutropenia, 58 per cent with leukemia or lymphoma, to determine the clinical course and infectious complications of granulocytopenia.[135] In this sample, 16 per cent presented with localized skin inflammation, 14 per cent with mucositis, 6 per cent with a new or increased chest roentgenogram infiltrate, and 5 per cent with a red or tender Hickman catheter exit site. In 57 per cent of the patients, the potential cause of fever could not be established, and 43 per cent had no microbiological evidence of infection (negative blood and urine cultures). Data demonstrated an increased risk of coagulase-negative *Staphylococcus* bacteremia in patients with indwelling central catheters, a finding consistent with other research. All patients began empirical broad-spectrum antibiotics upon admission. Fevers resolved in a median of 3 days and severe granulocytopenia in 6 days, and hospitalization was a median of 11 days. Results suggested that the prognostic significance of fever and neutropenia may differ, dependent on the extent of cancer.

Other studies examined infections in indwelling central venous catheters (CVC). During a year-long study of 452 patients with cancer, Benezra and associates documented a total of 142 episodes of infectious complications in 488 CVCs.[89] Of these episodes, 88 were identified as catheter-related sepsis, 34 as exit site infection, and 20 as tunnel infections. Catheter removal was required to achieve cure in most tunnel infections, particularly if *Pseudomonas* was cultured from the exit sites. Interestingly, infections occurring in neutropenic patients were associated with a similar outcome to those that developed in non-neutropenic patients. Armstrong and colleagues identified predictors of infection from data on 169 CVCs used for total parenteral nutrition in an adult medical-surgical population (n = 88).[136] Infection was associated with a positive insertion site skin culture taken close to the time of catheter removal and with erythema at the insertion site greater than 4 mm in diameter. Blood culture results, however, added little to the risk estimate. These researchers concluded that periodic insertion site cultures should be useful in evaluating subsequent fever in stable patients with CVCs.

Identification of risk factors can help clinicians prospectively define specific subgroups of immunocompromised patients (cancer patients) who would most benefit from receiving antimicrobial prophylaxis. Regarding varicella-zoster virus disseminated infection, Rusthoven and associates found Hodgkin's disease, non-Hodgkin's lymphoma, and head and neck cancer significantly correlated with dissemination of localized varicella-zoster.[83] In a study of 78 immunocompromised patients admitted for bone marrow transplantation, 12 had a detectable respiratory virus (confirmed by culture) before transplantation, with 11 exhibiting upper respiratory symptoms.[104] According to the investigators, infections with respiratory viruses are frequent and symptomatic in immunocompromised patients.

Since increasing age has been correlated with increasing postoperative infection, Penin and Ehrenkranz analyzed medical records randomly drawn from 17,500 postoperative patients to determine whether the cost-effectiveness of surveillance could be enhanced by selecting fewer classes of operation or by selecting subjects of older age in all operations.[137] Data revealed that in four of eight classes of designated operations (large bowel operations, hysterectomies, total hip replacement, other hip prosthesis), the mean ages of persons with major infection were no greater than those of uninfected persons. In this community hospital–based consortium study, the other elective operations were cholecystectomy, prostatectomy, laminectomy, and hip fracture. Among major infections, wound infection was most frequent at 47.5 per cent and then pneumonia at 36.4 per cent. According to these researchers, a decision to focus surveillance primarily on older patients or on wound infection alone would not result in an effective infection control program.

Research has also addressed problems related to the assessment and prevention of specific infections, such as oral or perirectal, and the effects of infection prevention strategies, including isolation. Weikel and associates examined the medical and dental records of 100 granulocytopenic cancer patients to determine the incidence of fever from prechemotherapy invasive dental procedures.[138] They found that although periodontal probing and dental scaling invade mucosal barriers, these procedures did not significantly affect the incidence of fever or bacteremia.

Eilers and associates explored the feasibility of the Oral Assessment Guide and the severity of oral problems in 20 patients undergoing bone marrow transplantation.[109] They concluded that intensive chemotherapy and radiation therapy have a two-phase effect on the oral cavity: an initial direct stomatotoxic effect and a secondary late effect due to myelosuppression and the general effects of the treatment. Kenny conducted a pilot study (n = 18) of two oral care protocols differing in the type of lip lubricant, toothette, and mouthwash on the incidence of stomatitis.[139] She did not find a significant difference between group mean oral assessments scores but did find a negative correlation between the degree of stomatitis and the leukocyte count. According to Yeomans and associates, using chlorhexidine gluconate in a prophylactic perirectal skin care regimen did not offer increased protection against perirectal infections in 40 patients undergoing intensive chemotherapy.[140] Their data, however, also showed a correlation between the severity of granulocytopenia and the incidence of infection. All of these investigators used assessment tools specifically designed for their studies.

ILLUSTRATIVE CASE STUDY

C.L., a 20-year-old female with multiple prior admissions, was admitted for treatment of low blood cell counts secondary to induction chemotherapy. Her acute lymphoblastic leukemia (ALL), diagnosed 10 months previously, was in remission. An initial course of intensive chemotherapy can produce marrow hypoplasia, allowing normal cells to repopulate and thus correct the massive infiltration of marrow with blast (immature) cells that occurs in ALL. The goal of her current chemotherapy was to consolidate the remission. C.L. had her third Hickman (tunneled) catheter in place, since two previous central venous catheters had been removed for infection. After completion of her initial chemotherapy and last catheter-related infection, an episode of hepatitis occurred.

On this admission, the patient presented with fever (38.5° C). Her lungs were clear. An oral examination revealed mucositis that included ulcerative mouth lesions and an infected molar. Petechiae were noted on her face, abdomen, and lower legs.

She appeared tired and pale and complained of mild malaise, fatigue, nausea, diarrhea, and headache. Laboratory studies revealed thrombocytopenia, anemia, and mild hypokalemia.

C.L. was being treated with trimethoprim-sulfamethoxazole prophylaxis for *P. carinii* pneumonia and nystatin to prevent candidal infections. Empiric antibiotic therapy consisted of tobramycin, an aminoglycoside, and the broad-spectrum antibiotics penicillin and ticarcillin. She received 10 units of random donor platelets and 2 units of packed red blood cells. Table 17–4 lists laboratory data showing the progress of C.L. over time.

For 3 days, C.L. could tolerate only a full liquid diet, owing partially to her mucositis and nausea. Prochlorperazine was prescribed for the nausea. Acetaminophen with codeine was used for the mucosal pain, and an oral care regimen was initiated. On day 4, an oral examination revealed less mucositis; however, the antifungal agent clotrimazole was prescribed. At this time, both rectal and perirectal areas were excoriated and C.L. complained of rectal pain. The nursing staff initiated sitz baths and an ointment developed by the hospital pharmacy to aid wound healing. After two as-needed (p.r.n.) intravenous doses, daily diphenhydramine was ordered to decrease extremity and trunk pruritus. The rectal lesions decreased in size by day 8, but the degree of rectal pain required p.r.n. intravenous morphine.

On day 9, the nursing staff identified C.L. as depressed and documented the length of the present hospitalization and the lack of visits by the family, who lived some

TABLE 17–4 LABORATORY DATA ILLUSTRATIVE OF IMMUNOSUPPRESSION

HOSPITAL DAY	1	2	3	4	5	6	10
WBC*	0.5	0.3	0.5	0.8			1
PMNs (%)	0				6	12	22
Total neutrophils*	0.15						
Hematocrit (%)	25	23	29				29
Platelets*	9	48	45	55			

*Thousands/mm³.

Normal values for age and sex: white blood cell count (WBC), 4500 to 13,200/mm³; polymorphonuclear neutrophils (PMNs), 25 to 70%; total neutrophils, 1800 to 8000/mm³; hematocrit 36 to 46%; platelets 140,000 to 450,000/mm³.

distance away, as contributing factors. Both rectal and mouth discomfort decreased by day 10. During the 10 days of hospitalization, all cultures of blood, urine, and oral secretions, and a cytology stain of an oral lesion for herpes were negative. The nursing staff had instituted unit infection prevention strategies for neutropenic patients, including a sign on the door of C.L.'s private room stating: "no entry if recent exposure to infection, wash hands at room sink, no plants or flowers, and dietary restrictions." The nurses also noted the importance of decreasing the patient's depression and encouraged nutritional intake when tolerated.

This case illustrates the phenomenon of immunosuppression. C.L.'s disease and its treatment, in addition to the infection and antimicrobials, contributed to the development of immunosuppression. Colonization due to multiple admissions can be an additional factor. C.L. exemplifies populations at risk for this phenomenon. She was chronically ill, hospitalized for a lengthy period, experienced stress (documented depression), and was nutritionally depleted. Mouth discomfort, nausea, malaise, and infection prevention strategies, such as dietary restrictions, can result in an inadequate dietary intake.

C.L. exhibited the most common manifestation of immunosuppression, infection, occurring in the usual sites (mucous membranes) and a history of infections. She was maintained on prophylactic antifungal and antiparasitic therapy. Opportunistic organisms, the endogenous fungus *Candida* and herpes, a latent virus, were suspected as causative agents. The staff identified C.L. as a compromised host and monitored her immune status through sequential testing of a daily differential white blood cell count. They prevented infection by reducing damage to her skin, a mechanical barrier, through medication for her pruritus. An antifungal agent plus oral care prevented further alterations in the oral mucosa, and the rectal area was treated as well. Infection prevention techniques helped to reduce the acquisition of new organisms. Selective microbials provided broad-spectrum coverage of organisms with minimal emergence of resistant strains.

Treating the infection, thrombocytopenia, anemia, and any nutritional deficits can augment the host defense.

IMPLICATIONS FOR FURTHER RESEARCH

Several aspects of immunosuppression support the feasibility and necessity of nurse researchers investigating this phenomenon. Of primary importance is the prevalence of immunocompromised hosts in clinical practice. Also, as noted throughout this chapter and as shown in Review of Research Findings, clinical studies either are few in number or have not adequately identified populations at risk for infection. This hinders infection prevention and treatment for a large group of patients. Nursing research can expand the knowledge base of this prevalent and clinically relevant phenomenon and improve the care of immunocompromised patients.

Many general questions germane to nursing and the phenomenon of immunosuppression identify areas that need further study. For instance, nurses need to identify immunocompromised patients. What identification measures would avoid a delay in the prevention or treatment of infectious complications? What surveillance methods need to follow identification? Also, nursing practices may decrease the risk of infection. How effective are current approaches in decreasing the acquisition of new organisms? What prophylactic approaches to infection prevention are needed? Nurses initiate infection prevention strategies for immunocompromised hosts, but it is not known what nursing protocols for the patient with neutropenia are the most effective and what facilitates staff compliance with such protocols. Additional work needs to explore problems of mucositis. Which oral care protocols are effective? What is the stomatotoxicity index of treatment protocols? What individuals are at risk for problems secondary to mucositis? In the area of patient education, nurses must explore what immunocompromised patients need to be taught upon discharge about the prevention or manifestations of infection.

In preparation for the twenty-first century, the American Nurses Association directs nurses to give immediate priority to nursing research that will generate knowledge that ensures the needs of particularly vulnerable groups are met through appropriate strategies.[141] Nurses have the clinical expertise and roles to effect practice changes in the care of immunocompromised hosts, a vulnerable patient population for many clinical specialties.

REFERENCES

1. Young, L. (1991). Opportunistic infections in the compromised host. In D. Stites & A. Terr (eds.), *Basic and Clinical Immunology* (7th ed., pp. 712–716). East Norwalk, CT: Appleton & Lange.
2. *Nursing: A Social Policy Statement*. (1980). (Publication No. NP-63). Kansas City: American Nurses Association.
3. Ammann, A. (1991). Antibody (B cell) immunodeficiency disorders. In D. Stites & A. Terr (eds.), *Basic and Clinical Immunology* (7th ed., pp. 322–334). East Norwalk CT: Appleton & Lange.
4. Anaissie, E., & Bodey, G. (1989). Nosocomial fungal infections: Old problems and new challenges. Infect Dis Clin North Am 3:867–881.
5. Rinaldi, M. (1989). Emerging opportunists. Infect Dis Clin North Am 3:65–76.
6. Garovoy, M., Melzer, J., Ascher, N., Magilligan, D., & Bozdech, M. (1991). Clinical transplantation. In D. Stites & A. Terr (eds.), *Basic and Clinical Immunology* (7th ed., pp. 747–765). East Norwalk, CT: Appleton & Lange.
7. Frank, M. (1987). Complement in the pathophysiology of human disease. N Engl J Med 316:1525–1530.
8. Stone, H. (1986). Infection in postoperative patients. Am J Med 81(Suppl. 1A):39–44.
9. *Cancer Facts & Figures—1992*. (1992). Atlanta: American Cancer Society.
10. Oleske, J. (1989). Immunologic disorders. J Allergy Clin Immunol 84:1078–1081.
11. *HIV/AIDS Surveillance* (1992). (February). Washington, D.C.: Department of Health and Human Services.
12. Ammann, A. (1987). Immunodeficiency diseases. In D. Stites, J. Stobo, & J. Wells (eds.), *Basic and Clinical Immunology* (6th ed., pp. 317–355). Los Altos, CA: Lange Medical.
13. Desal, M., Herndon, D., & Abston, S. (1987). Candida infection in massively burned patients. J Trauma 27:1186–1188.
14. Hansbrough, J., Zapata-Sirvent, R., & Peterson, V. (1987). Immunomodulation following burn injury. Burns 67:69–92.
15. Luterman, A., Dacso, C., & Curreri, P. (1986). Infections in burn patients. Am J Med 81(Suppl. 1A):45–52.
16. Shaw, J., & Print, C. (1989). Postsplenectomy sepsis. Br J Surg 76:1074–1081.
17. Brook, G., Butel, J., & Ornston, L. (1991). *Jawetz, Melnick & Adelberg's Medical Microbiology*. East Norwalk, CT: Appleton & Lange.
18. Landers, D., Bronson, R., Pavia, C., & Stites, D. (1991). Reproductive immunology. In D. Stites & A. Terr (eds.), *Basic and Clinical Immunology* (7th ed., pp. 200–216). East Norwalk, CT: Appleton & Lange.
19. Strober, W., & James, S. (1991). The mucosal immune system. In D. Stites, & A. Terr (eds.), *Basic and Clinical Immunology* (7th ed., pp. 175–186). East Norwalk, CT: Appleton & Lange.
20. Weigle, W. (1989). Effects of aging on the immune system. Hosp Pract (Dec. 15), 24:112–119.
21. Keasbery, P., & Ershler, W. (1989). The importance of immunesenescence in the incidence and malignant properties of cancer in hosts of advanced age. J Gerontol 41:63–66.
22. Jawetz, E., Melnick, J., Adelberg, E., Brooks, G., Butal, J., & Ornston, L. (1989). *Medical Microbiology* (18th ed.). East Norwalk, CT: Appleton & Lange.
23. Claman, H. (1989). The biology of the immune system. JAMA 258:2834–2840.
24. Bach, F. (1990). Cell-mediated immunity: Its basis and analysis. *Nutrition* 6(Suppl.)2–4.
25. Claman, H. (1989). Immune mechanisms: T cells and B cells. J Allergy Clin Immunol 84:1012–1014.
26. Coffman, R. (1989). T-helper heterogeneity and immune response patterns. Hosp Pract (Aug. 15), 24:101–133.
27. Faltynek, C., & Oppenheim, J. (1988). Interferons in host defense. J Natl Cancer Instit 80:151–153.
28. Roitt, I. (1988). *Essential Immunology* (6th ed.). Boston: Blackwell Scientific.
29. Heinzel, F. (1989). Infection in patients with humoral immunodeficiency. Hosp Pract (Sept. 15), 24:99–130.
30. Grady, C. (1988). Host defense mechanisms: An overview. Semin Oncol Nurs 4:86–94.
31. Kaufmann, S. (1988). CD8+ T lymphocytes in intracellular microbial infections. Immunol Today 9:168–173.
32. Herzenberg, L., & Herzenberg, L. (1989). Toward a layered immune system. Cell 59:953–954.
33. Rosenberg, Z., & Fauci, A. (1990). Immunopathogenic mechanisms of HIV infection: Cytosine induction of HIV expression. Immunol Today 11:176–180.
34. Lovejoy, N. (1988). The pathophysiology of AIDS. Oncol Nurs Forum 15:563–571.
35. Lewis, A. (1988). HIV: The basics. In A. Lewis (ed.), *Nursing Care of the Person with AIDS/ARC* (pp. 3–9). Rockville, MD: Aspen.
36. Levy, J. (1988). The human immunodeficiency virus and its pathogenesis. Infect Dis Clin North Am 2:285–297.
37. Grady, C. (1989). The immune system and AIDS/HIV infection. In J. Flaskerud (ed.), *AIDS/HIV Infection. A Reference Guide for Nursing Professionals* (pp. 37–57). Philadelphia: W. B. Saunders.
38. Deitch, E. (1988). Infection in the compromised host. Surg Clin North Am 68:181–197.
39. Christou, N., & Tellado, J. (1989). In vitro polymorphonuclear neutrophil function in surgical patients does not correlate with anergy but with "activating" processes such as sepsis or trauma. Surgery 106:718–724.
40. Faist, E., Ertel, W., Cohnert, T., Huber, V., Inthorn, D., & Heberer, G. (1990). Immunoprotective effects of cyclooxygenase inhibition in patients with major surgical trauma. J Trauma 30:8–18.
41. Lazarou, S., Barbul, A., Wasserkrug, H., & Efron, G. (1989). The wound is a possible source of posttraumatic immunosuppression. Arch Surg 124:1429–1431.
42. MacLean, L. (1988). Delayed type hypersensitivity

testing in surgical patients. Surg Gynecol Obstet *166*:285–293.

43. Tellado, J., Giannias, B., Kapadia, B., Chartrand, L., deSantis, M., & Christou, N. (1990). Anergic patients before elective surgery have enhanced nonspecific host-defense capacity. Arch Surg *125*:48–53.

44. Fye, K., & Sack, K. (1991). Rheumatic diseases. In D. Stites & A. Terr (eds.), *Basic and Clinical Immunology* (7th ed., pp. 438–463). East Norwalk, CT: Appleton & Lange.

45. Froelich, C., Guiffaut, S., Sosenko, M., & Muth, K. (1989). Deficient interleukin-2 activated killer cell cytotoxicity in patients with systemic lupus erythematosus. Clin Immunol Immunopathol *50*:132–145.

46. Pollack, R., & Roth, J. (1989). Cancer-induced immunosuppression: Implications for therapy. Semin Surg Oncol *5*:414–419.

47. Greenberg, P. (1991). Mechanisms of tumor immunology. In D. Stites & A. Terr (eds.), *Basic and Clinical Immunology* (7th ed., pp. 580–567). East Norwalk, CT: Appleton & Lange.

48. Gallucci, B. (1987). The immune system and cancer. Oncol Nurs Forum *14*(Suppl.):3–12.

49. Fahey, J. (1987). Immune interventions in disease. Ann Intern Med *106*:257–274.

50. Allison, A., & Lee, S. (1989). The mode of action of anti-rheumatic drugs. 1. Anti-inflammatory and immunosuppressive effects of glucocorticoids. Prog Drug Res *33*:63–81.

51. Hadden, J. (1987). Immunopharmacology. Immunomodulation and immunotherapy. JAMA *258*:3005–3010.

52. Hadden, J. (1987). Correction of secondary T-cell immunodeficiencies with biological substances and drugs. Cancer Detect Prevent (Suppl. 1):*11*:409–421.

53. Mokyr, M., & Dray, S. (1987). Interplay between the toxic effects of anticancer drugs and host antitumor immunity in cancer therapy. Cancer Ther *5*:31–38.

54. Groopman, J., & Broder, S. (1989). Cancer in AIDS and other immunodeficiency states. In V. DeVita, S. Hellman, & S. Rosenberg (eds.), *Cancer: Principles and Practice of Oncology* (pp. 1953–1970). Philadelphia: J. B. Lippincott.

55. Fraser, M., & Tucker, M. (1988). Late effects of cancer therapy: Chemotherapy-related malignancies. Oncol Nurs Forum *15*:67–77.

56. Chandra, R. (1990). Nutrition is an important determinant of immunity in old age. Prog Clin Biol Res *326*:321–334.

57. Daly, J., Reynolds, J., Sigal, R., Shou, J., & Liberman, M. (1990). Effects of dietary protein and amino acids on immune function. Crit Care Med *18* (Suppl.):S86–S93.

58. Lowell, J., Parnes, H., & Blackburn, G. (1990). Dietary immunomodulation: Beneficial effects on oncogenesis and tumor growth. Crit Care Med *18*:S145–S148.

59. Kinsella, J., Lokesh, B., Broughton, S., & Whelan, J. (1990). Dietary polysaturated fatty acids and eicosanoids: Potential effects on the modulation of inflammatory and immune cells: An overview. Nutrition *6*:45–52.

60. Terr, A., Dubey, D., Yunis, E., Slavin, R., & Waldman, R. (1991). Physiologic and environmental influences on the immune system. In D. Stites &

A. Terr (eds.), *Basic and Clinical Immunology* (7th ed., pp 187–200). East Norwalk, CT: Appleton & Lange.

61. Wan, J., Teo, T., Babayan, V., & Blackburn, G. (1988). Invited comment: Lipids and the development of immune dysfunction and infection. *J Parenter Enter Nutr 12* (Suppl.):43S–52S.

62. Alexander, J., & Gottschilch, M. (1990). Nutritional immunomodulation in burn patients. Crit Care Med *18*:S149–S153.

63. Cerra, F., Lehman, S., Konstantinides, N., Konstantinides, F., Shronts, E., & Holman, R. (1990). Effect of enteral nutrient on in vitro tests of immune function in ICU patients: A preliminary report. Nutrition *6*:84–87.

64. Chandra, R. (1989). Nutritional regulation of immunity and risk of infection in old age. Immunology *67*:141–147.

65. Bogden, J., Oleske, J. Laventar, M., Munves, E., Kemp, F., Breuning, K., Holding, K., Denny, T., Guarino, M., Krieger, L., & Holland, B. (1988). Zinc and immunocompetence in elderly people: Effects of zinc supplementation for 3 months. Am J Clin Nutr *48*:655–663.

66. Good, R., & Lorenz, E. (1988). Nutrition, immunity, aging and cancer. Nutr Rev *46*:62–67.

67. Goodwing, J., & Garry, P. (1988). Lack of correlation between indices of nutritional status and immunologic function in elderly humans. J Gerontol *43*:M46–M49.

68. Khansari, D., Murgo, A., & Faith, R. (1990). Effects of stress on the immune system. Immunol Today *11*:170–175.

69. Smith, E., & Blalock, J. (1988). Molecular basis for interactions between the immune and neuroendocrine systems. Int J Neurosci *38*:455–464.

70. Rabin, B., Ganguli, R., Cunnick, J., & Lysle, D. (1988). The central nervous system–immune system relationship. Clin Lab Med *8*:254–268.

71. Daruna, J., & Morgan, J. (1990). Psychosocial effects on immune function: Neuroendocrine pathways. Psychosomatics *31*:4–12.

72. Stein, M. (1989). Stress, depression, and the immune system. J Clin Psychiatry *50*(Suppl.):35–40.

73. Restak, R. (1989). The brain, depression, and the immune system. J Clin Psychiatry *50*(Suppl.):23–25.

74. Kiecolt-Glaser, J., & Glaser, R. (1988). Methodological issues in behavioral immunology research with humans. Brain Behav Immun *2*:67–78.

75. Farrar, W. (1988). Evidence for the common expression of neuroendocrine hormones and cytokines in the immune and central nervous systems. Brain Behav Immun *2*:322–327.

76. Weiss, J., Sundar, S., Becker, K., & Cierpial, M. (1989). Behavioral and neural influences on cellular immune responses: Effects of stress and interleukin-1. J Clin Psychiatry *50*(Suppl.):43–55.

77. Pizzo, P. (1989). Combating infections in neutropenic patients. Hosp Pract (July 15), *24*:93–110.

78. Hughes, W. (1990). Empiric antimicrobial therapy in the febrile granulocytopenic patient. Infect Control Hosp Epidemiol *11*:151–156.

79. Young, L. (1989). Infections in patients with cellular immunodeficiency. Hosp Pract (August 15), *24*:191–212.

80. Saral, R. (1988). Management of mucocutaneous herpes simplex virus infections in immunocompromised patients. Am J Med *85*:57–60.

81. Balfour, H. (1988). Varicella-zoster virus infections in immunocompromised hosts: A review of the natural history and management. Am J Med *85*:68–73.

82. Mandal, B. (1987). Herpes zoster and the immunocompromised. J Infect *14*:1–5.

83. Rusthoven, J., Ahlgren, P., Elhakim, T., Pinfold, P., Stewart, L., & Feld, R. (1988). Risk factors for varicella zoster disseminated infection among adult cancer patients with localized zoster. Cancer *62*:1641–1646.

84. Leoung, G., Chaisson, R., & Mills, J. (1987). Comparison of nosocomial infections due to *Staphylococcus aureus* and enterococci in a general hospital. Surg Gynecol Obstet *165*:339–342.

85. Khardori, N. (1989). Host-parasite interaction in fungal infections. Eur J Clin Microbiol Infect Dis *8*:331–351.

86. Pfaller, M. (1989). Infection control: Opportunistic fungal infections. The increasing importance of *Candida* species. Infect Control Hosp Epidemiol *10*:270–273.

87. Rostad, M. (1990). Management of myelosuppression in the patient with cancer. Oncol Nurs Forum *17* (Suppl.):4–8.

88. Kiehn, T. (1989). Bacteremia and fungemia in the immunocompromised patient. Eur J Clin Microbiol Infect Dis *8*:832–837.

89. Benezra, D., Kiehn, T., Gold, J., Brown, A., Turnbull, A., & Armstrong, D. (1988). Prospective study of infections in indwelling central venous catheters using quantitative blood cultures. Am J Med *85*:495–498.

90. Link, D. (1987). Antibiotic therapy in the cancer patient: Focus on third generation cephalosporins. Oncol Nurs Forum *14*:35–41.

91. Gold, J., & Armstrong, D. (1989). Opportunistic infections in AIDS patients. In P. Ma & D. Armstrong (eds.), *AIDS and Infections of Homosexual Men* (2nd ed., pp. 325–335). Boston: Butterworths.

92. Sande, M. (1989). Antimicrobial therapy of infections in patients with AIDS—an overview. J Antimicrob Chemother *23*:63–65.

93. Glatt, A., & Chirgwin, K. (1990). *Pneumocystis carinii* pneumonia in human immunodeficiency virus-infected patients. Arch Intern Med *150*:271–279.

94. Henry, K., & Thurn, J. (1990). The evolving challenge of pneumocystis carinii. Postgrad Med *87*:45–53.

95. Krumholz, H., Sande, M., & Lo, B. (1989). Community-acquired bacteremia in patients with acquired immunodeficiency syndrome: Clinical presentation, bacteriology, and outcome. Am J Med *86*:776–779.

96. Dinarello, C. (1989). The endogenous pyrogens in host-defense interactions. Hosp Pract (Nov. 15), *24*:111–128.

97. Stites, D. (1991). Laboratory evaluation of immune competence. In D. Stites & A. Terr (eds.), *Basic and Clinical Immunology* (7th ed., pp. 312–318). East Norwalk, CT: Appleton & Lange.

98. de Shazo, R., Lopez, M., & Salvaggio, J. (1987). Use and interpretation of diagnostic immunologic laboratory tests. JAMA *258*:3011–3031.

99. Hong, R. (1987). Evaluation of immunity. Immunol Invest *16*:453–499.

100. Ogle, C., Ogle, J., & Alexander, J. (1989). The basics of immunological tests. J Parenter Enter Nutr *13*:651–657.

101. Tellado-Rodriguez, J., & Christou, N. (1988). Clinical assessment of host defense. Surg Clin North Am *68*:41–55.

102. Brandt, B. (1990). Nursing protocol for the patient with neutropenia. Oncol Nurs Forum *17* (Suppl.):9–15.

103. Lipscomb, M. (1989). Lung defenses against opportunistic infections. Chest *96*:1393–1399.

104. Ljungman, P., Gleaves, C., & Meyers, J. (1989). Respiratory virus infection in immunocompromised patients. Bone Marrow Transplant *4*:35–40.

105. McNally, J., & Stair, J. (1991). Potential for infection. In J. McNally, E. Somerville, C. Miaskowski, & M. Rostad (eds.), *Guidelines for Oncology Nursing Practice* (2nd ed., pp. 191–202). Philadelphia: W. B. Saunders.

106. Oniboni, A. (1990). Infection in the neutropenic patient. Semin Oncol Nurs *6*:50–60.

107. Rostad, M. (1991). Current strategies for managing myelosuppression in patients with cancer. Oncol Nurs Forum *18*(Suppl.):7–15.

108. National Institutes of Health. (1990). Oral complications of cancer therapies: Diagnosis, preventions, and treatment. Clin Courier *8*:1–8.

109. Eilers, J., Berger, A., & Petersen, M. (1988). Development, testing, and application of the oral assessment guide. Oncol Nurs Forum *15*:325–330.

110. Poland, J. (1991). Prevention and treatment of oral complications in the cancer patient. Oncology *5*:45–62.

111. Sonis, S. (1989). Oral complications of cancer therapy. In D. DeVita, S. Hellman, & S. Rosenberg (eds.), *Cancer: Principles and Practice of Oncology* (pp. 2144–2152). Philadelphia: J. B. Lippincott.

112. Holmes, S. (1991). The oral complications of specific anticancer therapy. Int J Nurs Studies *28*:343–360.

113. Larson, E. (1989). Infection control. Annu Rev Nurs Res *7*:95–113.

114. Larson, E., McGinley, K., Grove, G., Leyden, J., & Talbot, G. (1986). Physiologic, microbiologic, and seasonal effects of hand-washing on the skin of health care personnel. Am J Infect Control *14*:51–59.

115. Gould, D. (1991). Nurses' hands as vectors of hospital-acquired infection: A review. J Adv Nurs *16*:1216–1225.

116. *CDC Guidelines for Hand-washing and Hospital Environmental Control.* (1985). Atlanta: Centers for Disease Control.

117. Rubin, M., Hathorn, J., & Pizzo, P. (1988). Controversies in the management of febrile neutropenic cancer patients. Cancer Invest *6*:167–184.

118. Meijer, K., van Saene, H., & Hill, J. (1990). Infection control in patients undergoing mechanical ventilation: Traditional approach versus a new development-selective decontamination of the digestive tract. Heart Lung *19*:11–20.

119. Holtzclaw, B., & Rutledge, D. (1990). Use of amphotericin B in immunosuppressed patients with cancer. Part two: Pharmacodynamics and nursing implications. Oncol Nurs Forum *17*:737–742.

120. Rutledge, D., & Holtzclaw, B. (1990). Use of amphotericin B in immunosuppressed patients with cancer. Part one: Pharmacology and toxicities. Oncol Nurs Forum *17*:731–736.

121. Niederman, M. (1987). Strategies for the prevention of pneumonia. Clin Chest Med *8*:543–556.

122. Craven, D., & Regan, A. (1989). Nosocomial pneu-

monia in the ICU patient. Crit Care Nurs Q *11*:28–44.

123. Klein, R. (1989). Prophylaxis of opportunistic infections in individuals infected with HIV. AIDS *3* (Suppl. 1):S161–S173.

124. Massanari, R. (1989). Nosocomial infections in critical care units: Causation and prevention. Crit Care Nurs Q *11*:45–57.

125. Craven, D., & Regan, A. (1989). Nosocomial pneumonia in the ICU patient. Crit Care Nurs Q *11*:28–44.

126. Haeuber, D. (1989). Recent advances in the management of biotherapy-related side effects: Flu-like syndrome. Oncol Nurs Forum *16*(Suppl.):35–41.

127. Mitsuyasu, R. (1989). The enhanced potential use of recombinant alpha interferon in the treatment of AIDS-related Kaposi's sarcoma. Oncol Nurs Forum *16*(Suppl.):5–7.

128. Terebelo, H. (1991). Alpha interferon: Perspectives in the biotherapy of chronic myelogenous leukemia. Oncol Nurs Forum *16*(Suppl.):5–10.

129. Parkinson, D. (1989). The role of interleukin-2 in the biotherapy of cancer. Oncol Nurs Forum *16* (Suppl.):16–20.

130. Rosenberg, S. (1991). Adoptive cellular therapy in patients with advanced cancer. An update. Biol Ther Cancer Update *1*:1–15.

131. Brogley, J., & Sharp, E. (1990). Nursing care of patients receiving activated lymphocytes. Oncol Nurs Forum *17*:187–193.

132. Gabrilove, J. (1989). Introduction and overview of hematopoietic growth factors. Semin Hematol *26* (Suppl. 2):1–4.

133. Vadhan-Raj, S. (1989). Clinical applications of colony-stimulating factors. Oncol Nurs Forum *16*(Suppl.):21–26.

134. *Biological Response Modifier Guidelines. Recommendations for Nursing Education and Practice*. (1989). Pittsburgh: Oncology Nursing Society.

135. Talcott, J., Finberg, R., Mayer, R., & Goldman, L. (1988). The medical course of cancer patients with fever and neutropenia. Arch Intern Med *148*:2561–2568.

136. Armstrong, C., Mayhall, C., Miller, K., Newsome, H., Sugerman, H., Dalton, H., Hall, G., & Hunsberger, S. (1990). Clinical predictors of infection of central venous catheters used for total parenteral nutrition. Infect Control Hosp Epidemiol *11*:71–78.

137. Penin, G., & Ehrenkranz, J. (1988). Priorities for surveillance and cost-effective control of postoperative infection. Arch Surg *123*:1305–1308.

138. Weikel, D., Peterson, D., Rubinstein, L., Samuels, C., & Overholser, C. (1989). Incidence of fever following invasive oral interventions in the myelosuppressed cancer patient. Cancer Nurs *12*:265–270.

139. Kenny, S. (1990). Effect of two oral care protocols on the incidence of stomatitis in hematology patients. Cancer Nurs *13*:345–353.

140. Yeomans, A., Davitt, M. Peters, C. Pastuszek, C., & Cobb, S. (1991). Efficacy of chlorhexidine gluconate use in the prevention of perirectal infections in patients with acute leukemia. Oncol Nurs Forum *18*:1207–1213.

141. *Directions for Nursing Research: Toward the Twenty-First Century*. (1985). Kansas City: American Nurses Association.

18

Impaired Wound Healing

Nancy Stotts

DEFINITION

Wound healing is tissue repair or regeneration that results in tissue continuity being re-established. Impaired healing is disruption of the normal biochemical repair or regeneration process. Abnormalities in healing are manifested in a variety of problems including separation of the wound edges, dehiscence, evisceration, hematoma or seroma formation, delayed wound healing, wound infection, and abnormal scar formation.

Wound healing is initiated whenever there is tissue damage. The process of repair is the same regardless of whether the tissue destruction is caused by trauma, heat, chemicals, or pressure. Most tissue is restored by replacement with scar tissue, although the skin and liver have some of the regenerative abilities seen in lower animals.[1]

Tissue injury is often classified by the depth of tissue damage: *partial-thickness injury*, involving the epidermis and possibly extending down to a portion of the dermis; and *full thickness injury* extending through the skin into the subcutaneous tissues below. Repair of a partial thickness injury occurs primarily by epithelialization. Repair of a full-thickness injury includes both the development of granulation tissue and epithelial closure. Repair of a full-thickness injury is classified as healing by primary, secondary, and tertiary intention.

Healing by primary intention results when the wound edges are closely approximated and little dead space is left in the wound. *Secondary intention healing* occurs when there is a loss of tissue or when the wound is left open for drainage, most often in heavy bacterial contamination or edema. Closure of a wound by tertiary intention, or *delayed primary closure*, is used when the wound is heavily contaminated. With this closure technique, the wound is left open for approximately 4 days after surgery or injury until the bacteria count drops to less than one million organisms per gram of tissue and then is closed primarily.[2]

PREVALENCE AND POPULATIONS AT RISK

The prevalence of impaired wound healing is not known, as statistics are not recorded under the heading "impaired healing." One approach to estimate its prevalence is to examine the rate of problems in repair among major groups of patients, such as those with pressure ulcers, vascular ulcers, and surgical wounds.

To examine the prevalence of pressure ulcers, the National Pressure Ulcer Advisory Panel (NPUAP) clustered data on pressure ulcers that had been generated across studies.[3] Although the NPUAP acknowledged methodological limitations of studies on ulcers in various health care settings, they concluded that the prevalence of pressure ulcers was as follows: 3 to 14 per cent among hospitalized patients; 15 to 25 per cent in clients on admission to skilled nursing facilities; and 7 to 12 per cent in persons in the home setting.

The cost of treatment of ulcers in the acute care setting is estimated as $2,000 to $30,000 per patient, in which the lower figure represents the cost of treatment in patients whose primary diagnosis is not a pressure ulcer.[3] Data are not available to estimate costs of ulcers in skilled nursing facilities and in home

443

care settings. The NPUAP speculates that prevention is less expensive than treatment of ulcers, although the figures that reflect the cost of surveillance and targeted intervention are not available. Also, treatment costs are difficult to assess because patient costs in many institutions are not divided into the fee for various services (e.g., nursing, supplies, dietary services), and they become part of the overall patient hospital charge; the specific cost of ulcers is lost.[3]

Impaired healing among patients with peripheral vascular disease is seen most frequently in venous stasis ulcers. They account for 90 per cent of the ulcers of the lower extremities and are estimated to affect 0.5 per cent of the population of the United States.[4] Valves in the venous system are disrupted, and high hydrostatic pressure eventually damages both the deep and superficial venous system. As the disease progresses, local tissue ischemia, chronic edema, and fibrosis interact to produce chronic venous insufficiency. Ulcers usually develop about 10 years after the initial valvular damage and often are associated with minor local trauma. Once these ulcers develop, the healing is often prolonged. In elderly patients with venous ulcers, approximately 50 per cent have arterial insufficiency.[5]

Diabetics are a subpopulation of patients with vascular disease who have a high incidence of indolent ulcers. The incidence of peripheral vascular disease is four to seven times greater in diabetics than in the general population. They have disease of both large and small vessels; often the large vessel disease can be repaired or bypassed, leaving them with flow problems in the microvasculature. As a result of the neuropathy associated with diabetes, these patients often unknowingly experience trauma to the feet, most often over bony prominences, that goes unnoticed and untreated for long periods of time. About 15 per cent of diabetics have an ulcer on the feet or ankles. Amputation is the most common sequela of these ulcers, accounting for 40 to 45 per cent of all non-traumatic amputations. This occurs in 60 out of 10,000 diabetics. Each year about 12,400 amputations are performed on medicare beneficiaries with diabetes at a cost of between $8,600 and $12,400 per patient, equaling $106.6 to $153.8 million per year.[6]

The primary problem seen in surgical wounds is wound infection. The rate of surgical wound infection is predictable, based on clinical estimate of the bacterial density, level of contamination, risk of subsequent wound infection, and the type of surgery performed. Surgical procedures are classified as "clean," "clean-contaminated," "contaminated," or "dirty," and infection rates vary from about 5 per cent for clean procedures to 40 per cent or more for those that are dirty (Table 18–1). Although limiting the infection rate is largely under the control of the surgeon in the intraoperative period, perioperative activities have been shown to influence patient outcomes.[7] For example, Cruse and Foord[7] found in a 10-year study of surgical patients that risk of wound infection increased as length of hospitalization increased. With a 1-day preoperative stay, the infection rate was 1.2 per cent, it increased to 2.1 per cent within a week and was 3.4 per cent when the hospital stay extended more than 2 weeks. Also, as length of time of the actual surgical procedure increased, the infection rate increased, doubling each hour that the operative procedure continued.

Preparation of the operative area prior to surgery also was found to be important in controlling infection.[7] In patients who showered immediately before surgery using a

TABLE 18–1 CLASSIFICATION OF RISK OF INFECTION OF SURGICAL PROCEDURES

Category	Description	Examples
Clean wound	Nontraumatic injury in which no inflammation is encountered and there is no break in sterile technique	Vascular surgery
Clean-contaminated wound	Gastrointestinal or respiratory tract is entered without significant contamination	Gastric or biliary surgery
Contaminated wound	Major break in sterile technique; gross spillage from gastrointestinal tract	Colon surgery with no preoperative preparation
Dirty or infected wound	Acute bacterial inflammation or pus encountered with devitalized tissue or contamination	Traumatic wounds

hexachlorophene soap, the infection rate was 1.3 per cent; in those who did not follow this practice, the rate was 2.3 per cent. Shaving and the use of a nonelectric razor to remove hair at the operative site resulted in a 2.5 per cent infection rate. This was considerably above that seen with unshaved patients with clipped pubic hair (infection rate of 1.7 per cent), those who were shaved with an electric razor (infection rate of 1.4 per cent), and those who neither shaved nor clipped (infection rate of 0.9 per cent). Differences in infection rates as a result of hair removal technique were explained by the authors as due to the microscopic skin damage caused by the razor or clipper.

Tissue injury that is not on the body surface is often ignored when healing is discussed; however, tissue repair and regeneration are basically the same whether injury is external or internal. An example of impaired healing that is not visible on the body surface is atherosclerosis, in which blood vessels are disrupted by mechanical injury caused by shear and high-driving pressures. Cellular processes necessary for repair of these tissues have been implicated in impairment in function of vessels.[8, 9] In 1980, more than 730,000 deaths in the United States were due to impaired healing of blood vessels, resulting in heart attack or stroke.[10] There is little question that heart attack and stroke, two examples of sequelae of impaired healing, produce significant threat to functional capacity, psychological well-being, and life itself.

This sampling of diseases and conditions indicates that wound impairment is a prevalent problem. It has the potential to result in significant physical, financial, and emotional cost to those affected.

SITUATIONAL STRESSORS

Stressors are factors in the internal and external environment that strain the normal healing process and place the patient at risk for impaired healing. Knowledge of the stressors that increase risk of wound impairment will allow the nurse to plan the assessment and therapies needed to optimize patient outcomes.

Established stressors are age;[11–13] concurrent conditions and treatments;[14–21] physiological status including perfusion and oxygenation[22–33]; glucose control[15–18]; and nutritional status.[34–46] Other stressors that increasingly are implicated in healing are preinjury status,[47] noise,[48–49] pain,[50–51] and stress[52–53] (Table 18–2).

The very old are at increased risk for impaired healing because the rate of replacement of cells is slowed. In addition, immunological response is delayed, increasing the risk of infection. The premature infant also is at increased risk for impaired healing because of an immature immunological system rather than a deficit that causes the increased vulnerability.

Concurrent diseases and treatments also place the patient at risk for impaired healing. Persons with cardiovascular disease are at increased risk because of perfusion problems. Diabetics have the triad of small vessel disease, neuropathy, and hyperglycemia that contribute to impaired perfusion and ineffective white blood cell (WBC) function. A number of drugs also affect healing, but the most notorious of these is the steroids, which impair all phases of healing.

Physiological states that place the patient at increased risk for impaired healing include impaired perfusion, inadequate oxygenation, and insufficient nutrient intake. All of these situations result in insufficient substrates for healing. Similarly, emerging stressors that result in sympathetic nervous system stimulation and therefore may impair delivery of substrates to the injured tissue are noise, pain, and emotional stress. Poor preinjury nutritional status in which cellular constituents are depleted prior to injury also has been implicated in impaired repair.

MECHANISMS

Partial Thickness Injuries

Understanding healing of partial-thickness injury requires an appreciation of the anat-

TABLE 18–2 STRESSORS: FACTORS CRITICAL TO IMPAIRED HEALING

Established stressors
Age
Concurrent conditions and treatments
Physiological status
Perfusion and oxygenation
Glucose control
Nutritional status
Emerging stressors
Preinjury status
Noise
Pain
Stress

omy (Fig. 18–1). The skin is composed of the epidermis, dermis, and subcutaneous tissue. The epidermis is an avascular layer composed of keratinocytes, squamous cells, basal cells, and melanocytes. Below the epidermis is the dermis, a vital, viable layer of the skin. It contains capillaries, hair follicles, sweat glands, sebaceous glands, and collagen fibers. Below the skin is the subcutaneous tissue, muscle, fascia, bone, and the internal organs.

Partial-thickness injuries heal primarily by epithelialization. Migration of epithelial cells from the edges of the wound is initiated soon after injury and occurs from cells surrounding the denuded area and those in the base of the hair follicles, sweat glands, and sebaceous glands. Coverage of an area with new epithelial cells occurs rapidly because of the short distance between cells. Epithelial migration continues until all sides of the epithelial cells are surrounded by other epithelial cells.

Epithelial growth occurs most rapidly in a moist environment.[54] When cells encounter a dry or scab-covered wound, they must bury under it. This uses energy that could be applied to epithelial growth, and also results in delayed sealing of the wound. The mechanism by which epithelization occurs is not entirely understood[55]; however, epithelial growth factor (EGF) is known to stimulate epidermal growth.[56] Whether this hormone becomes an important part of wound healing therapy remains to be established.[57]

Full-Thickness Injuries

With full-thickness injury, repair is focused on development of a new vasculature, syn-

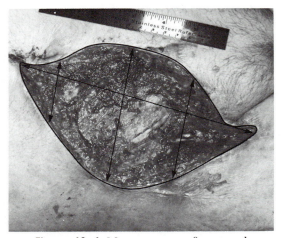

Figure 18–1. Measurement of a wound.

TABLE 18–3 MAJOR EVENTS THAT TAKE PLACE DURING NORMAL HEALING

Phase of Healing	Major Physiological Processes
Inflammatory phase	Contraction of small blood vessels
	Activation of platelets and coagulation cascade
	Growth factors released
	Mobilization of complement cascade and kinin system
	Transient vasoconstriction followed by vasodilation and increased capillary permeability
	White blood cells to the area
	Lymph channels blocked
	Epithelial cell migration
Proliferative phase	New blood vessels form
	Granulation tissue develops
	Collagen fills defect
	Epithelial migration continues
Remodeling phase	Collagen is reorganized
	Tensile strength increases

thesis of scar tissue to fill in the tissue defect, and generation of epithelial cells to cover the area denuded by injury. The process of repair has been divided into three phases: inflammatory or exudative phase, proliferative or connective tissue phase, and scar maturation or remodeling phase (Table 18–3). Each phase has characteristic physiological events, and the phases are sequential yet overlapping.[58]

Inflammatory Phase

The inflammatory phase begins immediately after injury and is characterized by preparation of the site of injury for growth of new tissue. A loose clot is formed at vessel ends because of activation of factor IV and platelets. Hageman's factor (Factor XII) is also activated and mobilizes the intrinsic pathway. The extrinsic pathway has been mobilized with the tissue damage. These two pathways work together to convert the loose platelet plug at the vascular site into a strong clot to stop bleeding. The thrombin produced as part of this clot process causes the platelets to release growth factors. These include platelet-derived growth factor (PDGF), platelet-derived angiogenesis factor (PDAF), platelet-derived epidermal growth factor (PDEGF), transforming growth factor-beta (TGF-β), and platelet factor 4 (PF-4).[56, 57, 59–61] The growth factors were named as they were discovered, explaining to some extent why their names do not describe either the tissues that they affect or all of the sites where they are found. Frequently cited growth factors are listed in Table 18–4. These factors have important effects on the subsequent phases of healing, although controversy exists about the mechanisms by which the growth factors influence healing. Currently accepted data indicate that PDGF is a mitogenic chemoattractor. Its actions include stimulation of fibroblast migration and mitosis at various concentrations. Platelet-derived angiogenesis factor is a nonmitogen chemoattractant for capillary endothelial cells that stimulates migration and mitosis of epidermal cells. The growth factor TGF-β is a potent chemoattractant for monocytes, inhibits fibroblast mitosis, and stimulates collagen synthesis by fibroblasts. Neutrophils are attracted by PF–4. The macrophage is another important site of production of the growth factors.

The injured vessels attract leukocytes that line the vessels, the phenomenon of neutrophilic margination. From this location neutrophils move through the endothelial walls to the area of injury.

Activation of the complement cascade also is critical to healing. During the inflammatory process, complement factors are released that are chemotactic and cause vasodilation. They also directly lyse bacteria and opsonize or mark other bacteria for later phagocytosis by white blood cells. Complement C5a and C3a are the most important complement fractions to healing.

Kinins are another important factor in the inflammotory phase of healing. They cause vasodilation and increased capillary permeability, thus allowing intravascular factors to come in contact with the tissues where they are required for healing. Histamine, released from mast cells immediately after injury, is the most well known of the kinins, and its effects last about an hour after injury. The vasodilation seen in the vasculature after that time is thought to be brought about by the prostaglandins, especially prostaglandin E_2.

Within hours after injury, polymorphonu-

TABLE 18–4 FREQUENTLY CITED GROWTH FACTORS

Platelet-derived growth factor
Fibroblast growth factor–basic
Epidermal growth factor
Transforming growth factor–alpha
Transforming growth factor–beta

clear leukocytes (PMNs) are concentrated in the area of injury where they phagocytize foreign material and clean the wound. The primary PMN present is the neutrophil. Prior opsonization of organisms by complement makes phagocytosis possible. Chemotactic substances have attracted the WBCs to the site of injury, and foreign material and debris are readily removed from the tissue.

When the bacteria are phagocytized, the WBCs have a respiratory burst.[58] The oxygen consumption at this time is up to 20 times the resting oxygen consumption of the cell. The by-products of the respiratory burst are oxygen metabolites (called free radicals in the older literature) that are effective in killing anaerobes. For example, superoxide dismutase catalyzes the reduction of superoxide radical to hydrogen peroxide in the phagosome, resulting in the death of the organism. These effects are augmented in the presence of substances such as myeloperoxidase and halide ions. In addition, other high energy derivatives are produced during phagocytosis and participate in bacteriocidal activity. The oxygen metabolites produced also cause damage to surrounding tissue; their role in tissue repair and destruction is not yet fully understood.

During the early postinjury period, neutrophils are the WBCs that predominate. They are short-lived, and when they die, effete WBCs are phagocytized by other WBCs. White blood cells function in an anaerobic environment, but they are not nearly as effective as in an aerobic environment. A hypoxic environment thus lends itself to proliferation of organisms. Neutrophils are critical to early cleansing of the wound after injury and protecting it from infection. However, wounds heal in patients who are neutropenic.[62]

Monocytes also arrive in the wound soon after injury and predominate 48 to 72 hours after injury. They are thought to arise from the nearby tissue and are transformed into macrophages. Macrophages act to phagocytize bacteria, mobilize fibroblasts to release collagen, and release factors that stimulate angiogenesis. Wounds will not heal without macrophages.[63]

In the wound healing by primary intention, the inflammatory phase lasts about 3 or 4 days. This is an important period in the healing of a wound because during this phase the environment is created in which repair can occur. It prepares the area for the formation of new vessels, collagen to fill the wound defect, and epithelial tissue to cover the denuded tissue. In situations in which the inflammatory response is absent or suppressed (e.g., malnutrition, immunosuppressive drug therapy), healing often is delayed or disrupted by infection.

Proliferative Phase

The inflammatory phase is followed by the proliferative phase, so called because cell mitosis is the predominant activity during this period. It begins 1 to 5 days after injury and continues for up to about 3 weeks in wounds healing by primary intention. Major processes during this period are the development of new blood vessels by the process of angiogenesis, formation of proteoglycans and collagen for the production of granulation tissue, and epithelialization. Also during this period, wounds healing by secondary intention begin to contract or shrink in size.

Tissue injury causes impaired blood flow and results in a hypoxic wound.[64-66] Dead space oxygen is 0 to 3 mm Hg, and the PO_2 in the growing edge of the capillary is thought to be 5 to 15 mm Hg. Hypoxia and lactate, produced through the Krebs cycle under anaerobic conditions, stimulate the release of growth factors from macrophages that support angiogenesis. If oxygen is provided so that hypoxia is ablated in the early postinjury period, angiogenesis is inhibited. When provided 24 hours after injury, increasing the oxygen concentration sharply increases capillary budding. Angiogenesis is slowed naturally as healing is completed.[26] These findings indicate that in the immediate postinjury phase, hypoxia at the wound is a stimulus to repair; after this phase, increased oxygen serves as a stimulus for healing and hypoxia may result in impaired capillary budding.

With angiogenesis, new capillary buds come out of the ends of the cut vessels and grow into the wound space. When the capillary buds from one side of the wound meet those from the opposite side, blood flow occurs, bringing oxygen dissolved in plasma and oxygen bound to hemoglobin. The acidotic tissue fluid is reabsorbed as flow occurs through new vessels and the stimulus for angiogenesis is gradually dissipated and angiogenesis stops.

Fibroblasts are essential for healing. With injury, they are activated and arise from surrounding tissue to manufacture collagen and deposit it in the wound space. Fibroblasts require a PO_2 of at least 20 to 30 mm Hg to function efficiently.[25, 26, 66] Collagen is of several types and is specific to different tissues (Table 18–5). Type III collagen is synthesized by granulation tissue of skin wounds, although it is usually present only in small amounts in normal skin.

Collagen, a triple helix structure, is continually formed in the wound space where it attaches to strands of fibronectin to form new tissue. The collagen that is produced is surrounded by glycoproteins, whose exact role in healing is not entirely understood. There is a continual synthesis and lysis of collagen in tissue that has been injured. The lysis of collagen is controlled by enzymes. Factors critical to the synthesis of collagen include proteins, nonprotein calories, vitamin C, zinc, oxygen, and alpha-ketoglutarate. If collagen synthesis is disrupted by conditions such as malnutrition, lysis continues, and wounds that were healing will not only be stopped in that process but will be broken down. The classic example of this occurred in the 1700s with British seamen whose old wounds opened when they were at sea. The seamen were not ingesting ascorbic acid, scurvy developed, and collagen lysis exceeded synthesis; thus, the wounds broke down.

Collagen formation depends on biochemical reactions, a major one of which is hydroxylation of the amino acids proline and lysine. The tensile strength of the wound is related to collagen deposition; it is not directly related to the amount of hydroxyproline laid down but rather to the cross-linking that occurs as the collagen matures.

Remodeling Phase

The third phase of healing begins about 3 weeks after injury and can still be in progress 6 months to 2 years later, depending on the extent and location of the injury and the patient's underlying condition. The remod-

TABLE 18–5 TYPES OF COLLAGEN

Type	Location
I	Bone, tendon, skin
II	Hyaline cartilages
III	Skin, arteries, uterus
IV	Basement membranes

eling phase is characterized by a change in the nature of the scar from the simultaneous synthesis by fibroblasts and lysis by the collagenases. The resultant architecture of the scar is more organized as the scar matures; the bulk of the scar decreases, and the color of the scar changes from pink to pearly white.[54, 60] Incisional strength also builds during this period after injury. Three weeks after injury, it is approximately 20 per cent of original strength, by 5 weeks it is nearly 40 per cent and at 8 weeks it is just over 70 per cent; however, it never reaches preinjury strength.[58]

Impaired Healing

The situational and developmental stressors that alter normal healing and its trajectory, as previously described, include age, concurrent conditions and treatments, impaired perfusion and oxygenation, glucose control, altered nutritional status, and the emerging stressors of preinjury status, noise, pain, and stress. Understanding the mechanism by which the various risk factors affect healing helps the nurse to identify high-risk patients and to develop strategies to mitigate impairment.

Age

People of all ages are at risk for impaired healing, and the cause of the increased risk varies among them by age. Of all the age groups, the older population is at greatest risk. With aging, there are physiological changes in tissues, decreased rate of replacement of cells, changes in the nature of new tissue, and motor-sensory losses.[20] The immune system is often implicated in impaired healing because its function has declined over time and microorganisms proliferate before they can be removed. In addition, the rate of cell replication is decreased, so that when injury occurs, repair is delayed owing to alterations in fibroblast function, decreased rate of capillary budding, and slowed epithelialization. Decreased function of the cardiovascular, gastrointestinal, and pulmonary systems may result in lack of substrates for healing.[11, 12] Other alterations in the skin and connective tissue of older adults (e.g., less elastin and a different type of collagen replacing damaged tissues) influence the nature and rate of healing, but data about the effect

of these changes on wound healing are sparse. Finally, sensory-motor timing and coordination begin to deteriorate and result in increased rate of accidents and injuries. The combination of these factors may cause increased injuries, delayed wound repair, and infection.[11, 12] This is illustrated with data from a study of cardiac surgical patients in whom sternal wound infection in patients 80 years of age or older was more than double that of all adult cardiac surgical patients.[13]

The very young (i.e., preterm infants and neonates) also theoretically are at increased risk because of their immature immune systems and lack of cells for aggressive immune function. Neutrophil chemotaxis, antibody production ability, and bactericidal activities are decreased when the neonate is compared with the child or adult. In addition, the neonate's stores of glycogen and fat are limited; therefore, substrates needed for energy are quickly depleted in the face of increased energy demands that occur in illness, injury, or surgery.[36] Clinically impaired healing is not frequently seen in this population, perhaps because of the high level of growth hormone and the rapid rate of cell replacement.

Concurrent Conditions and Treatments

The presence of diseases, conditions, and treatments can also increase the risk of impaired healing. Cardiovascular disease is a risk factor for impaired healing. It is characterized by alteration in perfusion to end organs resulting in impairment in blood flow; this is often associated with the vascular disease. These patients have a high rate of wound complications, amputation failure, and overall complications, including infection.[13, 14]

Diabetics are another population at risk for impaired healing. They have a combination of small vessel disease, neuropathy, and problems in glucose control that interact to predispose them to disrupted healing.[15–18]

Also at increased risk are patients who are immunocompromised, whether from aging, cancer, malnutrition, Cushing's syndrome, diabetes, uremia, or genetic defects.[19, 20] The immune system plays a pivotal role in healing, and impairment of it results in increased risk of disruption of the normal course of healing.

Medications frequently disrupt the normal healing process at the cellular level. Steroids are particularly significant, as they inhibit all phases of healing.[20] Other anti-inflammatory compounds, such as aspirin, phenylbutazone, and vitamin E, also disrupt healing. Their effects are seen primarily during the inflammatory phase.

Antimitotic agents inhibit healing by interfering with cell mitosis. Radiation therapy has an effect similar to that of the antimitotic agents and thus is frequently the cause of impaired healing.[20, 21] The pathological effects of radiation therapy have been categorized as "acute" (first 6 months), "subacute" (second 6 months), chronic (second to the fifth year), and late (after the fifth year).

The acute period is characterized by organ damage that is clinically silent unless the tolerance limits are exceeded. In the subacute period, recovery from acute damage is completed and vascular deterioration may develop. This includes vascular damage that is fibrotic, especially at the arteriocapillary junction. The chronic period reflects a continuation of the vascular deterioration, and the most serious problems are related to hypoperfusion of the irradiated tissue. Clinically, the chronic period is characterized by premature involution of tissues with hypoplasia, atrophy and fibrosis. Dose and dose-rate determine to a large extent the extent of damage and rapidity with which it occurs. Radiation cancer may also occur during this period.[21] The chronic period blends into the late period, which is characterized by parenchymal degeneration.

Perfusion and Oxygenation

Perfusion and oxygenation are interlinked in the healing process. Problems of perfusion and oxygenation may be present without cardiovascular disease (e.g., hypovolemia). These problems may be overt and rapidly corrected, or they may be subtle[22] and contribute substantially to wound healing impairment. Bedside measurements of arterial blood gases, transcutaneous oxygen, and oxygen saturation are not sensitive indicators of tissue perfusion,[23] so problems may go undetected. Treatment cannot be precisely titrated for perfusion problems so clinicians either overhydrate patients in an effort to perfuse them or underhydrate them in an attempt to prevent iatrogenic complications. Either of these extremes in treatment may contribute to the development of wound impairment in patients.

Oxygen, an essential component for cellular processes, is critical for wound healing. It is needed for all phases of healing and also is a marker of perfusion.[24] Angiogenesis, new vessel formation, takes place in the wound space where vessels have been disrupted by injury. Initially after injury, the wound becomes hypoxic. The hypoxia is important in the release of growth factors that support angiogenesis. After the first day of injury, increasing oxygen to the injured tissue is important in increasing capillary budding.

Another important component in the repair process that is sensitive to oxygen is the fibroblast. Fibroblasts secrete collagen, which provides the tensile strength of the wound. Tensile strength is the ability of tissue to resist breaking when tension is applied. Fibroblasts are sensitive to oxygen and function well at a PO_2 of 20 to 30 mm Hg.[25-26] It is been shown that fibroblast proliferation requires more oxygen than does collagen formation. Also, increased oxygen tension significantly augments the collagen synthesis rate, collagen accumulation, and tensile strength.[26]

Epithelial tissue is also responsive to oxygen levels.[27] Mitotic activity of epithelial cells has a linear relationship with oxygen tension; that is, hypoxia depresses epithelial activity while hyperoxia stimulates it. These findings have been substantiated in research studies using both hyperbaric oxygen[28] and exposure to varying oxygen tensions at 1 atmosphere of pressure.[29, 30]

Infection rate is a function of hypoxia. When environments that were hypoxic, normoxic, and hyperoxic were compared, wound contamination and infection were highest in the hypoxic group and lowest in the hyperoxic groups. Oxygen supports leukocyte activity and therefore suppresses infection rate.[31]

Because the majority of oxygen content in the blood is carried bound to hemoglobin, anemia and impaired healing have been linked conceptually. Research, however, supports this connection only when the anemia is severe (hematocrit < 20 g/dl) or when anemia is accompanied by hypovolemia.[32, 33]

Glucose Control

Generally, type I diabetics are at higher risk for wound healing problems than type II diabetics or people without diabetes. Diabetic wound healing problems include infection, failure or delay in epithelialization, impaired or delayed collagen formation, slowed wound contraction, and wound closure. Cellular effects are seen as delayed chemotaxis and impaired phagocytic function.[15–18]

An interesting study by Hjortrup and associates compared diabetic surgical patients with a nondiabetic control group that was matched for age, sex, weight, concurrent diseases, and a number of other factors.[67] They concluded that risk of morbidity was not greater when diabetics were compared with the control group. No follow-up studies have been reported to support or contradict these findings.

Glucose control in the postinjury period probably is the major factor that influences healing in the diabetic. Insulin resistance after injury is amplified in the diabetic. In diabetic rats, glucose concentration in the wound fluid was high immediately after injury, although slightly less so than in the blood. Over time in the rat model, the hyperglycemia was accompanied by a decreased rate of collagen formation and decreased wound tensile strength.[17] Also, exogenous insulin given to rats restored normal healing parameters, and insulin given early in the course of healing produced significantly better results than when supplements were given later in the postinjury phase.[18] These data indicate that blood glucose levels need to be monitored frequently in the postinjury period and insulin supplements should be provided as needed to control blood glucose levels. Sliding-scale insulin coverage has little basis in the scientific literature and in fact may not be the optimal method to control glucose in these patients.[68] In addition, because of the high renal threshold for glucose (about 180 mg/dl), urine glucose levels are not sensitive enough to provide good control of blood glucose. Therefore, the use of a more sensitive measure of blood glucose, such as that provided with a glucometer, is an essential assessment strategy.

Glycosylated hemoglobin (HgbA$_{1c}$) provides information about the patient's control over the last 120 days. Regardless of whether lack of control was caused by inattention or a concurrent underlying condition (e.g., infection), patients who lack good control require close monitoring. For patients with wounds, the recommended zone of control in serum glucose is 100 to 250 mg/dl.[16] Studies need to be undertaken to define the optimal frequency and duration for blood glucose monitoring in these individuals to reduce healing impairment due to hyperglycemia.

Other adjuncts to support healing must be used in the diabetic. Supplemental zinc, vitamin A, and a well-balanced nutritional and activity plan have been shown to be important in maximizing healing in these patients.[18, 69]

Nutrition

Nutrients are essential for normal healing. They provide the building blocks for cellular repair and regeneration. Nutrients that have a role in healing include protein, fat, carbohydrate, vitamins (A, B, C, D, E, and K) and minerals (zinc, iron, magnesium, copper, and others). In addition, malnutrition results in disruption of normal healing but the rate of repair can be returned to normal with refeeding.[35, 36]

Protein. Protein is needed in wound healing for repair and regeneration. Amino acids are basic components of protein and are an integral part of deoxyribonucleic acid (DNA) and ribonucleic acid (RNA), providing the template for mitosis and control of enzyme systems.[36] Amino acids essential to wound healing include methionine, cystine (especially for premature and newborn infants), and lysine. Deficiencies result in impaired neovascularization, fibroblast proliferation, collagen synthesis, and wound remodeling. Immune defenses are also impaired in the presence of protein deficiency, and the body's ability to resist infection may be decreased.

Amino acids from exogenous protein intake and the continuous turnover of endogenous protein form an amino acid pool. When there is inadequate intake of protein, body mass is catabolized to provide needed amino acids. With severe injury, catabolism of body tissues cannot occur at a rate adequate to provide sufficient substrates for repair and regeneration; thus, severe protein starvation results in depletion of body stores and, when prolonged, results in impaired healing.[34–38]

Carbohydrates and Fats. Metabolism of carbohydrate and fat supplies most of the energy needed for cell function. When these substances are not provided in sufficient quantities by ingestion or endogenous means, the energy needs of cells are met by catabolism of body protein. Protein is needed for structural and visceral integrity. Glucose balance must be maintained so that available carbohydrate can be used for energy.

Fat is an essential component of the membranes of the cell and the substructures within the cell. It also is part of the structure of prostaglandin, an important substance in the control of inflammation and circulation.

Prolonged undernutrition may result in deficiencies of fat but especially important are insufficient quantities of linoleic, linolenic, and arachidonic acids. Because of the accelerated needs of the impaired tissue immediately after injury, these essential fatty acids cannot be synthesized fast enough to meet wound healing needs. Premature infants and newborns as well as cachectic individuals are especially vulnerable to fatty acid deficiencies because they lack body stores of fat.[36]

Vitamins and Minerals. Vitamins are an integral part of cell metabolism and all are important in repair. Those recognized at this time as especially important to healing are vitamins A, B, C, D, E, and K.

Vitamin A is a fat-soluble vitamin necessary for healing. It appears to be active in stimulating and supporting epithelialization, capillary budding, and collagen formation. It also supports the inflammatory phase of healing and is important because it may be used in chronic steroid users to override the anti-inflammatory action of long-term steroid use. In fact, all aspects of healing that are inhibited by corticosteroids can be restored by administration of vitamin A, except wound contraction.[40–42]

The B vitamins are important as cofactors in enzymatic reactions.[36] All are water-soluble and must be provided daily in the diet, except vitamin B_{12}; it is stored in the liver and the reserve can last for several years. Injury increases the use of specific B vitamins, and yet clinically significant healing problems have not been associated with such deficiencies.

Vitamin C is required for angiogenesis as well as for the hydroxylation of proline and lysine in the formation of collagen. Fibroblasts, necessary for production of collagen, can be produced without increased concentration of vitamin C, but their function is markedly impaired. In addition, vitamin C is a reducing agent that participates in the conversion of oxygen to superoxide, which acts as an antibacterial substance in the wound. Vitamin C deficiencies result in poor quality wound healing and increased capillary fra-

gility. In wound healing and infection, increased metabolic demands markedly accelerate the use of vitamin C, and the dose administered in situations such as burns or severe injury may need to be augmented.[39–41]

Vitamin D is important to absorption of calcium and the healing of bone. It controls the uptake of calcium and phosphorus. In addition, calcium is important in many enzyme systems, including collagenases and formation of peroxide. Vitamin D is fat-soluble and stored in the body; however, prolonged starvation or metabolic demands may lead to deficiencies.

Vitamin E is needed for normal fat metabolism. Although regarded by the lay public as a healing agent, in fact it retards healing and fibrosis. Unless otherwise indicated, doses should not exceed the Recommended Daily Allowance.

Vitamin K is important to healing because it controls coagulation and prevents bleeding and hematoma formation.[34] Bleeding into the wound increases the distance across which new vessel formation, development of the collagen matrix, and epithelialization must occur and hence delays healing. The hematoma that forms with bleeding into the wound space also serves as a nidus for infection.

Minerals needed for normal repair include zinc, iron, and other trace minerals. Zinc deficiencies result in delayed healing, probably because of the important role of zinc in enzyme systems. Healing is not accelerated with zinc supplementation in individuals with normal serum zinc levels; however, supplemental zinc in deficient individuals will return healing to its normal rate.[43]

Iron is another mineral that is essential to normal healing. It participates in the chemical reaction leading to collagen formation and formation of superoxide, and a severe deficiency in available iron results in derangement of this process. Deficiencies that affect wound healing have been reported in children[34] but not in adults or the elderly. Anemia is the most frequent hematological problem in the elderly, occurring in 12 to 20 per cent of the healthy elderly and presumably more frequently in those with chronic or acute disease.[44] With the high incidence of anemia in the elderly, wound healing problems due to insufficient iron are theoretically possible but have not been documented.

Trace elements such as magnesium and

copper also play an important role in wound repair. Magnesium is needed for adenosine triphosphate (ATP) reactions as well as protein synthesis. Copper is used for red blood cell (RBC) and collagen formation. Other trace minerals (e.g., cobalt, selenium) function as part of normal cell synthesis; no specific roles for them have been identified in wound healing.

Preinjury Status

Preinjury condition has been shown to be a risk factor for impaired healing. Studies indicate that patients who experience longer periods of acute preoperative illness[13] and those who have poor nutritional status before surgery[43] exhibit less hydroxyproline formation (a measure of collagen formation) than controls who have shorter periods of preoperative illness or better preoperative nutritional status. Also, recent food intake in the preoperative period can be more important in preventing impairment in hydroxyproline deposition than absolute losses of protein and fat from body stores.[46] Thus, preliminary data indicate that preinjury status is an emerging factor in risk of impaired healing.

Noise

Noise is a stress factor that has been shown to increase epinephrine levels in animals,[45] causing vasoconstriction of blood vessels in the skin and subcutaneous tissue. Wounded rats exposed to noise demonstrated significantly less healing than the control group not exposed to noise.[49] Although Wysocki is careful to indicate that because of differences in healing in animals and humans findings cannot be generalized to wounded humans,[49] results are highly suggestive and pave the way for studies on the effect of noise on healing in humans.

Pain

Therapies to reduce the pain associated with dressing changes have also have been examined. The effects of transcutaneous electrical nerve stimulation (TENS) on the pain associated with cleaning and packing an abdominal surgical wound have been studied. A group receiving TENS, a group receiving a TENS placebo, and a group receiving no treatment were asked to rate their pain at the time of dressing change 2 days after surgery. The TENS group reported a significantly lower level of pain than subjects in the other two groups.[50] Healing was not measured in this study.

The effect of music on reducing pain during dressing change also was examined in patients with open surgical wounds. Specifically, Angus and Faux examined the effects of music on postoperative abdominal surgery pain during wound packing.[51] They found pain to be less while music was played than when no music was played. This study needs to be extended to include a measure of healing as an additional outcome variable.

Stress

Stress has been examined in relation to the development and healing of wounds. Braden examined the effects of the stress of transfer to a nursing home on the development of pressure ulcers. She studied patients shortly after admission to the nursing home and found those with the greatest stress, measured with cortisol levels, developed pressure ulcers.[52]

The effect of relaxation and guided imagery on surgical stress and wound healing was studied in patients who had undergone cholecystectomy surgery. Findings show that those who had received the relaxation and guided imagery treatment demonstrated significantly less anxiety, lower cortisol levels, and less inflammatory response than the control group.[53] These data show that the inflammatory response can be mediated by this intervention; yet because inflammatory response is critical to initiating repair processes, more information is needed concerning the effects of decreased inflammation on wound healing before clinicians undertake interventions to manipulate inflammation. Extension of this study is warranted to address more sensitive measures of inflammation and other indices of healing.

PATHOLOGICAL CONSEQUENCES

Several pathological consequences result from disruption of the normal biochemical sequence in healing. Generally, these can be clustered under the headings of delayed healing, infection, dehiscence, and abnormalities of collagen formation. Most frequently these conditions are due to inadequate substrates for healing, overwhelming contamination by microorganisms, and metabolic defects.

Delay in Healing

A delay in the usual rate of healing may be seen in all types of wounds. For those healing by primary intention, delay is often related to lack of substrates needed for healing or an overwhelming contaminant load so that energy that would normally be spent in healing is shunted to WBCs for the process of phagocytosis to remove organisms from the area. The formation of new granulation tissue, development in wound tensile strength, epithelial migration, and wound contraction are affected by delay in healing.

Wound Infection

Wound infection frequently is an impairment seen with injury. It occurs secondary to tissue contamination from endogenous and exogenous sources. The risk of infection is related to the number, type, and virulence of the contaminants, the amount of debris present in the wound, the nature and location of the wound, and the immunocompetence of the host.[70]

The diagnosis of infection is made on the basis of the presence of greater than 10^5 organisms and signs of infection, specifically, increased inflammation, development of pus, and the occurrence of fever.[70] In the immunocompromised host, these signs may be subtle or absent, and only with vigilant observation can infection be detected.

The most accurate means of obtaining a quantitative bacterial evaluation is by tissue biopsy; however, such a biopsy necessitates removal of intact tissue, resulting in disruption of the healing process. Swab cultures are often used in clinical practice as an alternative to this method. The swab technique is subject to variation, depending on the nature of the wound and the technique of the individual performing the culture; thus, the reliability and validity of the results are sometimes questionable. There are guidelines for the swab technique that if followed consistently will increase the accuracy of the results.[71]

Infection occurs when host defenses are overcome by the invading organisms. The immunocompetence of the host and the number and type of invading organisms, bacterial or viral, are factors that greatly influence the development of wound infection. Defects in the immune system, such as major abnormalities in complement, polymorphonucleocytes, monocytes, or macrophages, may predispose the individual to infection and, ultimately, impairment of healing.

Normally, invading organisms are eliminated from the wound by polymorphonucleocytes and monocytes. Polymorphonucleocytes predominate immediately after injury and have phagocytic functions but a short half-life. Monocytes predominate from about the third day until approximately 30 days after injury; they act as phagocytes. In addition, monocyte-derived macrophages stimulate endothelial angiogenesis and mitosis as well as fibroblast activity.[72]

The ability of leukocytes to destroy organisms is directly proportional to their ability to locate foreign organisms and interfere with their cellular processes. The complement system is pivotal in lysing bacteria or marking them with opsonins so that the bacteria are recognizable to the leukocyte for later phagocytosis.

Using energy arising from aerobic or anaerobic metabolism, WBCs phagocytize organisms and kill them. One of the factors controlling this bactericidal action of leukocytes is the amount of available dissolved oxygen in the blood. White blood cells consume more oxygen and produce more peroxidase and hydrogen peroxide as the Po_2 rises; concomitantly, the bacteria count falls and the infection rate decreases. Hypoxia inhibits the leukocyte's ability to kill and supports growth of bacteria, causing an increase in infection rate. Adequate pulmonary function, intravascular volume, hemoglobin, and local wound perfusion provide oxygen to support host defenses in order to prevent wound infection.[73]

Therapeutic treatment with corticosteroids in moderate to large doses in the first several (2 to 3) days after injury may potentiate the development of wound infection. Steroids have serious deleterious effects on all phases of healing. In the inflammatory phase, corticosteroids delay the arrival of leukocytes so that inflammation is delayed and markedly less potent. If a significant level of contamination with organisms has occurred, the leukocytes present in the wound may not be sufficient to protect the wound from overgrowth of organisms and infection may develop.

Dehiscence

Dehiscence, breaking open of a previously closed wound, is a complication of healing. It may or may not be accompanied by evisceration. A sign of impending dehiscence is the leakage of serous or serosanguineous fluid from an incision line several days after injury. This indicates that the wound has not been sealed, that collagen is not being properly formed, and that the tensile strength of the wound is impaired. Dehiscence occurs more often with obese individuals because of poor tissue perfusion and with those receiving steroids because collagen formation and epithelialization are suppressed. In addition, dehiscence may be anticipated in patients who fail to form a healing ridge on a well-approximated wound by the seventh to ninth day after closure. The healing ridge is a palpable accumulation of collagen, which fills the wound space and holds the wound together.[74] In cosmetic surgery, the surgeon uses subcutaneous surgical techniques to avoid the build-up of collagen in order to provide a specific cosmetic effect and minimize the healing ridge.

Abnormal Collagen Formation

Abnormal collagen formation and the resulting side effects have received increased attention in developed countries in recent years. Hypertrophic scar tissue and keloid formation as well as impairments in functional capacity secondary to scar tissue are included in this category.

Hypertrophic scar is characterized by bulky, rigid scar tissue that arises from wounds that extend down to the reticular dermis but do not extend beyond the edges of the original wound.[75] It usually occurs in joints or in areas on the body with motion but can be created on any surface; for example, some African tribes purposefully create decorative hypertrophic scar on their faces and bodies. Hypertrophic scar normally increases in bulk up to a specific point and then regresses in size, often creating mobility or functional problems secondary to contraction. The collagen in the hypertrophic scar forms in large whorls, often centering on a cluster of cells, such as macrophages or fibroblasts, with a limited vascular system. The exact cause of hypertrophic scar tissue is

unknown. It is thought to be caused by tension, inflammation, or infection of the suture line, such that collagen synthesis is stimulated and lysis inhibited.

Keloids are itchy, rigid, bulky tissue that are larger than the wound they cover and darker than the surrounding tissue.[75] The tissue of the keloid is composed of eosinophilic bands of collagen with a thin atrophic epidermal layer. Keloids are thought to be caused by tension on the wound or by melanocyte-stimulating hormone. The stimulus causes both synthesis and lysis of collagen to be accelerated beyond that in adjacent tissue but with the synthesis stimulus being slightly greater than lysis. Keloids are more common in dark skinned persons (i.e., those with increased melena). Most people who are prone to keloids form them in all injuries they receive, regardless of how trivial or major.

Scar tissue that causes cosmetic disfigurement or functional limitation is an important wound-healing problem. Scarring after burns, facial trauma, and radical neck surgery are examples of this type of problem. Scar formation can limit mobility as a result of contractures or may cause severe psychological problems because of changes in body image.

Scarring that is seen in pulmonary fibrosis, resulting in restrictive lung disease, and in bacterial endocarditis, producing scarring of cardiac valves, is a defect in healing. Exploring the scientific basis of healing will no doubt aid in understanding the mechanisms that cause these conditions.

RELATED PATHOPHYSIOLOGICAL CONCEPTS

Concepts of concern to healing are immunocompetence, ischemia, malnutrition, stress, clotting, edema, fatigue, infection, and hypoxia. Each of these concepts has independent characteristics and needs to be studied in relation to wound healing. None of these concepts can be totally subsumed under impaired healing, and impaired healing cannot be entirely subsumed under any one of these concepts.

ASSOCIATED PSYCHOSOCIAL CONCEPTS

Psychosocial concepts related to impaired healing have not been examined extensively.

Impaired healing has been shown to be related to self-concept; Anderson and Andberg found that self-concept was an important factor in accounting for the development of pressure sores in paraplegics and quadriplegics.[76] Early studies have linked stress and stress reduction techniques with wound healing.[52, 53] Nonetheless, overall the relationship between healing and psychosocial concepts, such as loss, depression, hope, and coping, has not been examined sufficiently. Understanding this relationship will provide a more holistic perspective on healing impairment.

MANIFESTATIONS

Subjective Manifestations

Physiological data indicative of impaired healing may have subjective psychological or behavioral correlates. Studies in which psychological and behavioral correlates of impaired healing have been examined are lacking.

Objective Manifestations

In wounds healing by primary intention, a number of impairments may be seen. One of the important but more subtle impairments in primarily closed wounds is a decreased inflammatory response. This is manifested in the first 3 days after injury by a lack of redness, heat, pain, and induration along the incision. It is somewhat problematic to determine the "normal" amount of inflammation along an incision line, as induration, heat, pain, and redness are part of the normal response to mechanical trauma to tissues and are dependent on the amount and duration of the trauma. In persons with darkly pigmented skin, the problem of detection of decreased inflammation is augmented by the fact that a change in temperature and induration may be the only signs of inflammation.

The inflammatory response may continue after 3 to 4 days, and this is also a sign of impairment. Usually, a continued inflammatory response is associated with a high level of wound contamination.[70]

Drainage along the incision line (in a wound that has no drain) after 24 to 48 hours also indicates that healing is not progressing normally. Usually, a wound is sealed within 24 hours of primary closure so continued drainage suggests impairment. Most frequently, this drainage is serous or serosanguineous.

The third sign of impaired healing in a wound closed by primary intention is lack of a healing ridge by 7 to 9 days after injury. When the healing ridge is not present, there is an increased risk of dehiscence.

In wounds healing by secondary intention, manifestations of impairment are related to a delay in tissue repair or regeneration and the presence of wound drainage or exudate. Lack of an inflammatory response is also important in these patients, but observation of this is difficult.

Tissue color has characteristic patterns. Fresh granulation tissue is pale pink and progresses to a beefy red as the depth of the vascular supply increases. Delay in development is a subjective evaluation but one that can be made by a clinician who has developed expertise in assessment of wounds. Color changes may indicate wound healing problems. Overall lack of flow may slow the rate of development of granulation tissue. Also, impaired arterial circulation to the wound area results in a pale pink to blanched tissue color. Venous obstruction results in decreased flow through tissue; the blood becomes deoxygenated, and the wound looks ruddy.

Epithelial tissue development along the edges of the wound may also be delayed with impairment. Delayed healing is observed when the epithelial edge is not complete around the wound and when it does not move into the bed of the wound. Epithelial tissue migrates most readily over healthy granulation tissue and is delayed by unhealthy granulation tissue and a dry environment. Also, epithelial tissue is quite fragile and may be disrupted with friction to the wound, which occurs when a dressing is not secure and rubs against the wound with movement.

The presence of exudate indicates an impairment in the individual's ability to resist infection. The color of the wound exudate varies, depending on the degree of wound moisture or dryness and the organisms present. As the wound becomes excessively dry, the color of its exudate darkens. The presence of specific microorganisms determines the nature of the exudate; for example, *Pseudomonas* produces a thick, green drainage. Odor of the exudate is also related to the type of organisms present. Consistent assessment of odor is important in detecting changes in the predominant type of organism in the wound.

Scarring is another major category of impairment that may be present. It may limit mobility and cause disfigurement. Observations of impairment are related to the function that has been impaired. Scar tissue may also cause limitation of function in internal organs, for example, restrictive lung disease due to asbestosis and renal failure secondary to renal tubular necrosis.

SURVEILLANCE AND MEASUREMENT

Systematic assessment and evaluation of the wound is essential in providing information about the status of wound repair. A systematic approach to wound assessment helps provide a consistent and comprehensive evaluation of wound status (Tables 18–6 and 18–7). The location of the wound is noted first. This may be important, as in some types of illness there is progression of the disease and development of new wounds (e.g., gas gangrene and pemphigus).

The size and shape of the wound are then measured. In the low-risk individual with a surgical incision healing by primary intention, this step may be omitted; however, for persons with wounds healing by secondary intention, these measurements are important because progression in healing can be evaluated by changes in them. If possible, the wound shape should be traced. When tracing is not possible, wound size can be estimated by measuring the wound at several points along the length, width, and depth (Fig. 18–1). Because a wound is rarely uniform in shape, these dimensions need to be recorded at various points along the wound.

One of the important parts of measuring the wound is noting the presence of pockets or tracts in the wound. Such areas need to be recognized and treated so that they do not become walled off and form localized

TABLE 18–6 SYSTEMATIC ASSESSMENT OF WOUNDS HEALING BY PRIMARY INTENTION

Location
Approximation of edges
Inflammatory response
Drainage along incision line
Healing ridge

TABLE 18–7 SYSTEMATIC ASSESSMENT OF WOUNDS HEALING BY SECONDARY INTENTION

Location	Position on body diagram
Size and shape	Length, depth, width
Tracts	Size and shape
Inflammatory response	Pain, redness, induration, temperature
Granulation tissue	Color, rate of formation
Exudate	Color, consistency, odor
Epithelialization	Continuity around edge, migration into wound
Contraction	Decrease in size over time

abscesses. On the line drawing of the wound as well as in the narrative portion of the permanent record, the location, size, and shape of these areas need to be well described.

Surveillance then is a systematic approach to document the manifestations of wound healing and its improvement (Tables 18–6 and 18–7). The rate of wound contraction is noted with a decrease in size of the wound. Healing wounds need systematic evaluation at regular intervals. To date, there are no instruments with adequate validity and reliability that can be used to assess wounds healing either by primary or secondary intention. There remains a need for such instruments in clinical practice as well as in research.[77]

Several methods have been developed to evaluate various aspects of wound healing. Bohannon and Pfaller reported the reliability of three techniques used to estimate wound size from tracings of the wound parameter with transparent film.[78] Specifically, they evaluated the reliability of measuring the size of a wound tracing in three ways: using graph paper to quantitate the area (number of square millimeters), weighing the paper on a gram scale, and measuring the area with a planimeter. Although the standard error of measurement with these techniques cannot be known because of the study design, the error reported among the techniques was less than 6 per cent. The greatest percentage of differences was seen with small wounds. The authors did not measure the difference in areas of tracings of the wound by different individuals, and this needs to be done before the validity and reliability of the techniques are established.

Kundin has developed a tool for measuring wound volume.[79] This tool may be used throughout healing to document the rate and direction of healing of open wounds. Progression is usually noted when the wound volume decreases in size. One of the theoretical problems of such a measure is that when used on open debris-filled wounds, the wound's volume increases in size as the exudate and debris are removed. To some, this may be seen as a deterioration in the healing process because the wound volume is increasing as opposed to decreasing; however, these substances must be removed for healing to occur. The tool does not provide a means to indicate whether the volume measured reflects viable tissue or wound debris, and progress cannot be appraised accurately by wound volume alone. In addition, research has challenged the validity of measuring volume with this method,[80] and this discrepancy needs to be resolved.

Another method has been proposed to measure wound size. It uses the change in wound area divided by the perimeter of the wound to measure the distance the wound margin advances over time.[81] This approach is more accurate than measuring size using the wound perimeter, absolute area, or percentage of reduction in area. It is especially helpful in comparing the rate of closure of wounds of various sizes, where other approaches tend to overestimate the rate of closure of large wounds when compared with smaller wounds. Currently, measurement of the area and the perimeter have not been customized for use in daily care, although it is a technique that is used in research. If used in research, one of the ongoing issues remains where to measure the wound edge while measuring the perimeter and area.

Another measure that has been used to predict healing time is the greatest dimension of the wound (depth, breadth). In a study of laparotomy wounds (n = 37) and pilonidal sinus repairs (n = 26), linear regressions of healing time against wound size were determined. The authors considered the impact of varying levels of *Bacteroides* species in the pilonidal sinus series. The correlations were significant ($P < .001$; r = .863 in laparotomy series, r = .899 in pilonidal sinus series with low counts of *Bacteroides* species, r = .842 in pilonidal series with high counts of *Bacteroides* species). The authors acknowledged the difficulty in measuring wound size in shallow wounds. For this reason, they omitted wounds with any dimension less than 5 mm. They recommended that data not be extrapolated from this series to estimate healing rate in another set of patients but that data should be collected in the setting. The rationale provided was that generalization is not possible because many aspects of wound care are not well understood at this time.[82]

A mold of the wound, formed with dental impression material (alginate), has also been used to measure wound volume. When used over time, this approach can show healing with a decrease in wound size. Difficulties in use of this technique are related to positioning the patient and determining where the top edge of the wound is in the measurement. Validity of the technique is dependent on the specific product used.[83–85]

Methods also have been proposed to evaluate overall wound status. One such method was designed for wounds healing by primary intention.[53] The three dimensions of healing assessed are edema, erythema, and exudate. Each is categorized on a scale of 1 to 3 and summed to reach a total score that is divided by the number of categories scored. Preliminary validity and reliability are within an acceptable range.

Other systems have been devised to assess healing in wounds closing by secondary intention. Rank and associates'[86] and Thompson's[87] classification of wounds as either "tidy" or "untidy," the grading of pressure sores,[3, 88, 89] a wound severity score,[90] an instrument developed to assess wound healing and the need for additional treatment,[91] and an instrument developed by Stotts and Cooper[92] and revised by Cooper[77] to describe open surgical wounds are available.

Rank and associates[86] and Thompson[87] developed a system to classify a hand injury as (1) a tidy wound, (2) an untidy wound, (3) a wound with tissue loss, or (4) an infected wound. Each category is defined and a protocol for treatment of each type of wound is described. Because the same categories of criteria are not used to address all classifications, the progression of healing between categories is not clear. In addition, because the authors do not operationally define the criteria for various categories (e.g., infected or significant tissue damage), each criterion is open to subjective interpretation. The validity and reliability of this system were not addressed.

The grading of pressure sores on a scale of I to IV was devised to assist the clinician in determining the degree of injury by identifying the depth of the wound and associated symptoms.[3, 88, 89] This system has been used to report the incidence and severity of pressure sores as well as to provide a basis for making such decisions as when skin grafting will be needed. Progression within each grading classification has not been addressed, nor has any means to assess movement between the grades been noted. Although this system seems to be a good beginning for classifying pressure sores, it lacks the refinement needed to identify discrete improvement or deterioration in the healing process.

The Wound Severity Score is designed from clinical practice to be used with chronic open wounds.[90] The scale has three dimensions: general wound parameters, anatomical considerations, and wound measurements. Various aspects of the tool are weighted; the reason for the specific weighing of items is not described. The instrument has a possible score of 0 to 97, with higher scores indicating greater severity. Preliminary data indicate the score decreases as healing occurs.

Stotts and Cooper[92] developed an instrument to measure healing in open surgical wounds. A 31-item paper-and-pencil Likert instrument was designed to be used by the bedside nurse to guide evaluation of wound status. Using preliminary work on that instrument, Cooper developed the Wound Characteristics Instrument. This is a 17-item criterion-referenced clinical evaluation tool. Content and construct validity were established and validity and reliability testing are ongoing.[77]

THERAPIES

Therapeutic Goals

The goal of therapy for impaired wound healing is to restore healing to its normal rate and pattern. This goal is actualized by manipulating local and systemic factors that optimize wound healing. In addition, attention is directed at minimizing the etiological factors that precipitate impairment.

At the local level, this goal is translated into practice by manipulating (1) the moisture of the environment, (2) debris and exudate, and (3) antiseptic solutions and ointments. At the systemic level, the goals of therapy related to healing are to provide (1) adequate perfusion and oxygenation, (2) sufficient nutrition, and (3) glucose control. The goal of minimizing etiological factors precip-

itating wounds and their impairment is directly related to understanding the pathophysiology of the specific wound and intervening in the factors that can be manipulated. For example, pressure ulcers are due to ischemia from excess pressure, and interventions that lower local pressure reduce the incidence of ulcers. In addition, a number of issues in therapy must be resolved.

Local Care

Moist Environment

Research in the past 30 years has laid the foundation for significant changes in wound care. Perhaps one of the most important findings was that wound healing progresses best in a moist environment. In fact, in a moist environment, wounds epithelialize twice as fast as in a dry environment.[54, 93] Changes in practice that are consistent with providing for moist wound healing were slow to be adapted because it also was recognized that moisture supported the growth of microorganisms. The fear that bacteria proliferation would lead to an increased incidence of wound infection resulted in a resistance to accept therapies based on moist healing.[94, 95]

The scientific foundation for moist wound healing was initially conducted on partial-thickness injuries.[54] The primary type of healing of this type of wound is epithelialization. Subsequently the importance of this concept for all healing was recognized (i.e., cells cannot live in a desert). Many new types of dressings have been developed. They vary in their porosity, adsorptiveness, effects on various cellular processes, and cost.[96-101] For a more detailed discussion of the various types of dressings available, see one of the review articles.[102-105]

Attempts to apply the concept of moist wound healing to wounds healing by primary intention are very limited. Early work on the use of transparent dressings in wounds healing by primary intention showed that tensile strength was delayed in incisions covered with a transparent dressing during the first week after injury.[106] Because the wound is vulnerable to dehiscence during this period and there are not additional data about the effect of these dressings on tensile strength over time, it seems premature to use them on wounds healing by primary intention. This is a conservative approach, however, because none of the clinical trials using transparent dressings in wounds healing by primary intention demonstrated an increased incidence of dehiscence.[106–108]

One of the ongoing issues that has been created by the wide range of dressings available is determining which product to use for a specific wound. For wounds healing by primary intention, one of the issues has been whether or not a dressing is needed in the early postoperative period. Studies show that the sutured incision with good hemostasis is sealed from external contamination within 6 to 24 hours of closure.[109] Also, a prospective study has been reported on the use of dressings (versus no dressing) on the infection rate of patients who have undergone clean and clean-contaminated surgeries. Subjects were randomly assigned to a group that had a dressing until time of suture removal (n = 633) and to a group with a dressing in place only for the first postoperative day (n = 569). All patients took showers from the first postoperative day onward (dressings were covered with plastic). Results showed no difference in infection rate between the two groups.[110] These data indicate that treating primarily closed clean or clean-contaminated wounds with and without dressings is equally safe. Because no dressing after 24 hours would require fewer supplies and less dressing change time, the no dressing technique might be adapted in practice. Follow-up studies are needed to assess the stress and anxiety associated with the patient and the family viewing the incision. Theoretically, it may be very stressful to see the incision, the stress may cause catecholamines to be released, perfusion to the area may be compromised, and healing may be impaired.

With wounds healing by secondary intention, the gold standard for comparison of the newer dressings is coarse mesh gauze that has been moistened with a solution. This type of dressing has been called a "wet-to-dry" or "wet-to-damp" dressing, in which the dressing inserted into the wound is damp and the outer layer of it is dry to protect the wound from external contaminants. The damp dressing keeps the granulating tissue as well as peripheral epithelial tissue moist and yet provides a means to facilitate removal of wound exudate or necrotic tissue. The dry outer dressing protects the wound from external contamination. An intermediate layer may be used for absorption of excessive exudate.

Moist gauze dressings continue to be the mainstay of clinical practice for many wounds today. As the population of patients continues to change (i.e., hospitalized patients are increasingly ill and patients are discharged to the home or nursing home with wounds that previously would have required them to be hospitalized), the use of coarse gauze will require continued re-evaluation. Issues of concern include the fact that this type of dressing requires changing several times a day, and although the gauze is inexpensive, the expertise needed to change a dressing often is quite costly. Coarse mesh gauze may result in greater patient pain, an increased potential for contamination with dressing change, and added caregiver burden when compared with use of a more expensive product (e.g., Sorbsan, DuoDerm) that can be left in place for several days and therefore will require less manipulation. The ability to observe the wound and note subtle change in wound status must also be considered and data generated to answer this concern before one approach is universally adopted.

Debris and Exudate

Debris and exudate slow the healing process. Substrates that might be used for energy by the advancing capillary edge or in epithelialization instead provide nutrients for the phagocytic action of WBCs. Additionally, the debris and exudate act as irritants, causing the inflammatory process to be continued. Thus, excessive wound debris and exudate need to be removed from the wound for healing to occur.

A loosely inserted moist coarse gauze dressing frequently is used to débride the exudate from the wound surface.[103] This dressing makes use of the principle that (1) exudate will move into the interstices of gauze and be absorbed and trapped by the dressing, (2) coarser gauze is more absorbent and better for drainage of exudate than is finer gauze,[111] (3) the exudate and organisms are removed with the dressing,[112] and (4) wetting or dampening the dressing with an anti-infective agent at the time the dressing is placed in the wound provides the pharmacological effects of that agent. This dressing should accomplish the purpose of débridement while producing minimal disruption (i.e., bleeding of granulation tissue) when the dressing is changed. While there is conflict in the literature over whether the dressing is allowed to dry completely, even for purposes of débridement,[111] several authorities support removal of the dressing when it is moist and not stuck to the tissue.[113–115]

Because of the problems associated with coarse gauze used for débridement, hydrophilic beads, powders, and gels were developed to remove exudate and bacteria from open wounds. These have been effective in promoting granulation and decreasing exudate, inflammation, and pain in patients whose diagnoses included leg ulcers, infected traumatic wounds, wounds following local infection, and superficial decubitus ulcers.[116–119] The primary disadvantage of these agents is their high cost. This disadvantage needs to be weighed against the advantages of shortened healing time in situations of impaired healing.

Wound irrigation is another means that has been used alone or in conjunction with dressings to mechanically débride the wound. Microorganisms, dirt, exudate, and devitalized tissues are removed from the wound when the pressure of the irrigation fluid exceeds the adhesive forces of the foreign material in the wound. High-pressure irrigation at 8 pounds per square inch or more was found to be more effective than low pressure irrigation in removing debris from wounds.[120–123] Pulsatile irrigation was more effective in cleansing the wound than continuous low-pressure irrigation but damaged wound defenses.[123] Thus, the use of high-pressure nonpulsatile irrigation is recommended for removal of debris from open wounds, with the recognition that such high-pressure irrigation may cause mechanical damage to exposed blood vessels, bowel, or other friable tissue.[124] An 18-gauge angiocatheter with a 35-cc syringe can be used to provide safe and effective irrigation. Clinically, a shower has been used to irrigate wounds and remove debris; however, no studies document the effects of showering on patient outcomes.

Antiseptic Solutions and Ointments

Antiseptics are used to inhibit the growth and development of organisms on the wound surface. They also must promote a moist environment favorable to capillary budding, collagen formation, and epithelialization, while minimizing the possibility of superinfection. There are conflicting reports regarding the effects of various agents.[125, 126] The literature on the available solutions must be

carefully evaluated to determine both the local effects of the agent on infection and healing and also the potential systemic effects.

For example, povidone-iodine has both therapeutic and iatrogenic effects. It has been described as a safe, nonselective antigermal aerosol spray, surgical scrub, and antiseptic agent.[127, 128] Conversely, the scrub form of povidone-iodine has been found to increase the wound's susceptibility to infection.[129] This effect was attributed to its detergent content, which was thought to alter the activity of WBCs in the wound. Despite the antigermal qualities of povidone-iodine in the scrub, it was not potent enough to overcome the deleterious effects of the detergent content when applied to a wound. Another study demonstrated that concentrations of 5% povidone-iodine in both the aerosol spray and the solution resulted in a higher infection rate than the 1 per cent concentration.[13] This effect was attributed to inhibition of leukocyte activity by the higher concentration of the agent. Povidone-iodine as a 1 per cent solution also has been shown to be toxic to human fibroblasts.[130, 131] As an irrigant, it does not lower the infection rate more than normal saline or pluronic F–68 (Shurcleans).[132] When used as a soak solution for 10 minutes, the organisms may increase significantly more than when no soak is performed.[133]

Thus, the benefits and risks of each antiseptic that may be used with the wound must be evaluated.[134] The patient's physiological status and the specific goals of therapy will indicate whether a trial of a specific agent is warranted.

Another issue in the care of wounds is whether the suture line in wounds healing by primary intention should have a specific type of care. Data are not available to substantiate how to care for the incision line. Various practices are used clinically (e.g., do nothing, clean with various strengths of hydrogen peroxide or povidone-iodine, shower, apply antibiotic ointment), and a strong physiological rationale can be provided for each approach. Yet no studies have been reported on the effect of various cleaning approaches that indicate how they affect outcome.

Systemic Support for Healing
Perfusion and Oxygenation

Systemic therapies that maximize perfusion, oxygenation, and adequate wound substrates are important to wound healing. Adequate volume must be provided as measured by classical parameters of hydration.

Studies have shown that hypovolemia or hemorrhage producing clinical signs of volume depletion have resulted in impaired healing.[32–34] It also has been established that decreased volume, rather than anemia, is the critical factor in precipitating impaired healing.[32, 33] In volume-depleted patients, specific therapy to correct the hemorrhage or hypovolemia is indicated. Minimizing the duration of the low-flow state will mitigate the effects of healing impairment.

Another group of individuals of concern are those who have subclinical hypovolemia (i.e., signs and symptoms of hypovolemia are not visible). Chang and associates, as part of a larger study, examined the effects of a bolus of fluid on wound oxygenation of individuals who were clinically normovolemic but hypoxic and refractory to oxygen treatment.[22] A bolus of fluid increased wound PO_2, indicating that (1) local wound hypovolemia occurs prior to or unrelated to the classic signs of hypovolemia; (2) wound PO_2 could be monitored clinically, and (3) perfusion and oxygenation could be factored out separately, with therapy planned to treat each of these problems and evaluated using a subtle clinical index of perfusion. Although an ideal instrument is not available to detect changes in tissue perfusion, several new instruments are available at the bedside that increase our understanding of tissue oxygenation including transcutaneous oxygen, conjunctival oxygen, and subcutaneous oxygen measurement.[23]

Oxygen is an important substrate in the healing process. It is crucial to support the cellular processes needed as a defense against pathological wound microorganisms and for repair and regeneration of tissues. Providing increased levels of inhaled oxygen increased wound and tissue PO_2, with tissue PO_2 always remaining higher than wound PO_2.[22]

Wound oxygen tension can be raised by increasing the fraction of inspired oxygen.[22, 135] Controlled studies have not been reported on the effects of varying modes of treatment and on concentrations of oxygenation on healing in the acutely ill patient; completion of such research will add to the scientific basis of clinical management of these individuals. Until such data are available, it is important to use our existing knowledge of the means to increase tissue oxygenation, such as maximal inspiratory maneuvers, early ambulation, and regular turning for bed-bound patients.[78]

Studies have examined the effects of various stressors on healing. Stress causes catecholamine release that reduces perfusion and oxygenation to subcutaneous tissue and wounds. Data show that music[48] and TENS[47] reduce the pain associated with dressing changes in open surgical wounds. Because adaptation of a proposed change in intervention cannot be based on findings from a single study, these research studies need to be repeated before their results can be used in practice. Quantitative data about the relationship of analgesics, and these treatments need to be reported to enhance our understanding of the interaction of pain, analgesics, and various therapies.

Manipulation of the environment to reduce external stressors seems to be an area that holds promise for affecting healing. Early studies have been conducted that show that noise reduces the rate of wound closure in animals[48, 49] and that high stress correlates with the development of pressure ulcers in long-term care.[52] Also, one study has shown that relaxation and guided imagery promote healing and reduce stress in postoperative surgical patients.[53] These studies are timely and need to be replicated and extended to establish a basis for a change in practice. Related phenomena that affect healing, such as sleep and social support, need to be considered as part of these stress-related studies.[136]

Glucose Control

Control of serum glucose levels is important with injury. Therapy in the early postinjury period in the diabetic must be planned to carefully titrate glucose levels to prevent complications in wound healing. Using glucometer readings or serum glucose levels provides for early identification of hyperglycemia, allows rapid reporting of this problem, and aids in maximizing healing potential.

Nutrition

Nutrients are also a concern in healing, and a sufficient quantity must be administered to support wound healing. The protein needs of the adult with healing wounds are estimated to be as much as 1.5 to 2.0 g/kg.

Nonprotein calories required are estimated to be 25 to 30 kcal/kg.[137] In addition, a multivitamin supplement should be routinely administered to patients with wounds and provision of extra vitamin C considered.[36] Depending on the resources of a specific institution, assistance in determining the patient's nutritional needs may be available from a dietitian or nutritionist. Quantitating the patient's needs and goals of therapy is critical to therapy. Once specific goals are set and prescription planned, interventions to actualize the goals can be undertaken.

Nutrients are provided by the usual routes, that is, orally or enterally and parenterally if no other route is available *or* if aggressive therapy is needed immediately because the individual is critically ill and would be seriously compromised if not given immediate nutritional support. Information on the administration of these therapies is readily available in the literature on nutrition.[137–139]

The need for nutrients continues throughout the healing process. Recent research on patients at home with surgical wounds healing by secondary intention indicates that patients do not take sufficient nutrients for healing[140] and this may contribute to their impaired healing.

Innovative Therapies

New therapies to promote healing are continuously being introduced. Growth factors, tested in the laboratory for a number of years, have been shown in clinical studies to accelerate healing in chronic wounds.[55, 56, 59, 141] Their use has the potential to revolutionize care. At present, use of this therapy is expensive and available only through specialized agencies. For patients with chronic debilitating wounds, this new therapy holds much hope.

A new approach to wound closure being tested clinically is the use of cultured skin grafts.[142, 143] Skin is grown in the laboratory from cells obtained by biopsy or from an allogenic source such as neonatal foreskin. The tissue culture grows to a confluent sheet in about 3 weeks. The tissue then is "grafted" onto the wound. Early research in this area was conducted with burn victims, but now the technology is being applied in selected centers on patients with chronic wounds such as pressure ulcers, vascular ulcers, and amputation sites.[142, 143] Wound healing appears to be stimulated because the cultured epider-

mal cells release growth factors into the wound environment as well as function as a skin substitute.

Another new therapy that has local and systemic effects is the use of electrical therapy.[144, 145] Electrical current has been used to support healing in patients with delayed or retarded wound healing. With this method, electrodes are placed on the skin and a small voltage is passed through them. Electrical stimulation results in accelerated intracellular biosynthesis of granulation tissue in the healing wound and in increased circulation.

Special Considerations

Care of specific types of wounds requires attention to their cause and underlying pathology. For example, pressure ulcers are a serious problem that demand attention. Identification of patients at increased risk for ulcers is critical to early intervention, to therapy applied at the time risk is identified, and before tissue damage has occurred. A number of instruments can assess risk of pressure ulcer development, the most frequently cited being the Norton scale, the Gosnell scale, and the Braden scale.[146–148] Preliminary work indicates that all three scales are able to predict risk of ulcer development. Additional work is in progress to verify validity with specific patient populations.

Excess scar formation is another type of impairment that warrants special consideration. This impairment can be mitigated during its formation with the use of elastic garments that place pressure on the wound.[149, 150] After keloids or hypertrophic scars occur, the symptomatic treatment of the concomitant itching is provided with antihistamines. In some cases, intrakeloid injection with a steroid has resulted in softening and regression of the lesion.[151] Surgical excision remains an option for persons with keloids or hypertrophic scar; however, it cannot be predicted which patients will experience recurrence of abnormal scar tissue after this procedure.

ILLUSTRATIVE CASE STUDIES

CASE STUDY NO. 1

A 62-year-old man had undergone axillofemoral bypass graft for arteriosclerosis obliterans, and dehiscence developed at the groin incision line approximately 14 days postoperatively. On hospital admission, albumin was 2.8 g/100 ml (normal, 3.5 to 5.5 g/100 ml); total protein, 5.6 g/100 ml (normal, 6 to 8 g/100 ml); serum transferrin 154 mg/100 ml (normal 250 to 350 mg/100 ml), and total WBC count 10,100/mm³ (normal 6 to 900/mm³). The patient was 5 feet, 7 inches tall, weighed 124 pounds, and had lost approximately 20 pounds in the past month.

He was taken to surgery, where his wound was débrided and dressed with a moist-to-moist half-strength povidone-iodine dressing. After débridement the wound was 4 x 8 x ½ inches, a diamond-shaped wound located in the left groin. The tissue on the floor and walls of the wound was dry and pinkish-yellow. The pink coloration represented new granulation tissue, and the yellow was a result of Betadine staining. The graft was visible on the floor of the wound, differentiated from the tissue or exudate by the fact that it was cream colored, moist, and visible as an indentation in the granulation tissue. Exudate was evident throughout the floor and walls of the wound. The yellow-brown color of the exudate was due to dryness and discoloration by the povidone-iodine. A thin, pale pink epithelial border surrounded the wound. Peripheral tissue within 2 inches of the wound was pale and dry, with povidone-iodine discoloration present. No scars were visible. The dressing was changed to a normal saline coarse gauze dressing, and the yellow-orange color and dryness of the wound for the most part abated.

The patient's nutritional status was supported with oral and enteral feedings. A high-protein, 2500-calorie diet was prescribed. In addition, nasogastric feedings were provided at night using a small bore (No. 7 French) feeding tube. Multivitamins were also provided. The patient did not gain weight or have an appreciable improvement in plasma proteins, but the granulation tissue in the floor and walls of the wound became thicker over the next week and the epithelial edge increased. The wound was almost ready for grafting when a concomitant problem caused the patient to die.

CASE STUDY NO. 2

A 37-year-old woman underwent a colectomy after a stab wound to the abdomen. Eight days after surgery, the colectomy incision was healing by secondary intention. This woman was 60 inches tall and weighed 300 pounds; her albumin was 4.5 g/100 ml (normal, 3.5 to 5.5 g/100 ml), total protein, 7.2 g/100 ml (normal, 6 to 8 g/100 ml), and WBC count, 12,000/mm³ (normal, 6 to 9,000/mm³).

The abdominal wound was a transverse incision 14 x 3 x 2 inches. The entire floor of the wound was covered with thin yellow to beige exudate. No floor tissue was visible. The walls of the wound were very light red and moist. In addition, a coating of pale yellow exudate covered the walls. The edge of the wound had no epithelial tissue. The peripheral tissue was pale pink and was intact around the entire wound.

The wound was treated with hydrophilic beads two to three times per day until the exudate was removed. The treatment was then changed to moist-to-moist dressings with quarter-strength Dakin's solution, three times per day. The patient was supported systemically with a vigorous activity regimen, using a binder on her wound when she walked. In addition, she was maintained on oxygen per nasal prongs at 2 L/minute while in bed. An oral diet high in protein (1.5 g/kg) was provided, and the patient was maintained in positive nitrogen balance. When she was discharged 20 days postoperatively, moist-to-moist dressing changes at home were required for the open granulating wound.

IMPLICATIONS FOR FURTHER RESEARCH

There is a need for research into many facets of healing. Of particular concern to nursing is the individual's response to wounds and to treatment of the wound; this research must include biological as well as psychosocial dimensions. Both new wounds and chronic wounds are of concern to health care providers.

Some of the areas in the biological realm to be addressed are development of instruments to measure healing in wounds, the effects of specific types of dressings on healing, the impact of various irrigation regimens on wound infection, the relationship of post-operative mobilization and activity to rate of healing, how nutrient repletion approaches affect healing, the therapeutic and iatrogenic effects of various topical and systemic agents on healing, and identification of accelerators of healing.

In the psychosocial realm, research needs to examine the effect of chronic open wounds on self-concept, coping styles in persons with chronic wounds, adaptation profiles in persons with abnormalities of collagen that limit activities or function, the relationship between affective response (e.g., depression) and rate of healing, and the effect of impaired healing on family dynamics.

In addition, studies are also needed that explore the relationship of healing to the psychophysiological phenomena of stress that results from tissue injury, hospitalization, life-threatening illness, and psychological adjustment. Because healing and stress are complex psychophysiological phenomena, it might be hypothesized that the potential benefit from understanding and being able to manipulate this interaction could be quite important.

There continues to be a need for use of study designs that control for threats to internal validity and that have a sufficient number of subjects. Lastly, there is an important place for both basic and applied research in wound healing. Basic research serves to build the theoretical framework or foundation for future applied research. Applied research tests and modifies theory to solve clinical problems. Thus, each type of research has an important role in development of our knowledge for high-quality care of patients with impaired healing.

REFERENCES

1. Hunt, T. K., & Van Winkle, W. (1979). *Normal Repair*. In T. K. Hunt & J. E. Dunphy (eds.), *Fundamentals of Wound Management* (p. 4). New York: Appleton-Century-Crofts.
2. Dimick, A. R. (1988). Delayed wound closure: Indications and techniques. Ann Emerg Med *17*:1303–1304.
3. National Pressure Ulcer Advisory Committee. (1989). Pressure ulcers: Prevalence, cost and risk assessment: Consensus development conference statement. Decubitus 2:24–28.
4. Cutler, B. S., Dodson, T. F., Silva, W. E., & Vandersalm, T. J. (1988). *Manual of Clinical Problems in Surgery*. Boston: Little, Brown & Co.
5. Callam, M. J., Harper, D. R., Dale, J. J., & Ruckley, C. V. (1987). Arterial disease in chronic leg ulcer-
ation: An underestimated hazard? Lothian and Forthe Valley leg ulcer study. Br Med J *294*:929–931.
6. Doucette, M. M., Fylling, C., & Knighton, D. R. 1989). Amputation prevention in a high-risk population through comprehensive wound healing protocol. Arch Phys Med Rehabil *70*:780–785.
7. Cruse, P. J. E., & Foord, R. (1980). The epidemiology of wound infection: A ten-year prospective study of 62,939 wounds. Surg Clin North Am *60*:27–40.
8. Heughan, C., Niinikoski, J., & Hunt, T. K. (1973). Oxygen tension in lesions of experimental atherosclerosis of rabbits. Atherosclerosis *17*:361–367.
9. Ross, R., & Glomet, J. A. (1973). Atherosclerosis and the arterial smooth muscle cell. Science *180*:1332–1339.
10. *Heart Facts* (1983). Dallas: American Heart Association.
11. Goodson, W. H. III, & Hunt, T. K. (1979). Wound healing and aging. J Invest Dermatol *73*:88–91.
12. Eaglstein, W. H. (1989). Wound healing and aging. Clin Geriatr Med *5*:183–188.
13. Tsai, T., Matloff, S., & Gray, R., et al. (1986). Cardiac surgery in the octogenarian. J Thorac Cardiovasc Surg *91*:924–928.
14. Kay, S. P., Moreland, J. R., & Schmitter, E. (1987). Nutritional status and wound healing in lower extremity amputations. Clin Orthop *217*:253–256.
15. Rosenberg, C. S. (1990). Wound healing in the patient with diabetes mellitus. Nurs Clin North Am *25*:247–261.
16. Pearl, S. H., & Kanat, I. O. (1988). Diabetes and healing: A review of literature. J Foot Surg *27*:268–270.
17. Goodson, W. H., III, & Hunt, T. K. (1977). Studies of wound healing in experimental diabetes mellitus. J Surg Res *22*:221–227.
18. Goodson, W. H., III, Radolf, J., & Hunt, T. K. (1980). Wound healing and diabetes. In T. K. Hunt (ed.), *Wound Healing and Wound Infection: Theory and Surgical Practice* (pp. 106–117). New York: Appleton-Century-Crofts.
19. Shukla, V. K., Roy, S. K., Kumar, J., & Vaidya, M. P. (1985). Correlation of immune and nutritional status with wound complications in patients undergoing abdominal surgery. Am Surg *51*:442–445.
20. Hotter, A. N. (1990). Wound healing and immunocompromise. Nurs Clin North Am *25*:193–203.
21. Heimbach, R. D. (1988). Radiation effects on tissue. In J. C. Davis & T. K. Hunt (eds.), *Problem Wounds: The Role of Oxygen*. New York: Elsevier.
22. Chang, N., Goodson, W. H., III, Gottrup, F., & Hunt, T. K. (1983). Direct measurement of wound and tissue oxygen tension in postoperative patients. Ann Surg *197*:470–478.
23. Gottrup, F., Gellett, S., Kirkegaard, L., Stender Hansen, E., & Johannsen, G. (1988). Continuous monitoring of tissue oxygen tension during hyperoxia and hypoxia: Relation of subcutaneous, transcutaneous, and conjunctival oxygen tension to hemodynamic variables. Crit Care Med *16*:1229–1234.
24. Knighton, D. R., Silver, I. A., & Hunt, T. K. (1981). Regulation of wound-healing angiogenesis—effect of oxygen gradients and inspired oxygen concentration. Surgery *90*:262–270.
25. Niinikoski, J., Hunt, T. K., & Dunphy, J. E. (1972).

Oxygen supply in healing tissue. Am J Surg *123*:247–252.

26. Hunt, T. K., & Pai, M. P. (1972). The effect of varying ambient oxygen tensions on wound management and collagen synthesis. Surg Gynecol Obstet *135*:561–567.

27. Bullough, W. S., & Johnson, M. (1951). Epidermal mitotic activity and oxygen tension. Nature *167*:488.

28. Winter, G. D., & Perrins, D. J. D. (1970). Effects of hyperbaric oxygen treatment on epidermal regeneration. In J. Wada & T. Iwa (eds.), *Proceedings of the Fourth International Congress on Hyperbaric Medicine* (p. 363). Tokyo: Igaku-Shoin.

29. Pai, M. P., & Hunt, T. K. (1972). Effect of varying oxygen tensions on healing of open wounds. Surg Gynecol Obstet *135*:756–758.

30. Hunt, T. K., Linsey, M., Sonne, M., & Jawetz, E. (1972). Oxygen tension and wound infection. Surg Forum *23*:47–49.

31. Hunt, T. K., Linsey, M., Grislis, G., Sonne, M., & Jawetz E. (1975). The effect of differing ambient oxygen tensions on wound infection. Ann Surg *181*:35–39.

32. Heughan, C., Chir, B., Grislis, G., & Hunt, T. K. (1974). The effect of anemia on wound healing. Ann Surg *179*:163–167.

33. Hunt, T. K., Zederfeldt, B. H., Goldstick, T. K., & Conolly, W. B. (1967). Tissue oxygen tension during controlled hemorrhage. Surg Forum *18*:3–4.

34. Modolin, M., Bevilacqua, R. G., Margarido, N. F., & Lima-Goncalcaves, E. (1985). Effects of protein depletion and repletion on experimental open wound contraction. Ann Plast Surg *15*:123–126.

35. Haydock, D. A., Flint, M. H., Hyde, K. F., Reilly, H. C., Poole, C. A., & Hill, G. L. (1988). The efficacy of subcutaneous Goretex implants in monitoring wound healing response in experimental protein deficiency. Connect Tissue Res *17*:159–169.

36. Levenson, S., Seifer, E., & Van Winkle, W., Jr. (1979). Nutrition. In T. K. Hunt & J. E. Dunphy (eds.), *Fundamentals of Wound Management* (pp. 286–363). New York: Appleton-Century-Crofts.

37. Levine, M. (1986). New concepts in the biology and biochemistry of ascorbic acid. N Engl J Med *314*:892–902.

38. Greenhalgh, D. G., & Gamelli, R. L. (1987). Is impaired wound healing caused by infection or nutritional depletion?. Surgery *102*:306–312.

39. Olson, J. A., & Hodges, R. E. (1987). Recommended dietary intakes (RDI) of vitamin C in humans. Am J Clin Nutr *45*:693–703.

40. Hunt, T. K., Ehrlich, H. P., Garcia, J. A., & Dunphy, J. E. (1969). Effect of vitamin A on reversing the inhibitory effect of cortisone on healing in open wounds in animals and man. Ann Surg *170*:633–641.

41. Ehrlich, H. P., & Hunt, T. K. (1968). Effects of cortisone and vitamin A on wound healing. Ann Surg *167*:324–641.

42. Seifter, E., Crowley, L. V., Rettura, G., Nakao, K., Gruber, C., Kan, D., & Levenson S. M. (1975). Influence of vitamin A on wound healing in rats with femoral fracture. Ann Surg *181*:836–841.

43. Prasad, A. S. (1985). Clinical manifestations of zinc deficiency. Annu Rev Nutr 341–363.

44. Calkins, E., Davis, P. J., & Ford, A. B. (1986). *The Practice of Geriatrics*. Philadelphia: W.B. Saunders.

45. Haydock, D. A., & Hill, G. L. (1987). Improved wound healing response in surgical patients receiving intravenous nutrition. Br J Surg *74*:320–323.

46. Windsor, J. A., Knight, G. S., & Hill, G. L. (1988). Wound healing response in surgical patients: Recent food intake is more important than nutritional status. Br J Surg *75*:135–137.

47. Goodson, W. H., Jensen, J. A., Granja-Mena, L., Lopez-Sarmiento, A., West, J., & Bhavez-Estrella, J. (1987). The influence of brief preoperative illness on postoperative healing. Ann Surg *205*:250–255.

48. Schmid, P., Horejsi, R. C., Mlekusch, W., & Paletta, B. (1989). The influence of noise stress on plasma epinephrine and its binding to plasma protein in the rat. Biomed Biochim Acta *48*:453–456.

49. Wysocki, A. B. (1986). The effect of intermittent noise exposure on the rate of wound healing in albino rats. Unpublished doctoral dissertation. Austin: The University of Texas.

50. Hargreaves, A., & Lander, J. (1989). Use of transcutaneous electrical nerve stimulation for postoperative pain. Nurs Res *38*:159–161.

51. Angus, J. E., & Faux, S. (1989). The effect of music on adult postoperative patients' pain during a nursing procedure. In S. G. Funk, E. M. Tournquist, M. T. Champagne, L. A. Copp, & R. A. Weise (eds.), *Key Aspects of Recovery: Management of Pain, Fatigue and Nausea* (pp. 166–172). New York: Springer.

52. Braden, B. J. (1990). Emotional stress and pressure sore formation among the elderly recently relocated to a nursing home. In S. G. Funk, E. M. Touruquist, M. T. Champagne, & R. A. Weise (eds.), *Key Aspects of Recovery: Improving Mobility, Rest, and Nutrition*. New York, Springer.

53. Holden-Lund, C. (1988). Effects of relaxation with guided imagery on surgical stress and wound healing. Res Nurs Health *11*:235–244.

54. Winter, G. D., & Scales, J. T. (1963). Effect of air drying and dressings on the surface of a wound. Nature *197*:91–92.

55. Sprugel, K., McPherson, J. M., Clowes A. W., & Ross, R. (1987). The effects of different growth factors in subcutaneous wound chambers. Am J Pathol *129*:601–613.

56. Brown, G. L., Nanny, L. B., Griffen, J., Cramer, A. B., Yancey, J. M., Curtsinger, L. J., III, Holtzin, L., Schultz, G. S., Jurkiewicz, M. J., & Lynch, J. B. (1989). Enhancement of wound healing by topical treatment with epidermal growth factor. N Engl J Med *321*:76–79.

57. Hunt, T. K., & La Van, F. B.(1989). Enhancement of wound healing by growth factors. N Engl J Med *321*:111–112.

58. Orgill, D., & Demiling, R. H. (1988). Current concepts and approaches to wound healing. Crit Care Med *16*:899–908.

59. Knighton, D. R., Siegel, V. D., Doucette, M. M., Fylling, C. P., & Cerra, F. B. (1989). The use of typically applied platelet growth factors in chronic nonhealing wounds: A review. Wounds *1*:72–78.

60. Nemeth, G. G., Bolander, M. E., & Martin, G. R. (1988). Growth factors and their role in fracture healing. In *Growth Factors and Other Aspects of Wound Healing: Biological and Clinical Implications* (pp. 1–17). New York: Alan R. Liss.

61. Jackson, D. S., & Rovee, D. T. (1988). Current concepts in wound healing: Research and theory. J Enterostom Ther *15*:133–137.

62. Simpson, D. M., & Ross, R. (1972). The neutrophilic leukocytes in wound repair: A study with antineutrophil serum. J Clin Invest 51:2009–2014.

63. Leibovich, S. J., & Ross, R. (1975). The role of macrophages in wound repair. Am J Pathol 78:71.

64. Hunt, T. K., Twomey, P., Zederfeldt B., & Dunphy, J. E. (1967). Respiratory gas tensions and pH in healing wounds. Am J Surg 114:302–307.

65. Ehrlich, H. P., Grislis G., & Hunt, T. K. (1972). Metabolic and circulatory contributions to oxygen gradients in wounds. Surgery 72:578–583.

66. Silver, I. A. (1969). The measurement of oxygen tension in healing tissue. Prog Respiration 3:124–128.

67. Hjortrup, A., Rasmussen, B. F., & Kehlet, M. (1983). Morbidity in diabetic and non-diabetic patients after major vascular surgery. Br Med J 287:1107.

68. Shagon, B. P. (1990). Does anyone here know how to make insulin work backwards? Pract Diabetol 9:1–4.

69. Engel, E. D., Erlick, N. E., & Davis, R. H. (1981). Diabetes mellitus, impaired healing from zinc deficiency. J Am Pod Assoc 71:536–544.

70. Garner, J. S., Jarvis, W. R., Emori, T. G., Horan, T. C., & Hughes, J. M. (1988). CDC definitions for nosocomial infections. Am J Infect Control 16:128–140.

71. Crow, S. (1990). Infection control perspectives, chronic wound care. In D. Krasner (ed.), Chronic Wound Care: A Clinical Source Book for Health Care Professionals. (pp. 367–377). King of Prussia, PA: Health Management Publications.

72. Banda, M. J., Knighton, D. R., Hunt, T. K., & Werb, Z. (1982). Isolation of a nonmitogenic angiogenesis factor from wound fluid. Proc Natl Acad Sci 79:7773–7777.

73. Whitney, J. D. (1989). Physiologic effects of tissue oxygenation on wound healing. Heart Lung 18:466–474.

74. Hunt, T. K., & Goodson, W. H., III. (1991). Wound healing. In L. W. Way (ed.), Current Surgical Diagnosis and Treatment (pp. 95–108). Norwalk, CT: Appleton & Lange.

75. Hunt, T. K. (1979). Disorders of repair and their management. In T. K. Hunt & J. E. Dunphy (eds.), Fundamentals of Wound Management (pp. 68–169). New York: Appleton-Century-Crofts.

76. Anderson, T. P., & Andberg, M. M. (1979). Psychosocial factors associated with pressure sores. Arch Phys Med Rehabil 60:341–346.

77. Cooper, D. M. (1990). Human wound assessment: Status report and implications for clinicians. AACN Clin Issues Crit Care Nurs 1(3):553–565.

78. Bohannon, R. W., & Pfaller, B. A. (1983). Documentation of wound surface area of tracing of wound parameter. Phys Ther 63:1622–1664.

79. Kundin, J. I. (1989). A new way to size up a wound. Am J Nurs 89:206–207.

80. Thomas, A. C., & Wysocki, A. B. (1989). The healing wound: A comparison of three clinically useful methods of measurement. Decubitus 3:18–25.

81. Gilman, T. H. (1990). Parameter for measurement of wound closure. Wounds 2:95–101.

82. Marks, J., Hughes, L. E., Harding, K. G., Campbell, H., & Ribeiro, C.D. (1983). Prediction of healing time as an aid to the management of open granulating wounds. World J Surg 7:641–645.

83. Resch, C. S., Kerner E., Robson, M. C., Heggers, J. P., Scherer, M., Boertman, J. A., & Schileru, R. (1988). Pressure sore volume measurement: A technique to document and record wound healing. J Am Geriatr Soc 36:444–446.

84. Covington, J. S., Griffin, J. W., Mendius, R. K., Tooms, R. E., & Clifft, J.K. (1989). Measurement of pressure ulcer volume using dental impression materials: Suggestion from the field. Phys Ther 69:690–694.

85. Peutzfeldt, A., & Asmussen, E. (1989). Accuracy of alginate and elastomeric impression materials. Scand J Dent Res 97:375–379.

86. Rank, B. K., Wakefield, A. R., & Hueston, J. T. (1968). Surgery of Repair As Applied to Hand Injuries (3rd ed., pp. 88–89, 90–91, 126–179). London: Churchill Livingstone.

87. Thompson, R. V. S. (1969). Primary Repair of Soft Tissue Injuries (pp. 3–9). Victoria, Australia: Melbourne University Press.

88. Sather, M. R., Weber, C. E., Jr., & George, J. (1977). Pressure sores and the spinal cord injury patient. Drug Intell Clin Pharm 11:154–169.

89. Shea, J. D. (1975). Pressure sores—classification and management. Clin Orthop 112:89.

90. Knighton, D. R., Fiegel, V. D., Austin, L. L., Ciresi, K. F., & Butler, E. L. (1986). Classification and treatment of chronic nonhealing wounds. Ann Surg 204:322–329.

91. Wilson, A. P. R., Treasure, T., Sturridge, M. F., & Gruneberg, R. N. (1986). A scoring method (ASEPSIS) for postoperative wound infections for use in clinical trials of antibiotic prophylaxis. Lancet 1:311–313.

92. Stotts, N. A., & Cooper, D. M. (1984). Development of an instrument to measure wound healing. Abstract, 12th Annual Nursing Research Conference, University of Arizona, Tucson, Arizona.

93. Hinman, C. D., & Maibach, H. (1963). Effect of air exposure and occlusion on experimental human skin wounds. Nature 200:377–378.

94. Buchan, I. A., Andrews, J. K., Land, S. M., Boorman, J. G., Harvey Kemble, J. V., & Lamberty, B. G. H. (1981). Clinical and laboratory investigation of the composition and properties of human skin wound exudate under semi-permeable dressings. Burns 7:326–334.

95. Mulder, G., Kissil, M., & Mahr, J. J. (1989). Bacterial growth under occlusive and non-occlusive wound dressings. Wounds 1:63–69.

96. Pickworth, J. J., & De Souda, N. (1988). Angiogenesis and macrophage response under the influence of Duoderm. Proceedings of the Second International Forum on Fibrinolysis and Angiogenesis, San Antonio (pp. 44–48).

97. Chvapil, M., Chvapil, T. A., & Owen, J. A. (1987). Comparative study of four wound dressings on epithelialization of partial-thickness wounds in pigs. J Trauma 27:278–282.

98. Silverman, R. A., Lender, J., & Elmets, C. A. (1989). Effects of occlusive and semiocclusive dressings on the return of barrier function to transepidermal water loss in standardized human wounds. J Am Acad Dermatol 5:755–760.

99. Myers, R. B., Moore, K., Mulder, G. D., Pike, R. A., & Kissil, M. T. (1988). Report of a multicenter clinical trial on the performance characteristics of two occlusive hydrocolloid dressings in the treat-

ment of noninfected, partial thickness wounds. J Enterostom Ther *15*:158–161.

100. Watts, C., & Shipes, E. (1988). A study to compare the overall performance of two hydrocolloid dressings on partial thickness wounds. Ostomy Wound Manage *21*:28–31.

101. Oot-Giromini, B., Bidwell, F. C., Heller, N. B., Parks, M. L., Prebish, E. M., Wicks, P., & Williams, P. M. (1989). Pressure ulcer versus treatment, comparative product case study. Decubitus *2*:52–54.

102. Wheeland, R. G. (1987). The newer surgical dressings and wound healing. Adv Dermatol Surg *5*:393–407.

103. Cuzzell, J. Z. (1990). Choosing a wound dressing: A systematic approach. AACN Clin Issues Crit Care Nurs *1*:566–577.

104. Falanga, V. (1988). Occlusive wound dressings: Why, when, which? Arch Dermatol *124*:872–877.

105. Alvarez, O., Rozint, J., & Meehan, M. (1990). Principles of moist wound healing: Indications for chronic wounds. In D. Krasner (ed.), *Chronic Wound Care* (pp. 266–281). King of Prussia, PA: Health Management Publications.

106. Linsky, C. B., Rovee, D. T., & Dow, T. (1981). Effects of dressings on wound inflammation and scar tissue. In P. Dineen & G. Hildick-Smith (eds.), *The Surgical Wound* (pp. 191–205). Philadelphia: Lea & Febiger.

107. Moshakis, V., Fordyce, M. J., Griffiths, J. D., & McKinna, J. A. (1984). Tegaderm versus gauze dressing in breast surgery. Br J Clin Pract *38*:149–152.

108. Gardezi, S. A. R., Chaudhary, A. M., Sial, G. A. K., Ahmad, I., & Rashid, M. (1983). Role of "polyurethene membrane" in postoperative wound management. JPMA *33*:219–222.

109. Heifetz, C. J., Lawrence, M. S., & Richards, O. F. (1952). Comparison of wound healing with and without dressings. Arch Surg *65*:746–751.

110. Chrintz, H., Vibits, H., Cordtz, T. O., Harreby, J. S., Waaddengaard, P., & Larsen, S. O. (1989). Need for surgical wound dressings. Br J Surg *76*:204–205.

111. Noe, J. M., & Kalish, S. (1983). Dressing materials and their selection. In R. Rudolph & J. M. Noe (eds.), *Chronic Wounds* (pp. 37–46). Boston: Little, Brown & Co.

112. Levine, N. S., Lindberg, R. A., Salisbury, R. E., Mason, A. D., & Pruitt, B. A., Jr. (1976). Comparison of coarse mesh gauze with biologic dressings on granulating wounds. Am J Surg *131*:727–729.

113. Winter, G. D. (1971). Healing of skin wounds and the influence of dressings on the repair process. In K. V. Karkiss (ed.), *Surgical Dressings and Wound Healing* (pp. 46–60). London: Bradford University Press.

114. Sawyer, P. N., Bergan, J., Dagher, F. J., Degreef, H., Haeger, K., Hunt T. K., Jacobsson, S., & Winter, G. D. (1980). Treatment alternatives for pressures sores. Mod Med *48*:49–56.

115. Pollock, A. (1987). *Surgical wound infection* (pp. 201–204). Baltimore: Williams & Wilkins.

116. Thomas, S., & Tucker, C. A. (1989). Sorbsan in the management of leg ulcers. Pharm J *243*:706–709.

117. Floden, C. H., Wikstrom, K. (1978). Controlled clinical trial with dextranomer (Debrisan) on venous leg ulcers. Curr Ther Res *24*:753–760.

118. Jacobson, S. Rothman, U., Arturson, G., Ganrot, K., Haeger, K., Juhlin, I. (1976). A new principle for the cleansing of infected wounds. Scand J Plast Reconstr Surg *10*:65–72.

119. Pace, W. E. (1978). Beads of a dextran polymer for the local treatment of cutaneous ulcers. J Dermatol Surg Oncol *4*:678–682.

120. Rodeheaver, G. T., Petty, D., Thacker, J. G., Edgerton, M. T., & Edlich, R. F. (1975). Wound cleansing by high pressure irrigation. Surg Gynecol Obstet *141*:357–362.

121. Hamer, M. L., Robson, M. C., Krizek, T. J., & Southwick, W. O. (1975). Quantitative bacterial analysis of comparative wound irrigations. Ann Surg *181*:819–822.

122. Brown, L. L., Shelton, H. T., Bornside, G. H., & Cohn, I. (1978). Evaluation of wound irrigation by pulsatile jet and conventional methods. Ann Surg *187*:170–173.

123. Wheeler, C. B., Rodeheaver, G. T., Thacker, J. G., Edgerton, M. T., & Edlich, R. F. (1976). Side-effects of high pressure irrigation. Surg Gynecol Obstet *143*:775–778.

124. Stotts, N. A. (1983). The most effective method of wound irrigation. Focus Crit Care *10*:45–48.

125. Rodeheaver, G. (1989). Controversies in topical wound management. Wounds *1*:19–27.

126. Lineaweaver, W., Howard, R., Soucy, D., McMorris, S., Freeman, J., Crain, C., Robertson, J., & Rumley, T. (1985). Topical antimicrobial toxicity. Arch Surg *120*:267–270.

127. Connell, J. F., & Rousselot, L. M. (1964). Povidone-iodine: Extensive surgical evaluation of a new antiseptic agent. Am J Surg *108*:849–855.

128. Gruber, R. P., Vistnes, L., & Pardoe, R. (1975). The effect of commonly used antiseptic on wound healing. Plast Reconstr Surg *55*:472–476.

129. Custer, J., Edlich, R. F., Prusak, M., Madden, J., Panek, P., & Wangenstein, O. H. (1971). Studies in the management of the contaminated wound: V. An assessment of the effectiveness of phisohex and Betadine surgical scrub solutions. Am J Surg *121*:572–575.

130. Viljanto, J. (1980). Disinfection of surgical wound without inhibition of normal wound healing. Arch Surg *115*:253–256.

131. Lineaweaver, W., McMorris, S., & Howard, R. (1982). Effects of topical disinfectants and antibiotics on human fibroblasts. Surg Forum *33*:37–39.

132. Dires, D. J. (1990). A comparison of wound irrigation solutions used in the emergency department. Ann Emerg Med *19*:704–708.

133. Lammers, R. L., Fourre, M., Callaham, M. L., & Boone, T. (1990). Effect of povidone-iodine and saline soaking on bacterial counts in acute, traumatic, contaminated wounds. Ann Emerg Med *19*:709–714.

134. Kwan, M. R., & Hunt, T. K. (1973). Continuous tissue oxygen tension measurements during acute blood loss. J Surg Res *14*:420–425.

135. Goodson, W. H., III, Andrews, W. S., Thakral, K. K., & Hunt, T. K. (1979). Wound oxygen tension of large vs. small wounds in man. Surg Forum *30*:92–95.

136. Lee, K. A., & Stotts, N. A. (1990). Support of the growth hormone-somatomedin system to facilitate healing. Heart Lung *19*:157–163.

137. Berger, R., & Adams, L. (1989). Nutritional sup-

port in the critical care setting (Part 1). Chest *96*:139–150.

138. Kinney, J. M., Jeejeebhoy, K. N., Hill, G. L., & Owen, O. E. (1988). *Nutrition and Metabolism in Patient Care*. Philadelphia: W.B. Saunders.

139. Berger, R., & Admas, L. (1989). Nutritional support in the critical care setting (Part 2). Chest *96*:372–380.

140. Stotts, N. A., & Whitney, J. D. (1990). Nutritional intake and status of clients in the home with open surgical wounds. J Comm Health Nurs 7:777–786.

141. Knighton, D. R., Ciresi, K., Fiegel, V. D., Schmerth, S., Bulter, E., & Cerra, F. (1990). Stimulation of repair in chronic, nonhealing, cutaneous ulcers using platelet-derived wound healing formula. Surg Gynecol Obstet *170*:56–60.

142. Phillips, T. J., Kehinde, O., Green, H., & Gilchrest, B. A. (1989). Treatment of skin ulcers with cultured epidermal allografts. J Am Acad Dermatol *21*:191–199.

143. Phillips, T. J. (1988). Cultured skin grafts: Past, present, future. Arch Dermatol *124*:1035–1038.

144. Carey, L. C., & Lepley, D. (1962). Effect of contin-uous direct electric current on healing wounds. Surg Forum *13*:33–35.

145. Biedebach, M. C. (1989). Accelerated healing of skin ulcers by electrical stimulation and the intracellular mechanisms involved. Acupuncture and Electro-Therapeutics Research, International Journal *14*:43–60.

146. Norton, D. (1989). Calculating the risk: Reflections on the Norton Scale. Decubitus *2*:24–31.

147. Bergstrom, N., Demuth, P. J., & Braden, B. J. (1987). A clinical trial of the Braden Scale for predicting pressure sore risk. Nurs Clin North Am *22*:417–428.

148. Gosnell, D. J. (1989). Pressure sore risk assesment: A critique. Part I. The Gosnell Scale. Decubitus *2*:32–38.

149. Robson, M. C. (1988). Disturbances of wound healing. Ann Emerg Med *17*:1274–1278.

150. Becker, B. E. (1980). Hypertrophic burn scarring: Control of chest deformities with a new device. Arch Phys Med Rehabil *61*:187–189.

151. Cohen, I. K., McCoy, B. J. (1981). Keloid: Biology and treatment (pp. 123–131). In P. Dineen (ed.), *The Surgical Wound*. Philadelphia: Lea & Febiger.

19

Altered Clotting

Cheryl Hubner

DEFINITION

Altered clotting is a state of imbalance in the normal mechanisms of hemostasis. Hemostasis is the regulation of the formation, retraction, and dissolution of clot. It is dependent on the dynamic interplay of platelets, plasma proteins, and the characteristics of the blood vessel wall.[1] The consequences of an alteration in any of these factors may be as insignificant as a transient shift in laboratory values or as dramatic as uncontrolled hemorrhage. Bleeding disorders and abnormal clot formation are the extreme pathological consequences of altered clotting. Both extremes are presented in this chapter.

PREVALENCE

Conditions leading to an alteration in clotting may be inherited or acquired. Inherited conditions are relatively uncommon in the general population. Hemophilia A, the most common inherited bleeding disorder, occurs in 10 to 20 persons per 100,000.[2] Von Willebrand's disease, a bleeding disorder, occurs in only 1 per 100,000, with significant manifestations occurring in one person per million.[2] Antithrombin III (AT III) and protein C and protein S deficiencies are inherited disorders that result in a state of hypercoagulability.[3] Although exact prevalence is unknown, protein C deficiencies may occur in 1 person per 200 to 300.[4]

Acquired disorders account for most clinically significant abnormalities. Deep vein thrombosis (DVT), pulmonary embolism, spontaneous bleeding, and disseminated intravascular coagulation (DIC) are clinical phenomena resulting from altered clotting.

The incidence of DVT is estimated to be 170,000 new cases annually and 90,000 recurrent cases.[5] The mortality rate from pulmonary embolism is 12 per cent in patients admitted for DVT.[5] Thromboembolic phenomena continue to be a leading cause of maternal death in the postpartum period.[6, 7] Disseminated intravascular coagulation manifests itself systemically as both profuse bleeding and thrombosis. The incidence of DIC in hospitalized patients is difficult to quantify owing to variability in diagnostic criteria and reporting mechanisms. In a classic retrospective study, a 10 per cent incidence of DIC was noted among 3400 hospitalized patients.[8] Activated by many primary diseases, DIC is a major threat to critically ill patients.

SITUATIONAL STRESSORS AND POPULATIONS AT RISK

Altered clotting occurs in all age groups and many disease states. Its timing is unpredictable, and its course is difficult to manage. The consequences of altered clotting are major contributors to the morbidity and mortality of hospitalized patients.

Clinical States or Diagnoses

Situational stressors of altered clotting are clinical states that alter the velocity of blood flow, alter the availability of coagulation factors, or injure the vascular endothelium. Several examples of situational stressors are illustrated in Table 19–1.

Stasis of blood increases the patient's risk of clot formation by diminishing circulation to the liver and reticuloendothelial system,

TABLE 19–1 SITUATIONAL STRESSORS IN CLOTTING

Alterations in Velocity of Blood Flow	Alterations in Platelets and Coagulation Factors	Vessel Wall Injury
Bedrest	Pathogens: bacterial and viral	Hypertension
Intrinsic luminal narrowing (i.e., ASOD*)	Chemotherapy	Intravenous drugs (i.e., potassium chloride, cocaine)
Extrinsic luminal narrowing (i.e., tumors, improper body position)	Radiation therapy	Tobacco smoking
Hypovolemia	Acidosis	Trauma to the vessels
Hypotension	Obesity	Burns
Pregnancy	Anticoagulation therapy	Surgery, especially vascular surgery
Increased venous pressures	Antiplatelet therapy	Hyperlipidemia
Venous dilation	Induction of anesthesia	
Varicose veins	Hypothermia	
Immobility	Liver disease	
Shock	Vitamin K deficiency	
Arterial or venous clamping during surgery	Pregnancy	
Obesity	Extracorporeal bypass (for open heart surgery)	
	Hyperlipidemia	

*ASOD, atherosclerotic occlusive disease.

which clear activated clotting factors from the blood stream. Stasis also allows activated clotting factors to cluster in one area and form a clot. Common stressors that decrease the velocity of blood flow are bed rest, immobility, hypovolemia, and hypotension.

The availability of platelets and clotting factors for hemostasis is determined by their rate of production, consumption, and inactivation. Production of coagulation factors is impaired in states of hepatitis, cirrhosis, and vitamin K deficiency. Platelet production is compromised by bone marrow abnormalities. Intrinsic bone marrow disease, such as leukemia, replacement of bone marrow by multiple myeloma, radiation therapy to the pelvic region or long bones, and folic acid deficiency may result in thrombocytopenia (a platelet count less than 100,000/mm^3).[9, 10]

Consumption of coagulation factors and platelets occurs during clot formation and fibrinolysis. Clinical states that activate the coagulation system are anoxia, acidosis, infections, induction of anesthesia, extracorporeal bypass, obstetrical complications, trauma, mucin-secreting adenocarcinomas, and disseminated malignancies.[9] A relative

loss of platelets occurs when they are pooled in the spleen, such as in severe congestive heart failure and hepatic failure. A dilutional thrombocytopenia may occur in critically ill patients who receive massive transfusions of platelet-poor blood (stored blood) to treat acute hemorrhage.[10, 11]

Inactivation of platelets is caused primarily by medications. Platelet function is affected by aspirin, dextran, nonsteroidal anti-inflammatory agents, some penicillins, amitriptyline, and ethanol.[12] Hypothermia inhibits platelet and coagulation factor function. The exact mechanism is unclear, but proposed theories include decreased platelet aggregation and enhanced fibrinolysis due to the release of a heparin-like factor.[13]

Pregnancy is a situational stressor that alters the availability of coagulation factors and promotes venous stasis. During the third trimester, there is an increase in procoagulation factors, a decrease in protein S levels, a decrease in fibrinolytic activity, and a decrease in the velocity of venous blood flow in the lower extremity veins.[6] Stasis of venous blood flow is related to the action of estrogen on water retention and to the physical obstruction to venous outflow by the uterus pressing on the iliac veins.[6]

The third category of situational stressors in altered clotting is vessel wall injury. Vessel wall injury may be induced by trauma, sheer stress, and vessel wall irritants. Trauma exposes blood products to the subintimal layer of the artery or vein, activating the coagulation system. The degree of vessel wall injury is related to the magnitude and recurrence of the stressor.

Developmental Dimensions

Infants and the elderly are at greater risk for experiencing an alteration in hemostasis than the rest of the population. At birth a healthy term baby has normal fibrinogen activity and decreased activity of procoagulant plasma proteins II, VII, IX, X, XI, XII, ATIII, prekallikrein, high-molecular-weight (HMW) kininogen, and proteins C and S (see Mechanisms).[6, 14] Premature infants and seriously ill infants have more profound abnormalities in their coagulation factors and platelet counts. When the neonate is stressed by illness, thrombocytopenia and bleeding are likely to occur. Sepsis, intravascular coagulation, necrotizing enterocolitis, and infant respiratory distress syndrome are clinical states associated with neonatal bleeding disorders.[6]

Although advanced age is frequently cited as a risk factor for thrombotic disorders,[11] the exact mechanism is not known. Age-related decreased spontaneous fibrinolytic activity, pooling of blood in the soleal veins during periods of immobility, and chronic illness may contribute to the increased incidence of thrombotic disorders associated with the aged.[11, 15]

MECHANISMS

Normal hemostasis is contingent on coagulation factors, the fibrinolytic system, the complement system, the kinin system, and their inhibitors.[1] When a stressor injures the vascular endothelium, platelets begin to aggregate over the injury and degranulate. Plasma coagulation factors are activated, and a thrombus is formed. Activation of the coagulation factors sets the fibrinolytic system into motion, which limits the size of the thrombus and eventually dissolves it. The complement system mediates the inflammatory response to injury; the kinin system potentiates the activation of the coagulation proteins. Coagulation proteins are commonly referred to by Roman numerals: factor I (fibrinogen), factor II (prothrombin), factors V, VII, VIII, IX, X, XI, and XII (Hageman's factor). The coagulation proteins circulate in the blood stream in a neutral state until they are activated. Activated procoagulant plasma proteins are designated by Roman numeral with the suffix "a" added (i.e., factor XIIa or activated factor XII).

The processes leading to clot formation are extremely complex and not fully understood. For simplicity, they are traditionally described in terms of the intrinsic, extrinsic, and common pathways of the coagulation cascade (Fig. 19–1). Contact with collagen or a foreign surface, such as a prosthetic cardiac valve, activates the intrinsic pathway by activating factor XII. Factor XIIa activates factor XI to XIa; factor XIa, in the presence of calcium, activates factor IX to IXa. A bond is then formed among factors IXa, VIIIa, and Xa on the surface of a platelet. Factor Xa is the gate to the common pathway. Factor Xa binds phospholipids to convert prothrombin to thrombin.

The formation of thrombin is the central focus of the coagulation processes. Thrombin converts fibrinogen to fibrin monomers that aggregate or polymerize to form fibrin polymers (fibrin strands). The gelatinous soluble clot is susceptible to dissolution by the fibri-

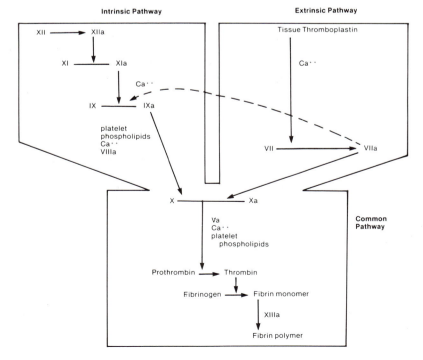

Figure 19–1. Coagulation processes: intrinsic, extrinsic, and common pathways. (Adapted from Hirsh, J., Brain, E. A. [1983]. Homeostasis and Thrombosis: A Conceptual Approach [2nd ed.]. New York: Churchill Livingstone, with permission.)

nolytic protein, plasmin.[1] Factor XIIIa (the fibrin-stabilizing factor) and calcium cross-link the fibrin polymers or strands to form an insoluble clot. Alpha$_2$-plasmin inhibitor is trapped within the insoluble clot. It increases the clot's resistance to fibrinolysis by inhibiting plasmin.[1] Thrombin accelerates the activation of factors IX, X, XI, and XII. The formation of thrombin is accelerated by activated factors V and VIII. Thrombin is also responsible for activating a feedback system that slows the coagulation processes. Thrombin attaches to thrombomodulin on the surface of endothelial cells. This thrombin-thrombomodulin complex activates protein C to break down factors Va and VIIIa.[16]

Another important interaction in the coagulation process is the formation of the thromboplastin–factor VIIa complex (extrinsic pathway). When tissue cells are injured, they release an intracellular lipoprotein called thromboplastin. Thromboplastin activates factor VII and binds with it in the presence of calcium to activate factor X of the common pathway. The thromboplastin–factor VIIa complex may also directly activate factor IX of the intrinsic pathway. Therefore, one stimulus, such as a brain injury, may rapidly activate both the extrinsic and intrinsic pathways. Thromboplastin is abundant in brain, lung, and placental tissue.

In addition to the plasma proteins active in the coagulation processes, plasma proteins are key to the fibrinolytic system. The fibrinolytic system, composed of plasminogen, plasminogen activators, and antiplasmins, dissolves clot by digesting fibrin (Fig. 19–2).[16]

Plasminogen, a beta-globulin produced by the liver, is converted to plasmin (a proteolytic enzyme). Conversion is controlled by factor XIIa, thrombin, and plasminogen ac-

tivators.[1] When plasminogen is activated to plasmin, it digests fibrin, along with factors V and VIII. It also cleaves polypeptide chains from the intact fibrinogen degradation products (FDP). The FDP bind to fibrin monomers, preventing polymerization and further clot formation. Tissue-type plasminogen activator (t-PA) is produced by and secreted from endothelial cells as a result of local or systemic stimuli.[1] The release of t-PA is stimulated by DVT, physical exercise, epinephrine, and thrombin.[1]

Modulators of coagulation and fibrinolysis are plasminogen activator inhibitor 1 (PAI-1), alpha$_2$-plasmin inhibitor (alpha$_2$-PI), antithrombin III (AT-III), alpha$_2$-macroglobulin, alpha$_1$-antitrypsin, C1 inactivator and prostacyclin (prostaglandin I$_2$, or PGI$_2$), protein C and protein S.[16] PAI-1 and alpha$_2$-PI inhibit the activity of plasmin. AT-III blocks the activation of factors II and X. PGI$_2$ inhibits coagulation by preventing platelet adhesion. Protein C inactivates factors Va and VIIIa. It also stimulates fibrinolysis by inhibiting PAI-1.[16]

Mechanisms of altered clotting refer to disruption of the normal mechanisms of hemostasis brought on by deficiencies in the coagulation factors, abnormal platelet activity, abnormal fibrinolytic activity, and chronic defects in the vascular endothelium. Patients with defective coagulation factors have a delayed response to initiation of the coagulation cascade and a tendency to bleed. The severity of the manifestations depends on the activity level of the abnormal clotting factor. For example, severe hemophiliacs have factor VIIIC levels less than 1 per cent of normal whereas mild hemophiliacs have activity levels 6 to 30 per cent of normal.[10]

Deficiencies in the coagulation factors may also be acquired through repeated activation of the coagulation system, hemorrhage, the development of an antigen-antibody response, anticoagulant or fibrinolytic therapy for dissolution of a clot, or decreased synthesis of coagulation factors, such as in liver disease. The continual activation of the coagulation cascade may lead to depletion of the coagulation factors at a rate greater than they are able to be replaced. The balance between coagulation and fibrinolysis is upset and bleeding results, such as in disseminated intravascular coagulation (DIC).

Platelet deficiencies interfere with normal hemostasis by preventing the binding of fac-

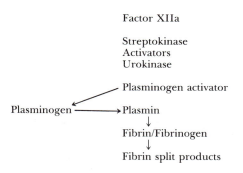

Figure 19–2. Fibrinolytic pathway.

tors VIIIa and IXa with X, and the binding of Xa and Va to change prothrombin to thrombin.[16] Platelet hyperaggregability interferes with normal hemostasis by promoting the activation of the coagulation factors. Hyperaggregability of platelets has been associated with diabetes mellitus, myocardial infarction, hyperlipidemic states and smoking.

Pathological Consequences

Dramatic pathological consequences of altered clotting are hemorrhage, venous thrombosis, embolic phenomena, and DIC. Hemorrhage may be caused by a deficiency in the coagulation factors or by a lack of vascular wall integrity. Patients with hemophilia lack sufficient levels of factor VIIIC to maintain normal hemostasis.[2] Hemophilia A is characterized by extensive bruising and hemarthrosis. Prolonged bleeding into the knees, elbows, ankles, wrists, shoulders, and hips eventually causes weakening of joint structures, atrophy of the muscles, increased vascularization of the synovial membranes, and a tendency for rebleeding. Massive bleeding in the early postoperative period may be due to suture defects, inherited or acquired coagulation defects, platelet abnormalities, or DIC.[17, 18]

Another frequent cause of altered clotting is liver disease. Liver disease results in decreased synthesis of factors II, V, VII, IX, X, ATIII, alpha$_2$-plasmin inhibitor, thrombocytopenia, and abnormal fibrinolysis.[19] Increased congestion in the liver slows the clearance of activated clotting factors and FDP from the circulation. Vitamin K deficiency, common in liver disease, contributes to plasma protein abnormalities. Although abnormal clot formation may occur, bleeding episodes are more frequently encountered.[19]

Venous thromboembolism is a serious, and sometimes fatal, consequence of altered clotting. Activated clotting factors and platelets accumulate in vein valve cusps, in the soleal sinuses of the calf, and in venous segments exposed to trauma (Fig. 19–3).[15] A platelet-fibrin mesh develops, which captures red blood cells. The thrombus begins to extend out of the valve pocket and propagates in the direction of blood flow. Eventually, the lumen of the vessel is occluded and more red blood cells are trapped by the fibrin mesh. Naturally occurring inhibitors of coagulation and proteolytic enzymes attempt to limit the

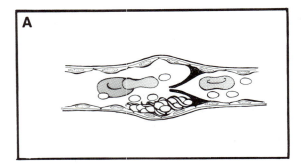

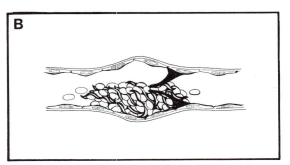

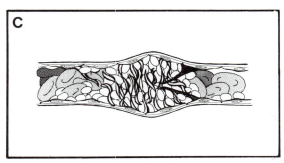

Figure 19–3. Formation of a vein thrombosis. *A,* A thrombus nidus. A nidus composed of platelets and fibrin grows out of a valve pocket in the direction of flow. *B,* A propagating thrombus. The growing thrombus starts to occlude the lumen. As blood is slowed, the thrombus propagates both proximally and distally. *C,* An occluding thrombus. When the lumen becomes totally occluded, propagation of the thrombus continues in the form of a red coagulation thrombus that is composed of red blood cells with interspersed fibrin. (Adapted from Hirsh, J., Genton, E., Hull, R. [1981]. *Venous Thromboembolism* [p. 45]. New York: Grune & Stratton, with permission.)

size of the thrombus. In a few cases, complete lysis of the clot may occur. Thrombi that are only partially dissolved form intraclot channels through which blood can flow.[15] Although blood flow resumes through the traumatized vein, the function of the valve is lost and venous hypertension results. Chronic venous insufficiency characterized by ankle edema, discoloration of the ankle area, and venous stasis ulcers may develop. Deep vein thrombosis in the popliteal, femoral, and iliac veins is a major cause of pulmonary emboli.[15]

Pulmonary emboli formed from blood clots are the result of dislodged or reorganized pieces of deep vein thrombosis,[15] right heart mural thrombus or, sleeve thrombus from a subclavian vein catheter. The pulmonary embolism mechanically blocks part of the pulmonary arterial tree and chemically induces arterial and bronchial constriction. Thrombin within the embolism activates circulating platelets, which release thromboxane A_2 and serotonin.[20] Thromboxane A_2 is a potent vasoconstrictor. Serotonin is a potent vasoconstrictor and bronchoconstrictor. It may be a major mediator in the pulmonary hypertension, bronchoconstriction, and hypoxia that follows pulmonary embolism.[20]

Pulmonary emboli lodged in an arterial bed stimulate the arterial endothelium to secrete plasminogen activator, which enhances the fibrinolytic system. The clot begins to autolyse. The lysis of the clot produces secondary emboli, which also may lodge in the distal pulmonary vasculature. The consequences of pulmonary emboli depend on the size and the location of the clot and range from no clinical significance to sudden death.

Acute DIC is a dramatic illustration of the interplay between the coagulation and fibrinolytic systems in response to disease or injury. A trigger event activates the coagulation and fibrinolytic pathways, resulting in systemic circulating thrombin and plasmin. Thrombin accelerates the production of fibrin monomers, which polymerize to macroemboli and microemboli, evident in the kidneys, liver, lungs, adrenal glands, brain, and peripheral tissues. The platelet-fibrin emboli decrease the number of circulating platelets, which results in thrombocytopenia.[16] Plasmin degrades fibrinogen and fibrin monomers to FDP. FDP inhibit platelet function by coating the platelet surface. Plasmin biodegrades factors V, VII, IX, and XI. The marked "consumption" of coagulation factors by the coagulation system, breakdown of coagulation factors by plasmin, loss of platelet number and function, and unbalanced production of plasmin lead to hemorrhage. The activation of the complement and kinin systems by plasmin causes vasodilatation and increased capillary permeability. Plasma proteins and fluid shift into the interstitial space, blood pressure falls, and shock ensues. Although hemorrhage is the more common expression of DIC, the irreversible organ damage produced by diffuse microthromboemboli and macrothromboemboli is a major cause of the morbidity and mortality associated with DIC.[8, 16, 21]

RELATED PHYSIOLOGICAL CONCEPTS

The physiological concept most closely related to altered clotting is ischemia. Either hemorrhage or the formation of microthromboemboli or macrothromboemboli in the circulation may cause tissue ischemia, a condition in which insufficient oxygen is available to meet the metabolic demands of the tissue involved. The characteristics of ischemia are presented in Chapter 2.

EXAMPLES OF RELATED PSYCHOSOCIAL CONCEPTS

Patients who experience one or more episodes of altered clotting may also experience anxiety, altered body image, social isolation, a sense of loss, and altered role performance. Many of the pathological consequences of altered clotting lead to temporary or permanent disfigurement and disability. Repeated absence from work may impair employment opportunities. Patients may also worry about future episodes of bleeding or clotting.

MANIFESTATIONS

The manifestations of altered clotting range from abnormal laboratory values with no clinically apparent signs and symptoms to profound evidence of bleeding and thrombosis. The manifestations of bleeding are listed in Table 19–2.

Subdermal bleeding manifests itself as petechia, purpura, and ecchymosis. Petechiae and purpura (defined in Table 19–3) are signs of increased vascular permeability. The vascular permeability allows red blood cells to leak out of the intact blood vessels. Ecchymosis reflects bleeding under the skin from ruptured capillaries.

TABLE 19–2 MANIFESTATIONS OF BLEEDING

Objective	Subjective
Spontaneous bleeding	Dizziness, orthostatic
Ecchymosis	Fatigue
Epistaxis	Pain, abdominal and joint
Decreased hemoglobin	Weakness
Hemarthrosis	
Hematemesis	
Decreased hematocrit	
Hematoma	
Hematuria	
Hemoptysis	
Hypotension	
Melena	
Oozing from intravascular sites	
Pallor	
Petechiae	
Purpura	
Tachycardia	

Frank bleeding is easily identified and may occur from multiple sites. Internal bleeding is more difficult to identify. Indirect indicators of internal bleeding are hypotension, tachycardia, tachypnea, cutaneous pallor, pale mucous membranes, orthostatic dizziness, fatigue, altered mental status, and general malaise.[22] The suspicion of bleeding is confirmed by a concurrent drop in the serum hemoglobin and hematocrit.

Manifestations of acute arterial occlusion vary widely in the population and are dependent on the size of the occluded vessel, the amount of available collateral circulation, and the rate of lumen occlusion. Sudden occlusion of a large vessel, such as the femoral artery, manifests itself as pain, pallor, pulselessness, paralysis, and paresthesia in the

TABLE 19–3 TERMS ASSOCIATED WITH ALTERED CLOTTING

Ecchymosis	Flat discoloration of skin caused by subdermal bleeding
Epistaxis	Spontaneous bleeding from the nares
Hemarthrosis	Bleeding into the joint space
Hematemesis	Blood in emesis
Hematoma	Swelling and discoloration of the skin due to subcutaneous bleeding
Hematuria	Blood in the urine
Hemoptysis	Blood in the sputum
Melena	Black, tarry stools, indicative of old blood in the stool
Petechiae	Small red dots occurring in patches over various parts of the body
Purpura	Petechial patches

lower extremity.[23] Although pain is absent in a small percentage of patients with sudden arterial occlusion, most patients experience pain that is sudden in onset, excruciating in intensity, and continuous. The color of the extremity below the level of occlusion pales rapidly, then becomes mottled and bluish. The skin is cool, and there are no palpable pulses below the level of occlusion. Loss of sensation and decreased ability to move the extremity are subtle at first, but then worsen as the ischemic time increases.

Sudden occlusion of a vessel already narrowed by atherosclerosis produces different symptoms. An individual thus affected frequently has a history of claudication, muscle pain brought on by exercise and relieved by rest. With the sudden occlusion of a narrowed vessel, claudication may worsen or progress to rest pain. Rest pain is defined as severe pain in the toes, dorsum of the foot, and heel. If blood flow is not restored, tissue necrosis will occur.[23]

Color is an indicator of the severity of the thrombotic episode. Uniform pallor implies large vessel occlusion. Patchy pallor or mottling implies diffuse occlusion of more than one distal vessel. Small purplish-red or black gangrenous lesions on the toes and plantar surface of the foot represent discrete occlusion of vessels at the microvascular level.

Pulse amplitude is a measure of the patency of the vessel. Sudden loss of a pulse that has been gradually diminishing in amplitude over time implies thrombosis of a vessel narrowed by atherosclerosis. Sudden loss of a pulse that was normal in amplitude or the combination of purplish-red (pre-gangrenous) or black (gangrenous) lesions on the foot, with normal pedal pulses, indicates an embolic phenomenon.

The peripheral manifestations of embolic and thrombotic disorders are the manifestations of ischemia. Since the manifestations of atherosclerotic occlusive disease may overshadow the manifestations of a hypercoagulable state, it is important that the clinician differentiate the causes of the symptoms and assess the integrity of the coagulation and fibrinolytic systems.

The signs and symptoms of DVT vary widely from patient to patient. Many patients are asymptomatic; other patients experience calf pain but have no other indicators of venous thrombosis. The pain associated with thrombophlebitis is caused by inflammation and distention of the vein wall. If the thrombosis does not cause vein wall inflammation, the patient will be free of pain.

Increased girth of the extremity is the most common manifestation in patients with venous occlusion.[5] Extravasation of fluid may present as a slight increase in limb circumference, or it may manifest as pitting edema in the pedal and pretibial areas. Swelling of the extremity implies extension of the clot above the popliteal fossa. If the clot is extensive or involves the iliofemoral region, a slight elevation in body temperature may be noted.

Color changes are dependent on the extent of the venous thrombosis. A slight increase in color and warmth of the extremity may be noted in deep calf vein thrombosis, as the superficial veins dilate and transport the blood around the occlusion and back to the heart. Iliofemoral vein thrombosis may cause redness, mottling, and marked edema as blood is trapped in the lower extremity venous system. In the presence of profound edema, increased interstitial pressure may impede arterial flow, resulting in a dusky bluish color in the extremity. If the situation is not resolved, venous gangrene may develop.

The manifestations of thrombosis or embolism in the pulmonary vasculature depends on the size and number of vessels occluded and the presence of pre-existing cardiopulmonary disease. An embolism to a small pulmonary arteriole may be clinically undetectable. A large thrombus that lodges in a major vessel or breaks down to shower the pulmonary vasculature with microemboli may present as sudden pleuritic pain, dyspnea, apprehension, and alterations in hemodynamic measurements. Dyspnea and tachypnea are the most commonly occurring symptoms.[5]

The most common cardiac abnormality after massive pulmonary embolism is an increase in intensity of the pulmonic component of the second heart sound. If the embolism is large enough, pulmonary artery hypertension, right-sided heart failure, and shock may occur.[20] Bronchospasm may occur, leading to crackles, rhonchi, wheezes, and dyspnea.

The manifestations of DIC are highly variable (Table 19–4) but commonly include bleeding from at least three unrelated sites, fever, hypotension, acidosis, shock, proteinuria, and hypoxia.[9, 21] Signs of bleeding include petechiae, purpura, hemorrhagic bul-

TABLE 19–4 MANIFESTATIONS OF DISSEMINATED INTRAVASCULAR COAGULATION

Bleeding
  Petechiae
  Purpura
  Subcutaneous hematomas
  Hemorrhagic bullae
  Oozing (surgical site, wounds, intravascular lines)

Hemodynamic instability
  Hypotension
  Shock

Pulmonary complications
  Hypoxemia
  Acidosis

Other
  End-organ ischemia (lungs, kidneys, pituitary glands)
  Acral cyanosis
  Gangrene

lae, and general oozing from wounds, incisions, intravascular line sites, and venipuncture sites. Microthrombi manifest as acral cyanosis, gangrene, and end-organ ischemia. The most common tissues affected by microthrombi are the skin, lungs, kidneys, and pituitary glands.[9, 21]

SURVEILLANCE

Assessment and surveillance of alterations in clotting are managed through careful history and physical examination, ongoing patient assessment, and monitoring of laboratory and diagnostic studies. The history is the most critical piece of information against which the clinical symptomatology and laboratory data are interpreted. The onset, location, duration, intensity, and frequency of the patient's prominent symptoms are explored. Aggravating and alleviating factors as well as related symptomatology are elicited.

The patient's past history of bleeding or thrombotic disorders is queried, especially as it relates to prior surgeries or trauma, dental procedures, childhood illnesses, or family history. Clues to an inherited defect in coagulation factors include a history of prolonged bleeding from the incised umbilical cord at birth or from a tonsillectomy or early trauma. A family history of bleeding or DVT may also indicate an inherited coagulopathy.

Acquired bleeding disorders tend to manifest themselves as generalized bleeding, with onset in adulthood, no family history of bleeding disorders, and no past history of abnormal bleeding associated with surgery or trauma. Acquired disorders are associated with ongoing situational stressors, such as chemotherapy. Acute DIC is an acquired disorder brought on by situational stressors such as leukemia, septicemia, obstetrical accidents, solid tumor malignancy, intravascular hemolysis, viremia, acidosis-alkalosis, burns, crush injuries, and vascular disorders.[21]

The physical examination provides a careful scrutiny of the patient for the manifestations of bleeding and thrombosis (see Manifestations). The extremities and trunk of the body are inspected for color, petechiae, purpura, hematomas, and abnormal venous patterns. Bleeding from intravenous sites, surgical incisions, and body cavities is noted. The major arteries and veins are palpated for rigidity, nodularity, and tenderness. In addition, pulse amplitude over the major arteries is palpated.

Auscultation over the carotid, subclavian, renal, femoral, and popliteal arteries as well as the abdominal aorta may reveal the presence of a bruit, indicating turbulent flow. The lungs are also auscultated for quality of breath sounds and presence of adventitious sounds.

As the clinician identifies indicators of altered clotting, laboratory screening tests are needed to define the precise nature and extent of the disease process. A bleeding time, blood smear, and platelet count may confirm the clinician's suspicion of a platelet disorder in a person with petechiae or purpura. The normal platelet count is 150,000 to 350,000/mm^3.[10] Although severe spontaneous bleeding generally occurs when the platelet count is less than 10,000/mm^3, spontaneous bleeding may occur at platelet levels greater than 40,000/mm^3 if there are platelet function defects or coagulation factor defects.[16] The presence of large platelets on a blood smear indicates rapid platelet turnover. A blood smear is also useful as a crude indicator of the platelet count. Unusually large clumps of platelets suggest an above average number of platelets. Absence of clumps indicates thrombocytopenia.[10]

The bleeding time measures platelet function and the ability of the vasculature to respond to injury. The normal value is less than or equal to 9 minutes. Prolongation of the bleeding time suggests platelet disorders.[16] Screening tests to detect abnormalities in the coagulation factors include prothrombin time (PT), activated partial thromboplastin time (PTT), and activated blood clotting time (ACT).

The PT reflects activity of the extrinsic pathway. A prolonged PT time (> 10 to 12 seconds) may indicate congenital deficiencies of factors I, II, V, VII, and X; acquired multiple deficiencies of factors II, VII, and X; or circulating anticoagulants.[10] The effects of oral anticoagulants and vitamin K deficiency are reflected in the PT level.[10]

A prolonged PTT may reflect circulating anticoagulants or abnormalities in factors VIII, IX, X, XI, and XII and in prothrombin and fibrinogen. Heparin, dextran, diphenylhydantoin, asparaginase, and naloxone hydrochloride prolong PTT.

The activated clotting time causes maximal contact activation of factor XII. It is sensitive to mild and severe abnormalities in the coagulation factors.

When initial screening test results are abnormal, special studies may be ordered. Special studies include the presence of fibrinogen degradation products, antithrombin III activity, protein C and S levels, specific coagulation factor assays (especially factors VIII and IX), and platelet aggregation studies. Laboratory findings of DIC vary, depending on the pathological phenomenon occurring. The PT and activated PTT are generally prolonged but are unreliable as measures to assess treatment effectiveness. More reliable indicators are elevated FDP levels, protamine sulfate test, AT-III levels, platelet count, blood smears for schistocytes, platelet function and count, fibrinopeptide A levels, B-beta 15–42 related peptide levels, and D-dimer measurements.[21] The combination of tests to measure FDP and D-dimers have a high predictive value for diagnosing DIC.[24]

Platelet adhesiveness and platelet aggregation studies are useful in determining hypercoagulability. These studies include platelet count, platelet aggregation with dilute collagen, thrombin generation time test (TGTT), platelet retention in adeplat T columns to detect increased adhesiveness, and serum AT-III activity. Although no clear picture of hypercoagulability has been identified, several abnormalities may contribute to a hypercoagulable state[10] (Table 19–5).

CLINICAL THERAPIES
Bleeding

Prevention of a bleeding episode is the primary goal in the management of patients

TABLE 19–5 CLINICAL ABNORMALITIES CONTRIBUTING TO A HYPERCOAGULABLE STATE

Increased numbers of circulating platelets
Increased adhesiveness of platelets
Spontaneous aggregation of platelets, platelet
  aggregation with low concentrations of aggregating
  agents, delayed disaggregation of platelets in the
  presence of weak levels of ADP
Accelerated coagulation, as detected by TGTT
Decreased levels of AT-III

ADP, adenosine diphosphate; AT-III, antithrombin III; TGTT, thrombin generation time test

at risk for altered clotting. Therapeutic goals for patients in which an episode of bleeding has already occurred are arrest of the underlying cause, replacement of blood components, prevention of tissue damage, maintenance of the patient's body image and support systems, and timely return of the patient to an active, productive life.

Prophylactic vitamin K administration in newborns, genetic counseling in families with bleeding disorders, and replacement of coagulation factors are therapeutic measures to prevent bleeding episodes. All critically ill newborn infants are given vitamin K at birth.[6] The role of vitamin K in preventing bleeding episodes in healthy full-term babies is less well defined. Despite controversies in the literature, Hathaway and Bonner recommend that all newborns receive 0.5 to 1.0 mg of vitamin K as soon as possible after delivery.[6] Nursing management of high-risk newborns includes surveillance for signs and symptoms of bleeding and monitoring of the newborn's laboratory values.

Prevention of inherited deficiencies in factor VIII and IX is becoming possible through full genetic counseling, amniocentesis, and fetoscopy.[25] Hemophilia A, a disorder of factor VIII deficiency, is an X-linked recessive trait, affecting one in two male fetuses if the mother is a carrier.[25] If amniocentesis establishes the sex of the fetus as male, fetoscopy may be scheduled for the 19th week of gestation. Fetal blood samples are withdrawn from the umbilical vessel just above the placental insertion of the cord, and factor VIII levels are assayed. The nurse monitors the mother's vital signs and complete blood cell count to detect bleeding and infection. This is an emotionally charged time for the family. Partners need time to discuss their feelings and support for their decisions to retain or terminate the pregnancy. Nurses play a key role in providing this emotional support. Through the advent of prenatal diagnosis, mothers who may have remained childless out of fear of producing a hemophiliac son are now able to plan a family.

The key to hemostasis in inherited bleeding disorders is component replacement. Coagulation factor replacement is available in the forms of fresh frozen plasma, cryoprecipitate, clotting factor concentrates, and platelet preparations. Plasma is rarely used to replace specific factors in inherited bleeding disorders. Cryoprecipitate is fractionated plasma containing only about 3 per cent of the original plasma proteins, 20 to 85 per cent of factor VIII levels, and large amounts of fibrinogen. It is more efficient than fresh frozen plasma in arresting acute bleeding diathesis even though concentrations of factor VIII vary considerably from one bag of cryoprecipitate to the next.[26] Clotting factor concentrates represent the most efficient means of raising plasma levels of specific factors. To prevent intraoperative bleeding in a patient with hemophilia, plasma levels of factor VIII should be raised to 40 per cent of normal. Inhibitors to factor VIIIC develop in 5 to 15 per cent of hemophiliacs receiving replacement therapy.[27] Plasmapheresis and factor VIIIC replacement in high concentrations may overcome the inhibitors.[28] Platelet transfusions are available to sustain serum platelet number and function in thrombocytopenia until the bone marrow function is able to keep up with demand.

Nursing management of patients receiving plasmapheresis treatments includes patient surveillance to detect and manage bleeding episodes and sepsis. Nurses monitor total protein and albumin levels, hematocrit values, serum electrolytes, and coagulation studies. Major shifts in intravascular fluid volume are preventable by maintaining albumin and total protein levels. Emotional support and fostering independence are key to the patient's care. Group sessions may promote open exchange of patients' fears, hopes, successes, and disappointments with managing chronic illness.[29]

Severe traumatic or postsurgical bleeding may be caused by a suture defect, acquired deficiencies in coagulation factors and platelets, and massive transfusions of stored blood. Re-exploration of the traumatized area may be necessary for local control of bleeders. When multiple units of packed red blood cells (PRBC) are necessary to maintain a hematocrit level, it is important to warm the blood and to supplement missing clotting factors with fresh frozen plasma or cryoprecipitate.[11, 17, 22, 30] Platelet therapy may also be necessary, especially in patients with prolonged bleeding after cardiopulmonary bypass. Complications specific to massive blood transfusions include infection, immunological reaction, impaired oxygen delivery, coagulation defects, acid-base abnormalities, citrate toxicity, hypothermia, and microembolism.[11, 30]

Nursing management of the patient with a bleeding disorder focuses on surveillance of laboratory values, prevention of new bleeding episodes, prevention of tissue damage from immobility, and evaluation of sensitivity to blood products. The frequency of surveying laboratory values is determined by the patient's situation. Hemoglobin and hematocrit levels, PT, PTT, platelet count, and electrolyte levels may be determined every 4 hours during the critical period. Blood gas analysis is performed every 1 to 4 hours, depending on the patient's respiratory status and acid-base balance.

To prevent tissue breakdown, the patient is turned every 1 to 2 hours. Even a slight rotation of the body decreases pressure on bony prominences. Careful mouth care with saline soaked gauze will refresh the patient without stimulating oral bleeding. Lip balm or petroleum jelly may be used to protect the lips from cracking. Although soft wrist restraints may be necessary to protect a patient with altered mental status from self-injury, care must be taken to prevent wrist bruising.

The major types of transfusion reactions are febrile, hemolytic, bacterial, allergic, and circulatory overload.[31] The symptoms include fever, chills, rash, shortness of breath, crackles, wheezing, tachycardia, headache, altered level of consciousness, nausea, vomiting, and flank pain. If a transfusion reaction is suspected, the transfusion must be stopped and the physician and the blood bank called. The transfusion reaction report usually indicates which blood and urine specimens will be necessary for analysis. It is important to monitor the patient's vital signs and provide supportive care as needed.

Psychosocial support for the patient and family is a major nursing function in individuals with altered clotting. Most bleeding disorders are chronic and require considerable adjustments to changes in body image, financial considerations, and role changes.[31] Providing continuity and coordination of care relieve some of the patient's stress.

Thrombosis

The goals of therapy in thrombotic disorders are similar to those in bleeding disorders. Prevention of thrombotic episodes involves identification of high-risk groups and initiation of preventive measures. If a thrombotic episode has occurred, the goals are to ameliorate the underlying cause and initiate anticoagulant therapy.

Prevention of thrombotic disorders incorporates general principles of patient care such as hydration, frequent positioning, and physical activity. Leg elevation, foot dorsiflexion, elastic compression stockings, and hydration decrease stasis in the lower extremity venous system.[15] Their effects on prevention of DVT are not well documented. Antithrombotic agents and pneumatic compression stockings may be needed, especially in the high-risk population. Low-dose heparin (5000 units) administered two to three times a day subcutaneously reduces the incidence of DVT and pulmonary embolism after general surgery, gynecological surgery, and neurosurgery.[32] It is also effective in preventing pulmonary embolism in patients with chronic obstructive lung disease.[33] Results of prophylaxis, measured by fibrinogen I 125 testing, are less convincing in patients undergoing urologic surgery[32] and in patients who have experienced a myocardial infarction.[34, 35] Low-dose heparin is not effective in reducing the risk of thromboembolism in high-risk orthopedic or oncology patients.[36]

In low doses, heparin effectively inhibits the coagulation system if it has not already been activated.[35] To be effective, preventive measures must be instituted prior to activation of the coagulation system, for example, before induction of anesthesia and surgery. Adverse effects of heparin therapy include hemorrhage, thrombocytopenia, allergic reactions, and, rarely, skin necrosis.[37] The risk of bleeding from low-dose heparin is increased when it is administered with dextran, since the actions of the two agents are synergistic.

When low-dose heparin is used to prevent DVT, the nurse should monitor the occurrence and size of ecchymotic areas around injection sites and any disruption of wound healing. Intramuscular injections are avoided to prevent hematoma formation. Patients receive special instructions on the purpose of heparin and possible side effects.

Other antithrombotic agents used to prevent thromboembolism are oral anticoagulants, antiplatelet drugs, and dextran. Anticoagulation therapy inhibits blood clotting by direct action on plasma proteins. Warfarin (Coumadin) alters the synthesis of vitamin K–dependent coagulation factors II, VII, IX, and X by the liver.[35] Although production of factors continues to occur, the factors have no coagulative effect. Pumphrey and associates recommend the use of oral anticoagulants for the prevention of systemic embolization in patients with a combination of atrial fibrillation and mitral valve disease, in patients with an enlarged left atrium (greater than 55 mm), and in patients with prosthetic heart valves.[38] The risk for embolus formation in patients with mitral valve disease and atrial fibrillation is most pronounced in the first 12 months after onset of fibrillation. The first month after surgery is the time of greatest risk for patients with mechanical prosthetic valves, as the Dacron on the valve cusp is not fully endothelialized.[38]

Antiplatelet agents used to block platelet deposition and aggregation are acetylsalicylic acid, dipyridamole, and dextran. Acetylsalicylic acid (aspirin) depresses platelet aggregation by inhibiting the release of adenosine diphosphate (ADP) from platelets and by blocking adhesion of platelets to exposed collagen fibers.[39] The aspirin-platelet surface reaction persists as long as the platelet response does; thus, a single dose of aspirin can alter platelet function for about 7 days.[39] The combination of aspirin and dipyridamole has a synergistic effect on thrombus inhibition. Dipyridamole (Persantine) suppresses platelet aggregation by inhibiting ADP release.

Dextran 40 acts as a volume expander in the vascular space. It interferes with clotting by coating the surface of platelets and by blocking platelet phospholipid-coagulation factor coupling. Dextran coats the surface of blood vessels and decreases surface contact of coagulation factors with injured endothelium. It may also cause defective fibrin bonding, resulting in unstable clot formation and increased susceptibility to fibrinolysis.[39] The increased fluid volume in the vascular space decreases blood viscosity and increases venous return. Side effects of dextran include hypersensitivity reaction, fluid overload, oozing from surgical wounds, and renal failure.

Nursing management of patients receiving anticoagulant therapy includes surveillance for signs of bleeding, monitoring of laboratory values for adequate anticoagulation, and patient education. Because hematuria is an early indication of overanticoagulation, the patient's urine should be tested daily for the presence of red blood cells. Epistaxis, bleeding from the gums, hemoptysis, and melena may also be noted. Laboratory values important to monitor are PT, PTT, and hematocrit values.

Patient education includes proper administration and recording of medication dosage and time, possible drug side effects, precautionary measures, and drug interaction with other substances, such as clofibrate, chloral hydrate, and ethyl alcohol. Patients should mark their calendars after each dose of heparin or warfarin because missing a dose or taking extra medication may have serious consequences.[40] Precautionary measures include ordering a medical alert band and encouraging the patient to notify physicians and dentists about the anticoagulation therapy. Patients are also instructed to take their medication at the same time each day to avoid fluctuation in blood levels.

Sequential pneumatic cuff compression devices are effective in preventing DVT in certain populations. Pneumatic compression devices increase pulsatile flow in the femoral vein by intermittently inflating and deflating leg cuffs. Compression is effective in emptying calf veins and the area behind valve leaflets.[36] The pulsatile pressure compresses the soleal plexus and increases venous return to the heart. It is an effective form of prophylaxis in major abdominal surgery,[41, 42] urological surgery,[43] and neurosurgery.[44] Pneumatic compression devices have not proved effective in high-risk patients with a malignancy or who have undergone orthopedic surgery. Oral anticoagulants and dextran are still the "front runners" in effective prophylaxis in these high-risk groups.

Pneumatic compression devices are cumbersome and may be uncomfortable for the patient. Excessive calf sweating may be diminished by having the patient use noncompressive stockings under the compression cuffs. Patients who understand the purpose of the compression devices may experience less anxiety and discomfort with them. Compression devices to the level of the knees are less cumbersome than those that extend to the thigh. They are necessary only while the patient is maintained on bed rest and should be removed before the patient gets out of bed. Pneumatic compression devices are an important adjunct to antithrombotic measures. They produce no serious side effects and are useful in a variety of populations. Similar to other preventive measures, pneumatic compression must be initiated in the preoperative period prior to activation of the coagulation system.

Antithrombotic therapy for the management of thromboembolism encompasses anticoagulant therapy, thrombolytic therapy, and surgical removal of the clot (embolectomy).[45] Balloon catheter embolectomy is the treatment of choice for removing a fresh thrombus from a large-caliber artery; it is less effective for removal of smaller clots or for removal of a thrombus superimposed on atherosclerotic plaque.[46] Venous thrombectomy and pulmonary embolectomy are rarely indicated because the survival rate of patients after pulmonary embolectomy is 35 to 50 per cent.[47]

An indication for pulmonary embolectomy is a massive pulmonary embolism with rapid cardiopulmonary deterioration. Cardiopulmonary deterioration is defined as systolic blood pressure less than 90 mm Hg, urine output less than 20 ml per hour, arterial oxygen level less than 60 mm Hg, and signs of peripheral vasomotor collapse that remain unresponsive to maximal medical therapy (oxygen therapy, isoproterenol, and heparin) after 1 hour.[47] Patients who have undergone pulmonary embolectomy demand close surveillance of respiratory status, detection of pulmonary hemorrhage, increased dyspnea, and pulmonary edema.

Recent developments in thrombolytic therapy may decrease the need for pulmonary embolectomy. In June 1990, recombinant tissue-type plasminogen activator (rt-PA) was approved by the Food and Drug Administration for use in the treatment of pulmonary embolism.[48] Thrombolytic therapy with 50 to 90 mg of rt-PA administered over 2 to 6 hours has been shown to lyse pulmonary emboli in up to 94 per cent of patients.[48] Although exact criteria for patient selection have not been established for rt-PA, the National Institutes of Health published general guidelines for the use of thrombolytic therapy in 1980.[49]

Thrombolytic therapy enhances the fibrinolytic system and lyses clots. The three most common agents are urokinase, streptokinase, and rt-PA. Although their modes of action differ, all three agents have been shown to effectively lyse clot in specific situations.[46, 47, 49–51] The goal of thrombolytic therapy is lysis of the thrombus with minimal complications of therapy. Although indications for use lack precise definition, thrombolytic therapy has been recommended for treatment of extensive iliofemoral thrombosis,[46] massive pulmonary emboli,[49–51] and acute arterial lesions in patients who do not have limb-threatening ischemia or surgically accessible thrombi.[46] It is used as an adjunct to percutaneous transluminal angioplasty and has also been used to lyse arterial thrombi in order to more clearly visualize distal blood flow by arteriography. Thrombolytic therapy is contraindicated for patients with recent strokes, advanced cerebrovascular disease, intracranial neoplasms, recent surgery, hepatic or renal insufficiency, severe allergy to thrombolytic agents, active internal bleeding, subacute bacterial endocarditis, limb-threatening ischemia, and septic thrombophlebitis.[46]

The major side effect of thrombolytic therapy is hemorrhage, especially from skin incisions and puncture sites. In the event of hemorrhage, the thrombolytic infusion is stopped and clotting factors and red blood cells are replaced with fresh whole blood, packed red blood cells, cryoprecipitate, and fresh-frozen plasma. Intracranial bleeding, hematuria, cardiac arrhythmias, anaphylaxis, and fever may also occur.[52] Because the effects of therapy last only a few hours, intravenous heparin is frequently started concurrently or shortly after the thrombolytic treatment is completed. Special considerations include monitoring the patient closely for bleeding, especially intracranial hemorrhage. The insertion of a Foley catheter and venipuncture should be withheld for at least 4 hours after the completion of thrombolytic therapy. Intravenous sites are immobilized to prevent trauma and bleeding. The intravascular catheter used for fibrinolytic therapy is frequently left in place for several hours after therapy is terminated, especially if the femoral approach has been used.[48] The patient should be monitored for signs of rethrombosis as the coagulation values return to normal. Fever, if it occurs, is treated with acetaminophen, because aspirin products may increase the patient's risk of bleeding.

Vena caval interruption may be indicated for patients who have experienced multiple episodes of pulmonary emboli. Approaches to vena caval interruption include transvenous insertion of a filter in the inferior vena cava (IVC), partial interruption of the IVC by plication with clips, or total interruption by ligation.[53] Severe lower extremity edema may result from partial or total occlusion of the inferior vena cava. Pulmonary emboli may recur as collateral channels around the interrupted vena cava dilate and carry larger thrombi to the lungs.[53]

Anticoagulant therapy is recommended for use in the treatment of acute arterial occlusion, systemic embolic phenomenon, acute venous thromboembolism, and pulmonary embolism. Therapeutic levels of heparin and warfarin prevent clot extension and the formation of new clots by inhibiting the coagulation system.[34] It is important to overlap intravenous heparinization for full anticoagulation with the onset of oral anticoagulants. At subtherapeutic levels, warfarin increases procoagulant activity by suppressing protein C function.[45]

Complications from heparin therapy include hypersensitivity reaction, hemorrhage, thrombocytopenia, and osteoporosis.[37] Hypersensitivity reaction is characterized by fever, bronchospasm, giant urticaria, rhinitis, and lacrimination. Hematuria, hemarthrosis, gastrointestinal bleeding, and wound hematomas may result from heparinization. Thrombocytopenia has been associated with beef lung heparin and is quickly reversed after the heparin is discontinued. Osteoporosis has been associated with long-term therapy, i.e., after 6 months of intravenous therapy.

DIC is a challenging disorder of hemostasis with clinical evidence of hemorrhage, thrombosis, or both. It is potentially life-threatening and difficult to treat. General principles in the treatment of DIC are to arrest the underlying cause, support the body systems, control bleeding, and avoid thrombus formation (Table 19–6).[21] Antibiotic therapy for sepsis, removal of necrotic tissue, and antineoplastic therapy are examples of treating or removing the triggering process. Fluid resuscitation and vasoconstrictive agents

TABLE 19–6 SEQUENTIAL THERAPY OF ACUTE DISSEMINATED INTRAVASCULAR COAGULATION

Treat or remove the triggering process
  Evacuate uterus
  Antibiotics
  Control shock
  Volume replacement
  Maintain blood pressure
  Steroids (?)
  Antineoplastic therapy
  Other indicated therapy

Stop intravascular clotting process
  Subcutaneous heparin
  Intravenous heparin(?)
  Antiplatelet agents
  AT-III concentrate therapy

Component therapy as indicated
  Platelet concentrates
  Packed red blood cells (washed)
  AT-III concentrates
  Fresh-frozen plasma
  Cryoprecipitate (fibrinogen)
  Prothrombin complex

Inhibit residual fibrino(geno)lysis
  Aminocaproic acid (?)

Adapted from Bick, R.L.: (1988). Disseminated intravascular coagulation: A clinician's point of view. Semin Thromb Hemost 14:324, with permission.

counter circulatory collapse. Acute respiratory failure is treated with oxygen therapy and mechanical ventilation, if needed.

Component therapy remains controversial for DIC. Although many clinicians use fresh whole blood, fresh frozen plasma, and cryoprecipitate for component replacement,[54] Bick recommends using only components free of fibrinogen, such as washed PRBC, platelet concentrates, and AT-III concentrates.[21] The fibrinogen in fresh frozen plasma, cryoprecipitate, and whole blood may enhance hemorrhage and thrombosis.[21]

Antithrombotic therapy in DIC includes heparin and AT-III concentrates. Low-dose heparin is being studied as an alternative to intravenous heparin.[21] The use of AT-III concentrates is investigational. Preliminary research indicates that the addition of AT-III to ongoing therapy may improve hemostatic parameters and shorten the duration of DIC.[55, 56]

ILLUSTRATIVE CASE STUDIES

The following case studies illustrate the presentation and management of two conditions of altered clotting.

CASE STUDY NO. 1

A.C. is a 46-year-old woman with acute myelomonocytic leukemia (AMML). One year after diagnosis she was admitted to the hospital with severe bilateral knee pain and swelling, multiple ecchymosis, intermittent gingival bleeding, and a 3-day episode of epistaxis. The white blood cell count was 66,700/mm³ (normal range is 6000 to 9000/mm³) and the platelet count was 22,000/mm³ (normal range is 150,000 to 350,000/mm³). A.C.'s past history is significant for three chemotherapy treatment sessions using the DAT protocol (daunorubicin, cytarabine [Ara-C], 6-thioguanine) in the past 12 months. After A.C.'s last series of treatments, she required packed red blood cells and platelet transfusion for suppressed bone marrow function.

A.C. is married and has two teenage children. She was forced to resign her executive position the previous year when frequent hospitalizations interfered with her ability to be productive.

A patient care conference was called to coordinate A.C.'s care. On the basis of her history of bleeding episodes, physical evidence of severe bleeding and abnormal laboratory values, the staff categorized A.C.'s condition as high risk for the development of further bleeding episodes. Goals of therapy were outlined as control of the thrombocytopenia, prevention of bleeding, and support of her physical and emotional needs. Platelet replacement therapy was required every 3 to 4 days to maintain the platelet count above 20,000/mm³. Neurological status examinations were performed twice daily to monitor for cerebral hemorrhage. Protection of mucous membranes was provided by gentle oral care with mouth swabs and saline rinses. Harsh mouthwashes and toothbrushes were avoided. A high Fowler's position and avoidance of nose blowing usually controlled the epistaxis. Amenorrhea was induced to prevent profound menstrual bleeding. Despite the use of lip balm, A.C.'s lips continued to bleed. Stools, urine, emesis, and sputum were examined for occult blood. Although the staff were unable to totally prevent the episodes of bleeding, their vigilant efforts to protect A.C. from skin breakdown were successful.

Emotional support was provided by the primary nurse, family members, and clergyman. The primary nurse met with A.C. for at least 10 minutes each day to allow A.C. time to express her feelings and to discuss activities that would help A.C. feel productive and important. Her family visited daily. They focused on A.C. as an individual rather than as a sick person. The family enjoyed playing cards and Monopoly.

Gradually, the platelet count stabilized, and A.C. was able to return home. Discharge instructions included early warning signs of bleeding, proper administration and possible side effects of her medications; and a list of community resources that A.C. could contact if needed.

CASE STUDY NO. 2

L.N., a 75-year-old man, was hospitalized for repair of an ileofemoral aneurysm. His past medical history is significant for chronic bronchitis, emphysema, arrhythmias, and a 50 pack-year history of cigarette smoking. On the fifth postoperative day, L.N. experienced sharp pain behind his right knee. The nurse noted that his right leg was edematous (Table 19–7) and that the superficial veins were engorged. A diagnosis of DVT in the

TABLE 19–7 GIRTH MEASUREMENTS OF THE LOWER EXTREMITIES AFTER RIGHT POPLITEAL VEIN THROMBOSIS

Right Extremity	Dates of Measurements*		Left Extremity	Dates of Measurements*	
	11/9	*11/16*		*11/9*	*11/16*
5 inches above knee	16¼	14½	5 inches above knee	15	15
5 inches below knee	13⅛	11	5 inches below knee	11½	11½
Ankle level	7¾	7	Ankle level	7⅛	7⅛

*Measurements in inches.

popliteal vein was confirmed by impedance plethysmography.

Situational stressors contributing to the occurrence of L.N.'s DVT included arterial surgery, induction of anesthesia, bedrest, hypovolemia secondary to postoperative nausea and decreased fluid intake, and hypotensive episodes in the recovery room. Mr. N. had continued to smoke after surgery. His postoperative arrhythmias may have also promoted venous stasis in the extremities.

A bolus of 5000 units of heparin was given intravenously followed by 1000 units per hour continuous drip. The drip infusion was gradually increased to 1400 units. The activated clotting time (ACT) was stabilized at 2 minutes, 20 seconds. The nursing staff identified the goals of care as early detection of bleeding, especially wound hematomas and hematuria; protection against skin breakdown, especially over sacral area and heels; adequate hydration; pain relief; prevention of pulmonary embolism; and prevention of depression.

Warm, moist compresses were applied to the calf and knee area, and the extremity was elevated to decrease edema and promote patient comfort. The compresses were removed for 15 minutes at least every 6 to 8 hours to prevent skin maceration. Pulmonary status was assessed every shift. L.N. was evaluated daily for swelling and tenderness around the surgical incision. His urine was tested daily for blood. All stools were examined for occult blood. Activated clotting time and hematocrit and hemoglobin levels were determined daily. The second day after heparin therapy was initiated, minimal serous drainage was noted to be leaking from the proximal end of the surgical incision. The wound was painted with povidone-iodine (Betadine) and covered with dry sterile gauze pads. The primary nurse provided emotional support by informing L.N. of his progress and by encouraging his friends to visit or send cards.

Swelling and discomfort decreased within 24 hours. By the fourth day of heparin therapy, the patient stated there was almost no pain. Edema had resolved, but the superficial veins remained prominent. Warfarin therapy was initiated. Heparin therapy was continued until the PT

was twice the normal value. L.N. was fitted with a support stocking and the hot compresses were discontinued.

Prevention of a clinically significant pulmonary embolism was successful through the early detection of the venous thrombosis by the nurses and the prompt initiation of therapy. Mr. L.N. did not experience serious complications of anticoagulant therapy. Skilled wound management, pulmonary assessment, skin care, and awareness of daily laboratory values promoted L.N.'s safety. An identification card and medical alert band were ordered. Discharge instructions included information about signs and symptoms of bleeding, proper drug administration, charting of the daily warfarin dose, dates for PT to be checked, a list of over-the-counter medications to be avoided without physician approval, proper application and care of the support stocking, and referral for home care.

These two case studies demonstrate the physical and emotional needs of patients with bleeding or clotting disorders. Both cases emphasize the critical role nurses play in the early detection and management of complications of altered clotting. Vigilant assessment and care prevented further disability and prolonged hospitalizations for A.C. and L.N.

REVIEW OF RESEARCH FINDINGS

Therapeutic modalities for the prevention of thrombotic episodes are gaining acceptability as larger, well-controlled studies are reported. Moser and associates compared the effects of subcutaneous heparin plus dihydroergotamine, heparin alone, and pneumatic compression devices on 289 consecutive patients admitted for elective operations.[42] Subjects were randomized to three groups: group A received 5000 units of heparin subcutaneously (s.q.) every 8 hours for 6 days; group B received 5000 units of heparin s.q. every 12 hours plus 0.5 mg of dihydroergotamine; group C used foot exercises after surgery plus pneumatic compression during surgery for 1 hour every day for 6 days after surgery. Prophylactic meas-

ures were instituted in the preoperative period. The overall incidence of thrombosis was
19 cases of DVT and seven cases of pulmonary embolism. The results of the study
showed no statistical difference between the
three groups.

Pneumatic compression devices were as effective as heparin in preventing DVT, without placing the patient at risk for bleeding
or wound hematoma formation. The study
design would be strengthened by including a
control group and by comparing the overall
rate of occurrence of DVT in the study with
other published statistics on occurrence of
DVT. Because low-dose heparin appears to
be equally effective when given every 8 hours
or every 12 hours, it is difficult to determine
the beneficial effects of dihydroergotamine
on Group B's success. Reliability was
strengthened by obtaining presurgical fibrinogen I 125 studies and Doppler examinations
on all the patients. The chief complaints
about the pneumatic compression devices
from the health team staff and the patients
were that the devices were cumbersome and
uncomfortable. Several patients experienced
excessive calf sweating, which was relieved by
noncompressive stockings worn under the
device.

Despite numerous research studies that
categorize patients as low, medium, and high
risk for thromboembolic phenomena, some
patients continue to receive no prophylactic
measures or receive measures inappropriate
for their risk factors. In 1982 Conti published
the results of a national questionnaire surveying physicians' general attitudes and practices in using antithrombotic protective measures.[57] Questionnaires were randomly mailed
to 978 physicians; 288 forms were returned.
In the high-risk population of patients, the
most common prophylactic measures were
low-dose heparin (35 per cent) and elastic
compression stockings (21 per cent), even
though these methods have been shown to
be ineffective in high-risk patient populations. No prophylaxis was chosen by 21 per
cent of the physicians. Seventy-three per cent
of the physicians believed that the effectiveness of available preventive measures had
not been well established. Thirty-six per cent
of the physicians reported bleeding risks as
a major deterrent to using antithrombotic
agents. Other frequently cited reasons for
not using preventive measures were lack of
familiarity with use, cost, and difficulty in

using equipment (pneumatic compression
devices).

Results of the study were weakened by the
low return rate (29 per cent). The study
provided valuable insights into possible reasons why prophylactic measures were not
consistently used. It would be valuable to
repeat this study now to document any
change in physicians' attitudes and practices.

Nursing research in altered clotting has
focused on identifying techniques for the
administration of subcutaneous heparin,
which will reduce the number and size of
ecchymotic areas at the puncture site. Several
techniques for administering heparin are described in nursing textbooks. Sites of injection, needle size, angle of injection, speed of
injection of heparin, whether or not to aspirate prior to injection, use of a tiny air bubble
to clear the needle after injection of heparin,
utilization of ice to massage the injection site
before and after injections, and the method
of gentle massage versus sustained pressure
to prevent bleeding after injection have been
described. Few studies exist to support any
of the techniques.

In 1981 Brenner and associates studied 33
patients receiving subcutaneous low-dose
heparin twice daily.[58] Each patient served as
his or her own control, receiving one injection by the standard technique and one injection by the modified technique every day.
The standard technique included using a 5/8-
inch tuberculin syringe. A cushion of flesh
was grasped at the iliac or abdominal site.
The needle was inserted at a 45-degree angle.
The plunger was pulled back, the fluid was
injected slowly, and the needle was quickly
removed. The site was wiped or gently mas-
saged with an alcohol sponge. The modified
technique also included the use of a tuberculin syringe. The needle was changed after
the heparin was drawn up, so no heparin
would be available on the needle to track
down the injection site. A small cushion of
fatty tissue was pinched at the abdominal site.
The needle was inserted at a 90-degree angle,
the tissue fold was released, the heparin was
injected without aspiration, and the needle
was quickly removed. The area was pressed
for a few seconds with an alcohol sponge.

Hematomas were classified as large (>1.0
cm in diameter), medium (0.2 to 1.0 cm),
and pinpoint. Thirty-three hematomas were
noted for both groups; 15 pinpoints, eight
medium, and ten large. The standard

method produced seven large hematomas, and the modified method produced three. Using chi-square test analysis, the authors found no statistical significance for either method.

The study design would be strengthened by using more subjects. The techniques were so diverse it was difficult to know which part of the technique, if any, accounted for the hematoma formation.

Vancree and associates studied the effects of three techniques for administering subcutaneous low-dose heparin on hematoma formation in 43 adult postoperative cardiothoracic surgery patients.[59] All patients received a prepackaged unit dose of 5000 units of heparin into a roll of abdominal tissue with a 25-gauge needle via a metal cartridge-type syringe at a 90-degree angle to skin. Postinjection skin preparation consisted of pressing the site lightly with an alcohol swab. Technique 1 included releasing the tissue and pulling back on the plunger to check for blood return before injecting the heparin. In technique 2, the heparin was injected without releasing the skin and without pulling back on the plunger. Technique 3 was the same as technique 2 with the addition of injecting 0.2 cc of air behind the heparin to clear the needle of medicine. Three injections were given to each patient, encompassing the three techniques. Forty-eight hours after the third injection the sites were observed for ecchymotic areas; any present were measured. Ecchymosis occurred in 72 of the 129 injections (55.8 per cent). Using the Friedman test for data analysis, a 0.569 level of significance was obtained. It was concluded that none of the three techniques was clearly superior for ensuring smaller sites or less frequent episodes of ecchymosis. The authors suggested replicating the study using tuberculin syringes rather than metal cartridge syringes, which may be more traumatic to the patient. They also suggested exploring the use of ice at the injection site. Hematomas are uncomfortable, unsightly, and mentally distressing for the patient. Further investigation into methods to prevent hematoma formation are needed.

IMPLICATIONS FOR RESEARCH

Research is still needed to define effective prophylactic therapy for thrombotic disorders. Health professionals frequently fail to identify high-risk populations and begin the prophylactic measures before a thrombotic episode occurs. The unwillingness to institute prophylactic measures appears to be due to lack of knowledge about pneumatic compression equipment and skepticism that the benefits of treatment outweigh the cost and the potential hazards.[57] Hemorrhage and wound hematomas are critical concerns to the practitioner. More studies are needed to weigh the benefits of therapy against the cost and the risk of therapy. Patient populations need to be defined better, since "abdominal surgical patients" cross the age span and a variety of illnesses. Pneumatic cuff compression offers promising results; however, it is not well accepted and the purchase of equipment is an additional expense for hospitals to bear. New treatments must be identified for the prophylaxis of high-risk groups, such as orthopedic patients and oncology patients. Research studies are needed to re-evaluate the role of compression stockings and foot dorsiflexion exercise in the prevention of DVT in low-risk populations. Dorsiflexion foot exercises are low-cost, easy to perform, and low-risk and may prove effective in decreasing the incidence of DVT and pulmonary emboli.

Therapeutic methods for controlling extension of clot and for lysis of thrombus need to be standardized for a variety of populations and clinical situations. Bleeding complications too frequently constitute a side effect of therapy. Methods to increase the rate of clot lysis are also needed, since the long duration of time before initiation of therapy and clot lysis limits its usefulness.

Genetic counseling for patients with hemophilia needs further refinement. Equipment necessary for fetoscopy and factor VIII assays are not available at all hospitals. Hemostasis would be more effective in these populations if concentrations of plasma proteins were more standardized. Treatment of inhibitors is still in an embryonic stage of development. Research studies need to focus on how to prevent the antigen-antibody reaction.

The morbidity and mortality related to DIC remain high. Multicenter controlled experiments are needed to investigate component replacement and heparin therapy in the treatment of DIC.

The pathological consequences of altered clotting continue to challenge the skills of health care professionals. As the incidence of conditions of altered clotting increases, individuals and society bear the physical, psychological, and financial consequences. Nurses help patients adapt to these consequences by mobilizing the patient's own strength and resources, identifying resources in the family and community that can provide services, utilizing multiple health care disciplines, and providing emotional support and reinforcement throughout the process.[60] Future research must more sharply define methods of prevention, early detection, and tertiary management of bleeding and clotting disorders as well as methods of optimizing adaptive processes.

REFERENCES

1. Saito, H. (1991). Normal hemostatic mechanisms. In O.D. Ratnoff & C.D. Forbes (eds.), *Disorders of Hemostasis* (2nd ed., pp. 18–47). Philadelphia: W.B. Saunders.
2. Miller, C. (1989). Genetics of hemophilia and von Willebrand's disease. In M. Hilgartner & C. Pochedly (eds.), *Hemophilia in the Child and Adult* (pp. 295–345). New York: Raven Press.
3. Kwaan, H.C. (1989). Protein C and protein S. Semin Thromb Hemost 15:353–355.
4. Miletich, J.P. (1990). Laboratory diagnosis of protein C deficiency. Semin Thromb Hemost 16:169–176.
5. Anderson, F.A., Wheeler, H.B., Goldberg, R.J., Hosmer, D.W., Patwardh, N.A., Jovanovic, B., Forcier, A., & Dalen, J.A. (1991). A population-based perspective on the hospital incidence and case-fatality rates of deep vein thrombosis and pulmonary embolism. Arch Intern Med 151:933–938.
6. Hathaway, W.E., & Bonner, J. (1987). *Hemostatic Disorders of the Pregnant Woman and Newborn Infant.* New York: Elsevier.
7. Hirsh, J., Ginsberg, J., Turner, C., & Levine, M.N. (1990). Management of thromboembolism during pregnancy: Risks to fetus. In M.M. Bern & F.D. Frigoletto, Jr. (eds.), *Hemotologic Disorders in Maternal-Fetal Medicine* (pp. 523–543). New York: Wiley-Liss.
8. Spero, J.A., Lewis, J.H., & Haseba, U. (1979). Disseminated intravascular coagulation: Findings in 346 patients. Thromb Hemost 42:983–993.
9. Baker, W.F., Jr., (1989). Clinical aspects of disseminated intravascular coagulation: A clinician's point of view. Semin Thromb Hemost 15:1–57.
10. Sirridge, M.S., & Shannon, R. (1983). *Laboratory Evaluation of Hemostasis and Thrombosis* (3rd ed.). Philadelphia: Lea & Febiger.
11. Idvall, J., & Hedner, U. (1988). Risks associated with massive blood transfusion. In E. Hans Renck (ed.), *Bleeding and Thrombotic Disorders in the Surgical Patient* (pp. 81–85). East Norwalk, CT: Appleton & Lange/Mediglobe.
12. Calandri, C., & Rand, J.H. (1991). Preoperative evaluation of hematologic status. Mt Sinai J Med 58:41–47.
13. Patt, A., McCroskey, B.L., & Moore, E.E. (1988). Hypothermia-induced coagulopathies in trauma. Surg Clin North Am 68:775–783.
14. Andrew, M., Paes, B., Milner, R., Johnston, M., Mitchell, L., Tollefsen, D.M., & Powers, P. (1987). Development of the human coagulation system in the full-term infant. Blood 70:165–172.
15. Hirsh, J., Genton, E., & Hill, R. (1981). *Venous Thromboembolism.* New York: Grune & Stratton.
16. Hirsh, J., & Brain, E.A. (1983). *Hemostasis and Thrombosis: A Conceptual Approach* (2nd ed.). New York: Churchill Livingstone.
17. Lampe, G.H. (1988). Blood loss and blood transfusion. Acta Chir Scand Suppl 550:88–94.
18. Newman, R.S. (1987). Excessive blood loss and its relationship to clotting system changes during and after major surgery. Crit Care Clin 3:417–427.
19. Ratnoff, O. (1991). Hemostatic defects in liver and biliary tract disease and disorders of vitamin K metabolism. In O.D. Ratnoff, & C.D. Forbes (eds.), *Disorders of Hemostasis* (2nd ed., pp. 459–479). Philadelphia: W.B. Saunders.
20. Hural, W.V., Mathieson, M.A., Stemp, L.I., Dunhan, B.M., Jones, A.G., Shepro, D., & Hechtman, H.B. (1983). Therapeutic benefits of 5-hydroxytryptamine inhibition following pulmonary embolism. Ann Surg 197:220–225.
21. Bick, R.L. (1988). Disseminated intravascular coagulation: A clinician's point of view. Semin Thromb Hemost 14:229–238.
22. Griffin, K.B. (1990). Postoperative bleeding: Current nursing management. Crit Care Nurs Clin North Am 2:549–557.
23. Spittell, J.A., Jr. (1990). Diagnosis and management of occlusive peripheral arterial disease. Curr Probl Cardiol 15:7–35.
24. Carr, J.M., McKinney, M., & McDonagh, J. (1989). Diagnosis of disseminated intravascular coagulation: Role of D-dimer. Am J Clin Pathol 91:280–287.
25. Mibashar, R., & Rodeck, C. (1982). Prenatal diagnosis of haemophilia A and Christmas disease. In C.D. Forbes & G.D.O. Lowe (eds.), *Unresolved Problems in Haemophilia.* Boston: MTP Press.
26. Nilsson, I. (1988). Congenital bleeding disorders. In E.H. Renck (ed.), *Bleeding and Thrombotic Disorders in the Surgical Patient* (pp. 20–31). Fribourg, Switzerland: Appleton & Lange.
27. Bloom, A.L. (1981). Current status and trends in the treatment of hemophilic patients with inhibitors. In D. Merache, D. Mac, N. Surgenoc, & H.D. Anderson (eds.), *Hemophilia and Hemostasis: Progress in Clinical and Biological Research* (Vol. 72, pp. 123–138). New York: Alan R. Liss.
28. Brinkhous, K.M. (1981). An overview: Hemophilia and hemostasis. In D. Merache, D. Mac, N. Surgenoc, & H.D. Anderson (eds.), *Hemophilia and Hemostasis: Progress in Clinical and Biological Research* (Vol. 72, pp. 259–275). New York: Alan R. Liss.
29. Lopez, L.A., & Hausz, M. (1982). Therapeutic apheresis. Am J Nurs 82:1572–1578.
30. Newman, R.S. (1987). Excessive blood loss and its relationship to clotting system changes during and after major surgery. Crit Care Clin 3:417–427.
31. Jennings, B.M. (1985). The hemolytic system. In I.G. Alspach & S.M. Williams (eds.), *AACN Core Curriculum for Critical Case Nursing* (pp. 495–562). Philadelphia: W.B. Saunders.
32. Russell, J.C. (1983). Prophylaxis of postoperative deep vein thrombosis and pulmonary embolism. Collective review. Surg Gynecol Obstet 157:89–102.

33. Lippman, M., & Fein, A. (1981). Pulmonary embolism in the patient with chronic obstructive pulmonary disease. A diagnostic dilemma. Chest 79:39–42.

34. Genton, E., & Turpie, A.G.G. (1983). Anticoagulant therapy following acute myocardial infarction. Part II. Antithrombotic therapy in acute myocardial infarction. Mod Concepts Cardiovasc Dis 52:49–51.

35. Kakkar, V. (1990). Prevention of venous thrombosis and pulmonary embolism. Am J Cardiol 65:50C–54C.

36. Halperin, J.L. (1991). Prevention of deep vein thrombosis and pulmonary embolism in surgical patients. Mt Sinai J Med 58:28–33.

37. Silver, D., Kapsch, D.N., & Tsai, E.K.M. (1983). Heparin-induced thrombocytopenia, thromboses and hemorrhage. Ann Surg 198:301–303.

38. Pumphrey, C.W., Fuster, V., & Chesebro, J.H. (1982). Systemic thromboembolism in valvular heart disease and prosthetic heart valves. Mod Con Cardiovasc Dis 51(12), 131–136.

39. Clagett, G.P., & Collins, G.J. (1978). Platelets, thromboembolism and the clinical utility of antiplatelet drugs. A collective review. Surg Gynecol Obstet 147:257–272.

40. Fahey, V. (1989). An in-depth look at deep vein thrombosis. Nursing 19:86–93.

41. Nicolaides, A.N., Miles, C., Hoare, M., Tury, P., Helmis, E., & Venniker, R. (1983). Intermittent sequential pneumatic compression of the legs and thromboembolism-deterrent stockings in the prevention of postoperative deep venous thrombosis. Surgery 94:21–25.

42. Moser, G., Krahenbuhl, B., Barroussel, R., Bene, J.J., Donath, A., & Rohner, A. (1981). Mechanical versus pharmacologic prevention of deep venous thrombosis. Surg Gynecol Obstet 152:448–450.

43. Coe, N.P., Collins, R.E.C., Klein, L.A., Bettmann, M.A., Skillman, J.J., Shapiro, R.M., & Salzman, E.W. (1978). Prevention of deep vein thrombosis in urological patients: A controlled, randomized trial of low-dose heparin and external pneumatic compression boots. Surgery 83:230–231.

44. Skillman, J.J., Collins, R.E.C., Coe, N.P., Goldstein, B.S., Shapiro, R.M., Zervas, N.T., Bettmann, M.A., & Salzman, E.W. (1978). Prevention of deep vein thrombosis in neurosurgical patients: A controlled randomized trial of external pneumatic compression boots. Surgery 83:354–358.

45. Trulock, E.P. (1988). Approaches to deep venous thrombosis and pulmonary embolism in aging patients. Geriatrics 43:101–113.

46. Berni, G.A., Bandy, K.D.F., Zierler, E., Thiele, B.L., & Strandress, E. (1983). Streptokinase treatment of acute arterial occlusion. Ann Surg 198:185–191.

47. Sasahara, A.A., Barsamian, E.M., Cella, G., Sharma, G.V.R.K., McIntyre, K.M., Parisi, A.F., & Tow, E. (1982). Acute pulmonary embolism. Part 2. Therapy. Vasc Diag Ther 3:19–26.

48. Goldhaber, S.Z. (1991). Recent advances in the diagnosis and lytic therapy of pulmonary embolism. Chest 99:1735–1795.

49. Goldhaber, S.Z. (1980). Thrombolytic therapy in thrombosis: A National Institutes of Health consensus development conference. Ann Intern Med 93:141–144.

50. Bresler, M.J. (1989). Future roles of thrombolytic therapy in emergency medicine. Ann Emerg Med 18:1331–1338.

51. Kessler, C.M., Druy, E., & Goldhabes, S.Z. (1988). Acute pulmonary embolism treated with thrombolytic agents: Current status of TPA and future implications for emergency medicine. Ann Emerg Med 17:1216–1220.

52. Comerota, A.J. (1988). Complications of thrombolytic therapy. In A.J. Comerato (ed.), Thrombolytic Therapy (pp. 255–281). Philadelphia: Grune & Stratton.

53. Falotico, J.B. (1981). Pulmonary embolism. Crit Care Update 28:5–15.

54. Feinstein, D.I. (1988). Treatment of disseminated intravascular coagulation. Semin Thromb Hemost 144:351–362.

55. Wisecarver, J.L., & Haire, W.D. (1989). Disseminated intravascular coagulation with multiple arterial thromboses responding to antithrombin III concentrate infusion. Thromb Res 54:709–717.

56. Vinazzer, H. (1989). Therapeutic use of antithrombin III in shock and disseminated intravascular coagulation. Semin Thromb Hemost 15:347–352.

57. Conti, S. (1982). Venous thromboembolism prophylaxis. Arch Surg 117:1036–1040.

58. Brenner, Z.R., Wood, R.M., & George, P. (1981). Effects of alternative techniques of low dose heparin administration on hematoma formation. Heart Lung 10:657–660.

59. Vancree, V.C., Hollerbach, A.D., & Brooks, G.P. (1984). Clinical evaluation of three techniques for administering low-dose heparin. Nurs Res 33:15–19.

60. Bondy, B. (1987). An overview of arterial disease. J Cardiovasc Nurs 1:1–11.

20

Impaired Sleep

Connie R. Robinson

DEFINITION

Sleep disorders, or alterations in the sleep-wake cycle, are many in number and vary across age groups and environmental situations. It is estimated that there are 100 million people in the United States who have some form of sleep disorder.[1] Sleep problems appear invariant across countries and cultures as well. Sleep-wake cycle disruptions are defined by patterns that occur outside the normal range for the developmental age group or that are in conflict with environmental and sociocultural expectations.

Impaired sleep is a global and nonspecific term used to indicate that a person has an alteration in sleep architecture and daytime functioning. Impaired sleep is a more inclusive term than the concept of sleep disorders. For example, sleep disturbance that may occur after anesthesia or fragmented sleep as a result of nursing interventions in an intensive care unit (ICU) would not necessarily be classified as sleep disorders. Another difference between the two concepts is the duration of the changes in sleep. Persons with impaired sleep may exhibit a variety of alterations in the sleep-wake cycle. Impaired nocturnal sleep may consist of longer latency to sleep onset, reduced total time asleep, reduced sleep efficiency (time asleep versus time spent trying to sleep), increased time spent awake and in light sleep, and many other combinations. Changes in daytime functioning and an altered sense of well-being are important components of impaired sleep.

Impaired sleep may result in a wide range of problems, from an occasional "bad day" to complete disruption of work and social and family life to death. These disorders may be short-term (a few days) to totally incapacitating. Initially, daytime functioning may become slightly impaired. If the sleep problem continues to exist, it progresses along a continuum from slight cognitive and behavioral disruptions (e.g., slowness in getting work done and a sense of tiredness) to profound sleepiness or profound alertness, severe memory difficulties, and autonomic and other organ system physiological disorders. The socioeconomic consequences of impaired sleep are largely unresearched. However, the impact of industrial accidents, automobile accidents, and decreased productivity associated with impaired sleep is likely to be enormous.

Normal Sleep

Because it is important to be able to differentiate normal sleep from biobehavioral changes exhibited in impaired sleep, a brief review of normal sleep is presented. In the mammalian sleeping brain, two states of sleep can easily be recognized by polygraphic techniques. The first state is characterized by the sleeping posture, with the eyes closed and the pupils myotic. A degree of tonus remains in some muscle groups. Electrical activity of the cortex is characterized by spindles and slow waves. There are four stages of sleep (non–rapid eye movement [NREM]) in this state (Figs. 20–1 to 20–6).

The second state of sleep has been called "paradoxical" sleep but is now more commonly called rapid eye movement (REM) sleep.[2, 3] Cortical activity is similar to that of waking and is associated with the regular

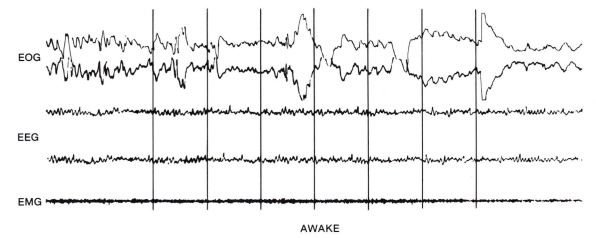

EOG

EEG

EMG

AWAKE

Figure 20–1. Awake. Frequent and fast eye movements, low voltage, mixed frequency EEG. (Alpha rhythm, 8–12 Hz, and Beta, 13–35 Hz), high frequency muscle activity. (Channels 1 and 2—right and left EOG. Channels 3 and 4—EEG, C2, Channel 5—EMG, submental.)

theta rhythm of the hippocampus; electromyographic activity is decreased. Rapid eye movements (50 to 60 per minute) occur in a pattern that differs from that of waking. In REM sleep there are cortical and subcortical components of activity, ponto-geniculo-occipital activity, seen in research animals when electrodes are placed in the lateral geniculate nucleus of the thalamus. High-voltage waves can be recorded from the reticular formation of the pons, the lateral geniculate nucleus of the thalamus, and the occipital cortex. These waves always precede REM sleep by about 30

to 45 seconds and accompany REM at about 60 per minute.

In addition to the states of sleep, human sleep is further defined by five stages: the four NREM stages of sleep and one stage of REM sleep. The muscle tone varies significantly from NREM to REM sleep stages. See Table 20–1 for the stages and characteristics of each stage.

The polygraphic criteria of sleep include the cortical sleep electroencephalogram (EEG). Frequency and amplitude of waveforms and other identifying characteristics

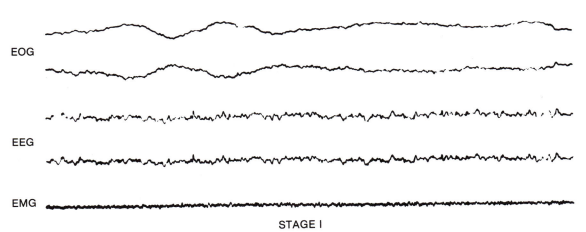

EOG

EEG

EMG

STAGE I

Figure 20–2. Stage 1 sleep. Rolling eye movements, low voltage, mixed frequency EEG. (Channels 1 and 2—right and left EOG. Channels 3 and 4—EEG, C2. Channel 5—EMG, submental.)

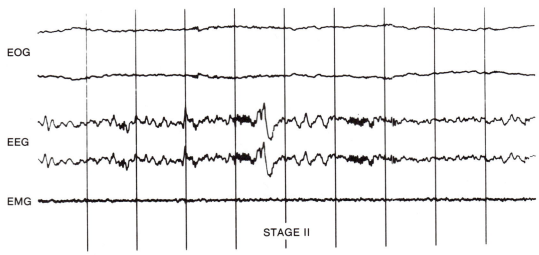

EOG

EEG

EMG

STAGE II

Figure 20–3. Stage 2 sleep. Rolling eye movements. Spindles 12–14 Hz and K complexes. (Channels 1 and 2—left and right EOG. Channels 3 and 4—EEG, C2. Channel 5— EMG, submental.)

are used in staging sleep, stages 1 to 4 and REM. Also, the electromyogram (EMG) and electro-oculogram (EOG) are necessary components for staging sleep. Standardized terminology, techniques, and a scoring system for sleep stages of human subjects have been developed.[4] Because infant sleep is very different from that of the child and adult, separate criteria for scoring the sleep of infants have been developed.[5] The frequency

of waveforms observed during sleep and used in staging sleep are alpha, which consists of 8 to 13 hertz (Hz) or cycles per second and arises primarily from the occipital cortex; beta, 13 to 35 Hz, characteristic of the awake state; delta, defined by less than 4 Hz, beginning in the frontoparietal cortex and spreading to other areas of the cortex during sleep recording; and theta, 4 to 8 Hz, which arises from the hippocampus in the temporal lobe.

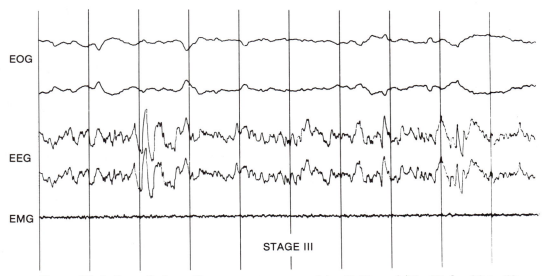

EOG

EEG

EMG

STAGE III

Figure 20–4. Stage 3 sleep. Few eye movements, delta (4 Hz and 75 μV) for 20 to 50 per cent of the page. (Channels 1 and 2—left and right EOG. Channels 3 and 4—EEG, C2. Channel 5—EMG, submental.)

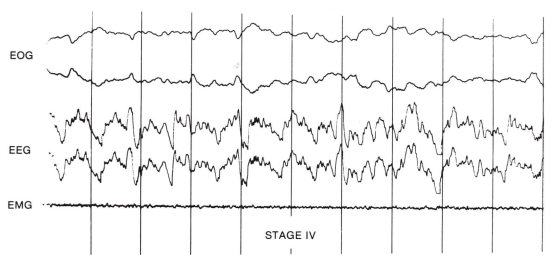

Figure 20–5. Stage 4 sleep. Few eye movements, delta (4 Hz and 75 μV) for more than 50 per cent of the page. (Channels 1 and 2—left and right EOG. Channels 3 and 4—EEG, C2. Channel 5—EMG, submental.)

Spindles are characteristic of certain stages of sleep (stage 2 primarily) and are defined by 12- to 14-Hz bursts of activity lasting at least 0.5 seconds.[4]

The sleep EEG is clearly different from the electrocortical activity of the awake state.[6–9] Initially, research in sleep focused on the sleeping individual. Within the last decade, there has been growing recognition that psychophysiological aspects of the awake state are an indicator of the quantity and quality of sleep and also influence sleep.

Nosology

While new findings have emerged from research, the classification system has been necessarily built on symptoms rather than causes of sleep-wake disorders. The causes of sleep-wake disorders are not currently

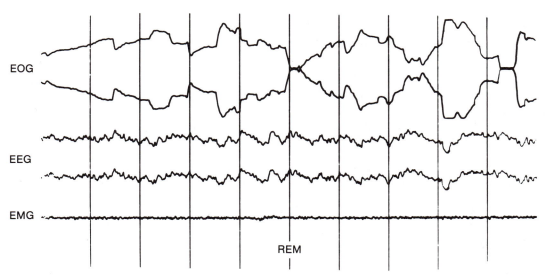

Figure 20–6. REM sleep. Frequent and rapid eye movements, theta rhythm (4–8 Hz), muscle tone drops. (Channels 1 and 2—left and right EOG. Channels 3 and 4—EEG, C2. Channel 5—EMG, submental.)

TABLE 20–1 STAGES AND CHARACTERISTICS OF ADULT SLEEP

Stage	Characteristics	Total Recording Time (%)
Stage 1	Low voltage Mixed frequency Rolling eye movements Muscle, high frequency and amplitude	1–2
Stage 2	Spindles 12–14 Hz and K complexes Rolling eye movements	50
Stage 3	Delta, <4 Hz and 75 μV or greater, occurring in 20%-50% of epoch Few eye movements	10–15
Stage 4	Delta, <4 Hz and 75 μV or greater, occurring in 50% or more of epoch Few eye movements	10–15
REM	Theta, 4–8 Hz Frequent eye movements Muscle tone drops	20–25
Awake	Alpha, 8–12 Hz Beta, 13–35 Hz Frequent eye movements Muscle, high frequency and amplitude	.04

are classified under two subgroups: (1) dyssomnias, which include disorders producing complaints of insomnia and excessive sleepiness, and (2) parasomnias, including disorders that intrude into or occur during sleep but do not produce a primary complaint of insomnia or excessive sleepiness. The dyssomnias are further divided into the intrinsic, extrinsic, and circadian rhythm sleep disorders. The intrinsic and extrinsic groupings separate the major insomnias and excessive sleepiness disorders into those caused primarily by factors within the body from those caused by factors outside the body. Interestingly, the 1990 nosology committee noted that this grouping had been proposed as early as 1939.[12] The primary sleep disorders are separated from the medical/psychiatric sleep disorders, the third grouping. The latter include disorders of primary medical or psychiatric origin but have either sleep disturbance or excessive sleepiness as a major component. A fourth group, proposed sleep disorders, includes those for which there is insufficient information available to confirm the unequivocal existence of the disorder. See the manual by the American Sleep Disorders Association for more detailed information on each disorder.[11]

PREVALENCE AND POPULATIONS AT RISK

Studies indicate that the problem of impaired sleep is widespread. Impaired sleep can occur in the very young. Infant sleep apnea is a severe problem and is discussed in Chapter 8. Most sleep disturbances in childhood are associated with behavioral issues.[11] Five to ten per cent of children older than 3 years of age have limit-setting sleep disorders in which the parent or caretaker sets inadequate limits on bedtime.[48] In one large study, infant and toddler sleep disturbances manifested themselves as resistance to going to bed (42 per cent) and in waking and crying during the night (35 per cent).[13] Of children aged 6 months to 3 years, 15 to 20 per cent experience a sleep-onset association disorder in which a familiar set of circumstances or a certain object is absent.[11] Children of this age may also experience nocturnal eating or drinking disorders in which they awaken from sleep and are unable to return to sleep without food or drink. Infants may experi-

known. However, a nosological system allows communication among health care workers and researchers for upgrading and refining the system.

Sleep disorders originally were grouped by symptom into four major categories.[10] These included disorders in initiating and maintaining sleep (DIMS) and disorders of excessive somnolence (DOES), respectively. This 1979 classification became unsatisfactory, since many patients had more than one sleep-related symptom and fell into more than one category of disorder. For example, persons unable to maintain sleep throughout the night may also be excessively sleepy during their normal waking hours. The revised nosology of 1990[11] is necessarily still based on symptomatology, since the pathology of a majority of sleep disorders remains unknown, but the categories are more discrete. The major categories are discussed and listed in Table 20–2. The primary sleep disorders

TABLE 20–2 DIAGNOSTIC CLASSIFICATION OF SLEEP-WAKE DISORDERS

I. Dyssomnias
  A. Intrinsic sleep disorders
    1. Psychophysiological insomnia
    2. Sleep-state misperception
    3. Idiopathic insomnia
    4. Narcolepsy
    5. Recurrent hypersomnia
    6. Idiopathic hypersomnia
    7. Post-traumatic hypersomnia
    8. Obstructive sleep apnea syndrome
    9. Central sleep apnea syndrome
    10. Central alveolar hypoventilation syndrome
    11. Periodic limb movement disorder
    12. Restless legs syndrome
  B. Extrinsic sleep disorders
    1. Inadequate sleep hygiene
    2. Environmental sleep disorder
    3. Altitude insomnia
    4. Adjustment sleep disorder
    5. Insufficient sleep syndrome
    6. Limit-setting sleep disorder
    7. Sleep-onset association disorder
    8. Food allergy insomnia
    9. Nocturnal eating (drinking) syndrome
    10. Hypnotic-dependent sleep disorder
    11. Stimulant-dependent sleep disorder
    12. Alcohol-dependent sleep disorder
    13. Toxin-induced sleep disorder
  C. Circadian rhythm sleep disorders
    1. Time zone change (jet lag) syndrome
    2. Shift work sleep disorder
    3. Irregular sleep-wake pattern
    4. Delayed sleep phase syndrome
    5. Advanced sleep phase syndrome
    6. Non–24-hour sleep-wake disorder
II. Parasomnias
  A. Arousal disorders
    1. Confusional arousals
    2. Sleepwalking
    3. Sleep terrors
  B. Sleep-wake transition disorders
    1. Rhythmic movement disorder
    2. Sleep starts
    3. Sleep talking
    4. Nocturnal leg cramps
  C. Parasomnias usually associated with REM sleep
    1. Nightmares
    2. Sleep paralysis
    3. Impaired sleep-related penile erections
    4. Sleep-related painful erections
    5. REM sleep-related sinus arrest
    6. REM sleep behavior disorder
  D. Other parasomnias
    1. Sleep bruxism
    2. Sleep enuresis
    3. Sleep-related abnormal swallowing syndrome
    4. Nocturnal paroxysmal dystonia
    5. Sudden unexplained nocturnal death syndrome
    6. Primary snoring
    7. Infant sleep apnea
    8. Congential central hypoventilation syndrome
    9. Sudden infant death syndrome
    10. Benign neonatal sleep myoclonus
III. Medical/psychiatric sleep disorders
  A. Associated with mental disorders
    1. Psychoses
    2. Mood disorders
    3. Anxiety disorders
    4. Panic disorder
    5. Alcoholism
  B. Associated with neurological disorders
    1. Cerebral degenerative disorders
    2. Dementia
    3. Parkinsonism
    4. Fatal familial insomnia
    5. Sleep-related epilepsy
    6. Electrical status epilepticus of sleep
    7. Sleep-related headaches
  C. Associated with other medical disorders
    1. Sleeping sickness
    2. Nocturnal cardiac ischemia
    3. Chronic obstructive pulmonary disease
    4. Sleep-related asthma
    5. Sleep-related gastroesophageal reflux
    6. Peptic ulcer disease
    7. Fibrositis syndrome
IV. Proposed sleep disorders
    1. Short sleeper
    2. Long sleeper
    3. Subwakefulness syndrome
    4. Fragmentary myoclonus
    5. Sleep hyperhidrosis
    6. Menstrual-associated sleep disorder
    7. Pregnancy-associated sleep disorder
    8. Terrifying hypnagogic hallucinations
    9. Sleep-related neurogenic tachypnea
    10. Sleep-related laryngospasm
    11. Sleep choking syndrome

From American Sleep Disorders Association (1990). *The International Classification of Sleep Disorders: Diagnostic and Coding Manual.* Lawrence, KS: Allen Press. Used with permission.

ence sleep disorders caused by food allergy. Children often experience parasomnias such as confusional arousals (usually before age 5), sleepwalking (peaks between ages 4 and 8), sleep terrors (3 per cent of all children and usually those between ages 4 and 12), nightmares (10 to 50 per cent of children between ages 3 and 5), and sleep enuresis (30 per cent of 4-year-olds, 10 per cent of 10-year-olds, 3 per cent of 12-year-olds, 1 to 3 per cent of 18-year-olds, and rare in adulthood).[11]

Insufficient sleep syndrome may be found often in the teenager and college-age young adults at a time of life when they restrict their sleep time purposely because of involvement in many awake activities. The onset of narcolepsy is thought to occur in the second decade of life and affects 0.03 to 0.16 per cent of the general population.[11]

Impaired sleep is a common disorder in adults. Approximately 38 per cent of the general population complains of a current sleep problem, and 52 per cent state that they have current or have had past problems with sleep.[1] About 5 per cent of all persons complaining of insomnia have no objective evidence of sleep disturbance. Among the intrinsic sleep disorders, in sleep disorders centers learned sleep-preventing associations (psychophysiological insomnia) accounts for about 15 per cent of all persons complaining of insomnia. Among those complaining of hypersomnia, about 0.03 to 0.16 per cent are found to have narcolepsy. For 5 to 10 per cent of those evaluated in sleep clinics for hypersomnia, no cause can be found. One to two per cent of the population is suspected of having obstructive sleep apnea.[11]

Periodic limb movement disorder increases with age and may account for impaired sleep in up to 34 per cent of patients with insomnia over age 60 years. "Restless legs syndrome" has been identified in 5 to 15 per cent of normal subjects, 11 per cent of pregnant women, 15 to 20 per cent of uremic patients, and up to 30 per cent of patients with rheumatoid arthritis.[1] Restless legs may therefore account for a large number of complaints related to sleep in these groups.

Among the extrinsic sleep disorders, poor sleep hygiene is thought to account for a large number of complaints of sleep disturbances. Transient sleep disturbances related to environmental causes are likely to be very common. Twenty-five per cent of those who ascend to 2000 meters will have sleep disturbances, and virtually all who ascend to 4000 meters or higher will experience sleep difficulties.[11] Situational episodes of insomnia may be experienced by almost all individuals throughout the course of their lifetime. Insufficient sleep has become more common with the advent of the electric light and changes in lifestyle. Though no statistics are available, many people experience sleep problems with tolerance to or withdrawal from hypnotics.

In addition to the intrinsic and extrinsic sleep dyssomnias, circadian rhythm disruptions also occur. Sleep-wake rhythm disorders result from many external influences and, possibly, from some primary neurological disorders. Jet lag is becoming a more prevalent disorder, although the exact incidence is not available. Shift workers account for 5 to 8 per cent of the population of various countries, and a prevalence of shift work sleep disturbance of 2 to 5 per cent has been estimated. Among severely brain-impaired persons who are institutionalized, irregular sleep-wake patterns may account for a large percentage of impaired sleep. Five to ten per cent of those in sleep clinics who complain of insomnia probably have "delayed sleep phase syndrome," in which the major sleep episode occurs after the desired clock time.[11]

Parasomnias in adults include sleep starts in 60 to 70 per cent of the population. These sudden and brief contractions of the legs at sleep onset are often not recalled and in extreme cases can cause sleep-onset difficulties. Sleep talking is thought to be very common, nocturnal leg cramps occur in up to 16 per cent of healthy individuals, sleep paralysis occurs at least once in a lifetime in 40 to 50 per cent of normal subjects, and rare REM sleep behavior disorders are present. Other parasomnias include bruxism in 85 to 90 per cent of the population and primary snoring in 40 to 50 per cent of men and women older than age 65. Fewer than 1 per cent of adults have sleep terrors. Some few adults experience sleepwalking.[1, 11]

Impaired sleep associated with medical and psychiatric disorders includes psychosis, almost always associated with some degree of sleep disturbance; mood disorders (depression or depression-mania), 90 per cent of which are associated with sleep disturbance; anxiety with sleep impairment; panic disorder, with an associated sleep disturbance occurring in 0.5 to 1.0 per cent of the population; and alcohol abuse (occurs in about 10 per cent of the population) with disturbed sleep. In neurological disorders, "sundown syndrome" has been estimated to occur in 12 per cent of mixed demented and nondemented institutionalized patients, and dementia occurs in 5 per cent of the population older than 65 years of age and in approximately 15 per cent older than 85 years of age. The incidence of Parkinson's disease in persons older than 60 years of age may reach 20 per cent. In Parkinson's disease, 60 to 90 per cent of patients have sleep impairments. Twenty-five per cent of those with epilepsy have sleep-related epilepsy. Although the prevalence is unknown, nocturnal cardiac ischemia is a serious problem. The majority of patients with chronic obstructive pulmonary disease have sleep impairments. Persons with low awake arterial oxygen pressure (<60 mm Hg) may have 5 per cent or greater drops in oxygen saturation during sleep. Of persons with asthma, 61 to 74 per cent report awakenings due to the asthma. Gastroesophageal reflux occurs in 7 to 10 per cent of the population on a daily basis and can account for sleep disturbances.[11]

Though very few data have been collected on incidence and prevalence of impaired sleep in the hospital settings, it is commonly believed to be a widespread problem. These disorders include intrinsic and iatrogenic sleep-wake dysrrhythmic sleep disorders, drug-induced sleep impairment (many analgesics alter the architecture of sleep), anesthesia-related impaired sleep, environmental noise disturbances, and many other impairments. In a study ranking stressors in an ICU by patients and nurses, it was found that patients' perception of not being able to sleep ranked fourth, just below pain, needles, and tubes. Nurses also listed the patients' not being able to sleep as a significant ICU stressor.[14]

SITUATIONAL STRESSORS

Impaired sleep in the child is usually due to an event in the category of parasomnias, that is, sleepwalking, sleep talking, bed wetting, and nightmares. These disorders usually disappear with maturation.[15] Sleeplessness in the child often is related to habits associated with sleep transition, lack of self-soothing behaviors, and excessive nighttime feeding. In the older child, impaired sleep is more often related to parents' poor and inconsistent limit setting.[16, 17]

Circadian function is closely related to the establishment and maintence of appropriate sleep patterns throughout life. Consistent light-dark cycles, sleep-wake cycles, and somewhat regular social cues, such as eating times, act as Zeitgebers, or time givers, to assist in establishing and maintaining temperature and cortisol and hormone levels and many other biological rhythms. Disruptions or abnormal responses to rhythms produce impaired sleep; for example, the occurrence of asthmatic attacks in early morning hours

as a response to normal histamine rhythms causes major disruptions in sleep maintenance and architecture.

Other situational stressors are related to disease entities such as chronic obstructive lung disease or obesity predisposing to sleep apneas, psychiatric conditions resulting in insomnia of some type, gastrointestinal disorders and reflux with awakenings, and brain injury or Alzheimer's disease with sleeplessness.

Normal developmental processes sometimes act as stressors, precipitating impaired sleep in individuals with certain predispositions. The onset of puberty interacting with genetic predisposition to narcolepsy results in the occurrence of the impairment in adolescence.[18] Normal aging is coupled with multiple miniature or brief arousals during sleep and with less robust biological rhythms, resulting in sleep that is less restful, less consolidated to certain times of day, and potentially harmful.[19]

DEVELOPMENTAL DIMENSIONS

The length of each cycle of sleep has been studied in a cross-section of all age groups and in both sexes. Each sleep cycle in infants lasts for 50 to 60 minutes. In adult humans it is 90 minutes long. In addition to developmental variations, sleep cycles vary across species as well. For example, the rat, mouse, cat, and elephant have sleep cycles of 9 minutes, 4 minutes, 25 minutes, and 120 minutes, respectively. For a summary and comparison of sleep across different age groups, see Table 20–3[20] and Figure 20–7.

Throughout this chapter, the reader is to assume that all data on norms, disorders, and impairments are the result of studies in subjects who normally sleep during the dark period of the day and usually spend their waking time during the light period. The sleep norms change across age groups and reflect the ontogeny, or developmental, characteristics of sleep.

Spontaneous electrical activity associated with sleep has been recorded from the lower pons beginning on the seventh day of fetal life in the human. Three-month-old fetuses have waves of 0.5 to 2.0 cycles per second of electrical activity.[21] Term neonates and infants experience two stages of sleep: active sleep and quiet sleep, with eye movements and without eye movements, respectively,

TABLE 20–3   A COMPARISON OF SLEEP ACROSS THE LIFE SPAN

Age Groups	Awake	Sleep	Stage 1	Stage 2	Stage 3	Stage 4	REM	Sleep Stages	Sleep Efficiency	Arousals	Other Comments
Neonates and infants	17 of 24 hr; 14–15 hr 4th to 8th months			Spindles 3–4 months; 20–45% quiet sleep			55–80% active sleep	Cycle 50–60 minutes long			
6 months to 1 yr 3–5 yr		14–15 hr gradual → 10 hr boys > girls		70% quiet sleep 48% boys; 41% girls	Higher for girls		30% 31%		Girls > boys; changes completed in girls		
6–9 yr		↓ in boys to < that of 3–5 yr					Changes begin in boys; changes completed in girls		Changes completed in boys		
10–12 yr		Boys = girls			More SWS in boys			Greater number in boys; abrupt changes in stage shifts in boys not experienced in girls until old age			
Adolescents—13–15 yr											More homogeneous across all aspects than any other time
16–19 yr							Decline in REM Men ↑ REM				
Early adult—29 years	Number of awakenings men > women; percentage rapidly increases with age	↓ TIB			Women ↓ in SWS						Men show effects of aging

498

Age					
30–39 yr	Men and women exhibit similar patterns				
40–49 yr	Men > women			Women sleep more restfully	
50–59 yr	Women > men	Men ↓ REM	Women ↓ to level in men in 40–49 yr group	Women exhibit sleep changes that occurred in men 20 yr earlier	Fall asleep faster
60+ yr	Multiple miniature arousals	Women > men	↓ in men and women by amplitude and frequency criteria; women retain more than men	None in one third of men	More disturbed sleep for men
70–79 yr	None in men	Women retain more than men	More time in bed without changes in sleep time		

SWS, slow-wave sleep

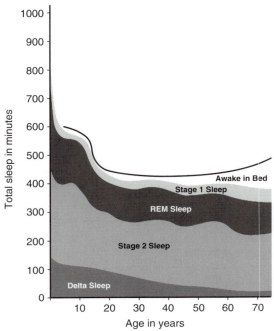

Figure 20–7. Development of sleep across the life span. (From Hauri, P. [1982]. *The Sleep Disorders, Current Concepts,* p. 14. Kalamazoo, MI: Upjohn. Used with permission.)

with bursts of large-amplitude slow waves superimposed on the fast rhythm. Cyclic organization appears at only what would be term in premature infants (see Chapter 8). Active sleep (or REM sleep in the adult) declines from 55 to 80 per cent in a neonate or infant, to 35 to 45 per cent during the first 6 months, and to 30 per cent by the end of the first year of life when it then stabilizes.

Spindle development occurs between the end of the second month and the end of the fourth month. During the first 6 months of life, sleep becomes condensed into fewer periods of longer duration, with a higher probability of wakefulness during the day and sleep at night. NREM sleep becomes differentiated into stages 1, 2, 3, and 4 and is redistributed over the 24 hours.[22] The time from birth to 3 months of age is the most vulnerable period for respiratory adaptation during sleep.[23]

There is evidence that girls complete the process of sleep development earlier than boys. Girls in the 3- to 5-year age group show slightly greater sleep efficiency (time asleep divided by time in bed). Boys in the 6- to 9-year age group are completing processes finished by girls in the 3- to 5-year group. In the 10- to 12-year group, boys have more

sleep stages during the night than girls; that is, they change from one stage to another more frequently than girls. An increase in stage shifts is not seen in females until old age. Boys also have more slow-wave sleep in the 10- to 12-year age group.[21]

Adolescents have more homogeneous sleep patterns than at any other time. REM in older adolescents is significantly decreased over the younger group. As a result of societal and environmental pressures, the older adolescent generally restricts nighttime sleep and is sleepier during the day and has a generally decreased performance level.[18]

By early adulthood, there is a decrease in time in bed, in percentage of sleep time, and in total sleep time. Women who are 20 to 29 years old have less slow-wave sleep than they did in adolescence. Men increase their REM time and decrease REM latency. Awakenings are higher for men than for women, and this trend continues throughout the life span. After 29 years of age, awake time rapidly increases. In the 30- to 39-year age group, sleep patterns are again more alike than different between sexes. Women have more slow-wave sleep than men. From age 20 to 39 men show effects of aging not seen in women.[21]

In middle age (40 to 59 years), all changes are in the direction of more disturbed sleep. From 40 to 49 years, men experience an increase in awake time and a decrease in REM time, as seen in aging. Women experience a decrease in REM time in the 50- to 59-year age group but maintain more slow-wave sleep than men. In old age, sleep is also more disturbed for men than for women. Men continue to have less slow-wave sleep. By 70 to 79 years, one third of men have lost stage 3 sleep and none have stage 4 sleep by the amplitude criteria (greater than 75 μ). Men have a longer latency to sleep; i.e., they take longer to get to sleep after going to bed. Men and women in old age experience multiple miniature arousals (to stage 1 sleep or awake) during the normal night's sleep.[19] This, then, may in part account for the disturbed sleep of the older age group. Women have a higher number of stage shifts, probably because they have retained a greater number of absolute stages during sleep time.

The elderly have less consolidation of sleep-wake cycles. There is some flattening of the amplitude of their circadian rhythms—robustness of rhythms is decreased. Sleep cycles are distributed across the 24 hours, resulting in day-time napping and less efficiency in nighttime sleep.

MECHANISMS OF NORMAL AND IMPAIRED SLEEP

The physiological and anatomical (functional and structural) mechanisms of sleep are incompletely known. Certain aspects of sleep, however, are well researched. Alterations in these mechanisms (whether intrinsic, extrinsic, or a combination) result in impaired sleep. Note that the mechanisms of sleep do not explain the purpose or function of sleep. These are yet to be fully elucidated even though researchers have studied for many years the purpose of human sleep.[24]

At least three major neurotransmitters have been implicated in the physiology of sleep. These are norepinephrine (NE, a catecholamine), serotonin (5-hydroxytryptamine, or 5-HT), and acetylcholine (ACH). Other transmitters, putative or proven, that play major roles in the sleep process are gamma-aminobutyric acid (GABA), dopamine (DA, also a catecholamine), and the neuropeptides. Some neuropeptides acting as modulators of neurotransmission may serve major roles in the sleep processes. GABA is involved in the pharmacology of hypnotics, anxiolytics, and anticonvulsants and in the treatment of impaired sleep. Hypnogenic substances and sleep factors have not yet been substantiated.[25] Neurotransmitters do not cross the blood-brain barrier, and the study of peripheral substances can only indirectly indicate brain activity.

By 1958, neuroanatomists working with the fluorescent microscope had located the neurons in which serotonin and catecholamines are stored. They stated with little doubt that the green and yellow fluorescence was due to the accumulation of a primary catecholamine and of serotonin, or 5-HT, respectively. The fact that reserpine markedly reduced or abolished the fluorescence was further evidence.[26]

Pharmacological and neuroanatomical manipulations of certain areas of the brain (such as those where serotonin and catecholamine-containing cell bodies are located) have been shown to be responsible for the observable electrical phenomena in the various stages of sleep. See Table 20–4 for a summary of transmitter-active neurons and anatomical sites involved in sleep.

The compound parachlorophenylalanine (PCPA) selectively decreases the concentration of serotonin in the brain without altering the concentration of NE or DA. PCPA does this by inhibiting tryptophan formation.[2, 3, 27–30] The administration of the drug produces complete wakefulness in animals. This effect can be reversed by injecting 5-hydroxytryptophan, which readily crosses the blood-brain barrier and restores the synthesis of serotonin. Sleep then returns to normal. From this and other similar work it has been concluded that serotonin is necessary for sleep onset. Variations in this may then result in sleep-onset insomnia.

TABLE 20–4 TRANSMITTER-ACTIVE NEURONS AND ANATOMICAL SITES INVOLVED IN SLEEP

Sleep State	Transmitter-Active Neurons	Anatomical Site
Stage 1		
2	Serotonin	Midbrain raphe
SWS 3		and cortex
4		
REM	Acetylcholine	Hippocampus
Awake	Norepinephrine	Locus ceruleus

REM, rapid eye movement.

In research using animals it was found that after 10 minutes of NREM sleep or slow-wave sleep, the serotonin content of the cerebral cortex decreased from the awake value.[31] Other brain areas demonstrated the same trend. The serotonin values of all areas approximated the awake levels after 5 minutes of REM sleep. The decrease may be brought about by a massive release of serotonin, most likely caused by an increase in impulse traffic over serotonergic synapses during the specified time of sleep.

The fact that serotonin is necessary for the priming of REM is further substantiated by the finding that a minimum of 16 per cent of daily slow-wave sleep is necessary for the appearance of REM sleep in the cycle.[30] Figures 20–8 and 20–9 show the anatomical locations of NE- and serotonin-containing neurons.

Almost nothing is known about what triggers the serotonin system. Blood tryptophan levels may be involved in the triggering. Tryptophan is the amino acid precursor of serotonin. It has been found that in normal subjects the concentration of free (unbound) tryptophan in serum was about 45 per cent higher at midnight than it was at noon.[32] In addition, others found that among human subjects who ate three meals a day, tryptophan levels were highest in late morning or early afternoon and lowest between 2 and 4 a.m.[33] The circadian variation is related to the transport into the brain and the priming of the mechanisms for sleep onset in late evening and perhaps for the sleepiness experienced in mid-afternoon as well.

Oral administration of L-tryptophan to young adult males caused sedation or decreased levels of anxiety before sleep, de-

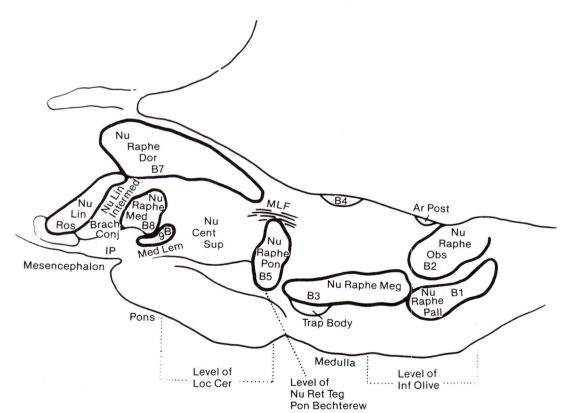

Figure 20–8. Midbrain raphe in sagittal section showing cell bodies of the serotonin system. Trap body = trapezoid body; Ar Post = area postrema; MLF = medial longitudinal fasciculus; Med Lem = Medial lemniscus; Nu Lin Intermed = nucleus linearis intermedius; Brach Conj = brachium conjunctivum; IP = interpeduncular nucleus. (From Morgane, P. J., & Stern, W. C. [1974]. Monoaminergic systems in the brain and role in the sleep states. In Weitzman, E. [ed.], *Advances in Sleep Research* [vol. I, p. 20]. New York: Spectrum Publishing.)

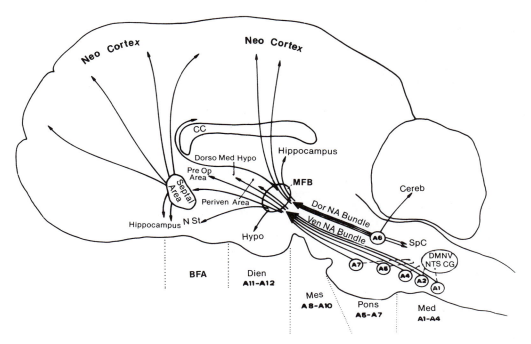

Figure 20–9. Sagittal section of rat brain showing norepinephrine (NE)-containing neuronal cell bodies with projections. Dor NA = dorsal noradrenergic; Ven NA = ventral adrenergic; periven = periventricular; Dorso Med Hypo = dorsal medial hypothalamic; CC = corpus callosum; Cereb = cerebellum; Preop = preoptic; NSt = nucleus of stria terminalis; MFB = medial forebrain bundle; A6 = locus coeruleus area; Med = medulla; Mes = mesencephalon; Dien = diencephalon; BFA = basal forebrain area; SpC = spinal cord; DMNV = dorsal motor nucleus of vagus; NTS = nucleus of tractus solitarius; CG = central gray; A1, 2, 4, 5, 6, 7 = noradrenergic cell groupings. (From Morgane, P. J., & Stern, W. C. [1974]. Monoaminergic systems in the brain and their role in the sleep states. In Weitzman, E. [ed.], *Advances in Sleep Research* [vol. I, p. 28]. New York: Spectrum Publishing.)

creased total awake time, reduced frequency of brief movement arousals, and increased slow-wave sleep. This was accompanied by a trend toward early onset of REM and significant shortening of the REM-to-REM cycle. Larger doses produced an increase in percentage and absolute amount of REM sleep.[34, 35]

In animal research, by surgical or pharmacological destruction of the neurons of the raphe system, insomnia results in proportion to the extent of the destruction of the serotonin-producing neurons located in the system. Also, a correlation between extent of destruction and decrease in serotonin has been demonstrated.[2, 3, 30] Serotonin is, therefore, necessary for the sleep process, namely sleep onset and sleep maintenance.

Serotonin becomes a candidate for being

at least one of the transmitters stimulating hippocampal cells to discharge during REM sleep. Data implicating the raphe nuclei in REM sleep come from studies done in animals with tungsten electrodes implanted in the median and magnus raphe (serotonin-containing neurons) of unrestrained, freely behaving cats.[36] It was found that these neurons fired slowly during slow-wave sleep, faster during awake states, and fastest during REM sleep. Also, during REM sleep, the raphe units tended to fire in bursts. Twelve units from the raphe magnus began to discharge more rapidly, about 10 to 20 seconds, before the onset of the hippocampal theta rhythm characteristic of REM sleep. This activity decreased concomitantly with cessation of theta activity of REM sleep.

Conversely, insomnia may be produced by

a reduction in serotonin. Nonspecific stress increases adrenal cortisol, which in turn induces the enzyme tryptophan pyrrolase and shunts tryptophan down an alternate pathway, so that serotonin is depleted.[37, 38]

A summary of the animal data that strongly favor the serotonin-containing neurons of the raphe system being involved in sleep mechanisms is given as follows:

1. The inhibition of the synthesis of serotonin leads to insomnia, which is quickly reversed by small doses of the immediate precursor of serotonin.
2. The destruction of the serotonin-containing cell bodies, in the raphe system leads to insomnia.
3. The hypersomnia that follows the destruction of the NE bundle at the level of the isthmus is accompanied by an increase in serotonin turnover.

The locus ceruleus has been implicated in REM sleep. Bilateral destruction produces total suppression of REM sleep. These nuclei contain NE and thus may play a role in REM sleep. One patient with an infarction of the basis pontis, in which the serotonin neurons were destroyed, but the NE neurons preserved, had a decreased sleep time but a normal percentage of REM sleep.[39] Blocking synthesis of catecholamines selectively suppresses REM sleep;[2] therefore, NE is implicated in that stage of sleep and may be very necessary for the cycling through the various stages of sleep throughout the sleep period.

The noradrenergic input to the raphe complex from the locus ceruleus may well be a link relating REM sleep to slow-wave sleep.[40] The locus ceruleus is primarily noradrenergic and may modulate activity rather diffusely in the raphe complex. It is possible that the medial and posterior raphe complex may interact with the locus ceruleus to affect or trigger REM sleep. Because the locus ceruleus system also innervates the geniculate bodies, this pathway may be involved in the regulation of geniculate discharges found during REM sleep.

One cannot make straightforward conclusions about the impairments that may result with an above or below normal level of NE in the brain. In vivo human brain studies cannot be done. It is, however, believed that early morning awakenings and truncated sleep periods may be associated with a decrease in NE levels during the prior sleep

time. Early morning awakening is also associated with some types of depressive illness.

Because acetylcholine is a transmitter found in the hippocampus and the hippocampus is the origin of theta activity found during REM sleep, acetylcholine becomes implicated in sleep as well. Changes in NE levels may result in sleep stage abnormalities.

Sleep maintenance and NREM sleep are probably determined by feedback mechanisms between the hemispheres and the brain stem as well as by the absence of arousal stimuli. REM sleep is usually dependent on previous NREM sleep. Arousal is primarily dependent on the duration of the previous sleep period.[28]

The monoamines (serotonin and NE) are biologically active through the following: the effect at the receptor, the effect of the receptor through neural feedback mechanisms on the synthesis and release of the amine, the interaction with other amines, and chemical or neural sequences of receptor events. Impaired sleep may result from any event that alters any one or more of the above. For example, a decrease in serotonin may result from stress, which changes the amount of the neurotransmitter available at its receptor site, and may then result in sleep-onset insomnia. The alteration of sleep by pharmacological agents (hypnotics, sedatives, analgesics) may be due to changes in any of the three biologically active sites listed above.

Other hormones have been implicated in sleep. For example, melatonin, the principal hormone of the pineal gland, appears to be a potent sleep inducer.[41] Similarly, other anatomical structures and their neurotransmitters play a role in the mechanisms of sleep. For example, the thalamus is responsible for the generation of sleep spindles seen in stage 2 sleep and for the synchronization of cortical firing (theta rhythm) during REM sleep.

Research has linked the biological rhythms of sleep-wake cycles and others to the suprachiasmatic nuclei of the hypothalamus (SCN)[42–44] (see also Chapter 4). There are thought to be two circadian drivers associated with the SCN and are termed x and y. The x driver is more powerful and more stable and is thought to be the driver establishing the time of day in which REM sleep occurs as well as being responsible for other of the robust biological rhythms (e.g., temperature and cortisol). Because it is not so easy to disrupt the x driver and because REM sleep tends to occur in the late period of the nighttime sleep (early morning hours), many night workers who fall asleep in the morning may normally experience sleep-onset REM—an otherwise abnormal finding in the adult. The y driver is linked to slow-wave sleep and is not as robust a mechanism.[45–47] Therefore, slow-wave sleep may be more easily displaced around the 24-hour day.

Although the mechanisms of sleep and impaired sleep are complex, some models have been proposed. A global view of the interaction of three systems—serotonergic, adrenergic, and cholinergic transmitter systems—has been proposed.[48] It is suggested that sleep onset is due primarily to the serotonin system; REM sleep onset is an adrenergic quiescence state in which the locus ceruleus cells of origin discharge highest during wakefulness, decline during NREM sleep, and discharge even less frequently early during REM sleep. The cholinergic system, primarily located in the mesencephalic, medullary, and pontine gigantocellular tegmental fields, discharges during the sleep-wake cycle in reverse order of frequency of the above. Modifications of this model are being made.[49, 50]

In contrast to the anatomical-physiological model, a phenomenological one has been postulated.[51] In this model, it is thought that sleep is the functional result of a set of reflex mechanisms. Sleep is viewed as an actively induced and homeostatically controlled, organized function. Impaired sleep, therefore, can result from a breakdown at any one or more of the many steps in the processes (anatomical, physiological, phenomenological) of sleep. The result is an alteration in the actively induced and homeostatically controlled, organized function.

PATHOLOGICAL CONSEQUENCES

The normal physiology of a person during sleep differs significantly from that of the person in the awake state. As a result of the physiological differences during sleep, certain pathological consequences are likely to occur in subsets of vulnerable persons. Systems most affected include cardiovascular, respiratory, and gastrointestinal. Cerebral blood flow and metabolism, temperature regulation, and endocrine and renal function also are altered during sleep. There may be pathological changes in each of the systems

mentioned as well. An example of this is sleep apnea—a pathological, rather than physiological, alteration.

Arterial blood pressure (BP) declines during stages 3 and 4 of sleep. Variability of BP and heart rate are increased during REM sleep. This may be due to a combination of decreased cardiac output and vasodilatation in peripheral resistance vessels. Pulmonary arterial pressure may increase during sleep but rises to harmful levels only in pathological sleep states (for example, sleep apnea). Phasic REM activity is associated with bursts of eye movements, muscle twitches, and brief tachycardias followed by bradycardia.[52, 53]

Other phasic changes during REM sleep include marked, brief cutaneous vasoconstrictions, a reduction in urine volume, and possibly an increased level of plasma catecholamines. These phasic events acting on the heart and coronary circulation may trigger nocturnal angina or infarction. The early morning hours are a time of vulnerability to these phasic changes, since the preponderance of REM sleep occurs at that time (around 5 or 6 a.m. in normal sleep).

Many physiological changes occur in the respiratory system during NREM and REM sleep. During NREM sleep, respiratory rate and minute ventilation decrease (although tidal volume increases) because of a reduced need. Metabolic rate declines and neural control of respiration changes with the loss of wakefulness. The behavioral (cortical) component is lost, and metabolic control of respiration predominates.[53] There is a small increase in arterial PCO_2. Greater changes in respiration occur during REM sleep than in other sleep stages. Breathing is partially driven by REM-related processes that stimulate or inhibit respiration. The respiratory rate is rapid and irregular. Studies indicate that response to hypercapnia and hypoxia vary. There appear to be competitive controlling influences. The metabolic control systems compete with medullary control during REM sleep. Respiration resembles that seen in the awake person. Intercostal and upper airway muscles are atonic during REM, but the diaphragm maintains normal activity. In some individuals, there may be significant reduction of the airway diameter in the oropharyngeal region, causing an increase in airway resistance that can lead to snoring and obstructive apnea. Respiratory secretions are cleared less readily during sleep, and the cough reflex is diminished. Aspiration can occur with esophageal reflux. In experimental animal research, stimulation of the cough reflex produces apnea. This mechanism may be related to sudden infant death. Smooth muscle tone in the airways decreases during sleep and becomes phasic in REM sleep. The increase in phasic activity and the decrease in tone may be related to nocturnal asthma attacks. During sleep, there is normally a decreased response to airway occlusion, hypoxia, hypercapnia, laryngeal stimulation, and airway irritation. Arousal is the mechanism by which the sleeping individual becomes more responsive. In prolonged sleep deprivation, arousal during sleep becomes progressively difficult.[52, 53]

Changes occur in gastrointestinal function during sleep. Swallowing and esophageal motility decline; motility of the remaining gastrointestinal tract may or may not be altered. Research findings are not definitive. An increase in esophageal reflux is associated with the position of sleep. In normal individuals, gastric acid secretion decreases during sleep; in those with active duodenal ulcer disease, it may increase.[52]

Cerebral blood flow (CBF) increases during REM sleep. Flow may increase even more with phasic REM events. An increase in CBF is associated with an increase in cerebral metabolism. Whether the changes in flow are due to changes in metabolism first or due to neurogenic changes in control of CBF is unclear. Electrophysiological studies show an increase, in general, in neuronal activity during REM sleep. While REM sleep is occurring, large intracranial pressure waves are seen. These changes normally do not exceed the compensatory capacity of the intracranial space. Brain temperature and total body oxygen consumption increase during REM sleep.[52]

Core body temperature is closely linked with the sleep-wake cycle. Body temperature usually peaks before sleep onset. When sleep onset occurs at a time when body temperature is highest, the total duration of sleep is longer. Body temperature falls throughout the night of sleep. There is a close relationship between ambient temperature and body temperature during REM sleep, indicating that the body does not thermoregulate during REM sleep. Thermoregulation does occur in NREM sleep. Also, sweating and shivering (and panting in animals) do not occur during REM.[52]

A number of normal endocrine functions are linked to the sleep-wake cycle. Growth hormone (GH) secretion peaks during stages 3 and 4 early in the night.[40, 52] The amplitude and peak patterns of GH secretion change with age. GH secretion is almost exclusively associated with sleep in prepubescent children, increases in puberty, decreases in amplitude in adults, and declines or is lost in the elderly during sleep. Other peaks occur throughout the day in pubescence and adulthood. Another hormone that is coupled with sleep is prolactin. Levels increase 30 to 90 minutes after sleep onset and peak in the early morning hours. Alternatively, thyroid-stimulating hormone reaches a maximum in the evening and is inhibited by sleep. The adrenocorticotropic-cortisol rhythm is independent of sleep-wake cycles but can be modified by sleep. Sleep onset is associated with a reduction in cortisol level. Cortisol rhythms can gradually be re-entrained if sleep is shifted around the clock.

Glomerular filtration, renal plasma flow, and excretion of sodium, chloride, potassium, and calcium decrease during the night. Plasma aldosterone levels increase during sleep. This, along with variations in autonomic activity and possible variations in parathyroid hormone secretion, accounts for some changes seen in renal function.[40, 52]

Reproductive system changes occur during sleep as well. Episodes of penile tumescence occur during REM sleep (and during NREM sleep to a lesser extent) in males of all ages. In females, clitoral erections also occur during sleep.

See Tables 20–5 and 20–6 for a summary of the physiological characteristics of sleep and a description of the alteration in physiological systems during sleep.

RELATED PATHOPHYSIOLOGICAL CONCEPTS

Although the causes and pathology of impaired sleep are largely unknown and often related to secondary disorders, and although the sleep disorders are still categorized by symptoms and signs, much research is being done and new data are available.

There is normally a loss or diminution of homeostatic mechanisms during REM sleep that particularly affects circulation and

TABLE 20–5 PHYSIOLOGICAL CHARACTERISTICS OF NREM AND REM SLEEP

NREM	Baseline REM	During Phasic REM Activity
Hypotension Bradycardia Decreased cardiac output Vasodilation	Hypotension Bradycardia Decreased cardiac output General vasodilation Vasoconstriction of red muscle	Increased blood pressure Tachycardia Decreased cardiac output Vasoconstriction
Intact baroreflexes	Intact baroreflexes (man); impaired baroreflexes (cat)	Intact baroreflexes (man) Impaired baroreflexes (cat)
Cerebral blood flow changes heterogeneously.	Cerebral blood flow increases. Increased intracranial pressure	Further increases in cerebral blood flow
Brain temperature decreases.	Brain temperature increases.	
Total body O_2 consumption decreases.	Total body O_2 consumption increases.	Total body O_2 consumption increases.
Thermoregulatory mechanisms are functional; sweating, shivering, tachypnea, and thermoregulatory vasomotion occur when needed.	Thermoregulation is impaired; sweating, shivering, tachypnea, and thermoregulatory vasomotion do not occur.	Thermoregulation is impaired; sweating, shivering, tachypnea, and thermoregulatory vasomotion do not occur.
Respiratory rate decreases.	Respiratory rate increases.	Further increases in respiratory rate
Minute ventilation decreases.	Minute ventilation is variously reported to increase or decrease.	Minute ventilation is variously reported to increase or decrease.
Respiratory muscles maintain their tone or show a small decrease in tone.	Diaphragmatic activity persists; intercostals are atonic; genioglossus and other upper airway muscles are atonic or hypotonic.	Transient inhibition of diaphragmatic activity; other respiratory muscles show twitches.
Ventilatory responses to hypoxia intact; slope of the response to CO_2 is reduced, and the curve is shifted to higher CO_2 levels.	Ventilatory responses to hypercapnia and hypoxia are intact.	Ventilatory responses to hypercapnia and hypoxia are impaired.
Mucociliary clearance is reduced; coughing does not occur; laryngeal stimulation produces apnea.	Mucociliary clearance is reduced; coughing does not occur; laryngeal stimulation produces apnea.	Mucociliary clearance is reduced; coughing does not occur; laryngeal stimulation produces apnea.
Airway smooth-muscle tone decreases.	Airway smooth-muscle tone generally decreases.	Airway smooth-muscle tone increases.
Pulmonary stretch receptor reflexes are intact.	Pulmonary stretch receptor reflexes are intact.	Pulmonary stretch receptor reflexes are absent.
Arousal response to airway occlusion hypoxia, hypercapnia, laryngeal stimulation, and airway and intrapulmonary irritation occurs with a shorter latency than during REM sleep.	Arousal response to airway occlusion hypoxia, hypercapnia, laryngeal stimulation, and airway and intrapulmonary irritation has a longer latency than during NREM sleep.	Arousal response to airway occlusion hypoxia, hypercapnia, laryngeal stimulation, and airway and intrapulmonary irritation has a longer latency than during NREM sleep.
Growth hormone is secreted in the early part of the night.		
Prolactin secretion peaks in the early morning hours; circadian episodes of thyrotropin secretion are inhibited by sleep; gonadotropin secretion occurs during sleep in puberty; sleep inhibits the ACTH-cortisol circadian rhythm; plasma aldosterone levels increase.		
Parathyroid hormone concentration increases.		
Gastric acid secretion, water secretion, and fractional rate of emptying decrease; swallowing and esophageal motility decrease.		
Penile tumescence occurs infrequently.	Penile tumescence; clitoral tumescence	Penile tumescence; clitoral tumescence
Glomerular filtration rate, renal plasma flow, filtration fraction, and excretion of Na^+, Cl^-, K^-, and Ca^{++} decrease.	Excretion of smaller amounts of more concentrated urine	Excretion of smaller amounts of more concentrated urine

From Orem, J., & Barnes, C.D. (1980). *Physiology in Sleep.* (pp. 330–334). Orlando: Academic Press. Used with permission.

breathing. This can be considered a crisis in regulation and may result in significant problems for some individuals, such as those with insufficient myocardial blood flow or with chronic obstructive lung disease. The decrease in regulatory influence occurs at the hypothalamic level, and brain stem and reflex control mechanisms drift out of the normal range of homeostasis.[54]

In sleep apnea, whether central or obstruc-

TABLE 20–6   DESCRIPTIONS OF PHYSIOLOGICAL SYSTEMS DURING SLEEP

Cardiovascular Physiology in Sleep
Blood pressure decreases during sleep.

Heart rate slows during sleep.

Cardiac output decreases and peripheral conductance increases during sleep.

Vasoconstrictions occur in association with phasic REM events.

Sinoaortic reflexes prevent a severe vasodilation during REM sleep in cats.

Baroreflexes are diminished during REM sleep in cats.

Cerebral Blood Flow, Intracranial Pressure, and Cerebral Metabolism During Sleep
Cerebral blood flow increases during REM sleep.

Phasic increases in cerebral blood flow are superimposed on the tonically increased cerebral blood flow in REM sleep.

The mechanisms for the changes in cerebral blood flow in sleep are unknown.

Some evidence indicates that there is a neurogenic cerebral vasodilation.

Intracranial pressure increases in REM sleep.

Brain temperature increases in REM sleep.

Total body oxygen consumption is greater in REM sleep than in NREM sleep, but lower in REM sleep than in wakefulness.

Temperature Regulation in Sleep
Body temperature falls throughout the night.

Increases in body temperature that coincide with REM sleep periods are superimposed on this decline.

Thermoregulatory sweating is suspended during REM sleep.

Temperature regulation is absent in REM sleep.

Respiration in Sleep
Respiration rate and minute ventilation decrease during NREM sleep.

Respiration is rapid and irregular in REM sleep.

The ventilatory response to carbon dioxide decreases in slope and shifts to higher CO_2 pressures during NREM sleep.

Ventilatory responses to hypercapnia and hypoxia are variable during REM sleep.

Some upper airway dilating muscles are hypotonic during sleep.

Snoring is more frequent in males than in females and the incidence of snoring increases with age.

Lung secretions are retained during sleep.

Airway reflexes are altered in sleep.

Airway smooth-muscle tone changes during sleep.

Pulmonary stretch receptor reflexes are intact in NREM sleep, but they are altered in REM sleep.

The arousal response to airway occlusion, hypoxia, hypercapnia, laryngeal stimulation, and airway and intrapulmonary irritation is delayed in REM sleep.

Endocrine Function During Sleep
Growth hormone is secreted during NREM sleep early in the night.

Prolactin secretion peaks during late sleep.

Secretion of thyroid-stimulating hormone peaks in the evening and is inhibited in sleep.

Gonadotropin secretion occurs during sleep in puberty.

Sleep inhibits the ACTH-cortisol circadian rhythm.

Renal Function During Sleep
Urine volume and the excretion of sodium, potassium, chloride, and calcium decrease during sleep.

Variations in the level of antidiuretic hormone do not account for the sleep-related changes in renal function.

Plasma aldosterone levels increase during sleep and may account for the reduced urine sodium excretion.

The sleep-related increase in plasma prolactin concentration may potentiate the actions of aldosterone.

Increases in parathyroid hormone may be a factor in the reduced calcium excretion during sleep.

Variations in autonomic activity may account for REM-related decreases in urine volume and increases in urine osmolality.

Alimentary Function in Sleep
Some studies report increased gastric acid secretion during sleep in patients with duodenal ulcer disease.

Reflux esophagitis is associated with reflux during sleep.

Swallowing frequency and esophageal motility decrease during sleep.

Studies of intestinal motility during sleep have obtained conflicting results.

Penile Tumescence During Sleep
Penile tumescence occurs during sleep.

Tumescence during sleep varies with age.

From Orem, J., & Barnes, C.D. (1980). *Physiology in Sleep* (pp. 332–334). Orlando: Academic Press. Used with permission.

tive, cyclical changes in heart rate occur.[55] Typically, during the apneic episode the heart rate decreases, with asystoles sometimes reaching 12 seconds. At the end of the apneic episode, the heart rate increases abruptly. Through studies of cardiac transplant patients, it was concluded that these changes in heart rate are mediated via the autonomic nervous system during sleep. Although research findings are conflicting regarding the incidence of arrhythmias during sleep, it is clear that some individuals experience more arrhythmias during sleep than during wakefulness.[56] Sleep apnea is a classic example of this phenomenon. Persons with chronic obstructive lung disease and those with conduction disturbances experience an increase in arrhythmias during sleep. Presumably, these arrhythmias are caused by oxygen desaturation. However, in some studies of patients with arrhythmias without sleep apnea or chronic lung disease, sleep may actually suppress the arrhythmias.[55, 56]

Obstruction of the upper airway is a common occurrence during sleep.[54–56] Under normal sleeping conditions, the size of the airway becomes smaller in all individuals. This is explained by the interaction of atmospheric pressure on persons in the supine position and physiological changes occurring in the structures of the passage. If a person then has an anomalous, anatomically smaller airway, a chain of events occurs to further reduce the airway diameter. Also, if there happens to be a defect in the timing or action of respiratory reflexes, as seen in chronic obstructive pulmonary disease, soft tissue collapse occurs with the resulting sleep apnea. As a result of the sleep apnea syndrome, hemodynamic changes exist from the beginning to the end of the sleep period. Systemic arterial pressure may reach dangerously high levels (up to 300/220 mm Hg), and pulmonary arterial and wedge pressures increase significantly as well.

Other changes may occur. For example, chronically impaired sleep may impair reproductive function. Gonadal corticosteroids are significantly reduced by 24 to 48 hours of sleep loss.[57] Sleep loss may heighten epileptiform activity in persons with some history of epilepsy. Elevated corticosteroid output associated with sleep loss does appear to facilitate paroxysmal EEG activity. Impaired sleep may seriously impair concentration, may produce visual illusions, and can lead to irritability with other behavioral changes. These changes are reversible with the restoration of normal sleep.

RELATED PATHOPHYSIOLOGICAL CONCEPTS

Impaired sleep differs from other physiological concepts such as coma, rest, and fatigue. For example, the EEG of the sleeping brain, normal or impaired, as defined by one of the four previously outlined categories, differs significantly from the EEG recorded during stupor or coma. In coma there may be large delta waves, spikes, or other abnormal activity—clearly different from the delta sleep of stages 3 and 4. The overall architecture of the sleep EEG is generally lost. It also is thought that if the comatose patient experiences patterns of sleep breaking through, the prognosis is more favorable. Coma and sleep have some characteristics in common, particularly during changes in the level of consciousness. When coma deepens or when patients fall asleep, the intracranial pressure rises. At the time of awakening from sleep and from coma, the intracranial pressure drops.[58]

Sleep as a restorative process is debated in the literature. Convincing arguments are made for sleep protein synthesis and body renewal as a result of the sleep-wake cycle.[59, 60] Others suggest that sleep may have its major effects on the central nervous system and that total sleep deprivation affects body renewal processes such as protein synthesis, mitosis, and immunity only as a result of stress factors leading to sleep loss rather than the loss itself.[57] Primary sleep deprivation does affect thermoregulation, shifting the daily average temperature downward, and affects energy metabolism through central mechanisms. These changes co-vary with self-assessed fatigue ratings as well. Fatigue is often an outcome of impaired sleep that is especially noted by those who have trouble initiating or maintaining sleep.

RELATED PSYCHOSOCIAL CONCEPTS

Sleep that does not conform to the polygraphic criteria, as defined across the age groups, may lead to severe consequences. For example, sleep-onset REM is normal in the infant but is not normal in the adult. The person who frequently falls asleep at inappropriate times and goes immediately into REM sleep and who also experiences cataplexic episodes, has hypnagogic hallucinations, and sleep paralysis is said to have narcolepsy. Because of the inappropriate daytime sleepiness, a belief may develop that the person is lazy, is not ambitious, cannot function adequately in school or work, or is generally a social misfit. By the time a diagnosis is made, a constellation of psychosocial problems exists. These may include severe problems relating to family and friends, academic failure, and inability to maintain work.

Decreased daytime functioning and increased sleepiness may account for decreased work productivity and increased industrial and automobile and other transportation accidents.

Depression is often accompanied by a

phase shift of the sleep cycle. In addition, the latency to the first REM period of the night is shorter and the overall percentage of REM is increased. The impaired sleep may then be an important indicator of the depressed state of the individual. Anxiety can also lead to a state of impaired sleep.

MANIFESTATIONS

Impaired sleep manifests itself in many objective and subjective, behavioral, and physiological symptoms and signs. For this discussion, the classification shown in Table 20–2 is used. The four major groupings of sleep disorders or impaired sleep are (1) the dyssomnias, (2) the parasomnias, (3) sleep problems associated with major medical and psychiatric problems, and (4) proposed disorders. Each major type of disorder has many subcategories, with a corresponding constellation of signs and symptoms. From those categories, the following have arbitrarily been selected for discussion on the basis of prevalence and severity of the problem and in the domain of adult impaired sleep.

The management of each type of disorder depends on careful diagnosis and is highly individualized. Patients often talk freely with nurses and may describe their symptoms in detail; nurses uniquely spend 24 hours observing and caring for patients throughout the entire sleep-wake cycle. It is incumbent on the nurse to observe and identify disorders, to be aware that the patient (especially the hospitalized one) may have disrupted sleep-wake cycles, and to construct an environment to maintain or return to normal the sleep-wake cycles.*

Dyssomnias

Intrinsic Sleep Disorders

The sleep disorders occurring as a result of some primary intrinsic mechanism include the various types of insomnia, hypersomnia, apnea syndromes, and motor or movement disorders that impair sleep.

Insomnia. Insomnia is a perception of in-

adequate sleep and includes difficulty in initiating sleep, frequent awakenings from sleep, short sleep, and nonrestorative sleep. The complaint of insomnia is more prevalent than any other complaint about sleep. *Idiopathic insomnia* may and usually does date from childhood.[61] It may be due to a neurochemical imbalance of the arousal system or the sleep-onset mechanisms or the sleep-maintenance system. This serious and lifelong insomnia cannot be explained by medical problems or psychological trauma. There is generally associated a decreased feeling of well-being during the day, a deterioration of mood and motivation, decreased attention and vigilance, low levels of energy and concentration, and increased fatigue.[11] If the insomnia is mild, the patient may adapt to the chronic sleep loss and learn not to focus on the sleep distrubance. When insomnia is severe, the psychological status of the individual may be markedly altered. Polysomnography shows the characteristics of the sleep stages described above to be intermixed. Sleep spindles are poorly formed, sleep latencies are long, and sleep efficiency is very poor (see Case Study No. 1).

Psychophysiological insomnia also accounts for a large proportion of those with sleep complaints. It is the consequence of two mutually reinforcing factors: somatized tension and learned sleep-preventing behavior.[11] The individual typically denies and represses the meaning of stressful events and manifests increased physiological arousal, such as increased muscle tension and increased vasoconstriction. The learned associations further increase the arousal. The associations may be related to internal cognitions or external stimuli. These patients are not sleepy during the day but function poorly in other ways, that is, with decreased cognitive skills and fatigue. Many are marginal, light sleepers at the outset and are possibly more vulnerable to psychophysiological changes.

About 15 per cent of all insomniacs in sleep disorders centers are said to have such insomnia. It typically starts in young adulthood and is more frequently found in females. Often there is excessive use of hypnotics or alcohol, possibly as a result of the disorder. There is increased stage 1 sleep and often a decrease in stages 3 and 4 sleep. Time from lights out to sleep onset (sleep latency) is long—greater than 20 minutes to hours. There may be increased alpha wave production (see Case Study No. 2).

---

*A list of accredited sleep diagnosis and treatment centers may be obtained from the American Sleep Disorders Association, 604 2nd St. S.W., Rochester, MN 55902.

Narcolepsy. This disorder is characterized by a set of clinical symptoms, including abnormal sleep, overwhelming episodes of sleep that may occur at inappropriate times, excessive daytime sleepiness, hypnagogic hallucinations, disturbed nocturnal sleep, paroxysmal muscle weakness, cataplexy, and sleep paralysis.[11, 62] Narcolepsy commonly begins in the second decade, peaking at 14 years of age. Excessive sleepiness appears first with cataplexy occurring simultaneously or delayed for a period of 1 to 30 years. Human leukocyte antigen (HLA) typing in persons with narcolepsy and studies of first-degree relatives of narcoleptics suggest that there is a strong genetic component that is related to the HLA, DR2 or Dw2.[11, 63] It is thought that there is a two-threshold, multifactorial model of inheritance, excessive daytime sleepiness being the more prevalent and less severe and narcolepsy being the most severe and less prevalent manifestation. Sleep attacks may occur when the individual is fully engaged in an activity as well as during monotonous activity. Hallucinations occur at sleep onset and are a disturbing and unpleasant experience. Cataplexy is an abrupt and reversible decrease or loss of voluntary muscle tone. It may range from a state of absolute powerlessness that involves the total voluntary muscle system to a fleeting sensation of weakness throughout the body. Cataplexy may be triggered by emotions such as laughter, anger, and surprise or by abrupt strain. These attacks may last from a few seconds to 30 minutes. In cataplexy, motor neurons are inhibited at the brain stem level, much as occurs in REM sleep.

Sleep paralysis occurs on falling asleep or on awakening and is described as a terrifying experience in which the patient is unable to speak, move, or even breathe deeply but is fully aware of the condition. Sleep paralysis and hypnagogic hallucinations almost always are associated with sleep-onset REM periods. Sleep-onset REM does not occur in the normal adult unless there is substantial sleep deprivation or unless sleep onset occurs in the morning hours when the tendency to REM is a potent drive. (Shift workers who sleep in the daytime may have sleep-onset REM which is considered normal.) In the narcoleptic individual, cataplexy, hypnagogic hallucinations, and sleep paralysis decrease in frequency over time. However, excessive daytime sleepiness seems to be lifelong. Both periodic limb movement disorder and sleep apnea are more prevalent in narcolepsy than in the population in general. These disorders may account for the increased sleepiness over time seen in some individuals with narcolepsy. Some researchers report memory problems in these individuals; others, more commonly, report no impairment of memory and learning.[64] This is a disorder that presents considerable risk to the individual and others working in industry or while driving. The patient must continually be assisted in developing ways to increase vigilance (see Case Study No. 3).

Sleep Apnea. This disorder was first identified in the late 1970s and has since become a major sleep disorder or impairment of sleep because of its prevalence and risks to the individual.[65–73] Sleep apnea syndrome may be obstructive or central or, more commonly, have characteristics of both. Obstructive sleep apnea (OSA) is characterized by repetitive episodes of upper airway obstruction that occur during sleep. Respiration during awake states may be normal. The obstructive episodes are usually associated with loud snores or gasps followed by silence that last 20 to 30 seconds. After a short time the patient demonstrates arousal on EEG studies. Termination of the episode is associated with vocalizations such as gasps, moans, or mumblings and with whole-body movements.

Most patients are aware of their sleep disturbance, as is the bed partner. The apnea develops over years and is associated with increased loudness in snoring. Subjects may be groggy upon awakening, experience mental dullness and incoordination, complain of morning headache, and be excessively sleepy during the day. They may awaken suddenly with chest discomfort, choking, or feeling of suffocation associated with anxiety. Secondary disorders often include depression, anxiety, irritability, and loss of libido. Severity of symptoms increases with weight; most patients are overweight at the time of seeking medical care. Sinus arrhythmia, premature ventricular contractions, atrioventricular block, and sinus arrest may occur during sleep. Bradycardia alternates with tachycardia, which occurs at the time of termination of the apneic episode. These patients commonly also have mild hypertension with elevated diastolic blood pressures. A decrease in oxygen saturation, sometimes to less than 50 per cent, commonly occurs. Carbon dioxide levels are usually only transiently elevated. During sleep, apneic episodes are typically 20 to 40 seconds in duration. Anything over 20 seconds is clinically significant. Respiratory effort continues in the absence of oral and nasal airflow. Arterial blood gases measured in awake states are usually normal. Polycythemia may be present. Gastroesophageal reflux may occur in some patients.

Although obstructive apnea may spontaneously resolve with weight reduction, it usually progresses and may lead to premature death. Nasopharyngeal abnormalities with narrowing of the upper airway are frequently found in these individuals. Some patients may have neurological abnormalities of the airway muscles. Obesity is common, but some patients are not overweight. These patients may have craniofacial abnormalities.

Obstructive sleep apnea occurs most commonly in middle-aged, overweight males. It is suspected to occur in 1 to 2 per cent of the population. More females are being diagnosed with OSA. An all-night polysomnogram reveals more than five obstructive apneic episodes of greater than 10 minutes duration per hour of sleep and evidence of frequent arousals from the apnea, bradycardia, arterial oxygen desaturation, or a mean Multiple Sleep Latency Test score of less than 10 minutes.[11] The total number of apneic episodes per night may be in the hundreds. REM sleep apnea is typically longer than NREM sleep apnea. Because of the blunting of arousability response during REM, the REM apneas necessitate a more potent stimulus to terminate. Carotid chemoreceptors may play a crucial role in terminating obstructive apneas.

Central sleep apnea is a pattern of sleep—not a disease process. There is a decrease or cessation of ventilatory effort usually accompanied by oxygen desaturation. There are two groups: (1) patients who have alveolar hypoventilation while awake and asleep and have poor responses to carbon dioxide and hypoxia and (2) patients who have normal or low arterial carbon dioxide levels while awake and asleep but have abnormally high ventilatory responses to hypercapnia and to hypoxia. Patients in the second group may be an extension of the obstructive sleep apnea group.[74] Patients with only OSA are uncommon. Usually, patients with sleep apnea have periods of central apnea and periods of mixed apnea throughout the night. It is thought that the presence of obstructive apnea with hypoxic episodes may produce an abnormally brisk ventilatory response to hypoxia and hypercapnia. The increase in ventilatory response with oscillating ventilation may result in central apnea. Patients with predominately mixed and central apnea who use continuous positive airway pressure (CPAP) have a fall toward normal in ventilatory response to hypoxia.[74] The patients complain of insomnia and somtimes are sleepy during their normal awake hours. They may also have systemic hypertension, cardiac arrhythmias, pulmonary hypertension, and cardiac failure. Cognitive difficulties may result from the excessive sleepiness. They may have other symptoms similar to those of OSA.[11] (See Chapter 8 for a further discussion of apnea in children.)

Other Dyssomnias. Other intrinsic dyssomnias are of importance, but space precludes thorough discussion. *Periodic limb movement disorder* and *restless legs syndrome* are two categories that arose with the advent of the polysomnogram when anterior tibilis monitoring was instituted. Researchers and clinicians listened to the patients who complained of awakenings in the night and to their bed partners, who noted excessive limb movement in the patients. Monitoring of the anterior tibialis muscle was begun. The power of astute, informed observation by the clinician and researcher cannot be underestimated. Similar observations have led to identification and treatment and thus improved quality of life for a large number of people (see Case Study No. 4).

Extrinsic Sleep Disorders

Impaired sleep due to environmental or extrinsic factors occurs as a result of inadequate sleep hygiene; noisy environments, such as a busy floor in the hospital or neighborhoods close to airports; drug dependency; and insufficient sleep.

In this category, external factors are integral in producing the impairment in sleep. Generally, when the environmental stimuli are removed, the disorder or impairment is resolved. Intrinsic factors are important in this category but would not have produced the problem without the environmental factor.[11]

Circadian Rhythm Disorders

Although these impairments may have their origin in both intrinsic and extrinsic factors, their common linkage is in the chronobiological and pathophysiological mechanisms, resulting in a problem with the timing of sleep in the 24-hour day. The appearance of these disorders as a separate category in the 1990 revision of *The International Classification of Sleep Disorders: Diagnostic and Coding Manual*[11] indicates a growing recognition of the severity and importance of circadian rhythm disorders. These disorders are discussed in depth in Chapter 4. Three of these disorders have both intrinsic and extrinsic causes: (1) delayed sleep phase syndrome, (2) advanced sleep phase syndrome, and (3) non–24-hour sleep-wake syndrome.

Subjects with *delayed sleep phase syndrome* have difficulty falling asleep at the desired time and may report ability to fall asleep only between 2 and 6 a.m., for example. Awakening and arising are difficult if work and social obligations demand an early morning time. These people may have little ability to advance their sleep time and may adjust by taking evening work.

Advanced sleep phase syndrome is a stable pattern in which there is extreme sleepiness in the evening and early morning awakening without sleepiness during the other times of day. These subjects are said to be extreme larks.[11] The terms owl and lark have been coined to describe individual tendencies to morningness and eveningness in human circadian rhythms.[75]

Non–24-hour sleep-wake syndrome occurs in people who experience a steady pattern of 1- to 2-hour delays in sleep onset and wake times. Their temperature rhythm shows a progressive delay as well.[11] These individuals tend to run on a different clock and are a constant mismatch with societal norms.

Jet lag and *shift work disorders* are other troublesome impairments. Jet travel moves the individual rapidly into a new time zone while the biological clock lags behind. Rapidly rotating shift work forces one to be awake during the usual sleep hours and vice versa. Sleep-wake cycles are in part regulated by an internal pacemaker. The internal circadian pacemaker is probably the suprachiasmatic nucleus (SCN) of the hypothalamus.[76] The SCN establishes and maintains the endogenous rhythm but can be re-entrained by exogenous factors, such as altered sleep-wake cycles or changes in light-dark cycles, or by drugs. Health care providers with abnormal shifts in rhythms of sleep complain of changes in alertness and judgments as well as other health problems. There is some evidence that night-shift work may result in an increase in stomach and respiratory problems, in low back pain, in an elevation of cardiovascular risk factors, and in reproductive dysfunction as well as in disorders of sleep.[77]

Some estimate that 20 per cent of the working population is engaged in permanent shift work.[78] Alterations in sleep time of day and other rhythms are frequently accompanied by fatigue, leading to a feeling of discomfort and reduced well-being and to concerns related to safety. Subjects with sleep disorders demonstrate no difference between morning and evening scores on a visual analogue scale, whereas subjects with no complaints of a sleep disorder do show a circadian difference.[79]

Rhythms in plasma cortisol levels and temperature provide the best indicator of endogenous circadian rhythms in normal people. With regard to altered sleep-wake schedules, it is important to know that the biological clocks can be phase-advanced or phase-delayed only about 2 hours each day. Therefore, to reverse sleep-wake time and re-establish cortisol and temperature rhythms (as well as numerous other associated rhythms), 1 to 2 weeks is required. For example, a person who rotates shifts of work each week is in constant change of biological rhythms.

Parasomnias

The parasomnias are disorders of arousal, partial arousal, and sleep-stage transition. They are not abnormalities of the processes responsible for sleep-wake states per se. Many of these impairments are manifestations of nervous system activation with autonomic system changes and skeletal muscle activity. For example, REM sleep behavior disorder is characterized by intermittent loss of REM atonia and the appearance of elaborate motor activity associated with dream mentation. These patients act out their dreams. Violent episodes may occur as often as once a week. In animals with lesions of the peri–locus ceruleus area similar behavior has been observed.[11] Technology and general awareness of the sleeping brain as anything but quiescent have made the identification of this and other sleep disorders or impairments possible. The parasomnias occur during sleep exclusively or are exaggerated by sleep. These include bruxism, sleepwalking, sleep talking, and enuresis (bed wetting). Most patients with these impairments are seen in outpatient or sleep disorders clinics.

Sleep Disorders Related to Medical or Psychiatric Conditions

Persons with impaired sleep may have some other underlying condition and seek help only when sleep becomes disrupted. For example, persons with parkinsonism are often first seen for medical help in a sleep disorders clinic. The patient's muscle rigidity and inability to place the head on a pillow when preparing for sleep sometimes alerts a bed partner to a problem.

In addition, many of the disorders related to medical or psychiatric conditions are associated with sleep because other biological rhythms are changing during that time of the 24-hour day as well. For example, histamine rhythms may be associated with nocturnal or *sleep-related asthma* or with *gastrointestinal symptoms* during sleep. Common sleep disturbances among persons with asthma include early morning awakening, difficulty in maintaining sleep, and daytime sleepiness.[80] Arthritis may result in marked alterations in the circadian variation in sleep-wake cycles and sleep architecture in human and animal studies. Sleep is fragmented, lighter, and less

consolidated at the appropriate times of the 24-hour day[81-84] (see Case Study No. 5).

Proposed Sleep Disorders

In this category, inadequate or insufficient work exists to substantiate the unequivocal existence of the disorder. The category includes but is not limited to short sleeper, long sleeper, sleep-choking syndrome, menstrual- or pregnancy-related sleep disorders, and other possible disorders. For example, sleep changes in women in midlife have been studied.[85, 86] In a study of 76 women between ages 40 and 59 years and classified as premenopausal, perimenopausal, or postmenopausal, no vast differences in sleep occurred. There was a tendency toward reduced sleep efficiency in symptomatic individuals, and postmenopasual women experienced less stable sleep. In a sample of 82 mid-life women, 42 per cent experienced poor sleep patterns by either objective or subjective criteria, with overlap occurring in only seven subjects. Subjective psychological distress does not result in objectively defined poor sleep. Further work is needed in these areas.

SURVEILLANCE

A typical sleep record consists of recordings from cortical regions C_1 and C_2 referred to A_2 and A_1, respectively, using the 10-20 System standardized for clinical EEG recording[4] (Figs. 20–10 and 20–11). Surface

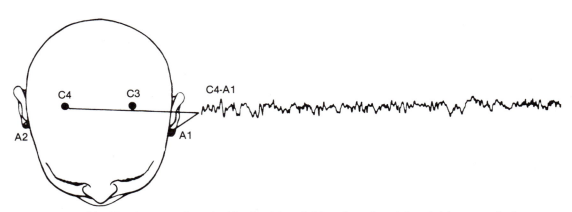

Figure 20–10. Diagram of cortical leads, C1 and C2, referred to A2 and A1, respectively. (From Rechtschaffen, A., & Kales, A. (eds.). (1973). *A Manual of Standardized Terminology, Techniques and Scoring System for Sleep Stages of Human Subjects.* University of California, Los Angeles: Brain Information Service, p. 15. Used with permission.)

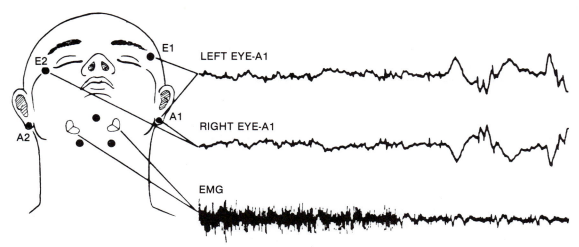

Figure 20–11. Placement of electrodes for EMG and EOG. (From Rechtschaffen, A., & Kales, A. (eds.). (1973). *A Manual of Standardized Terminology, Techniques and Scoring System for Sleep Stages of Human Subjects.* University of California, Los Angeles: Brain Information Service, p. 15. Used with permission.)

electrodes are placed at these sites with the appropriate reference, C_1A_2, C_2A_1. In order to record eye movements, the EOG electrodes are placed on the outer canthus of each eye with reference to the opposite ear or mastoid (A_1 or A_2). Muscle recording with the EMG is done by placing two electrodes over the submental (chin) muscles. For a full polysomnogram, respiratory and anterior tibialis (for leg movements) monitoring is also necessary. See Figures 20–12 and 20–13 for examples of respiratory and anterior tibialis muscle monitoring, respectively.

Examples of each stage of sleep using the EEG, the EOG, and the EMG are shown in Figures 20–1 to 20–6. A typical night's sleep in the young adult begins with lights out, followed by less than 20 minutes of awake time (Fig. 20–1), defined by low-amplitude, high-frequency beta rhythm. Drowsiness is indicated by rolling eye movements and a declining frequency of the EEG. Less than 1 to 5 per cent of the night is made up of this stage, stage 1 (Fig. 20–2). It is always the first stage of the night's sleep and may appear at intervals throughout the night, especially at

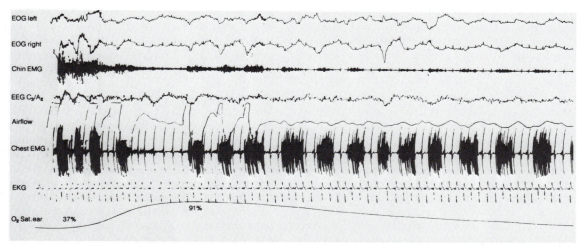

Figure 20–12. An example of a polygraph record from an all-night recording with monitoring for respiratory impairment. (From Hauri, P. [1982]. *The Sleep Disorders, Current Concepts* [pp. 41–42]. Kalamazoo, MI: Upjohn. Used with permission.)

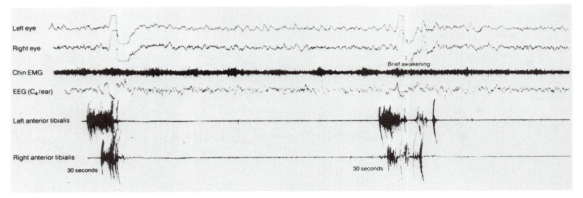

Left eye

Right eye

Chin EMG

EEG (C₄/ear)

Left anterior tibialis

Right anterior tibialis

Brief awakening

30 seconds

30 seconds

Figure 20–13. An example of a polygraph record from an all-night polysomnogram with monitoring of anterior tibialis muscle activity. (From Hauri, P. [1982]. *The Sleep Disorders, Current Concepts* [pp. 41–42]. Kalamazoo, MI: Upjohn. Used with permission.)

the end of a REM period. Stage 2 (Fig. 20–3) follows stage 1. Eye movements are almost absent. There is mixed-frequency, low-voltage corticoelectrical activity with bursts of sleep spindles and K complexes, a large-amplitude negative wave followed by a positive wave. After the appearance of two events marking stage 2, the epoch (page of recording) is scored as stage 2.

Stages 3 and 4, commonly called delta sleep, or slow-wave sleep (Figs. 20–4 and 20–5), are definded by their high-voltage (75 μV or greater), low-frequency waveform. When these waves appear in 20 to 50 per cent of the epoch or page (usually 15- or 20-second epochs, depending upon the type of polygraph used), the sleep is scored as stage 3. More than 50 per cent of this electrical activity per epoch is stage 4.

Finally, REM sleep on the EEG looks much like awake time in the human, with the exception that the muscle frequency of firing and amplitude decreases. It is characterized by low-voltage, mixed-frequency cortical activity, with a sawtooth waveform as well. Eye movements are both tonic and phasic (high number of movements and periods of fewer movements). Figure 20–6 shows as example of REM sleep electrical activity.

Throughout the night, the person cycles through the various stages approximately every 60 to 90 minutes. The initial latency to REM onset is the longest of the night with greater periods of slow-wave sleep early in the night's sleep and much denser REM sleep later in the sleep period, during the early morning hours.

If impaired sleep becomes a prolonged, chronic phenomenon, the patient should be referred to a major sleep disorders center at which an extensive description of the patient's sleep-wake cycle can be obtained.[87] Following this, a physical examination is done. Finally, in order to make a definitive decision with regard to the sleep problem, an all-night recording (polysomnogram) is needed.

After an all-night recording, the patient may be asked to spend the day in the sleep clinic, where daytime sleep tendency and characteristics may be defined using the Multiple Sleep Latency Test (MSLT). The patient is given five opportunities to nap: usually at 10 a.m., 12 p.m. (noon), 2 p.m., 4 p.m., and 6 p.m. Using standard polysomnographic techniques, the patient is given 10 minutes to go to sleep at each of the five times. If no sleep occurs within 10 minutes, the patient is not allowed to remain in bed. If sleep occurs, a maximum of another 10 minutes of sleep is allowed (a total of 20 minutes per nap trial), at which time the patient is asked to get out of bed. The average person requires 10 minutes or more to fall asleep after a good night's rest. Those with excessive daytime somnolence go to sleep in 5 minutes or less. In addition, those with narcolepsy have two or more sleep-onset REM periods.[88]

Surveillance of childhood sleep disorders, especially in infants, requires some modification of the techniques just described and is beyond the scope of this chapter. The reader is referred to the work of Guilleminault.[87]

The nurse in all settings, working with all ages and types of patients, is in a key position for case finding, referral, and education. Nurses frequently are employed by sleep centers and are directly responsible for obtaining the all-night recordings. In any setting the nurse can observe for apneic or hypopneic episodes during sleep. The patient must be observed for decreased oxygen saturation during sleep periods. Nurses can observe for abnormal movements of the legs (frequent periodic leg movements) during sleep. Also, do noises, medications, pain, or other phenomena, such as disordered schedules, keep the patient awake?

Surveillance of sleep in critical care units has been done by nurse researchers using a variety of techniques other than polysomnography. These include structured observation of sleep behaviors, cognitive behaviors, and nursing behaviors and activities. These techniques are summarized elsewhere.[89] The Verran and Snyder-Halpern Sleep Scale has been developed to measure sleep characteristics subjectively and is administered to the subject within 2 hours after arising in the morning.[90] Subjective measures of sleep are important, since perceptions of one's ability to sleep well influence daytime functioning. However, subjective and objective evidence of quality of sleep correlates poorly. A computer-compatible method for observing falling asleep behaviors of hospitalized children has also been developed.[91] One of the most widely used subjective self-rating scale of sleepiness is the Stanford Sleepiness Scale. It consists of seven statements ranked from (1) "feeling active and vital; alert; wide awake" to (7) "almost in reverie; sleep onset soon; lost struggle to remain awake." Ratings as frequently as every 15 minutes show discrete and sensitive changes in sleepiness.[92, 93] A modified version[94] of the St. Mary's Hospital Sleep Questionnaire[95] has been used to assess the quality of sleep and the relationship to sleep promotion methods of subjects from medical-surgical units of a private hospital. Auditory stimuli and sleep disturbance in preschool children in the pediatric care unit (PICU) have been studied by combining several techniques. The EEG, EMG, and EOG were recorded on the second postoperative night following open heart surgery in two children aged 3.6 years and 4.8 years. At the same time, tape recordings, sound pressure levels in decibels, and monitoring of sounds by the researcher were performed. Data revealed that although the children were able to sleep, they were in fact disturbed by sound events.[96]

In a few studies, attempts have been made to reliably and validly measure nocturnal sleep in ICU patients. One study was done to determine the reliability and validity of a sleep perception tool and a sleep observation instrument for the trauma patient in the critical care setting in which the sleep EEG was recorded and compared with results of the Patient's Sleep Behavior Observational Tool and the Verran and Snyder-Halpern Sleep Scale.[97] The multitrait-multimethod assessment and analysis of sleep-wake activity in patients is an important mechanism leading to better surveillance and thus sleep-promoting interventions.

The surveillance of other biological rhythms may result in sleep-wake linked findings. Time-series analysis of circadian rhythms in intracranial pressure produced findings of predominant peaks in rhythms from 14 to 40 hours in length. Some peaks were common in all subjects (all had both 48- and 72-hour rhythms), whereas others were specific to the subject and unchanged from day to day. Interestingly, 80 per cent of the peaks occurred between the hours of 12 a.m. (midnight) and 5 a.m. A second bimodal peak occurred at the time of the mid-afternoon sleep window.[98, 99] These types of data may be used to predict future biological response in a patient; that is, today's response may correlate highly with tomorrow's and will give the nurse clues in management of the patient. The surveillance of changes in other circadian biological rhythms, such as heart rate and temperature in head-injured patients,[100, 101] produces data helpful in planning care for the 24-hour day for all patients.

CLINICAL THERAPIES

The therapeutic goal is to maintain or restore the normal sleep-wake cycle. The therapies may vary with the type of sleep impairment identified. In insomnia, behavioral therapy plays a large role. This includes establishing a rigid routine of getting to bed and maintaining a set time of getting up for the day, usually with no naps. Daytime naps and support groups have been shown to be effective for persons with narcolepsy. In actual practice, drugs are indicated in narcolepsy and often are used to treat persons with other sleep impairments. Treatment for excessive daytime sleepiness includes stimulants such as amphetamine, methylphenidate, mazindol, and pemoline. Cataplexy is treated with antidepressants. Sleep medications are often indicated in short-term management of insomnia. Ideally, hypnotics should be used only for a brief period. They should have rapid onset, maintain effectiveness with consecutive administration, leave no alteration in daytime performance, produce no insomnia when stopped, and not alter significantly the stages of sleep (the sleep architecture). Because no drug meets all these criteria, it is best to deal with sleep impairments behaviorally, when possible. See Table 20–7 for some helpful suggestions.

The types of hypnotics used include the benzodiazepines, the barbiturates, drugs such as chloral hydrate and tricyclic antidepressants, and over-the-counter medications to induce sleepiness. The latter group includes antihistamines for their side effect of drowsiness and other drugs that induce relaxation and thus sleepiness.

The benzodiazepines are currently the hypnotic drugs of choice. Included in this group are flurazepam, temazepam, and triazolam. In Table 20–8, the most frequently

TABLE 20–8   COMMON BENZODIAZEPINE HYPNOTICS

Generic Name	Trade Name	Half-Life of Active Metabolites
Flurazepam	Dalmane	40–300 hr
Temazepam	Restoril	8–12 hr
Triazolam	Halcion	1–3 hr

used drugs are listed by generic and trade names, and the half-life of the active metabolites is given. None of these is ideal, innocuous, or effective for all insomniacs or for long periods of treatment. In addition, other benzodiazepines in the anxiolytic category are often used on a short-term basis for sleep impairments. No consistent treatment approach to idiopathic insomnia has evolved. However, some patients respond to treatment with tricyclic antidepressants and neuroleptics. In addition, supportive psychological care is very important, as is good sleep hygiene. Treatment for psychophysiological insomnia is varied and tailored to the individual and will consist of some components from three domains—sleep hygiene, behavioral treatment, and hypnotics.[61]

The therapies for other categories of impairments and disorders are tailored to the individual patient or subject. Some are discussed above in categories of disorders or impairments. For example, in obstructive and mixed sleep apnea, the goal is a patent airway during sleep. This may be obtained in one or a combination of ways: simple weight reduction, surgery, and CPAP.[102–105] The treatment of choice is CPAP, usually applied nasally during sleep. CPAP was first used in 1981, and by 1986 most major sleep disorders centers reported success with it. Pressures of 10 to 12 cm H_2O are usually used and well tolerated by the patient. Small, quiet, and portable CPAP units are available commercially. The positive pressure keeps the upper airway open by splinting. The most important problem is fitting a comfortable mask to ensure compliance. The patient should be observed for nasal congestion and sinus infections and other problems as well as for efficacy of treatment.

Surgical treatment of OSA includes tonsillectomy, adenoidectomy and nasal surgery, tracheostomy, uvulopalatopharyngoplasty, and maxillomandibular surgery.[106] Tracheostomy is permanent. The tracheostomy

TABLE 20–7   ELEVEN RULES FOR BETTER SLEEP HYGIENE

1. Sleep as much as needed to feel refreshed and healthy during the following day, but not more. Curtailing the time in bed seems to solidify sleep; excessively long times in bed seem related to fragmented and shallow sleep.
2. A regular arousal time in the morning strengthens circadian cycling and, finally, leads to regular times of sleep onset.
3. A steady daily amount of exercise probably deepens sleep; occasional exercise does not necessarily improve sleep the following night.
4. Occasional loud noises (e.g., aircraft flyovers) disturb sleep even in people who are not awakened by noises and cannot remember them in the morning. Sound-attenuated bedrooms may help those who must sleep close to noise.
5. Although excessively warm rooms disturb sleep, there is no evidence that an excessively cold room solidifies sleep.
6. Hunger may disturb sleep; a light snack may help sleep.
7. An occasional sleeping pill may be of some benefit, but their chronic use is ineffective in most insomniacs.
8. Caffeine in the evening disturbs sleep, even in those who feel it does not.
9. Alcohol helps tense people fall asleep more easily, but the ensuing sleep is then fragmented.
10. People who feel angry and frustrated because they cannot sleep should not try harder and harder to fall asleep but should turn on the light and do something different.
11. The chronic use of tobacco disturbs sleep.

Used with permission from Hauri, P. (1982). *The Sleep Disorders, Current Concepts.* Kalamazoo, MI: Upjohn.

stoma is plugged during the day and is open during sleep. Because of complications and problems of management over the years, whether or not to choose tracheostomy must be considered carefully and only after failure of CPAP or other interventions. Weight reduction is always indicated in those who are overweight[107–109] (see Case Study No. 6).

Since the parasomnias are a diverse category of impairments, the treatment is specific for each. For example, if sleepwalking endangers the patient, a drug may be given that will decrease stages 3 and 4 of sleep. Sleepwalking usually occurs during these stages. The nurse is uniquely able to assist in the identification of these disorders, in education of patients and families, and in management of medications. Often a childhood sleep disorder is best treated with counseling of parents, and sleep clinics are turning to nurses more frequently for assistance in this regard (see Case Study No. 7).

Treatment of circadian rhythm disorders may include drugs, such as lithium or antidepressants, or chronotherapy. In the latter case, for delayed-sleep phase syndrome, the patient is asked to delay sleep time even further, by 2 hours per night, until the desired sleep time is acheived. From that point forward, rigid adherence to the newly established bedtime is encouraged. It is thought that postponing sleep time is much easier than advancing the bedtime. One can force wakefulness but not sleep. Also, 2 hours is the maximum change that can occur in biological rhythms per 24 hours. See Chapter 4 for further discussion of treatments for circadian rhythm disorders.

In the acute care setting, nurses have the power to maintain, destroy, or re-establish the rhythms of patients. Manipulation of the environmental cues is important. Maintenance of a light-dark schedule similar to day-night rhythms is necessary, since light is a powerful Zeitgeber (time giver). Many of the medications administered by health care providers disrupt the biological rhythms and alter sleep architecture—distribution and percentage of sleep stages throughout the sleep period. For example, cortisol induces an enzyme that shunts tryptophan away from the serotonin pathway, and sleep-onset insomnia may result. Stress also leads to an increase in cortisol secretion and can result in insomnia by way of the same mechanisms. Many pain medications are REM-sleep de-

privers. When the patient is allowed normal sleep (when the drug is withdrawn), there may occur a REM-sleep rebound—a higher percentage of the total sleep time is spent in REM sleep. The patient is more vulnerable to phasic changes (described previously) during rebound REM sleep, since the normal catecholamine response is prolonged. The medications that alter sleep are numerous (see Case Studies Nos. 8 and 9).

Sleep latency is decreased in mid-afternoon and late evening. The tendency toward greater sleepiness at these times of day is independent of food intake and other cues and appears to be an intrinsic biological rhythm and independent of most other rhythms.[110–112] These findings have implications for planned rest periods and performance expectations.

In narcolepsy, a stimulant is indicated along with counseling and other techniques such as planned daytime naps. Since the hypothalamic-pituitary axis is influenced by both sleep and circadian rhythmicity, it is important for the person, whether in good health or poor health, to maintain the daily rhythms of life.[113] This includes a plethora of routines and daily adjustments from normal light-dark cycles in the ICU to good sleep hygiene in all persons. Simple but important considerations include observation of gastroesophageal reflux when nighttime feedings are given, more aggressive monitoring and treatment of nighttime increased intracranial pressure, preventing cognitive impairments and promoting wound healing by preventing sleep loss in patients, assisting new mothers with adjustments to sleep loss, helping the elderly to better consolidate their sleep times, more careful monitoring of arterial blood gases and arrhythmias during sleep of the patient, and finally recognizing when shift work and other rhythm disturbances in the nurse's own life may seriously disrupt judgments. Any sleep-wake disorder that results in daytime dysfunction must be considered, the specific impairment dictating the care.

Many therapies await further research in areas such as the effect of vitamins upon sleep. For example, it is thought that niacin (vitamin B_3) increases REM sleep and promotes sleep efficiency.[114–116] In other cases, nurses have known for many years that behavioral disturbances correlated with the amount of sleep deficit[117, 118] and that in ICUs about 50 to 60 per cent of the patient's sleep was obtained at night,[119] yet little has changed in practice in critical care areas.

For an up-to-date and clinically usefully handbook on sleep, the clinician is referred to *101 Questions about Sleep and Dreams.*[120]

REVIEW OF RESEARCH FINDINGS

The number of researchers in sleep-wake impairments and dysfunctions has grown enormously since the early 1970s when a small group of people began to consolidate their interests and findings. Sleep disorders medicine has become an established field. Pulmonologists, neuroscientists, pediatricians, and nurses and others have developed a growing interest in the field. In the mid-1970s, few nurses were involved in sleep research and related organizations and few nurse clinicians talked about this in their practice. Virtually no schools (neither nursing nor medical) included the topic in their curriculums. Now, however, the field has developed to the extent that the discussions in the preceding text are based on research findings.

IMPLICATIONS FOR RESEARCH

Sleep-wake cycles and circadian rhythms, normal and impaired, are experienced by all human beings throughout life and are one of the most basic human processes. Nurses are much more aware of this now than in the past. They are also aware of the basis for normal sleep-wake cycles and of the ways in which this becomes impaired. Research by nurses varies from basic science in the laboratory using animal models to clinical biological science to psychosocial and anthropological approaches. Basic measurement and instrumentation techniques have been developed in the area of nursing research. And readings and reports of research findings are much more exciting now than just 5 to 10 years ago. It is now possible for the nurse researcher to move quickly into studies ranging from physiological measurement to psychosocial measurement or to a combination of both.

With a bird's eye view of the field of sleep research in general and impaired sleep specifically, the areas least researched are those most appropiate to nurse researchers; that is,

much remains to be known about sleep in the hospitalized individual—all age groups, all types of illness. In addition, many nurses themselves fit into the category of workers who experience impaired sleep.

Questions to be asked and studied systematically are limited only by the questioner's creativity and sense of inquiry, matched with one's training in methodological approaches. Developing knowledge about the numerous factors that influence sleep, either contributing to impaired sleep or facilitating sleep, has important clinical implications for professional nursing practice.

ILLUSTRATIVE CASE STUDIES

The following case studies represent the most common types of sleep problems. They are slightly modified with permission of Peter Hauri, The Upjohn Company, and the WB Saunders Company.*

CASE STUDY NO. 1: IDIOPATHIC INSOMNIA

Mrs. I., a 45-year-old professional woman, was self-referred after reading a newspaper article on insomnia. On interview, she looked tired, grim, and worn out, and she gave the appearance that she held herself together by sheer willpower. She said that sleep had been her problem "forever." Indeed, her earliest memories were of incidents that occurred when she was about 3 years old, when her parents repeatedly discovered her playing "all night long" while the rest of her family slept.

Grade school was hard. Although not diagnosed at that time, she seems to have had some serious problem with attention or possibly some learning disability. She always felt tired and sickly. Nevertheless, she managed college and law school "by sheer force of will." She also noted during that time that even minor stimulations, such as an interesting evening of conversation or a book, would keep her awake most of the night and that even mild stimulants,

---

*Hauri, P. *The Sleep Disorder, Current Concepts* (1982), The Upjohn Co., and Hauri, P. (1989). Primary insomnia. In M. H. Kryger, T. Roth, & W. C. Dement (eds.), *Principles and Practice of Sleep Medicine*, W.B. Saunders.

such as chocolate or soft drinks with caffeine, did the same.

Over the past 20 years, Mrs. I. had undergone many medical evaluations at some of the country's leading medical centers. Nothing was ever found except a general lack of stamina despite her efforts to exercise. Psychological testing showed a generalized feeling of chronic malaise, but no noteworthy psychopathology. Specifically, there were no clear signs of either anxiety neurosis or depression. In spite of this, Mrs. I. had undergone two intensive courses of psychotherapy during the past 10 years "to get to the bottom of this," with no success.

In the past, Mrs. I. had been tried on most of the available hypnotics, some major tranquilizers, some daytime stimulants, and even some narcotics. Sleep typically improved for a few weeks with each new medication, but Mrs. I. habituated to each of them in turn. On a clinical course of tricyclic antidepressants (up to 200 mg of amitriptyline per day), she had slept much better but had been unable to function because of excessive fatigue during the day, headaches, and ataxia.

Studied in the laboratory for three nights, Mrs. I. slept fitfully for 2 to 5 hours each night, and she was easily aroused, even by faint noises from afar. When disturbed, she was immediately and fully awake. There was excessive stage 1 sleep, almost no delta sleep, and only very poorly defined, irregular sleep spindles that occurred rarely, no more than every 3 to 5 minutes. No respiratory or muscular abnormalities were found, and the alternations between REM and non-rapid eye movement (NREM) sleep seemed normal.

A discussion of sleep hygiene and an intensive course of EMG biofeedback improved sleep somewhat for Mrs. I., but not markedly so. She was then placed on minute doses of amitriptyline h.s., first 10 mg and later 25 mg. This practice improved her sleep markedly, and she has now been maintained on this medication for 6 years without any apparent decrease in efficacy. To assess her continuous need for amitriptyline, she withdraws from it once a year for 3 weeks during vacation, each time so far with disastrous results. The efficacy of such a low dose of amitriptyline

in this patient remains unexplained and deserves further investigation.

CASE STUDY NO. 2 BEHAVIORAL ISSUES

Mrs. S., 44, had been a somewhat poor sleeper all her life. However, four years ago her 19-year-old son became involved in drug trafficking. Mrs. S. was distraught and became "almost totally sleepless for at least 2 months." She never recovered and still reported extremely poor sleep when she entered the sleep disorders center 3 years after the scandal. By then her son had become rehabilitated and made a good adjustment.

To everybody's surprise, on the first night in the lab Mrs. S. fell asleep within five minutes of "lights out" and slept soundly throughout that night. There was an excess of delta sleep, as if Mrs. S. had been previously sleep-deprived. In the morning, Mrs. S. was embarrassed by her good sleep and claimed she had not slept that well in over a year. Sleep on nights two and three was poor by our standards (less than 80 per cent sleep of time-in-bed), but Mrs. S. rated both nights as "much better than my average night." Psychiatric evaluation and psychologic testing revealed a somewhat tense, slightly neurotic, and very anxious person, but without major psycho-pathology.

Mrs. S. was first treated with EMG biofeedback therapy. This enabled her to relax during the day and to cope. Although she slept somewhat more easily after biofeedback, she still had problems. She was then treated with Bootzin's stimulus-control behavior technique. This helped dramatically after some very difficult initial nights. Finally, Mrs. S. received a few sleeping pills, to be used only if she experienced two or three poor nights in a row.

Nine months later, Mrs. S. had returned to the "adequate" sleep that she had shown before the drug scandal. Although she still suffered a few poor nights each month, she took them in stride. Anxiety and agitation were no longer chronic but developed only when she was put under serious stress. She felt "cured."

CASE STUDY NO. 3: NARCOLEPSY

Mr. U. was a 52-year-old married Army officer referred to the sleep disorders center for evaluation of excessive daytime sleepiness. He dated the onset of his problem to the time when he was about 20 years old and had slept for two days without significant awakenings. Inappropriate sleep occurred mainly when driving, eating, and during sex. The problem had been a continuing embarrassment for him, particularly when he fell asleep at meetings with superior officers. To compensate, the patient held a set of keys in his hand when he absolutely had to stay awake. They fell to the floor when he dozed and woke him. A short nap offered considerable relief, and Mr. U. took two or three per day, despite adequate sleep at night.

A few years after Mr. U.'s problem with sleepiness began, he noticed that during periods of laughter or excitement he would sometimes collapse and fall. His first episode occurred while fishing with his daughter; he caught a fish and subsequently fell into the lake. Such cataleptic attacks had become increasingly bothersome; two or three episodes, with nearly complete collapse, occurred almost daily. Also, three or four times each week he either felt suddenly unable to move when in the process of falling asleep (sleep paralysis) or he vividly sensed the presence of other persons in the room even though he knew he was alone (hypnagogic hallucinations).

Mr. U.'s physical and neurologic examinations were essentially negative. Sleep in the lab was poor and fragmented with many awakenings. The MSLT revealed a mean sleep-onset latency of approximately two minutes; a sleep-onset REM period occurred with three of the five naps.

Following the evaluation, Mr. U. experienced considerable relief from a combination of methylphenidate 20 mg twice daily and imipramine 25 mg three times a day. However, he gradually adapted to this regimen. After numerous attempts to adjust the dosage, he was finally withdrawn from the chronic use of methylphenidate and now takes it only when needed, e.g., before long drives. Mr. U.'s narcolepsy was also discussed with his wife and his superiors, who then excused him from hazardous duties and allowed him to schedule two 20-minute naps per

day. Although Mr. U. still experiences one or two episodes of cataplexy, sleep paralysis, or hypnagogic hallucinations per week even while on imipramine 25 mg twice daily, these episodes frighten him less now that he understands their meaning as REM-related phenomena.

CASE STUDY NO. 4: PERIODIC LEG MOVEMENTS

Mr. M. was a 35-year-old electrician whose main complaint was that he felt "washed out" in the morning and that he had difficulties falling asleep because his "legs were nervous." By this he meant that he felt uncomfortable, but not painful, sensations creeping deep inside his calf when relaxing. The urge to move his legs became so strong that he usually had to get up and walk for 10 to 20 minutes before he could lie down again. Occasionally, this problem continued until 4 a.m. or 5 a.m. Even after sleeping an adequate number of hours, Mr. M. felt unrefreshed. Instead of a steady job commensurate with his training, Mr. M. sought jobs as a day laborer whenever he felt up to it.

Detailed neurologic and psychiatric evaluations were negative. A sleep evaluation was performed on two consecutive nights. On each of these nights, Mr. M. got up twice after "lights out" to "walk off his legs." When he finally fell asleep about 2 hours after "lights out," episodes of periodic leg movements (PLMs) were recorded. For periods of up to 1 hour, Mr. M.'s legs jerked every 30 to 40 seconds, and almost each time this happened the EEG showed a 5- to 15-second arousal. In the morning, Mr. M. was not aware that he had been aroused 300 to 400 times by PLMS, but he still felt tired, as if he "had not slept very much."

Mr. M. was placed first on 20 mg, later on 40 mg, diazepam at bedtime. Initially, he reported having fewer problems with his "nervous legs," and he experienced a more refreshing sleep on this medication. These effects soon wore off. Later, he was placed on 1 mg clonazepam to inhibit the myoclonus and on 4.5 mg oxycodone to calm the restless legs. Initial reaction to this regimen was favorable, but Mr. M. habituated to the medication within about 6 months. To restore potency, Mr. M. was then withdrawn from these drugs about twice yearly for "drug holidays" of 2 to 3 weeks' duration.

CASE STUDY NO. 5: MOOD DISORDER

Mrs. S. the 48-year-old wife of a local businessman, was referred to the sleep disorders center for serious and chronic insomnia of 18 months' duration. Trials with different hypnotics had been unsuccessful. Mrs. S. appeared for her first interview apparently weak from lack of sleep, with bloodshot eyes, but well in control of herself. She responded appropriately, with a polite, tired smile. She related that her sleep quality had fluctuated for years, but that during the past 1½ years it had deteriorated relentlessly. Mrs. S. could think of no reason for the sudden appearance of her insomnia.

A psychiatric history revealed that about 2 years ago a number of important life changes had occurred. Her youngest son had gone to college, and neighbors who had leaned on her for support had moved away. Mrs. S. felt that these events would have helped, not harmed, her sleep because she had always dreamt about the time when, freed from other duties, she could start a new career.

Mrs. S. was admitted for three nights of somnography. She averaged about 35 awakenings per night in the lab and less than 4 hours of total sleep. Much of it was stage 1; there was no delta sleep. REM latencies on all three nights were less than 30 minutes, and the first REM period was excessively long and intensive. In summary, Mrs. S.'s sleep was typical of depression.

Extended psychiatric interviews and psychologic testing over the next 2 weeks finally demonstrated a serious but extremely well-defended depression. According to her previously unconscious appraisal of her life, now verbalized for the first time, she felt incompetent and was only awaiting old age and death.

A sedating antidepressant improved sleep almost immediately. While undergoing psychotherapy, Mrs. S. explored reasons for her low self-esteem and ways of becoming useful again. Eventually she became involved almost full time in a charity organization.

On follow-up 9 months later, Mrs. S. was pronounced "remitted." She was off all drugs and functioned well. Repeat somnograms still revealed some insomnia. Although sleep had improved dramatically, Mrs. S. still showed more awakenings and more stage 1 sleep than expected from someone her age—and practically no delta sleep. However, she claimed to be satisfied: this was the way she had "always" slept since her early 20s.

CASE STUDY NO. 6: SLEEP-RELATED RESPIRATORY IMPAIRMENT

Mr. K. was a 45-year-old, severely obese (313 pounds) male with a primary complaint of excessive daytime sleepiness. His problem started when the patient was in his early 30s. Although Mr. K. seemed willing and intelligent and had made good grades in college, he had never held any job for more than 2 or 3 weeks since then, and he had usually been fired for "laziness" (falling asleep 5 to 10 times each day). He had sought numerous medical work-ups during the ensuing 15 years, work-ups involving most medical specialties from endocrinology to neurology and psychiatry. When he was first seen at the sleep disorders center, he had already spent more than $20,000 to find a cause for his sleepiness. However, except for finding gross obesity, essential hypertension, and some enlargement of the right ventricle, all of Mr. K.'s work-ups had been quite normal.

Although Mr. K. came from a relatively well-to-do family, he was destitute when seen in the lab because of his high medical bills and his inability to remain gainfully employed. His personal life was in ruins—two wives had left him, preferring divorce to living with a chronically sleeping, obese, heavy snorer. Also, he had been unable to maintain adequate social relationships with friends and peers because of his excessive sleepiness.

In the lab, Mr. K. was pleasant and polite. He fell asleep within five seconds after "lights out," but as soon as he fell asleep, his breathing stopped. He wakened 35 seconds later gasping for air. This cycle then repeated itself for the next 10 hours of "sleep." As soon as Mr. K showed signs of stage I sleep, he stopped breathing and then awakened 20 to 80 seconds later gasping for air. Throughout the night, he never slept for more than three uninterrupted minutes. By morning he had totaled 562 arousals from sleep, and more than 75 per cent of his "sleep" time had been spent in sleep apneas. Visual observation of the patient indicated that during the periods of sleep apnea his chest heaved, and although he was straining, no air passed through the upper airways. An ear oximeter indicated oxygen saturation of 92 per cent when awake. When sleeping, saturation fell repeatedly below 50 per cent.

In the morning, Mr. K. stated that he had experienced a normal night of sleep but that he was now more tired than when he had gone to bed. He guessed he had awakened "five to eight times" during the night, and he was totally unaware of his very labored breathing, the heavy snoring, and the more than 500 sleep-apnea awakenings. An MSLT indicated a mean daytime sleep latency of 2.6 minutes; twice Mr. K. was asleep before the machine could be turned on. There were no sleep-onset REM periods. Waking pulmonary function seemed normal, except for the effects of Mr. K.'s obesity. Hemoglobin was elevated, and there was some marginal impairment of liver and cardiac functioning.

Mr. K. was told that he suffered from upper airway apneas. Ear, nose, and throat consultations did not reveal any obvious obstructions such as swollen adenoids or an enlarged uvula, although Mr. K.'s otolarynx was described as "much smaller than average." Weight loss had been tried repeatedly in the past, never with any success. Based on this information, Mr. K. was then told that the only effective treatment for his condition was a special form of permanent tracheostomy, to be closed during the day but opened at night to allow breathing during sleep. Although the entire problem and its treatment were carefully explained to both Mr. K. and his private physician, both declined to consider a permanent tracheostomy for a "mere sleep problem."

In the 4 months that followed, Mr. K. became an alcoholic, and 7 months later he was caught in an armed robbery, attempting to steal liquor. Eleven months later, he died in a state prison during sleep "of unknown causes."

CASE STUDY NO. 7: SLEEPWALKING (SOMNAMBULISM)

Mr. S., a 34-year-old math teacher, sought help because of insomnia and because he was sleepwalking one to three times per week. Usually, these somnambulistic episodes were harmless: Mr. S. got up about 1 hour after he fell asleep, rummaged around for a while, then went back to sleep. He often slept the remainder of these nights in some unpredictable location such as the living room couch, the kitchen floor, or the bathtub. However, Mr. S.'s sleepwalking episodes were not always benign; he occasionally urinated on the living-room carpet, had severely hurt himself after stumbling over furniture, and twice had been found trying to climb out of a window in the couple's fourth-story apartment. His wife was terrified. She could not awaken him during the episodes, and she was not strong enough to control him physically. Hypnotics, tranquilizers, and antidepressants had been tried—to no avail.

In the laboratory, Mr. S. did not sleepwalk but showed extreme muscle tension, both during the day and when trying to sleep. Besides a long sleep latency and many awakenings, he showed high-voltage paroxysmal bursts of delta activity, especially during the early parts of the night; otherwise, his sleep was normal. During an interview, Mr. S. was anxious and nervous and claimed that he was barely keeping up with his teaching job. He felt that the students were "driving him insane." A clinical EEG and a thorough physical and neurologic evaluation were within normal limits.

Mr. S. was enrolled in an intensive psychotherapy program and encouraged to change his teaching job to a less demanding clerical one. Furthermore, he learned deep muscle relaxation through EMG biofeedback. For the sake of safety, the couple moved to a ground-level apartment. Door locks and window locks were installed in selected locations so that Mr. S. could sleepwalk only through the bedroom, hall, and bathroom, which were freed of all potentially dangerous objects. His wife kept the keys with her during sleep in case of fire.

Sleepwalking episodes first increased to four or five times a week as all these changes were instituted. However, 6 months later, sleepwalking episodes were decreased to two or three a month, and now, 2 years later, Mr. S. sleepwalks only two or three times a year.

CASE STUDY NO. 8: SCHEDULE DISORDER

Mr. E., 26, self-employed, was referred for an evaluation of insomnia. At the time of the evaluation, he went to bed at about 5 a.m. and slept until 3 p.m. Although he had slept well on this schedule a year earlier, his sleep had gradually deteriorated. Over the past few months, he had felt increasingly tired during his waking hours.

Mr. E. reported that since childhood he always went to bed late. In college, he arranged for his first classes to start during the afternoon, and he slept through most of the mornings. He also reported that occasionally he skipped a night of sleep and worked 30 to 40 continuous hours—not because of work pressure but because he "felt like it."

Mr. E. was suspected of being hypothyroid at the age of 15 and treated with thyroid supplements until age 23. When this treatment was stopped during an episode of depression, Mr. E. became chronically obese (250 pounds). Over the preceding 2 years before the evaluation, Mr. E. had also suffered from peptic ulcers, and his blood pressure rose to 145/110. Mr. E. had been hospitalized twice for depression, and he had received electroconvulsive therapy, with only temporary improvement.

Mr. E. was diagnosed as having delayed-sleep syndrome; chronotherapy was instituted, with initially excellent success. After 6 days of progressively later bed times, Mr. E. went to bed at 11 p.m. and slept until about 7:30 a.m. He then rigidly maintained this schedule and slept very soundly. However, after about 3 months on this schedule, insomnia redeveloped, together with excessive sleepiness during the day. Mr. E. was directed to repeat chronotherapy whenever this occurred, and he has successfully maintained the schedule for the past year. (This case history was provided by Dr. E. Phillips, Holy Cross Sleep Disorders Center.)

CASE STUDY NO. 9: NON–24-HOUR SLEEP-WAKE SYNDROME

Miss R., a 26-year-old, unmarried journalist, sought help for sleep-onset insomnia after she was recently fired because she overslept so regularly. She explained that she would often lie in bed 4 to 6 hours before falling asleep and then would have extreme difficulty getting up the next morning. Except for a certain defensiveness concerning her inability to arise on schedule, Miss R. seemed to be in good mental health.

Now unemployed, Miss R. kept a sleep log for 2 weeks. It revealed that her sleep-onset insomnia had disappeared after being fired. Now, each night she went to bed 4 to 6 hours later than she had on the previous day. Consequently, she would often stay up all night and sleep all day.

When consulting the sleep disorders center, Miss R. was writing a book. She was counseled to go to bed only when she felt sleepy and to sleep as long as she wished. A subsequent 1-month sleep log was astounding: Miss R. was healthy and alert, usually worked 20 to 22 consecutive hours, then relaxed for 1 or 2 hours before sleeping uninterruptedly for 10 to 12 hours. Realizing how well she felt under this new regimen, Miss R. decided to become a freelance writer and to continue "free running" on a 36-hour to 38-hour sleep/wake schedule. However, while feeling well on this regimen, her social life deteriorated.

To speed the circadian clock, lithium was later prescribed. Miss R. found that it was easier to maintain a 24-hour rhythm on this drug but still not always possible. For the past 3 years, she has settled into a normal sleep schedule (midnight to 8 a.m.) for about 3 weeks per month, then running freely around the clock for the last week of each month.

REFERENCES

1. Manfredi, R. L., Vgontzas, A., & Kales, A. (1989). An update on sleep disorders. Bull Menninger Clin *53*:25073.
2. Jouvet, M. (1967). Neurophysiology of the states of sleep. In G. C. Quarton, T. Melnechuk, & F. Schmitt (eds.), *Neurosciences* (pp. 522–544). New York: Rockefeller University Press.
3. Jouvet, M. (1969). Biogenic amines and the states of sleep. Science *163*:32–41.
4. Rechtschaffen, A., & Kales, A. (eds.). (1973). *A

Manual of Standardized Terminology, Techniques and Scoring System for Sleep Stages of Human Subjects. Los Angeles: University of California, Brain Information Service.

5. Anders, E. R., & Parmelee, A. (eds.). (1971). *A Manual of Standardized Terminology and Criteria for Scoring States of Sleep and Wakefulness in Newborn Infants.* Los Angeles: University of California, Brain Information Service.

6. Blake, H., Gerard, R. W., & Kleitman, N. (1939). Factors influencing brain potentials during sleep. J Neurophysiol 2:48–60.

7. Loomis, A. L., Harver, E. N., & Hobart G. A. (1937). Cerebral states during sleep as studied by human brain potentials. J Exp Psychol 21:127–144.

8. Gibbs, E. L. (1950). *Atlas of Encephalography* (vol. I, p. 324). Cambridge, MA: Addison-Wesley.

9. Dement, W., & Kleitman, N. (1957). Cyclic variations in EEG during sleep and their relation to eye movements, body motility, and dreaming. Electroencephalogr Clin Neurophysiol 9:673–690.

10. Sleep Disorders Classification Committee, Association of Sleep Disorders Centers. (1979). Diagnostic classification of sleep and arousal disorders. Sleep 2:137.

11. American Sleep Disorders Association. (1990). *The International Classification of Sleep Disorders: Diagnostic and Coding Manual.* Lawrence, KS: Allen Press.

12. Kleitman, N. J. (1939). *Sleep and Wakefulness.* Chicago: University of Chicago Press.

13. Johnson, C. M. (1991). Infant and toddler sleep: A telephone survey of parents in one community. J Dev Behav Pediatr 12:108–114.

14. Cochran, J., & Ganong, L. H. (1989). A comparison of nurses' and patients' perceptions of intensive care unit stressors. J Adv Nurs 14:1038–1043.

15. Klackenberg, G. (1987). Incidence of parasomnias in children in a general population. In C. Guilleminault (ed.), *Sleep and Its Disorders in Children.* New York: Raven Press.

16. Ferber, R. (1987). The sleepless child. In C. Guilleminault (ed.), *Sleep and Its Disorders in Children.* New York: Raven Press.

17. Ferber, R. (1987). Circadian and schedule disturbances. In C. Guilleminault (ed.), *Sleep and Its Disorders in Children.* New York: Raven Press.

18. Carskadon, M. A., & Dement, W. C. (1987). Sleepiness in the normal adolescent. In C. Guilleminault (ed.), *Sleep and Its Disorders in Children.* New York: Raven Press.

19. Carskadon, M. A., Brown, E. D., & Dement, W. C. (1982). Sleep fragmentation in the elderly: Relationship to daytime sleep tendency. Neurol Aging 3:321–327.

20. Parkes, J. D. (1985). *Sleep and Its Disorders.* Philadelphia: WB Saunders.

21. Williams, R. L., Karacan, I., & Hursch, C. J. (1974). *Electroencephalography (EEG) of Human Sleep: Clinical Applications.* New York: John Wiley.

22. Coons, S. (1987). Development of sleep and wakefulness during the first 6 months of life. In C. Guilleminault (ed.), *Sleep and Its Disorders in Children.* New York: Raven Press.

23. Gaultier, C. (1987). Respiratory adaptation during sleep from the neonatal period to adolescence. In C. Guilleminault (ed.), *Sleep and Its Disorders in Children.* New York: Raven Press.

24. Horne, J. (1988). *Why We Sleep.* New York: Oxford University Press.

25. Gaillard, J.-M. (1985). Neurochemical regulation of the states of alertness. Ann Clin Res 17:175–184.

26. Dahlstrom, A., & Fuxe, K. (1964). A method for the demonstration of monoamine-containing fibers in the central nervous system. Act Physiol Scand 60:293–294.

27. Dement, W., Henriksen, S., & Ferguson, J. (1973). The effect of the chronic administration of para-chlorophenylalanine (PCPA) on sleep parameters in the cat. In J. Barchas & E. Usdin (eds.), *Serotonin and Behavior.* Orlando: Academic Press.

28. King, C. D. (1974). 5-Hydroxytryptamine and sleep in the cat: A brief overview. Adv Biochem Psychopharm 11:211–216.

29. Ursin, R. (1974). Sleep after 5-HTP in the cat. Sleep Res 3:44.

30. Jouvet, M. (1973). Serotonin and sleep in the cat. In J. Barchas & E. Usdin (eds.), *Serotonin and Behavior.* Orlando: Academic Press.

31. Sinha, A. K. (1973). Cat brain serotonin content during sleep and wakefulness. In J. Barchas & E. Usdin (eds.), *Serotonin and Behavior.* Orlando: Academic Press.

32. Tagliamonte, A., Gessa, R., Biggio, B., Vargui, L., & Gessa, G. L. (1974). Daily changes of free tryptophan in humans. Life Sci 14:349–354.

33. Fernstron, J. D., & Wurtman, R. J. (1974). Control of brain serotonin levels by the diet. Adv Biochem Psychopharm 11:133–142.

34. Griffiths, W. J., Lester, B. K., Coulter, J., & Williams, H. L. (1971). Tryptophan and sleep. Biol Psychol Bull 1:20–23.

35. Hartmann, E., Cravens, J., & List, S. (1973). L-tryptophan as a natural hypnotic: A dose-response study in man. Sleep Res 2:59.

36. Sheu, Y.-S., Nelson, J. P., & Bloom, F. E. (1974). Discharge patterns of cat raphe neurons during sleep and waking. Brain Res 73:263–276.

37. Cho-Chung, R. S., & Pitot, H. C. (1967). Feedback control of rat liver tryptophan pyrrolase. J Biol Chem 242:1192–1198.

38. Cho-Chung, R. S., & Pitot, H. C. (1968). Regulatory effects of nicotinamide on tryptophan pyrrolase synthesis in rat liver in vivo. Eur J Biochem 3:401–406.

39. Freeman, F. R., Salinas-Garcia, R. F., & Ward, J. W. (1974). Sleep patterns in a patient with brain stem infarction involving the raphe nucleus. Electroencephalogr Clin Neurophysiol 36:657–660.

40. Morgane, P. J., & Stern, W. C. (1973). Monoaminergic systems in the brain and their role in the sleep states. In J. Barchas & E. Usdin (eds.), *Serotonin and Behavior.* Orlando: Academic Press.

41. Cramer, H., Rudolph, J., Consbruch, U., & Kendel, K. L. (1974). On the effects of melatonin on sleep and behavior in man. Adv Biochem Psychopharmacol 11:187–191.

42. Pickard, G. E., & Turek, F. W. (1983). The suprachiasmatic nuclei: Two circadian clocks? Brain Res 268:201–210.

43. Takahashi, J. S., & Zatz, M. (1982). Regulation of circadian rhythmicity. Science 217:1104–1111.

44. Czeisler, C. A., Kronauer, R., Allan, J. S., Duffy, J. F., Jewett, M. E., Brown, E. N., & Ronda, J. M. (1989). Bright light induction of strong (type O)

resetting of the human circadian pacemaker. Science *244*:1328–1333.

45. Moore-Ede, M. C., Sulzman, F. M., & Fuller, C. A. (1982). *The Clocks That Time Us.* Cambridge: Harvard University Press.

46. Moore-Ede, M. C., Czeisler, C. A., & Richardson, G. S. (1983). Circadian timekeeping in health and disease. Part I. Basic properties of circadian pacemaker. N Engl J Med *309*:469–476.

47. Moore-Ede, M. C., Czeisler, C. A., & Richardson, G. S. (1983). Circadian timekeeping in health and disease. Part 2. Clinical implications of circadian rhythmicity. N Engl J Med *309*:330–336.

48. Hobson, J. A. (1974). The cellular basis of sleep cycle control. Adv Sleep Res *1*:217–250.

49. Hobson, J. A., Lydic, R., & Baghdoyan, H. A. (1986). Evolving concepts of sleep cycle generation: From brain centers to neuronal populations. Behav Brain Sci *9*:371–448.

50. Steriade, M., & Hobson, J. A. (1976). Neuronal activity during the sleep-waking cycle. Prog Neurobiol *6*:155–376.

51. Koella, W. P. (1984). The organization and regulation of sleep: A review of the experimental evidence and a novel integrated model of the organizing and regulating apparatus. Experientia *40*:309–408.

52. Orem, J., & Barnes, C. D. (1980). *Physiology in Sleep.* Orlando: Academic Press.

53. Phillipson, E. A. (1978). Control of breathing during sleep. Am Rev Respir Dis *118*:909–939.

54. Parmeggiani, P. L. (1985). Regulation of circulation and breathing during sleep: Experimental aspects. Ann Clin Res *17*:185–189.

55. Motta, J., & Guilleminault, C. (1985). Cardiac dysfunction during sleep. Ann Clin Res *17*:190–198.

56. Guilleminault, C. (1985). Disorders of excessive sleepiness. Ann Clin Res *17*:209–219.

57. Horne, J. A. (1985). Sleep function, with particular reference to sleep deprivation. Ann Clin Res *17*:199–208.

58. Munari, C., & Calbucci, F. (1981). Correlations between intracranial pressure and EEG during coma and sleep. Electroencephalogr Clin Neurophysiol *51*:170–176.

59. Adam, K. (1980). Sleep as a restorative process and a theory to explain why. Prog Brain Res *53*:289–306.

60. Adam, K., & Oswald, I. (1983). Protein synthesis, body renewal and the sleep-wake cycle. Clin Sci *65*:561–567.

61. Hauri, P. (1989). Primary insomnia. In M. H. Kryger, T. Roth, & W. C. Dement (eds.), *Principles and Practice of Sleep Medicine.* Philadelphia, W. B. Saunders.

62. Guilleminault, C. (1989). Narcolepsy syndrome. In M. H. Kryger, T. Roth, & W. C. Dement (eds.), *Principles and Practice of Sleep Medicine.* Philadelphia, W. B. Saunders.

63. Billiard, M. (1985). Narcolepsy. Ann Clin Res *17*:220–226.

64. Rogers, A. E. (1987). Memory deterioration versus attentional deficits in patients with narcolepsy. Abst. Sleep Res *16*:418.

65. Guilleminault, C., & Dement, W. C. (1978). *Sleep Apnea Syndromes.* New York: Alan R. Liss.

66. Bradley, T. D. & Phillipson, E. A. (1985). Pathogenesis and pathophysiology of the obstructive sleep apnea syndrome. Med Clin North Am *69*:1169–1186.

67. Guilleminault, C. (1985). Obstructive sleep apnea: The clinical syndrome and historical perspective. Med Clin North Am *69*:1187–1204.

68. White, D. P. (1985). Central sleep apnea. Med Clin North Am *69*:1205–1220.

69. Kuna, S. T., & Remmers, J. E. Neural and anatomic factors related to upper airway occlusion during sleep. Med Clin North Am *69*:1221–1242.

70. Shepard, J. W. (1985). Gas exchange and hemodynamics during sleep. Med Clin North Am *69*:1243–1264.

71. Wittels, E. H. (1985). Obesity and hormonal factors in sleep and sleep apnea. Med Clin North Am *69*:1265–1280.

72. Kaplan, J., & Staats, B. A. (1990). Obstructive sleep apnea syndrome. Mayo Clin Proc *65*:1087–1094.

73. Fletcher, E. C. (1990). Chronic lung disease in the sleep apnea syndrome. Lung *168*(Suppl):751–761.

74. Sullivan, C. E., & Grunstein, R. R. (1989). Continuous positive airway pressure in sleep-disordered breathing. In M. H. Kryger, T. Roth, & W. C. Dement (eds.), *Principles and Practice of Sleep Medicine.* Philadelphia: W. B. Saunders.

75. Horne, J. A., & Ostberg, O. (1976). A self-assessment questionnaire to determine morningness eveningness in human circadian rhythms. Int J Chronobiol *4*:97–110.

76. Takahashi, J. S., & Zatz, M. (1982). Regulation of circadian rhythmicity. Science *217*:1104–1110.

77. Czeisler, C. A., Moore-Ede, M. C., & Coleman, R. M. (1983). Resetting circadian clocks: Applications to sleep disorders medicine and occupational health. In C. Guilleminault & E. Lugaresi (eds.), *Sleep/Wake Disorders: Natural History, Epidemiology, and Long-Term Evolution* (pp. 243–260). New York: Raven Press.

78. Akerstedt, T. (1985). Shifted sleep hours. Ann Clin Res *17*:273–279.

79. Lee, K. A., Hicks, G., & Nino-Murcia, G. (1991). Validity and reliability of a scale to assess fatigue. Psychiatry Res *36*:291–298.

80. Janson, C., Gislason, T., Boman, G., Hetta, J., & Roos, B. E. (1990). Sleep disturbances in patients with asthma. Respir Med *84*:37–42.

81. Landis, C. A., Robinson, C. R., & Levine, J. D. (1988). Sleep fragmentation in the arthritic rat. Pain *34*:93–99.

82. Landis, C. A., Levine, J. D., & Robinson, C. R. (1989). Decreased slow-wave and paradoxical sleep in a rat chronic pain model. Sleep *12*:167–177.

83. Landis, C. A., Robinson, C. R., Helms, C., & Levine, J. D. (1989). Differential effects of acetylsalicylic acid and acetaminophen on sleep abnormalities in a rat chronic pain model. Brain Res *488*:195–201.

84. Crosby, L. J. (1989). Fatigue, pain, depression, and sleep disturbance in rheumatoid arthritis patients. In S. G. Funk, E. M. Tornquist, M. T. Champagne, L. A. Copp, & R. A. Wiese (eds.), *Key Aspects of Comfort: Management of Pain, Fatigue, and Nausea.* New York, Springer.

85. Shaver, J., Giblin, E., Lentz, M., & Lee, K. (1988). Sleep patterns and stability in perimenopausal women. Sleep *11*:556–561.

86. Shaver, J. L. F., Giblin, E., & Paulsen, V. (1991). Sleep quality subtypes in midlife women. Sleep *14*:18–23.

87. Guilleminault, C. (ed.). (1982). *Sleeping and Waking Disorders: Indications and Techniques.* Menlo Park, CA: Addison-Wesley.

88. Richardson, G. S., Carskadon, M. A., Flagg, W., Van Den Hoed, J., Dement, W. C., & Mitler, M. M. (1978). Excessive daytime sleepiness in man: Multiple sleep latency measurement in narcoleptic and control subjects. Electroencephalogr Clin Neurophysiol 45:621–627.

89. Shaver, J. L. F., & Giblin, E. C. (1989). Sleep. In J. J. Fitzpatrick, R. L. Taunton, & J. Q. Benoliel (eds.), *Annual Review of Nursing Research* (vol. 7, pp. 71–93). New York: Springer.

90. Snyder-Halpern, R., & Verran, J. A. (1987). Instrumentation to describe subjective sleep characteristics in healthy subjects. Res Nurs Health 10:155–163.

91. White, M. A., Wear, E., & Stephenson, G. (1983). A computer-compatible method for observing falling asleep behavior of hospitalized children. Res Nurs Health 6:191–198.

92. Hoddes, E., Dement, W. C., & Larcone, V. (1972). The history and use of the Stanford sleepiness scale. Psychophysiology 8:150.

93. Hoddes, E., Zarcone, V., Smyth, H., Phillips, R., & Dement, W. C. (1974). Quantification of sleepiness: A new approach. Psychophysiology 11:133–146.

94. Mayer, B. L., & Robinson, C. R. (1987). Quality of sleep and the relationship to sleep promotion methods (abstr.). Sleep Res 16:490.

95. Ellis, B. W., Johns, M. W., Lancaster, R., Raptopoulos, P., Angelopoulos, N., & Priest, R. G. (1981). The St. Mary's Hospital Sleep Questionnaire: A Study of Reliability. Sleep 4:93–97.

96. Dunn, K. B., & Robinson, C. R. (1987). Auditory stimuli and sleep disturbance in preschool children in the pediatric intensive care unit (abstr.). Sleep Res 16:249.

97. Fontaine, D. K. (1989). Measurement of nocturnal sleep patterns in trauma patients. Heart Lung 18:402–410.

98. Robinson, C. R., McKay, T., Lanuza, D. L., & Patel, M. (1987). Circadian rhythms in intracranial pressure (abstr.). Sleep Res 16:632.

99. Robinson, C. R. Biological rhythms in intracranial pressure. Unpublished manuscript, 1987.

100. Lanuza, D. L., Robinson, C. R., McKay, T., Patel, M., & Marotta, S. F. (1987). Heart rate and temperature periodicities in head injured patients (abstr.). Sleep Res 16:623.

101. Lanuza, D. L., Robinson, C. R., Patel, M., & Marotta, S. (1989). Biological rhythms in blood pressure in head injury. J Appl Nurs 2:135–139.

102. Kaplan, J., & Staats, B. A. (1990). Obstructive sleep apnea syndrome. Mayo Clin Proc 65:1087–1094.

103. Fletcher, E. C. (1990). Chronic lung disease in the sleep apnea syndrome. Lung 168(Suppl.):751–761.

104. Stoohs, R., & Guilleminault, C. (1990). Obstructive sleep apnea syndrome or abnormal upper airway resistance during sleep? J Clin Neurophysiol 7:83–92.

105. Pelausa, E. O., & Tarshis, L. M. (1989). Surgery for snoring. Laryngoscope 99(10 Pt. 1):1006–1010.

106. Guilleminault, C., Riley, R. W., & Powell, N. B. (1989). Surgical treatment of obstructive apnea. In M. H. Kryger, T. Roth, & W. C. Dement (eds.), *Principles and Practice of Sleep Medicine.* Philadelphia: W. B. Saunders.

107. Meyer, J. B., & Knudson, R. C. (1990). The sleep apnea syndrome. Part II: Treatment. J Prosthet Dent 63:320–324.

108. Lombard, R. M., Jr., & Zwillich, C. W. (1985). Medical therapy of obstructive sleep apnea. Med Clin North Am 69:1317–1336.

109. Thawley, S. E. (1985). Surgical treatment of obstructive sleep apnea. Med Clin North Am 69:1337–1358.

110. Carskadon, M. A., & Dement, W. C. (1980). Distribution of REM sleep on a 90 minute sleep-wake schedule. Sleep 2:309–317.

111. Richardson, G. S., Carskadon, M. A., Orav, E. J., & Dement, W. C. (1982). Circadian variation of sleep tendency in elderly and young adult subjects. Sleep 5:S82–S94.

112. Lavie, P. (1986). Ultrashort sleep-waking schedule. III. "gates" and "forbidden zones" for sleep. Electroencephalogr Clin Neurophysiol 63:414–425.

113. Van Cauter, E. (1990). Diurnal and ultradian rhythms in human endocrine function: A minireview. Hormone Res 34:45–53.

114. Robinson, C. R., Pegram, G. V., Hyde, P. R., Beaton, J. M., & Smythies, J. R. (1977). The effects of nicotinamide upon sleep in humans. Biol Psychiatry 12:130–144.

115. Robinson, C. R., Pegram, G. V., & Christian, S. T. (1977). Some effects of nicotinamide administration upon mouse brain monoamines. Sleep Res 6:64.

116. Robinson, C. R., & Feinberg, I. (1984). Cortical and subcortical effects of phenylethylhydrazine, a monoamine oxidase inhibitor, on sleep in rats. Sleep Res 13:61.

117. Woods, N. F. (1972). Patterns of sleep in post cardiotomy patients. Nurs Res 21:347–352.

118. Woods, N. F., & Falk, S. A. (1974). Noise stimuli in the acute care area. Nurs Res 23:144–150.

119. Hilton, J. A. (1976). Quantity and quality of patients sleep disturbing factors in a respiratory intensive care unit. J Adv Nurs 1:453–468.

120. Mitler, E. A., & Mitler, M. M. (1992). *101 Questions About Sleep and Dreams.* La Jolla, CA: Wakefulness-Sleep Education and Research Foundation.

IV

ALTERATIONS IN MOTION

Motion is defined as the act or process of changing place with reference to the whole human body, its structures and parts, or its internal components. Thus, movement of the body from one place to another, changing the position or arrangement of the body or its parts, and the movement of ions, molecules, and substances from one side of a cell membrane to the other are all processes encompassed by this definition.

Examples of concepts related to motion include mobility, immobility, diffusion, transudation, circulation, contraction, extension, flexion, osmosis, and flow. The pathological alterations in motion can cause a variety of abnormalities, such as joint dislocations, muscle sprains, stasis of blood flow, remodeling of joint tissues, stasis of pulmonary secretions, cardiac deconditioning, skeletal muscle atrophy, hemorrhage, effusions, edema formation, fluid and electrolyte imbalances, and third space syndromes.

The two chapters in this section (Chapters 21 and 22) represent somewhat different perspectives on motion, that is, the effect of immobility on skeletal muscle size, strength, and endurance, as seen with skeletal muscle atrophy, and edema, the excess accumulation of fluid in tissues in response to altered hydrostatic or oncotic pressures or vascular permeability. The effects of either of these alterations in motion are impaired functional status of the person. Skeletal muscle atrophy results in decreased functional capacity and ability to perform activities of daily living, while edema can impede joint mobility, cause pain, impair gas exchange, or result in serious neurological deficits. Both of these phenomena are very prevalent in patients with acute and chronic illness and are encountered in a wide variety of clinical states and medical diagnoses.

These phenomena affect a wide variety of systems, such as cardiac, pulmonary, renal, and neurological, and are central concepts taught in all nursing programs. Maintenance of normal body motion is traditionally viewed as an important nursing function. Much nursing effort is spent in prevention of the effects of immobility and in support of tissues that have become immobilized, yet much remains unknown about the efficacy of many nursing actions related to these goals. At the same time, nursing research has shown that periods of quiet chair sitting or ambulation to the bathroom have important effects on preventing skeletal muscle atrophy and orthostatic hypotension and in reducing plasma volume losses in patients who otherwise stay in bed. Nursing research in edema has focused on the effects of various nursing activities and body positions on intracranial pressure in patients with cerebral edema. This remains a fruitful area for nursing research as newer and more valid measures of cerebral perfusion become available.

21

Skeletal Muscle Atrophy

Christine E. Kasper

DEFINITION

Skeletal muscle atrophy is defined as the decrease in the mass and cross-sectional area of a skeletal muscle that occurs when the average activities of daily living are decreased below normal levels (Table 21–1). Research suggests that atrophy of skeletal muscle is a major sequela of most pathophysiological phenomena, such as fatigue.[1]

Skeletal muscle function depends on intact proprioceptive activity, motor innervation, mechanical load, and mobility of joints.[1–5] If one of these factors is changed, the muscle then adapts to a new functional set-point that is dependent on its average daily level of activity. When either movement or weight-bearing is decreased, skeletal muscle adapts by reducing its mass and cross-sectional area.

Skeletal muscle mass is decreased by increasing protein degradation and decreasing protein synthesis.[6, 7] The muscle is unable to replace lost fibers and myofibrils, resulting in a decreased muscle size. A prolonged decrease in contractile activity, as seen in decreased movement and weight-bearing, is the principal stimulus for the occurrence of skeletal muscle atrophy.

Decreased contractile activity can be caused by decreased movement (hypokinesia, HK) or decreased weight-bearing (hypodynamia, HD). In the more extreme forms of decreased activity, a muscle may lose up to 50 per cent of its mass in 3 weeks.[8] Following a period of decreased contractile activity, subjects have impaired functional capacity and a reduced ability to perform their normal daily activities owing to a loss of skeletal muscle mass.

PREVALENCE AND POPULATIONS AT RISK

All hospitalized patients, bedfast and ambulatory, are subjected to some form of restricted mobility. Patients with activity restriction make up a major portion of both the short-term and long-term inpatient nursing case load. The hospital environment structures the amount of functional activity that a fully mobile patient is capable of performing and effectively decreases the level of daily activity. The incidence of disuse atrophy is not limited to inpatients; people in the community whose mobility is decreased by illness or symptoms such as pain, fatigue, and dysp-

TABLE 21–1 ETIOLOGY OF SKELETAL MUSCLE ATROPHY

Disuse
  ↓ Activities of daily living
  ↓ Weight-bearing
  ↓ Motion
Bed rest
Microgravity
Mechanical ventilation
Psychiatric
  Depression
  Schizophrenia
Physiological aging

Immobility
Orthopedic
  Casting
  Traction
  Joint immobilization
Paralysis
Pathological
  Paralytic poliomyelitis
  Guillain-Barré syndrome

Pharmacological
Glucocorticoids

nea are also at high risk for the development of disuse atrophy.

The major losses of skeletal muscle mass and contractile proteins occur during the first 3 to 13 days of inactivity.[9] It is important to note that this time frame is the same as that of the average number of days of restricted activity (14.2 days per person) due to chronic or acute illness or injuries.[10] Therefore, nearly all patient populations are at risk for the occurrence of skeletal muscle atrophy resulting from decreased levels of activity (Table 21–2).

SITUATIONAL STRESSORS

Situational stressors are those factors that act upon a patient to decrease the average activities of daily living. These factors may limit the activity of discrete anatomical segments or of the whole body. For example, orthopedic casting and traction of limbs are situational stressors that produce rapid and severe atrophy of skeletal muscle. Casting of a limb or joint is a true form of immobilization atrophy, as it prevents both range of motion and load on the muscle. A significant and rapid decline in the rates of protein synthesis occurs in immobilized muscle and begins by the sixth hour of cast immobilization.[11]

At the other end of the continuum of severity are patients who are limited in their activity by viral infections such as influenza. These patients experience a mild atrophy that occurs in proportion to their decrease in activity. These individuals continue to ambulate and conduct their normal activities of daily living but at a slower pace. Protein synthesis declines only mildly, and the resulting losses of skeletal muscle are minor. Research studies have not yet clearly defined the magnitude of skeletal muscle degradation that is necessary to produce symptomatology.

Decreasing activity during periods of illness is an adaptive and protective mechanism. It is during these periods of conservation of movement that skeletal muscle structure and function adapt to the new lower level of activity. Interventions, such as range of motion and ambulation, may decrease the magnitude of the atrophy to a small extent, but only activities that match the duration and intensity of prior daily activity will prevent the onset of disuse atrophy.[12–14] Unfortunately, it is often beyond the

TABLE 21–2 **HIGH RISK FOR SKELETAL MUSCLE ATROPHY**

High-Risk Populations	High-Risk Factors
Intensive care patients	Restriction of mobility due to bed rest
Orthopedic Patients Fractures Traction Pinning of joints	Immobilization, diminished muscle contraction
Patients with chronic low back pain	Pain, guarding of site, restriction of mobility
Elderly patients	Diminished mobility, restriction to chairs, surgical restriction of movement, medications, social isolation, depression
Patients with neurological disorders Closed head injury Cerebrovascular accident Spinal injury Neuromuscular disorder	Diminished or restricted movement and weight-bearing
Patients with nutritional deficiencies Anorexia Cachexia	Catabolism of lean body mass, diminished force generation
Astronauts	Weightlessness, decreased load on skeletal muscle and cardiovascular system, diminished weight-bearing
Patients with psychogenic disorders Depression Schizophrenia Organic brain syndrome	Decreased mobility and possible immobility
Postoperative patients	Altered mobility due to fatigue and pain
Pregnant women	High-risk pregnancies, antitocolytic therapy, bed rest
Cancer patients	Fatigue, diminished mobility, medication, pain
Respiratory patients Mechanical ventilation	Severe restriction of mobility, diminished contraction of respiratory muscles, drug-induced paralysis, dyspnea
Emphysema	Diminished mobility due to insufficient tissue perfusion of oxygen
Patients on corticosteroids	Drug-induced atrophy of skeletal muscle
Patients with unrelieved pain	Guarding of site, resulting in a restriction of movement

ability of the patient who is functionally limited by illness to maintain a high level of activity. The patient's movement, weight-bearing, and general activity can be increased only within the constraints of that pathological process. An awareness of the gap between these two different levels of activities of daily living will provide the nurse with the information necessary to plan the patient's recovery.

Clinical States

Until the 19th century, the bed was considered a place for sleeping. Only the terminally ill took to their beds during the daytime, and they did so with great aversion. As with the cowboys of the Old West, it was considered a sin to die with one's boots off. A change in this philosophy occurred between 1860 and 1862, when John Hilton, a surgeon at Guy's Hospital in London, gave a series of lectures on applied anatomy and physiology.[15] He proposed what appeared to be a coherent argument supporting the use of bed rest as a therapeutic measure. This series of lectures was published as "Rest and Pain: The Influence of Mechanical and Physiological Rest" and became a bestseller in 1863.[15] This popular book moved the bed from a place to sleep to the best form of medical therapy. To some extent, most patients are still encouraged to reduce their activities of daily living; however, they are not as strictly confined to supine bed rest as in the past. Certain categories of patients, such as those with myocardial infarction, are no longer strictly confined to their beds during treatment and are often encouraged to rapidly regain mobility.

Clinically, skeletal muscle atrophy can be caused by two major conditions: (1) inactivity, also known as disuse, and (2) immobilization (Table 21–1). Atrophy caused by pharmacological interventions forms a third minor category. Inactivity and immobilization are better understood as existing on a continuum of impaired mobility. Inactivity or disuse atrophy is defined as atrophy resulting solely from decreased movement and weight-bearing. The muscles in question have not been subjected to immobilization, denervation, or other pathological conditions.

Clinically, the most common forms of disuse atrophy are those caused by diminished activities of daily living and bed rest. Previously in the nursing literature, atrophy due to inactivity or disuse had been erroneously grouped with atrophy due to immobilization.[16] Atrophy due to immobilization is a subset of skeletal muscle atrophy and is specific only to those cases in which segments of the body are confined and immobilized by casts, traction, or motor neural defects.[17–19] On a continuum of severity, atrophy due to immobilization is severe and second only to that experienced in weightlessness or paralysis.[20–22]

The severity of skeletal muscle atrophy is directly related to two key variables: (1) the duration of decreased activity and (2) the magnitude of the restriction of activity. These variables affect the majority of patient populations regardless of diagnostic category and vary in prevalence in different patient populations (Table 21–2). This variation corresponds directly with the duration and magnitude of restriction of movement and weight-bearing. For example, a postoperative patient would have more mobility and less atrophy than a patient in bilateral leg traction.

The risk for skeletal muscle atrophy may be specific to one muscle group or may involve the total body muscle mass. It is the additive effect of the duration of decreased movement, decreased weight-bearing, and the individual's pathological condition that determines the severity of skeletal muscle atrophy. The risk of involving other organ systems, such as the cardiovascular system, is linearly related to the total percentage of skeletal muscle mass that is involved. For example, a highly mobile patient whose right arm is casted is at risk only for atrophy of the affected limb. Conversely, patients breathing with assisted ventilation and restricted to total bed rest and receiving glucocorticoids are at very high risk for severe skeletal muscle atrophy as well as all of the associated organ system sequelae.

In addition to restriction of mobility and movement, disease itself may exacerbate the magnitude of skeletal muscle protein loss. For example, certain cancer cells excrete tumor necrosis factor (TNF), which has been found to lyse skeletal muscle cells and produce severe forms of degeneration and atrophy.[23] This form of atrophy may contribute to the fatigue experienced by oncology patients.[24]

Alternate environments may also place certain populations at risk. It is currently rare for nurses to care for patients following prolonged microgravity exposure; however, this environment causes atrophy by removing the force of gravity or load from skeletal muscle. The microgravity of space flight produces atrophy of skeletal muscle that is as severe as that produced by casting. The mass of the leg muscles has been reported to atrophy 11 per cent during the Skylab missions.[25, 26]

Pharmacological intervention also produces skeletal muscle atrophy (Table 21–3). The development of skeletal muscle weakness and atrophy is a well-known complication of exogenous glucocorticoid administration.[27, 28] Specifically, it is the fluorinated glucocorticoids (triamcinolone, betamethasone, and dexamethasone) that cause this form of clinical myopathy.[29, 30] Glucocorticoids primarily inhibit protein synthesis and result in generalized atrophy of the muscles.[30–32]

Decreased protein synthesis reduces muscle size by decreasing the volume and density of myofibrils and is manifested as weakness due to atrophied muscles, especially in the leg and thigh. Chronic glucocorticoid therapy and Cushing's disease result in the preferential atrophy of type II (fast-twitch fiber) groups, while the type I (slow-twitch oxidative) fibers are not as severely affected.[33, 34] The characteristic type II atrophy is opposite that of atrophy due to disuse or immobilization, in which type I fibers are preferentially affected. Loss of muscle tissue in these patients can approach 30 per cent compared with normal populations.[35] The loss of type II fibers affects the ability to maintain contractile force, especially during anaerobic activity.

DEVELOPMENTAL DIMENSIONS

Development

Movement is fundamental to the development of mature skeletal muscle during the neonatal period.[36, 37] Restriction of normal patterns of movement may alter the growth and development of skeletal muscle. Immobilization of neonatal muscles in the shortened position decreases the longitudinal growth of the involved muscle.[38] Studies have demonstrated that reduced longitudinal growth results from the myofibrils failing to develop sarcomeres in series, that is, at the ends of the muscle. Skeletal muscle is able to recover to normal resting lengths following a period of time that is approximately equal to the duration of immobilization and occurs by the addition of sarcomeres in series to the ends of myofibrils.[38]

Clinically, adaptation of muscle length is seen following tendon transplantations. If the length of a muscle is increased owing to tendon transplantation of the distal end, the muscle will adapt to the new functional length within a few weeks.[39] Unlike developing muscle, the adult muscle has a remarka-

TABLE 21–3 EFFECTS OF GLUCOCORTICOIDS ON SKELETAL MUSCLE PROTEIN SYNTHESIS

Muscle	Drug	Duration (Days)	Change (%)
Soleus	Dexamethasone (25 mg/kg)	5	−7
Gastrocnemius, white	Dexamethasone (100 mg/kg)	2	−29
		4	−52
		8	−33
Gastrocnemius, red	Dexamethasone (100 mg/kg)	2	−25
		4	−34
Soleus	Cortisol acetate (100 mg/kg)	5	No change
Gastrocnemius, whole	Cortisol acetate (100 mg/kg)	5	−55
Extensor digitorum longus	Cortisol acetate (100 mg/kg)	3	−42

Data from Müller & Kugelberg, J Neurol Neurosurg Psychiatry 22:314, 1959[28]; Ruff et al, Am J Physiol 243:E512, 1982[30]; Askari et al, Am J Med 61:485, 1976[31]; Kelly & Goldspink, Biochem J 208:147, 1982[32]; Khaleeli et al, Clin Endocrinol 18:155, 1983[33]; Clarke, in Wilmore (ed.): *Exercise and Sport Science Reviews*, New York, Academic Press, 1973[125]; and Mayer & Rosen, Metabolism 26:937, 1977.[155]

ble ability to adapt to changes in length. If immobilized in the lengthened position, a muscle will add 25 per cent of its sarcomeres in series within 2 to 3 days. When the immobilization is removed, sarcomere length is recovered within 1 week.

Muscle cells are more susceptible to the modifying influences of reduced activity in the neonatal period.[40, 41] For example, if the weight-bearing muscles of the leg are prevented from normal movement during this period, they are unable to develop normal contractile characteristics and normal enzymatic properties.[42] The long-term consequences of these alterations are not yet known. Infants restrained or placed in traction or plaster casts for any prolonged period of time are at risk for alterations in skeletal muscle function. An example of restraint in this population would be spica casts or long-term restraint.

During early development, the action of insulin and growth hormones stimulates skeletal muscle growth and maturation. In the absence of these hormones, there is abnormal development and growth.[43] Testosterone has been shown to have a direct effect on skeletal muscle growth.[43] In adolescent males, continued muscle growth is stimulated by testosterone. When insufficient testosterone is present during adolescence, skeletal muscle growth will be severely limited. Therefore, skeletal muscle growth varies with the normal or abnormal variations in hormonal levels of individuals.

Aging

During the process of aging, a progressive loss of lean body mass occurs as a result of the gradual loss of the total number of muscle fibers. Between the ages of 30 and 80 there is a gradual loss of 40 per cent in the lean body mass with an associated increase in the spread of fiber sizes.[44] This loss of muscle mass is reflected in a decreased cross-sectional area of the muscle and parallels a drop in muscular strength.[44–46]

Isometric and dynamic maximal strength also functionally declines beyond age 50.[47] Aging and inactivity exert similar deleterious effects on skeletal muscle function; however, the rate of atrophy due to inactivity is far more rapid than that of aging. When inactivity or immobilization is superimposed on aging muscle, the resulting atrophy may be more severe and may require a longer period of recovery.

A significant factor in the recovery of skeletal muscle following atrophy is the satellite cell.[48] Satellite cells are found between the sarcolemma and basal lamina of all skeletal muscle fibers and are responsible for the regeneration of muscle. They are crucial in the regeneration of aging muscle because their ability to mitotically divide is finite. The ability of a damaged or atrophied aged skeletal muscle to regenerate is impaired owing to a decreased capacity of the satellite cells to divide and proliferate.[49–51]

The neuromuscular system is also capable of changing its structure to reflect altered function. During the human life span, the neuromuscular junction (NMJ) undergoes morphological remodeling from early development through maturity. Exercise and decreased activity are important mediators of this effect prior to the addition of new perturbations in the NMJ due to aging.[52] Aged NMJs have greater nerve terminal areas, branch numbers, and sprouts than young NMJs. The presence of significant morphological changes following only 5 days of subtotal disuse indicates that the NMJ is capable of a rapid anatomical remodeling in response to altered activity. It has been suggested that the simple increase in these structural parameters must underlie increased release of the acetylcholine transmitter in soleus muscle during aging. Acute inactivity also affects the morphology of the NMJ, creating an increase in neurotransmitter (acetylcholine) release. The changes in the NMJ due to decreased activity occur within 5 days of the start of subtotal disuse.

The structural and functional changes that occur in muscle during the process of aging place the inactive geriatric patient at very high risk. Not only will the magnitude of atrophy be more severe, but the ability of the individual to recover from atrophy is limited. If geriatric patients are subjected to cycles of atrophy and recovery, it is hypothetically possible that they will reach a point beyond which they can no longer recover skeletal muscle mass and function, resulting in confinement to the wheelchair and bed. Further research is needed to clarify this phenomenon.

MECHANISMS

Skeletal muscle is "plastic," or adaptable, and alters its structure, mechanical properties, and energy metabolism rapidly to adapt to an activity pattern.[53, 54] Skeletal muscle atrophy due to inactivity or immobilization primarily affects the antigravity muscles of the leg and back; however, all muscles of the body may be involved if their functional demands in the form of activity and muscle load are decreased (Fig. 21–1). The rate and magnitude of skeletal muscle atrophy are regulated by restriction of movement and the amount of weight-bearing or load on a muscle.[3, 9, 55–57]

Mass

Skeletal Muscle Mass

The immobilization of limbs has been shown to lead to muscular atrophy,[58] diminished muscular strength, and increased fatigability.[6, 9, 59, 60] Decreased loading of the weight-bearing muscles of the leg, especially the soleus, also produces a rapid loss of muscle mass. Three days following the start of hypodynamia, there is a decrease of 7 per cent in the muscle mass, with a further decline of 20 per cent after 5 days.[61] Losses have been reported as high as 35 per cent in the first 7 days, 45 per cent by 2 weeks of unloading,[62] and 55 per cent following 42 days of hypodynamia.[63]

Muscle atrophy begins rapidly, and the greatest losses are found early in the period of inactivity or immobilization. The onset of atrophy begins with rapid protein degradation, beginning within 6 hours of diminished activity.[6, 7, 9] Absolute losses of muscle mass and protein are greatest during days 3 to 7 of the period of inactivity or immobilization. The process of protein degradation results in a 14 to 17 per cent decrease in fiber and muscle size following the initial 72 hours.[55, 64]

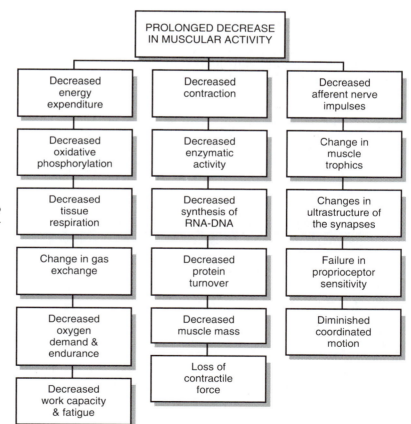

Figure 21–1. Adaptation to decreased skeletal muscle activity.

It is possible to calculate the rate at which a muscle or group of muscles will atrophy by the equation:

$$t\tfrac{1}{2} = \frac{\ln 2}{kd}$$

where $t\tfrac{1}{2}$ is the half-life; $\ln 2$, the natural logarithm of 2; and kd, the first-order rate constant for protein degradation.[55, 64, 65]

It remains unclear which molecular mechanisms are responsible for the regulation of protein synthesis and degradation in response to activity levels.[7, 66] It has been observed that changes in protein synthesis correlate with changes in ribonucleic acid (RNA) content in skeletal muscle following alterations in activity level.[7, 66] Likely regulatory sites for these alterations in muscle are changes in the phosphorylation state of eukaryotic initiation factor 2 (eIF-2).[67]

Total Body Mass

Total body mass decreases during limb immobilization or hypokinesia.[68] The loss of mass is due in part to muscle atrophy but also to alterations in eating habits. Body weight declines sharply during the first 3 days of hypokinesia, and thereafter body weight gradually increases[68] (Table 21–4). Studies have demonstrated that body weight loss in immobile patients with a relatively stable caloric intake of 2744 to 2796 kcal/day is a mean of 1.9 kg/day.[13, 69–72] Following removal of casts and the resumption of activity, body mass is rapidly regained.

Contractile Force

The loss of muscle mass results in a decreased cross-sectional area of muscle. The total cross-sectional area of a muscle is composed of bundles of individual muscle fibers. These fibers are normally 50 to 100 μm in diameter; during atrophy, fiber diameter significantly decreases. The volumetric change in the muscle is due to changes in fiber volume, which first occur by decreasing the size and later the number of the myofibrils within each fiber. During the initial weeks, skeletal muscle volume decreases by 25 to 30 per cent from decreased activity and 75 to 80 per cent in the same time period due to total denervation.[73] There is clear evidence that atrophy occurs in the first few months without a loss in the total number of fibers in the muscle.

The ability of a muscle to produce force is directly proportional to its cross-sectional area. When the cross-sectional area is reduced by the process of atrophy, the ability of a muscle to produce force is decreased. A muscle 1 cm² in cross-section can maximally contract a load of 3 to 4 g; therefore, strength is dependent on the cross-sectional area of muscle. When the cross-sectional area decreases because of atrophy, strength and ability to produce force decrease. Fatigue is a sequela of the process of atrophy and is seen as a limitation in the force-generating capacity or the inability to maintain the required force[1, 74] (Fig. 21–1).

Decreased contractile activity has two characteristic components: decreased mechanical loading and decreased movement. Mechani-

Table 21–4. PHYSIOLOGICAL ADAPTATIONS TO INACTIVITY AND DISUSE

Days 0–3	Days 4–7	Days 8–14	≥ 2 Weeks
↑ Diuresis	Hydroxyprolinuria	↑ Exercise hyperthermia	2° Increase in auditory threshold
↑ Venous compliance	Creatininuria	Pyrophosphaturia	Sensitivity to thermal stimuli
↑ Neutrophil activity	Negative nitrogen balance	↓ Red cell volume	Maximal hypercalciuria
↑ Glucose intolerance	↑ Blood fibrinogen	↓ Sweating	
↓ Gastric secretion	↑ Clotting	↓ Heat conductance	
↓ Peripheral blood flow	Vision changes		
↓ Plasma volume	↑ Auditory threshold		
↓ Interstitial volume	↑ blood flow and pressure in eyes		
↓ Extracellular fluid volume			

Adapted from Maloni, J. A., & Kasper, C. E. (1992). Physical and psychosocial effects of antepartum hospital bed rest: A review of the literature. Image 23(3):187–192.

cal loading occurs when the patient stands and increases the load of a muscle or bears weight. The decreased weight-bearing or mechanical loading component of disuse is known as hypodynamia.[62, 75, 76] Decreased movement or range of motion of the limbs causes decreased contractile activity and is known as hypokinesia. Patients may be subject to only one or both of these limitations.[77, 78]

Contractile and Biochemical Properties

The contractile and biochemical properties of skeletal muscle are altered by disuse atrophy. For example, cast immobilization has been shown to cause an increase in the maximal shortening velocity of normally slow-twitch muscles in the leg. Other changes that occur are a reduction in the isometric twitch contraction time and one-half relaxation time for the soleus muscle and a prolongation of these times for the extensor digitorum longus.[74, 79, 80]

The majority of human muscles can be characterized as fast-twitch or slow-twitch. The differences in the contractile speeds of these muscles are a function of the population of individual fibers of which these muscles are composed. For example, the classic slow-twitch muscle is the soleus, which contains predominantly slow fibers. The extensor digitorum longus and the flexor digitorum longus are faster muscles.

Slow and fast muscles are designed for functionally different purposes. Slow muscles are used for postural support and weight-bearing; fast muscles are used for rapid movement. Their functional uses also reflect two different forms of energy supply. Slow-contracting muscles use adenosine triphosphate (ATP) at a slow rate and have endurance capacities over long periods of time (Table 21–5). Conversely, fast muscle is used for rapid movements, burns ATP at a high rate, and is rapidly fatigued.[81] The energy sources for these two types of muscle are also different. Slow muscles are dependent on ATP synthesis associated with a good oxygen supply and mitochondria. This is known as the oxidative system. Fast muscles, on the other hand, are dependent on anaerobic phosphorylation and glycogen.

Characteristically, slow fibers within a muscle contain relatively high numbers of large mitochondria. Slow fibers are classified as slow oxydative (SO), or type I fibers (Table 21–5). Within the fast fibers, or type II fibers, there are subclassifications: the fast-twitch oxydative-glycolytic fibers (FOG, or type IIA), and the fast-twitch glycolytic fibers (FG, or type IIB). The type IIA fibers are intermediate fibers and contain fast contraction speeds with aerobic and anaerobic energetics, and the type IIB fibers have greater anaerobic capacities.[82]

Alterations in the speed of contraction of an atrophic muscle can be linked to shifts in the regulatory proteins of the muscle. The myosin heads contain ATPase and the actin-binding characteristics of myosin. There is a switch in protein composition during inactivity such that the amount of fast myosin isozymes relative to slow myosin increases markedly in slow muscle.[79] In fast muscle, there is an increase in the slow myosin isozymes. These changes in the myosin heavy chain regulatory proteins create a "regression toward the mean" effect. Slow-contracting endurance muscles become less able to sustain long-term aerobic activity, as inactivity has altered its function to act more like a fast-contracting muscle. The fast-contracting

TABLE 21–5 CLASSIFICATION OF MUSCLE FIBERS BASED ON PHYSIOLOGICAL, BIOCHEMICAL, AND HISTOCHEMICAL PROPERTIES

Property	Group I	Group II	
Twitch contraction time	Slow	Fast	Fast
Fatigability	Low	Intermediate	High
Oxidative enzymes	High	Moderate	Very low
Glycolytic enzymes	Very low	Moderate	High
Myosin ATPase activity	Low	High	High
Histochemical type	I	IIA	IIB

Reprinted from the *Oncology Nursing Forum*, with permission of the Oncology Nursing Press, Inc., St. Pierre, B. A., Kasper, C. E., & Lindsey, A. M. (1992). Fatigue mechanisms in patients with cancer: Effects of TNF and exercise on skeletal muscle. Oncol Nurs Forum 19(3):419–425.

ATPase, adenosine triphosphatase.

muscle also changes its speed and function to become more like a slow-twitch muscle.

The result of these shifts in contractile speed is that the original function of the muscle is altered. Postural muscles, such as the soleus and medial gastrocnemius, are primarily endurance muscles. Following inactivity and atrophy, the changes in their contractile proteins cause them to fatigue easily, as they are no longer predominantly aerobic muscles.[79]

Limbs are generally casted at a resting position to preserve function and prevent contracture. However, skeletal muscle adapts to an imposed static length. When a muscle is fixed in a lengthened position, sarcomeres are added in series to the muscle.[63] In effect, the muscle increases in length to adapt to its new function. Conversely, when muscles are fixed in the shortened position, sarcomeres are removed from the length of the muscle and the muscle decreases in length. These alterations in length occur in addition to the loss of strength and ability to maintain force production that is the result of decreased cross-sectional area with atrophy.[17, 18] Loss of a significant number of sarcomeres along the length of a muscle may permanently alter the length of a muscle. This alteration in length due to sarcomere loss is seen clinically as contracture.

PATHOLOGICAL CONSEQUENCES

The adaptations that occur to skeletal muscle during inactivity and immobilization are not pathological by themselves. They appear to represent a normal attempt of the homeostatic mechanisms to adapt to altered movement and decreased metabolic needs. Altered insulin resistance and injury are two consequences of skeletal muscle atrophy. The lack of recognition of these changes by health care professionals creates the potential for iatrogenesis.

Skeletal Muscle Injury

Injury to skeletal muscle recovering from atrophy is a potential problem. Evidence shows that running causes the degeneration of large segments of postural skeletal muscle. It appears that during the first 3 to 5 days following a period of decreased weight-bearing, strenuous exercise should not be done.[77] Heavy exercise, such as weight lifting or running, places a load in excess of the ability of the atrophied muscle to contract against. When contracting against the increased load, the muscle responds by "ripping" the myofibrils and degenerating.[37, 77, 83] The injured muscle will recover from this damage within 14 days in the absence of continued active exercise.[77]

Insulin Resistance

During inactivity, bed rest, and immobilization, skeletal muscle becomes characteristically diabetic-like. In other words, insulin is unable to stimulate glucose uptake and to activate glycogen synthase in human muscle. This insulin resistance occurs at the third day of inactivity and bed rest and, within 24 hours, in cast immobilization. Clinical studies have demonstrated that false-positive tests for glucose intolerance and diabetes mellitus can occur in humans as a result of inactivity and immobilization.[84, 85]

The administration of an oral glucose load following 3 days of inactivity or bed rest may cause hyperinsulinemia and hyperglycemia, which is indicative of altered carbohydrate metabolism. It has been demonstrated that the longer the period of inactivity and immobility, the greater the altered glucose tolerance responses.[86, 87] As previously discussed with other organ systems, the reduction in carbohydrate tolerance is directly proportional to the amount of restriction of activity.[88, 89] Daily range of motion or other exercise decreases but does not eliminate this response. Following a period of inactivity, it takes approximately 7 to 14 days to recover normal carbohydrate tolerance.[84] If mild exercise is done during this recovery period, only 7 days are needed for plasma glucose levels to return to normal.[89]

Previous studies indicate that some responses to insulin in unloaded hypokinetic muscle differ from those in denervated muscle.[90, 91] Denervated muscle shows insulin resistance of both 2-deoxyl[1,2-^{3}H]glucose and α-[methyl-^{3}H]aminoisobutyric acid uptake and unloaded hypokinetic muscle shows an increased or normal response, respectively.[92] The inhibition of protein degradation and the stimulation of protein synthesis by insulin are less in denervated than in unloaded hypokinetic muscle.[92]

RELATED PATHOPHYSIOLOGICAL CONCEPTS

Decreased activity and immobilization are known to cause alterations in every major organ system. They are the cause of a series of physiological adaptations that ultimately contribute to a deteriorating cardiovascular work capacity. The major adaptations include diminished plasma and blood volume, increased hemoglobin and hematocrit levels, increased resting heart rate, diminished cardiac output and stroke volume, and decreased maximal oxygen uptake.

Cardiovascular Function

Cardiovascular function is affected by intravascular fluid volume losses and changes in cardiac contractility. Parameters within the intravascular compartment that are affected during inactivity and immobilization include blood and plasma volume, hemoglobin hematocrit levels, and red blood cell volume.

Plasma Volume

The most significant changes in the vascular fluid compartment are reductions in plasma and blood volumes. Blood and plasma volumes are influenced by body position. The horizontal recumbent position leads to a decrease in the plasma volume of approximately 500 ml, or 7 per cent of the body weight during the first 24 to 48 hours. Blood pools in the thorax rather than in the lower extremities and creates a cephalic shift of blood volume (Fig. 21–2). The movement of blood into the thorax increases the venous volume, resulting in distention of the central veins and a stimulation of central blood volume receptors that trigger a decrease in antidiuretic hormone (ADH) secretion.[54, 93, 94] Increases in central blood volume induce inhibition of ADH release through left atrial receptors and aldosterone through the right atrial receptors. Inhibition of ADH and aldosterone results in diuresis of salt and water. Fortunately, ADH production follows a pattern of diurnal circadian variation; therefore, normal sleep patterns with the same thoracic pooling of blood do not cause a significant increase in the free water clearance. Table 21–4 shows that with at least 2 days of bed rest there is a significant decline in these volumes. These losses are progressive over

CARDIOVASCULAR ALTERATIONS DUE TO DECREASED ACTIVITY

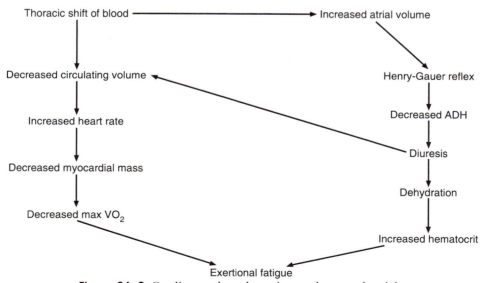

Figure 21–2. Cardiovascular adaptation to decreased activity.

time, with the greatest drop beginning with the second and reaching its nadir at the twentieth day of inactivity.[54, 69, 70, 93–96]

Vascular fluid volume loss is also dependent on the magnitude of the restriction of movement. Uncomplicated inactivity causes a plasma volume loss of 220 ml and blood volume loss of 340 ml in humans.[97] Severe losses of fluid volume were reported as a result of a 200-day period of confinement.[98] This study reported plasma volume losses of 600 ml at 70 days, 900 ml at 105 days, and 1000 ml from 180 to 200 days of continued bed rest.[99] Recovery of plasma and blood volumes is approximately 1.25 times the duration of inactivity.

Normal values for plasma volume are 42 ml/kg for adult men. Blood volume has a normal value of 64 to 69 ml/kg. A 10 to 20 per cent decrease in these values accompanied by increased hematocrit and hemoglobin levels would present a suspicious picture to the attending medical and nursing staff of any hospital. It has been observed that patients admitted for conditions that require decreased activity and result in confinement to bed are often the first to demonstrate signs of dehydration and abnormal laboratory values. These changes are uniformly followed by the regulation of intake and output along with intravenous infusion. The sudden, and unexplained, drop in hematocrit and hemoglobin levels that occurs 3 days after inactivity may also lead to unnecessary medication and treatment.

Red Blood Cell Volume

As the plasma and blood volume decreases during a period of horizontal inactivity, there is a corresponding increase in hemoglobin concentration and hematocrit level. Small increases in hematocrit and hemoglobin levels, usually nonsignificant, occur during the period of bed rest. However, after a period of inactivity and immobilization has ended, a significant drop in hemoglobin and hematocrit levels occurs in the first week of recovery.[70, 100, 101] Hemoglobin level decreases 1.7 g/dl, or 12 per cent, at the third day after bed rest.[101] The decrease in these values does not coincide with the return of plasma volume.

Hypodynamic states cause decreases in red blood cell volume.[70, 101, 102] Red blood cell mass is a more stable parameter than plasma vol-ume, as these cells cannot be stored or mobilized as plasma proteins can, and therefore losses are replaced slowly. Red blood cells have a fairly finite life span and live approximately 120 days. Inactivity and immobilization produce a consistent drop in red blood cell mass, which may be related to decreased erythropoietin production. No evidence for red cell hemolysis during inactivity and immobilization has been demonstrated. Recovery of the decreased red blood cell mass is incomplete 35 days after inactivity.[70, 101, 102]

Cardiac Output and Stroke Volume

Cardiac output and stroke volume are dependent on alterations in plasma volume and heart rate and are also affected by changes in body position. Movement from the upright to the supine position increases the cardiac output 25 to 30 per cent, while stroke volume is increased by 40 per cent.[71, 102–104] Conversely, when the position is changed from supine to standing or sitting, there is a decrease in the end-diastolic size of the heart and a decrease in stroke volume.

The stroke volume of the heart is affected by various factors; venous return to the heart, distensibility of the ventricles, and force of contraction in relation to pressure in the aorta or pulmonary arteries. Therefore, when the extracellular fluid is decreased by clinical states such as bed rest, a decrease in cardiac output may also occur[71, 102–104] (Fig. 21–2). Maximal cardiac output has been reported as 20 L/minute before and 14.8 L/minute following bed rest.[96, 105] Also, bed rest produces a marked decrease in stroke volume from 103 ml before bed rest and 86 ml following bed rest; with the patient in the sitting position, the stroke volume decreases 25 per cent.

In a normal individual in the recumbent position, the left ventricular stroke volume determined angiographically is approximately 60 to 70 per cent of volumes in upright control patients. Increased contractility may increase the ejection fraction and the stroke volume by producing a decreased end-systolic volume (ESV) with the end-diastolic volume (EDV) either decreasing or remaining the same. The heart compensates for the change in stroke volume by decreasing EDV 13 per cent and increasing ESV 13 per cent.[102] An increased stroke volume can also be produced by an increase in venous return, which increases the end-diastolic fiber length of the atria and ventricles. Following prolonged supine bed rest, the ability to increase the venous return is unlikely because of the decrease in plasma volume plus the tendency to pool blood in the legs in the upright position.

Heart Rate

As stroke volume and cardiac output decrease with inactivity or immobilization, the ability of the cardiovascular system to return blood to the heart is decreased. Heart rate increases to compensate, which is one of the simplest and most effective ways of increasing cardiac output. It is the most important and most frequently used mechanism for effecting rapid changes in cardiac output, particularly in untrained persons under conditions of moderately increased demands. An increase in heart rate by itself increases cardiac output threefold.

Resting supine heart rate can increase 2 to 5 beats per minute over 1 week of inactivity.[101, 106] Heart rate averages an increase of 0.5 beats per minute per day of decreased activity and immobilization.[107]

Increased heart rate upon rising from a horizontal position is indicative of orthostatic intolerance, and this phenomenon can be attributed to adaptation of the peripheral vasculature to the removal of hydrostatic pressure during supine bed rest.[107] The lack of hydrostatic pressure on lower body vasculature causes the smooth muscle to lose its tone; thus, these lower body blood vessels are unable to constrict and restrict the volume of blood that is delivered when the person returns to an upright position.[13, 102–104, 108]

Heart Size

Heart size has been investigated in an effort to clarify the relationship of stroke volume and inactivity. Heart size decreases following 14 days of supine bed rest.[102, 106] The mean control value was 869 ml and 770 ml ($P < .01$) after bed rest. The decrease of 90 ml corresponds to 11 per cent of the initial volume.

Recovery

Bed rest or supine immobilization appears to affect the ability of the cardiovascular system to respond to the increased demands of ambulation during the immediate post-recumbency period. During the period of confinement, the cardiovascular system adapts to a new relationship with gravity that does not require the hydrostatic column of blood that is a part of upright posture. Commonly, the normal homeostatic mechanisms that constitute the cardiac reserve regulate cardiac output to meet demands of the body and enable the heart to vary its output in response to demands. Most of these mechanisms are interrelated and affect one another, so that the contribution of one part depends on and alters with the addition of the other mechanisms. The decreased metabolic and cardiac needs of the immobile state alter and decrease the cardiac reserve so that it is unable to respond to the activities of daily living after a period of recumbency. The moment that this reserve is needed occurs when the patient begins to ambulate.

Pulmonary Function

Pulmonary function is also reduced following inactivity or immobilization. Secondary to decreased function is an impedance of maximal ventilatory gas exchange, which may be one of the mechanisms that cause $\dot{V}O_2$ max and exercise capacity to diminish following inactivity. Previous studies have demonstrated that the generalized effects of deconditioning do not change total lung capacity, forced vital capacity, 1-second forced expiratory capacity,[106] or residual lung volume.[70] Decreased activity and bed rest do decrease mean minute ventilation[106]; however, this variable is directly correlated to changes in the maximal oxygen uptake ($\dot{V}O_2$max).

Physical Work Capacity

For the skeletal muscle system, reuse damage and insulin resistance are significant conditions that contribute to the symptoms of deconditioning, weakness, and physiological fatigue. These symptoms originate not only with atrophy of skeletal muscle but also with changes in the cardiovascular, respiratory, and skeletal organ systems.

The concepts of deconditioning, weakness, and fatigue are the consequences of an altered ability to perform physical work. Many factors affect the relationship between workload and work capacity. The definitions of this concept are as follows:

1. Physical work, the ability to work, and the faculty of performing work are defined by the term "power."
2. "Capacity" is the maximum power output of the individual.
3. "Load" is the burden placed on the individual or the rate at which work is being performed.[109]

The ability to perform work is dependent on the ability of the muscle cell to transform energy into contractile force.[109] If the system is altered by decreased oxygen or energy delivery, work capacity will decrease.

Deconditioning

Deconditioning is a decrease in work capacity and is due to a loss of $\dot{V}O_2$max, lean body mass, and endurance. Each of these components contributes to the ability of an individual to perform work or exercise. Because oxygenation of the patient has been compromised by lowered oxygen uptake, circulating fluid volume, and cardiac output following inactivity, bed rest, and immobilization, the skeletal muscle is limited in its capacity to perform work. The skeletal muscle is also limited in ability to perform work by contracting against a load with smaller muscles. Because the strength of a muscle is directly related to its size, decreases in size decrease strength. This decrease in strength due to atrophy is perceived by the patient as "weakness" or "fatigue."

Alterations in Calcium Metabolism

In addition to alterations in the cardiovascular system, diminished weight-bearing has a significant effect on the skeleton. The absence of longitudinal weight-bearing on the skeleton during inactivity produces bone demineralization and calcium loss (Box 21–1). Inactivity and immobilization are associated with alterations in bone formation and reab-

---

BOX 21–1

Alterations in Calcium Metabolism During Inactivity

Osteoporosis
Hypercalciuria
Urinary calculi
Soft tissue calcification

---

sorption, which lead to a net negative calcium balance.[98, 110, 111] The magnitude of bone demineralization and calcium depletion is related to the duration and severity of the removal of weight-bearing.[112] These losses destabilize the skeleton and place the patient at risk for fracture (Box 21–1).

Urinary calcium losses during inactivity and bed rest are not related to the amount of calcium intake.[14, 112] Calcium is released from the skeleton during periods of inactivity and excreted.[14, 112, 113] During the growth process, diminished weight-bearing has been reported to decrease normal bone formation.[114, 115]

Patients remain in negative calcium balance even after ambulation has resumed. The duration of the recovery period is approximately equal to the duration of the decrease in weight-bearing.[98, 116] The return to positive calcium balance is time-dependent and is related to the amount of activity. Exercise speeds the recovery from negative calcium balance.[112] Weight-bearing exercise is more effective in restoring calcium retention after a period of inactivity than a sedentary mode of recovery. Following a 28-day period of inactivity, exercise decreases the duration of recovery from 25 days to 5 days.[112]

ASSOCIATED PSYCHOSOCIAL CONCEPTS

Inactivity and immobilization affect people by restraining their mobility and ability to interact with others.[117] Sensory deprivation may also occur in isolation because of inactivity or immobilization. Restriction of mobility has been shown to be a factor in psychological disturbances that occur during sensory deprivation.

Studies of patients confined to bed have shown that sensory deprivation decreases the ability to discriminate weight, temperature sensitivity, perceptions of patterns and forms, and speed of perception. The ability of patients to estimate time is also influenced by the extent of their restriction of activity. Time estimation is distorted so that there is a loss of orientation to person, place, and time. Subjects' estimates of set time intervals were exceeded by 10 to 13 per cent during a 3-day period of inactivity when compared with a control population.[117, 118]

Restriction of activity and immobilization result in sleep disturbances, neurological changes, increased emotional lability, and fatigue. Deterioration of motivation and cognitive performance is also linked to decreased mobility.[117] A number of these changes are due to the physiological impact of inactivity on neurological function; however, the effects of this system are compounded by the physical stress and sensory deprivation.[119] All of these alterations have been demonstrated to increase in magnitude as the duration of inactivity increases.

MANIFESTATIONS

Skeletal muscle atrophy produces a wide range of manifestations that are dependent on the severity and duration of inactivity or immobilization. The primary alterations that occur with skeletal muscle atrophy are decreased strength, decreased exercise capacity, and fatigue.

Strength

Muscular strength is defined as the maximum force or tension generated by a muscle or group of muscles. Human skeletal muscle is capable of generating 3 to 4 kg of force per square centimeter of muscle cross-section irrespective of gender.[120, 121] The greatest forces are exerted by muscles with the greatest cross-sectional areas. Therefore, an early sign of skeletal muscle atrophy is a report of weakness and fatigue as cross-sectional muscle area decreases.[86, 105, 122] Because these signs may also be attributed to medication or disease, they are difficult for the nurse to use in the assessment of strength without further objective data. Quantitative information may be obtained using (1) tensiometry, (2) dynamometry, or (3) computer-assisted force and work output determinations.

Tensiometry. Cable tensiometry is a simple and portable method of measuring the strength of large muscle groups. Tensiometers measure the pulling force of a limb during a static or isometric contraction when there is no change in the muscle's length. Batteries of strength tests have been developed using this device to measure the static force of the hand, fingers, thumb, wrist, forearm, elbow, shoulder, trunk, neck, hip, knee, and ankle.[86, 105, 122–125] These tests enable the nurse to evaluate the strength decrement as a result of skeletal muscle atrophy, and they are highly reproducible on repeated evaluations. The tensiometer may also be used to evaluate strength during various phases of movement and may give a more accurate assessment of patient weakness or strength than other methods.

Dynamometry. Hand-grip dynamometers are also used for the determination of patient strength. These devices work on the principle of compression. When force is applied to the handle of the dynamometer, a steel spring is compressed and moves a needle on a gauge. The resulting number is reflective of the strength applied.[125]

Computerized Dynamometers. Muscle strength may also be monitored using computerized dynamometers, which provide a rapid method of accurately quantifying muscular forces generated during movement. Dynamometers (e.g., Cybex II) assess strength by measuring isokinetic movement. The torque movement of muscle force is recorded during limb extension and flexion at maximal effort and constant angular velocity. This test permits a functional measurement of strength.[46, 126]

Muscle Volume

Different methods have been used to quantify atrophy (Table 21–6). Computed tomographic (CT) scans and magnetic resonance imaging (MRI) permit the visualization of the actual cross-sectional and volumetric areas of a muscle.[21, 127] Both methods also permit the measurement of the extremities to determine changes in leg volume and muscle size alterations following skeletal muscle atrophy. Muscle atrophy may be concealed by edema and increases in connective tissue that occur in conjunction with atrophy even when MRI or CT scans are used.[128–130]

TABLE 21–6   SELECTED CLINICAL METHODS OF ASSESSING MASS OF LEAN SKELETAL MUSCLE TISSUE

Method	Comments
Anthropometry	Fat, fat-free body mass, and muscle size can be calculated from skinfold thickness, body weight, and limb circumferences.
Isotopic methods	
Water	Total body water can be measured and fat and fat-free body mass can be calculated by use of ^3H_2O, D_2O, or $H_2^{18}O$.
Bromide-82	Can be used to measure extracellular fluid volume; when combined with total body water provides a measure of intracellular water.
Potassium	Naturally occurring ^{40}K or radioactive ^{42}K is used to measure body cell mass.
Sodium	Exchangeable-sodium technique permits calculation of body cell mass.
Neutron activation analysis	Measures elemental composition, which then can be used to calculate the mass of bone, skeletal muscle, and nonskeletal muscle tissues.
Photon absorptiometry	One of several methods that establish bone mass.
Densitometry	Fat and fat-free body mass can be calculated from total body density; available methods include underwater weighing, helium dilution, plethysmography, biostereometrics, body volume in water, and body volume in air.
Radiography	Fat, muscle, bone, liver, kidney, spleen, and brain size can be calculated from plain films and by computerized tomography.
Nuclear magnetic resonance (NMR)	Produces images without ionizing radiation; can calculate fat, muscle, bone, liver, kidney, spleen, and brain size from the images; potential for analyzing chemical composition of tissue.
Ultrasonography	Fat, muscle, bone, liver, and heart volume can be measured with modern ultrasonic and echocardiographic techniques.
Infrared interactance	Potentially useful for measuring fat and muscle thickness in the extremities.
Whole-body conductivity (TOBEC) and impedance (BIA)	Potentially useful for establishing total body fat and fat-free body mass.
Metabolic	
Creatinine/3-methylhistidine	Markers of skeletal muscle mass.
Nitrogen balance	Classic approach establishes daily change in total body nitrogen and thereby protein by measuring intake and losses of nitrogen. Method often abbreviated by measuring only losses of urinary urea nitrogen and then estimating the remaining urinary, stool, and integumental losses.
Oxygen consumption and energy expenditure	Fat-free body mass and body cell mass in the eumetaboic adult subject have well-defined oxygen consumption and heat release. Measuring oxygen uptake or heat release thus permits calculation of fat-free or body cell mass.
Serum proteins	Nutrition-sensitive serum proteins vary in rate of synthesis and breakdown, half-life, pool size, and compartmental distribution.

From Heymsfield, S.B. (1985). Clinical assessment of lean tissues: Future directions. In A. F. Roche (ed.), *Body-Composition Assessments in Youth and Adults* (p. 54). Columbus, OH: Ross Laboratories.

Methods have not yet been developed to account for the contribution of edema and increased connective tissue in the assessment of atrophy. Because this method of assessing skeletal muscle atrophy is expensive, it should be used only in patients with severe unexplained atrophy that occurs with complaints of extreme fatigue. These measures should be able to separate the complaints of fatigue due to atrophy from those originating with the concurrent pathological process. MRI and CT scans can also be used in conjunction with laboratory analyses that monitor skeletal muscle protein losses. An alternative assessment of muscle protein loss may be performed using a 24-hour urinalysis to detect creatinine loss which can be directly correlated.[65, 131]

Individuals with skeletal muscle atrophy and decreased exercise capacity also experience fatigue. Atrophic muscles are more prone to fatigue that is related to the anaerobic lactic acid processes of contraction. The ability of the atrophied muscle to buffer excess H^+ is less efficient.[53] This means that patients who must perform activities that require short-term bursts of strength will rapidly fatigue.

Skinfold thickness and limb circumference determinations are useful methods for monitoring the long-term changes in skeletal muscle (Box 21–2). However, special training in the accurate use of these techniques is necessary in order to produce valid and reliable results. Many new techniques have been demonstrated to provide accurate quantification

BOX 21–2

Measurement of Skinfold Thickness

Mid Arm Circumference

With the patient supine, place the left forearm palm down across the middle of the body so that the left elbow is at a 90° angle. Locate and mark half the distance between the left acromial and olecranon processes. Extend the left arm alongside the body with the palm of the hand facing upward. Measure the circumference to the upper arm at its midpoint, perpendicular to the long axis of the upper arm, while slightly supporting the upper arm off the surface of the bed.

Lateral Calf Circumference

With the patient supine and the left knee bent to a 90° angle, measure the maximum circumference of the calf in a plane perpendicular to the shaft of the tibia.

Triceps Skinfold Thickness

With the patient lying on the right side, the trunk in a straight line, and the left arm palm down along the trunk, use the left hand to grasp the skinfold and measure the skinfold with calipers. Make certain that a perpendicular line crosses the acromial processes to the surface of the bed and vertebral column.

of changes in lean body mass (see Table 21–6). Many of these methods have been previously described in Chapter 6, Cancer Cachexia. These methods provide additional tools to monitor skeletal muscle atrophy and changes in lean body mass; however, they need to be tested by nurses to establish their efficacy in the clinical environment.[132]

Work Capacity

The loss of skeletal muscle mass correlates with decreased exercise capacity of the patient. Clinical observation indicates that patients who have decreased their mean level of activities of daily living because of inactivity or immobility are less able to respond to the challenge of a given level of muscular exercise than a healthy ambulating person. Their ability to perform work will depend on the severity of restriction of mobility and the duration of decreased activity. Maximal oxygen uptake ($\dot{V}O_2$max) is the accepted standard by which the functional, or work, capacity of the cardiovascular and respiratory systems is measured.[109] The ability to perform work or exercise is measured by $\dot{V}O_2$max. Maximal oxygen uptake is defined as the greatest oxygen uptake an individual can achieve during a given exercise at an intensity that can be sustained for at least 2.5 to 3 minutes, but that causes complete exhaustion after 5 to 10 minutes. The highest levels of $\dot{V}O_2$max are attained with work that uses the largest groups of muscles.[109]

During training, physical adaptations occur that allow the body to adequately respond to various exercise loads. Following inactivity, bed rest, or immobility, patients are detrained and respond to an exercise challenge with great effort. They are unable to maintain that effort without fatigue.[109] The trained individual responds to the same stress with less effort and can maintain the activity for a much longer period before fatigue begins.

Submaximal oxygen uptake also decreases after prolonged inactivity or immobilization. There is a high correlation between cardiac output during exercise and oxygen uptake (in liters · min^{-1}); therefore, counting of the heart rate during exercise is all that is needed for the evaluation of exercise capacity.[109] During submaximal testing, the individual acts as his or her own control, and oxygen uptake can be predicted from the external power to which the person is subjected.

Inactivity in the form of chair rest has also been used in studies of oxygen uptake. In chair rest, patients are placed in the high Fowler's position in regular or cardiac chairs. This differs from the majority of bed rest studies in which patients are placed in the supine position in bed for the entire day. Following 30 days of chair rest, a 7 per cent decrease in maximal oxygen uptake was found. The large decrease was found by Saltin and associates, who observed an average reduction in maximal oxygen uptake of 26 per cent in healthy men who exercised following 20 days of supine bed rest.[106] It should be pointed out, however, that these subjects underwent 55 days of training prior to confinement in bed.

In most studies, the maximal work capacity tests were performed with the subjects in the upright position. When exercise tests are performed immediately after supine bed rest and in the upright position, the resultant orthostatic hypotension may result in a variable decrease in the maximal working time and $\dot{V}O_2$max. $\dot{V}O_2$max is approximately 15 per cent lower in the supine position than in the sitting position. Therefore, studies of subjects performing exercise tests in the supine position should have lower measures of $\dot{V}O_2$max.

A significant correlation exists between changes in body cell mass determined from isotope dilution and changes in the exercise capacity of large muscle masses. These are important considerations, as the major loss of protein during periods of stress and starvation is from skeletal muscle, thus depleting body cell mass and degrading function (exercise capacity).[95] Commonly used intravenous nutritional regimens affect the functional status of skeletal muscle and cause a form of disuse atrophy.[95]

SURVEILLANCE AND MEASUREMENT

The professional nurse has the responsibility for monitoring the physiological parameters and behavioral changes previously discussed. In addition, the professional nurse must monitor the changes in the patient's functional status over time, which is important in determining the development, the progression, and the recovery of atrophic skeletal muscle from periods of decreased activity, bed rest, or immobility. It is also crucial that the status of the initial activity and the severity of the restriction of mobility be considered as important factors in the nurse's evaluation of the patient. Specific surveillance parameters are similar to those used in the surveillance of cancer cachexia (see Chapter 6) and include weight; skinfold thickness of the triceps, quadriceps, and gastrocnemius; and mid arm and mid leg muscle determinations. In addition, the urinary excretion of creatinine and 3-methylhistidine (3-MH) may be used to monitor skeletal muscle atrophy. The laboratory standards for these excretion rates in patient populations have been previously described.[132, 133]

Alterations in heart rate, blood pressure, and orthostatic intolerance can be monitored during the standard daily vital signs checks. The staff would need instructions on the trends to follow indicating a deteriorating condition, such as increased heart rate of 1 beat per minute per day of bed rest and symptoms of orthostatic intolerance with standing. Routine laboratory analysis could be used to monitor the classic trends, such as

increased hematocrit and hemoglobin concentrations, that result from prolonged inactivity or immobility. These trends are gradual and can be differentiated from those of the existing pathological condition.[108] It must be remembered that some diseases will mask these trends.

Behavioral indicators of atrophy may precede the physiological parameters. The timing of behavioral alterations due to inactivity or immobilization have not been well defined in the literature. The predominant symptoms are associated with sensory deprivation, such as altered visual and auditory perception. These behavioral alterations are closely linked to confinement and isolation from normal social contact.[134] In addition, patients experience altered time perception.[134] Intervention should focus on prevention of social isolation and increasing visual and auditory stimulation. Patients confined to strict bed rest should be placed in multiple patient rooms near the nursing station. When possible, meals should be taken in group settings.

Prevention of severe skeletal muscle atrophy is most effective when there is an early recognition of a potential decrease in activity. Early recognition will enable the professional nurse to plan a schedule of activities of daily living that will permit the patient to maintain the highest activity level possible. Patient education is also essential to enlist the cooperation of the patient in the plan of activity. Research in the area of skeletal muscle atrophy has focused on normal adult populations; therefore, studies describing the course of atrophy in individual pathophysiological processes are not available.

Additional research is needed about the time course of skeletal muscle atrophy in disease processes. The rate and magnitude of the behavioral components of inactivity, bed rest, and immobility are also needed. However, the research base of skeletal muscle atrophy and its sequelae in control human populations is extensive and provides clear direction for nursing research. The role of the nurse is to continue monitoring activity levels and the patient's ability to perform self-care activities.

After the nurse has identified a patient at risk for skeletal muscle atrophy, key parameters must be assessed at least twice per day. These parameters include active and passive range of motion, anthropometric measurements, weight changes, changes in upper and lower extremity strength, work capacity, fatigue, and related biochemical measurements (see Manifestations). In addition, the monitoring of patient activity levels over time and range of motion must always be compared with initial assessments as well as projected to the levels of activity that will be needed when the patient is discharged to home. These observations will enable the nurse to respond rapidly and provide appropriate interventions and therapy.

THERAPIES

Decreases in the regular activities of daily living produce dramatic adaptations in both skeletal muscle and the cardiovascular system. The alteration in the composition of skeletal muscle is most pronounced in the weight-bearing muscles of the legs and postural muscles of the torso. The primary clinical goal is to encourage as much physical activity as is reasonable for the individual patient. Simple activities, such as performing self-care, eating in a group setting, and watching television in an activity room, encourage patients to move from their room and to exercise. Patients may participate in setting goals for walking the unit halls or simply increasing the time that they are able to bear weight at the bedside. The maintenance of activity is an effective method of diminishing the effects of disuse atrophy, even under the extreme conditions of orthopedic traction and weightlessness.[20–22, 60, 135] The maintenance of muscle strength by continuing activities of daily living and movement assists in the support of the capacity of the cardiovascular system to defend against orthostatic hypotension following inactivity.[21]

Countermeasures for cardiovascular alterations exist and have shown promise for clinical use; these are simply chair rest and standing.[29, 136] The simple method of placing subjects in a chair for 8 hours a day was found to slow the rate of decrease in orthostatic tolerance and work capacity.[29, 136] The rate of decrease in work capacity was less rapid in chair rest than in supine bed rest. Specifically, the effects of supine bed rest and sitting exercise were compared with quiet sitting on the circulatory and metabolic consequences of 24 days of bed rest.[29] Supine exercises did not prevent but diminished the decrease in orthostatic intolerance and work capacity. Sitting exercise (1 hour of bicycle ergometer exercise per day) minimized the effects in one of two subjects. In the final

comparison, 8 hours daily of quiet sitting in combination with 16 hours of supine bed rest resulted in only minor decreases in work capacity.

In a classic study of inactivity, Saltin and colleagues[106] demonstrated 3 hours per day of quiet standing during supine bed rest to be an effective rehabilitative measure for reversing bed rest–induced orthostatic hypotension and hypercalciuria in normal populations.

Exercise has been used as an intervening variable to prevent the loss of plasma and blood volumes. The use of exercise as a preventive measure resulted in the same pattern of plasma and blood volume losses as in other investigations.[70, 96, 106, 137] The exercise levels in these studies ranged from daily in-bed isometric exercise to 1 hour of cycling on a bicycle ergometer at 60 per cent of $\dot{V}O_2$max each day. It is obvious that hospitalized patients cannot be expected to engage in strenuous exercise while recuperating from surgery or other illness, thus yielding these measures clinically inappropriate. However, vigorous exercise may be a useful method of preventing fatigue and maintaining cardiovascular function in chronic disease. Research is needed to evaluate the effectiveness of increased exercise in these patient populations.

One intervention did impede the reduction of plasma volume with restricted activity. Vogt and Johnson found that 12 hours of quiet sitting in conjunction with 12 hours of bed rest reduced plasma volume loss to the insignificant amount of 95 ml in patients.[136] Birkhead and associates concurred, reporting that no significant change in plasma volume occurred during 42 days of unrestricted chair rest.[29] Subjects in this study, normal adult males, were restricted to quiet chair sitting for 8 hours per day.

Quiet chair rest is contraindicated in few instances in the hospital. At present, standard nursing procedure attempts to place most patients in a chair for some portion of every day. The length of time spent in the chair is very subjective and is controlled by the discretion of the primary nurse. The risk in implementing a procedure to maintain patients in a chair for timed duration would be small, as this is already used in clinical practice.[100, 138]

Studies of patients have shown that the pattern of deconditioning and its associated loss of $\dot{V}O_2$max, lean body mass, and endurance is similar to that in studies performed on healthy subjects. Most of these studies used orthopedic and surgical patients.[103, 139] One of the factors that may influence these vascular fluid volume losses is the amount of activity that persons perform during bed rest. When the supine position is maintained without periodic upright positioning, significant plasma and blood volume losses of approximately 15 per cent[70, 99, 113, 136] and 10 per cent,[71, 96, 99, 113] respectively, occur. In contrast, when a supine patient restricted to bed rest is granted bathroom privileges or can sit in a chair for 10 to 15 minutes per day, the plasma and blood volume losses are almost 50 per cent less than if the person had been restricted to bed rest alone.[106, 140] This change in posture may temporarily halt or slow down the deconditioning process because sitting or standing even for a short period of time causes some gravitational force to be exerted on the lower body. Thus, the effect on intravascular fluid volumes is minimized.

Fatigue in patients with skeletal muscle atrophy may be severe and is a result of the combined effects of decreased muscle mass, $\dot{V}O_2max$, and circulating plasma volume. Patient reports of fatigue will vary with the individual and may begin within 1 day of decreased levels of activities of daily living. Fatigue will increase, however, when the patient attempts greater mobilization and self-care activities. Slowly increasing activity in the patient with muscle atrophy will minimize the fatigue. Research is needed to determine the rate of remobilization that will minimize severe fatigue.

REVIEW OF RESEARCH FINDINGS

The promotion of mobility and maintenance of self-care activities has been recognized as one of the primary foci of nursing care. Skeletal muscle wasting has been a widely observed phenomenon in response to illness, decreased activities of daily living, and immobilization and bed rest. A better understanding of the process of skeletal muscle atrophy can serve as a substantive foundation for the development and testing of new approaches to the promotion of mobility.

Decreased motion (hypokinesia) and decreased weight-bearing (hypodynamia) have been implicated as causes of pathology in nearly every mammalian organ system. Hypokinesia and hypodynamia cause skeletal muscle atrophy,[141] increased fatigability,[142] alterations in skeletal muscle contraction time, decreases in plasma and blood volumes, orthostatic hypotension,[102] and pulmonary atelectasis.[96, 141] After prolonged hypokinesia or hypodynamia, patients have an impaired functional capacity and a reduced ability to perform their normal daily activities.[143]

Skeletal muscle atrophy is manifested by the exponential loss with time of muscle mass due to a decrease in the number of myofibrils in parallel,[144] the number of fibers per muscle, and muscle cell (fiber) diameter, as documented in rat skeletal muscle following hypokinesia.[6, 36, 68, 75, 77] Skeletal muscle with predominantly slowly contracting oxidative fibers (type I), such as the soleus muscle, has been reported to atrophy to a greater extent than muscle with a high proportion of fast-contracting (type II) fibers.[18] Mussacchia and associates report losses of 35 per cent in soleus muscle mass by 1 week and 45 per cent by 2 weeks of hypokinetic suspension; in the predominantly type II plantaris muscle, suspension restraint induced a 22 per cent loss of mass after 7 days. In both types of muscles, the onset of atrophy is rapid.

Disuse, or non-neurogenic atrophy, is commonly produced in a variety of experimental protocols, such as tenotomy and limb immobilization. Unlike tenotomy, limb immobilization allows the muscle to be fixed at resting or other specified lengths. Resting length is the length of choice, as it is less likely to produce contracture and maintains the normal passive load placed on the muscle throughout its tendons and skeletal attachments. Previous investigations immobilized the hindlimbs in bilateral casts at less than resting lengths[58, 59, 145] or by rigidly fixing the joints by pinning.[4, 146] These models are clinically appropriate for determining changes in immobile subjects but not for the general case of a mobile subject whose level of activity and weight-bearing has been compromised by hypokinesia or hypodynamia.

Animal models of inactivity, such as hindlimb suspension, are important in the study of disuse atrophy, as they closely resemble the degree of movement and lack of weight-bearing that[68, 75, 147] persons subjected to periods of bed rest and restricted activity experience. Furthermore, these models allow for study of fiber type distribution in atrophied muscle in a manner that is impossible in humans. A number of suspension models have been employed to simulate an environment of weightlessness.[68, 75, 147] A modification of Morey's model was introduced to examine the effects of hindlimb suspension on bone fracture healing.[75]

Slow-twitch fibers, predominant in the soleus and postural muscles, are recruited first during weight-bearing and have a tonic activity pattern that may be very sensitive to changes in their contraction frequency.[75, 148, 149] The functional weight-bearing role of these muscles is therefore significantly altered during suspension. Muscle mass rapidly declined during the first 7 days of suspension, continuing at a more gradual rate through the 28th day. This reflected an early atrophic response due to a more rapid rate of protein degradation and to a simultaneous decrease in protein synthesis.[75, 148, 149] Previous studies of hindlimb suspension and bed rest have shown that loss of muscle mass is associated with the development of a negative nitrogen balance, attributed to muscle protein catabolism.[76]

Changes in muscle mass give an estimate of the atrophic response of a particular muscle; however, the degree of fiber atrophy may be concealed to some extent by edema.[82, 129] Therefore, measurement of fiber cross-sectional area is considered a more accurate method of identifying the response of skeletal muscle to hypokinesia and/or hypodynamia.[129, 148] During inactivity, there is a marked decrease in type I mean cross-sectional area in contrast to type IIA fibers in which the cross-sectional area was maintained. Selective atrophy of soleus muscle type I fiber during a period of decreased activity is consistent in all previous reports using both bed rest and immobilization models.[36, 55] If the sample areas randomly chosen for analysis of fiber size and muscle composition are representative of the entire cross-sectional area, the changes in muscle composition produced by hindlimb suspension would seem to be similar, although not as profound as seen with immobilization.[59] Booth and Kelso, using the myosin ATPase technique, observed a significant reduction in the percentage of fibers staining as slow-twitch fibers in muscles of immobilized hindlimbs.[59] However, using fiber diameter as an estimate of fiber area, the postural muscle exhibits a type I selective atrophy in the soleus muscle, which is manifested as a progressive decrease in individual fiber cross-sectional area, and corresponding to the observed decrease in muscle mass during suspension.

Mild exercise or weight-bearing during the first 14 days of recovery from hypokinesia in rats produced skeletal muscle damage that appeared in the form of necrosis, the presence of phagocytosis and central nuclei, and fiber debris in the intrafascicular and interfibrillar spaces in postural muscles.[77, 83] The cause of exercise-induced muscle damage during recovery from hypokinesia is not known, although it most likely involves movement associated with exercise and an altered ability of the muscle fibers to bear the mechanical stress of external loads (weight-bearing). The functional load or tension per unit area required to maintain weight-bearing or exercise may exceed the reduced force-generating capacity of the atrophied muscle and may result in re-use injury. However, cellular defects, such as sarcomere length nonuniformities, dissociation of "Z" lines, loss of mitochondria, accumulation of redundant basement membrane, relative increases in the surface areas of the membrane systems (sarcoplasmic reticulum and T system), and evidence of secondary lysosomes,[146, 150] are also possible contributing factors.

With regard to the latter possibilities, the relationship of tension that a muscle can produce in response to a given level of calcium ion (tension-pCa relationship) in normal muscle is altered at long sarcomere lengths (3.00 to 3.25 μm), such that the development of tension at low Ca^{++} concentrations is increased. This provides structural stability during submaximal activations with Ca^{++}, since weaker sarcomeres will be stretched by stronger sarcomeres to a sarcomere length at which tension-generating capacity matches the functional load. Progressive alterations in the tension-pCa relationship as a function of sarcomere length could lead to longitudinal instability and eventually to muscle damage due to increased tension-generating capabilities along the fibers. For example, atrophy may alter the strength of Ca^{++} binding to the low-affinity sites on troponin C (Tn C) in skeletal muscle during force generation, resulting in damage of fibers even when normal weight-bearing does not load the muscle beyond its capacity to generate force as estimated by cross-sectional area. The underlying interaction between the tension-pCa relationship of individual fibers and atrophic damage has not been explored, particularly with regard to the time course of the development and the reversal of cellular contractile defects in the major types of skeletal muscle fibers (types I, IIA, IIB).

Loss of strength and mass in the lower extremities following inactivity, bed rest, and immobility can be severe in the human. The observation that 2.5 hours of daily cycling exercise in the patient on bed rest does not adequately prevent skeletal muscle atrophy is a significant finding.[12, 20, 151] Loss of strength in the lower limbs is twice that of the arms during maximal voluntary isometric exercise.[152] In order to further explore the relationship between skeletal muscle atrophy and strength, studies were done to examine force development following bed rest.[60] It was found that 30 days of inactivity significantly decreased the force output of the knee extensors of the leg but not the knee flexors.[60] Significant decreases in total cross-sectional area of the thigh and lower leg were found and accounted for the total loss of strength. However, skeletal atrophy was not the sole source of the loss of strength, as these changes were not affected by the type or speed of the muscle action.

Further research is needed to compare these findings from normal populations to human patient populations. As previous work has demonstrated, the mechanisms of atrophy may be influenced by drug therapy and disease. It may be hypothesized that the addition of the circumstances of the clinical environment may have an additional deleterious effect upon the progression of patient populations.

ILLUSTRATIVE CASE STUDY

George G., a 34-year-old accountant, had been an avid walker all of his adult life. Mr. G. was hospitalized for repair of the right patella due to chronic chondromalacia. Before admission, the patient's daily activity was gradually decreased over a 4-week period because of knee pain. At the time of admission, Mr. G. was unable to walk further than 50 feet at a speed of 10 meters per minute. Following surgical repair, Mr. G. commented that he was fearful of losing his ability to exercise and walk long distances because he experienced weakness, fatigue, and orthostatic hypotension when walking in the hospital.

Following surgical repair, physical assessment revealed an increased heart rate when the patient was standing, decreased range of motion in the affected limb, and decreased force production in both legs as measured by isokinetic dynamometry. Further studies revealed an increased hematocrit level and dehydration. MRI and measurements of calf size revealed a 30 per cent decrease in the size of the major weight-bearing muscle groups of the right leg, the gastrocnemius, soleus, extensor digitorum longus, and the plantaris.

A gradual program of increased exercise was devised for Mr. G. During the first 2 weeks he walked 100 feet at a pace of 10 m/minutes, rested, and repeated this three to four times per day. While in bed, he did exercises consisting of gently rolling from side to side and lower extremity extension. During week 3, he walked 100 feet at 15 m/minute, rested, and repeated this five to six times. During week 4, he walked 100 feet at 20 m/minute, rested, and repeated this five to six times. He also did bed exercises as described above plus lay supine on elbows and did unilateral straight leg raising. Also during the recovery period, Mr. G. was instructed to sit in a chair as much as possible and to do as many self-care tasks as possible.[109]

Mr. G.'s hematocrit level and heart rate returned to normal by week 4, and he no longer experienced orthostatic hypotension. Functional strength sufficient to perform activities of daily living was also recovered by week 4. Measurement of his lower extremities revealed the return of normal skeletal muscle mass. However, Mr. G. required another 4 weeks of gradual increased activity and walking to return to his prior level of rapid daily walking. At week 5, he began a program of walking one-quarter mile per day and ascending two flights of stairs. During weeks 6 and 7 he walked one-half to 1 mile per day and ascended three flights of stairs. Ultimately, additional mileage and stair climbing were incorporated into his exercise program.

To design an appropriate individualized exercise recovery program, a detailed physical assessment is required. This assessment should evaluate the patient's strength, level of fatigue, range of motion deficits, activities that cause pain, and balance and gait difficulties. The nurse should observe whether the assessment is causing fatigue for the patient. The plan should be structured to incorporate the individual's prior work history, leisure activities, and perception of activities that he is capable of performing. It is also important to determine how long the individual has participated in favorite activities without fatigue. All of this information provides a sound basis for nursing diagnosis and prescription of appropriate activities.

IMPLICATIONS FOR FURTHER RESEARCH

The vast majority of the research into disuse atrophy has centered on the effects of total immobility or weightlessness. Given that the majority of patients are not totally immobile or recovering from long-duration space flight, nursing research is needed to focus on the effects of decreased activities of daily living in patient populations specifically in relation to skeletal muscle atrophy, cardiovascular alterations, and physiological fatigue. Atrophy in patients is gradual and not as apparent as that seen in healthy individuals. Current clinical therapy is based on research done by the disciplines of kinesiology and sports medicine. Subjects in these studies are typically healthy athletic college males, and the research is focused on increasing human performance in relation to sports.

The measurement of exercise capacity or maximal oxygen uptake is based on a person's ability to cycle on a bicycle ergometer or run on a treadmill. The ability to evaluate this parameter is based on a person's mobility and exercise ability. To date, only one study has examined these parameters in a debilitated population consisting of burn patients.[153] Therefore, basic and applied research is needed to develop quantitative measures of exercise capacity in patient populations.

In addition, the effects of disuse atrophy need to be examined across the life span. Preliminary research has clearly demonstrated that the effects of restricted mobility on normal neonates and geriatric populations are vastly different. It is important for nurses to determine how the addition of pathology to the adaptive process of atrophy affects patient outcomes.

The rate and magnitude of recovery from atrophy have been examined only briefly in animal and human populations. Further studies are needed to determine the rates of recovery from skeletal muscle atrophy that can be expected in various patient populations. Additionally, there are few data as to the ability of the systems to recover without permanent or irreversible damage. Current research has been based on designs that measure the effects of a single acute occurrence of hypokinesia. The chronically ill are often subjected to repeated bouts of hypokinesia. Research designs should incorporate cyclical bouts of hypokinesia in order to mimic chronic populations. These studies are imperative prior to the initiation of work to determine the most effective methods of exercise prevention prior to disuse and those that are necessary to promote recovery.

Teach us to live that we may dread
Unnecessary time in bed.
Get people up and we may save
Our patients from an early grave.[154]

REFERENCES

1. Fell, R.D., Gladden, L.B., Steffen, J.M., & Musacchia, X.J. (1985). Fatigue and contraction of slow and fast muscle in hypokinetic/hypodynamic rats. J Appl Physiol 58:65–69.
2. Burke, R.E., & Edgerton, V.R. (1975). Motor unit properties and selective involvement in movement. In *Exercise and Sport Science Reviews* (pp. 31–81). New York: Academic Press.
3. Finol, H.S., Lewis, D.M., & Owens, R. (1981). The effects of denervation on contractile properties of rat skeletal muscle. J Physiol 319:82–92.
4. Fishback, G.D., & Robbins, N. (1969). Changes in contractile properties of disused soleus muscle. J Physiol 201:305–320.
5. Salvatori, S., Damiani, E., Zorzato, F., Volpe, P., Pierobon, D., Quaglino, D., Salviati, G., & Margreth, A. (1989). Denervation-induced proliferative changes of triads in rabbit skeletal muscle. Muscle Nerve 11:1246–1259.
6. Booth, F.W., & Seider, M.J. (1979). Early change in skeletal muscle protein synthesis after limb immobilization of rats. J Appl Physiol 47:974–977.
7. Tucker, K.R., Seider, M.J., & Booth, F.W. (1981). Protein synthesis rates in atrophied gastrocnemius muscles after limb immobilization. J Appl Physiol: Respirat Environ Exercise Physiol 51:73–77.
8. Boyes, G., & Johnson, J. (1979). Muscle fiber composition of rat vastus intermedius following immobilization. Pfluegers Arch. 381:195–200.
9. Booth, F.W. (1977). Time course of muscular atrophy during immobilization of hindlimbs in rats. J Appl Physiol: Respirat Environ Exercise Physiol 43:656–661.
10. *Vital and Health Statistics: National Hospital Discharge Survey: Annual Summary* (Series 13 No. 99). (1989). Washington, D.C.: National Center for Health Statistics. U.S. Department of Health and Human Services.

11. Howard, G., Steffen, J.M., & Geoghegan, T.E. (1989). Transcriptional regulation of decreased protein synthesis during skeletal muscle unloading. J Appl Physiol 66:1093–1098.

12. Graham, S.C., Roy, R.R., West, S.P., Thompson, D., & Baldwin, K.M. (1989). Exercise effects on the size and metabolic properties of soleus fibers in hindlimb-suspended rats. Aviat Space Environ Med 60:226–234.

13. Greenleaf, J.E. (ed.) (1982). *Physiological Consequences of Reduced Physical Activity During Bed Rest.* Philadelphia: Franklin Institute Press.

14. Issekutz, B., Blizzard, J.J., Birkhead, N.C., & Rohdahl, K. (1966). Effect of prolonged bed rest on urinary calcium output. J Appl Physiol 21:1013–1020.

15. Hilton, J. (1863). *Rest and Pain: On the Influence of Mechanical and Pathophysiological Rest.* London: Bell and Daldy.

16. Henderson, V., & Nite, G. (1978). *Principles and Practice of Nursing* (6th ed.). New York: Macmillan.

17. Booth, F.W., & Kelso, J.R. (1973). Effect of hindlimb immobilization on contractile and histochemical properties of skeletal muscle. Pflugers Arch 342:231–238.

18. Booth, F.W., & Seider, M.J. (ed.) (1980). *Effects of Disuse by Limb Immobilization on Different Muscle Fiber Types.* New York: Walter de Gruyter & Co.

19. Gossman, M.R., Rose, S.J., Sahrmann, S.A., & Katholi, C.R. (1986). Length and circumference measurements in one-joint and multijoint muscles in rabbits after immobilization. Phys Ther 66(4):516–520.

20. Buchanan, P., & Convertino, V.A. (1989). A study of the effects of prolonged simulated microgravity on the musculature of the lower extremities in man: An introduction. Aviat Space Environ Med 60:649–652.

21. Convertino, V.A., Doerr, D.F., Mathes, K.L., Stein, S.L., & Buchanan, P. (1989). Changes in volume, muscle compartment, and compliance of the lower extremities in man following 30 days of exposure to simulated microgravity. Aviat Space Environ Med 60:653–658.

22. Duvoisin, M.R., Convertino, V.A., Buchanan, P., Gollnick, P.D., & Dudley, G.A. (1989). Characteristic and preliminary observations of the influence of electromyostimulation on the size and function of human skeletal muscle during 30 days of simulated microgravity. Aviat Space Environ Med 60:671–678.

23. Cannon, J.G., Fielding, R.A., Fiatarone, M.A., Orencole, S.F., Dinarello, C.A., & Evans, W.J. (1989). Increased interleukin 1 beta in human skeletal muscle after exercise. Am J Physiol 257(2 Pt. 2):R451–R455.

24. St. Pierre, B.A., Kasper, C.E., & Lindsey, A.M. (1992). Fatigue mechanisms in cancer patients: TNF and exercise effects on skeletal muscle factors. Oncol Nurs Forum 19(3):419–425.

25. Oganov, V.S. (1981). Results of biosatellite studies of gravity dependent changes in the musculoskeletal system of mammals. Physiologist 24 (Suppl.):S55–S58.

26. Thornton, W.E., & Rummel, J.A. (1977). Muscular deconditioning and its prevention in space flight. In R.S. Johnston & L.F. Dietlein (eds.), *Biomedical Results from Skylab* (pp. 191–197). Washington D.C.: National Aeronautics and Space Administration.

27. Mastaglia, F.L. (1982). Adverse effect of drugs on muscle. Drugs 24:304–321.

28. Müller, R., & Kugelberg, E. (1959). Myopathy in Cushing's syndrome. J. Neurol Neurosurg Psychiatry 22:314–317.

29. Birkhead, N.C., Haupt, G.J., Issekutz, B.J., & Rohdahl, K. (1966). *Effect of Exercise, Standing, Negative Trunk and Positive Skeletal Pressure on Bedrest-induced Orthostasis and Hypercalciuria.* (Technical Report No. 66–6). Wright-Patterson Air Force Base, OH: Aerospace Medical Research Labs.

30. Ruff, R.L., Martyn, D., & Gordon, A.M. (1982). Glucocorticoid-induced atrophy is not due to impaired excitability of rat muscle. Am J Physiol 243:E512–E521.

31. Askari, A.P., Vignos, P.J., & Moskowitz, R.W. (1976). Steroid myopathy in connective tissue disease. Am J Med 61:485–492.

32. Kelly, F.J., & Goldspink, D.F. (1982). The differing responses of four muscle types to dexamethasone treatment in the rat. Biochem J 208:147–158.

33. Khaleeli, A.A., Edwards, R.H.T., Gohil, K., McPhail, G., Rennie, M.J., Round, J., & Ross, E.J. (1983). Corticosteroid myopathy: A clinical and pathological study. Clin Endocrinol 18:155–161.

34. Pleasure, D.E., Walsh, G.O., & Engel, W.K. (1970). Atrophy of skeletal muscle in patients with Cushing's syndrome. Arch Neurol 22:18–125.

35. Horber, F.F., Hoppeler, H., Herren, D., Claassen, H., Howald, H., Gerber, C., & Frey, F.J. (1986). Altered skeletal muscle ultrastructure in renal transplant patients on prednisone. Kidney Int 30:411–416.

36. Jaspers, S.R., & Tischler, M.E. (1984). Atrophy and growth failure of rat hindlimb muscles in tail-cast suspension. J Appl Physiol: Respirat Environ Exercise 57:1472–1479.

37. McCully, K.K., & Faulkner, J.A. (1986). Characteristics of lengthening contractions associated with injury to skeletal muscle fibers. J Appl Physiol 61:293–299.

38. Williams, P.E., & Goldspink, G. (1973). The effect of immobilization on the longitudinal growth of striated muscle fibers. J Anat 116:45–55.

39. Adler, A.B., Crawford, G.N.C., & Edwards, R.G. (1959). The effect of limitation of movement on longitudinal muscle growth. Proc R Soc Lond [Biol] 150:554–562.

40. Salmons, S., & Sreter, F.A. (1976). Significance of impulse activity in the transformation of skeletal muscle type. Nature 263:30–34.

41. Schiaffino, S., & Bormioli, S.P. (1973). Adaptive changes in developing rat skeletal muscle in response to functional overload. Exp Neurol 40:126–137.

42. Elder, G., & McComas, A. (1987). Development of rat muscle during short- and long-term hindlimb suspension. J Appl Physiol 62:1917–1923.

43. Papanicolau, G.N., & Falk, E.A. (1938). General muscle hypertrophy induced by androgenic hormone. Science 87:238–239.

44. Borkan, G.A., Hults, D.E., & Gerzof, S.G. (1983). Age changes in body composition revealed by computed tomography. J Gerontol 38:673–677.

45. Larson, L. (1978). Morphological and functional characteristics of aging skeletal muscle in man. Acta Physiol Scand Suppl 457:1–36.

46. Larson, L., Grimby, G., & Karlsson, J. (1979). Muscle strength and speed of movement in relation

to age and muscle morphology. J Appl Physiol *46*:451–456.

47. Kuta, I., Parizkova, J., & Dycka, J. (1970). Muscle strength and lean body mass in old men of different physical activity. J Appl Physiol *29*:168–171.

48. Mauro, A. (1961). Satellite cell of skeletal muscle fibers. J Biophys Biochem Cytol *9*:493–498.

49. Gibson, M.C., & Schultz, E. (1983). Age related differences in absolute numbers of skeletal muscle satellite cells. Muscle Nerve *6*:574–580.

50. Handel, S.E., Wang, S., Greaser, M.L., Schultz, E., Bulinski, J.C., & Lessard, J.L. (1989). Skeletal muscle myofibrillogenesis as revealed with a monoclonal antibody to titin in combination with detection of the α- and γ-isoforms of actin. *Dev Biol 132*:35–44.

51. Schultz, E., & Lipton, B.H. (1982). Skeletal muscle satellite cells: Changes in proliferation potential as a function of age. Mech Aging Dev *20*:377–383.

52. Fahim, M.A. (1987). Remodeling of the neuromuscular junction during aging and disuse. In M.J. Dowdall & J.N. Hawthorne (eds.), *Cellular and Molecular Basis for Cholinergic Function* (pp. 677–683). Chichester, England: Ellis Horwood Ltd.

53. Hainaut, K., & Duchateau, J. (1989). Muscle fatigue, effects of training and disuse. Muscle Nerve *12*:660–669.

54. Shepard, J.T. (1982). Reflex control of arterial blood pressure. Cardiovasc Res *16*:357.

55. Booth, F.W. (1982). Effect of limb immobilization on skeletal muscle. J Appl Physiol *52*:1113–1118.

56. Booth, F.W., & Gollnick, P.D. (1983). Effects of disuse on the structure and function of skeletal muscle. Med Sci Sports Exerc *15*:415–420.

57. Goldspink, D.F. (1977). The influence of immobilization and stretch on protein turnover of rat skeletal muscle. J Physiol *264*:267–282.

58. Holloszy, J.O., & Booth, F.W. (1976). Biochemical adaptations to endurance exercise in muscle. Ann Rev Physiol *38*:273–291.

59. Booth, F.W., & Kelso, J.R. (1972). Cytochrome oxidase of skeletal muscle: Adaptive reponse to chronic disuse. Can J Physiol Pharmacol *51*:679–681.

60. Dudley, G.A., Duvoisin, M.R., Convertino, V.A., & Buchanan, P. (1989). Alterations of the in vivo torque-velocity relationship of human skeletal muscle following 30 days exposure to simulated microgravity. Aviat Space Environ Med *60*:659–663.

61. Feller, D.D., Ginoza, H.S., & Morey, E.E. (1981). Atrophy of rat skeletal muscles in simulated weightlessness. Physiologist *24*(Suppl.):S9–S10.

62. Musacchia, X.J., Steffan, J., & Deavers, D.R. (1981). Suspension restraint: Induced hypokinesia and antiorthostasis as a simulation of weightlessness. Physiologist *24*(Suppl.):S21–S22.

63. Herbison, G.J., Jaweed, M.M., & Ditunno, J.F. (1978). Muscle fiber atrophy after cast immobilization in the rat. Arch Phys Med Rehab *59*:301–305.

64. Lindboe, C.F., & Platou, C.S. (1984). Effect of immobilization of short duration on the muscle fiber size. Clin Physiol *4*:183.

65. Schimke, R.T. (1975). Methods for analysis of enzyme synthesis and degradation in animal tissues. Methods Enzymol *40*:241.

66. Watson, P.A., Stein, J.P., & Booth, F.W. (1984). Changes in actin synthesis and actin-m RNA content in rat muscle during immobilization. Am J Physiol *247*:C39–C44.

67. Jagus, R., & Safer, B. (1981). Activity of eukaryotic initiation factor 2 is modified by processes distinct from phosphorylation. J Biochem *256*:1317–1323.

68. Musacchia, X.J., Deavers, D.R., Meininger, G.A., & Davis, T.P. (1980). A model for hypokinesia: Effects on muscle atrophy in the rat. J Appl Physiol: Respirat Environ Exercise Physiol *48*:479–486.

69. Greenleaf, J.E., Silverstein, L., Bliss, J., Langenheim, V., Rossow, H., & Chao, C. (1982). *Physiological Responses to Prolonged Bed Rest and Fluid Immersion in Man: A Compendium of Research (1974–1980).* (No. NASA Tech Memo 81324). Washington, D.C.: National Aeronautics and Space Administration.

70. Greenleaf, J.E., Bernauer, E.M., Young, H.L., Morse, J.T., Staley, R.W., Juhos, L.T., & Beaumont, W.V. (1977). Fluid and electrolyte shifts during bed rest with isometric and isotonic exercise. J Appl Physiol *42*:59–66.

71. Greenleaf, J.E., Greenleaf, C.J., Van Derveer, D., & Dorchak, K.J. (1976). *Adaptation to Prolonged Bed Rest in Man: A Compendium of Research.* (No. NASA Tech Memo X-3307). Washington, D.C.: National Aeronautics and Space Administration.

72. Medvedov, V.I., & Bagrova, N.D. (1977). Estimation of time during bedrest. Fiziologia Cheloveka *3*:288–294.

73. Nicks, D.K., Beneke, W.M., Key, R.M., & Timson, B.F. (1989). Muscle fiber size and number following immobilization atrophy. J Anat *163*:1–5.

74. Witzmann, F.A., Kim, D.H., & Fitts, R.H. (1983). Effect of hindlimb immobilization on fatigability of skeletal muscle. J Appl Physiol Respir Environ Exerc Physiol *54*:1242–1248.

75. Morey-Holton, E., & Wronski, J. (1981). Animal models for simulating weightlessness. Physiologist *24*(Suppl.):S45-S48.

76. Musacchia, X.J., Steffen, J., & Deavers, D. (1983). Rat hindlimb muscle responses to suspension hypokinesia/hypodynamia. Aviat Space Environ Med *54*:1015–1020.

77. Kasper, C., White, T., & Maxwell, L. (1990). Running during recovery from hindlimb suspension induces muscular injury. J Appl Physiol *68*:533–539.

78. Shepard, R.J., Bouhlel, E., Vandewalle, H., & Monod, H. (1988). Muscle mass as a factor limiting physical work. J Appl Physiol *64*:1472–1479.

79. Reiser, P., Kasper, C., & Moss, K. (1987). Myosin subunits and contractile properties of single fibers from hypokinetic rat muscles. J Appl Physiol *63*:2293–2300.

80. Witzmann, F.A., Kim, D.H., & Fitts, R.H. (1982). Hindlimb immobilization: Length-tension and contractile properties of skeletal muscle. J Appl Physiol *53*:335–345.

81. Close, R.I. (1964). Dynamic properties of fast and slow skeletal muscles of the rat during development. J Physiol *173*:74–79.

82. Brooke, M.H., & Kaiser, K.K. (1970). Muscle fiber types: How many and what kind? Arch Neurol *23*:369–379.

83. McNulty, A., Otto, A., Kasper, C., & Thomas, D. (1986). Use of the inverted cage suspension (ICS) model to induce skeletal muscle atrophy. Med Sci Sports Exerc *18*(Suppl.):55.

84. Lipman, R.L., Raskin, P., Love, T., Triebwasser, J., & Lecocq, F.R. (1972). Glucose intolerance during decreased physical activity in man. Diabetes *21*:101.

85. Nicholson, W.F., Watson, P.A., & Booth, F.W.

(1984). Glucose uptake and glucogen synthesis in muscles from immobilized limbs. J Appl Physiol *56*:431.

86. Blotner, H. (1945). Effect of prolonged physical inactivity on tolerance of sugar. Arch Intern Med *75*:39–44.

87. Bühr, P.A. (1963). On the influence of prolonged bodily inactivity on the blood sugar curves after oral glucose loading. Helv Med Acta *30*:156–175.

88. Günther, O., & Frenzel, R. (1969). Über den einfluss lüger andauernder køorperlicher inaktivität auf die kohlenhydrattoleranz. Z Gesamte Inn Med *24*:814–817.

89. Lutwak, L., & Whedon, G.D. (1959). The effect of physical conditioning on glucose tolerance. Clin Res *7*:143–144.

90. Henriksen, E.J., Tischler, M.E., & Johnson, D.G. (1986). Increased response to insulin of glucose metabolism in the six-day unloaded rat soleus muscle. J Biol Chem *261*:10707–10712.

91. Henriksen, E.J., & Tischler, M.E. (1988). Time course of the response of carbohydrate metabolism to unloading of the soleus. Metabolism *37*:201–208.

92. Tischler, M.E., Satarug, S., Eisenfeld, S.H., Henriksen, E.J., & Rosenberg, S.B. (1990). Insulin effects in denervated and non–weight-bearing rat soleus muscle. Muscle Nerve *13*:593–600.

93. Brown, A.M. (1979). Cardiac reflexes. In *The Cardiovascular System—The Heart; Section 2.* Bethesda, MD: American Physiological Society.

94. Brown, A.M. (1980). Receptors under pressure—an update on baroreceptors. Circ Res *46*:1.

95. Wood, C.D., Glover, J., McCune, M., Hendricks, J., & Johns, M. (1989). The effect of intravenous nutrition on muscle mass and exercise capacity in perioperative patients. Am J Surg *158*:63–67.

96. Greenleaf, J.E., Bernauer, E.M., Juhos, L.T., Young, H.L., Morse, J.T., & Staley, R.W. (1977). Effects of exercise on fluid exchange and body composition in man during 14-day bed rest. J Appl Physiol *43*(1):126–132.

97. Fortney, S.M., Beckett, W.S., Carpenter, A.J., Davis, J., Drew, H., LaFrance, N.D., Rock, J.A., Tankersley, C.G., & Vroman, N.B. (1988). Changes in plasma volume during bed rest: Effects of menstrual cycle and estrogen administration. J Appl Physiol *65*:525–533.

98. Donaldson, C.L., Hulley, S.B., McMillan, D.E., Hattner, R.W., & Bayers, J.H. (1970). Effect of prolonged bed rest on bone mineral. Metabolism *19*:1071–1084.

99. Taylor, H.L., Erickson, L., Henschel, A., & Keys, A. (1945). The effect of bed rest on the blood volume of normal young men. Am J Physiol *144*:227–232.

100. Browse, N.L. (1965). *The Physiology and Pathophysiology of Bed Rest.* Springfield, IL: Charles C Thomas.

101. Sandler, H., & Winter, D.L. (1978). *Physiological Responses of Women to Simulated Weightlessness.* (No. NASA SP-430). Washington, D.C.: National Aeronautics and Space Administration.

102. Sandler, H., Popp, R.L., & Harrison, D.C. (1988). The hemodynamic effects of repeated bed rest exposure. Aviat Space Environ Med *59*(11 Pt 1):1047–1054.

103. Oberfield, R.A., Ebaugh, F.G., Jr., O'Hanlon, E.P., & Schoaf, M. (1968). Blood volume studies during and after immobilization in human subjects as measured by sodium radiochromate (chromium 51) technique. Aerospace Med *39*:10–13.

104. Parin, V.V. (1970). Principle changes in the healthy human body after 120 days bed confinement. In *Space, Biology, Medicine.* Washington, D.C.: National Aeronautics and Space Administration.

105. Adolfsson, G. (1969). Circulatory and respiratory function in relation to physical activity in female patients before and after cholecystectomy. Acta Chir Scand Suppl *401*:5–106.

106. Saltin, B., Blomqvist, G., Mitchell, J.H., Johnson, R.L., Jr., Wildenthal, K., & Chapman, C.B. (1968). Response to exercise after bed rest and after training. Circulation *33*:VII-1–60.

107. Chase, G.A. (1966). Independence of changes in functional and performance capacities attending prolonged bed rest. Aerospace Med *37*:1232–1238.

108. Johnson, P.C. (1971). Vascular and extravascular fluid changes during six days of bed rest. Aerospace Med *42*:875–878.

109. Åstrand, P.-O., & Rohdahl, K. (1986). *Textbook of Work Physiology* (3rd ed.). New York: McGraw-Hill.

110. Dietrick, J.E., Whedon, G.D., & Shorr, E. (1948). Effects of immobilization upon various metabolic and physiologic functions of normal men. Am J Med *4*:3–36.

111. Evans, R.A., Bridgeman, M., Hills, E., & Dunstan, C.R. (1984). Immobilization hypercalcemia. Miner Electrolyte Metab *10*:244–248.

112. Lutz, J., Chen, F., & Kasper, C.E. (1987). Hypokinesia-induced negative net calcium balance reversed by weight-bearing exercise. Aviat Space Environ Med *58*:308–314.

113. Stremel, R.W., Convertino, E., Bernauer, E.M., & Greenleaf, J.E. (1976). Cardiorespiratory deconditioning with static and dynamic leg exercise during bed rest. J Appl Physiol *41*:905–909.

114. Globus, R.K., Bikle, D.D., & Morey-Holton, E. (1986). The temporal response to unloading. Endocrinol *118*:733–742.

115. Wronski, T.J., & Morey, E.R. (1983). Alterations in calcium homeostasis and bone during actual and simulated space flight. Metab Bone Dis Relat Res *15*:410–414.

116. Deitrick, J.E., Whedon, G.D., & Shorr, E. (1948). Effects of immobilization upon various metabolic and physiologic functions of normal men. Am J Med *4*:3–36.

117. Smith, S. (ed.) (1969). *Sensory Deprivation.* New York: Appleton-Century-Crofts.

118. Litman, T.J. (1961). *The influence of concept of self and life orientation factors upon the rehabilitation of orthopedic patients.* Dissertation, University of Minnesota, Minneapolis.

119. Vallbona, C., Spencer, W.A., Vogt, F.B., & Cardus, D. (1965). *The Effect of Bedrest on Various Parameters of Physiological Function.* (NASA No. NASA-CR-179). Houston: Texas Institute for Rehabilitation and Research.

120. Ikai, M., & Steinhaus, A.H. (1961). Some factors modifying the expression of human strength. J Appl Physiol *16*:157–160.

121. Ikai, M., & Fukinaga, T. (1968). Calculation of muscle strength per unit cross-sectional area of a human muscle by means of ultrasonic measurements. Int Z Angew Physiol *26*:26.

122. Sandler, H., & Vernikos, J. (ed.) (1986). *Inactivity: Physiological Effects.* Orlando: Academic Press.

123. Clarke, H.H. (1950). Improvements of objective

124. Clarke, H.H. (1952). New objective strength tests of muscle groups by cable tension methods. Res Q. *21*:399–404.

124. Clarke, H.H. (1952). New objective strength tests of muscle groups by cable tension methods. Res Q. *23*:136–141.

125. Clarke, D.H. (1973). Adaptations in strength and muscular endurance resulting from exercise. In J.H. Wilmore (ed.), *Exercise and Sport Science Reviews*. New York: Academic Press.

126. Haminrin, E., Eklund, G., Hillgren, A.-K., Borges, O., Hall, J., & Hellström, O. (1982). Muscle strength and balance in post-stroke patients. Upsala J Med Sci *87*:11–26.

127. Hägggmark, T., & Eriksson, E. (1979). Cylinder or mobile cast brace after knee ligament surgery. Am J Sports Med *7*:48–56.

128. Fischer, G.D., & Ramsey, V.W. (1946). Changes in protein content and in some physiologic-chemical properties of the protein during muscle atrophy of various types. Am J Physiol *145*:571–582.

129. Maxwell, L.C., Hyatt, G.J., & Layman, D. (1974). Adaptation of growing skeletal muscle fibers to immobilization, tenotomy, and training. Med Sci Sport *6*:75.

130. Williams, P.E., & Goldspink, G. (1974). Connective tissue changes in immobilized muscle. J Anat *138*:343–350.

131. Schutte, J.E., Longhurst, J.C., Gaffney, F.A., Bastian, B.C., & Blomqvist, C.G. (1981). Total plasma creatinine: an accurate measure of total striated muscle mass. J Appl Physiol: Respirat Environ Exercise Physiol *51*:762–766.

132. Heymsfield, S.B., Arteaga, C., McManus, C., & Smith, J. (1983). Measurement of muscle mass in humans: Validity of the 24-hour urinary creatinine method. Am J Clin Nutr *37*:478–494.

133. Buskirk, E.R., & Mendez, J. (1984). Sports science and body composition analysis: Emphasis on cell and muscle mass. Med Sci Sports Exerc *16*:584–593.

134. Winget, C.M., & Deroshia, C.W. (1986). Psychosocial and chronophysiological effects of inactivity and immobilization. In H. Sandler & J. Vernikos (eds.), *Inactivity: Physiological Effects* (p. 205). Orlando: Academic Press.

135. Deitlein, L.F. (1971). Spaceflight deconditioning: An overview of manned spaceflight results. In *Hypogravic and Hypodynamic Environments*. Houston: National Aeronautics and Space Administration.

136. Vogt, F.B., & Johnson, P.C. (1967). Effectiveness of extremity cuffs or leotards in preventing or controlling the cardiovascular deconditioning of bedrest. Aerospace Med *38*:702–707.

137. Gaffney, F.A., Fenton, B.J., Lane, L.D., & Lake, C.R. (1988). Hemodynamic, ventilatory, and biochemical responses of panic patients and normal controls with sodium lactate infusion and spontaneous panic attacks. Arch Gen Psychiatry, *45*:53–60.

138. Rusk, H.A. (1945). Convalescent care and rehabilitation in the Army Air Forces. Med Clin North Am, May 1945, p. 715.

139. Friden, J.M., Sjostrom, M., & Ekblom, B. (1983). Myofibrillar damage following intense eccentric exercise in man. Int J Sports Med *4*:170–176.

140. Friman, G. (1979). Effect of clinical bed rest for seven days on physical performance. Acta Med Scand *205*:389–393.

141. Dock, W. (1944). The evil sequlae of complete bedrest. JAMA *125*:1083–1085.

142. Roberts, D., & Smith, D.J. (1989). Biochemical aspects of peripheral muscle fatigue: A review. Sports Med *7*:125–138.

143. Hung, J., Goldwater, D., Convertino, V.A., McKillop, J.H., Goris, M.L., & DeBusk, R.F. (1983). Mechanisms for decreased exercise capacity after bed rest in normal middle-aged men. Am J Cardiol *51*:344–348.

144. Faulkner, J.A., Niemeyer, J.H., Maxwell, L.C., & White, T.P. (1980). Contractile properties of transplanted extensor digitorum longus muscle of the cat. J Appl Physiol *238*:C120–C126.

145. Booth, F.W., & Seider, M.J. (1979). Recovery of skeletal muscle after 3 months of hindlimb immobilization in rats. J Appl Physiol *47*:435–439.

146. Max, S.R. (1972). Disuse atrophy of skeletal muscle loss of functional activity of mitochondria. Biochem Biophys Res Commun *46*:1394–1398.

147. Fitts, R., Metzger, J., Riley, D., & Unsworth, B. (1986). Models of disuse: A comparison of hindlimb suspension and immobilization. J Appl Physiol *60*:1946–1953.

148. Appell, H.J. (1986). Skeletal muscle atrophy during immobilization. Int J Sports Med *7*:1–5.

149. Henneman, E., Somjen, C.G., & Carpenter, D.O. (1965). Functional significance of cell size in spinal motor neurons. J Neurophysiol *28*:599–620.

150. Tidball, J.G. (1984). Myotendinous junctions: Morphological changes and mechanical failure associated with muscle cell atrophy. Exp Molec Pathol *40*:1–12.

151. Goldspink, D. (1977). The influence of activity on muscle size and protein turnover. J Physiol *264*:283–296.

152. Greenleaf, J.E., Van Beaumont, W., Convertino, V.A., & Starr, J.C. (1983). Handgrip and general muscular strength and endurance during prolonged bedrest with isometric and isotonic leg exercise training. Aviat Space Environ Med *54*:696–700.

153. Black, S., Carter, G.M., Nitz, A.J., & Worthington, J.A. (1980). Oxygen consumption for lower extremity exercises in normal subjects and burned patients. Phys Ther *60*:10.

154. Asher, R.A. (1947). The dangers of going to bed. Br Med J *2*:967–968.

155. Mayer, M., & Rosen, F. (1977). Interaction of glucocorticoids and androgens with skeletal muscle. Metabolism *26*:937–962.

22

Edema

Phylita Skov
Marylou Muwaswes

DEFINITION

Edema is an excess accumulation of fluid in the interstitial component of the extracellular fluid compartment that results from disruption of the Starling forces.[1] As filtration of fluid out of the capillaries increases above the ability to return it to the venous circulation, swelling of the tissues occurs.[2–4] In addition, fluid may be sequestered from the effective extracellular fluid volume or overflow from the interstitium into body spaces such as the peritoneal cavity, intestinal lumen, and thoracic cavity.[5]

Alterations in sodium and water homeostasis resulting in hypo-osmolality of extracellular fluid cause fluid shift into the cells and intracellular edema.[6] Increased total body sodium and water may result from primary alterations in sodium and water homeostasis or from decreased intravascular volume exacerbating the edematous state.[7]

PREVALENCE, POPULATIONS AT RISK, AND SITUATIONAL STRESSORS

The overall prevalence of edema is not known. Edema is associated with primary diseases of all organ systems, local and disseminated neoplasms, surgical procedures, trauma, drowning, and infection. It also occurs secondary to congenital abnormalities of the cardiovascular, lymphatic, renal, gastrointestinal, and cerebral systems.

Edema can result from new pathological conditions, progression of existing pathological conditions, inadequate treatment, or noncompliance with treatment regimens. New pathological conditions, disease, or trauma can produce local edema in peripheral tissues or organs or in the entire organ. Inhalation of toxic gases produces edema throughout the lung, but a local tumor obstructing lymph flow produces edema of only that segment of the lung.

Progression of existing pathological conditions can overwhelm reserve mechanisms, which defend against edema. For example, in the patient with compromised cardiac function, further compromise of cardiac pumping ability by acute myocardial infarction may increase pulmonary blood volume and transcapillary fluid flux above the compensatory ability of the lymphatics to remove fluid. This results in acute fluid collection in the lung, that is, acute pulmonary edema.

Edema resulting from noncompliance with treatment regimens can also occur in the cardiac patient. Sodium and fluid restriction and diuretics are used to maintain fluid volume within the pumping capability of the compromised heart. Nonadherence to this regimen results in volume overload with pulmonary and peripheral edema.

Edema can result from conditions that alter cellular metabolism, such as ischemia, hypoxia, infarction, pus accumulation, and trauma. It also may arise from mechanical obstruction to fluid flow, such as venous occlusion, lymphatic obstruction, and obstructive hydrocephalus.

The rate and degree of edema formation and its resolution, and the degree to which vital functions are compromised, are modulated by the rate of development of the initial stressor, the developmental structure of organ systems, and the efficiency of compensatory mechanisms that defend against edema. An acute insult usually leads to a more rapid development of edema and compromise of vital functions. Conversely, the same level of insult developing more slowly allows for physiological adaptation by compensatory mechanisms; therefore, edema is less severe and function is less impaired. For example, a slow-growing cerebral hemispheric neoplasm causes less edema and fewer changes in neurological function than an acute cerebral infarction of comparable size.

In summary, situational stressors that place the person at risk to experience or extend edema or both are the type of insult, the degree and extent of the insult, the acuteness of the insult, and the body's ability to compensate for the insult.

Clinical States or Diagnoses

Edema is described in terms of the site of fluid accumulation (interstitial, intracavitary, or intracellular) and in terms of the initiating mechanism (Table 22–1). Vasogenic edema arises from primary disruptions of the Starling forces of the capillary, that is, alterations in microvascular pressure, protein concentration, or barrier permeability. Fluid collects in the interstitium and may overflow into body cavities. Cellular edema arises from conditions that decrease extracellular osmolality, alter permeability of the cell membrane, or impair metabolic function of active ion pumps that maintain cellular homeostasis. The capillary, the interstitium, and the tissue cells are a continuum, and factors that alter permeability of capillary cells may also alter permeability of tissue cells. For example, cerebral edema caused by focal ischemia may begin as vasogenic edema and may be followed by cellular (cytotoxic) edema. Lymphedema arises from obstruction of lymph return to the vascular system and results in protein accumulation in the interstitium.[8] In the brain, which does not have a lymph system, obstruction of the subarachnoid villi prevents reabsorption of cerebrospinal fluid (CSF) into the vasculature and results in an interstitial accumulation of water and sodium.[9] Renal retention of sodium and water can be a primary mechanism initiating the edematous state or can occur secondarily in existing edema. Vasogenic edema, cellular edema, lymphedema, and edema secondary

TABLE 22–1   CLASSIFICATION OF EDEMATOUS CONDITIONS ACCORDING TO INITIATING MECHANISM

Vasogenic and Cellular Edema
Capillary hypertension
  Cardiac dysfunction
    Left ventricular
    Right ventricular
    Biventricular
  Deep vein thrombosis
  Chronic venous insufficiency
  Cirrhosis
  Portal hypertension
  Intestinal obstruction
  Neurogenic pulmonary edema
  Angioneurotic edema
  Later stages of focal cerebral ischemia
Increased barrier permeability
  Inflammation
  Infection
    Viral pneumonia
    Brain abscess
    Pancreatitis
    Escherichia coli endotoxemia
  Smoke inhalation
  Aspiration pneumonia
  Shock
  Adult respiratory distress syndrome
  Surgical third space syndrome
  Cerebral vascular accident
  Cerebral contusion
  Brain tumor
  Initial stages of focal cerebral ischemia
Hypoproteinemia
  Nephrotic syndrome
  Hepatic disease
  Starvation
  Stress
  Burns
  Crystalloid fluid therapy

Lymphedema
Surgical interruption of lymph channels
Neoplasm
Infection and scarring of lymph channels
Hydrocephalus
Increased interstitial tissue pressure

Edema Secondary to Altered Sodium and Water Balance
Surgical or traumatic stress
Congestive heart failure
Cirrhosis
Nephrotic syndrome
Hypo-osmolar states

to altered sodium and water balance can occur concomitantly.

DEVELOPMENTAL DIMENSIONS

Both the infant and the aged adult have minimal reserve mechanisms and a decreased efficiency of homeostatic control mechanisms in comparison with the middle-aged adult. In the infant, this is due to immaturity of the organ systems, in the older adult, to senescence. Histological and functional characteristics are often similar. In these populations, then, edema may develop with a lesser insult because of the inefficiency of the control systems to defend against edema. Vital functions are compromised more rapidly and at a lower level of fluid accumulation.

The capillary system of the immature brain, that is, in infants under 6 months of age, is more permeable to substances than is the mature brain, resulting in a lack of protection. The factors responsible for this protection may be related to the development of capillary endothelial cells of the brain that in maturity have tight junctions or to a lack of effectiveness of cerebrospinal fluid absorption.[10] The same pathological processes that cause cerebral edema in adults also cause edema in children. Before closure of the cranial sutures, hydrocephalus in children produces enlargement of the skull.

Certain structural and functional differences in the respiratory system in the infant and the aged adult lead to more rapid compromise of oxygenation in the presence of edema. These differences are seen in the alveoli, the thorax, and the diaphragm. Alveolar development is incomplete at birth, and thus interstitial spaces are wide, diffusion distance is increased, and diffusing capacity and lung compliance are decreased.[11] Because of this structural difference, relatively large volumes of fluid can accumulate in the interstitial space. It has been proposed that alveolar membrane permeability is increased in infants, but the experimental studies needed to confirm this are conflicting.[12] Edema in early infancy can impede alveolar development and can result in lung dysplasia.[13] The thorax is unstable, and the diaphragm is undeveloped. This may potentially lead to fatigue, with an increase in the work of breathing.[13]

In the aged, coalescence of the alveoli decreases the gas exchange area and the diffusing capacity, and the loss of elastic tissue increases lung compliance, resulting in larger lung volumes at end-expiration and increased respiratory muscle work. The thorax becomes more rigid and the diaphragm less able to compensate for an increased respiratory demand.[14] This may also potentially lead to respiratory fatigue.

The ability of the cardiovascular system to compensate effectively for increased volume is limited in the infant and the aged, and thus edema occurs more rapidly and at a lower level of volume than in the middle-aged adult. In both populations, the heart has fewer contractile units and more fibrous tissue, with resultant decreased compliance.[15] In the infant, the heart is relatively unresponsive to increasing preload, stroke volume is relatively fixed, and cardiac output is increased primarily by an increase in heart rate.[15] In contrast, cardiac output in the aged is increased primarily through the Frank-Starling mechanism of increased preload and there is less increase in heart rate at any given workload than in younger individuals.[16] In addition, regulation by the endocrine system is less efficient.[16]

In both populations, fewer nephrons exist in the kidney and glomerular filtration rate and the ability to excrete sodium and water is decreased. As in the heart, there is less responsiveness to endocrine influence.[14]

MECHANISMS

Normal capillary dynamics provide the basis for understanding the mechanisms of edema and are reviewed here briefly. The Starling[1] hypothesis describes the mechanism of transcapillary fluid and solute exchange (Fig. 22–1) as a function of (1) the hydrostatic pressure gradient—microvascular pressure (P_{mv}) minus perimicrovascular pressure (P_{pmv})—and (2) the protein osmotic pressure gradient—plasma protein osmotic pressure (II_{mv}) minus perimicrovascular protein osmotic pressure (II_{pmv}). Normally, the sum of the forces of microvascular pressure, perimicrovascular pressure, and perimicrovascular protein osmotic pressure favoring outward movement is slightly greater than plasma protein osmotic pressure. Thus, there is a slight net fluid movement ($\dot{Q}$) into the tissue spaces that is equaled by lymph flow (L) returning this fluid to the vascular system. Specific values for P_{mv}, P_{pmv}, II_{mv}, and II_{pmv} may vary among tissues. The net rate of filtration per millimeters of mercury (mm Hg), or the hydraulic conductance, and the surface area perfused determine the filtration coefficient (K).[8] In addition, capillary membranes are not totally impermeable to proteins, as the relationships mentioned earlier suggest. The osmotic reflection coefficient (σ) expresses the degree of protein permeability and is 1 if the capillary is totally

A

CAPILLARY + TISSUE + LYMPHATIC SYSTEM

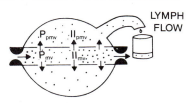

$$\begin{matrix} \text{VOLUME FLOW} \\ \text{ACROSS CAPILLARY} \\ \text{WALL} \end{matrix} = \frac{\text{LYMPH}}{\text{FLOW}} = K(P_{mv}-P_{pmv})-\sigma(II_{mv}-II_{pmv})$$

Examples: Muscle, Skin, Joints

B

CAPILLARY + TISSUE + LYMPHATIC + OVERFLOW SYSTEM

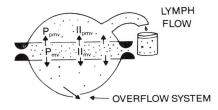

$$\begin{matrix} \text{VOLUME FLOW} \\ \text{ACROSS} \\ \text{CAPILLARY} \\ \text{WALL} \end{matrix} = \text{LYMPH FLOW} + \begin{matrix}\text{OVERFLOW}\\\text{SYSTEM}\end{matrix}$$

Examples: Lung—Alveoli; Intestine—Lumen;
Kidney—Urine; Liver—Ascites

Figure 22–1. Mechanism of transcapillary fluid and solute change. (From Taylor, A. [1981]. Capillary fluid filtration: Starling forces and lymph flow. Circ Res *49*:559. By permission of the American Heart Association, Inc.)

impermeable and 0 if the capillary is totally permeable.[17] Thus, the Starling equation is

$$\dot{Q} = K(P_{mv} - P_{pmv}) - \sigma(II_{mv} - II_{pmv})$$

The filtration coefficient and σ for individual tissues and organ system barriers are related to the capillary ultrastructure and its responsiveness to hormonal influences. The presence, type, and number of intercellular junctions, pinocytic vesicles, transendothelial channels, and the structure of the basement membrane (Fig. 22–2) affect the rate and degree of edema formation in various tissues.[2] Pinocytic vesicles and transendothelial channels are modes of molecular transport through the cells. Their presence in large numbers increases the filtration coefficient in that tissue. For example, in the hepatic sinusoids, intercellular junctions are quite loose and σ approaches 0. Pulmonary capillaries are moderately leaky to proteins, those in skeletal muscle less so, and in cerebral capillaries σ approaches 1. In general, more sites exist for fluid and solute movement on the venous end of the capillary than on the arterial end.[2]

As net fluid movement into the tissues rises, lymph flow rises concomitantly and the washout of proteins decreases perimicrovascular protein osmotic pressure, providing a safety factor against edema formation. When the maximum limit of $\dot{L}$ is reached, tissue pressure rises as free fluid or protein or both accumulate in the interstitium. The amount of fluid accumulation that occurs before there is a rapid increase in P_{pmv} depends on the compliance of the interstitial matrix in

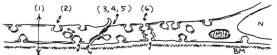

Figure 22–2. Schema showing all the real or imagined pathways for molecules across the lung's microvascular endothelium. The pathways are as follows: *1*, Cellular, directly through endothelial cell membranes and cytoplasm (water, small nonpolar solutes, lipid-soluble solutes). *2*, Vesicular, small cytoplasmic vesicles believed by some to shuttle back and forth between opposing cell surfaces and to exchange fluid and solutes by equilibrating contents at each surface. *3*, Lateral diffusion in cell membranes through junctional complexes may provide a pathway for water-insoluble lipids. *4*, Narrow junctions may provide pathways for diffusion and ultrafiltration exchange of water and lipid-insoluble solutes up to the size of plasma proteins. *5*, Wide junctions permit exchange of plasma proteins and other large molecules. The structure of the junctions appears to vary from arterial to venous regions of the microvascular bed. *6*, Transitory open channels, formed by the confluence of chains of micropinocytotic vesicles, may provide an additional extracellular transport pathway. N, nucleus; M, mitochondrion; BM, basement membrane. (From Renkin, E. [1977]. Multiple pathways of capillary permeability. Circ Res *41*:736. By permission of the American Heart Association, Inc.)

specific tissues. For example, in subcutaneous tissue pitting is seen. In major organ systems, overflow systems open.[17]

Regulation of solute exchange between the blood and extracellular fluid of the brain differs from the systemic circulation in several notable ways. The blood-brain barrier system prevents the passage of large macromolecules and highly ionized substances from the blood to the brain extracellular fluid. Brain endothelial cells contain tight junctions and few pinocytotic vesicles and are devoid of pores.[10] These morphological features provide the brain with a tight cellular barrier with a high membrane resistance.[10, 18] Although lipid-soluble molecules can cross the barrier by simple diffusion, water-soluble molecules are transported by facilitated diffusion and active transport. Joo and Klatzo state that in the brain the force with which edema spreads is influenced by the integrity of the capillary endothelial cells and the hydrostatic pressure of the intravascular volume. The brain also contains no lymphatic system, which functions as a safety factor of edema spread in the systemic circulation. Injuries may affect the blood-brain barrier system and produce edema, and, consequently, disturbance of the barrier may itself alter the regulation of substances that further enhance edema.[10]

The mechanisms of edema formation are described next in three major categories: vasogenic, lymphedema, and sodium and water imbalance. Vasogenic edema arises primarily from the alteration of Starling forces at the capillary and includes capillary hypertension, increased barrier permeability, and hypoproteinemia. Historically, these have been termed hydrostatic edema, permeability edema, and colloid edema. Lymphedema arises from the obstruction of lymph channels. Alteration in sodium and water balance may create or exacerbate the edematous state.

Vasogenic and Cellular Edema

Capillary Hypertension (Hydrostatic Edema)

Theoretically, capillary hypertension can arise from venous obstruction to outflow, arterial hypertension transmitted to the capillary bed, or arterial dilation, which increases flow at normal arterial pressures. The primary mechanism of capillary hypertension is an increase in pressure at the venous end of the capillary that increases P_{mv}, and thus $\dot{Q}$, above the limits of lymphatic capability without a concomitant rise in lymph protein concentration. The pressure rise can be due to increased venous volume, intravascular venous obstruction, extravascular venous compression, or active venous constriction. The P_{mv} required for acute edema formation is approximately 28 mm Hg in peripheral tissues and 21 mm Hg in the lung.[19] Theoretically, P_{mv} can also be elevated by arterial hypertension. However, myogenic autoregulation, in which stretch on arteriolar walls produces arteriolar constriction, minimizes transmission of pressure to the microcirculation and has relatively little effect on P_{mv} and $\dot{Q}$.[8]

The effect of arteriolar dilation on P_{mv} and edema formation has been studied using a variety of substances. In isolated limb preparations, isoproterenol and acetylcholine increase L without increasing lymph protein content owing to increased P_{mv}. Edema formation is slow, and fluid accumulation is minimal.[20] When these drugs are given systemically, however, the lowered arterial pressure and the induced baroreceptor response may actually lower P_{mv}.[21] Histamine, bradykinins, and prostaglandins also produce vasodilation and edema, but is it unclear to what degree the edema results from increased P_{mv} rather than from increased barrier permeability.

Increased Barrier Permeability (Permeability Edema)

Alterations in permeability can affect the capillary wall or the cellular membranes of the tissue or organ or both the capillary wall and cellular membranes. The primary mechanism of increased capillary permeability is widening of the intracellular junctions directly or secondarily through cellular disruption. The protein reflection coefficient is reduced, and II_{pmv} and lymph protein concentration rise as macromolecules sieve into the interstitium. The rate of filtration into the tissues rises rapidly until the increased P_{pmv} balances the decline in σ ($II_{mv} - II_{pmv}$) and a new steady state is reached. The ability to buffer changes in P_{mv} is lost, and a slight increase in P_{mv} produces a large transcapillary fluid flux.[11]

In the brain, the mechanism of increased

capillary permeability involves alterations in the blood-brain barrier endothelial transport systems and release of chemical factors that enhance edema with concomitant opening of intercellular junctions and enhanced vesicular transport.[10, 18, 22] The key events with this type of edema are that (1) vascular permeability increases; (2) driving forces to fluid flow increase, which moves fluid and large macromolecules into the interstitial space; and (3) fluid is retained.[18]

"Cytotoxic" or "cellular" edema is the term used to describe cerebral edema when the initial pathological process involves disruption of the brain's nonvascular cellular membranes.[10] The essential feature of cellular edema is the intracellular uptake of water such as occurs in association with severe ischemic injury. In this situation, failure of the adenosine triphosphate (ATP)–dependent sodium pump allows sodium to accumulate in the cell with subsequent increase in osmotic forces that move water into the cell.[10, 18] Cellular and vasogenic edema may occur together in response to specific insults.[10] Joo and Klatzo theorize that similar molecular mechanisms occur with cellular and vasogenic edema and the differences in the appearance of one versus the other depend on the sequence and the strength of activation of these mechanisms.[10]

Mechanical distention of the intercellular junctions by an acute rise in P_{mv}, called the "stretched pore phenomenon," has been produced in experimental conditions and has been demonstrated to increase permeability to macromolecules.[23] It is unclear whether similar elevations of P_{mv} actually occur in clinical conditions and, if so, to what degree they influence permeability. This mechanism has been proposed in cardiac failure, macroembolic or microembolic venous occlusion,[23] and neurogenic pulmonary edema.

Not all of the causes of widened intracellular junctions and blood-brain barrier dysfunction have been identified. In the brain, blood-brain barrier opening can occur with a variety of pathological states, such as incomplete ischemia, reperfusion after complete ischemia, trauma, infection, allergic diseases, and tumor.[18] A number of chemical agents have been proposed as mediators in edema formation and will be reviewed briefly.

Arachidonic acid is a polyunsaturated fatty acid that is normally protein-bound in cell membranes. Arachidonic acid, once released to free form by local injury, is converted either by cyclo-oxygenase to prostaglandins and lipid peroxides or by lipo-oxygenase to hydroxy fatty acids and leukotrienes.[4, 21, 23, 24] In an experimental model of brain edema,[24] release of these substances was believed responsible for the breakdown of membrane phospholipids and subsequent perioxidative damage to cellular membranes.

Wahl and associates concluded that bradykinin was a potent chemical mediator of cerebral edema in animal models because it increases vascular permeability and induces arterial dilation and venous constriction.[18] Although histamine opens the blood-brain barrier and H_2 receptors are involved in molecular transport,[10] its precise role as a chemical mediator is not well defined.

In the periphery, histamine and bradykinins are released in response to injury and widen intercellular junctions, primarily in the postcapillary venules, and increase vesicular transcellular transport of molecules. Their primary effect is in the initial local edema of injury; however, capillary junctions approach normal within several hours[8, 20] because of the counteractive effects of catecholamines.

Free radicals, such as superoxide ions, hydroxyl radicals, and singlet oxygen, are ions within cells that have a high degree of chemical reactivity and toxicity. Normally, they are rapidly converted to less reactive substances through cellular enzymes, such as superoxide dismutase and catalase. With cellular insult from ischemia, hypoxia, or toxins, they remain in the activated state and alter membrane lipids, increasing permeability with resultant swelling and loss of function of the cell and its organelles.[9] Inhibition of the sodium ATP pump and accumulation of calcium in the mitochondria result in further swelling. In the late stage, disintegration of lysosomes and release of proteolytic enzymes into the cytoplasm and further production of free radicals may contribute to cell death.[25] Other agents that have been implicated in permeability edema are complement in the presence of polymorphonuclear leukocytes, platelets, fibrin and fibrin degradation products, and artificial circulation and oxygenation devices.[4]

Hypoproteinemia (Colloid Edema)

An acute decrease in II_{mv}, primarily from reduction in serum albumin, increases transcapillary filtration of protein-poor fluid.

Lymph flow increases with washout of interstitial protein and a reduction of II_{pmv}. As the lymphatics are overwhelmed and fluid accumulates in the interstitium, P_{pmv} rises until it counterbalances P_{mv} and σ $(II_{mv} - II_{pmv})$ and a new steady state is reached.

Plasma protein concentration is decreased by external losses or by sequestration of proteins in ascites or burns. It is reduced also by inadequate protein intake, inadequate absorption in the gastrointestinal tract, decreased albumin synthesis in the liver, or increased protein utilization. Serum proteins also can be diluted as a consequence of water retention or iatrogenic therapy.[26]

Lymphedema

Complete or partial occlusion of the lymph channels increases pressure distal to the obstruction, producing incompetence of the lymphatic valves and of the endothelial junctions of lymphatic capillaries. Because vascular capillaries are not totally impermeable to protein, II_{pmv} begins to rise. Some of the excess protein can be ingested and metabolized by tissue macrophages. Over time, II_{pmv} will rise toward II_{mv}. Accumulation of protein-rich fluid in the interstitium will increase P_{pmv} toward P_{mv}, and $\dot{Q}$ will be minimal.[27]

Lymphedema can arise from primary malformation of the lymphatics in the extremities or intestine or secondarily from surgical interruption, obstruction of lymph flow into the venous system, or infection and scarring of the lymph channels.[3, 25] It can be either acute or chronic. For example, in radical mastectomy and organ transplantation, acute lymphedema occurs on the second or third postoperative day and resolves within 2 weeks owing to regeneration of lymph channels and formation of new connections with the venous system. Lymph return to the circulation can be impeded by venous hypertension from venous thrombosis or congestive heart failure. Scarring of the lymph channels, with closure of lymphatic intercellular junctions and thickening of the basement membrane, occurs in filariasis (elephantiasis) and chronic venous disease.[26, 27]

Chronic lymphedema can occur primarily, or it can follow acute lymphedema, with or without a latency period. The mechanism by which protein accumulation in the interstitium produces fibrosis is unclear but may be closely related to a chronic inflammatory process. In the extremities, the edema becomes nonpitting and is brawny edema. Chronic lymphedema is seen also in hepatic cirrhosis, chronic pancreatitis, and inflammatory bowel disease.

Edema Secondary to Altered Sodium and Water Balance

Paller and Schrier describe the afferent and efferent mechanisms of sodium and water retention common to the edematous states of cardiac failure, cirrhosis, and nephrotic syndrome.[7] Arieff and associates describe the mechanisms believed to be responsible for cerebral edema initiated by clinical disorders that produce hypo-osmolality.[28]

Fluid shift from the vascular to the extravascular spaces reduces the effective arterial blood volume (EABV). This signals the kidney to retain sodium (Na^+) and water (H_2O) by way of the baroreceptor pathways. On the other hand, decreased renal perfusion or function may directly decrease renal Na^+ and H_2O excretion. Both mechanisms may be operative at the same time.[7]

Decreased arterial pressure initiates the baroreceptor reflex, producing increased sympathetic stimulation and increased activity of the renin-angiotensin-aldosterone mechanism with Na^+ retention. In addition, increased secretion of antidiuretic hormone (ADH) promotes reabsorption of water. Alternatively, or in addition, decreased EABV in turn decreases renal perfusion pressure and renal blood flow and shifts perfusion to the juxtamedullary nephrons. A lowered glomerular filtration rate decreases sodium and water delivery to the renal tubules, and excretion is diminished. Secondarily, decreased renal perfusion pressure may also initiate the renin-angiotensin-aldosterone mechanism.

One or more of the preceding mechanisms may be operative in clinically identified edematous states. The mechanisms may be initiated together as a direct effect of the same initial stressor, or the presence of edema may initiate additional mechanisms that augment or perpetuate the edematous state. For example, in the situation of cerebral edema that results from altered sodium and water balance, the primary initiating injury may be direct, affecting the hypothalamic/pituitary secretion of ADH, or indirect, affecting brain osmoregulation through disruption of peripheral pathways. In either case, cellular (cytotoxic) edema results from a dysfunction of the ATP-supplied ion pump, which maintains cellular ion and water balance of neuronal and glial cells.

Edema may be more easily recognized and more life-threatening in some organ systems than in others,[26] such as pulmonary edema, third space syndrome, and cerebral edema. These three types of edema are the major prototypes discussed in the following text.

Pulmonary Edema

Edema formation in the lung usually follows the same sequence regardless of the specific cause. Fluid collects initially in the lung interstitium, the peribronchovascular space, and the alveolar interstitial space, producing interstitial pulmonary edema. As the quantity of fluid increases, fluid overflows into the alveoli, producing intra-alveolar edema. The rate of progression from interstitial to alveolar edema depends on the intensity of the stressful stimulus and the individual's compensatory mechanisms (Fig. 22–3). An exception to this sequence is the inhalation of toxic gases, in which alveolar epithelium is injured directly. In this instance, alveolar flooding may occur before there is appreciable interstitial edema.[29]

Pulmonary edema can arise from capillary hypertension or altered barrier permeability. Capillary hypertension is seen most frequently as pulmonary edema in acute or chronic congestive heart failure. Heart failure may be secondary to abnormalities of contractility, as in ischemic disease and cardiomyopathy, or abnormalities of ventricular filling, as in valvular and congenital heart disease.[30] In the lung there are two functional interstitial compartments. The alveolar interstitial pressure is directly affected by pressure in the alveoli and is relatively high compared with the pressure in the loose connective tissue of the peribronchovascular space. The latter acts as a sump, and fluid preferentially accumulates in this area. The low conductance of the alveolar wall to fluid, solute, and proteins defends against alveolar flooding until microvascular pressure is quite high. In chronic hypertensive pulmonary edema, increased size and number of lymphatic channels provide an additional margin of safety before overflow into the alveoli occurs.[4] In addition, the increased pressure results in recruitment of capillaries in the apical lung

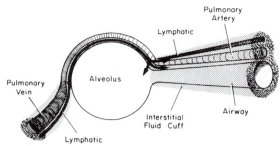

Figure 22–3. Schema of interstitial drainage pathways. Liquid filtering from the microcirculation in the terminal respiratory unit moves passively along a hydraulic pressure gradient to the initial lymphatics in the loose-binding connective tissue surrounding the pulmonary artery, airway, and vein. Normally, the lymphatics receive and pump all of the net filtered liquid and protein. When filtration increases, however, interstitial liquid and solute content increase. Some liquid bypasses the lymphatics and accumulates in the loose-binding connective tissue to form the interstitial fluid cuffs. As filtration increases, the volume and pressure of liquid in the interstitium rise. At some critical volume, the hydraulic pressure gradient from interstitium to alveolus is reversed from its normal condition, and liquid overflows into the gas compartment. See arrow at the bronchoalveolar junction. (From Staub, N.C. Alveolar flooding and clearance. Am Rev Respir Dis [1983]. *127* [Part 2]:S-46.)

segments (zone I) and a redistribution of ventilation/perfusion ratios ($\dot{V}/\dot{Q}$) across the lung.

If ventricular failure is severe enough to reduce forward flow, renal retention of sodium and water occurs. The increase in venous P_{mv} and decrease in II_{mv} increases $\dot{Q}$, and peripheral interstitial edema results. Also, severely compromised peripheral flow may alter barrier permeability in skeletal and subcutaneous tissue.

Permeability pulmonary edema may be secondary to an acute rise in microvascular pressure by way of the stretched pore phenomenon and has been proposed as the mechanism of neurogenic pulmonary edema. Massive sympathetic discharge shifts blood volume to the central circulation and may constrict postvenule sphincters in the lung, acutely increasing microvascular pressure.[4]

More commonly, permeability pulmonary edema arises by way of the chemical mediators described earlier that are released by local events in the lung or by systemic insult.

It is clinically described as adult respiratory distress syndrome, in which extravasation of protein, over time, produces fibrosis. Because this condition can exist in children as well as adults and may include a constellation of syndromes, the terms acute hypoxemic respiratory failure[31] and acute lung injury[32] have been introduced. The underlying cause may result in a decrease of II_{mv}, facilitating transcapillary fluid flux.[4] Interstitial edema is rapidly followed by alveolar flooding.

Surgical Third Space Syndrome

The mechanisms of surgical third space syndrome are increased barrier permeability with fluid sequestration and decreased effective arterial blood volume. These mechanisms may be augmented by external volume loss and additional volume conservation secondary to neuroendocrine response to tissue injury, hypothermia, and anesthesia.

Barrier permeability is increased at the surgical site by the direct trauma to the tissues involved. Retraction or manipulation of adjacent tissues also affects permeability in these structures. For example, procedures on the abdominal aorta or its major branches require manipulation of the intestine and postoperatively, 25 to 30 per cent of the extracellular fluid volume may be sequestered in the intestinal tract.[33]

Low-flow states may alter permeability in tissues distant from the surgical site and may be local or generalized. Local interruption of flow occurs during cross-clamping for vascular repairs and affects tissues distal to the occluded vessel. Generalized low-flow states or uneven distribution of flow in the microcirculation, with release of tissue metabolites and chemical mediators of permeability,[34] can occur from hypovolemia, anesthetic depression of cardiorespiratory function, and cardiopulmonary bypass. Both cellular and capillary membranes can be altered, resulting in interstitial and intracellular edema in muscle and subcutaneous tissue.[35]

Sodium and water retention occurs as a consequence of decreased EABV and is augmented by increased levels of aldosterone and vasopressin secondary to tissue trauma. Dilutional hyponatremia frequently results with additional fluid shift into the cells and intracellular edema.[34] Volume replacement with crystalloid solutions and increased protein utilization in the postoperative stressed state result in dilution of serum proteins, a decrease in II_{mv}, and an increase in Q̇.

Cerebral Edema

Cerebral edema is an increase in brain volume that results from an increase in its fluid content. It is differentiated from cerebral engorgement, in which there is an increase in brain blood volume caused by either arterial vasodilatation or blockage of the cerebral sinuses and veins.

The classification method of cerebral edema introduced by Klatzo[36] and expanded upon by Fishman[9] is the currently accepted way to discuss the pathogenesis, pathological features, and treatment of brain edema. This method differentiates three types of brain edema by pathogenesis: vasogenic, cytotoxic (or cellular), and interstitial (Table 22–2). It should be noted that more than one type of edema may occur in response to cerebral injury.[10]

Vasogenic edema represents the most common form of cerebral edema. It occurs in association with local brain lesions, such as tumor, abscess, and trauma; with more diffuse brain lesions, such as lead encephalopathy and purulent meningitis; or in the later stages of local ischemia. The pathogenesis of vasogenic edema is believed to be a defect in the normally tight junctions of the brain capillary endothelial cells and an increase in the number of vesicles responsible for the transport of macromolecules. Combined, these defects lead to an increase in the permeability of brain capillary endothelial cells, and the normal protective barrier function of these cells is impaired. Transudation of proteins, sodium, and other large molecular solutes are allowed to enter the brain. Water then follows its osmotic gradient into the extracellular spaces, and edema occurs.

Cellular (cytotoxic) edema involves swelling of all the cellular elements of the brain, the glia, and the astrocytes. With cellular edema, a reduction occurs in the volume of the brain's extracellular fluid space. In contrast to vasogenic edema, cellular edema does not involve leakage of proteins from the cell. The causes of cellular edema include pathological processes that alter cellular metabolism, such as anoxia, severe ischemia, hypo-osmolality, and diabetic coma.

Interstitial edema is an increase in the water and sodium content of cells of the

TABLE 22–2   CLASSIFICATION OF BRAIN EDEMA

	Vasogenic	Cellular (Cytotoxic)	Interstitial (Hydrocephalic)
Pathogenesis	Increased capillary permeability	Cellular swelling—glial, neuronal, endothelial	Increased brain fluid owing to block of CSF absorption
Location of edema in white matter	Chiefly white matter	Gray and white matter	Chiefly periventricular white matter in hydrocephalus
Edema fluid composition	Plasma filtrate including plasma proteins	Increased intracellular water and sodium	CSF
Extracellular fluid volume	Increased	Decreased	Increased
Capillary permeability to large molecules (RISA, insulin)	Increased	Normal	Normal
Clinical disorders			
	Brain tumor, abscess, infarction, trauma, hemorrhage, lead encephalopathy	Hypoxia, hypo-osmolality owing to water intoxication	Obstructive hydrocephalus
			Pseudotumor (?)
		Disequilibrium syndromes Ischemia	
	Ischemia	Purulent meningitis (granulocytic edema)	Purulent meningitis (granulocytic edema)
	Purulent meningitis (granulocytic edema)	Reye's syndrome	
EEG changes	Focal slowing common	Generalized slowing	EEG often normal
Therapeutic Effects			
Steroids	Beneficial in brain tumor, abscess	Not effective (? Reye's syndrome)	Uncertain effectiveness (? pseudotumor, ? meningitis)
Osmotherapy	Reduces volume of normal brain tissue only, *acutely*	Reduces brain volume *acutely* in hypo-osmolality	Rarely useful
Acetazolamide	? Effect	No direct effect	Minor usefulness
Furosemide	? Effect	No direct effect	Minor usefulness

Modified from Fishman, R.A. (1992). *Cerebrospinal Fluid in Diseases of the Nervous System* (2nd ed., p. 122). Philadelphia: W.B. Saunders. Originally based on data from Klatzko, 1967; Manz, 1974; and Fishman, 1975.

RISA, radioactive iodinated serum albumin; CSF, cerebrospinal fluid; EEG, electroencephalogram.

periventricular white matter. This form of edema occurs when CSF moves forcefully across the walls of the ventricles, as in the clinical disorder of hydrocephalus.[9]

Fishman describes a form of severe edema (granulocytic cerebral edema) that occurs in association with conditions that produce pus, such as brain abscess and purulent meningitis.[9] Cellular, vasogenic, and interstitial edema may each develop in such cases.[9]

RELATED PATHOPHYSIOLOGICAL CONCEPTS

Edema is related to the concepts of ischemia, hypoxia, and inflammation. During ischemia, edema formation is restricted by the limited inflow. The accumulation of cellular metabolites alters barrier permeability, and with reperfusion, rapid edema formation may occur.

In hypoxia the lack of oxygen inhibits the sodium ATP pump, allowing cellular swelling to occur. Because inflow is not necessarily limited, intracellular edema formation occurs in parallel fashion with the reduction of oxygen. If cellular disruption occurs, widening intercellular capillary junctions, interstitial edema will also be present.

An integral part of inflammation is edema caused by the release of vasoactive substances. The edema is localized and time-limited unless the stimulus continues or recurs.

ASSOCIATED PSYCHOSOCIAL CONCEPTS

Psychosocial concepts related to edema have not been studied. However, the observable physical changes associated with ascites, chronic venous insufficiency, and chronic peripheral lymphedemas presumably have an impact on body image. Altered neurological function caused by cerebral edema may produce mental status changes and may interfere with the ability to care for and protect oneself from injury and insult.

MANIFESTATIONS

Pulmonary Edema

Objective Manifestations

Tachypnea and increased respiratory effort with the use of accessory muscles constitute the primary clinical signs that accompany interstitial pulmonary edema. Pulmonary function is minimally compromised in interstitial edema, and arterial blood gas (ABG) values and pulmonary function test (PFT) results are usually within normal limits.[37]

Interstitial changes are seen on the chest radiograph. In high-pressure edema of cardiac origin, vascular engorgement and hilar enlargement are present on the radiograph just before and early in the edematous state.[38]

Engorgement of the lymphatics is seen as Kerley's A and Kerley's C lines.[29] Kerley's A lines are short markings extending from the hila and are most prominent in the upper and midportion of the lung. Kerley's C lines are fine and interlacing and occur in the central and basal portion of the lung[38] and represent lymphatics surrounding the lobules and acini.[29] Kerley's B lines are short, straight, horizontal lines most frequently seen in the right costophrenic angle and represent fluid in the interlobular septa (Fig. 22–4). Kerley's B lines are more common in chronic high-pressure edema.[29, 38] On x-ray, fluid in the peribronchovascular space appears as vascular engorgement and bronchial cuffs. Vessels seen end-on appear as small white nodules, and a white ring surrounds air-filled bronchioles (Fig. 22–5). Fluid overflow into the pleural space is seen as widening of the interlobar fissures and pleural effusion.[38]

Perihilar haze occurs frequently in a butterfly or batwing pattern and represents a combination of interstitial edema and alveolar flooding (Fig. 22–6). Progressive alveolar flooding is seen as patchy, fluffy infiltrates

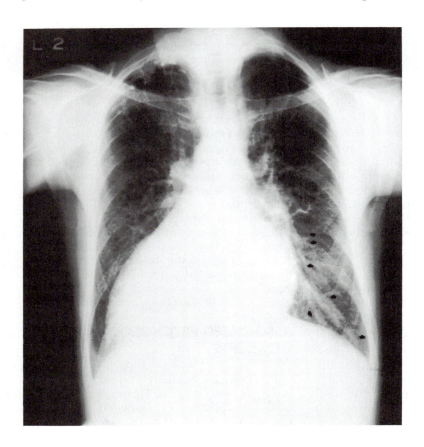

Figure 22–4. Kerley's A and B lines are indicated by arrows.

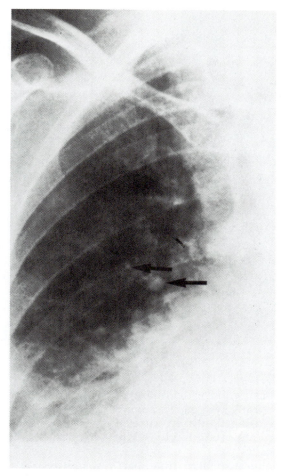

Figure 22–5. An engorged vessel seen end-on *(arrows)* just below the corresponding bronchus, which is visible owing to the bronchial cuff. (Reproduced by permission from Goodman, L., & Putnam, C. (eds.) [1978]. Intensive Care Radiology. St. Louis: C.V. Mosby.)

throughout the lung fields.[29] Cardiac enlargement is also visible on the radiograph. The cardiothoracic ratio is greater than 1:2. That is, the heart is greater than one-half the widest dimension of the thorax.[39]

X-ray findings in interstitial permeability edema are similar except for the vascular engorgement and cardiac enlargement.[38] With alveolar flooding, the densities have a more peripheral than hilar distribution. Because alveolar flooding occurs relatively early in permeability edema, the interstitial phase may not be seen clinically.[40] The sequence of radiographic changes are reversed in the inhalation of toxic agents or in near drown-

ing, with alveolar flooding at the site of injury occurring early.[29]

With progression to alveolar flooding, crackles (rales) are heard initially at the bases, or the most dependent portions of the lung, and then progress throughout the lung fields, and rhonchi appear.[30] The cough is dry in the early stages, and later large quantities of sputum are produced. In permeability edema, sputum is protein-rich, greater than 60 per cent of plasma concentration, and yellowish in color. In high-pressure edema, sputum protein concentration is less than 60 per cent of plasma and frothy and may be pink-tinged because of the rupture of pulmonary capillaries. Findings associated with underlying cardiac failure are displaced and diffuse apex impulse, S_3 or S_4, elevated pulmonary capillary wedge pressure (PCWP), loud P_2, decreased cardiac output, diaphoresis, decreased urine output, sodium and water retention, and peripheral edema occurring first in dependent areas. With alveolar flooding, ABG results become abnormal. Hypoxemia results from $\dot{V}/\dot{Q}$ imbalance and shunt ($\dot{Q}s/\dot{Q}t$). Arterial oxygen levels are decreased because of compromised oxygen uptake in poorly ventilated but perfused alveoli ($\dot{V}/\dot{Q}$ imbalance), and no oxygen is absorbed into blood flowing past nonventilated alveoli (shunt). Arterial carbon dioxide ($Paco_2$) initially is normal or low owing to the increased ventilation produced by the hypoxemia and the stimulation of the alveolar J receptors. With progressive edema, airway obstruction, alveolar flooding, and collapse, $Paco_2$ rises and respiratory acidosis ensues.[37] In cardiac failure, low cardiac output augments the $\dot{V}/\dot{Q}$ mismatch that worsens hypoxemia and CO_2 retention and inadequate forward flow may result in a superimposed metabolic acidosis.

Functional residual capacity (FRC) and compliance are reduced. Their reduction is thought to be due to airway compression, atelectasis, alveolar flooding, and inactivation of surfactant.[41] Wheezing, diminished or absent breath sounds, and bronchovesicular and bronchial breath sounds may appear.

Subjective Manifestations

The primary symptom of pulmonary edema is dyspnea, which may occur on exertion or at rest. Popa describes paroxysmal nocturnal dyspnea and orthopnea as being more frequent in high-pressure edema of cardiac origin than in permeability edema.[42]

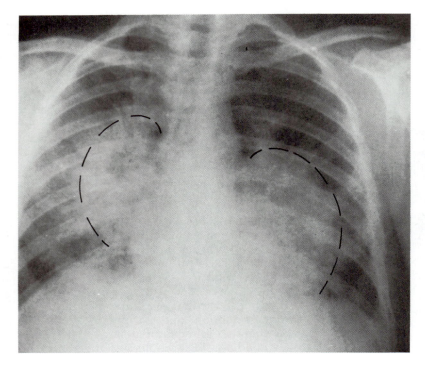

Figure 22–6. Perihilar haze in the "batwing pattern" (outlined). (From Barden, R. [1960]. Reflections of disease in the pulmonary medulla. Radiology 75:454. Reprinted with permission of the Radiological Society of North America.)

Anxiety, restlessness, combative behavior, confusion, and cerebral depression can also occur as pulmonary function deteriorates with decreasing levels of arterial oxygen.

Manifestations of pulmonary edema have been described here in a progressive nature as the stressor increases and compensatory mechanisms can no longer defend against edema. However, it may also present in an acute manner from a severe insult that overwhelms defense mechanisms. For example, an abrupt decrease in cardiac pumping ability, as in acute myocardial infarction, or an abrupt rise in left atrial pressure, as in acute mitral insufficiency, may result in rapid alveolar flooding, and the phase of interstitial pulmonary edema may not be seen clinically.

Surgical Third Space

Objective Manifestations

Early signs of decreased EABV result from the activation of physiological compensatory mechanisms. They are subtle and difficult to evaluate in the presence of immediate postoperative hypothermia and elevated catecholamine levels. Most circulatory parameters are within the limits defined as normal, and trends of increasing heart rate, decreasing pulse pressure, progressive peripheral constriction with cooling extremities and increasing systemic vascular resistance, and decreasing filling pressures and cardiac index are important to identify before hypotension occurs.[43]

Because increasing heart rate and systemic vascular resistance are mechanisms that maintain perfusion pressure at the expense of peripheral oxygen delivery and can compensate for an approximately 20 per cent loss of blood volume, mean arterial pressure or systolic blood pressure in this setting is an unreliable guide to EABV. In some cases, decreased EABV is manifested by erratic or sustained arterial hypertension. Central venous pressure may also be falsely elevated in relation to total blood volume owing to intense venous constriction.[44] ABG values frequently reflect respiratory alkalosis,[43] and mixed venous oxygen saturation (SvO_2) is 60 per cent or greater.

As temperature and tissue metabolic rates rise postoperatively, dilation of precapillary sphincters increases vascular space and facilitates washout of metabolites. If adequate fluid volume is not given, values for circulatory parameters become abnormal, ABG values reflect metabolic acidosis,[27] and SvO_2 decreases owing to increased tissue oxygen extraction. If low flow persists, postcapillary vasoconstriction predominates, increasing P_{mv} and facilitating transcapillary fluid flux.[45]

Parameters of clinical shock are usually defined as systolic blood pressure (SBP) less than 100 mm Hg or mean arterial pressure (MAP) less than 80 mm Hg (or less than 80 per cent of baseline in hypertensive patients), heart rate greater than 100 beats per minute, cardiac index (CI) less than 2.2 L/minute/m², central venous pressure (CVP) less than 4 cm H_2O, and urine output less than 30 ml/hour. However, significant maldistribution of microcirculatory flow may occur before these levels are reached, and early recognition and treatment are essential.[33] The earliest and most sensitive indicators of declining EABV and impending shock are those that are related to inadequate oxygen delivery (DO_2) to the tissues, increased oxygen extraction (VO_2), and lactate production.[46]

Sodium and water retention is manifested by urine output less than 30 ml/hr and urine Na^+ less than 20 mEq/L if Na^+-wasting diuretics have not been given. Although Na^+ is being retained by the kidney and total body Na^+ is increased, serum Na^+ over time is usually low to low normal. This occurs as a result of Na^+ shift to the intracellular space and water retention in excess of Na^+, diluting serum concentration.[47] Dilutional effects can also be seen as low hematocrit, low serum proteins, and low colloid osmotic pressure. Increased tissue demand for nutrients may increase albumin utilization.[34] Dilutional effects may be augmented by intraoperative fluid administration.

Additional signs of third space syndrome include increased body weight, especially occurring in conjunction with signs of inadequate circulating volume, and overflow into body cavities such as ascites or pleural effusions. The duration of this syndrome is variable and depends on re-establishing microcirculatory flow and the waning of the neuroendocrine response to stress.

Subjective Manifestations

Subjective and behavioral manifestations of third space syndrome have not been studied. In the immediate postoperative period, many patients are unable to communicate clearly owing to endotracheal intubation. Cognitive and psychomotor function may be depressed owing to anesthesia and pharmacological therapy.

Cerebral Edema

Objective Manifestations

Clinical measurement of cerebral edema involves specific neurodiagnostic studies: CSF analysis, computed tomographic (CT) scans, magnetic resonance imaging (MRI) isotope studies, and evaluation of the functional status of the patient through a neurological examination. The neurological examination is the method used to measure the objective manifestations of the effects of cerebral edema on the functional status of the patient, including behavioral disturbances. This, combined with evaluation of the individual in the remainder of the physical examination, forms the basis for decision-making and evaluation. Vasogenic edema produces focal neurological changes and alterations in consciousness and can lead to increased intracranial pressure (ICP).[9, 48] Vasogenic edema can be severe enough to displace the intracranial contents and produce cerebral herniation syndromes.[13, 49] The manifestations associated with the conditions that produce cellular edema include severe alterations in consciousness from stupor leading to coma and increased risk for seizures.[9] The more acute the underlying pathological process, such as with rapidly occurring hyponatremia that leads to hypo-osmolality, the more severe the neurological changes.[28]

The neurological changes that occur with the interstitial edema associated with chronic hydrocephalus may be minor, such as mental slowness and memory impairment. When the ventricular enlargement and periventricular edema is advanced and prolonged, dementia and gait disturbances occur.[9, 50]

CT scanning is a radiographic technique that measures the variations in x-ray absorption capabilities of brain tissue. The CT scan is a picture of the brain that has been calculated from the distribution differences in absorption. The picture shows the spatial relationship of intracranial structures and tissue densities in varying shades of black, white, and gray.[48] The CT scan can be completed with or without injecting iodinated contrast. Vasogenic edema is recognized as an area of diminished density with contrast enhancement on the CT scan.[48] Because capillary permeability is usually not affected in cellular edema, the CT scan does not show the presence of this type of edema. With interstitial (hydrocephalic) edema that accompanies conditions that cause obstruction of the circulation of CSF or absorption of CSF, the CT scan shows enlargement of the ventricles and edema of the periventricular white matter.[9] In conditions that produce ischemia,[51] such as arterial occlusion, first cellular edema and then vasogenic cerebral edema occur and overlap. Within 24 hours of cerebral infarction, an irregular area of reduced density is visualized on the CT scan, and at the time of maximum swelling the majority of the lesions are well defined.[51] In approximately 30 per cent of patients, the CT scan shows evidence of generalized edema after cerebral hemorrhage.[51]

Magnetic resonance imaging constructs an image of the brain through detection of the differences in the way hydrogen nuclei (protons) vibrate in the brain's tissue by an externally applied magnetic field. MRI provides greater contrast resolution of tissue, is sensitive to changes in tissue, and water content of body structures does not obstruct the image produced, as in the CT scan. Because of this latter factor, MRI is superior to CT scan in demonstrating brain structures of the posterior fossa and brain stem. In the clinical situation, because the CT scan can be completed more rapidly than MRI, it is the preferred method of evaluating an individual with an acutely expanding lesion.[52]

The changes in CSF composition, specifically protein, and isotope studies are (like the CT scan) reflective of the effect that each type of edema has on cellular structure and intracranial dynamics.[9] With isotope studies such as the brain scan, the patient is injected with a radioactive isotope, the head is placed in a scanning device, and an image of the brain and areas of isotope uptake are produced. With normal brain function, the isotope is excluded from brain tissue by the blood-brain barrier. A change in uptake reflects a change in permeability. Interstitial edema is associated with normal isotope studies.

Analysis of CSF protein in cerebral edema reflects the integrity of the brain's cellular membranes to protect its environment. CSF analysis for ionic and metabolic composition is routine in neurological medicine, and the findings are specific to the clinical disorder. In cerebral edema, elevated protein levels in CSF are indicative of a disruption in the capillary cellular membrane. With vasogenic edema, there is a characteristic increase in CSF protein; in cellular edema, the CSF protein is normal because the capillary usually maintains its normal permeability.[9] In granulocytic edema, because it represents a combination of edema forms, protein levels are elevated and isotope studies are abnormal.[9]

The signs and symptoms of cerebral edema may resemble those of the primary lesion and coexist with the primary lesion. For example, a brain tumor may result in mild focal deficits of function, such as limb hemiparesis and sensory disturbance. An enlarging area of cerebral edema surrounding the tumor may precipitate and worsen these symptoms and signs. There is not one neurological change or clinical sign that is specific for cerebral edema. Generally, the manifestations of cerebral edema can be thought of as a spectrum of neurological changes reflecting the severity and extent of cerebral edema. Cerebral edema may be mild and well localized within the tissue, in which case there is little or no change in neurological function. On the other end of the spectrum, it may be severe, in which case the neurological changes are produced by intracranial hypertension with subsequent signs and symptoms of herniation. Preservation of neurological function in conjunction with demonstrated edema may be due to the maintenance of a favorable ionic environment in the brain.[9, 48]

Subjective Manifestations

The awake individual may complain of bitemporal headache because of the mass effects of edema. The subjective manifestations of edema may relate to a change in the individual's neurological function specific to the underlying disorder. In edema associated with benign intracranial hypertension, a condition characterized by increased intracranial pressure without signs of focal neurological change,[9] the subjective complaints include headache and vision disturbances, such as blurring caused by papilledema.

In this disorder, as in other mass lesions that produce papilledema without focal neurological signs, the edema of the optic disc is related to the secondary effects of cerebral edema that produce increased ICP. Fully developed papilledema is characterized by a swollen and elevated optic disc, engorged and pulseless veins, and increased vascularity of the disc margins. In severe cases, hemorrhage and exudates may appear. Vision blurring, which may be episodic in nature, occurs during the late stage.

An earlier indicator than visual blurring is the loss of venous pulsations seen on examination with an ophthalmoscope. This is not a consistent indicator, however, since other factors, such as glaucoma, may delay the appearance of papilledema associated with increased ICP.[53]

SURVEILLANCE AND MEASUREMENT

Pulmonary Edema

One primary method in clinical surveillance of pulmonary edema is comparison of serial chest radiographs for exacerbation or resolution of the findings described under Manifestations. However, the radiographic appearance in relation to the actual amount of extravascular lung water (EVLW) can be altered by changes in lung volumes, inability of the patient to take a deep breath and hold it, and technical aspects, particularly in portable radiographic films taken in critical care units. In addition, a "lag" time has been reported between actual changes in capillary dynamics and their appearance on the chest radiograph.[39]

Sibbald and colleagues measured EVLW by a thermal-dye technique in 79 patients and compared measured volumes with radiographic findings, PCWP, and calculated shunt.[54] They found that EVLW was 5.6 ± 1.8 ml/kg and PCWP was 11.3 ± 5.3 mm Hg in patients without radiological evidence of pulmonary edema and suggested that this may represent the normal level of EVLW. Patients with high-pressure edema were characterized by lower EVLW (10.2 ml/kg), higher PCWP (20.5 mm Hg), and fewer radiographic findings compared with patients with permeability edema in whom EVLW was 15.8 ml/kg, PCWP was 11.6 mm Hg, and radiographic findings were of greater severity. Calculated shunt did not correlate with EVLW in either group. The authors concluded that clinical measurement of EVLW may be helpful in differentiating patients with high-pressure edema from those with permeability edema and in evaluating the effects of therapeutic interventions. Current techniques for the clinical measurement of EVLW are cumbersome; however, technological improvements may improve the ease of clinical application in the future.[30]

ABG determinations are the standard method of monitoring alterations in pulmonary status and the efficacy of therapy. Blood samples can be obtained by arterial puncture or by way of indwelling arterial catheters, and sampling is usually episodic, drawn at regular intervals, at specific intervals after alterations in therapy, or as indicated by changes in the patient's clinical status. Thus, the clinician must monitor respiratory frequency, depth, lung sounds, use of accessory muscles, skin color, and behavior as indicators of change in pulmonary status and the need for additional data.

Continuous monitoring of oxygen levels can be done transcutaneously in critically ill patients. The degree to which this method accurately reflects PaO_2, and thus pulmonary function, depends on the adequacy of regional blood flow and cardiac index (CI).[55] Tremper and Shoemaker compared PaO_2 and transcutaneous oxygen ($PtcO_2$) values in 106 adult patients grouped according to cardiac index: group 1, CI greater than 2.2 L/minute/m²; group 2, CI from 1.5 to 2.2 L/minute/m²; and group 3, CI less than 1.5 L/minute/m².[56] They found that $PtcO_2$ was 80 per cent of PaO_2 in group 1 with relatively normal flow, $PtcO_2$ was 50 per cent of PaO_2 in group 2 with moderate shock, and there was little correlation in group 3 with severe shock. Thus, $PtcO_2$ obtained under normal, stable hemodynamic conditions reflects primarily alterations in pulmonary function and oxygen uptake and is a useful, noninvasive method of monitoring pulmonary status and response to therapy. Conversely, in abnormal hemodynamic states $PtcO_2$ reflects not PaO_2 and oxygen uptake in the lung but altered oxygen delivery and extraction in the tissues.

A continuous, but invasive, method of monitoring tissue oxygen delivery and extraction is mixed venous oxygen saturation (SvO_2) obtained from a pulmonary artery catheter.[57] Mixed SvO_2 may reflect circulatory changes sooner than the usual monitoring parameters of arterial pressure, filling pressures, heart rate, physical findings, urine output, and skin temperature familiar to the clinician.[37] Baele and associates evaluated the usefulness of SvO_2 monitoring in 16 critically ill patients.[57] They found that SvO_2 reflected alterations in cardiac index and indicated changes in O_2 delivery to tissues that required immediate clinical response. In addition, SvO_2 monitored therapeutic interventions effectively and demonstrated the oxygen cost of turning, bathing, linen changes, and suctioning (Fig. 22–7). Like $PtcO_2$, decreases in SvO_2 indicate an alteration in the balance of oxygen delivery and extraction but do not, in themselves, differentiate between pulmonary or hemodynamic change.

Extensive pulmonary function tests are usually tolerated poorly by the patient with acute pulmonary edema. Bedside monitoring parameters that can be used in ventilated patients include level of inspired oxygen (FIO_2), tidal volume (V_T), minute volume (V_E), dynamic compliance or peak inspiratory pressure (PIP), and levels of positive end-expiratory pressure (PEEP). Intrapulmonary shunt (Qs/Qt) can be calculated.

Surgical Third Space Syndrome

Consistent evaluation of cardiorespiratory parameters for early detection of decreased EABV and for response to therapy is essential, since prospectively, the rate or total quantity of fluid alterations for individual patients cannot be identified. Fluid administration is titrated directly in response to the individual's degree and direction of circulatory response.

A variable rate of fluid administration is frequently prescribed to achieve or maintain

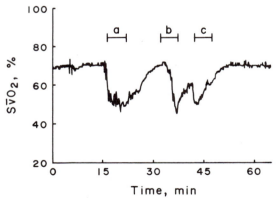

Figure 22–7. Effect on venous oxygen saturation (SvO_2) of suctioning tracheal tube (a), bathing and weighing (b), and turning patient and changing bed linen (c). Note prolonged duration of SvO_2 <60 per cent. (Reprinted with permission from the International Anesthesia Research Society from Continuous monitoring of mixed venous oxygen saturation in critically ill patients, by Baele, P., McMichan, J., Marsh, H., Sill, J., & Southorn, P. [1983]. Anesth Anal *61*:513–517.)

circulatory parameters within the fairly wide range of normal values, and the nurse must titrate the rate and the amount of fluid given. The specific hemodynamic values and the rate at which they need to be achieved to promote optimal recovery for specific populations or individuals are areas of current research.

Shoemaker and colleagues suggest that normal resting values in unstressed, healthy individuals measured in an experimental setting may not represent optimal therapeutic end points for critically ill postoperative patients but that optimal values would be better quantified by the median values of the survivors in this population (Table 22–3).[58] In 300 critically ill patients, they compared the median values between survivors and nonsurvivors of numerous cardiorespiratory variables. From these data they established preferred values and calculated the degree to which each variable predicted survival. In a subsequent study, patients managed with the preferred values of CI above 4.5 L/minute/m², systemic vascular resistance (SVR) > 1450 dynes/second/cm⁵, oxygen delivery > 600 ml/minute/m², and oxygen consumption > 170 ml/minute/m² as therapeutic end points had a higher survival rate than the control group in which normal values were the therapeutic end points.[59] The authors suggest that the better survival rate at these values may reflect the ability to meet the increased metabolic demands of the postoperative stressed state.[56] The population in this study comprised high-risk patients, representing 2 to 3 per cent of the general surgical population. For this subset, the findings do support that normal values and optimal values may be different. The authors suggest that these values may not be appropriate for the elderly or patients with primary cardiac disease.

Serum values of sodium, protein, colloid osmotic pressure, and hematocrit are evaluated periodically. Total external losses, including insensible loss, and total fluid intake are measured, and the patient is weighed at least daily. Serum potassium values are also evaluated, since the mechanisms that retain sodium promote potassium wasting, and hypokalemia requiring potassium supplementation usually is encountered in the postoperative period.

Excessive fluid administration is indicated by rising filling pressures associated with de-

TABLE 22–3   CARDIORESPIRATORY VARIABLES

Variable	Unit	Measurement or Calculation	Normal Value	Preferred Value	Per Cent Correct
Volume-related					
Mean arterial pressure (MAP)	mm Hg	Direct measurement	82–102	84	76
Central venous pressure (CVP)	cm H_2O	Direct measurement	1–9	5	62
Stroke index (SI)	ml/m^2	SI = CI/HR	30–50	48	67
Hemoglobin	g/dl	Direct measurement	12–16	12	66
Mean pulmonary artery pressure (MPAP)	mm Hg	Direct measurement	11–15	19	68
Wedge pressure (WP)	mm Hg	Direct measurement	0–12	9.5	70
Blood volume (BV)	ml/m^2	BV = PV (1 − Hct) × surface area	Men 2.74 Women 2.37	3.0	76
Red cell mass (RCM)	ml/m^2	RCM = BV − PV	Men 1.1 Women 0.95	1.1 0.95	85
Flow-related					
Cardiac index (CI)	L/minute/m^2	Direct measurement	2.8–3.6	4.5	70
Left ventricular stroke work (LVSW)	g/M/m^2	LVSW = SI × MAP × 0.0144	44–68	55	74
Right ventricular stroke work (RVSW)	g/M/m^2	RVSW = SI × MPAP × 0.0144	4–8	13	70
Stress-related					
Systemic vascular resistance (SVR)	dynes/second/cm^5	SVR = 79.92 (MAP − CVP)/CI	1760–2600	1/450	62
Pulmonary vascular resistance (PVR)	dynes/second/cm^5	PVR = 79.92 (MPAP − WP)/CI	45–225	226	77
Heart rate (HR)	beats/min	Direct measurement	72–88	100	60
Rectal temperature	°F	Direct measurement	97.8–98.6	100.4	64
Oxygen-related					
Hemoglobin saturation	%	Direct measurement	95–99	95	67
Arterial CO_2 tension	torr	Direct measurement	36–44	30	69
Arterial pH		Direct measurement	7.36–7.44	7.47	74
Mixed venous O_2 tension	torr	Direct measurement	33–53	36	68

Adapted from Shoemaker, W., Appel, P., & Bland, R. (1983). Use of physiologic monitoring to predict outcome and to assist in clinical decisions in critically ill postoperative patients. Am J Surg *146:*43–50.
PV, plasma volume; Hct, hematocrit..

clining cardiac index and oxygen levels. Pulmonary edema may ensue and is seen clinically (see Manifestations).[33]

The postoperative trajectory of abnormal fluid distribution follows a time course dependent on the degree of insult, the restoration of microcirculatory function, the reversal of barrier permeability, and the waning of the neuroendocrine stress response. Sodium retention and weight gain continue for 1 to 5 days postoperatively and may be seen as periorbital or dependent edema. After this period, spontaneous diuresis begins, and sequestered fluid returns to the intravascular space. If fluid is reabsorbed more rapidly than it is excreted, signs of intravascular volume overload may appear.[60]

Cerebral Edema

The clinical surveillance of cerebral edema initially includes a thorough neurological evaluation and diagnostic work-up to establish a baseline for comparison. The neurological examination provides the first line of evaluation for the patient with cerebral edema. The frequency of evaluation depends on the status of the patient, evaluation of any change in the patient's clinical condition, and knowledge about the time factor in presentation of edema. After brain surgery, edema reaches its maximum 48 to 72 hours after the procedure and usually manifests as a change in cognition or arousal or an increase in a neurological defect. Vasogenic edema associated with head injury worsens the first several days after injury as well.[61] Ropper and Shafran studied 12 patients after cerebral infarction and found the appearance of drowsiness between the second and fifth day after insult after an initial period of alertness was positively correlated to CT scan evidence of edema.[62] Posner and Plum provide a classic description of the clinical signs and symptoms that accompany the herniation syndromes associated with the increased intracranial pressure.[63]

The nursing considerations in surveillance of the patient with cerebral edema are to determine the nature of the change in the patient's condition in order to evaluate the clinical significance of any change and to plan intervention and treatment accordingly. The goals of nursing management for the patient with cerebral edema are (1) to identify changes in the patient's condition, (2) to plan evaluation based upon the patient's condition, and (3) to prevent complications that may result from cerebral edema or its effects through proper nursing interventions.

THERAPIES

Pulmonary Edema

Goals of therapy are to maintain adequate arterial oxygen levels and adequate delivery of oxygen to the tissues. An additional goal is to modify the effects of edema on lung mechanics.

Increasing FIO_2 through oxygen administration can improve hypoxemia resulting from $\dot{V}/\dot{Q}$ imbalance and impaired diffusion but not that resulting from shunt. In $\dot{V}/\dot{Q}$ imbalance only a modest change in PaO_2 may occur in response to increased FIO_2 owing to relief of hypoxic vasoconstriction and increased blood flow to poorly ventilated alveoli (increased shunt), usually in dependent portions of the lung. Oxygen administration does not change the restrictive effects of pulmonary edema on lung mechanics and the work of breathing. As FIO_2 approaches 100 per cent, absorption atelectasis in well-perfused alveoli may further decrease FRC and compliance.[37]

Position changes alter the distribution of the extravasation of fluid in the lung, which is most prominent in the dependent segments, because these segments receive relatively more blood flow and have higher microvascular pressure. Ray and colleagues demonstrated in animal and human subjects with increased EVLW that extravasation of fluid in dependent lung, with subsequent airway narrowing and alveolar collapse, occurred within 1 hour and could be minimized by hourly position changes.[64]

Optimum cardiac performance is achieved by interventions that alter preload, contractility, afterload, and heart rate. In high-pressure edema of cardiac origin, preload is excessive, contractility is depressed, afterload is increased, and heart rate is elevated in the absence of underlying bradyarrhythmias.

Preload can be acutely reduced by the sitting position, rotating tourniquets, and vasodilators that produce peripheral venous pooling and reduce central volume. Reduction of total volume is achieved by interrupting the feedback mechanisms of volume retention through the use of diuretics.

Decreasing preload to a PCWP of 15 to 18 mm Hg may of itself improve contractility and stroke volume, thus decreasing left ventricular end diastolic pressure (LVEDP) and intrapulmonary microvascular pressure. In addition, vasodilators that affect arteriolar as well as venous beds reduce afterload, further augment stroke volume, and decrease LVEDP.

Contractility, stroke volume, and thus cardiac index can be further enhanced by the use of inotropic agents. These agents also increase myocardial oxygen consumption, however, and must be used with caution in patients with ischemic disease.[65] Improved cardiac index improves renal perfusion and facilitates excretion of Na^+ and H_2O, and the effect can be augmented by Na^+ and H_2O restriction. As stroke volume improves, heart rate decreases reflexly through the baroreceptor mechanism. Underlying arrhythmias are treated with appropriate medications.

With increased barrier permeability, the ability of the lung to defend against increases in microvascular pressure, such as that due to increased PCWP, is reduced. Plasma protein osmotic pressure may be decreased by crystalloid resuscitation. Thus, fluid administration and preload levels must be sufficient to maintain organ perfusion with minimal increase in PCWP.[55] A prospective study in which patients were categorized by EVLW and PCWP and randomized to routine care or a protocol in which EVLW was the therapeutic end point demonstrated a significant decrease in mortality in patients with permeability edema in the protocol group. These patients were managed with fluid restriction or diuresis to maintain a PCWP less than 18 mm Hg; hypotension was managed with vasopressors.[66]

No direct agents have been clearly shown to restore barrier permeability to normal, although research is currently being conducted in this area. The use of high-dose corticosteroids remains controversial. It has been proposed that steroids prevent complement activation and stabilize lysosomal membranes, thus reducing the degree of alteration in barrier permeability.[55] In animal experiments, pretreatment or early treatment with corticosteroids in some models of lung injury decreases lymph protein concentration below that for injury alone.[67] There is some clinical evidence to suggest that corticosteroids are most useful in patients at risk for acute lung injury but have no effect in patients with sepsis and worsen the condition in postoperative patients. Furthermore, corticosteroids enhance cardiac contractility and may lower P_{mv} secondarily to an increase in stroke volume.[67] Clinically, the appropriate time for administration to best minimize increased barrier permeability remains elusive. Other agents that are under investigation in animal models include those that reduce polymorphonuclear leukocyte–mediated injury, inhibitors of arachidonic acid metabolites, free radical scavengers, and exogenous replacement of surfactant.[31]

In either capillary hypertension or increased permeability pulmonary edema, the presence of edema can produce a cycle of further decrease in lung volumes, more edema formation, more volume loss, further decreased compliance, and increasing fatigue that requires mechanical support of ventilation.[41] Ventilation with high tidal volumes (10 to 15 ml/kg) and low rates has been most effective in reversing or preventing atelectasis. However, in patients with acute lung injury (acute respiratory distress syndrome [ARDS]), there is evidence to suggest that high volumes accompanied by high airway pressure may overdistend the functional and more compliant areas of the lung, worsening the condition and increasing the risk of barotrauma.[68] Hickling recommends starting with tidal volumes of 7 to 10 ml in this population and reducing them if peak airway pressure exceeds 30 to 35 cm H_2O.[68]

PEEP increases FRC primarily by distending small airways, maintaining airway patency, and improving alveolar inflation. Improved ventilation of alveolar areas with low $\dot{V}/\dot{Q}$ or shunting improves hypoxemia. Furthermore, the increase in lung volume overcomes the elastic recoil of the lung and increases compliance. In some instances, PEEP conserves surfactant, thus maintaining alveolar surface forces and preventing collapse.[37]

The effect of PEEP on EVLW remains somewhat controversial. More complete alveolar expansion thins the layer of intraalveolar fluid and improves the diffusion pathway. There is little evidence that PEEP forces fluid from the alveoli to the interstitium.[69] It has been proposed that increased alveolar pressure is directly transmitted to the alveolar interstitium, raising P_{pmv} and opposing filtration. This may be opposed by a concomitant increase in P_{mv}.[23] The increase in lung volume may decrease P_{pmv} in the peribronchovascular tissue space, relative to the alveolar perivascular space, thus facilitating the drainage of fluid from the blood-gas interface and improving the diffusion pathway.[21]

PEEP may adversely affect cardiac performance by impeding venous return, thus reducing preload, increasing pulmonary vascular resistance, and decreasing pulmonary and systemic flow. Optimal PEEP is identified for individual patients by correlating PCWP, CI, and PaO_2 for increasing increments of PEEP. At low filling pressures volume loading may be necessary to maintain adequate preload as shown in Table 22–4.

The depression of cardiac performance is minimized, and the level of PEEP can be maximized with spontaneous ventilation. The use of intermittent mandatory ventilation (IMV) is recommended whenever possible.[70]

Interruption of PEEP for suctioning to remove edematous fluid and mucus from the airway may compromise the patient with minimal reserves. During this procedure airway pressure can be maintained by use of a special valve[71] or by an in-line suction catheter.

Surgical Third Space Syndrome

Goals of therapy are to provide fluids to normalize the microcirculation and in sufficient quantity to maintain EABV before significant hemodynamic deterioration occurs[72] and without acute circulatory overload. This, then, supports cardiorespiratory function and tissue oxygen needs.

Fluid therapy to restore EABV includes blood and blood products, crystalloids, and colloids. These fluids may be given alone or in combination. Controversy exists regarding

their theoretical and actual effects on the microcirculation and overall cardiorespiratory status.

Administration of red blood cells to maintain a hematocrit value of 30 to 35 per cent is the least controversial therapy. At this level, adequate oxygen-carrying capacity is maintained and the decreased blood viscosity may improve flow in the microcirculation. In some cases, the hematocrit value may be allowed to drop to 20 to 25 per cent if sufficient cardiac reserve is present, owing to concerns about blood-borne infections, interactions of multiple units of blood, and cost.[73]

Controversies surrounding the use of crystalloid and colloid solutions relate to the theoretical and demonstrated effects on microvascular fluid flux, the total volume of fluid required, the occurrence of pulmonary and peripheral edema, the duration and degree of clinical shock, and the rate at which therapeutic end points for cardiorespiratory variables can be achieved. Few well-controlled clinical studies are available.

Increased permeability of skeletal muscle cells and intracellular edema from inhibition of the Na^+ ATP pump has been demonstrated in acute hemorrhagic shock due to ischemia resulting from hypotension. Fluid shift from the interstitial to the intracellular space, and thus from the intravascular to the interstitial space, is isotonic and considered to be obligatory.[74] Thus, restoration of EABV with isotonic solutions such as Ringer's lactate or normal saline replenishes the extracellular fluid volume, which will be translocated, and normalizes cardiorespiratory parameters.[33]

The total volume of fluid required to restore or maintain hemodynamic parameters with crystalloid alone is approximately two to four times that required when colloid is also used and maybe as much as 6 to 12 L.[75, 76] The resultant decrease in II_{mv} would theoretically be expected to increase the rate and amount of transcapillary fluid flux. This may, in part, explain the quantity of fluid required and the relatively short time that crystalloids remain intravascular.

Increased lymph flow and washout of interstitial protein would tend to oppose the decrease in II_{mv} and maintain the σ ($II_{mv} - II_{pmv}$) gradient. This may explain the experimental and clinical results that show minimal change in EVLW with crystalloid resuscitation.[75] Peripheral edema in the absence of pulmonary edema may result from the initial

TABLE 22–4   VARIABLES CORRELATED TO DETERMINE OPTIMUM PEEP

PEEP (cm H_2O)	PCWP (mm Hg)	CI (L/minute/m²)	PaO_2 (mm Hg)
5	8	1.8	58
8	10*	2.2	74
12†	12*	2.8	92
14	12	2.0	88

*Volume expansion.
†Best PEEP.
CI, cardiac index; PCWP, pulmonary capillary wedge pressure; PEEP, positive end-expiratory pressure.

maldistribution of flow and greater tissue insult or from differences in lymphatic capability or both.[77] Additionally, alteration in σ ($\text{II}_{mv} - \text{II}_{pmv}$) may be, to a degree, mitigated by the concomitant decrease in P_{mv}.

The Starling equation predicts that administration of colloid to maintain II_{mv} would decrease transcapillary fluid flux, thus restoring EABV more rapidly with less total volume. Also, in the postresuscitative phase, sequestered interstitial fluid would be returned more rapidly to the vascular space.[33]

Colloid, in a 1:2 to 1:4 ratio with crystalloid, has been recommended when administration of 1 to 2 L of crystalloid has not achieved the desired cardiorespiratory variables or when interstitial fluid volume is already excessive. This combination has been shown to achieve therapeutic end points for cardiorespiratory variables more rapidly than crystalloid alone, improving tissue oxygen delivery and utilization.[27]

Conversely, it has been proposed that in low-flow states capillary membranes become more permeable to protein. Thus, maintaining II_{mv} only facilitates transcapillary protein flux, which then draws more fluid from the vascular space and increases interstitial edema. Also, as σ approaches normal, the increased II_{pmv} decreases the rate of fluid reabsorption into the circulation.[78] Some evidence suggests that translocation of albumin from the vascular space is due to increased protein utilization by the tissues rather than a major alteration in the capillary permeability to protein.[43]

A point of agreement in the controversy is that in any individual patient the amount of fluid given must be titrated to the individual's response to therapy. This is frequently operationalized by using an algorithm in which interventions for a set of variables are given and desired therapeutic end points are stated. Ley and colleagues studied the effects of colloid versus crystalloid therapy on total fluid requirements, hemodynamic stability, peripheral edema, and pulmonary edema in postoperative cardiac surgery patients randomly assigned to two treatment groups.[79] Fluid was given by the same specific protocol in both groups so that between-group differences, particularly in hemodynamic stability, could be related to the type of fluid rather than the manner in which it was given. The subjects receiving hetastarch required less total fluid and had superior hemodynamic performance as compared with the subjects receiving normal saline, although chest tube drainage and urine output were not significantly different between groups. Peripheral edema, measured by change in thigh and ankle circumference from the preoperative baseline, occurred in both groups but was not significantly different between groups. Pulmonary edema, evaluated by chest radiograph, demonstrated equal perfusion of upper and lower zones and minimal interstitial edema and did not differ between groups. The length of intensive care unit stay was significantly shorter in the group receiving colloid. Further studies to relate the effects of the types of fluid given and the method of administration in specific subsets of patients need to be undertaken.

Cerebral Edema

The goals of all the treatment modalities used to manage cerebral edema are (1) to reduce edema formation through correction of the causative agent and (2) to reduce the volume components of the intracranial cavity to prevent increased intracranial pressure or spread of the edema or both.[61, 80]

The goal of pharmacological treatment of cerebral edema is reduction of the fluid volume of the brain. This is achieved by using agents that act on the cell, such as glucocorticoids, produce osmotic diuresis, and reduce the formation of CSF fluid. Hyperventilation, hypothermia, barbiturate therapy, and positioning techniques are treatments geared toward prevention of increased ICP and facilitation of a favorable internal environment for brain metabolism. Surgical intervention for cerebral edema involves either excision or decompression of an intracranial mass or placement of an intracranial shunt to drain CSF.[61]

Glucocorticoids

The adrenal glucocorticoids have been successfully used in treatment of cerebral edema caused by brain tumor for more than 20 years.[81] The most commonly used glucocorticoid for reduction of cerebral edema and management of increased ICP is dexamethasone, a high-potency, long-acting steroid. Although glucocorticoids influence cellular function in a number of ways, the primary mechanism proposed to be responsible in reducing vasogenic cerebral edema is that glucocorticoids directly affect endothelial cell function to restore altered permeability to normal.[9, 18] Glucocorticoids also inhibit the release of arachidonic acid, possibly through inhibition of the enzyme phospholipase from cellular membranes.[18, 22] Dexamethasone has been shown to be effective in the treatment of vasogenic edema associated with brain tumor, brain abscess, and in some cases of head injury associated with mass effects.[9, 82]

The therapeutic benefit of steroids in edema caused by ischemia and hypoxia has not been proven. This may be because the cellular damage that occurs in these conditions outweighs the effects of the edema.[9] In edema associated with cerebral malaria, use of dexamethasone has been shown to be deleterious.[83] In a controlled clinical study, administration of megadose steroids (dexamethasone) to 161 head-injured patients was found to have no statistically significant effect on mortality and morbidity; survival at 1 month was the criterion used to measure effectiveness.[84] The clinical use of glucocorticoids is indicated in conditions that demonstrate mass effects and enhancement on CT scan.[9, 84]

Osmotherapy

Use of hyperosmolar agents, such as mannitol, urea, and glycerol, is standard therapy in the treatment of cerebral edema associated with increased ICP.[9, 61] Infusion of these agents increases the osmolality of the extracellular volume components, thereby creating an osmotic gradient between the intracellular and extracellular compartments that results in a net loss of intracranial water.[9] Reduction of ICP is achieved by reducing intracranial volume and not reduction of cerebral edema.[9] In fact, it has been shown that the major reduction in fluid volume is from normal cells, not edematous cells.

Mannitol is currently the most common solute used in neurosurgical practice for the treatment of increased ICP. Mannitol is usually given in a single dose "bolus" of 1 to 1.5 g/kg and is favored over urea and glycerol for several reasons. Although both mannitol and urea enter brain tissue, mannitol has a less toxic effect on that tissue than urea and may act as an oxygen radical scavenger.[18] It is also believed to have less "rebound" effect than urea. As the hyperosmolar substances are cleared from the systemic circulation, the concentration of solutes in the serum falls below the concentration in cerebral tissue, thereby causing water to move back into cerebral tissue—the rebound effect. Because mannitol penetrates brain tissue less readily than urea, serum concentration does not fall below brain concentration for more than 24 hours. Continuous use of mannitol with frequent successive doses is not recommended in patients without intracranial pressure monitoring because the brain adapts to sustained hyperosmolality and systemic dehydration is a risk.[61] Because of this, mannitol is used primarily as a palliative measure to reduce ICP secondary to cerebral edema until other treatment interventions can be instituted.

Because glycerol must be administered orally and is metabolized rapidly, it is not useful if rapid reduction of intracranial pressure is necessary.[32]

Diuretics

Acetazolamide is a carbonic-anhydrase inhibitor that reduces the formation of CSF within the ventricles by 50 per cent.[61] This agent is not effective in the management of cytotoxic edema. It has been recommended with some success in interstitial edema caused by obstructive hydrocephalus. Furosemide and acetazolamide have some usefulness in treating vasogenic edema by facilitating drainage of edematous fluid through reduction of CSF formation, although further clinical study with these drugs would elucidate this.[9]

Hyperventilation

The known responsiveness of cerebral vessels to $Paco_2$ levels forms the theoretical basis for use of controlled hyperventilation to produce arterial vasoconstriction, reduction of brain volume, and a decrease in ICP. Controlled hyperventilation, $Paco_2$ levels between 27 and 30 mm Hg, is ineffective on cerebral vessels that have lost their reactivity to $Paco_2$, a condition known as vasomotor paralysis, which may occur with severe head injury.[81] With acute cerebral ischemia, controlled hyperventilation has not shown benefit.[51]

Hypothermia and Barbiturates

The institution of iatrogenic coma with barbiturates to ameliorate the detrimental effects of ischemia induced by brain injury has been a clinical protocol in selected settings since 1970. In addition to the beneficial effects on cerebral metabolism related to ischemia, several studies have suggested that reduction of ICP is an added benefit when used in patients with head injury.[85-87] Results are inconclusive about the long-term benefits of barbiturate coma in improving patient outcome after head injury. Barbiturate coma has been shown to improve outcome in cases of Reye's syndrome.[88, 89] Whether this is due to the effects of the drug on ICP or on cerebral metabolism is not known. The role of barbiturates in the treatment of cerebral edema remains to be defined.

Fishman suggested that although hypothermia has been used to manage brain injury and edema in environments in which the physiological state of the patient is controlled, such as the operating room and critical care unit, its use in other clinical settings has not been well defined.[9] The effectiveness of hypothermia is based on the physiological principle that reduced cerebral blood flow results in reduced cerebral volume; its precise role in relation to its effect on cerebral edema is unknown. The clinical literature suggests that maintenance of normothermia is a standard therapy for patients with brain injury.[61]

ILLUSTRATIVE CASE STUDY

CASE STUDY NO. 1: SURGICAL THIRD SPACE SYNDROME

Data for a patient after coronary artery bypass grafting are presented in Table 22–5 to show the manifestations and trajectory of surgical third space syndrome. Mr. J., a 58-year-old white man, had a 3-month history of increasing angina from one episode a day relieved by sublingual nitroglycerin to four episodes a day, relieved by nitroglycerin, and 10 minutes of rest. He had no history or evidence of previous myocardial infarction. Cardiac catheterization demonstrated three-vessel disease and normal hemodynamic values at rest. The surgery was uncomplicated, and he received 2500 ml of Ringer's lactate during the 3-hour surgical period.

On admission from surgery, hemodynamic values were within normal limits and serum values reflected moderate hemodilution. Over the next hour, Mr. J. had two momentary episodes of arterial hypertension, a declining SvO$_2$, and mild compensatory changes in other

TABLE 22–5   CLINICAL DATA SHOWING TRAJECTORY OF THIRD SPACE SYNDROME

Variables	Admit From Surgery	1 Hour	4 Hours	20 Hours	Totals
HR (beats/minute)	90	104	92	94	
BP (mm Hg)	110/70	100/80, 140/90 × 2	116/76	122/70	
MAP (mm Hg)	84	86	89	87	
CVP (mm Hg)	6	5	9	10	
PCWP (mm Hg)	8	7	11	12	
CI (L/minute/m^2)	2.3	2.1	2.9	3.4	
SVR (dynes/second/cm^3)	1560	1620	1280	1120	
SvO$_2$ (%)	70	65	70	68	
Temperature (° C)	35	35.2	37.5	38.4	
Urine (ml/hour)	—	80	60/hour	65/hour	
Fluids (ml)	—	500 RL +250 Alb	1500 RL +250 Alb	2000 RL +250 Alb	4000 RL 750 Alb
Serum values					
Na$^+$ (mEq/L)	132		132	133	
K$^+$	3.5	20 mEq given	4.0	4.3	
Albumin (g/dl)	3.5		3.3	3.4	
Hematocrit (%)	35		32	33	

HR, heart rate; BP, blood pressure; MAP, mean arterial pressure; CVP, central venous pressure; PCWP, pulmonary capillary wedge pressure; CI, cardiac index; SVR, systemic vascular resistance; SvO$_2$, mixed venous oxygen saturation; RL, Ringer's lactate; Alb, albumin hemodynamic variables. These changes suggest extravascular fluid shift in excess of the 500 ml of Ringer's lactate he received during this time as external losses were minimal. The patient was given a fluid challenge of an additional 250 ml of 5 per cent albumin, which returned hemodynamic parameters to admission values.

Therapeutic end points were defined as pressures, CI, and SvO$_2$ in the high normal range, heart rate below 100 beats per minute, SVR between 1000 and 1450 dynes/second/cm^5, and urine output greater than 50 ml per hour. To achieve these therapeutic goals, he required 1500 ml of Ringer's lactate and 250 ml of 5 per cent albumin in the subsequent 3 hours. Hematocrit and albumin levels reflected additional dilutional effects. Although the hematocrit value was low, it remained within the acceptable range, and blood products were not given. Serum Na$^+$ levels were maintained by the Na$^+$ content of Ringer's lactate. Supplemental potassium was also required. To maintain these values, Mr. J. required an additional 2000 ml of Ringer's lactate and 250 ml of 5 per cent albumin before the next morning. Breath sounds were slightly diminished at the bases bilaterally, without adventitious sounds.

On the first postoperative day, Mr. J. was 6 kg above his preoperative weight and had slight puffiness of his hands, ankles, and sacrum. During this day, intake equaled output plus estimated insensible losses and hemodynamic values remained stable.

Spontaneous diuresis began on the second postoperative day and continued through the third day. Mr. J. was transferred from the intensive care unit on the morning of the third postoperative day. By the fourth postoperative day, he had returned to his preoperative weight and serum values had returned to normal. He was discharged home on the seventh postoperative day.

CASE STUDY NO. 2: CEREBRAL EDEMA

A 65-year-old man was admitted to the hospital with a 1-month history of right-sided headache and increasing drowsiness over the past week. The past medical history was significant for a left lower lobectomy 5 months prior to admission for large cell anaplastic carcinoma.

The admission examination revealed an emaciated man who was lethargic, opened his eyes spontaneously, moved all extremities to command (the right side stronger than the left side), and was oriented to name only. Both pupils were 3 mm in diameter and demonstrated both direct and consensual light reflex. Testing of cranial nerves III, IV, and V was normal, except for a decreased corneal reflex in the left eye; testing of cranial nerves IX and X revealed a depressed gag reflex. The motor examination was normal on the right side; the left limb reflexes were hyperactive with a positive Babinski's sign and sustained clonus of the left foot. Visualization of the optic discs revealed papilledema of both discs. CT scan of the skull demonstrated a large bifrontal mass with surrounding edema. The patient was started on intravenous administration of dexamethasone (10 mg every 6 hours) and prepared for surgery the next day.

A right frontal craniotomy was performed the day after admission, with partial tumor removal. Anesthetic induction was achieved using nitrous oxide, isoflurane (Forane), and fentanyl. Intraoperative events included systemic hypertension managed with nitroprusside and propranolol. Twelve hours after surgery the patient was extubated. His respiratory status was stable. Neurological examination at this time showed spontaneous eye opening, the patient was restless and moved all extremities, the right limbs continued to be stronger than the left limbs, and he spoke incomprehensible sounds. There were no other focal neurological signs.

Approximately 20 hours after surgery, the patient's left pupil (4 mm) reacted to light slightly and his right (5 mm) did not react to light. He demonstrated bilateral extension of his extremities to painful stimulation. Respiratory rate was 12 and irregular. The patient was intubated and hyperventilated; drug management at this time included furosemide (20 mg), mannitol (100 g), and dexamethasone (20 mg). He was positioned with his head elevated to 30 degrees. After stabilization of the patient's condition, a CT scan revealed herniation secondary to edema formation.

Both focal and global neurological changes were demonstrated. It is likely that the papilledema was related to the mass effects of cerebral edema. The focal changes in the motor examination were probably related to effects of a space-occupying lesion in the motor cortex, but the mass effect of the edema producing secondary changes in ICP could also be a factor.

Surgical intervention and medical management to treat cerebral edema improved the patient's preoperative status slightly. Within 24 hours after surgery, the patient's signs were of the classic neurological changes indicative of transtentorial herniation, a secondary complication precipitated by cerebral edema and subsequent intracranial hypertension. The CT scan confirmed the presence of edema and herniation. The treatment protocol outlined in this case illustrates standard procedure.

REVIEW OF RESEARCH FINDINGS

Increased Intracranial Pressure and Position

The development over the past 20 years of safe and reliable intracranial pressure monitoring devices has accelerated the enthusiasm for research in this area. The techniques have provided direct methods to measure the results of various medical and nursing management interventions. Direct measurement of intracranial pressure has provided a needed supplement to the indirect use of clinical signs and symptoms as the means to evaluate treatment for intracranial hypertension.[90, 91] Systematic studies have evaluated the effects of osmotic diuretics,[92] drug treatment,[84, 93, 94] and respiratory factors on intracranial hypertension.[95] Anecdotal information has accumulated, pointing out the effects of routine bedside activities on intracranial pressure in patients who are monitored. In addition, a lively interest in the study of patient position led to the development of studies that described the ICP response to varying patient positions in an attempt to understand position as a therapeutic modality as well as to understand the cardiovascular influences on varying positions and how these influence ICP. Comprehensive reviews by Mitchell,[80]

and Fontaine and McQuillan[96] evaluated studies of nursing care activities on intracranial hypertension and studies on positioning and cerebrovascular parameters, respectively. This review focuses on clinical studies that investigated the effects of head elevation on intracranial dynamics.

Head Elevation

Elevation of the head of the bed to 30 or 45 degrees is a standard, routine position protocol for patients who demonstrate, or who are at risk for, intracranial hypertension. Evidence that head elevation reduces ICP has been accumulated from clinical case reports and research studies.[93–105] A logical, physiological mechanism has been proposed that explains the therapeutic effect of head elevation on ICP.[9]

Data from studies have demonstrated that the reduction of ICP with head elevation is not consistent for all patients with intracranial hypertension and that head elevation has been associated with abnormal pressure waves.[106, 107] The inclusion of the measurement of critical cardiovascular parameters in studies of the ICP response to head elevation demonstrated that cerebral perfusion pressure (CPP), the driving force for cerebral blood flow, was adversely affected in certain circumstances as well. Table 22–6 provides information about the population studies, methods, and procedures of research about the ICP response to varying head positions. The following text discusses the results.

Although the procedures varied in the experimental protocols reviewed, the measurement of the independent variable—head elevation—was well described usually. Head elevation was measured with patients in bed and on their backs, and the degree of head and trunk elevation was measured in relation to the hips and lower extremities. Because of the possible effects on jugular venous pressure, the head was kept in a neutral non-flexed position. The responses of the dependent variables to changes in head elevation were recorded and comparison of different degrees of elevations, that is, supine, 45 to 60 degrees, were performed. The exception to this measurement of the independent variable was found in the study by Magnaes in which rapid sitting up from the supine position was the independent variable.[98] Magnaes established the normal ventricular and lumbar pressure response to changes in posture

TABLE 22–6 INTRACRANIAL PRESSURE RESPONSE TO VARYING HEAD ELEVATION

Author/Year*	Population	Method of Measurement	Procedure
Magnaes, 1976[98]	N = 72 controls noncerebral disease N = 48 nontraumatic brain injury: hydrocephalus, SAH, PF tumor, AVM, aqueductal stenosis	LP, N = 120 VFP, N = 14 LP & VFP, N = 4 AP, N = 11	Lateral position → upright → lateral Pressure recorded at each position
Kenning et al., 1981[108]	N = 24 traumatic and nontraumatic brain injury with and without increased ICP Age = 7–79 GCS = < 8 in 16 patients	SAS IVC	Head and trunk moved from supine → 45° → 90° 43 recordings for each position change
Ropper et al., 1982[106]	N = 19 supratentorial, traumatic, and nontraumatic brain injury	SAS, N = 19 IVC, N = 4	Head and trunk moved from supine → 60° Mean ICP values calculated from four consecutive recordings reported for each head elevation change
Durward et al., 1983[110]	N = 11 acute brain injury, near drowning, and MVA GCS = < 8 in all patients ICP > 25 mm Hg at least one time prior to study	IVC CV parameters, SAP, PAP, PCWP, CVP, HR, CO, CI	Group I (N = 4): consecutive measurements at 0°, 30°, 60° Group II (N = 7): consecutive measurements at 0°, 15°, 30°, 60° 31 separate recordings
Parsons & Wilson, 1984[105]	N = 18, severe head injury age = 5–67 years GCS = 3–10 ICP = 15 mm Hg resting CPP = > 50 mm Hg	SAB CV parameters, CPP, MAP HR	Head elevation to 35°, head lowering from 35°–0° (part of six movements) Values measured prior to, during, and 1 minute after change
Rosner & Coley, 1986[107]	N = 18 traumatic and nontraumatic brain injury with ICH	IVC CV parameters, SAP, CVP, calculated CPP	Head elevation 0° → 50° consecutive
March et al., 1990[109]	N = 4 comatose, head injured patients age = >16 years	SAB SAP, referenced to the head and heart Transcranial Doppler to measure CBF	Three position changes for each patient: 0° → 30°, 0° → 30° with knee gatch raised, 0° → reverse Trendelenberg ICP and other variables sampled at specific times

*For complete reference citation, see the reference list at the end of this chapter.

LP = lumbar pressure; VFP = ventricular fluid pressure; AP = arterial pressure; SAS = subarachnoid screw; SAB = subarachnoid bolt; IVC = interventricular catheter; SAH = subarachnoid hemorrhage; PF = posterior fossa; AVM = arteriovenous malformation; MVA = motor vehicle accident; GCS = Glasgow Coma Scale; ICP = intracranial pressure; ICH = intracranial hypertension; CV = cardiovascular; SAP = systemic arterial pressure; PAP = pulmonary artery pressure; PCWP = pulmonary capillary wedge pressure; CVP = central venous pressure; HR = heart rate; CO = cardiac output; CI = cardiac index; CPP = cerebral perfusion pressure; CBF = cerebral blood flow.

because of the inclusion of a control group with noncerebral disease in this study. Magnaes documented that patients with intracranial hypertension demonstrated different ICP responses to posture changes. These changes included a larger transient wave amplitude and less fall in ICP with resumption of the lying down position. In addition, in three patients with posterior fossa tumor, sitting up produced a stationary secondary rise in ICP. Subsequent investigations confirmed the finding that ICP does not always decrease with head elevation.[106, 107] Only in the study by Kenning and associates[108] was the degree of head elevation comparable to that of Magnaes. Kenning and associates elevated the head of the bed to 90 degrees,[108] and March and associates to 30 degrees and found that the ICP was always reduced.[109] Because the recording procedures were different and visualization of a continuous ICP response was not performed by Kenning and associates, it is difficult to state whether the findings of these studies were contradictory.

The small sample size in the studies reviewed makes comparison of the findings across studies difficult to interpret. Small sample size is a problem because the studies included patients with various clinical conditions and patients with and without intracranial hypertension. This last fact may explain why Kenning and associates[108] and Rosner and Coley[107] found ICP to always be reduced in response to head elevation from supine and other investigators did not. Almost half of the patients in the study by Kenning and associates had a normal ICP, while more than 60 per cent of those patients studied by Ropper and associates[106] and all of the patients studied by Durward and associates[110] had evidence of intracranial hypertension greater than 15 to 20 mm Hg. Rosner and Coley also suggested that CPP may be enhanced in the supine position. March and associates found no significant difference in CPP in the supine position, although the absolute CPP did change.[109] The small number of subjects in the study of March and associates may account for this finding.

Measurement of systemic arterial pressure (SAP), measured level with ICP, provides the clinician with additional information about the neurological status of the patient and allows calculation of global CPP. Because this is a gross estimation of cerebral blood flow and does not provide information about local blood flow changes, the use of CPP measurements to determine therapeutic intervention is not common. More frequently, the duration and level of ICP elevations are used to guide therapy. This does not negate the importance of considering the hemodynamic parameters in evaluation of neurological status. The results of the studies showed that ICP was reduced in some patients while CPP also decreased. Durward and associates point out that a decision must be made concerning which physiological variable—ICP or CPP—will be used to determine therapeutic intervention.[110]

The findings of the studies reviewed document that elevation of the head of the bed to 30 degrees does not reduce ICP in all patients. Although data are not conclusive, it appears that patients with pre-existing intracranial hypertension represent those who have the most varied ICP response to head elevation. Although a physiological ideal pressure for patients with diseased brains is not established, it is clear that in patients with head injuries, intermittently sustained pressures greater than 20 mm Hg are associated with a poor neurological outcome.[111] In addition, the appearance of plateau waves are interpreted to indicate poor cerebral autoregulation.

None of the studies reviewed make specific recommendations regarding which degree of head elevation is best for patients with specific neurological conditions. The need to recognize that there may be individual patient variation in the ICP response to head elevation was emphasized by the researchers. Awareness of this necessitates continued evaluation of each patient's clinical response. Proper positioning of the head is necessary to evaluate ICP response accurately. Avoidance of rotation of the head and forward flexion of the neck can be achieved by placing rolled towels on each side of the head and by placing a 2- to 3-inch pillow under the head. Compression of the intrathoracic cavity, which commonly occurs when the patient slides down in bed, should be avoided. In addition, when the patient is turned from side to side, the position of the head should be readjusted to maintain proper alignment to avoid compression on the jugular veins.

Evaluation of the patient's clinical response to changes in head elevation is achieved by monitoring for the signs of increased ICP and, for patients with an ICP monitor, by evaluating the peak pressure during the following position change, the duration of ICP elevations, whether the ICP returns to baseline values, and whether position change induces abnormal pressure waves. Intracranial pressure treatment protocols may vary, depending upon the patient's condition. Elevations greater than 15 to 20 mm Hg lasting for 3 minutes or longer usually require medical intervention. The cardiovascular stability of the patient is also a consideration. The hydration status of the patient, ventricular function, use of cardiac drugs, and level of systemic arterial pressure can also influence the patient's clinical response to head elevation. These factors may not affect ICP directly but could influence cerebral perfusion and therefore neurological status.

IMPLICATIONS FOR FURTHER RESEARCH

The recognition of the influence of cardiovascular dynamics on ICP and CPP and the technical capabilities to measure multiple cardiovascular parameters in critical care settings generated studies that included these physiological variables. These studies highlight the importance of including cardiovascular parameters in the design of studies that investigate the ICP response to positional changes as well as their relevance in evaluating the patient's overall clinical condition.

The practical problems of implementing clinical research with patients who are hemodynamically and neurologically unstable is appreciated. Yet it is the less stable group that challenges the bedside ingenuity of the nurse. This problem may be remedied by designing studies that include accurate and complete descriptions of the clinical status and course of the population studied, or the study design could include patients with similar clinical characteristics that would provide a more homogeneous population. The cardiovascular characteristics as well as neurological characteristics of patients should be considered when determining homogeneity.

The ultimate goal of research in this area is to define nursing care interventions that will prevent or ameliorate the potentially harmful effects of increased ICP, to develop knowledge of which patient characteristics place the patient at most risk to respond unfavorably to increases in ICP, and to define as precisely as possible the relationship between nursing care activities and increased intracranial pressure.

REFERENCES

1. Starling, E. (1896). On absorption of fluid from the connective tissue spaces. J Physiol 19:312–326.
2. Granger, D., & Barrowman, J. (1983). Microcirculation of the alimentary tract. I. Physiology of transcapillary fluid and solute exchange. Gastroenterology 84:846–868.
3. Ruschhaupt, W. (1983). Differential diagnosis of edema of the lower extremities. Cardiovasc Clin 15:307–320.
4. Staub, N. (1980). The pathogenesis of pulmonary edema. Prog Cardiovasc Dis 23:53–80.
5. Groer, M., & Shekelton, M. (1983). Basic Pathophysiology: A Conceptual Approach. St. Louis: C.V. Mosby.
6. Mitchell, P.H., & Loustau, A. (1981). Concepts Basic to Nursing (3rd ed.). San Francisco: McGraw-Hill.
7. Paller, M., & Schrier, R. (1982). Pathogenesis of sodium and water retention in edematous disorders. Am J Kidney Dis 2:241–251.
8. Granger, H., Laine, G., Barnes, G., & Lewis, R. (1984). Dynamics and control of transmicrovascular fluid exchange. In N. Staub & A. Taylor (eds.), Edema (pp. 189–228). New York: Raven Press.
9. Fishman, R.A. (1980). Cerebrospinal Fluid in Diseases of the Nervous System. Philadelphia: W.B. Saunders.
10. Joo, F., & Klatzo, I. (1989). Role of cerebral endothelium in brain edema. Neurol Res 11:67–75.
11. Korones, S., & Lancaster, J. (1981). High Risk Newborn Infants: The Basis for Intensive Care Nursing (3rd ed.). St. Louis: C.V. Mosby.
12. Wagensteen, D., & Goodman, B. (1983). Developmental changes in alveolar epithelial permeability. Am Rev Respir Dis 127:540–544.
13. Robotham, J. (1984). Maturation of the respiratory system. In W. Shoemaker, W. Thompson, & P. Holbrook (eds.), Textbook of Critical Care Medicine (2nd ed.). Philadelphia: W.B. Saunders.
14. Knudsen, R. (1991). Physiology of the aging lung. In R. Crystal & J. West (eds.), The Lung: Scientific Foundation (pp. 1749–1759). New York: Raven Press.
15. Hazinski, M.F. (1984). Nursing Care of the Critically Ill Child. St. Louis: C.V. Mosby.
16. Walsh, R. (1987). Cardiovascular effects of the aging process. Am J Med 82(Suppl. 1B):34–40.
17. Taylor, A., Parker, J., & Allison, R. (1984). Capillary exchange of fluid and protein. In W. Shoemaker, W. Thompson, P. Holbrook (eds.), Textbook of Critical Care Medicine (2nd ed.). Philadelphia: W.B. Saunders.
18. Wahl, M., Unterberg, A., Baethman, A., & Shilling, L. (1988). Mediators of blood-brain barrier dysfunction in the formation of vasogenic brain edema. J Cereb Blood Flow Metab 8:621–634.
19. Guyton, A. (1991). Textbook of Medical Physiology (8th ed.). Philadelphia: W.B. Saunders.
20. Grega, G., & Svensjo, E. (1984). Pharmacology of water and macromolecular permeability in the forelimb of the dog. In N. Staub & A. Taylor (eds.), Edema (pp. 405–424). New York: Raven Press.
21. Sparks, H., Korthuis, R., & Scott, J. (1984). Pharmacology of hemodynamic factors in fluid balance. In N. Staub & A. Taylor (eds.), Edema (pp. 425–435). New York: Raven Press.
22. Baethman, A., Maier-Hauff, K., Kempski, O., Unterberg, A., Wahl, M., & Schurer, L. (1988). Mediators of brain edema and secondary brain damage. Crit Care Med 16:972–978.
23. Staub, N. (1978). Pulmonary edema due to increased microvascular permeability to fluid and protein. Circ Res 43:143–151.
24. Chan, P.H., Fishman, R.A., Caronna, J., Schmidley, J.W., Prioleau, G., & Lee, J. (1983). Induction of brain edema following intracerebral injection of arachidonic acid. Ann Neurol 13:625–632.
25. Macknight, A. (1984). Cellular response to injury. In N. Staub & A. Taylor (eds.), Edema (pp. 489–520). New York: Raven Press.
26. Granger, D., & Bowman, I. (1983). Microcircula-

tion of the alimentary tract. II. Pathophysiology of edema. Gastroenterology *84*:1035–1049.

27. Foldi, M. (1984). Lymphedema. In N. Staub & A. Taylor (eds.), *Edema* (pp. 657–678). New York: Raven Press.

28. Arieff, A.I., Llack, F., & Massry, S.G. (1976). Neurological manifestations and morbidity of hyponatremia: Correlation with brain water and electrolytes. Medicine *55*:121–129.

29. Prichard, J.S. (1982). *Edema of the Lung*. Springfield, IL: Charles C Thomas.

30. Aherns, T. (1989). Extravascular lung water: Concepts in clinical application. Crit Care Nurs Clin North Am *1*:681–688.

31. Zuker, A. (1988). Therapeutic strategies for acute hypoxemic respiratory failure. Crit Care Clin *4*:813–830.

32. Murray, J., Matthay, J., Luce, J., & Flick, M. (1988). An expanded definition of the adult respiratory distress syndrome. Am Rev Respir Dis *138*:720–723.

33. Jenkins, M. (1983). History of sequestered edema associated with surgical operations and trauma. In B. Brown (ed.), *Fluid and Blood Therapy in Anesthesia* (pp. 1–32). Philadelphia: F.A. Davis.

34. Shoemaker, W. (1984). Pathophysiology and therapy of shock syndromes. In W. Shoemaker, W. Thompson, & P. Holbrook (eds.), *Text of Critical Care Medicine* (2nd ed., pp. 52–72). Philadelphia: W.B. Saunders.

35. Carrico, C.J., & Majer, R. (1983). Balanced salt solutions in massive trauma. In B. Brown (ed.), *Fluid and Blood Therapy in Anesthesia* (pp. 57–86). Philadelphia: F.A. Davis.

36. Klatzo, I. (1967). Neuropathological aspects of brain edema: Presidential address. J Neuropathol Exp Neurol *26*:1–14.

37. West, J. (1982). *Pulmonary Pathophysiology: The Essentials* (2nd ed.). Baltimore: Williams & Wilkins.

38. Pistolesi, M., & Giuntini, C. (1978). Assessment of extravascular lung water. Radiol Clin North Am *16*:551–574.

39. Squire, L. (1982). *Fundamentals of Radiology*. Cambridge: Harvard University Press.

40. Miniati, M., Pistolesi, M., Milne, E., & Guintini, C. (1990). Detection of lung edema. Crit Care Med *15*:1146–1155.

41. Hopewell, P. (1979). Adult respiratory distress syndrome. Basics Respir Disease *7*:1–6.

42. Popa, V. (1984). Noncardiac and cardiac pulmonary edema. Chest *85*:838–839.

43. Shoemaker, W. (1987). Physiology, monitoring, outcome prediction and therapy of shock states. Crit Care Clin *3*:307–357.

44. Shoemaker, W. (1990). Circulatory mechanisms of shock and their mediators. Crit Care Med *15*:787–794.

45. Wallace, A. (1981). Shock. In L. Smith & S. Thier (eds), *Pathophysiology, the Biological Principles of Disease* (pp. 1259–1264). Philadelphia: W.B. Saunders.

46. Edwards, J. (1990). Practical application of oxygen transport principles. Crit Care Med *18*:S45–S48.

47. Shoemaker, W. (1989). Fluids and electrolytes in the acutely ill adult. In W. Shoemaker, W. Thompson, & P. Holbrook (eds.), *Textbook of Critical Care Medicine* (2nd ed.). Philadelphia: W.B. Saunders.

48. Penn, R.D. (1980). Cerebral edema and neurological function: CT, evoked responses, and clinical examination. In J. Cervos & R. Ferszt (eds.), *Advances in Neurology: Brain Edema*. New York: Raven Press.

49. Seisjo, B.K. (1984). Cerebral circulation and metabolism. J Neurosurg *60*:883–908.

50. Frank, E., & Tew, J.M. (1982). Normal-pressure hydrocephalus: Clinical symptoms, diagnosis, pathophysiology, and treatment. Heart Lung *11*:321–326.

51. Katzman, R., Clasen, R., Klatzo, I., Meyer, J.S., Pappius, H.M., & Waltz, A.G. (1977). Brain edema in stroke. Stroke *8*:512–540.

52. Langfitt, T.W., Obrist, W.D., Alavi, A., Grossman, R.I., Zimmerman, R., Jaggi, J., Uzzell, B., Reivich, M., & Patton, D.R. (1986). Computerized tomography, magnetic resonance imaging, and positron emission tomography in the study of brain trauma. J Neurosurg *64*:760–767.

53. Reeves, A.G. (1981). *Disorders of the Nervous System*. Chicago: Year Book Medical.

54. Sibbald, W., Warshawski, F., Short, A.K., Harris, J., Lefcoe, M., & Holiday, R. (1983). Clinical studies measuring extravascular lung water by the thermal dye technique in critically ill patients. Chest *83*:725–731.

55. Ledingham, I., Macdonald, A., & Douglas, I. (1989). Monitoring of ventilation. In W. Shoemaker, W. Thompson, & P. Holbrook (eds.), *Text of Critical Care Medicine* (2nd ed.). Philadelphia: W.B. Saunders.

56. Tremper, K.K., & Shoemaker, W.C. (1981). Transcutaneous oxygen monitoring of critically ill adults with and without low flow shock. Crit Care Med *9*:706.

57. Baele, P., McMichan, J., Marsh, H., Sill, J., & Southorn, P. (1983). Continuous monitoring of mixed venous oxygen saturation in critically ill patients. Anesthes Analg *61*:513–517.

58. Shoemaker, W., Appel, P., & Bland, R. (1983). Use of physiologic monitoring to predict outcome and to assist in clinical decisions in critically ill postoperative patients. Am J Surg *146*:43–50.

59. Shoemaker, W., Appel, P., Kram, H., Waxman, K., & Lee, T. (1988). Prospective trial of supranormal values of survivors as therapeutic goals in high-risk surgical patients. Chest *94*:1176–1186.

60. Neville, W. (1983). *Intensive Care of the Surgical Cardiopulmonary Patient* (2nd ed.). Chicago: Year Book Medical.

61. Marshall, S., Marshall, L., Vos, H., & Chesnut, R. (1990). *Neuroscience Critical Care, Pathophysiology and Patient Management*. Philadelphia: W.B. Saunders.

62. Ropper, A.H., & Shafran, B. (1984). Brain edema after stroke. Arch Neurol *41*:26–29.

63. Posner, J., & Plum, F. (1980). *The Diagnosis of Stupor and Coma* (3rd ed.). Philadelphia: F.A. Davis.

64. Ray, J., Yost, L., Moallem, S., Sanoudos, G., Villamena, P., Paredes, R., & Clauss, R. (1974). Immobility, hypoxemia and pulmonary arteriovenous shunting. Arch Surg *109*:537–541.

65. Witte, C.L., Witte, M.H., & Dumont, A.E. (1984). Pathophysiology of chronic edema, lymphedema and fibrosis. In N. Staub & A. Taylor (eds.), *Edema* (pp. 521–542). New York: Raven Press.

66. Eisenberg, P., Hansbrough, J., Anderson, D., & Shuster, D. (1987). A prospective study of lung water measurements during patient management in an intensive care unit. Am Rev Respir Dis *136*:662–668.

67. Staub, N. (1984). Pathophysiology of pulmonary edema. In N. Staub & A. Taylor (eds.), *Edema* (pp. 719–746). New York: Raven Press.

68. Hickling, K. (1990). Ventilatory management of ARDS: Can it affect the outcome. Intensive Care Med *16*:219–226.

69. Boysen, P., & Modell, J.H. (1989). Pulmonary edema. In W. Shoemaker, W. Thompson, & P. Holbrook (eds.), *Textbook of Critical Care Medicine* (2nd ed.). Philadelphia: W.B. Saunders.

70. Douglas, M., & Downs. J. (1989). Respiratory therapy for ventilatory failure. In W. Shoemaker, W. Thompson, & P. Holbrook (eds.), *Textbook of Critical Care Medicine* (pp. 301–309). Philadelphia: W.B. Saunders.

71. Bodai, B. (1982). A means of suctioning without cardiopulmonary depression. Heart Lung *11*:172–176.

72. Shoemaker, W., Kram, H., & Appel, P. (1990). Therapy of shock based on pathophysiology, monitoring, and outcome prediction. Critical Care Medicine *18*:519–525.

73. Steinbronn, K., & Heustis, D. (1983). Rationale for blood therapy. In B. Brown (ed.), *Fluid and Blood Therapy in Anesthesia* (pp. 151–167). Philadelphia: F.A. Davis.

74. Shires, G.T., Cunningham, J.N., & Barker, C.R.F. (1972). Alterations in cellular membrane function during hemorrhagic shock in primates. Ann Surg *176*:288.

75. Shires, G., Peitzman, A., Albert, S., Illner, H., Silane, M., Perry, M., & Shires, G. (1983). Response of extravascular lung water to intraoperative fluids. Ann Surg *197*:515–519.

76. Viriglio, R., Rice, C., Smith, D., James, D., Zarins, C., Hobelmann, C., & Peters, R. (1979). Crystalloid vs. colloid resuscitation: Is one better? Surgery *85*:129–139.

77. Wisner, D., Street, D., & Demling, R. (1983). Effect of colloid versus crystalloid resuscitation on soft tissue edema formation. Curr Surg Jan–Feb:32–35.

78. Rodman, G., & Kirby, R. (1983). Posttraumatic respiratory failure: Role of fluid therapy. In B. Brown (ed.), *Fluid and Blood Therapy in Anesthesia* (pp. 119–136). Philadelphia: F.A. Davis.

79. Ley, S., Miller, K., Skov, P., & Preisig, P. (1990). Crystalloid versus colloid fluid therapy after cardiac surgery. Heart and Lung *19*:31–40.

80. Mitchell, P.H. (1986). Intracranial hypertension: Influence of nursing care activities. Nurs Clin North Am *21*:563–567.

81. Galicich, J.H., French, L.A., & Melby, J.C. (1961). Use of dexamethasone in treatment of cerebral edema associated with brain tumors. Lancet *81*:46–53.

82. Teasdale, G., & Jennett, B. (1981). *The Management of Head Injury*. Philadelphia: F.A. Davis.

83. Warrell, D., Looareesuwan, S., Warrell, M., Kasemsarn, P., Inatraprasert, R., Bunnag, D., & Harinasuta, T. (1982). Dexamethasone proves deleterious in cerebral malaria. N Engl J Med *306*:313–319.

84. Braakman, R., Schouten, J.H.A., Blaauw van-Dishoeck, M., & Minderhoud, J.M. (1983). Megadose steroids in severe head injury. J Neurosurg *58*:326–330.

85. Marshall, L., Smith, R., & Shapiro, H. (1978). Pentobarbital therapy for intracranial hypertension in metabolic coma: Reye's syndrome. Crit Care Med *6*:1–5.

86. Shapiro, H., Wyte, S., & Loeser, J. (1974). Barbiturate augmented hypothermia for reduction of persistent intracranial hypertension. J Neurosurg *40*:90.

87. Shapiro, H.M. (1975). Intracranial hypertension: Therapeutic and anesthetic considerations. Anesthesiology *43*:445–471.

88. Trauner, D., Brown, F., Ganz, E., & Huttenlocher, P. (1978). Treatment of elevated intracranial pressure in Reye's syndrome. Ann Neurosurg *4*:275–278.

89. Venes, J., Shaywitz, B., & Spencer, D. (1978). Management of severe cerebral edema in the metabolic encephalopathy of Reye-Johnson syndrome. J Neurosurg *48*:903–915.

90. Noce, J.P. (1990). Intracranial pressure monitoring. Biomed Instrum Technol *24*:54–55.

91. Lehman, L.B. (1990). Intracranial pressure monitoring and treatment: A contemporary view. Ann Emerg Med *19*:295–303.

92. Miller, J.D., & Leech, P. (1975). Effects of mannitol and steroid therapy on intracranial pressure. J Neurosurg *42*:274–281.

93. Kullberg, G., & Sundbarg, G. (1976). Reduction of raised intracranial pressure following infusion of mannitol. A review of clinical pressure recording. In J. W. Beks, D. A. Bosch, & M. Brock (eds.), *Intracranial Pressure III* (pp. 224–230). New York: Springer-Verlag.

94. Saul, T.G., & Ducker, T.B. (1982). Effect and intracranial pressure monitoring and aggressive treatment on mortality in severe head injury. J Neurosurg *56*:498–503.

95. Lordini, S., Montolivo, M., Pluchino, F., & Borroni, V. (1989). Positive end expiratory pressure in supine and sitting positions: Its effects on intrathoracic and intracranial pressures. Neurosurgery *24*:873–877.

96. Fontaine, D.K., & McQuillan, K. (1989). Positioning as a nursing therapy in trauma care. Crit Care Nurs Clin North Am *1*:105–112.

97. Lundberg, N. (1960). Continuous recording and control of ventricular fluid pressure in neurosurgical practice. Acta Psychiatr Neurol Scand *36*(Suppl. 149):1–193.

98. Magnaes, B. (1976). Body position and cerebrospinal fluid pressure, Part I: Clinical studies on the effect of rapid postural changes. J Neurosurg *44*:687–697.

99. Lipe, H.P., & Mitchell, P.H. (1980). Positioning the patient with intracranial hypertension: How turning and head rotation affect the internal jugular vein. Heart Lung *9*:1031–1037.

100. Shalit, M.N., & Umansky, R. (1977). Effect of bedside procedures on intracranial pressure. Israel J Med Sci *13*:881–886.

101. Hulme, A., & Cooper, R. (1976). The effects of head position and jugular vein compression (JVC) on intracranial pressure (ICP). A clinical study. In J. Bekss, D.A. Bosch, & M. Brock (eds.), *Intracranial Pressure III*. New York: Springer-Verlag.

102. Mitchell, P., & Mauss, N.K. (1978). Relations of patient-nurse activity to intracranial pressure variations, a pilot study. Nurs Res *27*:4–10.

103. Mitchell, P.H., Ozuna, J., & Lipe, H. (1981). Moving the patient in bed: Effects on intracranial hypertension. Nurs Res *30*:212–218.

104. Snyder, M. (1983). Relation of nursing activities to

increases in intracranial pressure. J Adv Nurs *8*:273–279.

105. Parsons, L.C., & Wilson, M.M. (1984). Cerebrovascular status of severe closed head injured patients following passive position changes. Nurs Res *33*:68–75.

106. Ropper, A.H., O'Rourke, D., & Kennedy, S.K. (1982). Head position, intracranial pressure, and compliance. Neurology *32*:1288–1291.

107. Rosner, M.J., & Coley, I.B. (1986). Cerebral perfusion pressure, intracranial pressure, and head elevation. J Neurosurg *65*:636–641.

108. Kenning, J.A., Toutant, S.M., & Saunders, R.L. (1981). Upright patient positioning in the management of intracranial hypertension. Surg Neurol *15*:148–152.

109. March, K., Mitchell, P., Grady, S., & Winn, R. (1990). Effect of backrest position on intracranial and cerebral perfusion pressures. J Neurosci Nurs *22*:375–381.

110. Durward, Q., Amacher, A., Del Maestro, R., & Sibbald, W. (1983). Cerebral and cardiovascular response to changes in head elevation in patients with intracranial hypertension. Neurosurg *58*:938–944.

111. Ropper, A.H. (1985). In favor of intracranial pressure monitoring and aggressive therapy in neurologic practice. Arch Neurol *42*:1194–1195.

Index

Note: Page numbers in *italics* refer to illustrations. Page numbers followed by b refer to boxed material; those followed by t refer to tables.

ISBN 0-7216-3494-X

90038